Prescription for NUTRITIONAL HEALING

SECOND EDITION

JAMES F. BALCH, M.D. • PHYLLIS A. BALCH, C.N.C.

Avery Publishing Group

Garden City Park, New York

Cover designers: Martin Hochberg, William Gonzalez, and Rudy Shur
In-house editors: Amy C. Tecklenburg, Joanne Abrams, and Marie Caratozzolo
Typesetters: Bonnie Freid and Evan Schwartz

Cataloging-in-Publication Data

Balch, James F., 1933–
   Prescription for nutritional healing : a practical A to Z
reference to drug-free remedies using vitamins, minerals, herbs &
food supplements / James F. Balch, Phyllis A. Balch.—2nd ed.
   p. cm.
   Includes index.
   ISBN 0-89529-727-2

   1. Nutrition—Popular works. 2. Diet therapy—Popular works. 3.
Vitamins—Therapeutic use. 4. Herbs—Therapeutic use. I. Balch,
Phyllis A.,   II. Title.

RA784.B248 1997   615.8′54
                                   QBI96-40260

Printed in the United States of America

SECOND EDITION

Contents

Part Three Remedies And Therapies

Appendix

Preface

"A wise man should consider that health is the greatest of human blessings."

—*Hippocrates*

Socrates once said, "There is only one good, knowledge, and one evil, ignorance." This statement should guide us in all of our actions, especially where our health is concerned. Too many of us do not have the slightest idea of how to maintain good health. When illness strikes, we rely on our doctors to cure us. What we fail to realize is that "the cure" comes from within. Nature has provided us with a wondrous immune system, and all we have to do is take proper care of this inner healing force.

Does this sound too simple? Basically, it is simple; our modern lifestyles have gotten us off the right track, with fast foods, alcohol abuse, drug dependencies, a polluted environment, and high-tech stress. Nature intended to fuel our inner healing force with the right natural substances to enable the body to function up to its fullest potential. Nature's resources—whole foods, vitamins, minerals, enzymes, amino acids, phytochemicals, and other natural bounties—are designed for use in our immune systems. However, because most of us have a profound lack of knowledge as to what our bodies need to function properly, we find ourselves out of balance and susceptible to all sorts of illnesses.

All individuals should take an active part in the maintenance of their health and in the treatment of their disorders with the guidance of a health care professional. The more we take it upon ourselves to learn about nutrition, the better prepared we will be to take that active role. Attitude is also an important factor in the processes of health maintenance and healing. We must have a positive state of mind in order to bring harmony to the body. The realization that body (lifestyle), spirit (desire), and mind (belief) must come together is the first step to better health.

This new edition has taken over twenty-five years of study, work, and research to put together. It is intended to provide you and your health care professional with a more natural approach to healing, which may be used in conjunction with your current medical treatment. A number of the suggestions offered, such as intravenous therapy, can be administered only by or under the supervision of a licensed physician. Also, because our body chemistries differ, some of us may have allergic reactions to certain supplements. Before taking any nutritional supplement, check with your health care professional regarding its appropriateness. Should you experience an allergic reaction to any supplement, immediately discontinue use of the supplement. You should never attempt to treat yourself without professional advice.

No statement in this publication should be construed as a claim for cure, treatment, or prevention of any disease. It is also important to point out that you should not reject mainstream medical methods. Learn about your condition, and don't be afraid to ask questions. Feel free to get second and even third opinions from qualified health professionals. It is a sign of wisdom, not cowardice, to seek more knowledge through your active participation as a patient.

Every effort has been made to include the latest research available on nutritional healing. We have also added new sections on many health disorders at the suggestions of our readers. All the information in this book has been carefully researched, and the data have been reviewed and updated throughout the production process. Because this body of knowledge promises to continue growing and changing, we suggest that when questions arise, you refer to other current sources of information to verify textual material. We will strive to keep abreast of new scientific information, treatments, and supplements, and make this information available to you in future editions of this book.

Over 800 years ago, Moses Maimonides said, "The physician should not treat the ailment, but the patient who is suffering from it." This book was designed to meet the differing needs of individuals and to help each person create his or her own nutritional program.

How to Use This Book

This is a comprehensive in-home guide that will help you achieve and maintain the highest level of health and fitness through careful dietary planning and nutritional supplementation. Even if you are free from so-called disorders you will benefit from this book, because it gives advice on how to achieve optimum health, build up your immune system, and increase your energy level. Written by a certified nutritionist and a medical doctor, this book blends the latest scientific research with traditional treatments. It provides all the information you need to design your own personal nutritional program. In addition, the authors offer traditional and up-to-date home remedies, and suggest healthful modifications in diet and lifestyle.

It is important to stress that the suggestions offered in this book are not intended to replace appropriate medical investigation and treatment. The supplements and medications recommended for a particular disorder should be approved and monitored by your medical doctor or trained health care professional. If surgery or other conventional medical interventions are crucial and cannot be avoided, the nutritional supplements can shorten healing time.

The book is divided into three parts. Part One discusses the basic principles of nutrition and health, and lists and explains the various types of nutrients, food supplements, and herbs found in health food shops and drugstores. Part Two is divided into sections on common disorders, from acne to cancer to yeast infection, arranged in alphabetical order. Each section discusses how to identify the symptoms, and suggests ways to correct or treat the disorder through dietary guidelines and a supplementation program. Some contain helpful diagnostic self-tests to help you determine whether or not you have the condition in question. Part Three offers descriptions and explanations of traditional therapies and conventional treatments that can be used in conjunction with a nutritional program. In addition, there are insets throughout the book providing in-depth coverage of important topics. The ramifications of different drug therapies are discussed and the latest medical updates are provided.

Also included, in an appendix, are information on how to find some of the products recommended in this book; a recommended reading list; and a list of health organizations and the addresses and/or phone numbers at which they can be reached for information. A glossary is provided for easy reference.

The supplementation programs recommended in this book should be followed for three to twelve months, depending upon your individual needs and the recommendations of your health care provider. Start by taking nutrients classified "essential" and "very important" for the relevant disorder. Many times, the nutrients recommended for a particular disorder can be found in a single product. Before you start taking them on a regular basis, test the supplements one at a time to find out if you have a reaction to any of them. If you do not find relief within thirty days, add the supplements from the "helpful" list to your program. Each of us is unique; you may need all the nutrients listed, or you may be deficient in only a few. If you still do not notice an improvement after a month, consult your health care provider. You may suffer from malabsorption.

Always take supplements with a full glass of water. Nutritional supplements are concentrated and can overburden the liver if not enough liquid is consumed with the supplements. Water enhances absorption and is needed to aid in carrying the nutrients to the cells.

If you follow a nutritional supplementation program for longer than a year, change brands periodically so that you do not develop an intolerance or build up a resistance to one or more of the ingredients in one supplement. Remember, you can develop an intolerance to the ingredients in vitamins and other supplements just as you can to foods. Learn to listen to your body. Given time, you will notice changes in your body and be able to identify their cause. After the supplementation period is completed, decrease supplement dosages gradually so that the body has a chance to adjust.

PART ONE

UNDERSTANDING THE ELEMENTS OF HEALTH

INTRODUCTION

The human body is a complex organism with the ability to heal itself—if only you listen to it and respond with proper nourishment and care. In spite of all the abuse our bodies endure—whether through exposure to environmental toxins, poor nutrition, cigarette smoking, alcohol consumption, or inactivity—they still usually serve us well for many years before they start to break down. Even then, with a little help, they respond and continue to function.

Think of your body as being composed of millions of tiny little engines. Some of these engines work in unison, some work independently; they all are on call twenty-four hours a day. In order for the engines to work properly, they require specific fuels. If the type of fuel given is the wrong blend, the engine will not perform to its maximum capacity. If the fuel is of a poor grade, the engine may sputter, hesitate, and lose power. If the engine is given no fuel at all, it will stop.

The fuel we give our bodies' engines comes directly from the things we eat. The foods we eat contain nutrients. These nutrients come in the form of vitamins, minerals, enzymes, water, amino acids, carbohydrates, and lipids. It is these nutrients that allow us to sustain life by providing us with the basic materials our bodies need to carry on their daily functions.

Individual nutrients differ in form and function, and in the amount needed by the body; however, they are all vital to our needs. The actions that involve nutrients take place on microscopic levels, and the specific processes differ greatly. Nutrients are involved in all body processes, from combating infection to repairing tissue to thinking. Although nutrients have different specific functions, their common function is to keep us going.

If we do not give ourselves the proper nutrients, we can impair the body's normal functions and cause ourselves great harm. Even if we show no signs of illness, we may not necessarily be healthy. It simply may be that we are not yet exhibiting any overt symptoms of illness. One problem most of us have is that we do not get the nutrients we need from our diets because most of the foods we consume are cooked and/or processed. Cooking and processing destroy vital nutrients the body needs to function properly. The organic raw foods that supply these elements are largely missing from today's diet.

The past decade has brought to light much new knowledge about nutrition and its effects on the body and the role it plays in disease. *Phytonutrients* are one example of the results of this research. Phytonutrients are chemicals present in plants that make the plants biologically active. They are not nutrients in the classic sense, but they are what determines a plant's color, flavor, and ability to resist disease. Researchers have identified literally thousands of phytochemicals and have also developed the technology to extract these chemical compounds and concentrate them into pills, powders, and capsules. These are called *nutraceuticals*—the newest type of dietary supplement.

By understanding the principles of holistic nutrition, and knowing what nutrients you need, you can improve the state of your health, stave off disease, and maintain a harmonious balance in the way nature intended. Part One should provide you with a clear understanding of the vitamins, minerals, amino acids, enzymes, and other nutrients you need, as well as important information on natural food supplements, herbs, and products that enhance nutrient activity.

Nutrition, Diet, and Wellness

UNDERSTANDING THE BASICS OF NUTRITION

Good nutrition is the foundation of good health. Everyone needs the four basic nutrients—water, carbohydrates, proteins, and fats—as well as vitamins, minerals, and other micronutrients. To be able to choose the proper foods, and to better understand why those foods should be supported with supplements, you need to have a clear idea of the components of a healthy diet.

The Four Basic Nutrients

Water, carbohydrates, proteins, and fats are the basic building blocks of a good diet. By choosing the healthiest forms of each of these nutrients, and eating them in the proper balance, you enable your body to function at its optimal level.

Water

The human body is two-thirds water. Water is an essential nutrient that is involved in every function of the body. It helps transport nutrients and waste products in and out of cells. It is necessary for all digestive, absorption, circulatory, and excretory functions, as well as for the utilization of the water-soluble vitamins. It is also needed for the maintenance of proper body temperature. By drinking an adequate amount of water each day—at least eight 8-ounce glasses—you can ensure that your body has all it needs to maintain good health. (For details on choosing the best water, *see* WATER in Part One.)

Carbohydrates

Carbohydrates supply the body with the energy it needs to function. They are found almost exclusively in plant foods, such as fruits, vegetables, peas, and beans. Milk and milk products are the only foods derived from animals that contain a significant amount of carbohydrates.

Carbohydrates are divided into two groups—simple carbohydrates and complex carbohydrates. *Simple carbohydrates*, sometimes called simple sugars, include fructose (fruit sugar), sucrose (table sugar), and lactose (milk sugar), as well as several other sugars. Fruits are one of the richest natural sources of simple carbohydrates. *Complex carbohydrates* are also made up of sugars, but the sugar molecules are strung together to form longer, more complex chains. Complex carbohydrates include fiber and starches. Foods rich in complex carbohydrates include vegetables, whole grains, peas, and beans.

Carbohydrates are the main source of blood glucose, which is a major fuel for all of the body's cells and the only source of energy for the brain and red blood cells. Except for fiber, which cannot be digested, both simple and complex carbohydrates are converted into glucose. The glucose is then either used directly to provide energy for the body, or stored in the liver for future use. When a person consumes more calories than the body is using, a portion of the carbohydrates consumed may also be stored in the body as fat.

When choosing carbohydrate-rich foods for your diet, always select unrefined foods such as fruits, vegetables, peas, beans, and whole-grain products, as opposed to refined, processed foods such as soft drinks, desserts, candy, and sugar. Refined foods offer few, if any, of the vitamins and minerals that are important to your health. In addition, if eaten in excess, especially over a period of many years, the large amounts of simple carbohydrates found in refined foods can lead to a number of disorders, including diabetes and hypoglycemia (low blood sugar). Yet another problem is that foods high in refined simple sugars often are also high in fats, which should be limited in a healthy diet. This is why such foods—which include most cookies and cakes, as well as many snack foods—are usually loaded with calories.

A word is in order regarding fiber, a very important form of carbohydrate. Referred to in the past as "roughage," dietary fiber is the part of a plant that is resistant to the body's digestive enzymes. As a result, only a relatively small amount of fiber is digested or metabolized in the stomach or intestines. Instead, most of it moves through the gastrointestinal tract and ends up in the stool.

Although most fiber is not digested, it delivers several important health benefits. First, fiber retains water, resulting in softer and bulkier stools that prevent constipation and hemorrhoids. A high-fiber diet also reduces the risk of colon cancer, perhaps by speeding the rate at which stool passes through the intestine and by keeping the digestive tract clean. In addition, fiber binds with certain substances that would normally result in the production of cholesterol, and eliminates these substances from the body. In this way, a high-fiber diet helps lower blood cholesterol levels, reducing the risk of heart disease.

It is recommended that about 60 percent of your total

daily calories come from carbohydrates. If much of your diet consists of healthy complex carbohydrates, you should easily fulfill the recommended daily minimum of 25 grams of fiber.

Protein

Protein is essential for growth and development. It provides the body with energy, and is needed for the manufacture of hormones, antibodies, enzymes, and tissues. It also helps maintain the proper acid-alkali balance in the body.

When protein is consumed, the body breaks it down into amino acids, the building blocks of all proteins. Some of the amino acids are designated *nonessential*. This does not mean that they are unnecessary, but rather that they do not have to come from the diet because they can be synthesized by the body from other amino acids. Other amino acids are considered *essential*, meaning that the body cannot synthesize them, and therefore must obtain them from the diet.

Whenever the body *makes* a protein—when it builds muscle, for instance—it needs a variety of amino acids for the protein-making process. These amino acids may come from dietary protein or from the body's own pool of amino acids. If a shortage of amino acids becomes chronic, which can occur if the diet is deficient in essential amino acids, the building of protein in the body stops, and the body suffers. (For more information about amino acids, *see* AMINO ACIDS in Part One.)

Because of the importance of consuming proteins that provide all of the necessary amino acids, dietary proteins are considered to belong to two different groups, depending on the amino acids they provide. *Complete proteins*, which constitute the first group, contain ample amounts of all of the essential amino acids. These proteins are found in meat, fish, poultry, cheese, eggs, and milk. *Incomplete proteins*, which constitute the second group, contain only some of the essential amino acids. These proteins are found in a variety of foods, including grains, legumes, and leafy green vegetables.

Although it is important to consume the full range of amino acids, both essential and nonessential, it is not necessary to get them from meat, fish, poultry, and other complete-protein foods. In fact, because of their high fat content—as well as the use of antibiotics and other chemicals in the raising of poultry and cattle—most of those foods should be eaten in moderation. Fortunately, the dietary strategy called *mutual supplementation* enables you to combine partial-protein foods to make *complementary protein*—proteins that supply adequate amounts of all the essential amino acids. For instance, although beans and brown rice are both quite rich in protein, each lacks one or more of the necessary amino acids. However, when you combine beans and brown rice with each other, or when you combine either one with any of a number of protein-rich foods, you form a complete protein that is a high-quality substitute for meat. To make a complete protein, combine *beans* with any one of the following:

- Brown rice.
- Corn.
- Nuts.
- Seeds.
- Wheat.

Or combine *brown rice* with any one of the following:

- Beans.
- Nuts.
- Seeds.
- Wheat.

Most Americans eat too much protein, largely as the result of a diet high in meat and dairy products. However, if you have reduced the amount of meat and dairy foods in your diet, you should make sure to get about 50 grams of protein a day. To make sure that you are getting a great enough variety of amino acids in your diet, add protein-rich foods to meals and snacks as often as possible. Eat bread with nut butters, for instance, or add nuts and seeds to salads and vegetable casseroles. Be aware that a combination of any grains, any nuts and seeds, any legumes (such as beans, peanuts, and peas), and a variety of mixed vegetables will make a complete protein. In addition, cornmeal fortified with the amino acid L-lysine makes a complete protein.

All soybean products, such as tofu and soymilk, are complete proteins. They contain the essential amino acids plus several other nutrients. Available in health food stores, tofu, soy oil, soy flour, soy-based meat substitutes, soy cheese, and many other soy products are healthful ways to complement the meatless diet.

Yogurt is the only animal-derived complete-protein source recommended for frequent use in the diet. Made from milk that is curdled by bacteria, yogurt contains *Lactobacillus acidophilus* and other "friendly" bacteria needed for the digestion of foods and the prevention of many disorders, including candidiasis. Yogurt also contains vitamins A and D, and many of the B-complex vitamins.

Do not buy the sweetened, flavored yogurts that are sold in supermarkets. These products contain added sugar and, often, preservatives. Instead, either purchase fresh unsweetened yogurt from a health food store or make the yogurt yourself, and sweeten it with fruit juices and other wholesome ingredients. Yogurt makers are relatively inexpensive and easy to use, and are available at most health food stores.

Fats

Although much attention has been focused on the need to reduce dietary fat, the body does need fat. During infancy and childhood, fat is necessary for normal brain development. Throughout life, it is essential to provide energy and support growth. Fat is, in fact, the most concentrated source of energy available to the body. However, after about two years of age, the body requires only small amounts of fat—much less than is provided by the average American diet. Excessive fat intake is a major causative factor in obesity, high blood pressure, coronary heart disease, and colon cancer, and has been linked to a number of other disorders as well. To understand how fat intake is related to these health problems, it is necessary to understand the different types of fats available and the ways in which these fats act within the body.

Fats are composed of building blocks called fatty acids. There are three major categories of fatty acids—saturated, polyunsaturated, and monounsatured. These classifications are based on the number of hydrogen atoms in the chemical structure of a given molecule of fatty acid.

Saturated fatty acids are found primarily in animal products, including dairy items, such as whole milk, cream, and cheese, and fatty meats like beef, veal, lamb, pork, and ham. The fat marbling you can see in beef and pork is composed of saturated fat. Some vegetable products—including coconut oil, palm kernel oil, and vegetable shortening—are also high in saturates.

The liver uses saturated fats to manufacture cholesterol. Therefore, excessive dietary intake of saturated fats can significantly raise the blood cholesterol level, especially the level of low-density lipoproteins (LDLs), or "bad cholesterol." (For more information about cholesterol, *see* Understanding Cholesterol on page 326.) Guidelines issued by the National Cholesterol Education Program (NCEP), and widely supported by most experts, recommend that the daily intake of saturated fats be kept below 10 percent of total caloric intake. However, for people who have severe problems with high blood cholesterol, even that level may be too high.

Polyunsaturated fatty acids are found in greatest abundance in corn, soybean, safflower, and sunflower oils. Certain fish oils are also high in polyunsaturates. Unlike the saturated fats, polyunsaturates may actually lower your total blood cholesterol level. In doing so, however, large amounts of polyunsaturates also have a tendency to reduce your high-density lipoproteins (HDLs)—your "good cholesterol." For this reason—and because, like all fats, polyunsaturates are high in calories for their weight and volume—the NCEP guidelines state that an individual's intake of polyunsaturated fats should not exceed 10 percent of total caloric intake.

Monounsaturated fatty acids are found mostly in vegetable and nut oils such as olive, peanut, and canola. These fats appear to reduce blood levels of LDLs without affecting HDLs in any way. However, this positive impact upon LDL cholesterol is relatively modest. The NCEP guidelines recommend that intake of monounsaturated fats be kept between 10 and 15 percent of total caloric intake.

Although most foods—including some plant-derived foods—contain a combination of all three types of fatty acids, one of the types usually predominates. Thus, a fat or oil is considered "saturated" or "high in saturates"

when it is composed primarily of saturated fatty acids. Such saturated fats are usually solid at room temperature. Similarly, a fat or oil composed mostly of polyunsaturated fatty acids is called "polyunsaturated," while a fat or oil composed mostly of monounsaturated fatty acids is called "monounsaturated."

One other element, *trans-fatty acids,* may also play a role in blood cholesterol levels. Also called trans fats, these substances occur when polyunsaturated oils are altered through hydrogenation, a process used to harden liquid vegetable oils into solid foods like margarine and shortening. One recent study found that trans-monounsaturated fatty acids raise LDL cholesterol levels, behaving much like saturated fats. Simultaneously, the trans-fatty acids reduced HDL cholesterol readings. Much more research on this subject is necessary, as studies have not reached consistent and conclusive findings. For now, however, it is clear that if your goal is to lower cholesterol, polyunsaturated and monounsaturated fats are more desirable than saturated fats or products with trans-fatty acids. Just as important, your total calories from fat should not constitute more than 20 to 25 percent of daily calories.

The Micronutrients: Vitamins and Minerals

Like water, carbohydrates, protein, and fats, vitamins and minerals are essential to life. They are therefore considered nutrients, and are often referred to as *micronutrients* simply because they are needed in relatively small amounts compared with the four basic nutrients.

Because vitamins and minerals are so necessary for health, the U.S. Food and Drug Administration (FDA) has formulated recommended consumption levels for vitamins called recommended daily allowances (RDAs). But, as we will see in VITAMINS in Part One, these allowances do not account for the amount needed to maintain maximum health rather than borderline health, only the amount needed to prevent deficiency diseases. Therefore, the average adult who is not suffering from any specific disorder should obtain more than the RDAs of vitamins and minerals from food sources and/or from supplements. The table on page 6—which includes not just vitamin and mineral supplements, but other supplements as well—should be used as a guideline. Although the amounts listed are safe (they will not cause toxicity), they should be varied according to size and weight. People who are active and exercise; those who are under great stress, on restricted diets, or mentally or physically ill; women who take oral contraceptives; those on medication; those who are recovering from surgery; and smokers and those who consume alcoholic beverages all need higher than normal amounts of nutrients.

In addition to a proper diet, exercise and a positive attitude are two important elements that are needed to prevent sickness and disease. If your lifestyle includes each of these, you will feel good and have more energy—something we all deserve.

Nutrients and Dosages for Maintaining Good Health

The nutrients listed below are recommended for good health. Daily dosages are suggested; however, before using any supplements, you should consult with your health care provider. The dosages given here are for adults and children weighing 100 pounds and over. Appropriate dosages for children vary according to age and weight. A child weighing between 70 and 100 pounds should be given three-fourths the adult dose; a child weighing under 70 pounds (and *over* the age of six) should be given half the adult dose. A child under the age of six years should be given nutritional formulas designed specifically for young children. Follow the dosage directions on the product label.

Vitamins	Daily Dosages
Vitamin A	10,000 IU
Beta-carotene	15,000 IU
Vitamin B_1 (thiamine)	50 mg
Vitamin B_2 (riboflavin)	50 mg
Vitamin B_3 (niacin)	100 mg
(niacinamide)	100 mg
Pantothenic acid (vitamin B_5)	100 mg
Vitamin B_6 (pyridoxine)	50 mg
Vitamin B_{12}	300 mcg
Biotin	300 mcg
Choline	100 mg
Folic acid	800 mcg
Inositol	100 mg
Para-aminobenzoic acid (PABA)	50 mg
Vitamin C with mineral ascorbates	3,000 mg
Bioflavonoids (mixed)	500 mg
Hesperidin	100 mg
Rutin	25 mg
Vitamin D	400 IU
Vitamin E	600 IU
Vitamin K (use natural sources such as alfalfa, green leafy vegetables)	100 mcg
Essential fatty acids (EFAs) (primrose oil, flaxseed oil, salmon oil, and fish oil are good sources)	As directed on label.

Minerals	Daily Dosages
Calcium	1,500 mg
Chromium (GTF)	150 mcg
Copper	3 mg
Iodine (kelp is a good source)	225 mcg
Iron*	18 mg
Magnesium	750–1,000 mg
Manganese	10 mg
Molybdenum	30 mcg
Potassium	99 mg
Selenium	200 mcg
Zinc	50 mg

Optional Supplements	Daily Dosages
Coenzyme Q_{10}	30 mg
Garlic	As directed on label.
L-Carnitine	500 mg
L-Cysteine	50 mg
L-Lysine	50 mg
L-Methionine	50 mg
L-Tyrosine	500 mg
Lecithin	200–500 mg
Pectin	50 mg
RNA-DNA	100 mg
Silicon	As directed on label.
Superoxide dismutase (SOD)	As directed on label.

*Iron should be taken only if a deficiency exists. Always take iron supplements separately, rather than in a multivitamin and mineral formula. Do not take iron with a supplement containing vitamin E.

Other supplements that you may wish to take for increased energy are:

- Bee pollen.
- Bio-Strath from Bioforce of America.
- Floradix Iron + Herbs from Salus Haus.
- Free-form amino acids.
- Kyo-Green from Wakunaga of America.
- N,N-Dimethylglycine (DMG).
- Octacosanol.
- Siberian ginseng.
- Spirulina.

Synergy and Deficiency

Data compiled by the U.S. Department of Agriculture indicate that at least 40 percent of the people in this country routinely consume a diet containing only 60 percent of the RDA of each of ten selected nutrients. This means that close to half of the population (and very likely more) suffer from a deficiency of at least one important nutrient. A poll of 37,000 Americans conducted by Food Technology found that half of them were deficient in vitamin B_6 (pyridoxine), 42 percent did not consume sufficient amounts of calcium, 39 percent had an insufficient iron intake, and 25 to 39 percent did not obtain enough vitamin C. Additional research has shown that a vitamin deficiency may not affect the whole body, but only specific cells. For example, those who smoke may suffer from a vitamin C deficiency, but only in the lung area.

Phytochemicals

For many years, researchers have recognized that diets high in fruits, vegetables, grains, and legumes appear to reduce the risk of a number of diseases, including cancer, heart disease, diabetes, and high blood pressure when compared with diets high in meat. More recently, it was discovered that the disease-preventing effects of these foods are partly due to antioxidants—specific vitamins, minerals, and enzymes that help prevent cancer and other disorders by protecting cells against damage from oxidation. Now, researchers have discovered that fruits, vegetables, grains, and legumes contain yet another group of health-promoting nutrients. Called *phytochemicals,* these substances appear to be powerful ammunition in the war against cancer and other disorders.

Phytochemicals are the biologically active substances in plants that are responsible for giving them color, flavor, and natural disease resistance. To understand how phytochemicals protect the body against cancer, it is necessary to understand that cancer formation is a multistep process. Phytochemicals seem to fight cancer by blocking one or more of the steps that lead to cancer. For instance, cancer can begin when a carcinogenic molecule—from the food you eat or the air you breathe—invades a cell. But if sulforaphane, a phytochemical found in broccoli, also reaches the cell, it activates a group of enzymes that whisk the carcinogen out of the cell before it can cause any harm.

Other phytochemicals are known to prevent cancer in other ways. Flavonoids, found in citrus fruits and berries, keep cancer-causing hormones from latching onto cells in the first place. Genistein, found in soybeans, kills tumors by preventing the formation of the capillaries needed to nourish them. Indoles, found in cruciferous vegetables such as Brussels sprouts, cauliflower, and cabbage, increase immune activity and make it easier for the body to excrete toxins. Saponins, found in kidney beans, chickpeas, soybeans, and lentils, may prevent cancer cells from multiplying. P-coumaric acid and chlorogenic acid, found in tomatoes, interfere with certain chemical unions that can create carcinogens. The list of

these protective substances goes on and on. Tomatoes alone are believed to contain an estimated 10,000 different phytochemicals.

Although no long-term human studies have shown that specific phytochemicals stop cancer, research on phytochemicals supports the more than 200 studies that link lowered cancer risk with a diet rich in grains, legumes, fruits, and vegetables. Moreover, animal and in vitro studies have demonstrated how some phytochemicals prevent carcinogens from promoting the growth of specific cancers. For instance, the phytochemical phenethyl isothiocyanate (PEITC), found in cabbage and turnips, has been found to inhibit the growth of lung cancer in rats and mice. Among other things, PEITC protects the cells' DNA from a potent carcinogen found in tobacco smoke.

Researchers have been able to isolate some phytochemicals, and a number of companies are now selling concentrates that contain phytochemicals obtained from vegetables such as broccoli. These may be used as supplemental sources of some of these nutrients. However, such pills should *not* be seen as replacements for fresh whole foods. Because several *thousand* phytochemicals are currently known to exist, and because new ones are being discovered all the time, no supplement can possibly contain all of the cancer-fighters found in a shopping basket full of fruits and vegetables.

Fortunately, it is easy to get a healthy dose of phytochemicals at every meal. Almost every grain, legume, fruit, and vegetable tested has been found to contain these substances. Moreover, unlike many vitamins, these substances do not appear to be destroyed by cooking or other processing. Genistein, the substance found in soybeans, for instance, is also found in soybean products such as tofu and miso soup. Similarly, the phytochemical PEITC, found in cabbage, remains intact even when the cabbage is made into cole slaw or sauerkraut. Of course, by eating much of your produce raw or only lightly cooked, you will be able to enjoy the benefits not just of phytochemicals, but of all of the vitamins, minerals, and other nutrients that fresh whole foods have to offer.

Whenever you seek to correct a vitamin or mineral deficiency, you must recognize that nutrients work synergistically. This means that there is a cooperative action between certain vitamins and minerals, which work as catalysts, promoting the absorption and assimilation of other vitamins and minerals. Correcting a deficiency in one vitamin or mineral requires the addition of others, not simply replacement of the one in which you are deficient. This is why taking a single vitamin or mineral may be ineffective, or even dangerous, and why a balanced vitamin and mineral preparation should always be taken in addition to any single supplements. The following table indicates which vitamins and minerals are necessary to correct certain deficiencies.

Vitamin Deficiency	Supplements Needed for Assimilation
Vitamin A	Choline, essential fatty acids, zinc, vitamins C, D, and E.
Vitamin B complex	Calcium, vitamins C and E.
Vitamin B_1 (thiamine)	Manganese, vitamin B complex, vitamins C and E.
Vitamin B_2 (riboflavin)	Vitamin B complex, vitamin C.
Vitamin B_3 (niacin)	Vitamin B complex, vitamin C.
Pantothenic acid (vitamin B_5)	Vitamin B complex, vitamins A, C, and E.
Vitamin B_6 (pyridoxine)	Potassium, vitamin B complex, vitamin C.

Biotin	Folic acid, vitamin B complex, pantothenic acid (vitamin B_5), vitamin B_{12}, vitamin C.
Choline	Vitamin B complex, vitamin B_{12}, folic acid, inositol.
Inositol	Vitamin B complex, vitamin C.
Para-aminobenzoic acid (PABA)	Vitamin B complex, folic acid, vitamin C.
Vitamin C	Bioflavonoids, calcium, magnesium.
Vitamin D	Calcium, choline, essential fatty acids, phosphorus, vitamins A and C.
Vitamin E	Essential fatty acids, manganese, selenium, vitamin A, vitamin B_1 (thiamine), inositol, vitamin C.
Essential fatty acids	Vitamins A, C, D, and E.

Mineral Deficiency	Supplements Needed for Assimilation
Calcium	Boron, essential fatty acids, lysine, magnesium, manganese, phosphorus, vitamins A, C, D, and F.
Copper	Cobalt, folic acid, iron, zinc.
Iodine	Iron, manganese, phosphorus.
Magnesium	Calcium, phosphorus, potassium, vitamin B_6 (pyridoxine), vitamins C and D.
Manganese	Calcium, iron, vitamin B complex, vitamin E.
Phosphorus	Calcium, iron, manganese, sodium, vitamin B_6 (pyridoxine).
Silicon	Iron, phosphorus.
Sodium	Calcium, potassium, sulfur, vitamin D.
Sulfur	Potassium, vitamin B_1 (thiamine), pantothenic acid (vitamin B_5), biotin.
Zinc	Calcium, copper, phosphorus, vitamin B_6 (pyridoxine).

GUIDELINES FOR SELECTING AND PREPARING FOODS

Clearly, a healthy diet must provide a proper balance of the four essential nutrients, as well as a rich supply of vitamins, minerals, and other micronutrients. However, it is not enough simply to purchase foods that are high in complex carbohydrates, fiber, and complementary proteins, and low in saturated fats. Food must also be free of harmful additives, and it must be prepared in a way that preserves its nutrients and avoids the production of harmful substances.

Avoid Foods That Contain Additives and Artificial Ingredients

Additives are placed in foods for a number of reasons: to lengthen shelf life; to make a food more appealing by enhancing color, texture, or taste; to facilitate food preparation; or to otherwise make the product more marketable. Certain additives, like sugar, are derived from natural sources. Other additives, like aspartame (NutraSweet), are made synthetically.

Although many additives are used in very small amounts, it has been estimated that the average American consumes about 5 pounds of additives per year. If you include sugar—the food-processing industry's most used additive—the number jumps to 135 pounds a year. Anyone whose diet is high in processed products clearly consumes a significant amount of additives and artificial ingredients.

At their best, additives and artificial ingredients simply add little or no nutritional value to a food product. At their worst, additives pose a threat to your health. The history of additive use includes a number of products that were once deemed safe but later were banned or allowed to be used only if accompanied by warnings. The artificial sweeteners cyclamate and saccharin are just two examples of such products. Other additives, like monosodium glutamate (MSG) and aspartame, are used without warnings, but have been known to cause problems ranging from headaches and diarrhea to confusion, memory loss, and seizures. (For more information on aspartame, *see* Is Aspartame a Safe Sugar Substitute? on page 9.)

The number of food additives now in use is staggering. To learn more about these substances, you can consult Michael Jacobson's *Safe Food: Eating Wisely in a Risky World* (Living Planet Press, 1991) or *Unsafe at Any Meal* by Earl Mindell (Warner Books, 1986).

Increase Your Consumption of Raw Produce

The most healthful fruits and vegetables are those that have been grown organically—without the use of insecticides, herbicides, artificial fertilizers, or growth-stimulating chemicals. Organic produce can be found in select health food stores, as well as in some supermarkets and greenmarkets and through food co-ops.

When choosing your produce, look for fruits and vegetables that are at the peak of ripeness. These contain more vitamins and enzymes than do foods that are underripe or overripe, or that have been stored for any length of time. Remember that the longer a food is kept in storage, the more nutrients it loses.

Once you get your organic produce home, running water and a vegetable brush are probably all that will be needed to get it ready for the table. If the produce is not organic, however, you will want to wash it more thoroughly to rid it of any chemical residues. Use a soft vegetable brush to scrub the foods, and then let them soak in

Is Aspartame a Safe Sugar Substitute?

Due to America's obsession with dieting, the popularity of aspartame (NutraSweet) has soared. Because it is about 200 times sweeter than sugar, much smaller amounts of aspartame are needed to sweeten the taste of foods. This artificial sweetener pervades supermarket shelves. It is especially prevalent in diet foods, and can be found in the following products:

- Instant breakfasts.
- Breath mints.
- Cereals.
- Sugar-free chewing gum.
- Cocoa mixes.
- Coffee beverages.
- Frozen desserts.
- Gelatin desserts.
- Juice beverages.
- Laxatives.
- Milk drinks.
- Multivitamins.
- Nonprescription pharmaceuticals.
- Shake mixes.
- Soft drinks.
- Tabletop sweeteners.
- Tea beverages.
- Instant teas and coffees.
- Topping mixes.
- Wine coolers.
- Yogurt.

Aspartame consists of three components: the amino acids phenylalanine and aspartic acid, and methanol, which is also known as methyl alcohol or wood alcohol.

Although it has been claimed that the amino acids in aspartame are metabolized in the same way that their natural counterparts, found in foods, are metabolized, research suggests otherwise. Consumption of aspartame in sodas, for instance, appears to cause a flooding of the amino acids in the bloodstream—a prompt rise that does not occur after the ingestion of dietary protein. This rise, it is believed, may cause problems.

No one disputes that aspartame should be avoided by people with phenylketonuria (PKU). People with PKU lack the enzyme need to convert phenylalanine into tyrosine, another amino acid. As a result, high concentrations of phenylalanine accumulate and can cause brain damage. It should be noted that a number of people who have disorders other than PKU—people with iron deficiencies and kidney disease, for instance—may also be prone to high levels of this amino acid. For such people, the consumption of aspartame may increase the risk of toxicity.

Methanol, the third ingredient in aspartame, is known to be poisonous even when consumed in relatively modest amounts. Disorders caused by toxic levels of methanol include blindness, brain swelling, and inflammation of the pancreas and heart muscle. Although the Food and Drug Administration (FDA) states that exposure to methanol through aspartame consumption is not of "sufficient quantity to be of toxicological concern," the cumulative effects of high doses of aspartame are unknown.

Regardless of any claims of the FDA, a significant number of people have reported suffering ill effects as a result of aspartame consumption. According to *Aspartame (NutraSweet): Is It Safe?* by H.J. Roberts (The Charles Press, 1990), reported reactions include headaches, mood swings, changes in vision, nausea and diarrhea, sleep disorders, memory loss and confusion, and even convulsions. Aspartame appears to be especially dangerous for children.

Needless to say, if you have experienced a reaction to aspartame, you should refrain from using foods that contain this additive. Better yet, avoid all additives, and enjoy a diet rich in fruits and fresh juices. These foods are naturally sweet, free of artificial coloring and preservatives, and full of the nutrients needed for good health.

---

water for ten minutes. You can also clean produce with nontoxic rinsing preparations, which are available in reputable health food stores. If the products are waxed, peel them, as wax cannot be washed away, but remove as thin a layer of peel as possible.

Most fruits and vegetables should be eaten in their entirety, as all of the parts, including the skin, contain valuable nutrients. When eating citrus fruits, remove the rinds, but eat the white part inside the skin for its vitamin C and bioflavonoid content.

Although most people usually cook their vegetables before eating, both fruits and vegetables should be eaten raw as much as possible. All enzymes and most vitamins are extremely sensitive to heat, and are usually destroyed in the cooking process.

If fresh produce is unavailable, use frozen foods instead. Do not use canned vegetables or boxed vegetable dishes, as they usually contain significant amounts of salt and other unhealthy additives. If raw produce does not agree with you, steam your vegetables lightly in a steamer, cooking pan, or wok just until slightly tender.

Avoid Overcooking Your Foods

As just discussed, cooking foods for all but brief periods of time can destroy many valuable nutrients. More alarming is that when foods are cooked to the point of browning or charring, the organic compounds they contain undergo changes in structure, producing carcinogens.

Barbecued meats seem to pose the worst health threat in this regard. When burning fat drips onto an open flame, polycyclic aromatic hydrocarbons (PAHs)—dangerous carcinogens—are formed. When amino acids and other chemicals found in muscle are exposed to high tempera-

Basic Nutritional Guide

A diet high in nutrients is the key to good health. Use the following table as a guide when deciding which types of food to include in your diet and which ones to avoid in order to maintain good health.

Types of Food	Foods to Avoid	Acceptable Foods
Beans	Canned pork and beans, canned beans with salt or preservatives, frozen beans.	All beans cooked without animal fat or salt.
Beverages	Alcoholic drinks, coffee, cocoa, pasteurized and/or sweetened juices and fruit drinks, sodas, tea (except herbal tea).	Herbal teas, fresh vegetable and fruit juices, cereal grain beverages (often sold as coffee substitutes), mineral or distilled water.
Dairy products	All soft cheeses, all pasteurized or artificially colored cheese products, ice cream.	Raw goat cheese, nonfat cottage cheese, kefir, unsweetened yogurt, goat's milk, raw or skim milk, buttermilk, rice milk, all soy products.
Eggs	Fried or pickled.	Boiled or poached (limit of four weekly).
Fish	All fried fish, all shellfish, salted fish, anchovies, herring, fish canned in oil.	All freshwater white fish, salmon, broiled or baked fish, water-packed tuna.
Fruits	Canned, bottled, or frozen fruits with sweeteners added; oranges.	All fresh, frozen, stewed, or dried fruits without sweeteners (except oranges, which are acidic and highly allergenic), unsulfured fruits, home-canned fruits.
Grains	All white flour products, white rice, pasta, crackers, cold cereals, instant types of oatmeal and other hot cereals.	All whole grains and products containing whole grains: cereals, breads, muffins, whole-grain crackers, cream of wheat or rye cereal, buckwheat, millet, oats, brown rice, wild rice. (Limit yeast breads to three servings per week.)
Meats	Beef; all forms of pork; hot dogs; luncheon meats; smoked, pickled, and processed meats; corned beef; duck; goose; spare ribs; gravies; organ meats.	Skinless turkey and chicken, lamb. (Limit meat to three 3-oz servings per week.)
Nuts	Peanuts; all salted or roasted nuts.	All fresh raw nuts (except peanuts).
Oils (fats)	All saturated fats, hydrogenated margarine, refined processed oils, shortenings, hardened oils.	All cold-pressed oils: corn, safflower, sesame, olive, flaxseed, soybean, sunflower, and canola oils; margarine made from these oils; eggless mayonnaise.
Seasonings	Black or white pepper, salt, hot red peppers, all types of vinegar except pure natural apple cider vinegar.	Garlic, onions, cayenne, Spike, all herbs, dried vegetables, apple cider vinegar, tamari, miso, seaweed, dulse.
Soups	Canned soups made with salt, preservatives, MSG, or fat stock; all creamed soups.	Homemade (salt- and fat-free) bean, lentil, pea, vegetable, barley, brown rice, onion.
Sprouts and seeds	All seeds cooked in oil or salt.	All slightly cooked sprouts (except alfalfa, which should be raw and washed thoroughly), wheatgrass, all raw seeds.
Sweets	White, brown, or raw cane sugar, corn syrups, chocolate, sugar candy, fructose (except that in fresh whole fruit), all syrups (except pure maple syrup), all sugar substitutes, jams and jellies made with sugar.	Barley malt or rice syrup, small amounts of raw honey, pure maple syrup, unsulfured blackstrap molasses.
Vegetables	All canned or frozen with salt or additives.	All raw, fresh, frozen (no additives), or home-canned without salt (undercook vegetables slightly).

tures, other carcinogens, called heterocyclic aromatic amines (HAAs), are created. In fact, many of the chemicals used to produce cancer in laboratory animals have been isolated from cooked proteins.

It is important to note, though, that cooked meats do not pose the only threat. Even browned or burned bread crusts contain a variety of carcinogenic substances.

The dangers posed by the practice of cooking foods at high temperatures or until browned or burned should not be dismissed. Although eating habits vary widely from person to person, it seems safe to assume that many people consume many grams of overcooked foods a day. By comparison, only half a gram of this same dangerous burned material is inhaled by someone who smokes two packs of cigarettes a day. Clearly, by eating produce raw or only lightly cooked, and by greatly limiting your consumption of meat, you will be doing much to decrease your risk of cancer and, possibly, other disorders.

Use the Proper Cooking Utensils

Although raw foods have many advantages over cooked, nourishing soups and a variety of other dishes can be made healthfully. One of the ways to ensure wholesome cooked food is the careful selection of cookware.

When preparing foods, use only glass, stainless steel, or iron pots and pans. Do not use aluminum cookware or utensils. Foods cooked or stored in aluminum produce a substance that neutralizes the digestive juices, leading to acidosis and ulcers. Worse, the aluminum in the cookware can leach from the pot into the food. When the food is consumed, the aluminum is absorbed by the body, where it accumulates in the brain and nervous system tissues. Excessive amounts of these aluminum deposits have been implicated in Alzheimer's disease.

Other cookware to be avoided includes all pots and pans with nonstick coatings. Too often, the metals and other substances in the pots' finish flakes or leaches into the food. Ultimately, these chemicals end up in your body.

Limit Your Use of Salt

Although some sodium is essential for survival, inadequate sodium intake is a rare problem. We need less than 500 milligrams of sodium a day to stay healthy. This is enough to accomplish all the vital functions that sodium performs in the body—helping maintain normal fluid levels, healthy muscle function, and proper acidity (pH) of the blood. Excessive sodium intake can cause fluid to be retained in the tissues, which can lead to hypertension (high blood pressure) and can aggravate many medical disorders, including congestive heart failure, certain forms of kidney disease, and premenstrual syndrome (PMS).

One of the best ways to limit the sodium in your diet is to limit your use of salt when cooking and dining. Just as important, stay away from processed foods, which often contain excessively high amounts of sodium.

VITAMINS

THE FUNCTION OF VITAMINS

Vitamins are essential to life. They contribute to good health by regulating the metabolism and assisting the biochemical processes that release energy from digested food. They are considered micronutrients because the body needs them in relatively small amounts compared with nutrients such as carbohydrates, proteins, fats, and water.

Enzymes are essential chemicals that are the foundation of human bodily functions. They are catalysts (activators) in the chemical reactions that are continually taking place within the body. As coenzymes, vitamins work with enzymes, thereby allowing all the activities that occur within the body to be carried out as they should.

Of the major vitamins, some are water soluble and some are oil soluble. Water-soluble vitamins must be taken into the body daily, as they cannot be stored and are excreted within one to four days. These include vitamin C and the B-complex vitamins. Oil-soluble vitamins can be stored for longer periods of time in the body's fatty tissue and the liver. These include vitamins A, D, E, and K. Both types of vitamins are needed by the body for proper functioning.

RDA VERSUS ODA

Recommended daily allowances (RDAs) were instituted over forty years ago by the U.S. Food and Nutrition Board as a standard for the daily amounts of vitamins needed by a healthy person. Unfortunately, the amounts they came up with give us only the bare minimum required to ward off deficiency diseases such as beriberi, rickets, scurvy, and night blindness. What they do not account for are the amounts needed to maintain maximum health, rather than borderline health.

Scientific studies have shown that larger dosages of vitamins help our bodies work better. The RDAs therefore are not very useful for determining what our intake of different vitamins should be. We prefer to speak in terms of *optimum daily allowances* (ODAs)—the amounts of nutrients needed for vibrant good health. This entails consuming larger amounts of vitamins than the RDAs. The nutrient doses recommended on page 6 are ODAs. By providing our bodies with an optimum daily allowance of necessary vitamins, we can enhance our health. The dosages outlined in this book will enable you to design a vitamin program that is custom-tailored for the individual.

BALANCE AND SYNERGY

The proper balance of vitamins and minerals is important to the proper functioning of all vitamins. Scientific research has proved that an excess of an isolated vitamin or mineral can produce the same symptoms as a deficiency of a vitamin or mineral. For example, high doses of isolated B vitamins have been shown to cause depletion of other B vitamins. Similarly, when zinc is taken in excess, symptoms of zinc deficiency can result. Studies have shown that an intake of up to 100 milligrams of zinc daily enhances the immune function, but an amount in excess of 100 milligrams daily may actually harm immune function.

Synergy is a phenomenon whereby two or more vitamins combine to create a stronger vitamin function. For example, in order for bioflavonoids to work properly (they prevent bruising and bleeding gums), they must be taken along with vitamin C. Recent studies show that bioflavonoids also may be a big factor in preventing cancer and many other diseases.

In addition, certain substances can block the absorption and effects of vitamins. For example, the absorption of vitamin C is greatly reduced by antibiotic drugs, so a person taking antibiotics requires a higher than normal intake of this vitamin.

SYNTHETIC VERSUS NATURAL

Ideally, all of us would get all of the nutrients we need for optimal health from fresh, healthful foods. In reality, however, this is often difficult, if not impossible. In our chemically polluted and stress-filled world, our nutritional requirements have been increasing, but the number of calories we require has been *decreasing,* as our general level of physical activity has declined. This means we are faced with needing somehow to get more nutrients from less food. At the same time, due to the cooking and processing of foods, which destroy most nutrients, getting even the RDAs of vitamins from today's diet has become quite hard to do. This means that to obtain the optimal amount of many nutrients, it is necessary to take them in supplement form.

Vitamin supplements can be divided into two groups: synthetic and natural. Synthetic vitamins are vitamins produced in laboratories from isolated chemicals that mirror their counterparts found in nature. Natural vitamins are derived from food sources. Although there are no major chemical differences between a vitamin found in food and one created in a laboratory, synthetic supplements contain the isolated vitamins only, while many natural supplements contain other nutrients not yet discovered. This is because these vitamins are in their natural state. If you are deficient in a particular nutrient, the chemical source will work, but you will not get the benefits of the vitamin as found in whole foods. Supplements that are not labeled natural may also include coal tars, artificial coloring, preservatives, sugars, and starch, as well as other additives. You should beware of such harmful elements. However, you should also note that a bottle of "natural" vitamins may contain vitamins that have not been extracted from a natural food source. It is necessary to read labels carefully to make sure the products you buy contain nutrients from food sources, with none of the artificial additives mentioned above.

Studies have shown that protein-bonded vitamins, as found in natural whole food supplements, are absorbed, utilized, and retained in the tissues better than supplements that are not protein-bonded. Chemical-derived vitamins are not protein-bonded. Vitamins and minerals in food are bonded to proteins, lipids, carbohydrates, and bioflavonoids. Dr. Abram Hoffer, one of the "founding fathers" of orthomolecular medicine, explains:

Components [of food] do not exist free in nature; nature does not lay down pure protein, pure fat, or pure carbohydrates. Their molecules are interlaced in a very complex three-dimensional structure which even now has not been fully described. Intermingled are the essential nutrients such as vitamins and minerals, again not free, but combined in complex molecules.

Using a natural form of vitamins and minerals in nutritional supplements is the objective of the protein-bonding process. Taking supplements with meals helps to assure a supply of other nutrients needed for better assimilation as well.

WHAT'S ON THE SHELVES

Over-the-counter vitamin supplements come in various forms, combinations, and amounts. They are available in tablet, capsule, gel-capsule, powder, sublingual, lozenge, and liquid forms. They can also be administered by injection. In most cases, it is a matter of personal preference as to how they are taken; however, due to slight variations in how rapidly the supplements are absorbed and assimilated into the body, we will sometimes recommend one form over another. These recommendations are given throughout the book.

Vitamin supplements are usually available as isolated vitamins or in combination with other nutrients. It is important to select your vitamins based upon what you really need. (See NUTRITION, DIET, AND WELLNESS in Part One.)

The amount of any vitamin you take should be based upon your own requirements. A program designed for health maintenance would be different from one designed to overcome a specific disorder. If you find one supplement that meets your needs, remember to take it daily. If it does not contain a large enough quantity of what you want, you may consider taking more than one. Just make sure that you are aware of the increased dosage of the other nutrients it may contain. If there is no single supplement that provides you with what you are looking for, consider taking a combination of different supplements. This book lists each supplement separately, so you will know what each does and the amount needed. You may find a supplement that contains several needed nutrients in one tablet or capsule.

Because the potency of most vitamins may be decreased by sunlight, make sure that the container holding your vitamins is dark enough to shield its contents properly. Some people may be sensitive to plastic, and may need to purchase vitamins in glass containers. Vitamin supplements should be kept in a cool, dark place.

All vitamin supplements work best when taken in combination with food. Unless specified otherwise, oil-soluble vitamins should be taken before meals, and water-soluble ones should be taken after meals.

VITAMINS FROM A TO Z

Vitamin A and the Carotenoids

Vitamin A prevents night blindness and other eye problems, as well as some skin disorders, such as acne. It enhances immunity, may heal gastrointestinal ulcers, protects against pollution and cancer formation, and is needed for the maintainence and repair of epithelial tissue, of which the skin and mucous membranes are composed. It is important in the formation of bones and teeth, aids in fat storage, and protects against colds, influenza, and infections of the kidneys, bladder, lungs, and mucous membranes. Vitamin A acts as an antioxidant, helping to protect the cells against cancer and other diseases (see ANTIOXIDANTS in Part One) and is necessary for new cell growth. This important vitamin also slows the aging process. Protein cannot be utilized by the body without vitamin A.

A deficiency of vitamin A may be apparent if dry hair or skin, dryness of the conjunctiva and cornea, poor growth, and/or night blindness is present. Other possible results of vitamin A deficiency include abscesses in the ears; insomnia; fatigue; reproductive difficulties; sinusitis, pneumonia, and frequent colds and other respiratory infections; skin disorders, including acne; and weight loss.

The carotenoids are a class of compounds related to vitamin A. In some cases, they can act as precursors of vitamin A; some act as antioxidants or have other important functions. The best known of the carotenoids is beta-carotene, but there are others, including alpha- and gamma-carotene, lutein, and lycopene. When food or supplements containing beta-carotene are consumed, the beta-carotene is converted into vitamin A in the liver. According to recent reports, beta-carotene appears to aid in cancer prevention by scavenging, or neutralizing, free radicals.

Taking large amounts of vitamin A over long periods can be toxic to the body, mainly the liver. Toxic levels of vitamin A are associated with abdominal pain, amenorrhea, enlargement of the liver and/or spleen, gastrointestinal disturbances, hair loss, itching, joint pain, nausea and vomiting, water on the brain, and small cracks and scales on the lips and at the corners of the mouth. No overdose can occur with beta-carotene, although if you take too much, your skin may turn slightly yellow-orange in color. Beta-carotene does not have the same effect as vitamin A in the body and is not harmful in larger amounts unless you cannot convert beta-carotene into vitamin A. People with hypothyroidism often have this problem. It is important to take only *natural* beta-carotene or a natural carotenoid complex. Betatene is the trade name for a type of carotenoid complex extracted from sea algae. It is used as an ingredient in various products by different manufacturers.

Sources

Vitamin A can be found in animal livers, fish liver oils, and green and yellow fruits and vegetables. Foods that contain significant amounts include apricots, asparagus, beet greens, broccoli, cantaloupe, carrots, collards, dandelion greens, dulse, fish liver and fish liver oil, garlic, kale, mustard greens, papayas, peaches, pumpkin, red peppers, spirulina, spinach, sweet potatoes, Swiss chard, turnip greens, watercress, and yellow squash. It is also present in the following herbs: alfalfa, borage leaves, burdock root, cayenne (capsicum), chickweed, eyebright, fennel seed, hops, horsetail, kelp, lemongrass, mullein, nettle, oat straw, paprika, parsley, peppermint, plantain, raspberry leaf, red clover, rose hips, sage, uva ursi, violet leaves, watercress, and yellow dock.

Comments

Antibiotics, laxatives, and some cholesterol-lowering drugs interfere with vitamin A absorption.

Cautions

If you have liver disease, do not take a daily dose of over 10,000 international units of vitamin A in pill form, or any amount of cod liver oil. If you are pregnant, do not take more than 10,000 international units of vitamin A daily. Children should not take more than 18,000 international units of vitamin A on a daily basis for over one month.

If you have hypothyroidism, avoid beta-carotene, be-cause your body probably cannot convert beta-carotene into vitamin A.

Vitamin B Complex

The B vitamins help to maintain the health of the nerves, skin, eyes, hair, liver, and mouth, as well as healthy muscle tone in the gastrointestinal tract and proper brain function. B-complex vitamins are coenzymes involved in energy production, and may be useful for alleviating depression or anxiety. Adequate intake of the B vitamins is very important for elderly people because these nutrients are not as well absorbed as we age. There have even been cases of people diagnosed with Alzheimer's disease whose problems were later found to be due to a deficiency of vitamin B_{12} plus the B complex. The B vitamins should always be taken together, but up to two to three times more of one B vitamin than another can be taken for a particular disorder. Although the B vitamins are a team, they will be discussed individually.

Vitamin B₁ (Thiamine)

Thiamine enhances circulation and assists in blood formation, carbohydrate metabolism, and the production of hydrochloric acid, which is important for proper digestion. Thiamine also optimizes cognitive activity and brain function. It has a positive effect on energy, growth, normal appetite, and learning capacity, and is needed for muscle tone of the intestines, stomach, and heart. Thiamine also acts as an antioxidant, protecting the body from the degenerative effects of aging, alcohol consumption, and smoking.

Beriberi, a nervous system disease, is caused by a deficiency of thiamine. (*See* BERIBERI in Part Two.) Other symptoms that can result from thiamine deficiency include constipation, edema, enlarged liver, fatigue, forgetfulness, gastrointestinal disturbances, heart changes, irritability, labored breathing, loss of appetite, muscle atrophy, nervousness, numbness of the hands and feet, pain and sensitivity, poor coordination, tingling sensations, weak and sore muscles, general weakness, and severe weight loss.

Sources

The richest food sources of thiamine include brown rice, egg yolks, fish, legumes, liver, peanuts, peas, pork, poultry, rice bran, wheat germ, and whole grains. Other sources are asparagus, brewer's yeast, broccoli, Brussels sprouts, dulse, kelp, most nuts, oatmeal, plums, dried prunes, raisins, spirulina, and watercress. Herbs that contain thiamine include alfalfa, bladderwrack, burdock root, catnip, cayenne, chamomile, chickweed, eyebright, fennel seed, fenugreek, hops, nettle, oat straw, parsley, peppermint, raspberry leaf, red clover, rose hips, sage, yarrow, and yellow dock.

Comments

Antibiotics, sulfa drugs, and oral contraceptives may decrease thiamine levels in the body. A high-carbohydrate diet increases the need for thiamine.

Vitamin B₂ (Riboflavin)

Riboflavin is necessary for red blood cell formation, antibody production, cell respiration, and growth. It alleviates eye fatigue and is important in the prevention and treatment of cataracts. It aids in the metabolism of carbohydrates, fats, and proteins. Together with vitamin A, it maintains and improves the mucous membranes in the digestive tract. Riboflavin also facilitates the use of oxygen by the tissues of the skin, nails, and hair; eliminates dandruff; and helps the absorption of iron and vitamin B_6 (pyridoxine). Consumption of adequate amounts of riboflavin is important during pregnancy, because a lack of this vitamin can damage a developing fetus even though the woman shows no signs of deficiency. Riboflavin is needed for the metabolism of the amino acid tryptophan, which is converted into niacin in the body. Carpal tunnel syndrome may benefit from a treatment program that includes riboflavin and vitamin B_6.

Deficiency symptoms include cracks and sores at the corners of the mouth, eye disorders, inflammation of the mouth and tongue, and skin lesions, a group of symptoms collectively referred to as *ariboflavinosis*. Other possible deficiency symptoms include dermatitis, dizziness, hair loss, insomnia, light sensitivity, poor digestion, retarded growth, and slowed mental response.

Sources

High levels of vitamin B_2 are found in the following food products: cheese, egg yolks, fish, legumes, meat, milk, poultry, spinach, whole grains, and yogurt. Other sources include asparagus, avocados, broccoli, Brussels sprouts, currants, dandelion greens, dulse, kelp, leafy greens, mushrooms, molasses, nuts, and watercress. Herbs that contain vitamin B_2 include alfalfa, bladderwrack, burdock root, catnip, cayenne, chamomile, chickweed, eyebright, fennel seed, fenugreek, ginseng, hops, horsetail, mullein, nettle, oat straw, parsley, peppermint, raspberry leaves, red clover, rose hips, sage, and yellow dock.

Comments

Factors that increase the need for riboflavin include the use of oral contraceptives and strenuous exercise. This B vitamin is easily destroyed by light, antibiotics, and alcohol.

Vitamin B₃ (Niacin, Niacinamide, Nicotinic Acid)

Vitamin B_3 is needed for proper circulation and healthy skin. It aids in the functioning of the nervous system; in the metabolism of carbohydrates, fats, and proteins; and in the production of hydrochloric acid for the digestive system. It is involved in the normal secretion of bile and stomach fluids, and in the synthesis of sex hormones. Niacin lowers cholesterol and improves circulation. It is helpful for schizophrenia and other mental illnesses, and is also a memory-enhancer.

Pellagra is a disease caused by niacin deficiency. (*See* PELLAGRA in Part Two.) Other symptoms of niacin deficiency include canker sores, dementia, depression, diarrhea, dizziness, fatigue, halitosis, headaches, indigestion, insomnia, limb pains, loss of appetite, low blood sugar, muscular weakness, skin eruptions, and inflammation.

Sources

Niacin and niacinamide are found in beef liver, brewer's yeast, broccoli, carrots, cheese, corn flour, dandelion greens, dates, eggs, fish, milk, peanuts, pork, potatoes, tomatoes, wheat germ, and whole wheat products. Herbs that contain niacin include alfalfa, burdock root, catnip, cayenne, chamomile, chickweed, eyebright, fennel seed, hops, licorice, mullein, nettle, oat straw, parsley, peppermint, raspberry leaf, red clover, rose hips, slippery elm, and yellow dock.

Comments

A flush, usually harmless, may occur after the ingestion of niacin supplements; a red rash appears on the skin and a tingling sensation may be experienced as well.

Cautions

People who are pregnant or who suffer from diabetes, glaucoma, gout, liver disease, or peptic ulcers should use niacin supplements with caution. Amounts over 500 milligrams daily may cause liver damage if taken for prolonged periods.

Vitamin B₅ (Pantothenic Acid)

Known as "the anti-stress vitamin," pantothenic acid plays a role in the production of the adrenal hormones and the formation of antibodies, aids in vitamin utilization, and helps to convert fats, carbohydrates, and proteins into energy. It is required by all cells in the body and is concentrated in the organs. It is also involved in the production of neurotransmitters. This vitamin is an essential element of coenzyme A, a vital body chemical involved in many necessary metabolic functions. Pantothenic acid is also a stamina enhancer and prevents certain forms of anemia. It is needed for normal functioning of the gastrointestinal tract and may be helpful in treating depression and anxiety. A deficiency of pantothenic acid may cause fatigue, headache, nausea, and tingling in the hands.

Sources

The following foods contain pantothenic acid: beef, brewer's yeast, eggs, fresh vegetables, kidney, legumes, liver, mushrooms, nuts, pork, royal jelly, saltwater fish, torula yeast, whole rye flour, and whole wheat.

Vitamin B6 (Pyridoxine)

Pyridoxine is involved in more bodily functions than almost any other single nutrient. It affects both physical and mental health. It is beneficial if you suffer from water retention, and is necessary for the production of hydrochloric acid and the absorption of fats and protein. Pyridoxine also aids in maintaining sodium and potassium balance, and promotes red blood cell formation. It is required by the nervous sytem, and is needed for normal brain function and for the synthesis of the nucleic acids RNA and DNA, which contain the genetic instructions for the reproduction of all cells and for normal cellular growth. It activates many enzymes and aids in the absorption of vitamin B_{12}, in immune system function, and in antibody production.

Vitamin B_6 plays a role in cancer immunity and aids in the prevention of arteriosclerosis. It inhibits the formation of a toxic chemical called homocysteine, which attacks the heart muscle and allows the deposition of cholesterol around the heart muscle. Pyridoxine acts as a mild diuretic, reducing the symptoms of premenstrual syndrome, and it may be useful in preventing oxalate kidney stones as well. It is helpful in the treatment of allergies, arthritis, and asthma.

A deficiency of vitamin B_6 may be recognized by anemia, convulsions, headaches, nausea, flaky skin, a sore tongue, and vomiting. Other possible signs of deficiency include acne, anorexia, arthritis, conjunctivitis, cracks or sores on the mouth and lips, depression, dizziness, fatigue, hyperirritability, impaired wound healing, inflammation of the mouth and gums, learning difficulties, weak memory, hair loss, hearing problems, numbness, oily facial skin, stunted growth, and tingling sensations. Carpal tunnel syndrome has been linked to a deficiency of vitamin B_6 as well.

Sources

All foods contain some vitamin B_6; however, the following foods have the highest amounts: brewer's yeast, carrots, chicken, eggs, fish, meat, peas, spinach, sunflower seeds, walnuts, and wheat germ. Other sources include avocado, bananas, beans, blackstrap molasses, broccoli, brown rice and other whole grains, cabbage, cantaloupe, corn, dulse, plantains, potatoes, rice bran, soybeans, and tempeh. Herbs that contain vitamin B_6 include alfalfa, catnip, and oat straw.

Comments

Antidepressants, estrogen therapy, and oral contraceptives may increase the need for vitamin B_6. Diuretics and cortisone drugs block the absorption of this vitamin by the body.

Vitamin B12 (Cyanocobalamin)

Vitamin B_{12} is needed to prevent anemia. It aids folic acid in regulating the formation of red blood cells, and helps in the utilization of iron. This vitamin is also required for proper digestion, absorption of foods, the synthesis of protein, and the metabolism of carbohydrates and fats. It aids in cell formation and cellular longevity. In addition, vitamin B_{12} prevents nerve damage, maintains fertility, and promotes normal growth and development by maintaining the fatty sheaths that cover and protect nerve endings. Vitamin B_{12} is linked to the production of acetylcholine, a neurotransmitter that assists memory and learning.

A vitamin B_{12} deficiency can be caused by malabsorption, which is most common in elderly people and in those with digestive disorders. Deficiency can cause abnormal gait, chronic fatigue, constipation, depression, digestive disorders, dizziness, drowsiness, enlargement of the liver, eye disorders, hallucinations, headaches, inflammation of the tongue, irritability, labored breathing, memory loss, moodiness, nervousness, neurological damage, palpitations, pernicious anemia, ringing in the ears, and spinal cord degeneration. Strict vegetarians must remember that they require vitamin B_{12} supplementation, as this vitamin is found almost exclusively in animal tissues. Although people adopting a strictly vegetarian diet may not see signs of the deficiency for some time—the body can store up to five years' worth of vitamin B_{12}—signs will eventually develop.

Sources

The largest amounts of vitamin B_{12} are found in brewer's yeast, clams, eggs, herring, kidney, liver, mackerel, milk and dairy products, and seafood. Vitamin B_{12} is not found in many vegetables; it is available only from sea vegetables, such as dulse, kelp, kombu, and nori, and soybeans and soy products. It is also present in the herbs alfalfa, bladderwrack, and hops.

Comments

Anti-gout medications, anticoagulant drugs, and potassium supplements may block the absorption of vitamin B_{12} from the digestive tract. Vegetarians need supplements of vitamin B_{12} because it is found mostly in animal sources.

Biotin

Biotin aids in cell growth; in fatty acid production; in the metabolism of carbohydrates, fats, and proteins; and in the utilization of the other B-complex vitamins. Sufficient quantities are needed for healthy hair and skin. One hundred milligrams of biotin daily may prevent hair loss in some men. Biotin also promotes healthy sweat glands, nerve tissue, and bone marrow. In addition, it helps to relieve muscle pain.

In infants, a condition called seborrheic dermatitis, or "cradle cap," which is characterized by a dry, scaly scalp, may occur as a result of biotin deficiency. In adults, deficiency of this B vitamin is rare because it can be produced in the intestines from foods such as those mentioned below. However, if a deficiency does occur, it can cause anemia, depression, hair loss, high blood sugar, inflammation or pallor of the skin and mucous membranes, insomnia, loss of appetite, muscular pain, nausea, and soreness of the tongue.

Sources

Biotin is found in brewer's yeast, cooked egg yolks, meat, milk, poultry, saltwater fish, soybeans, and whole grains.

Comments

Raw egg whites contain a protein called avidin, which combines with biotin in the intestinal tract and depletes the body of this needed nutrient. Fats and oils that have been subjected to heat or exposed to the air for any length of time inhibit biotin absorption. Antibiotics, sulfa drugs, and saccharin also threaten the availability of biotin.

Choline

Choline is needed for the proper transmission of nerve impulses from the brain through the central nervous system, as well as for gallbladder regulation, liver function, and lecithin formation. It aids in hormone production and minimizes excess fat in the liver because it aids in fat and cholesterol metabolism. Without choline, brain function and memory are impaired. Choline is beneficial for disorders of the nervous system such as Parkinson's disease and tardive dyskinesia. A deficiency may result in fatty buildup in the liver, as well as in cardiac symptoms, gastric ulcers, high blood pressure, the inability to digest fats, kidney and liver impairment, and stunted growth.

Sources

The following foods contain significant amounts of choline: egg yolks, lecithin, legumes, meat, milk, soybeans, and whole-grain cereals.

Folic Acid

Considered a brain food, folic acid is needed for energy production and the formation of red blood cells. It also strengthens immunity by aiding in the proper formation and functioning of white blood cells. Because it functions as a coenzyme in DNA and RNA synthesis, it is important for healthy cell division and replication. It is involved in protein metabolism, and has been used in the prevention and treatment of folic acid anemia. This nutrient may also help depression and anxiety. It may be effective in the treatment of uterine cervical dysplasia.

Folic acid is very important in pregnancy. It helps to regulate embryonic and fetal nerve cell formation, which is vital for normal development. Studies have shown that a daily intake of 400 micrograms of folic acid in early pregnancy may prevent the vast majority of neural tube defects such as spina bifida and anencephaly. It may also help to prevent premature birth. To be effective, this regimen must begin *before* conception and continue for at least the first three months of pregnancy; if a woman waits until she knows she is pregnant, it may be too late, because critical events in fetal development occur during the first six weeks of pregnancy— before most women know that they have conceived. This is why many experts recommend that every woman of childbearing age take a folic acid supplement daily as a matter of course. Folic acid works best when combined with vitamin B_{12} and vitamin C.

A sore, red tongue is one sign of folic acid deficiency. Other possible signs include anemia, apathy, digestive disturbances, fatigue, graying hair, growth impairment, insomnia, labored breathing, memory problems, paranoia, weakness, and birth defects in one's offspring. Folic acid deficiency may be caused by inadequate consumption of fresh fruits and vegetables; consumption of only cooked or microwaved vegetables (cooking destroys folic acid); and malabsorption problems.

Sources

The following foods contain significant quantities of folic acid: barley, beef, bran, brewer's yeast, brown rice, cheese, chicken, dates, green leafy vegetables, lamb, legumes, lentils, liver, milk, mushrooms, oranges, split peas, pork, root vegetables, salmon, tuna, wheat germ, whole grains, and whole wheat.

Comments

Oral contraceptives may increase the need for folic acid. Alcohol also can act as an enemy to folic acid absorption.

Cautions

Do not take high doses of folic acid for extended periods if you have a hormone-related cancer or convulsive disorder.

Inositol

Inositol is vital for hair growth. This vitamin has a calming effect and helps to reduce cholesterol levels. It helps prevent hardening of the arteries, and is important in the formation of lecithin and the metabolism of fat and cholesterol. It also helps remove fats from the liver. Deficiency can lead to arteriosclerosis, constipation, hair loss, high blood cholesterol, irritability, mood swings, and skin eruptions.

Sources

Inositol is found in brewer's yeast, fruits, lecithin, legumes, meats, milk, unrefined molasses, raisins, vegetables, and whole grains.

Comments

The consumption of large amounts of caffeine may cause a shortage of inositol in the body.

Para-Aminobenzoic Acid (PABA)

PABA is one of the basic constituents of folic acid and also helps in the assimilation of pantothenic acid. This antioxidant helps protect against sunburn and skin cancer, acts as a coenzyme in the breakdown and utilization of protein, and assists in the formation of red blood cells. PABA also aids in the maintenance of healthy intestinal flora. Supplementing the diet with PABA may restore gray hair to its original color if the graying was caused by stress or a nutritional deficiency.

A deficiency of PABA may lead to depression, fatigue, gastrointestinal disorders, graying of the hair, irritability, nervousness, and patchy areas of white skin.

Sources

Foods that contain PABA are kidney, liver, molasses, mushrooms, spinach, and whole grains.

Comments

Sulfa drugs may cause a deficiency of PABA.

Vitamin C (Ascorbic Acid)

Vitamin C is an antioxidant that is required for tissue growth and repair, adrenal gland function, and healthy gums. It also aids in the production of anti-stress hormones and interferon, and is needed for the metabolism of folic acid, tyrosine, and phenylalanine. It protects against the harmful effects of pollution, helps to prevent cancer, protects against infection, and enhances immunity. Vitamin C increases the absorption of iron. It also may reduce cholesterol levels and high blood pressure, and prevent atherosclerosis. Essential in the formation of collagen, vitamin C protects against blood clotting and bruising, and promotes the healing of wounds and burns.

New evidence indicates that vitamin C works synergistically with vitamin E—that is, when these vitamins work together, they have a greater effect than when they work separately. Vitamin E scavenges for dangerous free radicals in cell membranes, while vitamin C attacks free radicals in biologic fluids. These vitamins reinforce and extend each other's antioxidant activity.

Because the body cannot manufacture vitamin C, it must be obtained through the diet or in the form of supplements. Unfortunately, most of the vitamin C consumed in the diet is lost in the urine. When larger amounts of vitamin C are required due to serious illness, such as cancer, it is more effective to take vitamin C intravenously, under the advisement and supervision of a physician, than it is to take high doses orally.

Scurvy is a disease caused by vitamin C deficiency. It is characterized by poor wound healing, soft and spongy bleeding gums, edema, extreme weakness, and "pinpoint" hemorrhages under the skin. Fortunately, this condition is rare in Western societies. More common are signs of lesser degrees of deficiency, including gums that bleed when brushed; increased susceptibility to infection, especially colds and bronchial infections; joint pains; lack of energy; poor digestion; prolonged healing time; a tendency to bruise easily; and tooth loss.

Sources

Vitamin C is found in berries, citrus fruits, and green vegetables. Good sources include asparagus, avocados, beet greens, black currants, broccoli, Brussels sprouts, cantaloupe, collards, dandelion greens, dulse, grapefruit, kale, lemons, mangos, mustard greens, onions, oranges, papayas, green peas, sweet peppers, persimmons, pineapple, radishes, rose hips, spinach, strawberries, Swiss chard, tomatoes, turnip greens, and watercress. Herbs that contain vitamin C include alfalfa, burdock root, cayenne, chickweed, eyebright, fennel seed, fenugreek, hops, horsetail, kelp, peppermint, mullein, nettle, oat straw, paprika, parsley, pine needle, plantain, raspberry leaf, red clover, rose hips, skullcap, violet leaves, yarrow, and yellow dock.

Comments

Alcohol, analgesics, antidepressants, anticoagulants, oral contraceptives, and steroids may reduce levels of vitamin C in the body. Smoking causes a serious depletion of vitamin C.

Diabetes medications such as chlorpropamide (Diabinese) and sulfa drugs may not be as effective when taken with vitamin C. Taking high doses of vitamin C may cause a false-negative reading in tests for blood in the stool.

For maximum effectiveness, supplemental vitamin C should be taken in divided doses, twice daily. Esterified vitamin C (Ester-C) is a remarkably effective form of vitamin C, especially for those suffering from chronic illnesses such as cancer and AIDS. It is created by having the vitamin C react with a necessary mineral, such as calcium, magnesium, potassium, sodium, or zinc. This results in a form of the vitamin that is nonacidic and that contains vitamin C metabolites identical to those produced by the body. Esterified vitamin C enters the bloodstream and tissues four times faster than standard vitamin C, moves into the blood cells more efficiently, and also stays in the body tissues longer. The levels of vitamin C in white blood cells achieved by taking esterified vitamin C are four times higher than those achieved with standard vitamin C. Further, only one-third as much is lost through excretion in the urine. Natrol produces supplements of Ester-C in combination with other valuable nutrients: one with the antioxidants Pycnogenol and proanthocyanidins; another with the herb echinacea; and still another with garlic.

Cautions

If aspirin and standard vitamin C (ascorbic acid) are taken together in large doses, stomach irritation can occur, possibly leading to ulcers. If you take aspirin regularly, use an esterified form of vitamin C.

If you are pregnant, do not take more than 5,000 milligrams of vitamin C daily. Infants may become dependent on this supplement and develop scurvy when deprived of the accustomed megadoses after birth.

Avoid using chewable vitamin C supplements, as these can damage tooth enamel.

Vitamin D

Vitamin D, a fat-soluble vitamin, is required for the absorption and utilization of calcium and phosphorus by the intestinal tract. It is necessary for growth, and is especially important for the normal growth and development of bones and teeth in children. It protects against muscle weakness and is involved in regulation of the heartbeat. It is also important in the prevention and treatment of osteoporosis and hypocalcemia, enhances immunity, and is necessary for thyroid function and normal blood clotting.

The form of vitamin D that we get from food or supplements is not fully active. It requires conversion by the liver, and then by the kidneys, before it becomes fully active. This is why people with liver or kidney disorders are at a higher risk for osteoporosis. When the skin is exposed to the sun's ultraviolet rays, a cholesterol compound in the skin is transformed into a precursor of vitamin D. Exposing the face and arms to the sun for fifteen minutes three times a week is an effective way to ensure adequate amounts of vitamin D in the body.

Severe deficiency of vitamin D can cause rickets in children and osteomalacia, a similar disorder, in adults. Lesser degrees of deficiency may be characterized by loss of appetite, a burning sensation in the mouth and throat, diarrhea, insomnia, visual problems, and weight loss.

Sources

Fish liver oils, fatty saltwater fish, dairy products, and eggs all contain vitamin D. It is found in butter, cod liver oil, dandelion greens, egg yolks, halibut, liver, milk, oatmeal, salmon, sardines, sweet potatoes, tuna, and vegetable oils. Vitamin D is also formed by the body in response to the action of sunlight on the skin. Herbs that contain vitamin D include alfalfa, horsetail, nettle, and parsley.

Comments

Intestinal disorders and liver and gallbladder malfunctions interfere with the absorption of vitamin D. Some cholesterol-lowering drugs, antacids, mineral oil, and steroid hormones (cortisone) also interfere with absorption. Thiazide diuretics such as chlorothiazide (Diuril) and hydrochlorothiazide (Esidrix, HydroDIURIL, Oretic) disturb the body's calcium/vitamin D ratio.

Cautions

Do not take vitamin D without calcium. Toxicity may result from taking amounts over 65,000 international units over a period of years.

Vitamin E

Vitamin E is an antioxidant that is important in the prevention of cancer and cardiovascular disease. It improves circulation, is necessary for tissue repair, and is useful in treating premenstrual syndrome and fibrocystic disease of the breast. It promotes normal blood clotting and healing, reduces scarring from some wounds, reduces blood pressure, aids in preventing cataracts, improves athletic performance, and relaxes leg cramps. It also maintains healthy nerves and muscles while strengthening capillary walls. In addition, it promotes healthy skin and hair, and helps to prevent anemia and retrolental fibroplasia, an eye disorder that can affect premature infants.

As an antioxidant, vitamin E prevents cell damage by inhibiting the oxidation of lipids (fats) and the formation of free radicals. It protects other fat-soluble vitamins from destruction by oxygen, and aids in the utilization of vitamin A and protects it from destruction by oxygen. It retards aging and may prevent age spots as well.

Vitamin E deficiency may result in damage to red blood cells and destruction of nerves. Signs of deficiency can include infertility (in both men and women), menstrual problems, neuromuscular impairment, shortened red blood cell life span, spontaneous abortion (miscarriage), and uterine degeneration. Low levels of vitamin E in the body have been linked to both bowel cancer and breast cancer. Epidemiological links have been identified between the increase in the incidence of heart disease and the increasing lack of vitamin E in the diet due to our reliance on overprocessed foods.

Vitamin E is actually a family of eight different but related molecules that fall into two major groups: the tocopherols and the tocotrienols. Within each group, there are alpha beta, gamma, and delta forms. Of all eight of these molecules, it is the alpha-tocopherol form that is the most potent.

Sources

Vitamin E is found in the following food sources: cold-pressed vegetable oils, dark green leafy vegetables, legumes, nuts, seeds, and whole grains. Significant quantities of this vitamin are also found in brown rice, cornmeal, dulse, eggs, kelp, dessicated liver, milk, oatmeal, organ meats, soybeans, sweet potatoes, watercress, wheat, and wheat germ. Herbs that contain vitamin E include alfalfa, bladderwrack, dandelion, dong quai, flaxseed, nettle, oat straw, raspberry leaf, and rose hips.

Comments

The body needs zinc in order to maintain the proper level of vitamin E in the blood.

If you take both vitamin E and iron supplements, take them at different times of the day. Inorganic forms of iron (such as ferrous sulfate) destroy vitamin E. Organic iron (ferrous gluconate or ferrous fumarate) leaves vitamin E intact.

Cautions

If you are taking an anticoagulant medication (blood thinner), do not take more than 1,200 international units of vitamin E daily. If you suffer from diabetes, rheumatic heart disease, or an overactive thyroid, do not take more than the recommended dose. If you have high blood pressure, start with a small amount, such as 200 international units daily, and increase slowly to the desired amount.

Vitamin K

Vitamin K is needed for the production of prothrombin, which is necessary for blood clotting. It is also essential for bone formation and repair; it is necessary for the synthesis of osteocalcin, the protein in bone tissue on which calcium crystallizes. Consequently, it may help prevent osteoporosis.

Vitamin K plays an important role in the intestines and aids in converting glucose into glycogen for storage in the liver, promoting healthy liver function. It may increase resistance to infection in children and help prevent cancers that target the inner linings of the organs. It aids in promoting longevity.

A deficiency of this vitamin can cause abnormal and/or internal bleeding.

Vitamin K exists in three forms. Vitamin K_1 (phylloquinone or phytonactone) and vitamin K_2 (a family of substances called menoquinones) occur naturally; vitamin K_3 (menadione) is a synthetic substance.

Sources

Vitamin K is found in some foods, including asparagus, blackstrap molasses, broccoli, Brussels sprouts, cabbage, cauliflower, dark green leafy vegetables, egg yolks, liver, oatmeal, oats, rye, safflower oil, soybeans, and wheat. Herbs that can supply vitamin K include alfalfa, green tea, kelp, nettle, oat straw, and shepherd's purse. However, the majority of the body's supply of this vitamin is synthesized by the "friendly" bacteria normally present in the intestines.

Comments

Antibiotics increase the need for dietary or supplemental vitamin K. Because vitamin K is synthesized by bacteria in the intestines, taking antibiotics—which kill the bacteria—interferes with this process. Antobiotics also interfere with the absorption of vitamin K.

Cautions

Do not take large doses of synthetic vitamin K during the last few weeks of pregnancy. It can result in a toxic reaction in the newborn.

Megadoses of this vitamin can accumulate in the body and cause flushing and sweating.

Bioflavonoids

Although bioflavonoids are not true vitamins in the strictest sense, they are sometimes referred to as vitamin P. Bioflavonoids enhance the absorption of vitamin C, and the two should be taken together. There are many different bioflavonoids, including hesperetin, hesperidin, eriodictyol, quercetin, quercetrin, and rutin. The human body cannot produce bioflavonoids, so they must be supplied in the diet.

Bioflavonoids are used extensively in the treatment of athletic injuries because they relieve pain, bumps, and bruises. They also reduce pain located in the legs or across the back, and lessen symptoms associated with prolonged bleeding and low serum calcium. Bioflavonoids act synergistically with vitamin C to protect and preserve the structure of capillaries. In addition, bioflavonoids have an antibacterial effect and promote circulation, stimulate bile production, lower cholesterol levels, and treat and prevent cataracts. When taken with vitamin C, bioflavonoids also reduce the symptoms of oral herpes.

Quercetin, a bioflavonoid found in blue-green algae and available in supplement form, may effectively treat and prevent asthma symptoms. Activated Quercetin from Source Naturals is a good source of quercetin. It also contains two other ingredients that increase its efficacy: bromelain, an enzyme from pineapple, and vitamin C, in the nonacidic form of magnesium ascorbate. Bromelain and quercetin are synergists, and should be taken in conjunction to enhance absorption.

Sources

The white material just beneath the peel of citrus fruits, peppers, buckwheat, and black currants contain bioflavonoids. Sources of bioflavonoids include apricots, cherries, grapefruit, grapes, lemons, oranges, prunes, and rose hips. Herbs that contain bioflavonoids include chervil, elderberries, hawthorn berry, horsetail, rose hips, and shepherd's purse.

Comments

Extremely high doses may cause diarrhea.

Coenzyme Q10

Coenzyme Q_{10} is a vitaminlike substance whose actions in the body resemble those of vitamin E. It may be an even more powerful antioxidant. It is also called ubiquinone. There are ten common substances designated coenzyme Qs, but coenzyme Q_{10} is the only one found in human tissue. This substance plays a critical role in the production of energy in every cell of the body. It aids circulation, stimulates the immune system, increases tissue oxygenation, and has vital anti-aging effects. Deficiencies of coenzyme Q_{10} have been linked to periodontal disease, diabetes, and muscular dystrophy.

Research has revealed that supplemental coenzyme Q_{10} has the ability to counter histamine, and therefore is beneficial for people with allergies, asthma, or respiratory disease. It is used by many health care professionals to treat anomalies of mental function such as those associated with schizophrenia and Alzheimer's disease. It is also beneficial in fighting obesity, candidiasis, multiple sclerosis, and diabetes.

Coenzyme Q_{10} appears to be a giant step forward in the treatment and prevention of cardiovascular disease. A six-year study conducted by scientists at the University of Texas found that people being treated for congestive heart failure who took coenzyme Q_{10} in addition to conventional therapy had a 75-percent chance of survival after three years, compared with a 25-percent survival rate for those using conventional therapy alone. In a similar study by the University of Texas and the Center for Adult Diseases in Japan, coenzyme Q_{10} was shown to be able to lower high blood pressure without medication or dietary changes.

In addition to its use in fighting cardiovascular disease, coenzyme Q_{10} has been shown to be effective in reducing mortality in experimental animals afflicted with tumors and leukemia. Some doctors give their patients coenzyme Q_{10} to reduce the side effects of cancer chemotherapy.

Coenzyme Q_{10} is widely used in Japan. More than 12 million people in that country are reportedly taking it at the direction of their physicians for treatment of heart disease (it strengthens the heart muscle) and high blood pressure, and also to enhance the immune system. Research in Japan has shown that coenzyme Q_{10} also protects the stomach lining and duodenum, and may help heal duodenal ulcers.

The amount of coenzyme Q_{10} present in the body declines with age, so it should be supplemented in the diet, especially by people who are over the age of fifty. A sublingual form containing 50 milligrams of this vital nutrient, available from FoodScience Laboratories, is an especially assimilable supplement.

Sources

Mackerel, salmon, and sardines contain the largest amounts of coenzyme Q_{10}. It is also found in beef, peanuts, and spinach.

Comments

Coenzyme Q_{10} is oil soluble and is best absorbed when taken with oily or fatty foods, such as fish. Be cautious when purchasing coenzyme Q_{10}. Not all products offer it in its purest form. Its natural color is dark bright yellow to orange, and it has very little taste in the powdered form. It should be kept away from heat and light. Pure coenzyme Q_{10} is perishable and deteriorates in temperatures above 115°F. A liquid or oil form is preferable. Look for a brand that contains a small amount of vitamin E as this helps to preserve the coenzyme Q_{10}.

MINERALS

THE FUNCTION OF MINERALS

Every living cell on this planet depends on minerals for proper function and structure. Minerals are needed for the proper composition of body fluids, the formation of blood and bone, the maintenance of healthy nerve function, and the regulation of muscle tone, including that of the muscles of the cardiovascular system. Like vitamins, minerals function as coenzymes, enabling the body to perform its functions, including energy production, growth, and healing. Because all enzyme activities involve minerals, minerals are essential for the proper utilization of vitamins and other nutrients.

The human body, as all of nature, must maintain its proper chemical balance. This balance depends on the levels of different minerals in the body and especially the ratios of certain mineral levels to one another. The level of each mineral in the body has an effect on every other, so if one is out of balance, all mineral levels are affected. If not corrected, this can start a chain reaction of imbalances that leads to illness.

Minerals are naturally occurring elements found in the earth. Rock formations are made up of mineral salts. Rock and stone are gradually broken down into tiny fragments by erosion, a process that can take literally millions of years. The resulting dust and sand accumulate, forming the basis of soil. The soil is teeming with microbes that utilize these tiny crystals of mineral salts, which are then passed from the soil to plants. The plants are eaten by herbivorous animals. We obtain these minerals by consuming plants or herbivorous animals.

Nutritionally, minerals belong to two groups: bulk minerals (also called macrominerals) and trace minerals (microminerals). Bulk minerals include calcium, magnesium, sodium, potassium, and phosphorus. These are needed in larger amounts than trace minerals. Although only minute quantities of trace minerals are needed, they are nevertheless important for good health. Trace minerals include boron, chromium, copper, germanium, iodine, iron, manganese, molybdenum, selenium, silicon, sulfur, vanadium, and zinc.

Because minerals are stored primarily in the body's bone and muscle tissue, it is possible to develop mineral toxicity if extremely large quantities are consumed. Such situations are rare, however, because toxic levels of minerals generally accumulate only if massive amounts are ingested for a prolonged period of time.

WHAT'S ON THE SHELVES

As with vitamins, it can be difficult, if not impossible, to obtain the amounts of minerals needed for optimum health through diet alone. Mineral supplements can help you to make sure you are getting all the minerals your body requires.

Minerals are often found in multivitamin formulas. Minerals can also be sold as single supplements. These are available in tablet, capsule, powder, and liquid forms. Some are available in chelated form, which means that the minerals are bonded to protein molecules that transport them to the bloodstream and enhance their absorption. When mineral supplements are taken with a meal, they are usually automatically chelated in the stomach during digestion. There is some controversy over which mineral supplements are best, but we prefer the chelated preparations. Our experience with the various chelated formulas available has shown that, in general, orotate and arginate forms of minerals make the most effective supplements.

Once a mineral is absorbed, it must be carried by the blood to the cells and then transported across the cell membranes in a form that can be utilized by the cells. After minerals enter the body, they compete with one another for absorption. For example, too much zinc can deplete the body of copper; excessive calcium intake can affect magnesium absorption. Consequently, supplemental minerals should always be taken in balanced amounts. Otherwise, they will not be effective and may even be harmful. The absorption of minerals can also be affected by the use of fiber supplements. Fiber decreases the body's absorption of minerals. Therefore, supplemental fiber and minerals should be taken at different times.

THE ABC'S OF MINERALS

Boron

Boron is needed in trace amounts for healthy bones and for the metabolism of calcium, phosphorus, and magnesium. It also enhances brain function and promotes alertness. Most people are not deficient in boron. However, elderly people usually benefit from taking a supplement of 2 to 3 milligrams daily because they have a greater problem with calcium absorption. Boron deficiency accentuates vitamin D deficiency.

Boron helps to prevent postmenopausal osteoporosis and build muscle. A study conducted by the U.S. Department of Agriculture indicated that within eight days of supplementing their daily diet with 3 milligrams of boron, a test group of postmenopausal women lost 40 percent less calcium, one-third less magnesium, and slightly less phosphorus through their urine than they had before beginning boron supplementation.

Sources

Boron is found in apples, carrots, grapes, leafy vegetables, nuts, pears, and grains.

Cautions

Do not take more than 3 milligrams of boron daily.

Calcium

Calcium is vital for the formation of strong bones and teeth and for the maintenance of healthy gums. It is also important in the maintenance of a regular heartbeat and the transmission of nerve impulses. Calcium lowers cholesterol levels and helps prevent cardiovascular disease. It is needed for muscular growth and contraction, and for the prevention of muscle cramps. It may increase the rate of bone growth and bone mineral density in children. This important mineral is also essential in blood clotting and helps prevent cancer. It may lower blood pressure and prevent bone loss associated with osteoporosis as well. Calcium provides energy and participates in the protein structuring of RNA and DNA. It is also involved in the activation of several enzymes, including lipase, which breaks down fats for utilization by the body. In addition, calcium maintains proper cell membrane permeability, aids in neuromuscular activity, helps to keep the skin healthy, and protects against the development of preeclampsia during pregnancy, the number one cause of maternal death.

Calcium protects the bones and teeth from lead by inhibiting absorption of this toxic metal. If there is a calcium deficiency, lead can be absorbed by the body and deposited in the teeth and bones.

Calcium deficiency can lead to the following problems: aching joints, brittle nails, eczema, elevated blood cholesterol, heart palpitations, hypertension (high blood pressure), insomnia, muscle cramps, nervousness, numbness in the arms and/or legs, a pasty complexion, rheumatoid arthritis, rickets, and tooth decay. Deficiencies of calcium are also associated with cognitive impairment, convulsions, depression, delusions, and hyperactivity.

Sources

Calcium is found in milk and dairy foods, salmon (with bones), sardines, seafood, and green leafy vegetables. Food sources include almonds, asparagus, blackstrap molasses, brewer's yeast, broccoli, buttermilk, cabbage, carob, cheese, collards, dandelion greens, dulse, figs, filberts, goat's milk, kale, kelp, mustard greens, oats, prunes, sesame seeds, soybeans, tofu, turnip greens, watercress, whey, and yogurt. Herbs that contain calcium include alfalfa, burdock root, cayenne, chamomile, chickweed, chicory, dandelion, eyebright, fennel seed, fenugreek, flaxseed, hops, horsetail, kelp, lemongrass, mullein, nettle, oat straw, paprika, parsley, peppermint, plantain, raspberry leaves, red clover, rose hips, shepherd's purse, violet leaves, yarrow, and yellow dock.

Comments

The amino acid lysine is needed for calcium absorption. Food sources of lysine include cheese, eggs, fish, lima beans, milk, potatoes, red meat, soy products, and yeast. Lysine is also available in supplement form.

Female athletes and menopausal women need greater amounts of calcium than other women because their estrogen levels are lower. Estrogen protects the skeletal system by promoting the deposition of calcium in bone.

Heavy exercising hinders calcium uptake, but moderate exercise promotes it. Insufficient vitamin D intake, or the ingestion of excessive amounts of phosphorus and magnesium, also hinders the uptake of calcium.

Taking calcium with iron reduces the effect of both minerals. Too much calcium can interfere with absorption of zinc, and excess zinc can interfere with calcium absorption. A hair analysis can determine the levels of these minerals.

A diet that is high in protein, fat, and/or sugar affects calcium uptake. The average American diet of meats, refined grains, and soft drinks (which are high in phosphorus) leads to increased excretion of calcium. Consuming alcoholic beverages, coffee, junk foods, excess salt, and/or white flour also leads to the loss of calcium by the body. A diet based on foods such as vegetables, fruits, and whole grains, which contain significant amounts of calcium but lower amounts of phosphorus, is preferable.

Oxalic acid (found in almonds, beet greens, cashews, chard, cocoa, kale, rhubarb, soybeans, and spinach) interferes with calcium absorption by binding with calcium in the intestines and producing insoluble salts that cannot be absorbed. Casual consumption of foods with oxalic acid should not pose a problem, but overindulgence in these foods inhibits absorption of calcium.

Calcium supplements are more effective when taken in smaller doses spread throughout the day and before bedtime. When taken at night, calcium also promotes a sound sleep. This mineral works less effectively when taken in a single megadose.

Several vitamin companies use D_1-calcium-phosphate in their products, but do not list it on the label. This form of calcium is insoluble and interferes with the absorption of the nutrients in a multinutrient supplement. The level of electrolytes in the body also affects calcium absorption.

Antacids such as Tums are not recommended as a source of calcium. While they do contain calcium, if taken in sufficient quantities to serve as a source of this mineral, they would also neutralize the stomach acid needed for calcium absorption.

Cautions

Calcium may interfere with the effects of verapamil (Calan, Isoptin, Verelan), a calcium channel blocker sometimes prescribed for heart problems and high blood pressure. Calcium supplements should not be taken by persons with a history of kidney stones or kidney disease.

Chromium

Because it is involved in the metabolism of glucose, chromium (sometimes also called glucose tolerance factor or GTF) is needed for energy. It is also vital in the synthesis of cholesterol, fats, and protein. This essential mineral maintains stable blood sugar levels through proper insulin utilization, and can be helpful both for people with diabetes and those with hypoglycemia. Studies have shown that low plasma chromium levels can be an indication of coronary artery disease.

The average American diet is chromium deficient. Researchers estimate that two out of every three Americans are hypoglycemic, prehypoglycemic, or diabetic. The ability to maintain normal blood sugar levels is jeopardized by the lack of chromium in our soil and water supply and by a diet high in refined white sugar, flour, and junk foods.

A deficiency of chromium can lead to anxiety, fatigue, glucose intolerance (particularly in people with diabetes), inadequate metabolism of amino acids, and an increased risk of arteriosclerosis. Excessive intake can lead to chromium toxicity, which has been associated with dermatitis, gastrointestinal ulcers, and kidney and liver impairment.

Chromium is best absorbed by the body when it is taken in a form called *chromium picolinate* (chromium chelated with picolinate, a naturally occurring amino acid metabolite). Picolinate enables chromium to readily enter into the body's cells, where the mineral can then help insulin do its job much more effectively. Chromium picolinate has been used successfully to control blood cholesterol and blood glucose levels. It also promotes the loss of fat and an increase in lean muscle tissue. Studies show it may increase longevity and help to fight osteoporosis. Chromium polynicotinate (chromium bonded to niacin) is an effective form of this mineral as well.

Sources

Chromium is found in the following food sources: beer, brewer's yeast, brown rice, cheese, meat, and whole grains. It may also be found in dried beans, blackstrap molasses, calf liver, chicken, corn and corn oil, dairy products, dried liver, dulse, eggs, mushrooms, and potatoes. Herbs that contain chromium include catnip, horsetail, licorice, nettle, oat straw, red clover, sarsaparilla, wild yam, and yarrow.

Cautions

If you have diabetes, *do not* take supplemental chromium (especially chromium picolinate) without first consulting with a qualified health care provider. This supplement can affect insulin requirements, so you will have to monitor your blood sugar level very carefully.

Some people experience lightheadedness or a slight skin rash when taking chromium. If you feel lightheaded, stop taking the supplement and consult your health care provider. If you develop a rash, either try switching brands or discontinue use.

Copper

Among its many functions, copper aids in the formation of bone, hemoglobin, and red blood cells, and works in balance with zinc and vitamin C to form elastin. It is involved in the healing process, energy production, hair and skin coloring, and taste sensitivity. This mineral is also needed for healthy nerves and joints.

One of the early signs of copper deficiency is osteoporosis. Copper is essential for the formation of collagen, one of the fundamental proteins making up bones, skin, and connective tissue. Other possible signs of copper deficiency include anemia, baldness, diarrhea, general weakness, impaired respiratory function, and skin sores. A lack of copper can also lead to increased blood fat levels. (*See* COPPER DEFICIENCY in Part Two.)

Excessive intake of copper can lead to toxicity, which has been associated with depression, irritability, nausea and vomiting, nervousness, and joint and muscle pain. (*See* COPPER TOXICITY in Part Two.)

Sources

Besides its use in cookware and plumbing, copper is also widely distributed in foods. Food sources include almonds, avocados, barley, beans, beets, blackstrap molasses, broccoli, garlic, lentils, liver, mushrooms, nuts, oats, oranges, pecans, radishes, raisins, salmon, seafood, soybeans, and green leafy vegetables.

Comments

The level of copper in the body is related to the levels of zinc and vitamin C. Copper levels are reduced if large amounts of zinc or vitamin C are consumed. If copper intake is too high, levels of vitamin C and zinc drop.

The consumption of high amounts of fructose can significantly worsen a copper deficiency. In a study conducted by the U.S. Department of Agriculture, people who obtained 20 percent of their daily calories from fructose showed decreased levels of red blood cell superoxide dismutase (SOD), a copper-dependent enzyme critical to antioxidant protection within the red blood cells.

Germanium

Germanium improves cellular oxygenation. This helps to fight pain, keep the immune system functioning properly, and rid the body of toxins and poisons. Researchers have shown that consuming foods containing organic germanium is an effective way to increase tissue oxygenation, because, like hemoglobin, germanium acts as a carrier of oxygen to the cells. A Japanese scientist, Kazuhiko Asai, found that an intake of 100 to 300 milligrams of germanium per day improved many illnesses, including rheumatoid arthritis, food allergies, elevated cholesterol, candidiasis, chronic viral infections, cancer, and AIDS.

Sources

The following foods contain germanium: garlic, shiitake mushrooms, onions, and the herbs aloe vera, comfrey, ginseng, and suma.

Comments

Germanium is best obtained through the diet.

Iodine

Needed only in trace amounts, iodine helps to metabolize excess fat and is important for physical and mental development. It is also needed for a healthy thyroid gland and the prevention of goiter. Iodine deficiency in children may result in mental retardation. In addition, iodine deficiency has been linked to breast cancer and is associated with fatigue, neonatal hypothyroidism (cretinism), and weight gain. Excessive iodine intake (over thirty times the RDA) can produce a metallic taste and sores in the mouth, swollen salivary glands, diarrhea, and vomiting.

Sources

Foods that are high in iodine include iodized salt, seafood, saltwater fish, and kelp. It may also be found in asparagus, dulse, garlic, lima beans, mushrooms, sea salt, sesame seeds, soybeans, spinach (but see Comments, below), summer squash, Swiss chard, and turnip greens.

Comments

Some foods block the uptake of iodine into the thyroid gland when eaten raw in large amounts. These include Brussels sprouts, cabbage, cauliflower, kale, peaches, pears, spinach, and turnips. If you have an underactive thyroid, you should limit your consumption of these foods.

Iron

Perhaps the most important of iron's functions in the body is the production of hemoglobin and myoglobin (the form of hemoglobin found in muscle tissue) and the oxygenation of red blood cells. Iron is the mineral found in the largest amounts in the blood. It is essential for many enzymes, including catalase, and is important for growth. Iron is also required for a healthy immune system and for energy production.

Iron deficiency is most often caused by insufficient intake. However, it may result from intestinal bleeding, excessive menstrual bleeding, a diet high in phosphorus, poor digestion, long-term illness, ulcers, prolonged use of antacids, excessive coffee or tea consumption, and other causes. In some cases, a deficiency of vitamin B_6 (pyridoxine) or vitamin B_{12} can be the underlying cause of anemia. Strenuous exercise and heavy perspiration deplete iron from the body.

Iron deficiency symptoms include anemia, brittle hair, difficulty swallowing, digestive disturbances, dizziness, fatigue, fragile bones, hair loss, inflammation of the tissues of the mouth, nails that are spoon-shaped or that have ridges running lengthwise, nervousness, obesity, pallor, and slowed mental reactions.

Because iron is stored in the body, excessive iron intake can also cause problems. Too much iron in the tissues and organs leads to the production of free radicals and increases the need for vitamin E. High levels of iron have also been found in association with heart disease and cancer. The buildup of iron in the tissues has been associated with a rare disease known as hemochromatosis, a hereditary disorder of iron metabolism that causes bronze skin pigmentation, cirrhosis of the liver, diabetes, and heart disorders.

Sources

Iron is found in eggs, fish, liver, meat, poultry, green leafy vegetables, whole grains, and enriched breads and cereals. Other food sources include almonds, avocados, beets, blackstrap molasses, brewer's yeast, dates, dulse, kelp, kidney and lima beans, lentils, millet, peaches, pears, dried prunes, pumpkins, raisins, rice and wheat bran, sesame seeds, soybeans, and watercress. Herbs that contain iron include alfalfa, burdock root, catnip, cayenne, chamomile, chickweed, chicory, dandelion, dong quai, eyebright, fennel seed, fenugreek, horsetail, kelp, lemongrass, licorice, milk thistle seed, mullein, nettle, oat straw, paprika, parsley, peppermint, plantain, raspberry leaf, rose hips, sarsaparilla, shepherd's purse, uva ursi, and yellow dock.

Comments

There must be sufficient hydrochloric acid (HCl) present in the stomach in order for iron to be absorbed. Copper, manganese, molybdenum, vitamin A, and the B-complex vitamins are also needed for complete iron absorption. Taking vitamin C can increase iron absorption by as much as 30 percent.

Excessive amounts of zinc and vitamin E interfere with iron absorption. Iron utilization may be impaired by rheumatoid arthritis and cancer. These diseases can result in anemia despite adequate amounts of iron stored in the liver, spleen, and bone marrow. Iron deficiency is more prevalent in people with candidiasis or chronic herpes infections.

Cautions

Do not take iron supplements if you have an infection. Because bacteria require iron for growth, the body "hides" iron in the liver and other storage sites when an infection is present. Taking extra iron at such times encourages the proliferation of bacteria in the body.

Magnesium

Magnesium is a vital catalyst in enzyme activity, especially the activity of those enzymes involved in energy production. It assists in calcium and potassium uptake. A deficiency of magnesium interferes with the transmission of nerve and muscle impulses, causing irritability and nervousness. Supplementing the diet with magnesium can help prevent depression, dizziness, muscle weakness and twitching, and premenstrual syndrome (PMS), and also aids in maintaining the body's proper pH balance.

Magnesium is necessary to prevent the calcification of soft tissue. This essential mineral protects the arterial linings from stress caused by sudden blood pressure changes, and plays a role in the formation of bone and in carbohydrate and mineral metabolism. With vitamin B_6 (pyridoxine), magnesium helps to reduce and dissolve calcium phosphate kidney stones. Recent research has shown that magnesium may help prevent cardiovascular disease, osteoporosis, and certain forms of cancer, and it may reduce cholesterol levels. It is effective in preventing premature labor and convulsions in pregnant women. Magnesium combined with vitamin B_6 may prevent calcium oxalate kidney stones.

Possible manifestations of magnesium deficiency include confusion, insomnia, irritability, poor digestion, rapid heartbeat, seizures, and tantrums; often, a magnesium deficiency can be synonymous with diabetes. Magnesium deficiencies are at the root of many cardiovascular problems. Magnesium deficiency may be a major cause of fatal cardiac arrhythmia, hypertension, and sudden cardiac arrest, as well as asthma, chronic fatigue, chronic pain syndromes, depression, insom-

nia, irritable bowel syndrome, and pulmonary disorders. To test for magnesium deficiency, a procedure called an intracellular (mononuclear cell) magnesium screen should be performed. This is a more sensitive test than the typical serum magnesium screen, and can detect a deficiency with more accuracy. Magnesium screening should be a routine test, as a low magnesium level makes nearly every disease worse. It is particularly important for individuals who have, or who are considered at risk for developing, cardiovascular disease.

Sources

Magnesium is found in most foods, especially dairy products, fish, meat, and seafood. Other rich food sources include apples, apricots, avocados, bananas, blackstrap molasses, brewer's yeast, brown rice, cantaloupe, dulse, figs, garlic, grapefruit, green leafy vegetables, kelp, lemons, lima beans, millet, nuts, peaches, black-eyed peas, salmon, sesame seeds, soybeans, tofu, torula yeast, watercress, wheat, and whole grains. Herbs that contain magnesium include alfalfa, bladderwrack, catnip, cayenne, chamomile, chickweed, dandelion, eyebright, fennel seed, fenugreek, hops, horsetail, lemongrass, licorice, mullein, nettle, oat straw, paprika, parsley, peppermint, raspberry leaf, red clover, sage, shepherd's purse, yarrow, and yellow dock.

Comments

The consumption of alcohol, the use of diuretics, diarrhea, the presence of fluoride, and high levels of zinc and vitamin D all increase the body's need for magnesium.

The consumption of large amounts of fats, cod liver oil, calcium, vitamin D, and protein decrease magnesium absorption. Fat-soluble vitamins also hinder the absorption of magnesium, as do foods high in oxalic acid, such as almonds, chard, cocoa, rhubarb, spinach, and tea.

Manganese

Minute quantities of manganese are needed for protein and fat metabolism, healthy nerves, a healthy immune system, and blood sugar regulation. Manganese is used in energy production and is required for normal bone growth and for reproduction. In addition, it is used in the formation of cartilage and synovial (lubricating) fluid of the joints. It is also necessary for the synthesis of bone.

Manganese is essential for people with iron-deficiency anemias and is needed for the utilization of vitamin B_1 (thiamine) and vitamin E. Manganese works well with the B-complex vitamins to give an overall feeling of well-being. It aids in the formation of mother's milk and is a key element in the production of enzymes needed to oxidize fats and to metabolize purines.

A deficiency of manganese may lead to atherosclerosis, confusion, convulsions, eye problems, hearing problems, heart disorders, high cholesterol levels, hypertension, irritability, memory loss, muscle contractions, pancreatic damage, profuse perspiration, rapid pulse, tooth-grinding, tremors, and a tendency to breast ailments.

Sources

The largest quantities of manganese are found in avocados, nuts and seeds, seaweed, and whole grains. This mineral may also be found in blueberries, egg yolks, legumes, dried peas, pineapples, and green leafy vegetables. Herbs that contain manganese include alfalfa, burdock root, catnip, chamomile, chickweed, dandelion, eyebright, fennel seed, fenugreek, ginseng, hops, horsetail, lemongrass, mullein, parsley, peppermint, raspberry, red clover, rose hips, wild yam, yarrow, and yellow dock.

Molybdenum

This essential mineral is required in extremely small amounts for nitrogen metabolism. It aids in the final stages of the conversion of purines to uric acid. It promotes normal cell function, and is a component of the metabolic enzyme xanthine oxidase. Molybdenum is found in the liver, bones, and kidneys. A low intake is associated with mouth and gum disorders and cancer. A molybdenum deficiency may cause impotence in older males. Those whose diets are high in refined and processed foods are at risk for deficiency.

Sources

This trace mineral is found in beans, cereal grains, legumes, peas, and dark green leafy vegetables.

Comments

Heat and moisture can change the action of supplemental molybdenum. A high intake of sulfur may decrease molybdenum levels. Excess amounts of molybdenum may interfere with copper metabolism.

Cautions

Do not take over 15 milligrams of molybdenum daily. Higher doses may lead to the development of gout.

Phosphorus

Phosphorus is needed for bone and tooth formation, cell growth, contraction of the heart muscle, and kidney function. It also assists the body in the utilization of vitamins and the conversion of food to energy. A proper balance of magnesium, calcium, and phosphorus should be main-

tained at all times. If one of these minerals is present either in excessive or insufficient amounts, this will have adverse effects on the body.

Deficiencies of phosphorus are rare, but can lead to such symptoms as anxiety, bone pain, fatigue, irregular breathing, irritability, numbness, skin sensitivity, trembling, weakness, and weight changes.

Sources

Phosphorus deficiency is rare because this mineral is found in most foods, especially carbonated soft drinks. Significant amounts of phosphorus are contained in asparagus; bran; brewer's yeast; corn; dairy products; eggs; fish; dried fruit; garlic; legumes; nuts; sesame, sunflower, and pumpkin seeds; meats; poultry; salmon; and whole grains.

Comments

Excessive amounts of phosphorus interfere with calcium uptake. A diet consisting of junk food is a common culprit. Vitamin D increases the effectiveness of phosphorus.

Potassium

This mineral is important for a healthy nervous system and a regular heart rhythm. It helps prevent stroke, aids in proper muscle contraction, and works with sodium to control the body's water balance. Potassium is important for chemical reactions within the cells and aids in maintaining stable blood pressure and in transmitting electrochemical impulses. It also regulates the transfer of nutrients through cell membranes. This function of potassium has been shown to decrease with age, which may account for some of the circulatory damage, lethargy, and weakness experienced by older people.

Signs of potassium deficiency include abnormally dry skin, acne, chills, cognitive impairment, constipation, depression, diarrhea, diminished reflex function, edema, nervousness, insatiable thirst, fluctuations in heartbeat, glucose intolerance, growth impairment, high cholesterol levels, insomnia, low blood pressure, muscular fatigue and weakness, nausea and vomiting, periodic headaches, proteinuria (protein in the urine), respiratory distress, and salt retention.

Sources

Food sources of potassium include dairy foods, fish, fruit, legumes, meat, poultry, vegetables, and whole grains. It is specifically found in apricots, avocados, bananas, blackstrap molasses, brewer's yeast, brown rice, dates, dulse, figs, dried fruit, garlic, nuts, potatoes, raisins, winter squash, torula yeast, wheat bran, and yams. Herbs that contain potassium include catnip, hops, horsetail, nettle, plantain, red clover, sage, and skullcap.

Comments

Kidney disorders, diarrhea, and the use of diuretics or laxatives all disrupt potassium levels. Tobacco and caffeine reduce potassium absorption.

Potassium is needed for hormone secretion. The secretion of stress hormones causes a decrease in the potassium-to-sodium ratio both inside and outside the cells. As a result, stress increases the body's potassium requirements.

Selenium

Selenium's principal function is to inhibit the oxidation of lipids (fats). It is a vital antioxidant, especially when combined with vitamin E. It protects the immune system by preventing the formation of free radicals, which can damage the body. (See ANTIOXIDANTS in Part One.) It has also been found to function as a preventive against the formation of certain types of tumors. Selenium and vitamin E act synergistically to aid in the production of antibodies and to help maintain a healthy heart and liver. This trace element is needed for pancreatic function and tissue elasticity. When combined with vitamin E and zinc, it may also provide relief from an enlarged prostate. Selenium supplementation has been found to protect the liver in people with alcoholic cirrhosis.

Selenium deficiency has been linked to cancer and heart disease. It has also been associated with exhaustion, growth impairment, high cholesterol levels, infections, liver impairment, pancreatic insufficiency, and sterility. Symptoms of excessively high selenium levels can include arthritis, brittle nails, garlicky breath odor, gastrointestinal disorders, hair loss, irritability, liver and kidney impairment, a metallic taste in the mouth, pallor, skin eruptions, and yellowish skin.

Sources

Selenium can be found in meat and grains, depending on the selenium content of the soil where the food is raised. Because New Zealand soils are low in selenium, cattle and sheep raised there have suffered a breakdown of muscle tissue, including the heart muscle. However, human intake of selenium there is adequate because of imported Australian wheat. The soil of much American farm land is low in selenium, resulting in selenium-deficient produce.

Selenium can be found in Brazil nuts, brewer's yeast, broccoli, brown rice, chicken, dairy products, dulse, garlic, kelp, liver, molasses, onions, salmon, seafood, torula yeast, tuna, vegetables, wheat germ, and whole grains. Herbs that contain selenium include alfalfa, burdock root, catnip, cayenne, chamomile, chickweed, fennel seed, fenugreek, garlic, ginseng, hawthorn berry, hops, horsetail, lemongrass, milk thistle, nettle, oat straw, parsley, peppermint, raspberry leaf, rose hips, sarsaparilla, uva ursi, yarrow, and yellow dock.

Silicon

Silicon is necessary for the formation of collagen for bones and connective tissue; for healthy nails, skin, and hair; and for calcium absorption in the early stages of bone formation. It is needed to maintain flexible arteries, and plays a major role in preventing cardiovascular disease. Silicon counteracts the effects of aluminum on the body and is important in the prevention of Alzheimer's disease and osteoporosis. It stimulates the immune system and inhibits the aging process in tissues. Silicon levels decrease with aging, so elderly people need larger amounts.

Sources

Foods that contain silicon include alfalfa, beets, brown rice, the herb horsetail, bell peppers, soybeans, leafy green vegetables, and whole grains.

Comments

Boron, calcium, magnesium, manganese, and potassium aid in the efficient utilization of silicon.

Sodium

Sodium is necessary for maintaining proper water balance and blood pH. It is also needed for stomach, nerve, and muscle function. Although sodium deficiency is rare—most people have adequate (if not excessive) levels of sodium in their bodies—it can occur. This condition is most likely to affect people who take diuretics for high blood pressure, especially if they simultaneously adhere to low-sodium diets. Some experts estimate that as many as 20 percent of elderly people who take diuretics may be deficient in sodium. Symptoms of sodium deficiency can include abdominal cramps, anorexia, confusion, dehydration, depression, dizziness, fatigue, flatulence, hallucinations, headache, heart palpitations, an impaired sense of taste, lethargy, low blood pressure, memory impairment, muscular weakness, nausea and vomiting, poor coordination, recurrent infections, seizures, and weight loss. Excessive sodium intake can result in edema, high blood pressure, potassium deficiency, and liver and kidney disease.

Sources

Virtually all foods contain some sodium.

Comments

A proper balance of potassium and sodium is necessary for good health. Since most people consume too much sodium, they typically need more potassium as well. An imbalance of sodium and potassium can lead to heart disease.

Sulfur

An acid-forming mineral that is part of the chemical structure of the amino acids methionine, cysteine, taurine, and glutathione, sulfur disinfects the blood, helps the body to resist bacteria, and protects the protoplasm of cells. It aids in necessary oxidation reactions in the body, stimulates bile secretion, and protects against toxic substances. Because of its ability to protect against the harmful effects of radiation and pollution, sulfur slows down the aging process. It is found in hemoglobin and in all body tissues, and is needed for the synthesis of collagen, a principal protein that gives the skin its structural integrity.

Sources

Brussels sprouts, dried beans, cabbage, eggs, fish, garlic, kale, meats, onions, soybeans, turnips, and wheat germ contain sulfur, as do the herb horsetail and the amino acids cysteine, cystine, lysine, and methionine. Sulfur is also available in tablet and powder forms.

Comments

Moisture and heat may destroy or change the action of sulfur in the body. Sulfur is the key substance that makes garlic the "king of herbs."

Vanadium

Vanadium is needed for cellular metabolism and for the formation of bones and teeth. It plays a role in growth and reproduction, and inhibits cholesterol synthesis. A vanadium deficiency may be linked to cardiovascular and kidney disease, impaired reproductive ability, and increased infant mortality. Vanadium is not easily absorbed.

Sources

Vanadium is found in dill, fish, olives, meat, radishes, snap beans, vegetable oils, and whole grains.

Comments

There may be an interaction between vanadium and chromium. If you take supplemental chromium and vanadium, take them at different times. Tobacco use decreases the uptake of vanadium.

Zinc

This essential mineral is important in prostate gland function and the growth of the reproductive organs. Zinc may help prevent acne and regulate the activity of oil glands. It is required for protein synthesis and collagen formation, and promotes a healthy immune system and the healing of wounds. Zinc also allows acuity of taste and smell. It protects the liver from chemical damage and is vital for bone formation. It is a constituent of insulin and many vital enzymes, including the antioxidant enzyme superoxide dismutase (SOD). It also helps to fight and prevent the formation of free radicals in other ways. A form of zinc called zinc monomethionine (zinc bound with the amino acid methionine), sold under the trademark OptiZinc, has been found to have antioxidant activity comparable to that of vitamin C, vitamin E, and beta-carotene.

Sufficient intake and absorption of zinc are needed to maintain the proper concentration of vitamin E in the blood. In addition, zinc increases the absorption of vitamin A. For optimum health, a proper 1-to-10 balance between copper and zinc levels should be maintained.

A deficiency of zinc may result in the loss of the senses of taste and smell. It can also cause fingernails to become thin, peel, and develop white spots. Other possible signs of zinc deficiency include acne, delayed sexual maturation, fatigue, growth impairment, hair loss, high cholesterol levels, impaired night vision, impotence, increased susceptibility to infection, infertility, memory impairment, a propensity to diabetes, prostate trouble, recurrent colds and flu, skin lesions, and slow wound healing.

Sources

Zinc is found in the following food sources: brewer's yeast, dulse, egg yolks, fish, kelp, lamb, legumes, lima beans, liver, meats, mushrooms, pecans, oysters, poultry, pumpkin seeds, sardines, seafood, soy lecithin, soybeans, sunflower seeds, torula yeast, and whole grains. Herbs that contain zinc include alfalfa, burdock root, cayenne, chamomile, chickweed, dandelion, eyebright, fennel seed, hops, milk thistle, mullein, nettle, parsley, rose hips, sage, sarsaparilla, skullcap, and wild yam.

Comments

Zinc levels may be lowered by diarrhea, kidney disease, cirrhosis of the liver, diabetes, or the consumption of fiber, which causes zinc to be excreted through the intestinal tract. A significant amount of zinc is lost through perspiration. The consumption of hard water also can upset zinc levels. Compounds called phytates that are found in grains and legumes bind with zinc so that it cannot be absorbed.

If you take both zinc and iron supplements, take them at different times. If these two minerals are taken together, they interfere with each other's activity.

Cautions

Do not take a total of more than 100 milligrams of zinc daily. While daily doses under 100 milligrams enhance the immune response, doses of more than 100 milligrams can depress the immune system.

WATER

INTRODUCTION

The human body is composed of approximately 70 percent water. In fact, the body's water supply is responsible for and involved in nearly every bodily process, including digestion, absorption, circulation, and excretion. Water is also the primary transporter of nutrients throughout the body and so is necessary for all building functions in the body. Water helps maintain normal body temperature and is essential for carrying waste material out of the body. Therefore, replacing the water that is continually being lost through sweating and elimination is very important. To keep the body functioning properly, it is essential to drink at least eight 8-ounce glasses of quality water each day. While the body can survive without food for about five weeks, the body cannot survive without water for longer than five days.

Obtaining quality water would seem to be an easy matter. However, due to the numerous types of classifications water is given, the average consumer can easily be confused about what is available. This section is a guide to understanding what the most commonly used classifications of water mean and how these different kinds of water may help or harm the body.

TAP WATER

Water that comes out of household taps or faucets is generally obtained either from surface water—water that has run off from ponds, creeks, streams, rivers, and lakes, and is collected in reservoirs—or from ground water—water that has filtered through the ground to the water table and is extracted by means of a well.

Hard Versus Soft Water

Hard water, found in various parts of the country, contains relatively high concentrations of the minerals calcium and magnesium. The presence of these minerals prevents soap from lathering and results in filmy sediment being deposited on hair, clothing, pipes, dishes, washtubs, and anything else that comes into regular contact with the water. It also affects the taste. Hard water can be annoying, and though some studies have shown that deaths from heart disease may be lower in areas where the drinking water is hard, we believe that the calcium found in hard water is not good for the heart, arteries, or bones. Hard water

deposits its calcium and other minerals on the *outside* of these structures, while it is the calcium and magnesium found *within* these structures that are beneficial to the body.

Soft water can be naturally soft or it may be hard water that has been treated to remove the calcium and magnesium. One potentially serious problem with artificially softened water is that it is more likely than hard water to dissolve the lining of pipes. This poses an especially significant threat if pipes are made of lead. Another threat comes from certain plastic and galvanized pipes, which contain cadmium, a toxic heavy metal. These types of pipe are rarely used in construction today, but they may be present in older buildings that have not undergone extensive renovation. But leaching from pipes can be a problem with today's copper pipes as well. Dangerous levels of copper, iron, zinc, and arsenic can leach into softened water from copper pipes.

The Safety of Tap Water

Most people assume that when they turn on their kitchen tap, they are getting clean, safe, healthy drinking water. Unfortunately, this is often not the case. Regardless of the original source of tap water, it is vulnerable to a number of different types of impurities. Some undesirable substances found in water, including radon, fluoride, and arsenic, iron, lead, copper, and other heavy metals, can occur naturally. Other contaminants, such as fertilizers, asbestos, cyanides, herbicides, pesticides, and industrial chemicals, may leach into ground water water through the soil, or into any tap water from plumbing pipes. Still other substances, including chlorine, carbon, lime, phosphates, soda ash, and aluminum sulfate, are intentionally added to public water supplies to kill bacteria, adjust pH, and eliminate cloudiness, among other things. In addition, water can contain biological contaminants, including viruses, bacteria, and parasites.

A study conducted by the Natural Resources Defense Council found that 18,500 of the nation's water systems (serving some 45 million Americans) violated safe drinking water laws at some point during 1994 or 1995. The council's report blamed contaminated water for some 900,000 illnesses a year, including 100 deaths. Even if the levels of individual substances in water are well within "allowable" limits, the total of all contaminants present may still be harmful to your health.

The greatest concerns about water quality today focus on chlorine, pesticides, and parasites. Chlorine has long been added to public water supplies to kill disease-causing bacteria. However, the levels of chlorine in drinking water today can be quite high, and some byproducts of chlorine are known carcinogens. As a result, the U.S. Environmental Protection Agency (EPA) is considering steps to reduce the level of chlorine in drinking water, but is facing opposition from industry groups.

Pesticides pose a risk in any area where the tap water is extracted from an underground source. These chemicals are suspected of causing, or at least contributing to, an increased incidence of cancer, especially breast cancer. Some scientists believe this may be because certain pesticides can mimic the action of the female sex hormone estrogen in the body. Others point to the fact that toxins in the body tend to accumulate in fatty tissues, and the human breast is composed largely of fatty tissue. The pesticide problem is a particular concern in areas where agriculture is (or was) a major part of the economy. These chemicals are persistent. Residues from pesticides used decades ago may still be present in water coming out of the tap today, and may pose a risk to health.

Long considered a problem limited to poor, developing countries, the presence of bacteria and parasites in drinking water—especially a parasite called *cryptosporidium*—is becoming a serious problem in the United States today. In 1993, the residents of one of Wisconsin's largest cities were forced to boil their tap water after it was discovered to contain "unacceptable" levels of cryptosporidium, most likely from agricultural runoff. This outbreak was suspected of causing six deaths in the area. The same organism has created controversy over the safety of the water in New York City; many people with weakened immune systems have charged that cryptosporidium in the city water has made them sick, even though local officials insist that the water is safe to drink. For people with HIV or AIDS, cryptosporidium can be lethal. The chlorine added to water to kill bacteria is not effective at killing these parasites.

Whatever the source of your water, it is important to know some warning signs of bad water. Watch for cloudiness or murkiness in water. Chlorination causes some cloudiness that usually clears if the water is left to stand, but bacterial or sedimentary cloudiness will remain. Foaming may be caused by bacterial contamination, by floating particles of sediment, or by soaps or detergents. Bacteria can be destroyed by boiling water for at least five minutes, while sediment should settle out if you let the water stand for several hours. Strange smells or tastes in water that was previously fine could mean chemical contamination. However, many toxic hazards that work their way into water do not change its taste, smell, or appearance.

Fluoridation

For many years now, controversy has raged over whether fluoride should be added to drinking water. As early as 1961, as recorded in the Congressional Record, fluoride was exposed as a lethal poison in our nation's water supply. Proponents say that fluoride occurs naturally and helps develop and maintain strong bones and teeth. Opponents to fluoridation contend that when fluoridated water is consumed regularly, toxic levels of fluorine, the poisonous substance from which fluoride is derived, build up in the body, causing irreparable harm to the immune system. The Delaney Congressional Investigation Committee, the government body charged with monitoring additives and other substances in the food supply, has stated that "fluoridation is mass medication without parallel in the history of medicine."

Meanwhile, no convincing scientific proof has ever been generated that fluoridated water makes for stronger bones and teeth. It is known, however, that chronic fluoride use results in numerous health problems, including osteoporosis and osteomalacia, and also damages teeth, and leaves them mottled. The salts used to fluoridate our nation's water supply, sodium fluoride and fluorosalicic acid, are industrial byproducts that are never found in nature. They are also notoriously toxic compounds, so much so that they are used in rat poison and insecticides. The naturally occurring form of fluoride, calcium fluoride, is not toxic—but this form of fluoride is not used to fluoridate water.

Today, more than half the cities in the United States fluoridate their water supplies. In many states, it is required. Although many ailments and disorders—including Down syndrome, mottled teeth, and cancer—have been linked to fluoridated water, fluoridation has become the standard rather than the exception.

The fluoride added to tap water can be a problem. Individuals have different levels of tolerance for toxins such as fluoride. In addition, many water sources have levels of fluoride higher than one part per million, the level generally recognized as safe and originally set as the acceptable limit by the EPA. After the EPA learned that water in many towns had natural fluoride levels much higher than this, the permissible fluoride limit was raised—quadrupled, in fact—to four parts per million. And this is in addition to fluoride encountered from other sources. Fluoride is the thirteenth most widely distributed element on earth, so it can turn up just about anywhere—in vegetables and meats, for example. Since so many local water supplies are fluoridated, there is a good chance that virtually any packaged food product made with water, such as soft drinks and reconstituted juices, contains fluoride. Additional fluorides are widely used in toothpaste products, so it is easy to see how many Americans may be ingesting excessive amounts of this potentially toxic substance.

If your tap water contains fluoride, and you wish to remove it, you can use a reverse osmosis, distillation, or activated alumina filtration system to eliminate almost all of the fluoride from your water.

Water Analysis

Not all drinking water contains significant amounts of toxic substances. Some places rate higher in water safety than others. In addition, not all cities and towns process their water supplies the same way. Some do nothing at all to their water. Others add chemicals to the water to kill bacteria. Still others filter their water. It is up to the individual to find out how local drinking water is treated and to determine how safe the water coming out of the tap is.

The EPA has defined pure water as "bacteriologically safe" water, and it recommends—but does not require—that tap water have a pH between 6.5 and 8.5. This allows for a great deal of leeway in what passes as acceptable water. If you are concerned about the safety of the water coming out of your tap, you can contact your local water officials or local health department, which may test your tap water free of charge. In some cases, you may have to contact your state's water supply or health department. Typically, however, these agencies test the water only for bacteria levels, not for toxic substances. Therefore, you might want to contact a commercial laboratory or local state university laboratory to test your water for its chemical content. If you find that your tap water is unacceptable either because of its taste or because of its toxic chemical content, you may choose to use one of the alternative water supplies described in this section.

The Water Quality Association is prepared to answer questions about the various types of water and methods of water treatment. Their address is 4151 Naperville Road, Lisle, IL 60532; telephone 708–505–0160.

Improving Tap Water

Tap water can be improved in several ways. Heating tap water to a rolling boil and keeping it there for three to five minutes will kill bacteria and parasites. However, most people find boiling their drinking water too impractical and time-consuming. In addition, this procedure has the effect of concentrating whatever lead is present in the water, and the water must then be refrigerated if it is to be used for drinking. The taste of chlorinated tap water can be improved by keeping the water in an uncovered pitcher for several hours to allow the chlorine taste and odor to dissipate. Water can also be aerated in a blender to remove chlorine and other chemicals. Nevertheless, neither of these last two methods will improve the quality of the water—only the taste.

Filtration is a means by which contaminants in water are removed, rendering the water cleaner and better tasting. There are many different ways in which water can be filtered. Nature filters water as the water runs through streams and as it seeps down through the soil and rocks to the water table. As water passes through the earth or over the rocks in a stream, the bacteria in the water leech into the rocks and are replaced with minerals such as calcium and magnesium.

There are also man-made ways of filtering water. There are three basic types of filters available: absorbent types, which use materials such as carbon to pick up impurities; microfiltration systems, which run water through filters with tiny pores to catch and eliminate contaminants (the filter may be made of any of a number of different materials); and special media like ion-exchange resins that are designed to remove heavy metals. Water filtration systems vary in effectiveness. Two types that are considered good are reverse osmosis and ceramic filtration systems. However, no filter can remove absolutely all contaminants. Each pore of even the finest filter is large enough for some viruses to permeate. To remove parasites such as cryptosporidium, the EPA and CDC recommend purchasing a filter that has a National Sanitation Foundation (NSF) rating for parasite reduction *and* that has an absolute pore size of 1 micron or smaller.

BOTTLED WATER

Because of concerns over the safety and health effects of tap water, many people today are turning to bottled water. Bottled water is usually classified by its source (spring, spa, geyser, public water supply, etc.), by its mineral content (containing at least 500 parts per million of dissolved solids), and/or by the type of treatment it has undergone (deionized, steam-distilled, etc.). Because there is a lot of overlapping among these criteria, some water fits more than one classification. In addition, most states have no rules governing appropriate labeling, so some bottled water claims may be misleading or incorrect.

Deionized or Demineralized Water

When the electric charge of a molecule of water has been neutralized by the addition or removal of electrons, the resulting water is called *deionized* or *demineralized.* The deionization process removes nitrates and the minerals calcium and magnesium, in addition to the heavy metals cadmium, barium, lead, and some forms of radium.

Mineral Water

Mineral water is natural spring water, usually from Europe or Canada. To be considered mineral water, in addition to containing minerals, the water must flow freely from its source, cannot be pumped or forced from the ground, and must be bottled directly at the source. Depending on where the source is, the minerals contained will vary. If you are suffering from a deficiency of certain minerals and are drinking mineral water for therapeutic reasons, you must be aware of which minerals are in the particular brand of water you drink. If you are drinking mineral water containing minerals that you do not lack, you could be doing yourself more harm than good.

Most mineral waters are carbonated. However, some sparkling waters, such as club soda, are called mineral waters only because the manufacturer added bicarbonates, citrates, and sodium phosphates to filtered or distilled tap water.

Natural Spring Water

The number of gallons of "natural spring water" flowing through water coolers and from bottles has more than doubled in the last few years. The word "natural" on the label doesn't tell you where the water came from, only that the mineral content of the water has not been altered. It may or may not have been filtered or otherwise treated. Similarly, because there is no legal definition of the word "spring" as it is used on bottled water labels, a bottle of "natural spring water" may not have come from a spring. However, most companies that sell bottled water willingly list their water source on the label.

Spring water is water that rises naturally to the earth's surface from underground reservoirs. This water is unprocessed, and flavor or carbonation may be added.

If you use a water cooler for bottled spring water, you should be sure to clean the cooler once a month to destroy bacteria. Run a 50-50 mixture of hydrogen peroxide and baking soda through the reservoir and spigots, then remove the residue by rinsing the cooler with four or more gallons of tap water.

Sparkling Water

Sparkling water is water that has been carbonated. It can be a healthful alternative to soda and alcoholic beverages, but if it is loaded with fructose and other sweeteners, it may be no better than soda pop. Read labels before you buy.

Understanding where the carbonation in sparkling water comes from isn't always easy. A "naturally sparkling water" must get its carbonation from the same source as the water. If a water is "carbonated natural water," that means the carbonation came from a source other than the one that supplied the water. That doesn't mean the water is of poor quality. It can still be called "natural" because its mineral content is the same as when it came from the ground, even though it has been carbonated from a separate source. People suffering from intestinal disorders or ulcers should avoid drinking carbonated water because it may be irritating to the gastrointestinal tract.

Steam-Distilled Water

Distillation involves vaporizing water by boiling it. The steam rises, leaving behind most of the bacteria, viruses, chemicals, minerals, and pollutants from the water. The steam is then moved into a condensing chamber, where it is cooled and condensed to become distilled water.

Once consumed, steam-distilled water leaches inorganic minerals rejected by the cells and tissues out of the body. We believe that only steam-distilled water should be consumed.

Flavor can be added to distilled water by adding 1 to 2 tablespoons of raw apple cider vinegar (obtained from a health food store) per gallon of distilled water. Vinegar is an excellent solvent and aids in digestion. Lemon juice is another good flavoring agent, and has cleansing properties as well. For added minerals, you can add mineral drops to steam-distilled water. Concentrace from Trace Minerals Research is a good product for this purpose. Add 2 tablespoons of mineral drops to every 5 gallons of water.

AMINO ACIDS

THE FUNCTION OF AMINO ACIDS

Amino acids are the chemical units or "building blocks," as they are popularly called, that make up proteins. Amino acids contain about 16 percent nitrogen. Chemically, this is what distinguishes them from the other two basic nutrients, sugars and fatty acids, which do not contain nitrogen. To understand how vital amino acids are, you must understand how essential proteins are to life. It is protein that provides the structure for all living things. Every living organism, from the largest animal to the tiniest microbe, is composed of protein. And in its various forms, protein participates in the vital chemical processes that sustain life.

Proteins are a necessary part of every living cell in the body. Next to water, protein makes up the greatest portion of our body weight. In the human body, protein substances make up the muscles, ligaments, tendons, organs, glands, nails, hair, and many vital body fluids, and are essential for the growth of bones. The enzymes and hormones that catalyze and regulate all bodily processes are proteins. Proteins help to regulate the body's water balance and maintain the proper internal pH. They assist in the exchange of nutrients between the intercellular fluids and the tissues, blood, and lymph. A deficiency of protein can upset the body's fluid balance, causing edema. Proteins form the structural basis of chromosomes, through which genetic information is passed from parents to offspring. The genetic "code" contained in each cell's DNA is actually information for how to make that cell's proteins.

Proteins are chains of amino acids linked together by what are called peptide bonds. Each individual type of protein is composed of a specific group of amino acids in a specific chemical arrangement. It is the particular amino acids present and the way in which they are linked together in sequence that gives the proteins that make up the various tissues their unique functions and characters. Each protein in the body is tailored for a specific need; proteins are not interchangeable.

The proteins that make up the human body are not obtained directly from the diet. Rather, dietary protein is broken down into its constituent amino acids, which the body then uses to build the specific proteins it needs. Thus, it is the amino acids rather than protein that are the essential nutrients.

In addition to combining to form the body's proteins, some amino acids act as neurotransmitters or as precur-sors of neurotransmitters, the chemicals that carry information from one nerve cell to another. Certain amino acids are thus necessary for the brain to receive and send messages. Unlike many other substances, neurotransmitters are able to pass through the *blood-brain barrier*. This is a kind of defensive shield designed to protect the brain from toxins and foreign invaders that may be circulating in the bloodstream. The endothelial cells that make up the walls of the capillaries in the brain are much more tightly meshed together than are those of capillaries elsewhere in the body. This prevents many substances, especially water-based substances, from diffusing through the capillary walls into brain tissue. Because certain amino acids can pass through this barrier, they can be used by the brain to communicate with nerve cells elsewhere in the body.

Amino acids also enable vitamins and minerals to perform their jobs properly. Even if vitamins and minerals are absorbed and assimilated by the body, they cannot be effective unless the necessary amino acids are present. For example, low levels of the amino acid tyrosine may lead to iron deficiency. Deficiency and/or impaired metabolism of the amino acids methionine and taurine has been linked to allergies and autoimmune disorders. Many elderly people suffer from depression or neurological problems that may be associated with deficiencies of the amino acids tyrosine, tryptophan, phenylalanine, and histidine, and also of the *branched-chain amino acids*—valine, isoleucine, and leucine. These are amino acids that can be used to provide energy directly to muscle tissue. High doses of branched-chain amino acids have been used in hospitals to treat people suffering from trauma and infection.

There are approximately twenty-eight commonly known amino acids that are combined in various ways to create the hundreds of different types of proteins present in all living things. In the human body, the liver produces about 80 percent of the amino acids needed. The remaining 20 percent must be obtained from the diet. These are called the *essential amino acids*. The essential amino acids that must enter the body through diet are histidine, isoleucine, leucine, lysine, methionine, phenylalanine, threonine, tryptophan, and valine. The nonessential amino acids, which can be manufactured in the body from other amino acids obtained from dietary sources, include alanine, arginine, asparagine, aspartic acid, citrulline, cysteine, cystine, gamma-aminobutyric acid, glutamic acid, glutamine, glycine, ornithine, proline, serine, taurine, and tyrosine.

The fact that they are termed "nonessential" does not mean that they are not necessary, only that they need not be obtained through the diet because the body can manufacture them as needed.

The processes of assembling amino acids to make proteins, and of breaking down proteins into individual amino acids for the body's use, are continuous ones. When we need more enzyme proteins, the body produces more enzyme proteins; when we need more cells, the body produces more proteins for cells. These different types of proteins are produced as the need arises. Should the body become depleted of its reserves of any of the essential amino acids, it would not be able to produce the proteins that require those amino acids. If even one essential amino acid is missing, the body cannot continue proper protein synthesis. This can lead to lack of vital proteins in the body, which can cause problems ranging from indigestion to depression to stunted growth.

How could such a situation occur? More easily than you might think. Many factors can contribute to deficiencies of essential amino acids, even if you eat a well-balanced diet that contains enough protein. Impaired absorption, infection, trauma, stress, drug use, age, and imbalances of other nutrients can all affect the availability of essential amino acids in the body. If your diet is *not* properly balanced—that is, if it fails to supply adequate amounts of the essential amino acids—sooner or later, this will become apparent as some type of physical disorder.

This does not mean, however, that eating a diet containing enormous amounts of protein is the answer. In fact, it is unhealthy. Excess protein puts undue stress on the kidneys and the liver, which are faced with processing the waste products of protein metabolism. Nearly half of the amino acids in dietary protein are transformed into glucose by the liver and utilized to provide needed energy to the cells. This process results in a waste product, ammonia. Ammonia is toxic to the body, so the body protects itself by having the liver turn the ammonia into the much less toxic compound urea, which is then carried through the bloodstream, filtered out by the kidneys, and excreted.

As long as protein intake is not too great and the liver is working properly, ammonia is neutralized almost as soon as it is produced, so it does no harm. However, if there is too much ammonia for the liver to cope with—as a result of too much protein consumption, poor digestion, and/or a defect in liver function—toxic levels may accumulate. Strenuous exercise also tends to promote the accumulation of excess ammonia. This may put a person at risk for serious health problems, including encephalopathy (brain disease) or hepatic coma. Abnormally high levels of urea can also cause problems, including inflamed kidneys and back pain. Therefore, it is not the quantity but the quality of protein in the diet that is important (*see* DIET AND NUTRITION in Part One).

It is possible to take supplements containing amino acids, both essential and nonessential. For certain disorders, taking supplements of specific amino acids can be very beneficial. When you take a specific amino acid or amino acid combination, it supports the metabolic pathway involved in your particular illness. Vegetarians, especially vegans, would be wise to take a formula containing all of the essential amino acids to ensure that their protein requirements are met.

WHAT'S ON THE SHELVES

Supplemental amino acids are available in combination with various multivitamin formulas, as protein mixtures, in a wide variety of food supplements, and in a number of amino acid formulas. They can be purchased as capsules, tablets, liquids, and powders. Most amino acid supplements are derived from animal protein, yeast protein, or vegetable protein. Crystalline free-form amino acids are generally extracted from a variety of grain products. Brown rice bran is a prime source, although cold-pressed yeast and milk proteins are also used.

When choosing amino acid supplements, look for products that contain USP (U.S. Pharmacopoeia) pharmaceutical-grade L-crystalline amino acids. Most of the amino acids (except for glycine) can appear in two forms, the chemical structure of one being the mirror image of the other. These are called the D- and L- forms—for example, D-cystine and L-cystine. The "D" stands for *dextro* (Latin for "right") and the "L" for *levo* (Latin for "left"); these terms denote the direction of the rotation of the spiral that is the chemical structure of the molecule. Proteins in animal and plant tissue are made from the L- forms of amino acids (with the exception of phenylalanine, which is also used in the form of DL-phenylalanine, a mixture of the D- and L- forms). Thus, with respect to supplements of amino acids, products containing the L- forms of amino acids are considered to be more compatible with human biochemistry.

Free-form means the amino acid is in its purest form. Free-form amino acids need no digestion and are absorbed directly into the bloodstream. These white crystalline amino acids are stable at room temperature and decompose when heated to temperatures of 350°F to 660°F (180°C to 350°C). They are rapidly absorbed and do not come from potentially allergenic food sources. For best results, choose encapsulated powders or powder.

Each amino acid has specific functions in the body. The many functions and possible symptoms of deficiency of twenty-eight amino acids and related compounds are described below. When taking amino acids individually for healing purposes, take them on an empty stomach to avoid making them compete for absorption with the amino acids present in foods. When taking individual amino acids, it is best to take them in the morning or between meals, with small amounts of vitamin B_6 and vitamin C to enhance absorption. When taking an amino acid complex that includes all of the essential amino acids, it is best to take it one-half hour away from a meal, either before or after. If you are taking individual amino acids, it is wise also to take a full amino acid complex, including both essential and nonessential amino acids, at a different time. This is the best way to assure you have adequate amounts of all the necessary amino acids.

Individual amino acids should not be taken for long periods of time. A good rule to follow is to alternate the individual amino acids that fit your needs and back them up with an amino acid complex, taking the supplements for two months and then discontinuing them for two months. Researchers warn against taking large doses of amino acids for extended periods of time. Moderation is the key. Some amino acids have potentially toxic effects when taken in high doses (over 6,000 milligrams per day) and may cause neurological damage. These include aspartic acid, glutamic acid, homocysteine, serine, and tryptophan. Cysteine can be toxic if taken in amounts over 1,000 milligrams per day. Do not give supplemental amino acids to a child or take doses of any amino acid in excess of the amount recommended unless specifically directed to do so by your health care provider.

THE ABC'S OF AMINO ACIDS

Alanine

Alanine aids in the metabolism of glucose, a simple carbohydrate that the body uses for energy. Epstein-Barr virus and chronic fatigue have been associated with excessive alanine levels and low levels of tyrosine and phenylalanine. One form of alanine, beta-alanine, is a constituent of pantothenic acid (vitamin B5) and coenzyme A, a vital catalyst in the body.

Arginine

Arginine retards the growth of tumors and cancer by enhancing immune function. It increases the size and activity of the thymus gland, which manufactures T lymphocytes (T cells), crucial components of the immune system. Arginine may therefore benefit those suffering from AIDS and malignant diseases that suppress the immune system. It is also good for liver disorders such as cirrhosis of the liver and fatty liver; it aids in liver detoxification by neutralizing ammonia. Seminal fluid contains arginine. Studies suggest that sexual maturity may be delayed by arginine deficiency; conversely, arginine is useful in treating sterility in men. It is found in high concentrations in the skin and connective tissues, making it helpful for healing and repair of damaged tissue.

Arginine is important for muscle metabolism. It helps to maintain a proper nitrogen balance by acting as a vehicle for transportation and storage, and aiding in the excretion, of excess nitrogen. This amino acid aids in weight loss because it facilitates an increase in muscle mass and a reduction of body fat. It is also involved in a variety of

enzymes and hormones. It aids in stimulating the pancreas to release insulin, is a component of the pituitary hormone vasopressin, and assists in the release of growth hormones. Because arginine is a component of collagen and aids in building new bone and tendon cells, it can be good for arthritis and connective tissue disorders. Scar tissue that forms during wound healing is made up of collagen, which is rich in arginine. A variety of functions, including insulin production, glucose tolerance, and liver lipid metabolism, are impaired when the body is deficient in arginine.

This amino acid can be produced in the body; however, in newborn infants, production may not occur quickly enough to keep up with requirements. Foods high in arginine include carob, chocolate, coconut, dairy products, gelatin, meat, oats, peanuts, soybeans, walnuts, white flour, wheat, and wheat germ.

Those with viral infections such as herpes should *not* take supplemental arginine, and should avoid foods rich in arginine, as it appears to promote the growth of certain viruses. L-Arginine supplements should be avoided by pregnant and lactating women. Persons with schizophrenia should avoid amounts over 30 milligrams daily. Long-term use, especially of high doses, is not recommended. One study found that several weeks of large doses may result in thickening and coarsening of the skin.

Asparagine

Asparagine is needed to maintain balance in the central nervous system; it prevents you from being either overly nervous or overly calm. It promotes the process by which one amino acid is transformed into another in the liver. This amino acid is found mostly in meat sources.

Aspartic Acid

Because aspartic acid increases stamina, it is good for fatigue and plays a vital role in metabolism. Chronic fatigue may result from low levels of aspartic acid, because this leads to lowered cellular energy. It is beneficial for neural and brain disorders. It is good for athletes, and helps to protect the liver by aiding in the removal of excess ammonia. Aspartic acid combines with other amino acids to form molecules that absorb toxins and remove them from the bloodstream. It aids cell function and the function of RNA and DNA, which are the carriers of genetic information. It enhances the production of immunoglobulins and antibodies (immune system proteins). Plant protein, especially that found in sprouting seeds, contains an abundance of aspartic acid.

Carnitine

Carnitine is not an amino acid in the strictest sense (it is actually a substance related to the B vitamins). However, because it has a chemical structure similar to that of amino acids, it is usually considered together with them.

Unlike true amino acids, carnitine is not used for protein synthesis or as a neurotransmitter. Its main function in the body is to help transport long-chain fatty acids, which are burned within the cells to provide energy. This is a major source of energy for the muscles. Carnitine thus increases the use of fat as an energy source. This prevents fatty buildup, especially in the heart, liver, and skeletal muscles. Carnitine reduces the health risks posed by poor fat metabolism associated with diabetes; inhibits alcohol-induced fatty liver; and lessens the risk of heart disorders. Studies have shown that damage to the heart from cardiac surgery can be reduced by treatment with carnitine. It has the ability to lower blood triglyceride levels, aid in weight loss, and improve muscle strength in people with neuromuscular disorders. Conversely, it is believed that carnitine deficiency may be a contributor to certain types of muscular dystrophy, and it has been shown that these disorders lead to losses of carnitine in the urine. People with such conditions need greater than normal amounts of carnitine. Carnitine also enhances the effectiveness of the antioxidant vitamins E and C.

Carnitine can be manufactured by the body if sufficient amounts of iron, vitamin B_1 (thiamine), vitamin B_6 (pyridoxine), and the amino acids lysine and methionine are available. The synthesis of carnitine also depends on the presence of adequate levels of vitamin C. Inadequate intake of any of these nutrients can result in a carnitine deficiency. Carnitine can also be obtained from food, primarily meats and other foods of animal origin.

Many cases of carnitine deficiency have been identified as partly genetic in origin, resulting from an inherited defect in carnitine synthesis. Possible symptoms of deficiency include confusion, heart pain, muscle weakness, and obesity. Because of their generally greater muscle mass, men need more carnitine than women do. Vegetarians are more likely than nonvegetarians to be deficient in carnitine because it is not found in vegetable protein. Moreover, neither methionine nor lysine, two of the key constituents from which the body makes carnitine, are obtainable from vegetable sources in sufficient amounts. To ensure adequate production of carnitine, vegetarians should take supplements or should eat grains, such as cornmeal, that have been fortified with lysine.

Supplemental carnitine is available in different forms, including D-carnitine, L-carnitine, DL-carnitine, and acetyl-L-carnitine. L-carnitine is the preferred form.

Citrulline

Citrulline promotes energy, stimulates the immune system, is metabolized to form L-arginine, and detoxifies ammonia, which damages living cells. Citrulline is found primarily in the liver.

Cysteine and Cystine

These two amino acids are closely related; each molecule of cystine consists of two molecules of cysteine joined together. Cysteine is very unstable and is easily converted to L-cystine; however, each form is capable of converting into the other as needed. Both are sulfur-containing amino acids that aid in the formation of skin and are important in detoxification.

Cysteine is present in alpha-keratin, the chief protein constitutent of the fingernails, toenails, skin, and hair. Cysteine aids in the production of collagen and promotes the proper elasticity and texture of the skin. It is also found in a variety of other proteins in the body, including several of the digestive enzymes.

Cysteine helps to detoxify harmful toxins and protect the body from radiation damage. It is one of the best free radical destroyers, and works best when taken with selenium and vitamin E. Cysteine is also precursor to glutathione, a substance that detoxifies the liver by binding with potentially harmful substances there. It helps to protect the liver and brain from damage due to alcohol, drugs, and toxic compounds in cigarette smoke.

Since cysteine is more soluble than cystine, it is used more readily in the body and is usually best for treating most illnesses. This amino acid is formed from L-methionine in the body. Vitamin B_6 is necessary for cysteine synthesis, which may not take place as it should in the presence of chronic disease. Therefore, people with chronic illnesses may need higher than normal doses of cysteine, as much as 1,000 milligrams three times daily for a month at a time.

Supplementation with L-cysteine is recommended in the treatment of rheumatoid arthritis, hardening of the arteries, and mutogenic disorders such as cancer. It promotes healing after surgery and severe burns, chelates heavy metals, and binds with soluble iron, aiding in iron absorption. This amino acid also promotes the burning of fat and the building of muscle. Because of its ability to break down mucus in the respiratory tract, L-cysteine is often beneficial in the treatment of bronchitis, emphysema, and tuberculosis. It promotes healing from respiratory disorders and plays an important role in the activity of white blood cells, which fight disease.

Cystine or the N-acetyl form of cysteine (N-acetylcysteine) may be used in place of L-cysteine. N-acetylcysteine aids in preventing side effects from chemotherapy and radiation therapy. Because it increases glutathione levels in the lungs, kidneys, liver, and bone marrow, it has an anti-aging effect on the body—reducing the accumulation of age spots, for example. N-acetylcysteine has been shown to be more effective at boosting glutathione levels than supplements of cystine or even of glutathione itself.

People who have diabetes should be cautious about taking supplemental cysteine because it is capable of inactivating insulin. Persons with cystinuria, a rare genetic condition that leads to the formation of cystine kidney stones, should not take cysteine.

Dimethylglycine (DMG)

Dimethylglycine (DMG) is a derivative of glycine, the simplest of the amino acids. It acts as a building block for many important substances, including the amino acid methionine, choline, a number of important hormones and neurotransmitters, and DNA.

Low levels of DMG are present in meats, seeds, and grains. No deficiency symptoms are associated with a lack of DMG in the diet, but taking supplemental DMG can have a wide range of beneficial effects, including helping the body maintain high energy levels and boosting mental acuity. DMG has been found to enhance the immune system and to reduce elevated blood cholesterol and triglyceride levels. It improves oxygen utilization by the body, helps to normalize blood pressure and blood glucose levels, and improves the functioning of many important organs. It may also be useful for controlling epileptic seizures. Aangamik DMG from FoodScience Laboratories is a good source of supplemental DMG.

Gamma-Aminobutyric Acid

Gamma-aminobutyric acid (GABA) is an amino acid that acts as a neurotransmitter in the central nervous system. It is essential for brain metabolism, aiding in proper brain function. GABA is formed in the body from another amino acid, glutamic acid. Its function is to decrease neuron activity and inhibit nerve cells from overfiring. Together with niacinamide and inositol, it prevents anxiety- and stress-related messages from reaching the motor centers of the brain by occupying their receptor sites.

GABA can be taken to calm the body in much the same way as diazepam (Valium), chlordiazepoxide (Librium), and other tranquilizers, but without the fear of addiction. GABA has been used in the treatment of epilepsy and hypertension. It is good for depressed sex drive because of its ability as a relaxant. It is also useful for enlarged prostate, probably because it plays a role in the mechanism regulating the release of sex hormones. GABA is effective in treating attention deficit disorder.

Too much GABA, however, can cause increased anxiety, shortness of breath, numbness around the mouth, and tingling in the extremities.

Glutamic Acid

Glutamic acid is an excitatory neurotransmitter that increases the firing of neurons in the central nervous system. It is a major excitatory neurotransmitter in the brain and spinal cord and is the precursor of GABA.

This amino acid is important in the metabolism of sugars and fats, and aids in the transportation of potassium across the blood-brain barrier. Although it does not pass the blood-brain barrier as readily as glutamine does, it is found at high levels in the blood and may infiltrate the brain in small amounts. The brain can use glutamic acid as fuel. Glutamic acid can detoxify ammonia by picking up nitrogen atoms, in the process creating another amino acid, glutamine. The conversion of glutamic acid into glutamine is the only means by which ammonia in the brain can be detoxified.

Glutamic acid helps to correct personality disorders and is useful in treating childhood behavioral disorders. It is used in the treatment of epilepsy, mental retardation, muscular dystrophy, ulcers, and hypoglycemic coma, a complication of insulin treatment for diabetes.

Glutamine

Glutamine is the most abundant free amino acid found in the muscles of the body. Because it can readily pass the blood-brain barrier, it is known as brain fuel. In the brain, glutamine is converted into glutamic acid—which is essential for cerebral function—and vice versa. It also increases the amount of GABA, which is needed to sustain proper brain function and mental activity. It assists in maintaining the proper acid/alkaline balance in the body, and is the basis of the building blocks for the synthesis of RNA and DNA. It promotes mental ability and the maintenance of a healthy digestive tract.

When an amino acid is broken down, nitrogen is released. The body needs nitrogen, but free nitrogen can form ammonia, which is especially toxic to brain tissues. The liver can convert nitrogen into urea, which is excreted in the urine, or nitrogen may attach itself to glutamic acid. This process forms glutamine. Glutamine is unique among the amino acids in that each molecule contains not one nitrogen atom but two. Thus, its creation helps to clear ammonia from the tissues, especially brain tissue, and it can transfer nitrogen from one place to another.

Glutamine is found in large amounts in the muscles and is readily available when needed for the synthesis of skeletal muscle proteins. Because this amino acid helps to build and maintain muscle, supplemental glutamine is useful for dieters and bodybuilders. More importantly, it helps to prevent the kind of muscle-wasting that can accompany prolonged bed rest or diseases such as cancer and AIDS. This is because stress and injury (including surgical trauma) cause the muscles to release glutamine into the bloodstream. In fact, during times of stress, as much as one third of the glutamine present in the muscles may be released. As a result, stress and/or illness can lead to the loss of skeletal muscle. If enough glutamine is available, however, this can be prevented.

Supplemental L-glutamine can be helpful in the treatment of arthritis, autoimmune diseases, fibrosis, intestinal disorders, peptic ulcers, connective tissue diseases such as polymyositis and scleroderma, and tissue damage due to radiation treatment for cancer. L-glutamine can enhance mental functioning, and has been used to treat a range of problems including developmental disabilities, epilepsy, fatigue, impotence, schizophrenia, and senility. L-glutamine decreases sugar cravings and the desire for alcohol, and is useful for recovering alcoholics.

Many plant and animal substances contain glutamine, but it is easily destroyed by cooking. If eaten raw, spinach and parsley are good sources. Supplemental glutamine must be kept absolutely dry or the powder will degrade into ammonia and pyroglutamic acid. Glutamine should *not* be taken by persons with cirrhosis of the liver, kidney problems, Reye's syndrome, or any type of disorder that can result in an accumulation of ammonia in the blood. For such individuals, taking supplemental glutamine may only cause further damage to the body. Be aware that although the names sound similar, glutamine, glutamic acid (also sometimes called glutamate), glutathione, gluten, and monosodium glutamate are all different substances.

Glutathione

Like carnitine, glutathione is not technically one of the amino acids. It is a compound classified as a tripeptide, and the body produces it from the amino acids cysteine, glutamic acid, and glycine. Because of its close relationship to these amino acids, however, it is usually considered together with them.

Glutathione is a powerful antioxidant that is produced in the liver. The largest stores of glutathione are found in the liver, where it detoxifies harmful compounds so that they can be excreted through the bile. Some glutathione is released from the liver directly into the bloodstream, where it helps to maintain the integrity of red blood cells and protect white blood cells. Glutathione is also found in the lungs and the intestinal tract. It is needed for carbohydrate metabolism, and also appears to exert anti-aging effects, aiding in the breakdown of oxidized fats that may contribute to atherosclerosis.

A deficiency of glutathione first affects the nervous system, causing such symptoms as lack of coordination, mental disorders, tremors, and difficulty maintaining balance. These problems are believed to be due to the development of lesions in the brain.

As we age, glutathione levels decline, although it is not known whether this is because we use it more rapidly or produce less of it to begin with. Unfortunately, if not corrected, the lack of glutathione in turn accelerates the aging process.

Supplemental glutathione is expensive, and the effectiveness of oral formulas is questionable. To raise glutathione levels, it is better to supply the body with the raw materials it uses to make this compound: cysteine, glutamic acid, and glycine. The N-acetyl form of cysteine (N-acetylcysteine) is considered particularly effective for this purpose.

Glycine

Glycine retards muscle degeneration by supplying additional creatine, a compound that is present in muscle tissue and is utilized in the construction of DNA and RNA. Glycine is essential for the synthesis of nucleic acids, bile acids, and other nonessential amino acids in the body. It is used in many gastric antacid agents. Because high concentrations of glycine are found in the skin and connective tissues, it is useful for repairing damaged tissues and promoting healing.

Glycine is necessary for central nervous system function and a healthy prostate. It functions as an inhibitory neurotransmitter and as such can help prevent epileptic seizures. It has been used in the treatment of manic (bipolar) depression, and can also be effective for hyperactivity.

Having too much of this amino acid in the body can cause fatigue, but having the proper amount produces more energy. If necessary, glycine can be converted into the amino acid serine in the body.

Histidine

Histidine is an essential amino acid that is significant in the growth and repair of tissues. It is important for the maintenance of the myelin sheaths that protect nerve cells, and is needed for the production of both red and white blood cells. Histidine also protects the body from radiation damage, aids in removing heavy metals from the system, and may help in the prevention of AIDS.

Histidine levels that are too high may lead to stress and even psychological disorders such as anxiety and schizophrenia; people with schizophrenia have been found to have high levels of histidine in their bodies. Inadequate levels of histidine may contribute to rheumatoid arthritis and may be associated with nerve deafness. Methionine has the ability to lower histidine levels.

Histamine, an important immune system chemical, is derived from histidine. Histamine aids in sexual arousal. Because the availability of histidine influences histamine production, taking supplemental histidine—together with vitamins B_3 (niacin) and B_6 (pyridoxine), which are required for the transformation from histidine to histamine—may help improve sexual functioning and pleasure. Because histamine also stimulates the secretion of gastric juices, histidine may be helpful for people with indigestion resulting from a lack of stomach acid.

Persons with manic (bipolar) depression should not take supplemental histidine unless a deficiency has been identified. Natural sources of histidine include rice, wheat, and rye.

Isoleucine

Isoleucine, one of the essential amino acids, is needed for hemoglobin formation and also stabilizes and regulates blood sugar and energy levels. It is metabolized in muscle tissue. It is one of the three branched-chain amino acids. These amino acids are valuable for athletes because they enhance energy, increase endurance, and aid in the healing and repair of muscle tissue.

Isoleucine has been found to be deficient in people suffering from many different mental and physical disorders. A deficiency of isoleucine can lead to symptoms similar to those of hypoglycemia.

Food sources of isoleucine include almonds, cashews, chicken, chickpeas, eggs, fish, lentils, liver, meat, rye, most seeds, and soy protein. It is also available in supplemental form. Supplemental isoleucine should always be taken with a correct balance of the other two branched-chain amino acids, leucine and valine—approximately 2 milligrams each of leucine and valine for each milligram of isoleucine. Combination supplements that provide all three of the branched-chain amino acids are available and may be more convenient to use.

Leucine

Leucine is an essential amino acid and one of the branched-chain amino acids (the others are isoleucine and valine). These work together to protect muscle and act as fuel. They promote the healing of bones, skin, and muscle tissue, and are recommended for those recovering from surgery. Leucine also lowers elevated blood sugar levels, and aids in increasing growth hormone production.

Natural sources of leucine include brown rice, beans, meat, nuts, soy flour, and whole wheat. Supplemental L-leucine must be taken in balance with L-isoleucine and L-valine (see Isoleucine in this section), and it should be taken in moderation, or symptoms of hypoglycemia may result. An excessively high intake of leucine may also contribute to pellagra, and may increase the amount of ammonia present in the body.

Lysine

Lysine is an essential amino acid that is a necessary building block for all protein. It is needed for proper growth and bone development in children; it helps calcium absorption and maintains a proper nitrogen balance in adults. This amino acid aids in the production of antibodies, hormones, and enzymes, and helps in collagen formation and tissue repair. Because it helps to build muscle protein, it is good for those recovering from surgery and sports injuries. It also lowers high serum triglyceride levels.

Another very useful ability of this amino acid is its capacity for fighting cold sores and herpesviruses. Taking supplemental L-lysine, together with vitamin C with bioflavonoids, can effectively fight and/or prevent herpes outbreaks, especially if foods containing the amino acid arginine are avoided (see HERPESVIRUS INFECTION in Part Two).

Lysine is an essential amino acid, and so cannot be manufactured in the body. It is therefore vital that adequate amounts be included in the diet. Deficiencies can result in anemia, bloodshot eyes, enzyme disorders, hair loss, an inability to concentrate, irritability, lack of energy, poor appetite, reproductive disorders, retarded growth, and weight loss. Food sources of lysine include cheese, eggs, fish, lima beans, milk, potatoes, red meat, soy products, and yeast.

Methionine

Methionine is an essential amino acid that assists in the breakdown of fats, thus helping to prevent a buildup of fat in the liver and arteries that might obstruct blood flow to the brain, heart, and kidneys. The synthesis of the amino acids cysteine and taurine may depend on the availability of methionine. This amino acid helps the digestive system; helps to detoxify harmful agents such as lead and other heavy metals; helps diminish muscle weakness, prevent brittle hair, and protect against radiation; and is beneficial for people with osteoporosis or chemical allergies. It is useful also in the treatment of rheumatic fever and toxemia of pregnancy.

Methionine is a powerful antioxidant. It is a good source of sulfur, which inactivates free radicals. It is also good for people with Gilbert's syndrome, an anomaly of liver function, and is required for the synthesis of nucleic acids, collagen, and proteins found in every cell of the body. It is beneficial for women who take oral contraceptives because it promotes the excretion of estrogen. It reduces the level of histamine in the body, which can be useful for people with schizophrenia, whose histamine levels are typically higher than normal.

As levels of toxic substances in the body increase, the need for methionine increases. The body can convert methionine into the amino acid cysteine, a precursor of glutathione. Methionine thus protects glutathione; it helps to prevent glutathione depletion if the body is overloaded with toxins. Since glutathione is a key neutralizer of toxins in the liver, this protects the liver from the damaging effects of toxic compounds.

An essential amino acid, methionine is not synthesized in the body, and so must be obtained from food sources or from dietary supplements. Good food sources of methionine include beans, eggs, fish, garlic, lentils, meat, onions, soybeans, seeds, and yogurt. Because the body uses methionine to derive a brain food called choline, it is wise to supplement the diet with choline or lecithin (which is high in choline) to ensure that the supply of methionine is not depleted.

Ornithine

Ornithine helps to prompt the release of growth hormone, which promotes the metabolism of excess body fat. This effect is enhanced if ornithine is combined with arginine and carnitine. Ornithine is necessary for proper immune system and liver function. This amino acid also detoxifies ammonia and aids in liver regeneration. High concentrations of ornithine are found in the skin and connective tissue, making it useful for promoting healing and repairing damaged tissues.

Ornithine is synthesized in the body from arginine, and in turn serves as the precursor of citrulline, proline, and glutamic acid. Supplemental L-ornithine should *not* be taken by children, pregnant women, nursing mothers, or anyone with a history of schizophrenia, unless they are specifically directed to do so by a physician.

Phenylalanine

Phenylalanine is an essential amino acid. Once in the body, it can be converted into another amino acid, tyrosine, which in turn is used to synthesize two key neurotransmitters that promote alertness: dopamine and norepinephrine. Because of its relationship to the action of the central nervous system, this amino acid can elevate mood, decrease pain, aid in memory and learning, and suppress the appetite. It can be used to treat arthritis, depression, menstrual cramps, migraines, obesity, Parkinson's disease, and schizophrenia.

Phenylalanine is available in three different forms, designated L-, D-, and DL-. The L- form is the most common type, and is the form in which phenylalanine is incorporated into the body's proteins. The D- type acts as a painkiller. The DL-form is a combination of the D- and the L-. Like the D- form, it is effective for controlling pain, especially the pain of arthritis; like the L- form, it functions as a building block for proteins, increases mental alertness, suppresses the appetite, and helps people with Parkinson's disease. It has been used to alleviate the symptoms of premenstrual syndrome (PMS) and various types of chronic pain.

Supplemental phenylalanine should *not* be taken by pregnant women or by people who suffer from anxiety attacks, diabetes, high blood pressure, phenylketonuria (PKU), or preexisting pigmented melanoma, a type of skin cancer.

Proline

Proline improves skin texture by aiding in the production of collagen and reducing the loss of collagen through the aging process. It also helps in the healing of cartilage and the strengthening of joints, tendons, and heart muscle. It works with vitamin C to promote healthy connective tissue. Proline is obtained primarily from meat sources.

Serine

Serine is needed for the proper metabolism of fats and fatty acids, the growth of muscle, and the maintenance of a healthy immune system. It aids in the production of immunoglobulins and antibodies. Serine can be synthesized from glycine

in the body. It is included as a natural moisturizing agent in many cosmetics and skin care preparations.

Taurine

High concentrations of taurine are found in the heart muscle, white blood cells, skeletal muscle, and central nervous system. It is a building block of all the other amino acids as well as a key component of bile, which is needed for the digestion of fats, the absorption of fat-soluble vitamins, and the control of serum cholesterol levels. Taurine can be useful for people with atherosclerosis, edema, heart disorders, hypertension, or hypoglycemia. It is vital for the proper utilization of sodium, potassium, calcium, and magnesium, and it has been shown to play a particular role in sparing the loss of potassium from the heart muscle. This helps to prevent the development of potentially dangerous cardiac arrhythmias.

Taurine has a protective effect on the brain, particularly when the brain is dehydrated. It is used to treat anxiety, epilepsy, hyperactivity, poor brain function, and seizures. Taurine is found in concentrations up to four times greater in the brains of children than in those of adults. It may be that a deficiency of taurine in the developing brain is involved in epileptic attacks. Zinc deficiency also is commonly found in people with epilepsy, and this may play a part in the deficiency of taurine. Taurine is also associated with zinc in maintaining eye function; a deficiency of both may impair vision. Taurine supplementation may benefit children with Down syndrome and muscular dystrophy. This amino acid is also used in some clinics for breast cancer treatment.

Excessive losses of taurine through the urine can be caused by many metabolic disorders. Cardiac arrhythmias, disorders of platelet formation, intestinal problems, an overgrowth of candida, physical or emotional stress, a zinc deficiency, and excessive consumption of alcohol are all associated with high urinary losses of taurine. Excessive alcohol consumption also causes the body to lose its ability to utilize taurine properly. Diabetes increases the body's requirements for taurine; conversely, supplementation with taurine and cystine may decrease the need for insulin.

Taurine is found in eggs, fish, meat, and milk, but not in vegetable proteins. It can be synthesized from cysteine in the liver and from methionine elsewhere in the body, as long as sufficient quantities of vitamin B6 are present. For vegetarians, synthesis by the body is crucial. For individuals with genetic or metabolic disorders that prevent the synthesis of taurine, taurine supplementation is required.

Threonine

Threonine is an essential amino acid that helps to maintain the proper protein balance in the body. It is important for the formation of collagen and elastin, and aids liver and lipotropic function when combined with aspartic acid and methionine. Threonine is present in the heart, central nervous system, and skeletal muscle, and helps to prevent fatty buildup in the liver. It enhances the immune system by aiding in the production of antibodies.

Because the threonine content of grains is low, vegetarians are more likely than others to have deficiencies.

Tryptophan

Tryptophan is an essential amino acid that is necessary for the production of vitamin B_3 (niacin). It is used by the brain to produce serotonin, a necessary neurotransmitter that transfers nerve impulses from one cell to another and is responsible for normal sleep. Consequently, tryptophan helps to combat depression and insomnia and to stabilize moods. It helps to control hyperactivity in children, alleviates stress, is good for the heart, aids in weight control by reducing appetite, and enhances the release of growth hormone. It is good for migraine headaches, and may reduce some of the effects of nicotine. A sufficient amount of vitamin B_6 (pyridoxine) is necessary for the formation of tryptophan, which, in turn, is required for the formation of serotonin. A lack of tryptophan and magnesium may contribute to coronary artery spasms.

The best dietary sources of tryptophan include brown rice, cottage cheese, meat, peanuts, and soy protein. This amino acid is not available in supplement form in the United States. In November of 1989, the U.S. Centers for Disease Control (CDC) reported evidence linking L-tryptophan supplements to a blood disorder called eosinophilia-myalgia syndrome (EMS). Several hundred cases of this illness—which is characterized by an elevated white blood cell count and can also cause such symptoms as fatigue, muscular pain, respiratory ailments, edema, and rash—were reported, and at least one death was attributed to the outbreak. After the CDC established an association between the blood disorder and products containing L-tryptophan in New Mexico, the U.S. Food and Drug Administration first warned consumers to stop taking L-tryptophan supplements, then recalled all products in which L-tryptophan was the sole or a major component. Subsequent research showed that it was contaminants in the supplements, *not* the tryptophan, that was probably responsible for the problem, but tryptophan supplements are still banned from the market in the United States.

Tyrosine

Tyrosine is a precursor of the neurotransmitters norepinephrine and dopamine, which regulate mood, among other things. Tyrosine acts as a mood elevator; a lack of adequate amounts of tyrosine leads to a deficiency of norepinephrine in the brain, which in turn can result in depression. It suppresses the appetite and helps to reduce body fat. It aids in the production of melanin (the pigment responsible for skin and hair color) and in the functions of the adrenal, thyroid, and pituitary glands. It is also involved in the metabolism of the amino acid phenylalanine.

Tyrosine attaches to iodine atoms to form active thyroid hormones. Not surprisingly, therefore, low plasma levels of tyrosine have been associated with hypothyroidism. Symptoms of tyrosine deficiency can also include low blood pressure, low body temperature (such as cold hands and feet), and restless leg syndrome.

Supplemental L-tyrosine has been used for stress reduction, and research suggests it may be helpful against chronic fatigue and narcolepsy. It has been used to help individuals suffering from anxiety, depression, allergies, and headaches, as well as persons undergoing withdrawal from drugs. It may also help people with Parkinson's disease.

Natural sources of tyrosine include almonds, avocados, bananas, dairy products, lima beans, pumpkin seeds, and sesame seeds. Tyrosine can be also be produced from phenylalanine in the body. Supplements of L-tyrosine should be taken at bedtime or with a high-carbohydrate meal so that it does not have to compete for absorption with other amino acids.

Persons taking monoamine oxidase (MAO) inhibitors, commonly prescribed for depression, must strictly limit their intake of foods containing tyrosine and should *not* take any supplements containing L-tyrosine, as it may lead to a sudden and dangerous rise in blood pressure. Anyone who takes prescription medication for depression should discuss necessary dietary restrictions with his or her physician.

Valine

Valine, an essential amino acid, has a stimulant effect. It is needed for muscle metabolism, tissue repair, and the maintenance of a proper nitrogen balance in the body. Valine is found in high concentrations in muscle tissue. It is one of the branched-chain amino acids, which means that it can be used as an energy source by muscle tissue. It is good for correcting the type of severe amino acid deficiencies that can be caused by drug addiction. An excessively high level of valine may lead to such symptoms as a crawling sensation in the skin and even hallucinations.

Dietary sources of valine include dairy products, grains, meat, mushrooms, peanuts, and soy protein. Supplemental L-valine should always be taken in balance with the other branched-chain amino acids, L-isoleucine and L-leucine (*see* Isoleucine in this section).

ANTIOXIDANTS

INTRODUCTION

There is a group of vitamins, minerals, and enzymes called *antioxidants* that help to protect the body from the formation of free radicals. *Free radicals* are atoms or groups of atoms that can cause damage to cells, impairing the immune system and leading to infections and various degenerative diseases such as heart disease and cancer. Free radical damage is thought by scientists to be the basis for the aging process as well. (*See* Free Radicals on page 44.)

There are a number of known free radicals that occur in the body, including superoxide, hydroxy radicals, hydrogen peroxide, various lipid peroxides, hypochlorite radicals, nitric oxide, and singlet oxygen. They may be formed by exposure to radiation and toxic chemicals such as those found in cigarette smoke, overexposure to the sun's rays, or various metabolic processes, such as the process of breaking down stored fat molecules for use as an energy source.

Free radicals are normally kept in check by the action of *free radical scavengers* that occur naturally in the body. These scavengers neutralize the free radicals. Certain enzymes serve this vital function. Four important enzymes that neutralize free radicals are superoxide dismutase (SOD), methionine reductase, catalase, and glutathione peroxidase. The body makes these as a matter of course. There are also a number of nutrients that act as antioxidants, including vitamin A, beta-carotene, vitamins C and E, and the mineral selenium. Another antioxidant is the hormone melatonin, which is a powerful free radical neutralizer. Certain herbs have antioxidant properties as well.

Although many antioxidants can be obtained from food sources such as sprouted grains and fresh fruits and vegetables, it is difficult to get enough of them from these sources to hold back the free radicals constantly being generated in our polluted environment. We can minimize free radical damage by taking supplements of key nutrients. A high intake of antioxidant nutrients appears to be especially protective against cancer.

THE ANTIOXIDANTS

Alpha-Lipoic Acid

Alpha-lipoic acid helps to neutralize the effects of free radicals on the body by enhancing the antioxidant functions of vitamin C, vitamin E, and glutathione. An additional benefit of this nutrient is that it assures the proper functioning of two key enzymes that convert food into energy.

Bilberry

The herb bilberry is a strong antioxidant that keeps capillary walls strong and flexible. It also helps to maintain the flexibility of the walls of red blood cells and allows them to pass through the capillaries better. In addition, this herb supports and strengthens collagen structures, inhibits the growth of bacteria, acts as an anti-inflammatory, and has anti-aging and anticarcinogenic effects.

Coenzyme Q10

Coenzyme Q_{10} is an antioxidant similar to vitamin E. It also plays a crucial role in the generation of cellular energy, is a significant immunologic stimulant, increases circulation, has anti-aging effects, and is beneficial for the cardiovascular system.

Cysteine

This sulfur-containing amino acid is needed to produce the free radical fighter glutathione. It is used by the liver and the lymphocytes to detoxify chemicals and other poisons. Cysteine is a powerful detoxifier of alcohol, tobacco smoke, and environmental pollutants, all of which are immune suppressors. Taking supplemental L-cysteine can boost the levels of protective enzymes in the body, thus slowing some of the cellular damage that is characteristic of aging.

Ginkgo Biloba

Ginkgo biloba is a powerful antioxidant herb that is best known for its ability to enhance circulation. It has the ability to squeeze through even the narrowest of blood vessels to increase the supply of oxygen to the heart, brain, and all other body parts. This aids in mental functioning (ginkgo biloba is known as the "smart herb") and helps to relieve muscle pain. Ginkgo biloba also lowers blood pressure, inhibits blood clotting, and has anti-aging properties.

Glutathione

Glutathione is a protein that is produced in the liver from the amino acids cysteine, glutamic acid, and glycine. It is a powerful antioxidant that inhibits the formation of, and protects against cellular damage from, free radicals. It helps to defend the body against damage from cigarette smoking,

Free Radicals

A free radical is an atom or group of atoms that contains at least one unpaired electron. Electrons are negatively charged particles that usually occur in pairs, forming a chemically stable arrangement. If an electron is unpaired, another atom or molecule can easily bond with it, causing a chemical reaction. Because they join so readily with other compounds, free radicals can effect dramatic changes in the body, and they can cause a lot of damage. Each free radical may exist for only a tiny fraction of a second, but the damage it leaves behind can be irreversible.

Free radicals are normally present in the body in small numbers. Biochemical processes naturally lead to the formation of free radicals, and under normal circumstances the body can keep them in check. Indeed, not all free radicals are bad. Free radicals produced by the immune system destroy viruses and bacteria. Other free radicals are involved in producing vital hormones and activating enzymes that are needed for life. We need free radicals to produce energy and various substances that the body requires. If there is excessive free radical formation, however, damage to cells and tissues can occur. The formation of a large number of free radicals stimulates the formation of more free radicals, leading to even more damage.

The presence of a dangerous number of free radicals can alter the way in which the cells code genetic material. Changes in protein structure can occur as a result of errors in protein synthesis. The body's immune system may then see this altered protein as a foreign substance and try to destroy it. The formation of mutated proteins can eventually damage the immune system and lead to

leukemia and other types of cancer, as well as a host of other diseases.

In addition to damaging genetic material, free radicals can destroy the protective cell membranes. The formation of free radicals can also lead to retention of fluid in the cells, which is involved in the aging process. Calcium levels in the body may be upset as well.

Many different factors can lead to the production of free radicals. Exposure to radiation, whether from the sun or from medical x-rays, activates the formation of free radicals, as does exposure to environmental pollutants such as tobacco smoke and automobile exhaust. Diet also can contribute to the formation of free radicals. When the body obtains nutrients through the diet, it utilizes oxygen and these nutrients to create energy. In this oxidation process, oxygen molecules containing unpaired electrons are released. These oxygen free radicals can cause damage to the body if produced in extremely large amounts. A diet that is high in fat can increase free radical activity because oxidation occurs more readily in fat molecules than it does in carbohydrate or protein molecules. Cooking fats at high temperatures, particularly frying foods in oil, can produce large numbers of free radicals.

Substances known as antioxidants neutralize free radicals by binding to their free electrons. Antioxidants available in supplement form include the enzymes superoxide dismutase and glutathione peroxidase; vitamin A, beta-carotene, and vitamins C and E; the trace mineral selenium; and the hormone melatonin. By destroying free radicals, antioxidants help to detoxify and protect the body.

---

exposure to radiation, cancer chemotherapy, and toxins such as alcohol. As a detoxifier of heavy metals and drugs, it aids in the treatment of blood and liver disorders.

Glutathione protects cells in several ways. It neutralizes oxygen molecules before they can harm cells. Together with selenium, it forms the enzyme glutathione peroxidase, which neutralizes hydrogen peroxide. It is also a component of another antioxidant enzyme, glutathione-S-transferase, which is a broad-spectrum liver-detoxifying enzyme.

Glutathione protects not only individual cells but also the tissues of the arteries, brain, heart, immune cells, kidneys, lenses of the eyes, liver, lungs, and skin against oxidant damage. It plays a role in preventing cancer, especially liver cancer, and may also have an anti-aging effect. Glutathione can be taken in supplement form. The production of glutathione by the body can be boosted by taking supplemental N-acetylcysteine or L-cysteine plus L-methionine. Studies suggest that this may be a better way or raising glutathione levels than taking glutathione itself.

Grape Seed Extract

See under Oligomeric Proanthocyanidins in this section.

Green Tea

Green tea contains numerous compounds, including the flavonoid catechin, that have antioxidant and health-enhancing properties. It protects against cancer, lowers cholesterol levels, and reduces the clotting tendency of the blood. It also shows promise as a weight-loss aid that can promote the burning of fat and help to regulate blood sugar and insulin levels. Black tea is not effective for these purposes because valuable compounds are destroyed in processing.

Melatonin

Among the newest antioxidants to be discovered, the hormone melatonin may also be the most efficient free radical scavenger that has thus far been identified. While most antioxidants work only in certain parts of certain cells, melatonin can permeate any cell in any part of the body. In animal experiments, it has been shown to protect tissues from an amazing array of assaults. Within the cell, melatonin provides special protection for the nucleus— the central structure that contains the DNA. Thus, it protects the structure that enables a damaged cell to repair itself. Melatonin also stimulates the enzyme glutathione peroxidase, another antioxidant.

Oligomeric Proanthocyanidins

Oligomeric proanthocyanidins (OPCs) are naturally occurring substances present in a variety of food and botanical sources. They are unique flavonols that have powerful antioxidant capabilities and excellent bioavailability. Clinical tests suggest that OPCs may be as much as fifty times more potent than vitamin E and twenty times more potent than vitamin C in terms of bioavailable antioxidant activity. In addition to their antioxidant activity, they strengthen and repair connective tissue, including that of the cardiovascular system, and they moderate allergic and inflammatory responses by reducing histamine production.

OPCs are found throughout plant life, however, the two main sources are pine bark extract (Pycnogenol) and grape seed extract. Pycnogenol was the first source of OPCs discovered, and the process for extracting it was patented in the 1950s. As a result, even though Pycnogenol is a trademarked name for pine bark extract, the term is often used informally to refer to other OPC sources as well, most notably grape seed extract.

Pycnogenol

See under Oligomeric Proanthocyanidins in this section.

Selenium

A partner and synergist with vitamin E, selenium is also an essential component of the antioxidant enzyme glutathione peroxidase (each molecule of this enzyme contains four atoms of selenium). This enzyme targets harmful hydrogen peroxide in the body and converts it into water. It is a particularly important guardian of blood cells and of the heart, liver, and lungs. Selenium also stimulates increased antibody response to infection.

Superoxide Dismutase

Superoxide dismutase (SOD) is an enzyme. SOD revitalizes cells and reduces the rate of cell destruction. It neutralizes the most common, and possibly the most dangerous, free radical—superoxide. It also aids in the body's utilization of zinc, copper, and manganese. SOD levels tend to decline with age, while free radical production increases. Its potential as an anti-aging treatment is currently being explored.

There are two types of SOD: copper/zinc SOD (Cu/Zn SOD) and manganese SOD (Mn SOD). Each of these enzymes works to protect a particular part of the cell. Cu/Zn SOD protects the cytoplasm, where free radicals are produced as a result of various metabolic activities. Mn SOD is active in protecting the mitochondria of the cells, which contain the cells' genetic information and act as the site of cellular energy production.

SOD occurs naturally in barley grass, broccoli, Brussels sprouts, cabbage, wheatgrass, and most green plants. It is also available in supplement form. SOD supplements in pill form must be enteric coated—that is, coated with a protective substance that allows the pill to pass intact through the stomach acid into the small intestines to be absorbed. Cell Guard from Biotec Food Corporation is a good source of SOD.

Vitamin A and Beta-Carotene

Vitamin A and its precursor, beta-carotene, are powerful free radical scavengers. Vitamin A also is necessary for healthy skin and mucous membranes, the body's first line of defense against invading microorganisms and toxins, and promotes the immune response. Beta-carotene and vitamin A destroy carcinogens (cancer-causing substances), guard against heart disease and stroke, and lower cholesterol levels.

Vitamin C

Vitamin C is a very powerful antioxidant that also protects other antioxidants, such as vitamin E. The cells of the brain and spinal cord, which frequently incur free radical damage, can be protected by significant amounts of vitamin C. Vitamin C acts as a more potent free radical scavenger in the presence of a bioflavonoid called hesperidin.

In addition to its role as an antioxidant, vitamin C detoxifies many harmful substances and plays a key role in immunity. It increases the synthesis of interferon, a natural antiviral substance produced by the body, and stimulates the activity of certain key immune cells.

Vitamin E

Vitamin E is a powerful antioxidant that prevents the oxidation of lipids. Since cell membranes are composed of lipids, it effectively prevents the cells' protective coatings from becoming rancid as a result of the assault of free radicals. Vitamin E also improves oxygen utilization, enhances immune response, plays a role in the prevention of cataracts caused by free radical damage, and may reduce the risk of coronary artery disease. New evidence suggests that zinc is needed to maintain normal blood concentrations of vitamin E.

Selenium enhances vitamin E uptake. These two nutrients should be taken together.

Zinc

In addition to having antioxidant properties on its own, zinc is a constituent of the antioxidant enzyme superoxide dismutase (SOD). It is also needed for proper maintenance of vitamin E levels in the blood and aids in the absorption of vitamin A. Other important functions of this mineral include the promotion of glandular and reproductive health and proper functioning of the immune system.

Combination Antioxidant Supplements

There are also products available that combine two or more of these vital nutrients. It is now easy to find formulas that give you a balance of multiple antioxidants. Some recommended antioxidant combination products include the following:

• ACES + Zinc and ACES + Selenium from Carlson Laboratories.

• Advanced Carotenoid Complex from Solgar.

• Body Language Super Antioxidant from OxyFresh USA.

• Cell Guard from Biotec Food Corporation.

• Juice Plus from Kelco.

• Life Guard from Thompson Nutritional Products.

• Oxy-5000 Forte from American Biologics

    Using a combination supplement is often more convenient than taking many different products separately.

ENZYMES

WHAT ARE ENZYMES?

The late Dr. Edward Howell, a physician and pioneer in enzyme research, called enzymes the "sparks of life." These energized protein molecules play a necessary role in virtually all of the biochemical activities that go on in the body. They are essential for digesting food, for stimulating the brain, for providing cellular energy, and for repairing all tissues, organs, and cells. Life as we know it could not exist without the action of enzymes, even in the presence of sufficient amounts of vitamins, minerals, water, and other nutrients.

In their primary role, enzymes are catalysts—substances that accelerate and precipitate the hundreds of thousands of biochemical reactions in the body that control life's processes. If it were not for the catalytic action of enzymes, most of these reactions would take place far too slowly to sustain life. Enzymes are not consumed in the reactions they facilitate.

Each enzyme has a specific function in the body that no other enzyme can fulfill. The chemical shape of each enzyme is specialized so that it can initiate a reaction only in a certain substance, or in a group of closely related chemical substances, and not in others. The substance on which an enzyme acts is called the substrate. Because there must be a different enzyme for every substrate, the body must produce a great number of different enzymes.

THE FUNCTIONS OF ENZYMES

Enzymes assist in practically all bodily functions. Digestive enzymes break down food particles for storage in the liver or muscles. This stored energy is later converted by other enzymes for use by the body when necessary. Iron is concentrated in the blood by the action of enzymes; other enzymes in the blood help the blood to coagulate in order to stop bleeding. Uricolytic enzymes catalyze the conversion of uric acid into urea. Respiratory enzymes facilitate the elimination of carbon dioxide from the lungs. Enzymes assist the kidneys, liver, lungs, colon, and skin in removing wastes and toxins from the body. Enzymes also utilize the nutrients ingested by the body to construct new muscle tissue, nerve cells, bone, skin, and glandular tissue. One enzyme can take dietary phosphorus and convert it into bone. Enzymes prompt the oxidation of glucose, which creates energy for the cells. Enzymes also protect the blood from dangerous waste materials by converting these sub-

stances to forms that are easily eliminated by the body. Indeed, the functions of enzymes are so many and so diverse that it would be impossible to name them all.

Enzymes are often divided into two groups: digestive enzymes and metabolic enzymes. Digestive enzymes are secreted along the gastrointestinal tract and break down foods, enabling the nutrients to be absorbed into the bloodstream for use in various bodily functions. There are three main categories of digestive enzymes: amylase, protease, and lipase. Amylase, found in saliva and in the pancreatic and intestinal juices, breaks down carbohydrates. Different types of amylase break down specific types of sugars. For example, lactase breaks down milk sugar (lactose), maltase breaks down malt sugar (maltose), and sucrase breaks down cane and beet sugar (sucrose). Protease, found in the stomach juices and also in the pancreatic and intestinal juices, helps to digest protein. Lipase, found in the stomach and pancreatic juices, and also present in fats in foods, aids in fat digestion.

Metabolic enzymes are those enzymes that catalyze the various chemical reactions within the cells, such as energy production and detoxification. All of the body's organs, tissues, and cells are run by the metabolic enzymes. They are the workers that build the body from proteins, carbohydrates and fats. Metabolic enzymes are found in the blood, organs, and tissues doing their specific work. Each body tissue has its own specific set of metabolic enzymes.

Two particularly important metabolic enzymes are superoxide dismutase (SOD) and its partner, catalase. SOD is an antioxidant that protects the cells by attacking a common free radical, superoxide. (*See* Superoxide Dismutase *under* ANTIOXIDANTS in Part One.) Catalase breaks down hydrogen peroxide, a metabolic waste product, and liberates oxygen for the body to use.

FOOD ENZYMES

While the body manufactures a supply of enzymes, it can also obtain enzymes from food. Unfortunately, enzymes are extremely sensitive to heat. Even low to moderate heat (118°F or above) destroys most enzymes in food, so to obtain enzymes from the diet, one must eat raw foods. Eating raw foods or, alternatively, taking enzyme supplements, helps prevent depletion of the body's own enzymes and thus reduce the stress on the body.

Enzymes can be found in many different foods, from both plant and animal sources. Avocados, papayas, pineapples, bananas, and mangos are all high in enzymes. Sprouts are the richest source. Unripe papaya and pineapple are excellent sources of enzymes. The enzymes extracted from papaya and pineapple—papain and bromelain, respectively—are proteolytic enzymes.

Many fat-containing foods also supply lipase, which breaks down fats. In fact, fat in food exposed only to pancreatic lipase (the lipase produced by the body) in the intestines is not as well digested as fat that is first worked on in the stomach by food lipase. Pancreatic lipase digests fat in a highly alkaline environment (the intestines), whereas lipase found in food fats works in a more acidic environment (the stomach). The optimal extraction of nutrients from fats depends on the work of different fat-digesting enzymes in successive stages.

Superoxide dismutase occurs naturally in a variety of food sources, including barley grass, broccoli, Brussels sprouts, cabbage, wheatgrass, and most green plants.

COMMERCIALLY AVAILABLE ENZYMES

The majority of commercially available enzymes are digestive enzymes extracted from various sources. (Scientists are unable to manufacture enzymes synthetically.) Most commercial enzyme products are made from animal enzymes, such as pancreatin and pepsin, which help in the digestion of food once it has reached the lower stomach and the intestinal tract. Some companies make their supplements from enzymes extracted from aspergillus, a type of fungus. These enzymes begin their predigestive work in the upper stomach. All of these products are used primarily to aid the digestion of foods and absorption of nutrients, especially protein.

Proteolytic enzymes available in supplement form include pepsin, trypsin, rennin, pancreatin, and chymotrypsin. In addition to aiding digestion, proteolytic enzymes have been shown to be beneficial as anti-inflammatory agents. Pancreatin, derived from secretions of animal pancreas, is a focus of cancer research, because people with cancer are often deficient in this enzyme. Pancreatin is used in the treatment of pancreatic insufficiency, cystic fibrosis, digestive problems, food allergies, autoimmune disorders, viral infections, and sports injuries.

Also available in supplement form are the antioxidant enzymes superoxide dismutase (SOD) and catalase.

WHAT'S ON THE SHELVES

Enzymes are available over the counter in tablet, capsule, powder, and liquid forms. They may be sold in combination with each other or as separate items. Some enzyme products also contain garlic to help digestion.

For maximum benefit, any digestive enzyme supplement you choose should contain all of the major enzyme groups—amylase, protease, and lipase. Digestive enzymes should be taken after meals, unless you are eating processed and/or cooked foods, in which case it is best to take them during the meal. You can make your own digestive enzymes by drying papaya seeds, placing them in a pepper grinder, and sprinkling them on your foods. These have a peppery taste.

If you take supplemental superoxide dismutase, make sure to choose a product that is enteric coated—that is, coated with a protective substance that allows the SOD to pass intact through the stomach acid to be absorbed in the small intestine.

All forms of enzymes should be kept in a reasonably cool place to insure potency. Tablets and liquids can be stored in the refrigerator. However, powder and capsule forms should not be refrigerated because they are susceptible to moisture; they should be stored in a cool, dry place.

Research has shown that as we grow older, the body's ability to produce enzymes decreases. At the same time, malabsorption of nutrients, tissue breakdown, and chronic health conditions increase. Taking supplemental enzymes can help to ensure that you continue to get the full nutritional value from your foods. We believe that enzyme supplementation is vital for elderly persons.

The following are recommended enzyme complex products:

• *Infla-Zyme Forte from American Biologics.* This formula is a combination of enzymes and antioxidants for people requiring supplemental digestive enzymes to aid in the breakdown of proteins, fats, and carbohydrates. It may also be helpful for chronic or acute inflammation. Its ingredients include amylase, bromelain, catalase, chymotrypsin, L-cysteine, lipase, pancreatin, papain, rutin, superoxide dismutase, trypsin, and zinc. If taken as a digestive aid, the recommended dosage is 1 to 3 tablets following each meal; if you use it for other purposes, take 3 to 6 tablets one hour before each meal. Infla-Zyme Forte may be taken by persons on sodium-restricted diets.

• *Wobenzym N from Marlyn Nutraceuticals.* Wobenzym N contains a combination of enzymes designed to interact synergistically with each other. Its ingredients include bromelain, chymotrypsin, pancreatin, papain, rutosid, and trypsin.

Other sources for quality enzyme products include Prevail Corporation and National Enzyme Company. Both of these companies sell enzyme products derived from aspergillus that contain amylase, cellulase, lactase, lipase, maltase, protease, and sucrase.

NATURAL FOOD SUPPLEMENTS

INTRODUCTION

Natural food supplements include a wide variety of products. Almost all health food stores carry them, and a number of enlightened drug stores and supermarkets stock them on their shelves as well. In general, natural food supplements are composed of, derived from, or byproducts of foods that provide a multitude of health benefits. In some cases, health benefit claims made by manufacturers are based upon a supplement's use in traditional healing; in other cases, they are based on modern research and development.

Food supplements can be high in certain nutrients, contain active ingredients that aid digestive or metabolic processes, or provide a combination of nutrients and active ingredients. It is important to point out that some unscrupulous manufacturers make false promises. It is therefore vital to be an informed consumer. It is also necessary to be aware that many conservative "watchdog" organizations point to these few unsubstantiated products and label the whole industry as unreliable. This occurs in spite of the fact that many natural food supplements have been known to work for years; these products are only medically endorsed when they are "discovered" by researchers deemed acceptable by these groups. Such recent discoveries include garlic, aloe vera, fiber, fish oils, and bran—substances that have been used for centuries in many parts of the world.

WHAT'S ON THE SHELVES

Food supplements come in every shape and form—tablets, capsules, powders, liquids, jellies, creams, biscuits, wafers, granules, and more. Product packaging depends entirely on the nature of the food supplement's composition. The potency of these products varies. Because they are made up of perishable foods, food derivatives, or food byproducts, their potency may be affected by the length of time they sit on a shelf, or the temperature at which they are kept. If you don't understand how a product is to be used, ask questions or read the available literature on the particular supplement.

If you have never used a natural food supplement, you may be uncomfortable about buying and using one for the first time. This is normal. Keep in mind that once you become familiar with its use and benefits, you won't give the idea of using it a second thought.

The following are some of the food supplements that have been recommended for use in dealing with the various disorders discussed in Part Two of this book.

Acidophilus

See Lactobacillus Acidophilus in this section.

Alfalfa

One of the most mineral-rich foods known, alfalfa has roots that grow as much as 130 feet into the earth. Alfalfa is available in liquid extract form and is good to use while fasting because of its chlorophyll and nutrient content. It contains calcium, magnesium, phosphorus, potassium, plus all known vitamins. The minerals are in a balanced form, which promotes absorption. These minerals are alkaline, but have a neutralizing effect on the intestinal tract.

If you need a mineral supplement, alfalfa is a good choice. It has helped many arthritis sufferers. Alfalfa, wheatgrass, barley, and spirulina, all of which contain chlorophyll, have been found to aid in the healing of intestinal ulcers, gastritis, liver disorders, eczema, hemorrhoids, asthma, high blood pressure, anemia, constipation, body and breath odor, bleeding gums, infections, burns, athlete's foot, and cancer.

Aloe Vera

This plant is known for its healing effect and is used in many cosmetic and hair products. There are over 200 different species of aloe that grow around the world in dry regions.

Aloe vera is commonly known as a skin healer, moisturizer, and softener. It is dramatically effective on burns of all types, and is also good for cuts, insect stings, bruises, acne and blemishes, poison ivy, welts, skin ulcers, and eczema. Taken internally, 98- or 99-percent pure aloe vera is known to aid in the healing of stomach disorders, ulcers, constipation, hemorrhoids, rectal itching, colitis, and all colon problems. It can also be helpful against infections, varicose veins, skin cancer, and arthritis, and is used in the treatment of AIDS.

We have had excellent results using colon cleansers containing psyllium husks in combination with aloe vera juice. George's Aloe Vera Juice from Warren Laboratories is good, as it needs no refrigeration and tastes like plain water. We have found this combination to be good for food allergy and colon disorder sufferers. Psyllium keeps the folds and pockets in the colon free of toxic material that gathers there. The aloe vera not only has a healing effect, but if constipation or diarrhea is present, it will return the stools to normal. It takes a few weeks to cleanse the colon, but regular, periodic use will keep the colon clean. As with any substance, it is possible to develop an intolerance to aloe vera juice and/or psyllium husks, so this treatment should not be used on an ongoing basis.

Barley Grass

Barley grass is high in calcium, iron, all the essential amino acids, chlorophyll, flavonoids, vitamin B$_{12}$, vitamin C, and many minerals, plus enzymes. This food heals stomach, duodenal, and colon disorders as well as pancreatitis, and is an effective anti-inflammatory.

Bee Byproducts

See Bee Pollen, Bee Propolis, Honey, and Royal Jelly, all in this section.

Bee Pollen

Bee pollen is a powderlike material that is produced by the anthers of flowering plants and gathered by bees. It is composed of 10 to 15 percent protein and also contains B-complex vitamins, vitamin C, amino acids, essential fatty acids, enzymes, carotene, calcium, copper, iron, magnesium, potassium, manganese, sodium, plant sterols, and simple sugars.

Like other bee products, bee pollen has an antimicrobial effect. In addition, it is useful for combating fatigue, depression, cancer, and colon disorders. It is also helpful for people with allergies because it strengthens the immune system.

It is best to obtain bee pollen from a local source, as this increases its antiallergenic properties. Fresh bee pollen should not cling together or form clumps, and it should be sold in a tightly sealed container. Some people (an estimated 0.05 percent of the population) may be allergic to bee pollen. It is best to try taking a small amount at first and watch for a developing rash, wheezing, discomfort, or any other signs of a reaction. If such symptoms occur, discontinue taking bee pollen.

Bee Propolis

Bee propolis is a resinous substance collected from various plants by bees. Bees use propolis, together with beeswax, in the construction of hives. As a supplement, it is an excellent aid against bacterial infections. Bee propolis is believed to stimulate phagocytosis, the means by which white blood cells destroy bacteria.

Propolis is beneficial used as a salve for abrasions and bruises because of its antibacterial effect. Good results have been reported on the use of propolis against inflam-

mation of the mucous membranes of the mouth and throat, dry cough and throat, halitosis, tonsillitis, ulcers, and acne, and for the stimulation of the immune system.

Be sure that any bee products you use smell and taste fresh. All bee products should be in tightly sealed containers. It is best to purchase these products from a manufacturer who specializes in bee products. If you are using bee products for allergies, it is best to obtain products that are produced within a ten-mile radius of your home. This way, you get a minute dose of pollen to desensitize you to the local pollen in the area.

Brewer's Yeast

See Yeast in this section.

Bifidus

See Lactobacillus Bifidus in this section.

Bovine Cartilage

Cleaned, dried, and powdered bovine cartilage is a supplement that helps accelerate wound healing and reduce inflammation. Like shark cartilage, it has been shown to be helpful for psoriasis, rheumatoid arthritis, and ulcerative colitis. VitaCarte from Phoenix BioLabs contains pure bovine cartilage from range-raised, hormone-free cattle.

Cellulose

See under Fiber in this section.

Chlorella

Chlorella is a tiny, single-celled water-grown alga containing a nucleus and an enormous amount of readily available chlorophyll. It also contains protein (approximately 58 percent), carbohydrates, all of the B vitamins, vitamins C and E, amino acids, and rare trace minerals. In fact, it is virtually a complete food. It contains more vitamin B$_{12}$ than liver does, plus a considerable amount of beta-carotene. It has a strong cell wall, however, which makes it difficult to gain access to its nutrients. Consequently, it requires factory processing to be effective.

Chlorella is one of the few edible species of water-grown algae. The chlorophyll in chlorella can help speed the cleansing of the bloodstream. Chlorella is very high in RNA and DNA, and has been found to protect against the effects of ultraviolet radiation. Studies show that chlorella is an excellent source of protein, especially for people who cannot or who choose not to eat meat.

Chlorophyll

See Chlorella and "Green Drinks" in this section.

Citrin

Citrin is a trademarked name for a standardized herbal extract from the fruit of the *Garcinia cambogia* plant, also known as Indian berry. It inhibits the synthesis of fatty acids in the liver, promotes the burning of body fat as fuel, and suppresses the appetite. Its primary usefulness is in treating obesity, although it may also aid in preventing or slowing atherosclerosis and heart disease. It does not affect the nervous system or cause any known side effects. Citrin is an ingredient in a number of different products sold by various manufacturers.

Corn Germ

Corn germ is made by a process that isolates the embryo of the corn plant, which contains the most usable nutrients. Corn germ has a longer shelf life than wheat germ and is higher in some nutrients, especially zinc. Corn germ contains ten times the amount of zinc found in wheat germ. You can use corn germ to bread chicken or fish. It is also good when added to cereals and used as a topping.

Desiccated Liver

Desiccated liver is concentrated dried liver that is put into powdered or tablet form. This form of liver contains vitamins A, D, and C; the B-complex vitamins; and the minerals calcium, copper, phosphorus, and iron. Desiccated liver is good for anemia and aids in building healthy red blood cells. It is known to increase energy, aid in liver disorders, and help relieve stress in the body. Use only a product made from liver derived from beef that is raised organically.

Dimethylsulfoxide (DMSO)

Dimethylsulfoxide (DMSO) is a byproduct of wood processing for papermaking. It is a somewhat oily liquid that looks like mineral oil and has a slightly garlicky odor. Because it is an excellent solvent, it is widely used as a degreaser, paint thinner, and antifreeze. However, it also has remarkable therapeutic properties, especially for the healing of injuries. Applying DMSO on sprained ankles, pulled muscles, dislocated joints, and even at the site of simple fractures can virtually eliminate the pain. It also promotes immune system activity.

DMSO is absorbed through the skin and enters the bloodstream by osmosis through capillary walls. It is then distributed through the circulatory system, and ultimately is excreted through the urine. It has been used successfully in the treatment of brain and spinal cord damage; arthritis, Down syndrome, sciatica and other back problems, keloids, acne, burns, musculoskeletal problems, sports injuries, cancer, sinusitis, headaches, skin ulcers, herpes, and cataracts.

Essential Fatty Acids (EFAs)

Fatty acids are the basic building blocks of which fats and oils are composed. Contrary to popular myth, the body does need fat. It must be the right kind, however.

The fatty acids that are necessary for health and that cannot be made by the body are called essential fatty acids (EFAs). They are occasionally also referred to as vitamin F or polyunsaturates. EFAs must be supplied through the diet.

Essential fatty acids have desirable effects on many disorders. They improve the skin and hair, reduce blood pressure, aid in the prevention of arthritis, lower cholesterol and triglyceride levels, and reduce the risk of blood clot formation. They are beneficial for candidiasis, cardiovascular disease, eczema, and psoriasis. Found in high concentrations in the brain, EFAs aid in the transmission of nerve impulses and are needed for the normal development and functioning of the brain. A deficiency of essential fatty acids can lead to an impaired ability to learn and recall information.

Every living cell in the body needs essential fatty acids. They are essential for rebuilding and producing new cells. Essential fatty acids are also used by the body for the production of prostaglandins, hormonelike substances that act as chemical messengers and regulators of various body processes.

There are two basic categories of essential fatty acids, designated omega-3 and omega-6. Omega-6 EFAs, which include linoleic and gamma-linolenic acids, are found primarily in raw nuts, seeds, and legumes, and in unsaturated vegetable oils, such as borage oil, grape seed oil, primrose oil, sesame oil, and soybean oil. Omega-3 EFAs, including alpha-linolenic and eicosapentaenoic acid (EPA), are found in fresh deepwater fish, fish oil, and certain vegetable oils, among them canola oil, flaxseed oil, and walnut oil. In order to supply essential fatty acids, these oils must be consumed in pure liquid or supplement form and must not be subjected to heat, either in processing or cooking. Heat destroys essential fatty acids. Worse, it results in the creation of dangerous free radicals (see ANTIOXIDANTS in Part One). If oils are hydrogenated (processed to make the oil more solid, as is commonly done in the production of margarine), the linoleic acid is converted into trans-fatty acids, which are not beneficial to the body.

The daily requirement for essential fatty acids is satisfied by an amount equivalent to 10 to 20 percent of total caloric intake. The most essential of the essential fatty acids is linoleic acid.

A number of sources of essential fatty acids are recommended in this book, among them fish oils, flaxseeds and flaxseed oil, grape seed oil, and primrose oil.

Fish Oil

Fish oil is a good source of omega-3 essential fatty acids. Salmon, mackerel, menhaden, herring, and sardines are good sources of fish oil because they have a higher fat content and provide more omega-3 factors than other fishes. For instance, 4 ounces of salmon contains up to 3,600 milligrams of omega-3 fatty acids, while 4 ounces of cod (a low-fat fish) contains only 300 milligrams.

Carlson Laboratories markets a good Norwegian salmon oil that we recommend. Cod liver oil from Norway is the most commonly used fish oil, and is more mild tasting than other varieties. Author Dale Alexander claims it is excellent for arthritis. He has marketed an oil containing 13,800 international units of vitamin A and 1,380 international units of vitamin D per tablespoon. However, we do not recommend that you rely on cod liver oil as a source of the essential fatty acids. You would have to overdose on vitamins A and D to obtain the amount of fatty acids you need.

People with diabetes should not take fish oil supplements because of the high fat content, but they should consume fish for its essential fatty acids.

Flaxseeds and Flaxseed Oil

Flaxseeds are rich in omega-3 essential fatty acids, magnesium, potassium, and fiber. They are also a good source of the B vitamins, protein, and zinc. They are low in saturated fats and calories, and contain no cholesterol. The nutty taste of ground flaxseeds is pleasant, and they can be mixed with water or any fruit or vegetable juice. They can also be added to salads, soups, yogurt, cereals, baked goods, or fresh juices. You can grind these tiny seeds in a coffee grinder.

If you prefer not to eat the seeds, you can use flaxseed oil as an alternative. Like the seeds from which it is extracted, organic cold-pressed flaxseed oil is rich in essential fatty acids. Several studies have shown that it can reduce the pain, inflammation, and swelling of arthritis. It also has been found to lower blood cholesterol and triglyceride levels, and to help reduce the hardening effects of cholesterol on cell membranes.

Grape Seed Oil

Of the many natural sources of essential fatty acids, grape seed oil is among the highest in linoleic acid and among the lowest in saturated fats. It contains no trans-fatty acids, no cholesterol, and no sodium. It has a light, nutty taste that brings out the flavor in many foods. Unlike most other oils, it can be heated to temperatures as high as 485°F without producing dangerous and possibly carcinogenic free radicals. These features make it good for use in cooking. Buy only grape seed oil that is cold-pressed and contains no preservatives, such as Salute Santé Grapeseed Oil from Lifestar International.

Primrose Oil

Primrose oil (also known as evening primrose oil) contains the highest amount of gamma-linolenic acid (GLA) of any

food substance. This fatty acid is known to help prevent hardening of the arteries, heart disease, premenstrual syndrome, multiple sclerosis, and high blood pressure. It relieves pain and inflammation; enhances the release of sex hormones, including estrogen and testosterone; aids in lowering cholesterol levels; and is beneficial for cirrhosis of the liver.

Many women have found that primrose oil supplements relieve unpleasant menopausal symptoms such as hot flashes. Because it promotes the production of estrogen, women suffering from breast cancer that is estrogen related should avoid or limit their intake of primrose oil. Black currant seed oil is a good substitute.

Combination EFA Supplements

A product called Ultimate Oil, from Nature's Secret, contains a blend of cold-pressed organic oils that offers a good balance of both omega-3 and omega-6 fatty acids. A purely vegetable-based product, Ultimate Oil contains extra-virgin flaxseed oil, black currant seed oil, pumpkin seed oil, lecithin, and safflower oil. We also recommend Kyolic-EPA from Wakunaga of America, a blend of aged garlic extract and fish oil derived from northern Pacific sardines, and Cardiovascular Research's Essential Fatty Acid Complex.

Evening Primrose Oil

See Primrose Oil *under* Essential Fatty Acids in this section.

Fiber

Found in many foods, fiber helps to lower the blood cholesterol level and stabilize blood sugar levels. It helps prevent colon cancer, constipation, hemorrhoids, obesity, and many other disorders. Fiber is also good for removing certain toxic metals from the body. Because the refining process has removed much of the natural fiber from our foods, the typical American diet is lacking in fiber.

There are seven basic classifications of fiber: bran, cellulose, gum, hemicellulose, lignin, mucilages, and pectin. Each form has its own function. It is best to rotate among several different supplemental fiber sources. Start with small amounts and gradually increase your intake until your stools are the proper consistency. Also, be aware that while today's average diet is lacking in fiber, consuming excessive amounts may decrease the absorption of zinc, iron, and calcium. Always take supplemental fiber separately from other medications or supplements. Otherwise, it can lessen their strength and effectiveness.

In addition to using a fiber supplement, you should make sure to get fiber through your diet. Make sure your diet contains these high-fiber foods: whole-grain cereals and flours, brown rice, agar agar, all kinds of bran, most fresh fruit, dried prunes, nuts, seeds (especially flaxseeds), beans, lentils, peas, and fresh raw vegetables. Eat several of these foods daily. When eating organic produce, leave the skin on apples and potatoes. Coat chicken in corn bran or oats for baking. Add extra bran to cereals and breads. Unsalted, unbuttered popcorn is also excellent for added fiber.

Bran, Gums, and Mucilages

Both gums and mucilages help to regulate blood glucose levels, aid in lowering cholesterol, and help in the removal of toxins. They are found in oatmeal, oat bran, sesame seeds, and dried beans.

One of the following should be part of the daily dietary plan:

• *Fennel seed.* Fennel is an herb that is helpful for digestive purposes. The seeds of this plant help to rid the intestinal tract of mucus and aid in relieving flatulence.

• *Glucomannan.* Derived from the tuber of the amorphophallis plant, it picks up and removes fat from the colon wall. This substance is good for diabetes and obesity because it helps to get rid of fat. It has been recognized for normalizing blood sugar and is good for people with hypoglycemia. Glucomannan expands to sixty times its own weight, thereby helping to curb the appetite. Taking 2 to 3 capsules with a large glass of water thirty minutes before meals is helpful for reducing allergic reactions and some symptoms associated with high and low blood sugar disorders. Always be sure to drink a large glass of water when taking glucomannan in capsule or pill form, as capsules can lodge in the throat and expand there, causing breathing problems. Glucomannan is tasteless and odorless, and can be added to foods to help normalize blood sugar.

• *Guar gum.* Extracted from the seeds of the guar plant, guar gum is good for the treatment of diabetes and for curbing the appetite. It also has the ability to reduce the levels of cholesterol, triglycerides, and low-density lipoproteins in the blood, and binds with toxic substances and carries them out of the body. Guar gum tablets must be chewed thoroughly or sucked gradually, not swallowed whole, and should be taken with lots of water, because guar gum has a tendency to ball up in the throat when mixed with saliva. It should not be used by individuals who have difficulty swallowing or who have had gastrointestinal surgery. Some persons with colon disorders may have trouble using guar gum.

• *Oat bran and rice bran.* Bran is the broken coat of the seed of cereal grain that has been separated from the flour or meal by sifting or bolting. It helps to lower cholesterol.

• *Psyllium seed.* Psyllium is a grain grown in India that is utilized for its fiber content. A good intestinal cleanser and stool softener, it is one of the most popular fibers used. It thickens very quickly when mixed with liquid, and must be consumed immediately. Some doctors recommend

Metamucil, which contains psyllium hydrophilic mucilloid, as a laxative and fiber supplement. However, we prefer less processing and all-natural products.

Cellulose

Cellulose is an indigestible carbohydrate found in the outer layer of vegetables and fruits. It is good for hemorrhoids, varicose veins, colitis, and constipation, and for the removal of cancer-causing substances from the colon wall. It is found in apples, beets, Brazil nuts, broccoli, carrots, celery, green beans, lima beans, pears, peas, and whole grains.

Hemicellulose

Hemicellulose is an indigestible complex carbohydrate that absorbs water. It is good for promoting weight loss, relieving constipation, preventing colon cancer, and controlling carcinogens in the intestinal tract. Hemicellulose is found in apples, bananas, beans, beets, cabbage, corn, green leafy vegetables, pears, peppers, and whole grain cereals.

Lignin

This form of fiber is good for lowering cholesterol levels. It helps to prevent the formation of gallstones by binding with bile acids and removing cholesterol before stones can form. It is beneficial for persons with diabetes or colon cancer. Lignin is found in Brazil nuts, carrots, green beans, peaches, peas, potatoes, strawberries, tomatoes, and whole grains.

Pectin

Because it slows the absorption of food after meals, pectin is good for people with diabetes. It also removes unwanted metals and toxins, reduces the side effects of radiation therapy, helps lower cholesterol, and reduces the risk of heart disease and gallstones. Pectin is found in apples, bananas, beets, cabbage, carrots, citrus fruits, dried peas, and okra.

Combination Fiber Supplements

There are many products available that combine two or more different types of fiber, or that combine fiber with other ingredients. Two products of this kind that we recommend are:

• *Aerobic Bulk Cleanse (ABC).* This product, from Aerobic Life Industries, is an excellent source of fiber. It contains blond psyllium seed husks and the herbs licorice and hibiscus. This therapeutic drink aids in healing and cleansing the colon. It is excellent for diarrhea and constipation. Add it to a combination of one-half aloe vera juice and one-half fruit juice. Be sure to take this mixture on an empty stomach, first thing in the morning. Stir it well and drink it down quickly, before it thickens. Related products, also from Aerobic Life Industries, include 10-Day Colon Cleanse and 45-Day Cleanse for Colon, Blood and Lymph.

• *A.M/P.M. Ultimate Cleanse.* This formula combines gums with cellulose, hemicellulose, pectin, and lignin, plus herbs that support and cleanse the blood and internal organs. Sold by Nature's Secret, it is a two-part system for stimulating and detoxifying the entire body.

Fish Oil

See under Essential Fatty Acids in this section.

Flaxseeds and Flaxseed Oil

See under Essential Fatty Acids in this section.

Garlic

Garlic is one of the most valuable foods on this planet. It has been used since Biblical times, and is mentioned in the literature of the ancient Hebrews, Greeks, Babylonians, Romans, and Egyptians. The builders of the pyramids supposedly ate garlic daily for endurance and strength.

Garlic lowers blood pressure through the actions of one of its components, methyl allyl trisulfide, which dilates blood vessel walls. It thins the blood by inhibiting platelet aggregation, which reduces the risk of blood clots and aids in preventing heart attacks. It also lowers serum cholesterol levels and aids in digestion. Garlic is useful for many diseases and illnesses, including cancer. It is a potent immune system stimulant and a natural antibiotic. It should be consumed daily. It can be eaten fresh, taken in supplement form, or used to prepare garlic oil.

Garlic contains an amino acid derivative, alliin. When garlic is consumed, the enzyme alliinase, which converts alliin to allicin, is released. Allicin has an antibiotic effect; it exerts an antibacterial effect estimated to be equivalent to 1 percent of that of penicillin. Because of its antibiotic properties, garlic was used to treat wounds and infections and to prevent gangrene during World War I.

Garlic is also effective against fungal infections, including athlete's foot, systemic candidiasis, and yeast vaginitis, and there is some evidence that it may also destroy certain viruses, such as those associated with fever blisters, genital herpes, a form of the common cold, smallpox, and a type of influenza.

Garlic oil is good for the heart and colon, and is effective in the treatment of arthritis, candidiasis, and circulation problems. To make garlic oil, add peeled whole garlic cloves to a quart of olive or canola oil. Experiment to find the number of cloves that gives the degree of flavor you like. Be sure to wash your hands thoroughly and rinse the garlic after peeling and before placing it in the oil. The peel may contain mold and bacteria that can contaminate the oil. Keep this oil refrigerated. This mixture will keep for up to a month before you need to replace it with fresh oil. Garlic oil can be used for sautéing, in salad dressings, and in a variety of other ways. If you find the odor too strong after you eat garlic, chew some sprigs of parsley or mint, or caraway or fennel seeds.

An alternative to fresh garlic is Kyolic from Wakunaga of America. Kyolic is an odorless, "sociable" garlic product, and is available in tablet, capsule, and oil extract forms.

Ginkgo Biloba

The ornamental tree *Ginkgo biloba* originated in China thousands of years ago, and now grows in temperate climates throughout the world. The extract of its fan-shaped leaves is one of the world's most popular herbal products. It has been reported in scientific journals to enhance blood circulation and to increase the supply of oxygen to the heart, brain, and all bodily parts. This makes it useful for improving memory and relieving muscle pains. It also acts as an antioxidant, has anti-aging effects, reduces blood pressure, inhibits blood clotting, and is helpful for tinnitus, vertigo, hearing loss, impotence, and Raynaud's disease. Ginkgo biloba is widely known as the "smart herb" of our time. It has even been shown to slow the early progression of Alzheimer's disease in some individuals.

Ginseng

Ginseng is used throughout the Far East as a general tonic to combat weakness and give extra energy. There are a number of different types of ginseng: *Eleutherococcus senticosus* (Siberian ginseng), *Panax quinquefolium* (American ginseng), *Panax ginseng* (Chinese or Korean ginseng), and *Panax japonicum* (Japanese ginseng). *Panax ginseng* is the most widely used species.

Early Native Americans were familiar with ginseng. They called it *gisens* and used it for stomach and bronchial disorders, asthma, and neck pain. Russian scientists claim that the ginseng root stimulates both physical and mental activity, improves endocrine gland function, and has a positive effect on the sex glands. Ginseng is beneficial for fatigue because it spares glycogen (the form of glucose stored in the liver and muscle cells) by increasing the use of fatty acids as an energy source. It is used to enhance athletic performance, to rejuvenate and to increase longevity, and to detoxify and normalize the entire system.

In lower doses, ginseng seems to raise blood pressure, while higher amounts appear to reduce blood pressure. Research suggests that high doses of ginseng may be helpful for inflammatory diseases such as rheumatoid arthritis, without the side effects of steroids, and may also protect against the harmful effects of radiation. Ginseng is beneficial for people with diabetes because it decreases the level of the hormone cortisol in the blood (cortisol interferes with the function of insulin). However, people with hypoglycemia should avoid using large amounts of ginseng.

The root is sold in many forms: as a whole root or root pieces, which are either untreated or blanched; as a powder or powdered extract; as a liquid extract or concentrate; in granules for instant tea; as a tincture; in an oil base; and in tablets and capsules. These products should not contain sugar or added color, and should be pure ginseng. Many supplement manufacturers add ginseng to combination products, but these often contain such low amounts that they may not be effective. Wakunaga of America distributes several high-quality Korean and Siberian ginseng products.

We advise following the Russian approach to using ginseng: Take it for fifteen to twenty days, followed by a rest period of two weeks. Avoid long-term usage of high doses.

Glucomannan

See under Fiber in this section.

Glucosamine

This is one of a number of substances classified as an *amino sugar*. Unlike other forms of sugar in the body, amino sugars are components of carbohydrates that are incorporated into the structure of body tissues, rather than being used as a source of energy. Glucosamine is thus involved in the formation of the nails, tendons, skin, eyes, bones, ligaments, and heart valves. It also plays a role in the mucous secretions of the digestive, respiratory, and urinary tracts.

Glucosamine is made in the body from the simple carbohydrate glucose and the amino acid glutamine. It is also available as a supplement, in the form of glucosamine sulfate. GlucosaMend from Source Naturals, Glucosamine Plus from Food Science Laboratories, and Glucosamine Sulfate Complex from PhytoPharmica are recommended products. Supplemental glucosamine can be helpful for asthma, bursitis, candidiasis, food allergies, osteoporosis, respiratory allergies, tendinitis, vaginitis, and various skin problems. A related compound is N-acetylglucosamine (NAG), available as N-A-G from Source Naturals.

Grape Seed Oil

See under Essential Fatty Acids in this section.

"Green Drinks"

"Green drinks" are natural food formulas made from plants that are good detoxifiers and blood cleansers, as well as sources of chlorophyll, minerals, enzymes, and other important nutrients. Generally, they are sold in powdered form to be mixed just before use. Many different companies market green drink formulas. The following are some recommended products:

- *Barley Green from AIM International.* This product contains a combination of barley juice and kelp.

- *Earthsource Greens & More from Solgar.* This formula combines four organically grown grasses (alfalfa, barley, kamut, and wheat), Hawaiian blue-green spirulina, and Chinese chlorella with three potent immune-stimulating mushrooms (maitake, reishi, and shiitake), plus powdered broccoli, carrots, and red beets, which supply phytonutrients. Its fruit flavor comes from fresh fruit powders.

- *Green Magma from Green Foods Corporation.* Green Magma is a pure, natural juice of young barley leaves that are organically grown in Japan and are pesticide-free. Brown rice is added to supply vitamin B_1 and nicotinic and linoleic acids. Green Magma contains thousands of enzymes, which play an important role in the metabolism of the body (*see* ENZYMES in Part One), plus a high concentration of superoxide dismutase (SOD). The powdered product may be added to juice or quality water.

- *Kyo-Green from Wakunaga of America.* This is a combination of barley, wheatgrass, kelp, and the green algae chlorella. The barley and wheatgrass are organically grown. It is a highly concentrated natural source of chlorophyll, amino acids, vitamins and minerals, carotene, and enzymes. Chlorella is a rich natural source of vitamin A, and kelp supplies iodine and other valuable minerals. (*See* Chlorella and Kelp in this section.)

- *ProGreens from NutriCology.* ProGreens includes organic alfalfa, barley, oat, and wheatgrass juice powders; natural fiber; wheat sprouts; blue-green algae; sea algae; fructooligosaccharides (FOS); lecithin; standardized bioflavonoid extracts; royal jelly and bee pollen; beet and spinach extracts; acerola juice powder; natural vitamin E; and the herbs astragalus, echinacea, licorice, Siberian ginseng, and suma.

Guar Gum

See under Fiber in this section.

Hemicellulose

See under Fiber in this section.

Honey

Bees produce honey by mixing nectar, which is a sweet substance secreted by flowers, with bee enzymes. Honey is made up of 35 percent protein and contains half of all the amino acids, and is a highly concentrated source of many essential nutrients, including large amounts of carbohydrates (sugars), some minerals, B-complex vitamins, and vitamins C, D, and E.

Honey is used to promote energy and healing. It is a natural antiseptic and makes a good salve for burns and wounds. Honey is also used for sweetening other foods and beverages. It varies somewhat in color and taste depending on the origin of the flower and nectar, but in general it is approximately twice as sweet as sugar, so not as much is needed for sweetening purposes. People who have diabetes or hypoglycemia should be careful when consuming honey and its byproducts. These substances affect blood sugar levels in the same way that refined sugars do. Tupelo honey contains more fructose than other types of honey and it is absorbed at a slower rate, so some people with hypoglycemia can use this type sparingly without ill effects.

Buy only unfiltered, unheated, unprocessed honey, and *never* give honey to an infant under one year of age. In its natural form, honey can contain spores of the bacteria that cause botulism. This poses no problem for adults and older children, but in infants, the spores can colonize the digestive tract and produce the deadly botulin toxin there. Honey is safe for babies after age one.

Kelp

Kelp is a type of seaweed that can be eaten raw, but it is usually dried, granulated, or ground into powder. It is also available in a liquid form that can be added to drinking water. Granulated or powdered kelp can be used as a condiment and for flavoring, as a salt substitute. If you find the taste unappealing, you can purchase it in tablet form.

Kelp is a rich source of vitamins, especially the B vitamins, as well as of many valuable minerals and trace elements. It is reported to be very beneficial to brain tissue, the membranes surrounding the brain, the sensory nerves, and the spinal cord, as well as the nails and blood vessels. It has been used in the treatment of thyroid problems because of its iodine content, and is useful for other conditions as varied as hair loss, obesity, and ulcers. It protects against the effects of radiation and softens stools. Kelp is recommended as a daily dietary supplement, especially for people with mineral deficiencies.

Kombucha Tea

The kombucha, or Manchurian, "mushroom" has reputedly been used in Asian countries and in Russia for centuries. The "mushroom" itself is not eaten. Rather, a tea is made by fermenting the "mushroom" for about a week in a mixture of water, sugar, and green or black tea, with apple cider vinegar or a bit of previously made tea added. Kept in this mixture, the "mushroom" reproduces, and the "daughter mushrooms" can then be used to produce more tea (*see* MAKING KOMBUCHA TEA in Part Three).

Although commonly referred to as a mushroom, the kombucha is actually a combination of a number of different elements, including lichen, bacteria, and yeast. Kombucha tea contains a variety of different nutrients and other health-promoting substances. It is a natural energy booster and detoxifier that may also help slow or reverse the aging process and fight such serious diseases as AIDS, cancer, and multiple sclerosis.

Because of the way in which it has traditionally been propagated (one at a time, by individual users), kombucha may be difficult to find. Many people who have them received a daughter "mushroom" as a gift from a friend, although there are some herbal companies that sell both the "mushrooms" and the bottled tea commercially.

Lactobacillus Acidophilus

Lactobacillus acidophilus is a type of "friendly" bacteria that assists in the digestion of proteins, a process in which lactic acid, hydrogen peroxide, enzymes, B vitamins, and antibiotic substances that inhibit pathogenic organisms are produced. Acidophilus has antifungal properties, helps to reduce blood cholesterol levels, aids digestion, and enhances the absorption of nutrients.

The flora in the healthy colon should consist of least 85 percent lactobacilli and 15 percent coliform bacteria. However, the typical colon bacteria count today is the reverse. This can result in gas, bloating, intestinal and systemic toxicity, constipation, and malabsorption of nutrients, and is conducive to an overgrowth of candida. Taking an acidophilus supplement helps to combat all of these problems by returning the intestinal flora to a healthier balance. In addition, acidophilus may help to detoxify harmful substances.

There are many good acidophilus supplements available. Acidophilus products come in tablet, capsule, and powdered forms. We recommend using the powdered form. Natren markets quality products that contain very high numbers of organisms. Nondairy formulas are best for people who are allergic to dairy products, and they work well against candida. Kyo-Dophilus from Wakunaga of America is a milk-free product that remains stable at high temperatures. Other good nondairy acidophilus supplements include Primadophilus from Nature's Way and Neo-Flora from New Chapter. In general, we believe it is not advisable to buy a product containing a combination of different strains of lactobacilli, as one organism may be antagonistic to another. A single-strain product with a count of at least 1 billion organisms per gram is often better than a combination.

Acidophilus can die at high temperatures. Whatever product you choose, keep it in a cool, dry place—refrigerate but do not freeze it. Take acidophilus on an empty stomach in the morning and one hour before each meal. If you are taking antibiotics, do not take the antibiotics and acidophilus simultaneously.

Lactobacillus Bifidus

Lactobacillus bifidus aids in the synthesis of the B vitamins by creating healthy intestinal flora. *L. bifidus* is the predominant organism in the intestinal flora and establishes a healthy environment for the manufacture of the B-complex vitamins and vitamin K.

When you take antibiotics, the "friendly" bacteria in

your digestive tract are destroyed along with the harmful bacteria. Supplementing your diet with *L. bifidus* helps you maintain healthy intestinal flora. Unhealthy flora can result in the liberation of abnormally high levels of ammonia as protein-containing foods are digested. This irritates the intestinal membranes. In addition, the ammonia is absorbed into the bloodstream and must be detoxified by the liver, or it will cause nausea, a decrease in appetite, vomiting, and other toxic reactions. By promoting the proper digestion of foods, the friendly bacteria also aid in preventing digestive disorders such as constipation and gas, as well as food allergies. If digestion is poor, the activity of intestinal bacteria on undigested food may lead to excessive production of the body chemical histamine, which triggers allergic symptoms.

Yeast infections of the vaginal tract respond very favorably to douching with *L. bifidus* preparations. These microorganisms destroy the pathogenic organisms. When used as an enema, *L. bifidus* also helps establish a healthy intestinal environment. It improves bowel function by aiding peristalsis, and results in the production of a softer, smoother stool. Harmful bacteria are kept in check, and toxic wastes that have accumulated in the intestines are destroyed and/or eliminated from the body.

L. bifidus has proved useful in the treatment of cirrhosis of the liver and chronic hepatitis; by improving digestion, it reduces the strain on the liver. Many people who do not respond to *L. acidophilus* react positively to *L. bifidus*. Many experts consider *L. bifidus* to be preferable to *L. acidophilus* for use in children and for adults with liver disorders.

Lecithin

Lecithin is a type of lipid that is needed by every living cell in the human body. Cell membranes, which regulate the passage of nutrients into and out of the cells, are largely composed of lecithin. The protective sheaths surrounding the brain are composed of lecithin, and the muscles and nerve cells also contain this essential fatty substance. Lecithin consists mostly of the B vitamin choline, and also contains linoleic acid and inositol. Although lecithin is a lipid, it is partly soluble in water and thus acts as an emulsifying agent. This is why many processed foods contain lecithin.

This nutrient helps to prevent arteriosclerosis, protects against cardiovascular disease, improves brain function, and aids in the absorption of thiamine by the liver and vitamin A by the intestine. It is also known to promote energy and is needed to help repair damage to the liver caused by alcoholism. Lecithin enables fats, such as cholesterol and other lipids, to be dispersed in water and removed from the body. The vital organs and arteries are thus protected from fatty buildup.

Lecithin would be a wise addition to anyone's diet. It is especially valuable for elderly people. Anyone who is taking niacin for high serum cholesterol and triglycerides should also include lecithin in his or her program. Two tablespoons of lecithin granules can be sprinkled on cereals and soups or added to juices or breads. Lecithin also comes in capsule form. Taking one 1,200-milligram capsule before each meal helps in the digestion of fats and the absorption of fat-soluble vitamins.

Most lecithin is derived from soybeans, but recently egg lecithin has become popular. This type of lecithin is extracted from the yolks of fresh eggs. Egg lecithin may hold promise for those suffering from AIDS, herpes, chronic fatigue syndrome, and immune disorders associated with aging. Studies have shown that it works better for people with these disorders than soy lecithin does. Other sources of lecithin include brewer's yeast, grains, legumes, fish, and wheat germ.

Lignin

See under Fiber in this section.

Maitake

Maitake (*Grifola frondosa*) is a mushroom that has a long history of use in traditional Chinese and Japanese herbology and cooking. It grows wild in Japan, as well as in some wooded areas in eastern North America. Because maitake is difficult to cultivate, however, only relatively recently have the mushrooms become widely available.

Maitake is considered an adaptogen, which means that it helps the body adapt to stress and normalizes bodily fuctions. Its healing properties are thought to be related to its high content of a polysaccharide called beta-1.6-glucan, which is considered very powerful. In laboratory studies, this substance has been shown to prevent carcinogenesis, inhibit the growth of cancerous tumors, kill HIV, and enhance the activity of key immune cells known as T-helper cells or CD4 cells. Maitake may also be useful for diabetes, chronic fatigue syndrome, chronic hepatitis, obesity, and high blood pressure.

Research suggests that maitake is better absorbed than other mushrooms, such as shiitake, and it is almost as effective when taken orally as it is when taken intravenously. Maitake can be eaten in food or taken as a supplement. Buy organically grown dried mushrooms (to use them in cooking, soak them in water or broth for half an hour), or purchase maitake in capsule, extract, or tea form. Some of the capsule supplements contain a small amount of vitamin C, which enhances the effectiveness of the active ingredient in maitake by aiding in its absorption.

Melatonin

The hormone melatonin is naturally produced by the pineal gland, a cone-shaped structure in the brain. The body's pattern of melatonin production is similar to that of the other "anti-aging" hormones, human growth hormone (HGH) and

Maintaining Your Melatonin Level Naturally

As darkness falls at the end of each day, melatonin production rises. In the morning, when daylight hits the retina, neural impulses cause production of the hormone to slow. Clearly, light and darkness are the primary factors that set the rhythms of melatonin production. However, they are not the only factors involved. In fact, it has been found that a variety of regular daily routines can strengthen the rhythm of melatonin production. Here are a few simple ways in which you can help your body maintain high levels of this important hormone:

• Eat regular meals. The rhythm of melatonin production is strengthened by regular daily routines. Keep your mealtimes as regular as possible to keep your body in sync with the rhythms of the day.

• Keep your diet light at night. When melatonin production begins after nightfall, the digestive process is slowed. Thus, any heavy foods eaten close to bedtime may lead to digestive problems, which can make it difficult to sleep. To get the sleep you need, eat small, light meals in the late evening.

• Avoid stimulants. Stimulants like coffee, tea, and caffeine-containing medications and colas can interfere with melatonin production by interfering with your sleep. As much as possible, eliminate these stimulants from your diet and lifestyle.

• Avoid exercising late at night. Vigorous activity delays melatonin secretion. If you exercise in the morning, you will reinforce healthful sleeping habits that lead to regular melatonin production. For best results, do your morning exercise out of doors, in the morning light.

---

dehydroepiandrosterone (DHEA). Throughout early life, melatonin is produced in abundance. Shortly before puberty, though, the production of melatonin begins to drop, and then continues to decline steadily as we age.

Research has demonstrated that melatonin may have several profound long-term effects on the body. As one of the most powerful antioxidants ever discovered—with a greater range of effectiveness than vitamin C, vitamin E, or beta-carotene—melatonin helps prevent harmful oxidation reactions from occurring. In this way, melatonin may prevent the changes that lead to hypertension and heart attack, and may reduce the risk of certain kinds of cancer. Indeed, research has indicated that many age-related problems are caused by declining levels of melatonin, which leave the body less able to prevent and repair oxidative damage. Melatonin also has been found to stimulate the immune system; have a major role in the production of estrogen, testosterone, and possibly other hormones, helping to prevent cancers involving the reproductive system; and slow the growth of existing malignancies. Recent studies suggest that if melatonin is taken in the mornings, tumor growth may be stimulated, but if it is taken in the evenings, it has a retarding effect on tumor growth. In addition, as melatonin is secreted cyclically, in response to the fall of darkness at the end of each day, the hormone helps our bodies keep in sync with the rhythms of day and night. Thus, melatonin helps regulate sleep.

Research on melatonin continues, and with it, knowledge is increasing about the functions of melatonin in the body and the effects of melatonin supplementation. Both human research studies and anecdotal evidence indicate that melatonin supplements can be an effective and side-effect-free sleep aid both for adults suffering from insomnia and for children with autism, epilepsy, Down syndrome, cerebral palsy, and other problems that can cause sleep disorders. Animal and other laboratory research indicates that melatonin supplementation may help prevent age-related disorders, and perhaps extend life. Melatonin can be taken to ease PMS symptoms; stimulate the immune system; prevent memory loss, arteriosclerosis, and stroke; and treat cancer and Alzheimer's disease.

Although no toxic levels of melatonin have been found, some researchers feel that certain people probably should not use this supplement until further information is available. Included in this category are pregnant and nursing women; people with severe allergies or autoimmune diseases; people with immune system cancers, such as lymphoma and leukemia; and healthy children, who already produce sufficient amounts of the hormone. Since high doses of melatonin have been found to act as a contraceptive, women who wish to become pregnant might also want to avoid taking the supplement.

Melatonin should be taken two hours or less before bedtime. This schedule is designed to release the added hormone at the same time that natural production peaks. A sustained-release form is best if you frequently awaken after several hours' sleep; a sublingual form is best if you are very ill or suffer from malabsorption. When you awaken after melatonin-assisted sleep, you should feel refreshed—not tired or groggy. If you do experience grogginess, you should reduce the dosage. (To learn how you can maintain or increase your melatonin levels through daily routines, see Maintaining Your Melatonin Level Naturally, above.) For information on other anti-aging hormones, see DHEA THERAPY and GROWTH HORMONE THERAPY in Part Three.

Mucilage

See under Fiber in this section.

Oat Bran

See under Fiber in this section.

Octacosanol

Octacosanol is a naturally derived wheat germ oil concentrate. (Although it would be possible to extract octacosanol from whole wheat, 10 pounds of wheat would be needed to obtain just 1,000 micrograms of octacosanol.) Wheat germ has long been known for its many benefits. Today, extracts of wheat germ weighing only 2 milligrams offer remarkable benefits as well.

Octacosanol has been clinically proven to increase oxygen utilization during exercise and improve glycogen storage in muscle. As a result, it increases physical endurance, improves reaction time, reduces high-altitude stress, and aids in tissue oxygenation. This substance can greatly benefit those who experience muscle pain after exercise or who have a lowered endurance level, and is good for muscular dystrophies and other neuromuscular disorders as well. It also reduces blood cholesterol levels.

Pectin

See under Fiber in this section.

Primrose Oil

See under Essential Fatty Acids in this section.

Propolis

See Bee Propolis in this section.

Psyllium Seed

See under Fiber in this section.

Reishi

See Shiitake and Reishi in this section.

Rice Bran

See under Fiber in this section.

Royal Jelly

Royal jelly is a thick, milky substance that is secreted from the pharyngeal glands of a special group of young nurse bees between their sixth and twelfth days of life. When honey and pollen are combined and refined within the young nurse bee, royal jelly is naturally created. This substance contains all of the B-complex vitamins, including a high concentration of pantothenic acid (vitamin B_5) and vitamin B_6 (pyridoxine), and is the only natural source of pure acetylcholine. Royal jelly also contains minerals, enzymes, hormones, eighteen amino acids, antibacterial and antibiotic components, and vitamins A, C, D, and E. It is useful for bronchial asthma, liver disease, pancreatitis, insomnia, stomach ulcers, kidney disease, bone fractures, and skin disorders, and it strengthens the immune system.

This product must be combined with honey to preserve its potency. Royal jelly spoils easily. Keep it refrigerated and make sure it is tightly sealed when purchased.

Sea Cucumber

Sea cucumbers, also known as *bêche de mer* and *trepang*, are not actually cucumbers, but are marine animals related to starfishes and sea urchins. They have been used in China for thousands of years as a treatment for arthritis. Modern research has confirmed they are beneficial for musculoskeletal inflammatory diseases, especially rheumatoid arthritis, osteoarthritis, and ankylosing spondylitis, a rheumatic disease that affects the spine.

Researchers believe that sea cucumbers improve the balance of prostaglandins, which regulate the inflammatory process. They also contain substances known as mucopolysaccharides and chondroitins, which are often lacking in people with arthritis and connective tissue disorders. In addition, sea cucumbers provide vitamins A, B_1 (thiamine), B_2 (riboflavin), and B_3 (niacin), and C, as well as the minerals calcium, iron, magnesium, and zinc.

Sea Mussel

The green-lipped mussel (*Perna canaliculus*) is a species of edible shellfish. They contain numerous amino acids, the building blocks of body proteins, in addition to enzymes and essential trace elements. The minerals they contain are present in a balance similar to that in blood plasma, and these minerals are naturally chelated by the amino acids, making for better assimilation into the body.

Sea mussel aids in the functioning of the cardiovascular system, the lymphatic system, the endocrine system, the eyes, connective tissues, and mucous membranes. They help to reduce inflammation and relieve the pain and stiffness of arthritis. They also promote the healing of wounds and burns.

Shark Cartilage

The tough, elastic material that makes up the skeleton of the shark is dried and pulverized (finely powdered) to make this food supplement. Shark cartilage contains a number of active components, the most important of which is a type of protein that acts as an angiogenesis inhibitor—that is, it acts to suppress the development of new blood vessels. This makes it valuable in fighting a number of disorders. Many cancerous tumors, for instance, are able to grow only because they induce the body to develop new networks of blood vessels to supply them with nutrients. Shark cartilage suppresses this process, so that tumors are deprived of their source of nourishment and, often, begin to shrink. There are also certain eye disorders, such as diabetic retinopathy and macular degeneration, that are characterized by the growth of new blood vessels within the eye; because they grow in inappropriate places, the presence of these blood vessels can lead to blindness. Such diseases too may respond well to shark cartilage. Other conditions for which shark cartilage is useful include arthritis, psoriasis, and regional enteritis (inflammation of the lining of the bowels). In addition to angiogenesis-inhibiting protein, shark cartilage contains calcium (approximately 16 percent) and phosphorus (approximately 8 percent), which are absorbed as nutrients, and mucopolysaccharides that act to stimulate the immune system.

Shark cartilage is available in powder and capsule forms. Exercise caution when buying shark cartilage, as the purity and correct processing of the product are vital to its effectiveness. Not all shark cartilage products contain only 100-percent pure shark cartilage, so read labels carefully. Pure shark cartilage is white in color. If you find the odor and/or taste of pure shark cartilage to be stronger than you can tolerate, look for a product called BeneFin, which has significantly less fishy taste and smell than most other products. BeneFin is a trademarked name for naturally processed shark cartilage manufactured by Lane Labs-USA and marketed by various companies under license. If you are taking large quantities of shark cartilage, it may be wise to increase your supplementation of certain minerals, especially magnesium and potassium, to maintain a proper mineral balance in the body. Shark cartilage should *not* be taken by pregnant women or children, or by persons who have recently undergone surgery or suffered a heart attack.

Shiitake and Reishi

Shiitake and reishi are Japanese mushrooms with a delicate texture, strong stems, and well-defined undersides. They are attractive and have impressive health-promoting properties.

Shiitake (*Lentinus edodes*) contain a polysaccharide, lentinan, that strengthens the immune system by increasing T cell function. Shiitake mushrooms contain eighteen amino acids, seven of which are essential amino acids. They are rich in B vitamins, especially vitamins B_1 (thiamine), B_2 (riboflavin), and B_3 (niacin). When sun-dried, they contain high amounts of vitamin D. Their effectiveness in treating cancer has been reported in a joint study by the Medical Department of Koibe University and Nippon Kinoko Institute in Japan. These mushrooms are considered a delicacy and are entirely edible.

Reishi (*Ganoderma lucidum*) have been popular for at least 2,000 years in the Far East. They were rated number one on ancient Chinese lists of superior medicines, and were believed to give eternal youth and longevity.

Today, both shiitake and reishi mushrooms are used to treat a variety of disorders and to promote vitality. They are used to prevent high blood pressure and heart disease, to control and lower cholesterol, to build resistance to disease, and to treat fatigue and viral infections. They are also known to have anti-tumor properties valuable in treating cancer.

The mushrooms are available fresh or dried for use in foods (soak dried mushrooms in warm water or broth for thirty minutes before using), as well as in supplements in capsule, pill, and extract form.

Spirulina

Recognized the world over as the most promising of all microalgae, spirulina is an immediate food resource. Spirulina thrives in hot, sunny climates and in alkaline waters around the world. It represents a breakthrough in the production of food, producing twenty times as much protein as soybeans growing on an equal-sized area of land.

Spirulina contains concentrations of nutrients unlike any other single grain, herb, or plant. It contains gamma-linolenic acid (GLA), linoleic and arachidonic acids, vitamin B_{12} (needed, especially by vegetarians, for healthy red blood cells), iron, a high level of protein (60 to 70 percent), essential amino acids, the nucleic acids RNA and DNA, chlorophyll, and phycocyanin, a blue pigment that is found only in blue-green algae and that has increased the survival rate of mice with liver cancer in laboratory experiments.

Spirulina is a naturally digestible food that aids in protecting the immune system, in cholesterol reduction, and in mineral absorption. Spirulina is beneficial while fasting. It supplies the nutrients needed to help cleanse and heal, while also curbing the appetite. A person with hypoglycemia may benefit from using this food supplement between meals because its high protein content helps stabilize blood sugar levels.

Torula Yeast

See Yeast in this section.

Wheat Germ

Wheat germ is the embryo of the wheat berry. It is a good source of vitamin E; most of the B vitamins; the minerals calcium, magnesium, and phosphorus; and several trace elements.

One problem with wheat germ is that it becomes rancid easily. If you purchase wheat germ separately from the flour, make sure the product is fresh. It should be either vacuum packed or refrigerated, with a packing date or a label stating the date by which the product should be used.

Toasted wheat germ has a longer shelf life, but the raw product is better because it is unprocessed. Wheat germ oil capsules are also available.

Wheatgrass

Wheatgrass is a rich nutritional food that was popularized by Dr. Ann Wigmore, an educator and founder of the Hippocrates Health Institute in Boston. Wheatgrass contains a great variety of vitamins, minerals, and trace elements. According to Dr. Wigmore, 1 pound of fresh wheatgrass is equal in nutritional value to nearly 25 pounds of the choicest vegetables.

Dr. Wigmore reported that wheatgrass therapy, along with "living foods," helped to eliminate cancerous growths and helped many other disorders, including mental health problems. The molecular structure of chlorophyll resembles that of hemoglobin, the oxygen-carrying protein of red blood cells, and this may be the reason for the effectiveness of wheatgrass. The key difference between the two is that the metallic atom in the middle of each molecule of human hemoglobin is iron, while the metallic atom at the center of a molecule of chlorophyll is magnesium. In experiments on anemic animals, blood counts returned to normal after four to five days of receiving chlorophyll.

Yeast

Yeast are single-celled organisms that can multiply at extremely rapid rates, doubling in number in two hours. Yeast is rich in many basic nutrients, such as the B vitamins (except for vitamin B_{12}), sixteen amino acids, and at least fourteen different minerals. The protein content of yeast is responsible for 52 percent of its weight. Yeast is also high in phosphorus.

There are various media on which yeast may be grown. Brewer's yeast, also known as nutritional yeast, is grown on hops, a bitter herb that is also used as an ingredient in beer. Torula yeast is grown on blackstrap molasses or wood pulp. A liquid yeast product from Switzerland called Bio-Strath, distributed by Bioforce of America, is derived from herbs, honey, and malt. It is a natural product that we highly recommend.

Live baker's yeast should be avoided. Live yeast cells deplete the body of B vitamins and other nutrients. In nutritional yeast, these live cells are destroyed, leaving the beneficial nutrients behind.

Yeast may be consumed in juice or water, and is a good energy booster between meals. Yeast may also be added to the diet to aid in treating certain disorders. It helps in sugar metabolism and is good for eczema, heart disorders, gout, nervousness, and fatigue. By enhancing the immune system, yeast is useful for people undergoing radiation therapy or chemotherapy for cancer. Yeast also seems to increase mental and physical efficiency. Dr. William Crook, author of *The Yeast Connection* (Vintage Books, 1986), states that if a person with candida-related health problems is not specifically allergic to yeast, it is all right for him or her to take a food supplement containing yeast. However, we suggest avoiding yeast products if candidiasis is suspected. Because yeast contains significant amounts of phosphorus, people suffering from osteoporosis should avoid yeast products. (*See* OSTEOPOROSIS in Part Two.) Those who do take yeast should be sure to take extra calcium as well.

Specialty Supplements

In addition to the substances discussed above, there are many natural food supplements designed for specific circumstances. There are too many of these products to discuss them all here, but several that we feel are to be highly recommended are the following:

- *Body Language Essential Green Foods from Oxyfresh USA.* This is a combination that includes alfalfa, Atlantic kelp, kale, spinach, spirulina, bladderwrack, dulse, barley grass, chlorella, and wheatgrass, plus the enzymes maltase, amylase, protease, lipase, cellulase, dunaliella, and pectinase, to provide a green food concentrate rich in beta-carotene, chlorophyll, and trace minerals.

- *CamoCare cream from Abkit* contains chamomile and other active ingredients. It relieves pain associated with a variety of ailments involving the muscles and joints, such as backache, arthritis, and pain from inflamed joints. Chamomile acts similarly to cortisone in relieving pain, but without the side effects. Rub this cream onto the affected areas four times a day for best results.

- *Colostrum Specific from Jarrow Formulas.* This supplement contains freeze-dried bovine colostrum containing high levels of substances called *Cryptosporidium parvum* binding units (CPBUs), which are antibodies specific to *C. parvum*, a common parasite that can infect drinking water. Bovine colostrum also has immune-enhancing properties.

- *DynamO2 from En Garde Health Products.* This is a double-buffered stabilized oxygen product that releases oxygen in the digestive tract.

- *Jerusalem artichoke tablets.* Jerusalem artichoke whole tuber flour (JAF) tablets are a good source of fructooligosaccharides (FOS), which support the growth of healthy intestinal flora.

- *Smart Longevity from E'Ola Products.* This liquid supplement, distributed by Lifelines, is designed to bolster brain function. It contains nutrients to enhance brain function and antioxidants to protect against free radical damage. Ingredients include vitamin C, ginseng extract, schizandra extract, DMAE, choline, and vitamin E.

- *Sub-Adrene from American Biologics.* This is a highly concentrated whole adrenal-cortical extract of bovine origin.

Designed for sublingual administration, it has a peppermint taste and supplies a balance of natural steroids.

• *Wellness Formula from Source Naturals.* This supplement is designed to support optimal health in cold weather. Its ingredients include vitamins A and C, beta-carotene, and bioflavonoids; the immune-boosting mineral zinc; bee propolis; and the herbs angelica, astragalus, boneset, cayenne, echinacea, garlic, goldenseal, hawthorn berry, horehound, mullein, pau d'arco, and Siberian ginseng.

• *Whey to Go from Solgar.* Whey to Go is a powdered protein supplement. Its ingredients include three different types of whey protein concentrates, plus added free-form L-glutamine and branched-chain amino acids. Whey supplies beneficial elements such as calcium, the milk protein lactalbumin, and immunoglobulins, proteins that function as part of the immune system.

HERBS

INTRODUCTION

The medicinal benefits of herbs have been known for centuries. Records of Native American, Roman, Egyptian, Persian, and Hebrew medical practices show that herbs were used extensively to cure practically every known illness. Many herbs contain powerful ingredients that, if used correctly, can help heal the body. The pharmaceutical industry was originally based upon the ability to isolate these ingredients, and make them available in a purer form. Herbalists, however, contend that nature provides other ingredients in the same herbs to balance the more powerful ingredients. These other components, though they may be less potent, may help to act as buffers, synergists, or counterbalances working in harmony with the more powerful ingredients. Therefore, by using herbs in their complete form, the body's healing process utilizes a balance of ingredients provided by nature.

Many people believe that herbs are just as effective as drugs, but without the side effects. Most over-the-counter drugs should be used with caution. In addition, many of them are not particularly effective. Others can mask important symptoms, possibly leading to misdiagnoses and, ultimately, worse health problems. It is of interest to note that in many industrialized countries today, herbs are prescribed by physicians and prepared and sold through neighborhood drugstores. In developing countries, where access to hospitals and doctors is limited, herbal remedies often are the only generally available form of medicine.

Herbs do perform many healing functions in the body, but they must be used appropriately, not indiscriminately. Although herbal remedies are less likely than most conventional medicines to cause side effects, herbs nevertheless can be very potent. Moreover, not all plant life is beneficial. There are poisonous plants, and some of them are deadly, especially if used for long periods of time. In fact, it is important to point out that qualified herbalists use herbs with great care. Also, since herbs contain active ingredients, you should be aware that some of these elements may interact negatively with prescribed medications. It is therefore wise to consult a health professional when there is any question about safety.

As a general guideline, most of the bitter-tasting herbs are medicinal herbs. The pleasant-tasting herbs are potentially less toxic and can be used more often. All plant roots and bark are naturally fungicidal and bactericidal. (If they

were not, pathogens would destroy them in the ground.) Certain herbs should be used only for healing purposes, and not for extended periods of time. Also, the active ingredients in most herbs are more potent when the herbs are freshly picked. However, roots, bark, and other herb parts can retain their medicinal value for years if thoroughly dried and kept dry.

WHAT'S ON THE SHELVES

The fresh leaves, bark, and roots of herbs can be used in their natural form, or they can be found in the form of tablets, capsules, liquid beverages, bark pieces, powders, extracts, tinctures, creams, lotions, salves, and oils. The whole leaves, berries, seeds, roots, flowers, and bark of herbs are also dried and made available to consumers.

HOW TO USE HERBS

The many ways in which herbs can be used include:

• *Compresses.* A compress is a cloth soaked in a warm or cool herbal solution and applied directly on the injured area.

• *Decoctions.* A tea is made from the bark, root, seed, or berry of a plant. Decoctions should not be boiled; they should only be simmered for approximately twenty to thirty minutes, unless the product label states otherwise.

• *Essential oils.* Essential oils are derived from herbs or other plants through steam distillation or cold pressing. They are usually mixed with a vegetable oil or water, and used either as a mouth, ear, or eye wash, or as an inhalant, douche, or tea. These oils can also be used externally in massage or on burns and abrasions. Essential oils readily combine with the natural fats present in the skin. With a few exceptions, such as the use of camphor, eucalyptus, or tea tree oil for certain skin conditions, essential oils should always be diluted in either water or oil before being applied to the body, and they should not be taken internally except under the direction of a physician trained in their use.

• *Extracts.* Extracts are made by pressing herbs with a heavy hydraulic press and soaking them in alcohol or water. Excess alcohol or water is allowed to evaporate, yielding a concentrated extract. Extracts are the most effective form of herbs, especially for people with severe illnesses or malabsorption problems. Alcohol-free extracts, if available, are usually best. Herbal extracts should generally be diluted in a small amount of water before being ingested.

The following are some herbal extracts that are very beneficial in healing. They can be found in health food stores. Add these extracts to juices, and take them while fasting for greatest benefits:

Burdock	Ginkgo biloba	Red clover
Cat's claw	Goldenseal	Parsley
Celery	Hawthorn	Pau d'arco
Echinacea	Horsetail	Pumpkin
Fig	Licorice	Red beet crystals
Garlic	Milk thistle	Suma
Ginger	Nettle	Valerian root

• *Herbal vinegars.* Herbs are put into raw apple cider vinegar, rice vinegar, or malt vinegar and left to stand for two or more weeks.

• *Infusions.* Leaves, flowers, or other delicate parts of the plant are steeped, not boiled, for five to ten minutes in hot water, so that the benefits of the herbs are not destroyed. (*See* Herbal Teas and Their Effects, below.)

• *Ointments.* An extract, tea, pressed juice, or powdered form of an herb is added to a salve that is applied to the affected area.

• *Poultices.* A poultice is a hot, soft, moist mass of herbs, flour, mustard, or other substance spread on muslin or other loosely woven cloth and applied for up to twenty-four hours on a sore or inflamed area of the body to relieve pain and inflammation. Ground or granulated herbs are best. The cloth should be changed when it cools. (*See* USING A POULTICE in Part Three for further information on the uses of poultices.)

• *Powder.* The useful part of the herb is ground into a powder, which may then be made into capsules or tablets.

• *Syrup.* Herbs are added to a form of sugar and then boiled.

• *Salves.* Salves, creams, oils, and lotions are generally used on bruises, sores, and inflammations, and for poultices.

• *Tinctures.* Tinctures are a well-preserved form of previously fresh herbs. Most tinctures contain varying amounts of alcohol; however, there are now some on the market that contain less alcohol, and some that are alcohol-free.

If there are several herbs recommended for a certain disorder, it is best to alternate among the different herbs, so that you obtain the benefits of each. This may also help you to determine which herb agrees best with your body's chemistry and particular needs. Also, do not preserve herbs in clear glass jars; use colored glass or ceramic jars instead. The potency of herbs can be destroyed by exposure to light.

HERBAL TEAS AND THEIR EFFECTS

Herbal teas are the most convenient form of herbal remedy for long-term use. The powerful ingredients of the herb are diluted by water when made into tea. Mild teas may be used daily as tonics and for general well-being.

To prepare an herbal tea, use approximately 1 to 3 teaspoons of herbs per cup of boiling water. Boil water in a kettle as you would for ordinary tea, but do not use an aluminum kettle. Pour the water into a ceramic or glass (not metal) mug or teapot and leave the herbs to steep for at least five minutes (but don't leave them for longer than ten minutes or the tea may have a bitter taste). If you prefer a stronger tea, increase the amount of herbs used rather than steeping the tea for a longer period.

HERBS AND THEIR USES

The following table describes roughly 100 of the most commonly used medicinal herbs, including which parts of each herb are used, its chemical and nutrient content, and its various uses.

Herb	Parts Used	Chemical and Nutrient Content	Actions and Uses	Comments
Alfalfa	Flowers, leaves, petals, sprouts.	Alpha-carotene, beta-carotene, B-complex vitamins, calcium, chlorophyll, copper, essential amino acids, iron, magnesium, phosphorus, potassium, protein, sodium, sulfur, zinc, vitamins A, C, D, E, and K.	Alkalizes and detoxifies the body. Acts as a diuretic, eases inflammation, lowers cholesterol, balances hormones, and promotes pituitary gland function. Also contains an antifungal agent. Good for anemia, bleeding-related disorders, bone and joint disorders, colon and digestive disorders, skin disorders, and ulcers.	Must be used in fresh, raw form to provide vitamins. Sprouts are especially effective.

Herb	Parts Used	Chemical and Nutrient Content	Actions and Uses	Comments
Aloe vera	Pulp from insides of succulent leaves.	Anthroquinone, glucomannan, magnesium lactate, polysaccharides.	Applied externally, heals burns and wounds; stimulates cell regeneration; and has astringent, emollient, antifungal, and antibacterial and antiviral properties. Taken internally, soothes stomach irritation, aids in healing, and has laxative properties. Good for AIDS and for skin and digestive disorders.	Allergy, though rare, may occur in susceptible individuals. Before using, apply a small amount behind the ear or on the underarm. If stinging or rash occurs, do not use.
Anise	Seeds.	Alpha-pinene, creosol, dianethole, essential oils, proanethole.	Aids digestion, clears mucus from air passages, combats infection, and promotes milk production in nursing mothers. Good for indigestion and for respiratory infections such as sinusitis. Also helpful for menopausal symptoms.	Used in many popular products as a fragrance and flavoring.
Astragalus	Roots.	Betaine, B-sitosterol, choline, dimethoxyisoflavone, glucoronic acid, kumatakenin, sucrose.	Acts as a tonic to protect the immune system. Aids adrenal gland function and digestion. Increases metabolism, produces spontaneous sweating, promotes healing, and provides energy to combat fatigue. Increases stamina. Good for colds, flu, and immune-deficiency-related problems, including AIDS, cancer, and tumors. Effective for chronic lung weakness.	Also called huang qi. *Caution:* Should not be taken in the presence of a fever.
Barberry	Bark, berries, roots.	Berbamine, berberine, berberrubine, columbamine, hydrastine, jatrorrhizine, manganese, oxycanthine, palmatine, vitamin C.	Decreases heart rate, slows breathing, reduces bronchial constriction, kills bacteria on the skin, and stimulates intestinal movement.	*Caution:* Should not be used during pregnancy.
Bayberry	Root bark.	Acrid and astringent resins, albumin, berberine, essential oil, gum, lignin, mycricic acid, myricinic acid, starch, sucrose, tannic and gallic acids.	Helps clear congestion, aids circulation, reduces fever, acts as an astringent. Helpful for stopping bleeding. Good for circulatory disorders, fever, hypothyroidism, and ulcers. Also good for the eyes and immune system.	The wax of the berries is used to make fragrant candles.
Bilberry	Entire plant.	Fatty acids, flavonoids, hydroquinone, iron, loeanolic acid, neomyrtillin, sodium, tannins, ursolic acid.	Helps to control insulin levels and strengthen connective tissue. Acts as a diuretic and urinary tract antiseptic. Useful for hypoglycemia, inflammation, stress, anxiety, night blindness, and cataracts. May help halt or prevent macular degeneration.	Also known as blueberry. *Caution:* Interferes with iron absorption when taken internally.
Birch	Bark, leaves, sap.	Betulin, creosol, creosote, guaiacol, methyl salicylate, phenol.	Acts as a diuretic, lessens inflammation, and relieves pain. Good for joint pain and urinary tract infections. Applied externally, is good for boils and sores.	
Black cohosh	Rhizomes, roots.	Actaeine, cimicifugin, estrogenic substances, isoferulic acid, oleic acid, palmitic acid, pantothenic acid, phosphorus, racemosin, tannins, triterpenes, vitamin A.	Lowers blood pressure and cholesterol levels, and reduces mucus production. Helps cardiovascular and circulatory disorders; induces labor and aids in childbirth; relieves hot flashes, menstrual cramps with back pain, morning sickness, and pain. Helpful for poisonous snake bites. Good for arthritis.	Also known as black snakeroot. *Caution:* Should not be used during pregnancy until birth is imminent, or in the presence of chronic disease.
Black walnut	Husks, inner bark, leaves, nuts.	Ellagic acid, juglone, mucin.	Aids digestion and promotes healing of mouth or throat sores. Cleanses the body of some types of parasites. Good for bruising, fungal infection, herpes, poison ivy, and warts.	When boiled, the hulls produce a dye that is used to dye wool.

Herb	Parts Used	Chemical and Nutrient Content	Actions and Uses	Comments
Blessed thistle	Various parts.	Cincin, essential oils.	Increases appetite and stomach secretions. Heals the liver. Alleviates inflammation, improves circulation, purifies the blood, and strengthens the heart. May act as brain food. Good for female disorders. Also aids milk flow in the nursing mother.	*Caution:* Must be handled with care to avoid toxic skin effects.
Blue cohosh	Roots.	Calcium, coulosaponin, folic acid, gum, inositol, iron, leontin, magnesium, methyl-cystine, pantothenic acid, phosphoric acid, phosphorus, potassium, salts, silicon, starch, vitamins B_3 and E.	Relieves muscle spasms and stimulates uterine contractions for childbirth. Useful for memory problems, menstrual disorders, and nervous disorders.	*Caution:* Should not be used during the first two trimesters of pregnancy.
Boneset	Flower petals, leaves.	Essential oils, eupatroin, resin, sugar, tremetrol, wax.	Relieves congestion, loosens phlegm, reduces fever, increases perspiration, calms the body, acts as a laxative. Has anti-inflammatory properties. Useful for bronchitis and fever-induced aches and pains.	Also called white snakeroot. *Caution:* Long-term use is not advised, as toxicity may occur.
Borage	Leaves, seeds.	Calcium, essential oil, gamma-linolenic acid, linoleic acid, linolenic acid, mucilage, oleic acid, palmitic acid, potassium, tannins.	An adrenal tonic and gland balancer. Contains valuable minerals and essential fatty acids needed for proper cardiovascular function and healthy skin and nails.	The flowers of the borage plant are edible.
Buchu	Leaves.	Barosma camphor, diasmin, essential oils, l-enthone, hesperidin, mucilage, resin.	Decreases inflammation of the colon, gums, mucous membranes, prostate, sinuses, and vagina. Aids in controlling bladder and kidney problems, diabetes, digestive disorders, fluid retention, and prostate disorders. A specific for bladder infections.	Do not boil buchu leaves.
Burdock	Roots, seeds.	Arctiin, biotin, copper, essential oils, inulin, iron, manganese, sulfur, tannins, zinc, vitamins B_1, B_6, B_{12}, and E.	Purifies the blood, restores liver and gallbladder function, and stimulates the immune system. Helps skin disorders such as boils and carbuncles and relieves gout symptoms.	*Caution:* Interferes with iron absorption when taken internally.
Butcher's broom	Seeds, tops.	Alkaloids, hydroxytyramine, ruscogenins.	Relieves inflammation. Useful for carpal tunnel syndrome, circulatory disorders, edema, Ménière's disease, obesity, Raynaud's phenomenon, thrombophlebitis, varicose veins, and vertigo. Also good for the bladder and kidneys.	More effective if taken with vitamin C.
Calendula	Flower petals.	Carotene, calenduline, lycopine, saponin, resin, essential oil.	A natural anti-inflammatory and skin soother. Also helps to regulate the menstrual cycle and lessens fever. Useful for many skin disorders, such as rashes and sunburn, as well as for neuritis and toothache. Good for diaper rash and other skin problems in small children.	Generally nonirritating when used externally.
Cascara sagrada	Bark.	Anthraquinone, B-complex vitamins, calcium, cascarosides, essential oils, inositol, manganese, potassium.	Acts as a colon cleanser and as a laxative. Useful for colon disorders, constipation, and parasitic infestation.	Is very bitter in tea form.

Herb	Parts Used	Chemical and Nutrient Content	Actions and Uses	Comments
Catnip	Leaves.	Acetic acid, biotin, buteric acid, choline, citral, dipentene, essential oils, folic acid, inositol, lifronella, limonene, manganese, nepetalic acid, pantothenic acid, para-aminobenzoic acid, phosphorus, sodium, sulfur, valeric acid, vitamins A, B_1, B_2, B_3, B_6, and B_{12}.	Controls fever (catnip tea enemas reduce fever quickly). Aids digestion and sleep; relieves stress; stimulates the appetite. Good for anxiety, colds and flu, inflammation, pain, and stress.	
Cat's claw	Inner bark, roots.	Plant sterols, polyphenols, proanthocyanidins, oxindole alkaloids, quinovic acid glycosides, triterpenes.	Cleanses the intestinal tract, enhances the action of white blood cells, and acts as an antioxidant and anti-inflammatory. Good for intestinal problems and viral infections. May be helpful for people with AIDS, arthritis, cancer, tumors, or ulcers.	Also called uña de gato. *Caution:* Should not be used during pregnancy.
Cayenne	Berries.	Apsaicine, capsacutin, capsaicin, capsanthine, capsico, cobalt, folic acid, pantothenic acid, para-aminobenzoic acid, zinc, vitamins A, B_1, B_2, B_3, B_6, and C.	Aids digestion, improves circulation, and stops bleeding from ulcers. Acts as a catalyst for other herbs. Good for the heart, kidneys, lungs, pancreas, spleen, and stomach. Useful for arthritis and rheumatism. Helps to ward off colds, sinus infections, and sore throats. Good for pain when applied topically. Used with lobelia for nerves.	Also called capsicum, hot pepper, red pepper.
Cedar	Leaves, tops.	Borneal, bornyl acetate, camphor, flavonoids, isothujone, mucilage, tannins, thujone.	Has antiviral and antifungal properties, stimulates the immune system, and increases venous blood flow. Acts as an expectorant, lymphatic cleanser, and urinary antiseptic. Can be used externally for warts.	
Celery	Juice, roots, seeds.	B-complex vitamins, iron, vitamins A and C.	Reduces blood pressure, relieves muscle spasms, and improves appetite. Good for arthritis and kidney problems. Acts as an antioxidant and as a sedative.	*Caution:* Do not use in large amounts during pregnancy.
Chamomile	Various parts.	Antheme, anthemic acid, anthesterol, apigenin, calcium, chamazulene, essential oils, iron, magnesium, manganese, potassium, tannic acid, tiglic acid, vitamin A.	An anti-inflammatory, appetite stimulant, digestive aid, diuretic, nerve tonic, and sleep aid. Helps colitis, diverticulosis, fever, headaches, and pain. It is a traditional remedy for stress and anxiety, indigestion, and insomnia.	*Caution:* Should not be used for long periods of time, as this may lead to ragweed allergy. Should not be used by those who are allergic to ragweed.
Chaparral	Leaves.	Nordihydroquaiaretic acid, sodium, sulfur, zinc.	Bitter herb that acts as a free radical scavenger. Protects against harmful effects of radiation and sun exposure. Good for skin disorders. Protects against the formation of tumors and cancer cells and relieves pain.	*Caution:* Recommended for external use only. Taking it internally, especially in large doses and/or for prolonged periods, can cause liver damage.
Chickweed	Various parts.	Biotin, choline, copper, inositol, para-aminobenzoic acid, phosphorus, potash salts, rutin, silicon, sodium, vitamins B_6, B_{12}, C, and D.	Reduces mucus buildup in the lungs. May lower blood lipids. Useful for bronchitis, circulatory problems, colds, coughs, skin diseases, and warts. A good source of vitamin C and other nutrients.	Also called starweed.

Herb	Parts Used	Chemical and Nutrient Content	Actions and Uses	Comments
Cinnamon	Bark.	Cinnamic aldehyde, essential oils, eugenol, metholeugenol, mucilage, sucrose, starch, tannin.	Relieves diarrhea and nausea; counteracts congestion; aids the peripheral circulation of the blood. Warms the body and enhances digestion, especially the metabolism of fats. Also fights fungal infection. Useful for digestive problems, diabetes, weight loss, yeast infection, and uterine hemorraging.	*Caution:* Do not use in large amounts during pregnancy.
Clove	Flower buds, essential oil.	Caryophylline, eugenol, eugenyl acetate.	Has antiseptic and antiparasitic properties, and acts as a digestive aid. Essential oil is applied topically for relief of mouth pain.	*Caution:* Clove oil is very strong and can cause irritation if used in its pure form. Diluting the oil in olive oil or distilled water is recommended. Essential oil should not be taken internally except under the careful supervision of a health care professional.
Comfrey	Leaves, roots.	Allantoin, consolidine, mucilage, phosphorus, potassium, pyrrolizidine, starch, tannins, vitamins A, C, and E.	Speeds healing of wounds and skin conditions. Beneficial for many problems affecting the skin, including bedsores, bites and stings, bruises, inflamed bunions, burns, dermatitis, dry skin, bleeding hemorrhoids, leg ulcers, nosebleeds, psoriais, scabies, skin rashes, and sunburn.	Also called knitbone. *Caution:* May cause liver damage if taken internally. Not recommended for internal use except under the careful supervision of a health care professional. External use is generally considered safe. Should not be used during pregnancy.
Corn silk	Stamens.	Alkaloids, cryptoxanthin, fluorine, malic acid, oxalic acid, palmitic acid, panthothenic acid, resin, saponins, silicon, sitosterol, stigmasterol, tartaric acid, vitamin K.	Aids the bladder, kidneys, and small intestine. Acts as a diuretic. Good for bed-wetting, carpal tunnel syndrome, edema, obesity, premenstrual syndrome, and prostate disorders. Good used in combination with other "kidney herbs" to open the urinary tract and remove mucus from the urine.	
Cranberry	Juice from berries.	Alpha D-mannopyranoside, vitamin C.	Acidifies the urine and prevents bacteria from adhering to the bladder. Helpful for infections of the urinary tract. A good source of vitamin C.	Commercial cranberry juice cocktail products contain high amounts of sugar. It is best to buy pure, unsweetened cranberry juice concentrate and prepare it using as little sugar as possible.
Damiana	Leaves.	Arbutin, chlorophyll, damianian, essential oils, resin, starch, sugar, tannins.	Stimulates muscular contractions of the intestinal tract and brings oxygen to the genital area. Used as an energy tonic and aphrodisiac, as well as to remedy sexual and hormonal problems. A "sexuality tonic" for women.	*Caution:* Interferes with iron absorption when taken internally.

Herb	Parts Used	Chemical and Nutrient Content	Actions and Uses	Comments
Dandelion	Leaves, roots, tops.	Bioflavonoids, biotin, calcium, choline, fats, folic acid, gluten, gum, inositol, inulin, iron, lactupicrine, linolenic acid, magnesium, niacin, pantothenic acid, para-aminobenzoic acid, phosphorus, potash, proteins, resin, sulfur, zinc, vitamins A, B_1, B_2, B_6, B_{12}, C, and E.	Cleanses the bloodstream and liver, and increases the production of bile. Used as a diuretic. Also reduces serum cholesterol and uric acid. Improves functioning of the kidneys, pancreas, spleen, and stomach. Useful for abscesses, anemia, boils, breast tumors, cirrhosis of the liver, fluid retention, hepatitis, jaundice, and rheumatism. May aid in the prevention of age spots and breast cancer.	The roasted root can be used as a coffee substitute.
Dong quai	Roots.	Alcohols, cadinene, carotene, carvacrol, coumarin, essential oil, isosafrol, safrol, sesquiterpenes, sucrose, vitamins A, B_{12}, and E.	Increases the effects of ovarian and testicular hormones. Used in the treatment of female problems such as hot flashes and other menopausal symptoms, premenstrual syndrome, and vaginal dryness.	Also known as angelica.
Echinacea	Leaves, roots.	Arabinose, betaine, copper, echinacen, echinacin B, echinacoside, echinolone, enzymes, fructose, fatty acids, galactose, glucose, glucuronic acid, inulin, inuloid, iron, pentadecadiene, polyacetylene compounds, polysaccharides, potassium, protein, resin, rhamnose, sucrose, sulfur, tannins, xylose, vitamins A, C, and E.	Stimulates certain white blood cells and has anti-inflammatory and antiviral properties. Good for the immune system and the lymphatic system. Useful for colic, colds, flu, and other infectious illnesses. Also helpful for snakebite.	Also called coneflower. Available fresh, freeze-dried, dried, or as alcohol-based extract, liquid, tea, capsules, or salve. For internal use, the freeze-dried form or alcohol-free extract is recommended. *Caution:* Should not be used by those who are allergic to plants in the sunflower family.
Elder	Berries, flowers, inner bark, leaves, roots.	Anthocyanin, B-complex vitamins, calcium, carbohydrates, fat, itydrocyanic acid, potassium, protein, rutin, sambucine, tannic acid, tyrosin, vitamins A and C.	Builds the blood, cleanses the system, eases constipation, enhances immune system function, fights inflammation, increases perspiration, lowers fever, soothes the respiratory tract, and stimulates circulation. Also has powerful antioxidant properties. The flowers are used to soothe skin irritations.	*Caution:* Do not consume the stems of this plant. The stems contain cyanide, and can be very toxic.
Ephedra	Stems.	Essential oil, saponins, ephedrine and other alkaloids.	Acts as a decongestant, aids in the elimination of fluids, relieves bronchial spasm, and stimulates the central nervous system. Also may decrease appetite and elevate mood. Useful for allergies, asthma, colds, and other respiratory complaints, as well as for depression and obesity.	Also known as ma huang. *Caution:* Should not be used by persons who have anxiety disorder (panic attacks), glaucoma, heart disease, or high blood pressure, or who are taking monoamine oxidase (MAO) inhibitor drugs, commonly prescribed for depression.
Eucalyptus	Bark, essential oil, leaves.	Aldehyde, bitter resin, eucalyptol, tannins.	Clears congestion, has a mild antiseptic action, and reduces swelling by helping to increase blood flow. Relaxes tired and sore muscles. Good for colds, coughs, and other respiratory disorders.	Recommended for external use only. It should not be used on broken skin or open cuts or wounds.

Herb	Parts Used	Chemical and Nutrient Content	Actions and Uses	Comments
Eyebright	Entire plant, except the root.	Bitters, inositol, essential oils, pantothenic acid, para-aminobenzoic acid, sulfur, tannins, vitamins A, B_3, B_{12}, C, D, and E.	Used as an eyewash. Prevents secretion of fluids and relieves discomfort from eyestrain or minor irritation. Good for allergies, itchy and/or watery eyes, and runny nose. Also used to combat hay fever.	
False unicorn root	Roots.	Chamaelirin, fatty acids.	Balances sex hormones. Useful for treatment of infertility, menstrual irregularities and pain, premenstrual syndrome, and prostate disorders. May help prevent miscarriage.	Also called helonias.
Fennel	Berries, roots, stems.	Anethole, calcium, camphene cymene, chlorine, dipentene, essential oils, fenchone, limonene, oleic acid, petroselinic acid, phellandrene, pinene, 7-hydroxycoumarin, stigmasterol, sulfur, vitamins A and C.	Used as an appetite suppressant and as an eyewash. Promotes the functioning of the kidneys, liver, and spleen, and also clears the lungs. Relieves abdominal pain, colon disorders, gas, and gastrointestinal tract spasms. Useful for acid stomach. Good after chemotherapy and/or radiation treatments for cancer.	The powdered plant can be used as a flea repellant.
Fenugreek	Seeds.	Biotin, choline, essential oils, folic acid, inositol, iron, lecithin, mucilage, pantothenic acid, para-aminobenzoic acid, phosphates, protein, trigonelline, trimethylamine, vitamins A, B_1, B_2, B_3, B_6, B_{12}, and D.	Acts as a bulk laxative, lubricates the intestines, and reduces fever. Good for the eyes. Helps asthma and sinus problems by reducing mucus. Good for inflammation and lung disorders.	Oil of fenugreek has a maple-like flavor.
Feverfew	Bark, dried flowers, leaves.	Borneol, camphor, parthenolide, pyrethrins, santamarin, terpene.	Increases fluidity of lung and bronchial tube mucus, promotes menses, stimulates the appetite, and stimulates uterine contractions. Good for arthritis, colitis, fever, headaches, menstrual problems, muscle tension, pain.	Chewing the leaves is a folk remedy, but this may cause mouth sores. Also called featherfew, featherfoil. *Caution:* Should not be used during pregnancy.
Flax	Seeds, oil from seeds.	Beta-carotene, glycosides, gum, linamarin, linoleic acid, linolenic acid, mucilage, oleic acid, protein, saturated acids, tannins, wax, vitamin E.	Promotes strong bones, nails, and teeth, as well as healthy skin. Useful for colon problems, female disorders, and inflammation.	An excellent addition to diets that are low in fiber.
Garlic	Bulb.	Allicin, allyl disulfides, calcium, copper, essential oils, germanium, iron, magnesium, manganese, phosphorus, phytoncides, potassium, selenium, sulfur, unsaturated aldehydes, zinc, vitamins A, B_1, B_2, and C.	Detoxifies the body and protects against infection by enhancing immune function. Lowers blood pressure and improves circulation. Lowers blood lipid levels. Aids in the treatment of arteriosclerosis, arthritis, asthma, cancer, circulatory problems, colds and flu, digestive problems, heart disorders, insomnia, liver disease, sinusitis, ulcers, and yeast infections. Good for virtually any disease or infection.	Garlic contains many sulfur compounds, which give it its marvelous healing properties. Odorless garlic supplements are available. Aged garlic extract (such as Kyolic) is the best.
Gentian	Leaves, roots.	Gentiamarin, gentiin, gentisin, mesogentiogenin, protogentiogenin, sugar, xanthone pigment.	Aids digestion, boosts circulation, increases gastric secretions, kills plasmodia (organisms that cause malaria) and worms, and stimulates appetite. Good for circulatory problems, pancreatitis, and parasitic infection.	Also called bitter root.

Herb	Parts Used	Chemical and Nutrient Content	Actions and Uses	Comments
Ginger	Rhizomes, roots.	Acrid resin, bisabolene, borneal, borneol, camphene, choline, cineole, citral, essential oils, folic acid, ginerol, inositol, manganese, pantothenic acid, para-aminobenzoic acid, phellandrene, sequiterpene, silicon, zingerone, zingiberene, vitamin B_3.	Cleanses the colon, reduces spasms and cramps, and stimulates circulation. A strong antioxidant and effective antimicrobial agent for sores and wounds. Useful for bowel disorders, circulatory problems, fever, hot flashes, indigestion, morning sickness, motion sickness, nausea, and vomiting.	Can cause stomach distress if taken in large quantities.
Ginkgo	Leaves.	Ginkgolides, heterosides.	Improves brain functioning by increasing cerebral and peripheral blood flow, circulation, and oxygenation. Good for depression, headaches, memory loss, and tinnitis (ringing in the ears). May relieve leg cramps by improving circulation. Beneficial for asthma, eczema, and heart and kidney disorders.	Take for at least 2 weeks for best results.
Ginseng (Siberian, American, Korean [or Chinese])	Roots.	Arabinose, calcium, camphor, eleutherosides, gineosides, iron, mucilage, panaxosides, resin, saponin, starch, vitamins A, B_1, B_{12}, and E.	Strengthens the adrenal and reproductive glands. Enhances immune function, promotes lung functioning, and stimulates the appetite. Useful for bronchitis, circulatory problems, diabetes, infertility, lack of energy, and stress; to ease withdrawal from cocaine; and to protect against the effects of radiation exposure. Used by athletes for overall body strengthening.	Siberian ginseng belongs to a different botanical family than American and Korean ginseng, but the properties and uses of all three are similar, and all are generally referred to as ginseng. *Caution:* Should not be used by those with hypoglycemia, high blood pressure, or heart disorders.
Goldenseal	Rhizomes, roots.	Albumin, B-complex vitamins, berberine, biotin, calcium, candine, chlorine, choline, chologenic acid, essential oils, fats, hydrastine, inositol, iron, lignin, manganese, para-aminobenzoic acid, phosphorus, potassium, resin, starch, sugar, vitamins A, C, and E.	Acts as an antibiotic, cleanses the body, has anti-inflammatory and antibacterial properties, increases the effectiveness of insulin, and strengthens the immune system. Promotes functioning capacity of the colon, liver, pancreas, spleen, and lymphatic and respiratory systems. Cleanses mucous membranes, counters infection, improves digestion, and regulates menses. Also decreases uterine bleeding, reduces blood pressure, and stimulates the central nervous system. Good for inflammation, ulcers, and any infectious disease, as well as for disorders affecting the bladder, prostate, stomach, or vagina. Used at the first sign of possible symptoms, it can stop a cold, flu, or sore throat from developing.	Alternating goldenseal with echinacea or other herbs good for a particular disorder is recommended. Alcohol-free extract is the best form of this herb. *Caution:* Should not be used for prolonged periods or during pregnancy. Should be used under supervision by those with cardiovascular disease, diabetes, or glaucoma.
Gotu kola	Nuts, roots, seeds.	Catechol, epicatechol, magnesium, theobromine, vitamin K.	Aids in the elimination of excess fluids, decreases fatigue and depression, increases sex drive, shrinks tissues, and stimulates the central nervous system. May neutralize blood acids and lower body temperature, and is good for heart and liver function. Useful for cardiovascular and circulatory disorders, fatigue, connective tissue disorders, kidney stones, poor appetite, and sleep disorders.	May cause dermatitis if applied topically.

Herb	Parts Used	Chemical and Nutrient Content	Actions and Uses	Comments
Gravel root	Flowers, roots.	Euparin, eupurpurin.	Acts as a diuretic and urinary tract tonic. Good for combating prostate disorders and problems related to fluid retention.	Also called joe-pye weed, queen-of-the-meadow.
Green tea	Leaves.	Bioflavonoids, caffeine, catechins, epigallocatechin, flavonoids, fluoride, gallic acid, polyphenols, tannins, theophylline, vitamin C.	Combats mental fatigue. May lower the risk of esophageal, stomach, colon, and skin cancer, and delay the onset of arteriosclerosis.	*Caution:* Should not be used in large quantities during pregnancy or while nursing. Persons with anxiety disorder or irregular heartbeat should limit their intake to no more than 2 cups daily.
Hawthorn	Berries, flowers, leaves.	Anthocyanin-type pigments, choline, citric acid, cratagolic acid, flavone, flavonoids, folic acid, glycosides, inositol, pantothenic acid, para-aminobenzoic acid, purines, saponins, sugar, tartaric acid, vitamins B_1 (thiamine), B_2 (riboflavin), B_3 (niacin), B_6 (pyridoxine), B_{12}, and C.	Dilates the coronary blood vessels, lowers cholesterol levels, and restores heart muscle. Increases intracellular vitamin C levels. Useful for anemia, cardiovascular and circulatory disorders, high cholesterol, and lowered immunity.	
Hops	Berries, flowers, leaves.	Asparagine, choline, essential oil, humulene, inositol, lupulin, lupulinic acid, lupulon, manganese, para-aminobenzoic acid, picric acids, resin, vitamin B_6 (pyridoxine).	Good for anxiety, cardiovascular disorders, hyperactivity, insomnia, nervousness, pain, restlessness, sexually transmitted diseases, shock, stress, toothaches, and ulcers.	Placed inside a pillowcase, aids sleep.
Horehound	Flowers, leaves.	B-complex vitamins, essential fatty acids, essential oils, iron, marrubiin, potassium, resin, tannins, vitamins A, C, and E.	Decreases thickness and increases fluidity of mucus in the bronchial tubes and lungs. Useful for hay fever, sinusitis, and other respiratory disorders. Also boosts the immune system.	
Horsetail	Stems.	Aconitic acid, calcium, copper, equisitine, fatty acids, fluorine, nicotine, pantothenic acid, para-aminobenzoic acid, silica, sodium, starch, zinc.	Increases calcium absorption, which promotes healthy skin and strengthens bone, hair, nails, and teeth. Promotes healing of broken bones and connective tissue. Strengthens the heart and lungs and acts as a diuretic. Useful for the treatment of arthritis, bone diseases such as osteoporosis and rickets, bronchitis, cardiovascular disease, edema, gallbladder disorders, inflammation, muscle cramps, and prostate disorders. Used in poultice form to depress bleeding and accelerate healing of burns and wounds.	Also called bottle brush, shavegrass.
Hydrangea	Roots.	Essential oil, hydrangin, resin, saponin.	Acts as a diuretic and stimulates the kidneys. Good for bladder infection, kidney disease, obesity, and prostate disorders. Combined with gravel root, good for kidney stones.	*Caution:* Do not consume the leaves of this plant. They contain cyanide and can be toxic.

Herb	Parts Used	Chemical and Nutrient Content	Actions and Uses	Comments
Hyssop	Aerial parts.	Diosmine, essential oil, flavonoids, marrubin, tannins.	Relieves congestion, regulates blood pressure, and dispels gas. Used externally, helpful for wound healing. Good for circulatory problems, epilepsy, fever, gout, and weight problems. Poultices made from fresh green hyssop help to heal cuts.	
Irish moss	Entire plant.	Amino acids, bromine, calcium, carrageenan, chlorine, iodide, iron, manganese salts, mucins, protein, sodium.	Aids in the formation of stools and is good for many intestinal disorders. Also used in skin lotions.	Used in hair rinses for dry hair.
Juniper	Berries.	Alcohols, cadinene, camphene, essential oils, flavone, resin, sabinal, sugar, sulfur, tannins, terpinene.	Acts as a diuretic, helps to regulate blood sugar levels, and relieves inflammation and congestion. Helpful in treatment of asthma, bladder infection, fluid retention, gout, kidney problems, obesity, and prostate disorders.	*Caution:* May interfere with absorption of iron and other minerals when taken internally.
Kava kava	Roots.	Demethoxyangonin, dihydrokawin, dihydromethysticin, flavorawin A, kawain, methysticin, starch, yangonin.	Induces physical and mental relaxation. Acts as a diuretic and genitourinary antiseptic. Helpful for anxiety, depression, insomnia, stress-related disorders, and urinary tract infections.	Also called kava. *Caution:* Can cause drowsiness. If this occurs, use should be discontinued or the dosage reduced.
Lavender	Flowers.	Essential oil, geraniol, linalol 1-linalyl acetate.	Relieves stress and depression, and is beneficial for the skin. Good for burns, headaches, psoriasis, and skin problems.	Essential oil of lavender is very popular in aromatherapy.
Lemon-grass	Various parts.	Essential oils, citronellal, methylneptenone, terpene, terpene alcohol.	Has astringent and tonic properties. Good for the skin and nails.	Used in perfumes and other products as a fragrance.
Licorice	Roots.	Asparagine, biotin, choline, fat, folic acid, glycyrrhizin, gum, inositol, lecithin, manganese, pantothenic acid, para-aminobenzoic acid, pentacyclic terpenes, phosphorus, protein, sugar, yellow dye, vitamins B_1, B_2, B_3, B_6, and E.	Cleanses the colon, decreases muscular spasms, increases fluidity of mucus in the lungs and bronchial tubes, and promotes adrenal gland function. Has estrogen- and progesterone-like effects; may change the pitch of the voice. Also stimulates the production of interferon. Beneficial for allergic disorders, asthma, chronic fatigue, depression, emphysema, fever, herpesvirus infection, hypoglycemia, and inflammatory bowel disorders. Deglycyrrhizinated licorice may stimulate natural defense mechanisms that prevent the occurrence of ulcers by increasing the amount of mucus-secreting cells in the digestive tract. This improves the quality of mucus, lengthens intestinal cell life, and enhances microcirculation in the gastrointestinal lining.	Licorice derivatives have been recommended as a standard support for ulcer sufferers in Europe. *Caution:* Should not be used during pregnancy, or by persons with diabetes, glaucoma, heart disease, high blood pressure, severe menstrual problems, or a history of stroke. Also, should not be used on a daily basis for more than seven days in a row, as this can result in high blood pressure in persons with previously normal blood pressure.

Herb	Parts Used	Chemical and Nutrient Content	Actions and Uses	Comments
Lobelia	Flowers, leaves, seeds.	Alkaloids, chelidonic acid, isolobeline, lobelic acid, lobeline, selenium, sulfur.	A cough suppressant and relaxant that aids in hormone production and reduces cold symptoms and fever. Beneficial in the treatment of asthma, bronchitis, colds and flu, cardiovascular disease, epilepsy, pain, and viral infection.	Also called Indian tobacco. *Caution:* Should be used with caution, and should not be taken internally on an ongoing basis. Has nicotinelike effects on the body; taking more than 50 mg of dried lobelia can suppress breathing, depress blood pressure, and even lead to coma.
Marsh-mallow	Flowers, leaves, roots.	Asparagine, coumarin, fat, flavonoids, mucilage, pectin, polysaccharides, salicylic acid, tannins.	Soothes and heals skin, mucous membranes, and other tissues, externally and internally. Also acts as a diuretic and expectorant. Good for bladder infection, digestive upsets, fluid retention, headache, intestinal disorders, kidney problems, sinusitis, and sore throat.	Often used as a filler in the compounding of pills.
Milk thistle	Fruits, leaves, seeds.	The active component is silymarin, a unique type of flavonoid with antioxidant ability.	Contains some of the most potent liver-protecting substances known. Prevents free radical damage by acting as an antioxidant, protecting the liver. Also stimulates the production of new liver cells and prevents formation of damaging leukotrienes. Protects the kidneys. Good for adrenal disorders, inflammatory bowel disorders, weakened immune system, and all liver disorders, such as jaundice and hepatitis. Also beneficial for psoriasis.	Also called Mary thistle, wild artichoke.
Mullein	Leaves.	Aucubin, choline, hesperidin, magnesium, pantothenic acid, para-aminobenzoic acid, saponins, sulfur, verbaside, vitamins B_2, B_{12}, and D.	Acts as a laxative, painkiller, and sleep aid. Gets rid of warts. Useful for asthma, bronchitis, difficulty breathing, earache, hay fever, and swollen glands. Used in kidney formulas to soothe inflammation.	
Mustard	Seeds.	Myrosin, sinalbin, sinapine.	Improves digestion and aids in the metabolism of fat. Applied externally, helpful for chest congestion, inflammation, injuries, and joint pain.	*Caution:* Can be irritating when applied directly to the skin.
Myrrh	Resin from stems.	Acetic acid, essential oils, formic acid, myrrholic acids, resin.	Has antiseptic and disinfectant properties, and is a good deodorizer. Helps fight harmful bacteria in the mouth. Good for bad breath, periodontal disease, skin disorders, and ulcers.	Used in many perfumes and incense for its aromatic properties.
Nettle	Flowers, leaves, roots.	Calcium, chlorine, chlorophyll, formic acid, iodine, iron, magnesium, potassium, silicon, sodium, sulfur, tannin, vitamins A and C.	A diuretic, expectorant, pain reliever, and tonic. Contains vital minerals that are essential in many disorders. Good for anemia, arthritis, hay fever and other allergic disorders, kidney problems, and malabsorption syndrome. Improves goiter, inflammatory conditions, and mucous conditions of the lungs.	Also called stinging nettle.

Herb	Parts Used	Chemical and Nutrient Content	Actions and Uses	Comments
Oat straw	Whole plant.	Alkaloids, carotene, gluten, flavonoids, saponins, starch, steroidal compounds, vitamins B_1, B_2, D, and E.	Has antidepressant properties, acts as a restorative nerve tonic, and promotes sweating. Good for bed-wetting, depression, and skin disorders. Helps comfort insomnia.	
Oregon grape	Roots.	Alkaloids, berberine, oxycanthin.	Purifies the blood and cleanses the liver. Good for many skin conditions, from acne to psoriasis.	Can be used in place of goldenseal for some purposes.
Papaya	Fruit, inner bark, stems.	Amyolytic enzyme, caricin, myrosin, peptidase, vitamins C and E.	Stimulates the appetite and aids digestion. Good for heartburn, indigestion, and inflammatory bowel disorders.	Leaves can be used to tenderize meats.
Parsley	Berries, roots, stems.	Apiin (parsley camphor), apiol, bergaptein, calcium, fatty oil, essential oils, furanocumarin bergapten, iodine, iron, isoimperatorin, mucilage, myristicene, petroselinic acid, phosphorus, pinene, potassium, vitamins A and C.	Contains a substance that prevents the multiplication of tumor cells. Expels worms, relieves gas, stimulates normal activity of the digestive system, and freshens breath. Helps bladder, kidney, liver, lung, stomach, and thyroid function. Good for bed-wetting, fluid retention, gas, halitosis, high blood pressure, indigestion, kidney disease, obesity, and prostate disorders.	Contains more vitamin C than oranges, by weight.
Passion-flower	Plant, flower.	Aribine, ethylmaltol, flavonoids, harmaline, harman, harmine, harmol, loturine, maltol, passiflorine, yageine.	Acts as a gentle sedative. Helpful for anxiety, hyperactivity, insomnia, neuritis, and stress-related disorders.	Also called maypop. *Caution:* Should not be used in high doses during pregnancy.
Pau d'arco	Inner bark.	Lapachol.	A bitter herb that contains a natural antibacterial agent, cleanses the blood, and has a healing effect. Good for candidiasis, smoker's cough, warts, and all types of infection. Helpful for AIDS, allergies, cancer, cardiovascular problems, inflammatory bowel disease, rheumatism, tumors, and ulcers.	Also called lapacho, taheebo.
Peppermint	Flowering tops, leaves.	Essential oils, menthol, menthone, methyl acetate, tannic acid, terpenes, vitamin C.	Enhances digestion by increasing stomach acidity. Slightly anesthetizes mucous membranes and the gastrointestinal tract. Useful for chills, colic, diarrhea, headache, heart trouble, indigestion, nausea, poor appetite, rheumatism, and spasms.	*Caution:* May interfere with iron absorption.
Plantain	Leaves.	Glycosides, minerals, mucilage, tannins.	Soothing to the lungs and urinary tract; has a healing, antibiotic effect when used topically for sores and wounds. Taken internally, useful for preventing bed-wetting. Applied in a poultice, good for bee stings and any kind of bite.	Young leaves are tasty and can be eaten in salads.
Primrose	Oil from seeds.	Gamma-linolenic acid (GLA), linoleic acid.	Aids in weight loss and reduces high blood pressure. Helpful in treatment of alcoholism, arthritis, hot flashes, menstrual problems such as cramps and heavy bleeding, multiple sclerosis, skin disorders, and many other disorders.	A natural estrogen promoter. Also called evening primrose.
Pumpkin	Seed.	B vitamins, essential fatty acids, protein, zinc.	Useful for prostate disorders.	

Herb	Parts Used	Chemical and Nutrient Content	Actions and Uses	Comments
Red clover	Flowers.	Biotin, choline, copper, coumarins, folic acid, glycosides, inositol, isoflavonoids, magnesium, manganese, pantothenic acid, selenium, bioflavonoids, zinc, vitamins A, B_1, B_2, B_3, B_6, B_{12}, and C.	Acts as an antibiotic, appetite suppressant, blood purifier, and relaxant. Good for bacterial infections, HIV and AIDS, inflamed lungs, inflammatory bowel disorders, kidney problems, liver disease, skin disorders, and weakened immune system.	
Red raspberry	Bark, leaves, roots.	Calcium, citric acid, essential oils, iron, magnesium, malic acid, manganese, pectin, phosphorus, potassium, selenium, silicon, sulfur, tannic acid, vitamins B_1, B_3, C, D, and E.	Decreases menstrual bleeding, relaxes uterine and intestinal spasms, and strengthens the uterine walls. Also promotes healthy nails, bones, teeth, and skin. Good for diarrhea and for female disorders such as morning sickness, hot flashes, and menstrual cramps. Also heals canker sores. Combined with peppermint, good for morning sickness.	
Rhubarb	Roots, stalks.	Flavone, gallic acid, glucogallin, palmidine, pectin, phytosterol, rutin, starch, tannins.	Eliminates worms, enhances gallbladder function, and has antibiotic properties. Helps disorders of the colon, spleen, and liver. Promotes healing of duodenal ulcers. Good for constipation, malabsorption, and parasitic infection.	*Caution:* Should not be used during pregnancy.
Rose	Fruit (hips).	Bioflavonoids, citric acid, flavonoids, fructose, malic acid, sucrose, tannins, zinc, vitamins A, B_3, C, D, and E.	Good for all infections and bladder problems. A good source of vitamin C. Rose hip tea is good for diarrhea.	
Rosemary	Leaves.	Bitters, borneol, camphene, camphor, carnosic acid, carnosol, cineole, essential oils, pinene, resin, tannins.	Fights bacteria, relaxes the stomach, stimulates circulation and digestion, and acts as an astringent and decongestant. Improves circulation to the brain. Also helps prevent liver toxicity, and has anticancer and antitumor properties. Good for headaches, high and low blood pressure, circulatory problems, and menstrual cramps.	Makes a good food preservative.
Sage	Leaves.	Camphor, estrogenic substances, flavonoids, resin, salvene, saponins, tannins, terpene, thujone, volatile oils.	Stimulates the central nervous system and digestive tract, and has estrogenic effects on the body. Reduces sweating and salivation. Good for hot flashes and other symptoms of estrogen deficiency, whether in menopause or following hysterectomy. Beneficial for disorders affecting the mouth and throat, such as tonsillitis. In tea form, can be used as a hair rinse to promote shine (especially for dark hair) and hair growth. Also used to dry up milk when women wish to stop nursing.	*Caution:* Interferes with the absorption of iron and other minerals when taken internally, and decreases milk supply in lactating women. Should not be taken by individuals with seizure disorders.
St. Johnswort	Flowers, leaves, stems.	Essential oils, glycosides, hypericin, pseudohypericin, resins, rutin and other flavonoids, tannins.	May help to inhibit viral infections, including HIV and herpes. Good for depression and nerve pain.	*Caution:* When taken internally in large amounts, can cause heightened sun sensitivity, especially in fair-skinned people. Also interferes with the absorption of iron and other minerals.

Herb	Parts Used	Chemical and Nutrient Content	Actions and Uses	Comments
Sarsaparilla	Roots.	Copper, essential oil, fat, glycosides, iron, manganese, parillin, resin, saponins, sarsaponin, sitosterol stigmasterin, sodium, sugar, sulfur, zinc, vitamins A and D.	Increases energy, protects against harm from radiation exposure, regulates hormones, and has diuretic properties. Useful for frigidity, hives, impotence, infertility, nervous system disorders, premenstrual syndrome, and disorders caused by blood impurities.	Also called Chinese root, small spikenard.
Saw palmetto	Berries, seeds.	Capric, caproic, caprylic, lauric, oleic, and palmitic acids; resin.	Acts as a diuretic and urinary antiseptic. Stimulates the appetite. Inhibits the production of dihydrotestosterone, a hormone that contributes to enlargement of the prostate. Good for poor appetite and prostate disorders. May also enhance sexual functioning and desire.	Saw palmetto berry extracts have been approved in France and Germany for treatment of benign prostatic hypertrophy.
Skullcap	Aerial parts.	Fat, glycoside, iron, volatile oil, sugar, tannins, vitamin E.	Aids sleep, improves circulation, and strengthens the heart muscle. Good for anxiety, fatigue, cardiovascular disease, headache, hyperactivity, nervous disorders, and rheumatism. Relieves muscle cramps, pain, spasms, and stress. Useful in treating barbiturate addiction and drug withdrawal.	
Slippery elm	Inner bark.	Bioflavonoids, calcium, mucilage, phosphorus, polysaccharides, starch, tannins, vitamin K.	Soothes inflamed mucous membranes of the bowels, stomach, and urinary tract. Good for diarrhea and ulcers and for treatment of colds, flu, and sore throat.	Also called moose elm, red elm.
Squawvine	Leaves and stems.	Alkaloids, glycosides, tannins.	Relieves pelvic congestion and soothes the nervous system. Good for menstrual cramps and preparation for childbirth.	Also called partridgeberry.
Suma	Bark, berries, leaves, roots.	Albumin, allantoin, beta-ecdysome, germanium, malic acid, essential oils, pfaffic acid, six saponins (called pfaffosides A, B, C, D, E, and F), sitosterol, stigmasterol, tannins.	Combats anemia, fatigue, and stress. Acts as an immune system booster that may help to prevent cancer. Good for AIDS, cancer, liver disease, high blood pressure, and weakened immune system.	Also sometimes referred to as Brazilian ginseng. Research in Japan has shown that pfaffic acid is capable of inhibiting certain types of cancer.
Tea tree	Essential oil.	Antibacterial/antifungal agents.	Good for disinfecting wounds and healing virtually all skin conditions, including acne, athlete's foot, cuts and scrapes, fungal infection, herpes outbreaks, insect and spider bites, scabies, vaginitis, and warts. Can be added to water and used as a gargle for colds and sore throats, or as a douche for yeast infections.	*Caution:* If irritation occurs with topical use, use should be discontinued, or the tea tree oil diluted with distilled water or with primrose or vitamin E oil. Not recommended for internal use except under the careful supervision of a health care professional.
Thyme	Berries, flowers, leaves.	B-complex vitamins, borneol, cavacrol, chromium, essential oils, fluorine, gum, iron, silicon, tannins, thiamine, thyme oil, thymol, triterpenic acids, vitamins C and D.	Eliminates gas and reduces fever, headache, and mucus. Has strong antiseptic properties. Lowers cholesterol levels. Good for croup and other respiratory problems, and for fever, headache, and liver disease. Eliminates scalp itching and flaking caused by candidiasis.	

Herb	Parts Used	Chemical and Nutrient Content	Actions and Uses	Comments
Turmeric	Rhizomes.	A-atlantone, curcumin and related phenolic diarylheptanoids, curcuminoids, essential oils, turmerone, zingiberene.	Protects the liver against many toxins, inhibits platelet aggregation, and lowers cholesterol. Has antibiotic, anticancer, anti-inflammatory, and antioxidant properties.	Used as a seasoning and the main ingredient in curry powder. *Caution:* Should not be used in large quantities.
Uva ursi	Leaves.	Arbutin, chlorine, ellagic acid, ericolin, gallic acid, hydroquinolone, malic acid, methyl-arbutin, myricetin, volatile oils, quercetin, tannins, ursolic acid, ursone.	Acts as a diuretic and strengthens the heart muscle. Helps disorders of the spleen, liver, pancreas, and small intestine. Useful for bladder and kidney infections, diabetes, and prostate disorders.	Also called bearberry.
Valerian	Rhizomes, roots.	Acetic acid, butyric acid, camphene, chatinine, essential oils, formic acid, glycosides, magnesium, pinene, valeric acid, valerine.	Improves circulation and acts as a sedative. Reduces mucus from colds. Good for anxiety, fatigue, high blood pressure, insomnia, irritable bowel syndrome, menstrual cramps, muscle cramps, nervousness, pain, spasms, stress, and ulcers.	A water-soluble extract form is best.
White oak	Bark.	Calcium, cobalt, iron, phosphorus, potassium, sodium, sulfur, vitamin B_{12}.	Is an antiseptic and good for skin wounds. Good for bee stings, burns, diarrhea, nosebleed, poison ivy, and varicose veins. Also good for the teeth. Can be used in enemas and douches.	
Wild yam	Rhizomes.	Alkaloids, dioscin, diosgenin, phytosterols, starch, steroidal saponins, tannins.	Relaxes muscle spasms, reduces inflammation, promotes perspiration. Contains compounds similar to the hormone progesterone. Good for gallbladder disorders, hypoglycemia, kidney stones, and many female disorders, including premenstrual syndrome and menopause-related symptoms.	Many yam-based products are extracted from plants treated with fertilizers and pesticides, which may end up in the final products. The selection, cleansing, and processing of the raw materials is very important.
Willow	Bark.	Isorhamnetin, phenolic glycosides, quercetin, salicin, salicylic acid, salinigrin.	Relieves pain. Good for headache, backache, nerve pain, toothache, and injuries.	*Caution:* May interfere with absorption of iron and other minerals when taken internally.
Winter-green	Leaves, roots, stems.	Gaultherin (a compound composed of 90 percent methyl salicylate, a substance similar to aspirin), gaultherase, glycoside, mucilage, tannins, wax.	Relieves pain and inflammation. Good for arthritis, headache, toothache, muscle pain, and rheumatic complaints.	Oil distilled from the leaves is used in perfumes and as a flavoring.
Witch hazel	Bark, leaves, twigs.	Bitters, calcium oxalate, essential oils, gallic acid, hamamelitannin, hexose sugar, tannins.	Applied topically, has astringent and healing properties, and relieves itching. Good for hemorrhoids and phlebitis. Very useful in skin care.	
Wood betony	Leaves.	Magnesium, manganese, phosphorus, tannins.	Stimulates the heart and relaxes the muscles. Good for cardiovascular disorders, hyperactivity, and neuritis.	Also called betony.

Herb	Parts Used	Chemical and Nutrient Content	Actions and Uses	Comments
Wormwood	Leaves, tops.	Absinthol, acetylene, artemisic ketone, essential oils, flavonoids, lignin, phenolic compounds, pinene, thujone.	Acts as a mild sedative, expels worms, increases stomach acidity, and lowers fever. Useful for vascular disorders, including migraine, and for intestinal parasites.	Often used with black walnut for removal of parasites. *Caution:* Should not be used during pregnancy, as it can cause spontaneous abortion. Not recommended for long-term use, as it can be habit-forming.
Yarrow	Berries, leaves.	Achilleic acid, achilleine, caledivain, volatile oils, potassium, tannins, vitamin C.	Has healing effects on mucous membranes, reduces inflammation, improves blood clotting, increases perspiration. A good diuretic. Useful for fever, inflammatory disorders, colitis, and viral infections. Helps to alleviate bleeding problems.	Also called soldier's herb. *Caution:* Interferes with absorption of iron and other minerals.
Yellow dock	Leaves, roots.	Chrysarobin, iron, manganese, potassium oxalate, rumicin.	Acts as a blood purifier and cleanser, and tones the entire system. Improves colon and liver function. Good for anemia, liver disease, and skin disorders such as eczema, hives, psoriasis, and rashes. Combined with sarsaparilla, makes a tea for chronic skin disorders.	Also called curled dock, sad dock.
Yerba maté	All parts.	Chlorophyll, iron, pantothenic acid, trace minerals, vitamins C and E.	Cleanses the blood, controls the appetite, fights aging, stimulates the mind, stimulates the production of cortisone, and tones the nervous system. Is believed to enhance the healing powers of other herbs. Useful for allergies, constipation, and inflammatory bowel disorders.	Also called maté, Paraguay tea, South American holly.
Yohimbe	Bark.	Yohimbine hydrochloride.	A hormone stimulant. Increases libido and blood flow to erectile tissue. May increase testosterone levels.	Can be purchased in health food stores, but is also available by prescription. *Caution:* May induce anxiety, panic attacks, and hallucinations in some individuals. May also cause elevated blood pressure and heart rate, headache, dizziness, and skin flushing. Should not be used by women or by persons with kidney disease or psychological disorders.
Yucca	Roots.	Saponins.	Acts as a blood purifier. Beneficial in treatment of arthritis, osteoporosis, and inflammatory disorders.	Routinely prescribed for arthritis in some clinics. Can be cut up in water (1 cup of yucca in 2 cups of water) and used as a soap or shampoo substitute. Can also be added to shampoo.

PART TWO

THE DISORDERS

INTRODUCTION

Part One explored the nutritional and dietary needs of the body. In order to be well, the parts of the body must be fueled properly so that breakdown does not occur. With the growing number of stressors in the environment today, the body must obtain the proper nourishment in order to maintain a healthy immune system. If the immune system weakens, the body becomes susceptible to a number of harmful conditions.

Part Two offers an A-to-Z listing of disorders that can occur if the body is overcome by stress and suffering from insufficient nutritional intake due to poor eating habits. The descriptions of the conditions may help you identify whether you have a particular illness. If your symptoms match those given for a certain illness, confirm your suspicions by visiting your physician.

Your health care provider may recommend that certain diagnostic tests be performed to help in making a diagnosis. Some tests, such as amniocentesis or surgical biopsy, are invasive; others, such as urinalysis, are not. Many diagnostic tests—especially the newer ones such as magnetic resonance imaging (MRI) and computerized tomography (CAT) scans—can be quite expensive. Always be sure you understand exactly what a test involves before agreeing to it—how it is done, what it will show, why it is necessary in your case, what the potential risks are, how much it will cost, and anything else you need to know to feel confident in making a choice. You should also inform your health care provider about all medications (including natural medicines) and supplements you take regularly; any known allergies to foods, medications, anesthetics, x-ray materials, and/or other substances; pregnancy, if applicable; and any other special concerns you may have.

Once a diagnosis has been confirmed, refer to the appropriate dietary guidelines, recommendations, and supplementation program in this book to help speed your recovery. Always be sure to learn as much as possible about the use of any supplement you take. (*See* Part One for more detailed supplement information.) Most of the suggestions in Part Two can be utilized either alone or in conjunction with other therapies. However, if you have any questions about the appropriateness of any suggested nutrients or other therapy, speak to your physician.

Finally, a word about brand names. From time to time, we recommend specific products by specific manufacturers. These recommendations may appear on their own, or in parentheses following the generic term for the substance in question. This should not be taken to mean that these are the only such products available, or that they are the only ones that will work. There are many good supplements and other nutritional products available from many different manufacturers, and new products are being introduced to the market all the time. However, we occasionally choose to make specific recommendations for particular products because we have found them to be effective and of good quality.

Troubleshooting for Disorders

Some symptoms are indicative of a variety of illnesses. The following table lists some of the more common disorders that are associated with particular symptoms. It is *not* meant to serve as a substitute for professional diagnosis. Although you may experience one or more of the symptoms below, you may or may not have any of the illnesses cited.

Your body is simply sending a message that something may be wrong. Listening to your body can help stop a problem before it becomes serious. Moreover, the illnesses listed below are given in alphabetical order. This does not at all reflect your chances of having any of them. If you have any of these symptoms, consult with your health care provider.

Symptom	Possible Cause
Abdominal pain, cramping	Appendicitis; constipation; Crohn's disease; diarrhea; diverticulitis; endometriosis; food allergies; food poisoning; gallbladder disorders; hiatal hernia; indigestion; irritable bowel syndrome; lactose intolerance; miscarriage; pelvic inflammatory disease; peptic ulcer; premenstrual syndrome; prolapse of the uterus; stress; ulcerative colitis; uterine polyps or fibroids.
Anal bleeding itching, pain, swelling	Abscess; allergies; anal fissure; bruising; cancer; candidiasis; Crohn's disease; cysts; diverticulitis; food poisoning; genital warts; hemorrhoids; infection; muscle spasms; pinworms; polyps; sexually transmitted diseases; tumor; ulcers; ulcerative colitis.
Back pain	Aortic aneurysm; arthritis; awkward sleeping position; cancer; disk disease; endometriosis; gallbladder disorders; heart attack; improper lifting; injury; kidney disease; lack of exercise; menstrual cramps; muscle spasms; obesity; osteoporosis; overuse; Paget's disease of bone; pelvic inflammatory disease; peptic ulcer; pneumonia; poor posture; pregnancy; scoliosis; spinal tumor; sprain; strained muscle and/or ligament; urinary tract infection; uterine fibroids.
Bad breath	Abscessed tooth; diabetes; dry mouth; indigestion; infection; liver disease; lung disease; mouth ulcers; mouth-breathing; periodontal disease; poor oral hygiene; sinusitis; tooth decay.
Bleeding, menstrual, heavy or irregular	Blood clotting disorders; cancer; hormonal imbalance; menopause; miscarriage; obesity; overzealous dieting or exercise; urinary tract infection; use of improper oral contraceptives; uterine polyps or fibroids; vaginal infection; weight loss or gain.
Blinking, frequent	Anxiety; dry eyes; foreign body in the eye; injury; Parkinson's disease; stroke; use of contact lenses.
Bloating	Allergies; appendicitis; bowel or kidney obstruction; diverticulitis; edema; gallbladder disorders; heart failure; irritable bowel syndrome; kidney disease; lactose intolerance; peptic ulcer; tumor.
Blood in sputum, vomit, urine, or stools, or from vagina or penis	Blood clots and swelling of lung tissue; cancer; hemorrhoids; infection; nosebleed; peptic ulcer; polyps; prostatitis; ruptured blood vessel; tumor.
Body aches	Arthritis; infection; lupus; Lyme disease; overexertion.
Body odor	Diabetes; gastrointestinal abnormalities; indigestion; infection.
Breast lumps	Boils; cancer; fibrocystic disease; injury; infected milk duct; infected sweat gland or lymph node; premenstrual syndrome.
Breast tenderness	Breastfeeding-related problems; cancer; excessive consumption of fat, salt, and/or caffeine; hormonal imbalance; menopause; pregnancy; premenstrual syndrome; stress.
Breath, shortness of	Asthma; cardiovascular disease (especially in women); cystic fibrosis; emphysema; pneumonia.
Bruising, easy	AIDS; anemia; cancer; drug reaction; hemophilia; vitamin C deficiency; weakened immune system.
Chest pain	Angina; anxiety; bruised or broken rib; coronary artery disease; gas; heart attack; heartburn; hiatal hernia; hyperventilation; pleurisy; pneumonia; strained muscle; stress.
Chills	Acute infection; anemia; exposure to cold; fever; hypothermia; shock.
Cold sweats	AIDS; cancer; diabetes; influenza; menopause; mononucleosis; severe heart or circulatory disease; shock; tuberculosis.
Cough, persistent	Allergies; asthma; cancer; chronic bronchitis; emphysema; pneumonia; postnasal drip; tuberculosis.

Symptom	Possible Cause
Delirium	Alcohol abuse; appendicitis; diabetes; drug reaction; epilepsy; high fever; stroke.
Disorientation	Alcohol abuse; Alzheimer's disease; anemia; acute anxiety (panic attack); hypoglycemia; poor circulation; schizophrenia; seizure; stroke; transient ischemic attack (TIA, temporary interference with blood flow to the brain).
Dizziness, lightheadedness	Allergies; anemia; acute anxiety (panic attack); brain tumor; diabetes; drug reaction; heart disease; high blood pressure; hypoglycemia; impending stroke; infection; low blood pressure; Ménière's disease; motion sickness; stress; stroke; vertigo.
Double vision	Cataracts; concussion; eye disorders; hyperthyroidism.
Drooling	Drug withdrawal; ill-fitting dentures; Parkinson's disease; pregnancy-related problems; salivary gland disorders; seizure; stroke.
Drowsiness	Acute kidney failure; allergies; caffeine withdrawal; drug reaction; encephalitis; jet lag; narcolepsy; sleep disorders.
Dry mouth	Aging; diabetes; drug reactions; mouth-breathing; Sjögren's syndrome.
Ear discharge	Clogged eustachian tube; earwax buildup; immune system dysfunction; infection; ruptured eardrum; severe head injury; tumor.
Eye, bulging	Aneurysm; blood clot or hemorrhage; glaucoma; hyperthyroidism; infection.
Eyelid, drooping	Botulism; diabetes; head or eyelid injury; hypothyroidism; muscle weakness.
Fever, persistent	AIDS; autoimmune diseases; chronic bronchitis; cancer (especially leukemia, kidney cancer, lymphoma); diabetes; chronic infection; hepatitis; mononucleosis; rheumatic disorders.
Flushing	Alcohol consumption; anxiety; dehydration; diabetes; heart disease; high blood pressure; menopause; hyperthyroidism; pregnancy; use of high doses of niacin or of cholesterol-lowering medications.
Gas, frequent burping	Allergies; candidiasis; digestive problems; gallbladder disorders; intestinal obstruction; intestinal parasites; irritable bowel syndrome; lactose intolerance; stomach acid deficiency; swallowing air.
Hands and/or feet, cold	Exposure to cold; circulatory problems; Raynaud's phenomenon; stress.
Headaches, persistent	Allergies; asthma; brain tumor; cluster headaches; drug reaction; eyestrain; glaucoma; high blood pressure; sinusitis; stress; vitamin deficiency.
Heartbeat, irregular or rapid	Anemia; anxiety; arteriosclerosis; asthma; cardiovascular disease; caffeine, alcohol, or tobacco consumption; calcium, magnesium, and/or potassium deficiency; cancer; drug reaction; fever; heart attack; high blood pressure; hormonal imbalance; low blood pressure; obesity; overeating; overzealous exercising.
Incontinence	Advanced neurologic disease; aging; Alzheimer's disease; atrophic vaginitis; diabetes; loss of muscle tone; multiple sclerosis; prostatitis; psychological problems; restricted mobility; spinal cord trauma; stroke.
Intercourse, painful	Inflammation or infection of the vulva; muscle spasms; unaccustomed position during sex; urinary tract infection; vaginal dryness.
Irritability, mood swings	Alcohol or drug abuse; anxiety; Alzheimer's disease; brain tumor; depression; diabetes; drug reactions; food allergies; hyperthyroidism; hypothyroidism; nutritional deficiencies; premenstrual syndrome; schizophrenia; stress; stroke; virtually any chronic or disabling illness.
Joint pain, swelling	Arthritis; bone cancer; bone fracture; bone spur; bursitis; carpal tunnel syndrome; chronic overuse; cirrhosis of the liver; diabetes; edema; gout; hepatitis; hemophilia; hormonal imbalance; infection; injury; kidney disease; Lyme disease; lupus; neuritis; Paget's disease of bone; rheumatic fever; sprain; strained muscle and/or ligament; tendinitis.
Leg pain	Arteriosclerosis; bone fracture; cancer; injury; improper footwear; Lyme disease; osteomalacia; overuse; Paget's disease of bone; rickets; sciatica; tendinitis; thrombophlebitis; tumor or infection in intervertebral disk or spinal canal.

Symptom	Possible Cause
Lymph nodes, swollen	AIDS; any acute or chronic infection; lymphoma; metal toxicity.
Mouth sores	Canker sores; chickenpox; denture wearing; local trauma; measles; oral herpes; oral thrush; use of tobacco or aspirin.
Muscle control, loss of	Alcohol and/or drug abuse; extreme exhaustion; head injury; multiple sclerosis; muscular dystrophy; narcolepsy; overuse; Parkinson's disease; seizure; stroke.
Muscle cramps	Arthritis; calcium, magnesium, and/or potassium deficiency; dehydration; diabetes; hypothyroidism; injury; overuse; poor circulation.
Muscle pain, weakness	Anemia; arthritis; chronic fatigue syndrome; dehydration; diabetes; drug reaction; fever; fibromyalgia; infection; injury; lupus; multiple sclerosis; overuse.
Neck pain, stiffness	Awkward sleeping position; disk disease; injury; meningitis; strained muscle and/or ligament; stress.
Nausea	AIDS; alcohol consumption; anxiety; cancer; celiac disease; cirrhosis of the liver; copper toxicity; dehydration; drug withdrawal; endometriosis; extreme fatigue; food poisoning; gallbladder disorders; heart attack; hepatitis; hormonal imbalance; indigestion; influenza; kidney disease; kidney stones; Ménière's disease; migraine; morning sickness; motion sickness; pancreatitis; poisoning; sinusitis; stress; ulcerative colitis.
Night sweats	AIDS; anxiety; autoimmune disorders; bowel disease; cancer; cardiovascular disease; fever; hepatitis; menopause; sleep apnea; stress; weakened immune system.
Numbness	Carpal tunnel syndrome; diabetes; hyperventilation; multiple sclerosis; pinched nerve; poor circulation; rheumatoid arthritis; stroke; transient ischemic attack.
Pulse, weak	Blood loss; dehydration; drug reaction; heart attack; low blood pressure; malnutrition; shock; vomiting.
Seizure	Alcoholism; Alzheimer's disease; drug abuse; drug reaction; encephalitis; epilepsy; head injury; high fever; meningitis; stroke; tumor.
Swallowing, difficult	Bulimia; cancer; dehydration; dry mouth; hiatal hernia; stress; tumor.
Sweating, excessive	Alcohol consumption; anxiety; cardiovascular disease; consumption of hot and/or spicy foods; cystic fibrosis; food allergies; fever; hormonal imbalance; hyperthyroidism; infection; kidney disease; liver disease; lymphoma; malaria; menopause; overexertion; pneumonia; stress.
Swelling of ankles, feet, legs, hands, abdomen	Arthritis; bursitis; cardiovascular disease; chronic overuse; cirrhosis of the liver; diabetes; drug reaction; edema; food allergies; gout; improper footwear; joint infection; kidney disease; lupus; lymphatic disorders; pregnancy; premenstrual syndrome; poor circulation; sprain; strained muscle and/or ligament; varicose veins.
Thirst, excessive	Dehydration; diabetes; diarrhea; drug reaction; fever; menopause-related problems; any viral or bacterial infection.
Tremors	Alcoholism; anxiety; caffeine consumption; drug reaction; hyperthyroidism; multiple sclerosis; muscle fatigue; Parkinson's disease; stroke; tumor.
Urination, frequent	Aging; alcohol or caffeine consumption; bladder infection; cancer; diabetes; drug reaction; excessive liquid intake; kidney or bladder stones; pregnancy; prostatitis.
Vaginal discharge, itching	Cancer; chlamydia; genital herpes; polyps; pelvic inflammatory disease; sexually transmitted diseases; urinary tract infection; vaginitis; yeast infection.
Weight gain	Aging; congestive heart failure; depression; diabetes; drug reaction; edema; hormonal imbalance; hypothyroidism; kidney disease; overeating.
Weight loss	Aging; AIDS; Alzheimer's disease; anorexia nervosa; cancer; chronic infection; diabetes; hepatitis; hyperthyroidism; malabsorption syndrome; mononucleosis; Parkinson's disease; tuberculosis.
Wheezing	Any upper respiratory infection; allergies; asthma; cardiovascular disease; chronic bronchitis; croup; emphysema; lung cancer; pneumonia.

Abscess

When pus accumulates in a tissue, organ, or confined space in the body due to infection, an abscess forms. Abscesses may be located externally or internally, and may result from an injury or a lowered resistance to infection. The infected part becomes swollen, inflamed, and tender. The individual may also experience fatigue, loss of appetite, weight loss, and alternating bouts of fever and chills.

An abscess can form in the brain, lungs, teeth, gums, abdominal wall, gastrointestinal tract, ears, tonsils, sinuses, breasts, kidneys, prostate gland, or almost any other body part. Infections are the most common human diseases and can be produced by bacteria, viruses, parasites, and fungi.

NUTRIENTS

SUPPLEMENT	SUGGESTED DOSAGE	COMMENTS
Very Important		
Zinc	80 mg daily, in divided doses. Do not exceed a total of 100 mg daily from all supplements.	Powerful immune system stimulant. Necessary for T lymphocyte function, which is needed to fight infection. Needed for all skin disorders.
Important		
Colloidal silver	Take orally or apply topically as directed on label.	Acts as a natural antibiotic and disinfectant. Destroys bacteria, viruses, fungi, and parasites.
Garlic (Kyolic)	2 capsules 3 times daily, with meals.	Acts as a natural antibiotic and stimulates the immune system.
Superoxide dismutase (SOD) or	As directed on label.	A potent antioxidant. Use a sublingual form for best absorption.
Cell Guard from Biotec Foods	As directed on label.	An antioxidant complex that contains SOD.
Vitamin A	100,000 daily for 5 days, then 50,000 IU daily for 5 days, then reduce to 25,000 IU daily. If you are pregnant, do not exceed 10,000 IU daily.	Strengthens cell walls to protect against invasion by bacteria and promote tissue repair. Essential to the immune system. Use an emulsion form for easier assimilation and greater safety at high doses.
plus natural carotenoid complex (Betatene)	As directed on label.	Powerful antioxidants that promote healing.
Vitamin B complex	50 mg daily, with meals.	For repair and replacement of lost nutrients; aids in healing.
Vitamin C with bioflavonoids	5,000–20,000 mg daily, in divided doses. See ASCORBIC ACID FLUSH in Part Three.	Essential in immune function and tissue repair.
Vitamin E	400–600 IU daily. You can also open a capsule and apply it directly to the affected area.	Important in circulation and tissue oxygenation. Enhances the immune system and promotes healing.
Helpful		
Bromelain	500 mg 3 times a day.	Reduces inflammation and swelling; speeds healing.
Germanium	100 mg daily.	Enhances immune function.
Multivitamin and mineral complex	As directed on label.	All nutrients are needed for healing.
Proteolytic enzymes or Infla-Zyme Forte from American Biologics or Intenzyme Forte from Biotics Research	As directed on label. Take between meals. As directed on label. As directed on label.	To aid in cleanup of the abscess. Powerful free radical scavengers.

HERBS

❑ The following herbs are beneficial for healing abscesses and cleansing the blood: burdock root, cayenne (capsicum), dandelion root, red clover, and yellow dock root.

❑ Consuming distilled water with fresh lemon juice, plus 3 cups of echinacea, goldenseal, and astragalus or suma tea, every day is helpful. Goldenseal can also be made into a poultice and applied directly to the abscess. (*See* USING A POULTICE in Part Three.) Or apply alcohol-free goldenseal extract to sterile gauze and place the gauze over the abscess.

Caution: Do not use astragalus in the presence of a fever. Do not take goldenseal on a daily basis for more than one week at a time, and do not use it during pregnancy. If you have a history of cardiovascular disease, diabetes, or glaucoma, use it only under a doctor's supervision.

❑ A poultice that combines lobelia and slippery elm bark is soothing and fights infection. (*See* USING A POULTICE in Part Three.)

❑ Milk thistle, taken in capsule form, is good for the liver and aids in cleansing the bloodstream.

❑ Tea tree oil, applied externally, is a potent natural antiseptic that kills infectious organisms without harming healthy cells. Mix 1 part tea tree oil with 4 parts water and apply the mixture with a cotton ball three times a day. This will destroy the bacteria, hasten healing, and prevent the infection from spreading.

RECOMMENDATIONS

❑ Eat fresh pineapple daily. Pineapple contains bromelain, an enzyme that fights inflammation and aids healing.

❑ Add kelp to the diet for beneficial minerals.

❑ Perform a liquid fast using fresh juices for twenty-four to seventy-two hours. See FASTING in Part Three.

❑ For an external abscess, apply honey to the affected area. Honey destroys bacteria and viruses, apparently by drawing all the moisture out of them.

❑ To cleanse the affected area, apply chlorophyll liquid mixed with water several times a day.

❑ If you must take antibiotics, supplement your diet with the B vitamins and products containing "friendly" bacteria, such as acidophilus and yogurt.

CONSIDERATIONS

❑ Some abscesses need to be treated surgically, but most require only the administration of antibiotics. These drugs kill infectious bacteria, but they also destroy the "friendly" bacteria that normally inhabit the digestive tract. In addition, they deplete the body of the B vitamins.

❑ To heal an abscess, you may have to get plenty of bed rest, drink plenty of fluids, and either apply ice packs or take hot baths to alleviate the pain.

❑ To aid healing, the blood must be cleansed and vitamin deficiencies that accompany skin eruptions must be corrected.

Acidosis

Acidosis is a condition in which body chemistry becomes imbalanced and overly acidic. Symptoms associated with acidosis include frequent sighing, insomnia, water retention, recessed eyes, rheumatoid arthritis, migraine headaches, abnormally low blood pressure, dry hard stools, foul-smelling stools accompanied by a burning sensation in the anus, alternating constipation and diarrhea, difficulty swallowing, burning in the mouth and/or under the tongue, sensitivity of the teeth to vinegar and acidic fruits, and bumps on the tongue or the roof of the mouth.

Acidity and alkalinity are measured according to the pH (potential of hydrogen) scale. Water, with a pH of 7.0, is considered neutral—neither acid nor alkaline. Anything with a pH below 7.0 is acid, while anything with a pH above 7.0 is alkaline. The ideal pH range for the human body is between 6.0 and 6.8 (the human body is naturally mildly acidic). Values below pH 6.3 are considered on the acidic side; values above pH 6.8 are on the alkaline side.

Acidosis occurs when the body loses its alkaline reserve. Some causes of acidosis include kidney, liver, and adrenal disorders; improper diet; malnutrition; obesity; ketosis; anger; stress; fear; anorexia; toxemia; fever; and the consumption of excessive amounts of niacin, vitamin C, or aspirin. Diabetics often suffer from acidosis. Stomach ulcers are often associated with this condition.

ACID AND ALKALINE SELF-TEST

This test will determine whether your body fluids are either too acidic or too alkaline. An imbalance can cause illnesses such as acidosis or alkalosis.

Purchase pH paper, available at any drugstore, and apply saliva and/or urine to the paper. The paper will change color to indicate if your system is overly acidic or alkaline. Red litmus paper turns blue in an alkaline medium and blue litmus paper turns red in an acid medium. Always perform the test either before eating or at least one hour after eating.

Depending on the results of your test, you should alter your diet to help bring your body back into the normal range. If your test indicates that your body is too acidic, eat more alkaline-forming foods and omit acid-forming foods from your diet until another pH test shows that you have returned to normal. Conversely, if your body is too alkaline, eat more acid-forming foods and omit alkaline-forming foods. Use the list below as a guide to which foods are acid-forming and which are alkaline-forming. Low-level acid-forming and low-level alkaline-forming foods are almost neutral.

Acid-Forming Foods

Alcohol	Mustard
Asparagus	Noodles
Beans	Oatmeal
Brussels sprouts	Olives
Catsup	Organ meats
Chickpeas	Pasta
Cocoa	Pepper
Coffee	Plums
Cornstarch	Poultry
Cranberries	Prunes
Eggs	Sauerkraut
Fish	Shellfish
Flour; flour-based products	Soft drinks
Legumes	Sugar; all foods with
Lentils	sugar added
Meat	Tea
Milk	Vinegar

Aspirin, tobacco, and most drugs are also acid forming.

Low-Level Acid-Forming Foods

Butter	Grains (most)
Canned or glazed fruit	Ice cream
Cheeses	Ice milk
Dried coconut	Lamb's quarters
Dried or sulfured fruit (most)	Seeds and nuts (most)

Alkaline-Forming Foods

Avocados	Honey
Corn	Maple syrup
Dates	Molasses
Fresh coconut	Raisins
Fresh fruits (most)	Soy products
Fresh vegetables (most)	

Although it might seem that citrus fruits would have an acidifying effect on the body, the citric acid they contain actually has an alkalinizing effect in the system.

Low-Level Alkaline-Forming Foods

Almonds	Chestnuts
Blackstrap molasses	Lima beans
Brazil nuts	Millet
Buckwheat	Soured dairy products

NUTRIENTS

SUPPLEMENT	SUGGESTED DOSAGE	COMMENTS
Very Important		
Tri-Salts from Ecological Formulas	As directed on label.	For acid-alkaline balance.
Helpful		
Kelp	1,000–1,500 mg daily.	Reduces acid in the body. Aids in maintaining a proper balance of minerals.
Potassium	99 mg daily.	Increases metabolism. Aids in balancing the pH in the blood.
Vitamin A	50,000 IU daily for 1 month, then reduce to 25,000 IU daily. If you are pregnant, do not exceed 10,000 IU daily.	Helps to protect mucous membranes.
Vitamin B complex	100 mg twice daily.	Needed for proper digestion.

HERBS

❑ Use elder bark, hops, and willow for acidosis.

❑ Externally, apply ginger compresses to the kidney area.

RECOMMENDATIONS

❑ Eat a diet of 50 percent raw foods, such as apples, avocados, bananas, grapefruit, grapes, lemons, pears, pineapples, and all vegetables. Fresh fruits, especially citrus fruits, and vegetables reduce acidosis. Start with small amounts of citrus fruits and gradually add larger amounts.

❑ Drink potato broth every day. *See* THERAPEUTIC LIQUIDS in Part Three for the recipe.

❑ Avoid animal protein (especially beef and pork) and processed or junk foods, and reduce your intake of cooked food. When ingested, cooked and processed foods become acid in the body.

❑ Avoid beans, cereals, crackers, eggs, flour products, grains, oily foods, macaroni, and sugar. Plums, prunes, and cranberries do not oxidize and therefore remain acid to the body. Avoid these until the situation improves.

❑ Since excess vitamin C may lead to acidosis, reduce your intake of vitamin C for a few weeks. When taking vitamin C, use a non-acid-forming (buffered) variety.

❑ Practice deep breathing.

❑ Check your urine pH daily using pH paper. See the self-testing section for a list of acid-forming foods to avoid until your pH is corrected.

CONSIDERATIONS

❑ Phosphorus and sulfur act as buffers to maintain pH. Sulfur can be taken in supplement form.

Acne

Acne is an inflammatory skin disorder that to some degree afflicts about 80 percent of all Americans between the ages of twelve and twenty-four. Acne is more common in males because androgens (male sex hormones) like testosterone stimulate the production of keratin and sebum, which leads to clogged pores. During puberty, androgens increase in both sexes, making girls in this age group more susceptible as well. Hormones don't go away after adolescence, though. Many women suffer premenstrual acne flare-ups that are prompted by the release of progesterone after ovulation. Oral contraceptives high in progesterone can cause breakouts, too.

The sebaceous glands, located in each hair follicle or tiny pit of skin, produce oil that lubricates the skin. Sebaceous glands are found in large numbers on the face, back, chest, and shoulders. If some of the oil becomes trapped, bacteria multiply in the follicle and the skin becomes inflamed. Several of these spots can come and go over a period of months or years. Acne is not caused by "dirty" pores, but most likely by overactive oil glands; the excess oil makes the pores sticky, allowing bacteria to become trapped inside.

Blackheads form when sebum combines with skin pigments and plugs the pores. If scales below the surface of the skin become filled with sebum, whiteheads appear. In severe cases, whiteheads build up, spread under the skin, and rupture, which eventually spreads the inflammation.

The exact cause of acne is not known, but factors that contribute to the condition include heredity, oily skin, and androgens. Other factors are allergies; stress; the use of certain drugs (especially steroids, lithium, oral contraceptives, and certain antiepileptic drugs); overconsumption of junk food, saturated fats, hydrogenated fats, and animal products; nutritional deficiencies; exposure to industrial pollutants (machine oils, coal tar derivatives, chlorinated hydrocarbons); the use of cosmetics; monthly menstrual cycles; and overwashing or repeated rubbing of the skin.

The skin is the largest organ of the body. One of its functions is to eliminate a portion of the body's toxic waste products through sweating. If the body contains more toxins than the kidneys and liver can effectively discharge, the skin takes over. In fact, some doctors call the skin the "third kidney." As toxins escape through the skin, they disrupt the skin's healthy integrity. This is a key factor behind many skin disorders, including acne.

The skin also "breathes." If the pores become clogged, the microbes that are involved in causing acne flourish because they are protected against the bacteriostatic action of sunshine. Dirt, dust, oils, and grime from pollution clog the pores, but this can be eliminated by washing the skin properly. A body pH that is too high, or too alkaline, also fosters the nesting and breeding of acne-causing bacteria.

NUTRIENTS

SUPPLEMENT	SUGGESTED DOSAGE	COMMENTS
Very Important		
Chromium picolinate	As directed on label.	Aids in reducing infections of the skin.
Essential fatty acids (flaxseed oil and primrose oil are good sources)	As directed on label.	To supply essential gamma-linolenic acid, needed to keep the skin smooth and soft, repair damaged skin cells, and dissolve fatty deposits that block pores.
Vitamin B complex plus extra	100 mg 3 times daily.	Important for healthy skin tone. Use a high-potency formula.
vitamin B₃ (niacin)	100 mg 3 times daily. Do not exceed this amount.	Improves blood flow to the surface of the skin. *Caution:* Do not take niacin if you have a liver disorder, gout, or high blood pressure.
and pantothenic acid (vitamin B₅)	50 mg 3 times daily.	The anti-stress vitamin.
and vitamin B₆ (pyridoxine)	50 mg 3 times daily.	Involved in cellular reproduction. Deficiencies have been associated with acne.
Zinc	30–80 mg daily. Do not exceed a total of 100 mg daily from all supplements.	Aids in healing of tissue and helps to prevent scarring. A necessary element in the oil-producing glands of the skin.
Important		
Colloidal silver	Take orally or apply topically as directed on label.	Acts as a natural antibiotic and disinfectant.
Garlic (Kyolic)	2 capsules 3 times daily, with meals.	Destroys bacteria and enhances immune function.
Potassium	99 mg daily.	Deficiency has been associated with acne.
Vitamin A	25,000 IU daily until healed, then reduce to 5,000 IU daily. If you are pregnant, do not exceed 10,000 IU daily.	To strengthen the protective epithelial (skin) tissue. Use emulsion form for easier assimilation.
and natural carotenoid complex (Betatene) plus	As directed on label.	Antioxidants and precursors of vitamin A.
vitamin E	400 IU daily.	An antioxidant that enhances healing.
Helpful		
Acidophilus	As directed on label. Take on an empty stomach.	Replenishes essential bacteria.
Chlorophyll	As directed on label.	Aids in cleansing the blood, preventing infections. Also supplies needed nutrients.
GH3 cream from Gero Vita	Apply topically as directed on label.	Good for acne and any discoloration of the skin. Also helps prevent wrinkles.
Herpanacine from Diamond-Herpanacine Associates	As directed on label.	Contains antioxidants, amino acids, and herbs that promote overall skin health.
Multienzyme complex with hydrochloric acid (HCl)	As directed on label. Take with meals.	To aid digestion. *Caution:* Do not use HCl if you have a history of ulcers.
L-Cysteine	500 mg daily, on an empty stomach. Take with water or juice. Do not take milk. Take with 50 mg vitamin B₆ and 100 mg vitamin C for better absorption.	Contains sulfur, needed for healthy skin. *See* AMINO ACIDS in Part One.
Lecithin granules or capsules	1 tbsp 3 times daily, before meals. 1,200 mg 3 times daily, before meals.	Needed for better absorption of the essential fatty acids.
Proteolytic enzymes	As directed on label. Take with meals and between meals.	Free radical scavengers. Aid in breaking down undigested food particles in the colon.
Selenium	200 mcg daily.	Encourages tissue elasticity and is a powerful antioxidant.
Shark cartilage (BeneFin)	1 gm per 15 lbs of body weight daily, divided into 3 doses.	Reduces inflammation.
Tretinoin (Retin-A)	As prescribed by physician.	Acts as a gradual chemical peel; speeds up sloughing off of top layers of skin, leaving new, smoother skin. Available by prescription only. Takes around 6 months to show results.
Vitamin C with bioflavonoids	3,000–5,000 mg daily, in divided doses.	Promotes immune function and reduces inflammation. Use a buffered type.
Vitamin D	400 IU daily.	Promotes healing and tissue repair.

HERBS

❑ Burdock root and red clover are powerful blood cleansers. Milk thistle aids the liver in cleansing the blood.

❑ A poultice using chaparral, dandelion, and yellow dock root can be applied directly to the areas of skin with acne. (*See* USING A POULTICE in Part Three.)

Note: Chaparral is recommended for external use only.

❑ Lavender, red clover, and strawberry leaves can be used as a steam sauna for the face. Lavender kills germs and stimulates new cell growth. Using a glass or enameled pot, simmer a total of 2 to 4 tablespoons of dried or fresh herbs in 2 quarts of water. When the pot is steaming, place it on top of a thick potholder on a table, and sit with your face at a comfortable distance over the steam for fifteen minutes. You can use a towel to trap the steam if you wish. After fifteen minutes, splash your face with cold water. Allow your skin to air dry or pat it dry with a towel. If desired, you may follow this treatment with the use of a clay mask: Blend together well 1 teaspoon of green clay powder (available in health food stores) and 1 teaspoon raw honey, and apply the mixture to your face, avoiding the eye area. Leave it on for fifteen minutes, then rinse with lukewarm water.

Caution: If acne is extensive or badly inflamed, do not use steam treatments, as this may worsen the condition.

❑ Tea tree oil is a natural antibiotic and antiseptic. Dab full-strength tea tree oil (sparingly) on blemishes three times a day, or add 1 dropperful of tea tree oil to ¼ cup warm water and pat it on the affected area with a clean cotton ball (be sure to use 100-percent cotton). Tea tree oil soap also works well.

❑ Other beneficial herbs include alfalfa, cayenne (capsicum), dandelion root, echinacea, and yellow dock root.

RECOMMENDATIONS

❑ Eat a diet that is high in fiber. This is important for keeping the colon clean and ridding the body of toxins.

❑ Increase your intake of raw foods that contain oxalic acid, including almonds, beets, cashews, and Swiss chard. Exceptions are spinach and rhubarb; these contain oxalic acid, but should be consumed in small amounts only.

❑ Eat more foods rich in zinc, including shellfish, soybeans, whole grains, sunflower seeds, and a small amount of raw nuts daily. Zinc is an antibacterial agent and a necessary element in the oil-producing glands of the skin. A diet low in zinc may promote flare-ups.

❑ Eat plenty of soured products, such as low-fat yogurt, to maintain healthy intestinal flora.

❑ Avoid alcohol, butter, caffeine, cheese, chocolate, cocoa, cream, eggs, fat, fish, fried foods, hot and spicy foods, hydrogenated oils and shortenings, margarine, meat, poultry, wheat, soft drinks, and foods containing brominated vegetable oils.

❑ Try eliminating dairy products from your diet for one month. Acne may develop due to an allergic reaction to dairy products, and the fat content of the dairy products can worsen the condition. After the month is over, add dairy products back one at a time to see if the acne returns.

❑ Avoid all forms of sugar. Sugar impairs immune function. In addition, biopsies of individuals with acne have shown their tissues' glucose tolerance to be seriously flawed. One researcher calls this condition "skin diabetes."

❑ Eliminate all processed foods from the diet, and do not use iodized salt. These contain high levels of iodine, which is known to worsen acne. For the same reason, avoid fish, kelp, and onions.

❑ Follow a fasting program. See FASTING in Part Three.

❑ Use cleansing enemas to removing toxic buildup in the system and promote faster healing. See ENEMAS in Part Three.

❑ Keep the affected area as free of oil as possible. Shampoo your hair frequently. Use an all-natural soap with sulfur that is designed for acne (available at health food stores). Wash your skin thoroughly but gently; never rub hard. Vigorous scrubbing can make acne worse.

❑ Avoid wearing makeup. If you feel you must use cosmetics, use only natural, water-based products; do not use any oil-based formulas. Avoid any products containing harsh chemicals, dyes, or oils. Wash and dip makeup applicator brushes and sponges in alcohol after each use to avoid contamination.

❑ Friction makes pimples more likely to rupture, so avoid wearing tight clothing like turtlenecks. Carefully adjust straps on sports equipment such as bicycle or football helmets. Even using the telephone can exacerbate inflammation if you hold the receiver against your cheek for long periods.

❑ If you must shave an area of skin affected by acne, use a standard blade. Using an electric razor may lead to scarring. Always shave in the direction of hair growth.

❑ As much as possible, avoid stress. Stress can promote hormonal changes and cause flare-ups. Many dermatologists also recommend fifteen minutes of sunshine each day, regular exercise, and sufficient sleep for people with acne.

❑ Avoid the use of oral or topical steroids, which can aggravate acne.

❑ Do not squeeze the spots. To do so is to risk increasing the inflammation by causing breaks in the skin in which harmful bacteria can lodge. Do not touch the affected area unless your hands have been thoroughly cleaned.

CONSIDERATIONS

❑ For severe acne, the drug isotretinoin (Accutane) is the only reliable treatment. It disrupts plug formation and shrinks the sebaceous glands. Isotretinoin cures or greatly reduces acne in about 90 percent of the people who use it, but it can cause side effects like dry skin and nosebleeds. It can also be dangerous if a woman taking this drug becomes pregnant, because it can cause severe birth defects, such as fetal brain deformities.

❑ The weapon of choice against moderate cases of acne is topical tretinoin (Retin-A). It helps to keep the pores from becoming clogged by increasing the rate at which dead surface skin cells are shed. Like isotretinoin, tretinoin should not be taken during pregnancy. In addition, it renders the skin extremely vulnerable to sun damage.

❑ An antibiotic cream or an oral antibiotic is sometimes prescribed for acne. The long-term use of antibiotics often leads to candida infection. If you must take antibiotics, it is wise to take some form of acidophilus because antibiotics kill "friendly" bacteria along with "unfriendly" bacteria.

❑ Benzoyl peroxide is the active ingredient in many over-the-counter acne products. It can be helpful, particularly in mild cases, but it is extremely drying and allergic reactions can occur. It should not be applied around the eyes or mouth.

❑ A study conducted by the Department of Dermatology of the Royal Prince Alfred Hospital in New South Wales, Australia, found that a 5-percent solution of tea tree oil was as effective as a 5-percent benzoyl peroxide for most cases of acne, without the irritating side effects.

❑ Blackheads should be removed only with a specially designed instrument, a procedure best done by a professional. Picking, squeezing, or scratching the blemishes may cause scarring, according to dermatologists.

❑ Niacinamide is a major nutrient in the repair of any skin condition because it brings fresh, healthy blood to the surface of the skin. Niacinamide opens the vascular system, which supplies the skin with blood and nutrients.

❑ Kombucha tea, which has antibacterial and immune-boosting properties, has been found by many people to be beneficial for acne (*see under* NATURAL FOOD SUPPLEMENTS in Part One).

❑ Dimethylsulfoxide (DMSO), a byproduct of wood processing, can be applied to acne lesions to reduce inflammation and promote healing. If used regularly, it may also help minimize scarring from severe cystic acne.

Note: Only DMSO from a health food store should be used for therapeutic purposes. Commercial-grade DMSO such as that found in hardware stores is not suitable. The use of DMSO may result in a garlicky body odor. This is temporary, and is not a cause for concern.

❑ An acne treatment program called Derma-Klear from Enzymatic Therapy may be helpful.

❑ In rare cases, acne may be a sign of a potentially serious hormonal disorder caused by tumors in the adrenal glands or ovaries. Other symptoms of such problems include irregular menstrual periods and excess facial hair. If such symptoms develop, consult your health care provider.

❑ *See also* OILY SKIN and ROSACEA, both in Part Two.

Acquired Immune Deficiency Syndrome

See AIDS.

Addison's Disease

See under ADRENAL DISORDERS.

Adrenal Disorders

The adrenal glands are a pair of triangular-shaped organs that rest on top of the kidneys. Each gland normally weighs about 5 grams (slightly less than $1/5$ ounce) and is made up of two parts: the cortex, or outer section, which is responsible for the production of cortisone, and the medulla, or central section, which secretes adrenaline.

The adrenal cortex helps to maintain the salt and water balance in the body. It is also involved in the metabolism of carbohydrates and the regulation of blood sugar. In addition, the cortex produces a sex hormone similar to that secreted by the testes.

The adrenal medulla produces the hormone epinephrine, also called adrenaline, when the body is under stress. This hormone speeds up the rate of metabolism and produces other physiologic changes designed to help the body cope with danger.

Reduced adrenal function may be indicated by the following: weakness, lethargy, dizziness, headaches, memory problems, food cravings, allergies, and blood sugar disorders. If the adrenal cortex is seriously underactive, a rare condition called *Addison's disease* may develop. Symptoms include fatigue, loss of appetite, dizziness or fainting, nausea, moodiness, a decrease in the amount of body hair, and an inability to cope with stress. The individual may also constantly complain about feeling cold. Discoloration and darkening of the skin is common in people with Addison's disease; discoloration of knees, elbows, scars, skin folds, and creases in the palms are more noticeable when these body parts are exposed to the sun. The mouth, the vagina, and freckles may appear darker. This disease is also characterized by the development of bands of pigment running the length of the nails and by darkening of the hair. Addison's disease is a chronic condition that requires lifelong treatment.

Cushing's syndrome is a rare disorder caused by an overactive adrenal cortex. Persons with Cushing's syndrome take on a characteristic appearance: They generally are heavy in the abdomen and buttocks but have very thin limbs, and they have rounded "moon" faces. Muscular weakness and wasting of muscles are also characteristic of this syndrome. Round, red marks mimicking acne may appear on the face, and the eyelids may appear swollen. An increased growth of body hair is common, and women may grow mustaches and beards. People with Cushing's generally are more susceptible to illness and have trouble healing properly. Thinning of the skin from Cushing's syndrome often leads to stretch marks and bruising.

The functioning ability of the adrenal glands is most often impaired as a result of the extensive use of cortisone therapy for nonendocrine diseases, such as arthritis and asthma. The long-term use of cortisone drugs causes the adrenal gland to shrink in size, and can result in a "Cushinoid" appearance. Adrenocortical failure can also be caused by pituitary disease and tuberculosis. Poor nutritional habits, smoking, and alcohol and drug abuse can contribute to adrenal failure.

ADRENAL GLAND FUNCTION SELF-TEST

Normally, systolic blood pressure (the first number in the measurement of blood pressure—*120/80*) is approximately 10 points higher when you are standing than when you are lying down. If the adrenal glands are not functioning properly, however, this may not be the case.

Take and compare two blood pressure readings—one while lying down and one while standing. First, lie down and rest for five minutes. Then take your blood pressure.

Stand up and immediately take your blood pressure again. If your blood pressure reading is lower after you stand up, suspect reduced adrenal gland function. The degree to which the blood pressure drops upon standing is often proportionate to the degree of hypoadrenalism.

NUTRIENTS

SUPPLEMENT	SUGGESTED DOSAGE	COMMENTS
Essential		
Vitamin B complex plus extra	100 mg twice daily.	All B vitamins are necessary for adrenal function.
pantothenic acid (vitamin B$_5$)	100 mg 3 times daily.	The adrenal glands do not function adequately without pantothenic acid.
Vitamin C with bioflavonoids	4,000–10,000 mg daily, in divided doses.	Vital for proper functioning of the adrenals.
Very Important		
L-Tyrosine	500 mg daily, on an empty stomach. Take with water or juice. Do not take with milk. Take with 50 mg vitamin B$_6$ and 100 mg vitamin C for better absorption.	Aids adrenal gland function and relieves excess stress put on the glands. *See* AMINO ACIDS in Part One. *Caution:* Do not take tyrosine if you are taking an MAO inhibitor drug.
Important		
Raw adrenal and	As directed on label.	Protein derived from this adrenal gland substance helps to rebuild and repair the adrenal glands. *See* GLANDULAR THERAPY in Part Three.
raw adrenal cortex glandulars	As directed on label.	
Helpful		
Chlorophyll	As directed on label.	Cleanses the bloodstream.
Coenzyme Q$_{10}$	60 mg daily.	Carries oxygen to all glands.
Germanium	100 mg daily.	Enhances immune function.
Multivitamin and mineral complex with		All nutrients are needed to support proper adrenal function. Use a high-potency formula. If you have diabetes, use a formula without beta-carotene.
natural beta-carotene and	15,000 IU daily.	
copper plus	3 mg daily.	
potassium	99 mg daily.	Needed to balance with sodium. Potassium is lost with this disorder.
and zinc	50 mg daily. Do not exceed a total of 100 mg daily from all supplements.	Boosts immune function.
Raw liver extract	As directed on label.	Supplies natural B vitamins, iron, and enzymes.
Raw spleen and raw pituitary glandulars	As directed on label.	Boosts immune function and aids healing process. *See* GLANDULAR THERAPY in Part Three.

HERBS

❑ The herb astragalus improves adrenal gland function and aids in stress reduction.

Caution: Do not use this herb in the presence of a fever.

❑ China Gold from Aerobic Life Industries is a liquid herbal combination formula that helps to stimulate adrenal function and combat fatigue. It contains ten different varieties of ginseng plus twenty-six other valuable herbs.

❑ Using echinacea can increase white blood cell production and protect tissues from bacterial invasion.

❑ Milk thistle extract aids liver function, which in turn helps adrenal function.

❑ Siberian ginseng is an herb that helps the adrenal gland prepare the body for stressful situations.

Caution: Do not use this herb if you have hypoglycemia, high blood pressure, or a heart disorder.

RECOMMENDATIONS

❑ Consume plenty of fresh fruits and vegetables—particularly green leafy ones. Brewer's yeast, brown rice, legumes, nuts, olive and safflower oils, seeds, wheat germ, and whole grains are healthy additions to the diet as well.

❑ Eat deep-water ocean fish, salmon, or tuna at least three times a week.

❑ Include in the diet garlic, onions, shiitake mushrooms, and pearl barley. These foods contain germanium, a powerful stimulant of the immune system.

❑ Avoid alcohol, caffeine, and tobacco; these substances are highly toxic to the adrenal and other glands.

❑ Stay away from fats, fried foods, ham, pork, highly processed foods, red meats, sodas, sugar, and white flour. These foods put unnecessary stress on the adrenal glands.

❑ Get regular moderate exercise. This stimulates the adrenal glands and also helps to relieve stress.

❑ As much as possible, avoid stress. Continuous and prolonged stress from a troubled marriage, job-related problems, illness, or feelings of low self-esteem or loneliness can be detrimental to the adrenal glands. Take positive action to relieve stressful situations. *See* STRESS in Part Two.

CONSIDERATIONS

❑ A person with Addison's disease must take medication as prescribed and pay careful attention to diet. Nutritional supplements are recommended.

❑ Adrenocorticotropic hormone (ACTH), a hormone released by the pituitary gland when under stress, sets in motion a sequence of biochemical events that results in the activation of substances that raise blood pressure. The presence of this hormone leads to sodium retention and potassium excretion. As a result of this mechanism, stress not only puts strain on the adrenal glands, but may also cause the body to retain water, which can lead to hypertension.

❑ Distress—that is, unresolved stress—is the most important factor in "adrenal burnout," with all its manifestations, including immune deficiency and degenerative diseases.

Age Spots

Age spots are flat brown spots that can appear anywhere on the body as it ages. They are also called liver spots. Most age spots appear on the face, neck, and hands. These brown spots in themselves are harmless, but they can be a sign of more serious underlying problems. They are the result of a buildup of wastes known as *lipofuscin accumulation,* a byproduct of free radical damage in skin cells (*see* Free Radicals *under* ANTIOXIDANTS in Part One). These spots are actually signs that the cells are full of the type of accumulated wastes that slowly destroy the body's cells, including brain and liver cells. In other words, they are a surface sign of free radical intoxication of the body.

Factors that lead to the formation of age spots include poor diet, lack of exercise, poor liver function, the ingestion of oxidized oils over a period of time, and, above all, *excessive sun exposure.* Exposure to the sun causes the development of free radicals that damage the skin. Most people who have significant numbers of age spots have lived in sunny climates or otherwise had excessive sun exposure.

NUTRIENTS

SUPPLEMENT	SUGGESTED DOSAGE	COMMENTS
Very Important		
ACES + Zinc from Carlson Labs	As directed on label.	A combination of powerful antioxidants. Helps to protect against free radical damage.
Ageless Beauty from Biotec Foods	As directed on label.	A free radical destroyer.
Vitamin B complex	100 mg 3 times daily.	Needed by older people for proper assimilation of all nutrients.
plus extra pantothenic acid (vitamin B5)	50 mg 3 times daily.	Supports adrenal gland function.
Vitamin C with bioflavonoids	3,000–6,000 mg daily, in divided doses.	A powerful antioxidant and free radical scavenger that is necessary for tissue repair.
Important		
Lactobacillus bulgaricus (Digesta-Lac from Natren is a good source)	As directed on label.	Aids in liver regeneration and digestion.
Helpful		
Calcium and magnesium and vitamin D	1,500–2,000 mg daily. 750–1,000 mg daily. 400 IU daily.	Elderly people need these nutrients. Asporotate or chelate forms are best.
Herpanacine from Diamond-Herpanacine Associates	As directed on label.	To provide antioxidants, amino acids, and herbs that promote overall skin health.
L-Carnitine	As directed on label. Take between meals.	Aids in breaking up fat in the bloodstream so it can be removed from the body.
Lecithin granules or capsules	1 tbsp 3 times daily, with meals. 1200 mg 3 times daily, with meals.	Needed for proper brain function and healthy cell membranes. Works well as an antioxidant when taken with vitamin E.
Superoxide dismutase (SOD) plus selenium	As directed on label. As directed on label.	Powerful antioxidants. Good for brown age spots.
Tretinoin (Retin-A)	As directed by physician.	Acts as a gradual chemical peel; speeds up sloughing off of top layers of skin. Also removes fine wrinkles. Available by prescription only. Takes around 6 months to show results.

HERBS

❑ Burdock, milk thistle, and red clover aid in cleansing the bloodstream.

❑ Ginkgo biloba improves circulation and is a potent antioxidant.

❑ Other herbs beneficial for age spots include ginseng and licorice.
Caution: Both of these herbs can elevate blood pressure. Do not use them if you have high blood pressure.

RECOMMENDATIONS

❑ Eat a diet that is high in vegetable protein and that consists of 50 percent raw fruits and vegetables, plus fresh grains, cereals, seeds, and nuts. Be aware that seeds and nuts become rancid quickly when subjected to heat and/or exposed to the air; purchase only raw nuts and seeds that have been vacuum sealed.

❑ Omit all animal protein from the diet for one month.

❑ Avoid caffeine, fried foods, saturated fats, red meat, processed foods, sugar, and tobacco.

❑ Follow a fasting program to cleanse the liver and rid the body of toxins. A properly functioning liver and a clean colon are important. Use black radish extract or dandelion root and beet juice along with three days of fasting a month with distilled water and fresh lemon juice and fresh fruit and vegetable juices. *See* FASTING in Part Three. Use cleansing enemas while fasting. *See* ENEMAS in Part Three.

❑ Limit sun exposure.

❑ Do not use cleansing creams, especially hydrogenated, hardened creams. Cleanse your skin with pure olive oil and a warm wet washcloth, then rinse with lemon juice and water.

CONSIDERATIONS

❑ The prescription drug tretinoin (retinoic acid or Retin-A) is being used for age spots with good results.

❑ *See also* AGING in Part Two.

Aging

Growing older is not an illness, but the passing years do make the body more vulnerable to disease. Our genes dictate that the body's cells stop dividing after they have divided between twenty and thirty times. New cells must be made to replace those that die, a process that slows with age. In addition, cells are subject to premature death and damage. When there are no longer enough new cells to replace the ones that have died or suffered damage, the result is aging.

The free radical theory of aging has been the subject of a great deal of research in recent years, and has been gaining increasing acceptance. Free radicals are atoms or groups of atoms that are extremely unstable and highly reactive. If they are present in excessive amounts, they begin attacking the body on the cellular level. Free radicals attack the cells' protective membranes and genetic material (the nucleic acids DNA and RNA), causing cellular damage and malfunction. To make matters worse, the immune system may then attack the damaged cells as if they were foreign invaders.

Because they are so chemically reactive, free radicals exist for only a millionth of a second each. This has made it difficult for researchers to study them directly. But there are millions of them, and even with their short life span they do considerable damage to our cells. Denham Harman, M.D., Ph.D., of the University of Nebraska, is considered the founder of the free radical theory of aging. He postulated that many of the degenerative disorders we associate with aging, including cancer and hardening of the arteries, are not inevitable results of the passage of time, but rather are the result of the breakdown of nucleic acids, proteins, and cell structures caused by the presence of free radicals. He asserted that the phenomenon we refer to as aging is in fact nothing more than the ever-increasing accumulation of changes caused, or contributed to, by the presence of oxygen-based free radicals. Thus, though oxygen gives us life, it can also be our greatest enemy.

A significant number of problems faced by people over the age of sixty may also be attributable to nutritional deficiencies. Many elderly people have malabsorption problems, in which the nutrients in food are not properly absorbed from the gastrointestinal tract. In addition, as we age, our bodies do not assimilate nutrients as well as they once did. At the same time, as the body ages, its systems slow down and become less efficient, so the correct nutrients are more important than ever for the support, repair, and regeneration of the cells.

There are also problems with nutritional intake. One study of older people living in an urban area found that 90 percent of those examined had an inadequate intake of vitamins B_1 (thiamine) and B_6 (pyridoxine), and 30 to 40 percent demonstrated deficiencies of vitamin A, vitamin B_3 (niacin), vitamin B_{12}, vitamin C, calcium, and iron. Only 10 percent of the subjects consumed adequate amounts of protein. A diet that lacks essential nutrients over a long period of time leads to a greater risk of degenerative disease.

Vitamin B_{12} deficiency is a particular problem. A lack of vitamin B_{12} can lead to the development of neurologic symptoms ranging from tingling sensations, inability to coordinate muscular movements, weakened limbs, and lack of balance, to memory loss, mood changes, disorientation, and psychiatric disorders. Symptoms of vitamin B_{12} deficiency can easily be misinterpreted as signs of senility. Many older people become deficient in vitamin B_{12} because they do not produce adequate amounts of stomach acid for proper digestion. This creates a perfect environment for the overgrowth of certain bacteria that steal whatever vitamin B_{12} is extracted from protein in the digestive tract. Other people do not produce enough of a substance called *intrinsic factor*, without which vitamin B_{12} cannot travel from the stomach to the rest of the body, even if nothing else is standing in its way.

One can have vitality and a zest for living at any age. You should not assume that pain and illness are inevitable parts of aging. You can feel better at sixty than you did at thirty by making healthy changes in your diet and lifestyle. Adding the right supplements should give you the added power needed to boost immunity and prevent or cure most disorders—not to mention making you able to work or play longer than people much younger than you are. Looking youthful for your age is an added bonus. But remember: It takes years for these problems to develop, so it usually takes some time to resolve them as well. There are no silver bullets or magic potions, only the simple fact that if you give your body the correct fuel, it will perform for you.

NUTRIENTS

SUPPLEMENT	SUGGESTED DOSAGE	COMMENTS
Essential		
Coenzyme Q_{10}	100 mg daily.	Aids circulation, improves cellular oxygenation, and protects the heart.
Dimethylglycine (DMG) (Aangamik DMG from FoodScience Labs)	As directed on label.	Improves cellular oxygenation. Use a sublingual form.
Glutathione	500 mg daily, on an empty stomach.	A potent free radical scavenger and mental booster that acts as a mood elevator. Also destroys ammonia, which interferes with brain function.
L-Phenylalanine	500 mg daily, on an empty stomach.	An essential neurotransmitter that promotes vitality and alertness. *See* AMINO ACIDS in Part One. *Caution:* Do not take this supplement if you are pregnant or nursing, or if you suffer from panic attacks, diabetes, high blood pressure, or PKU.

Supplement	Suggested Dosage	Comments
L-Arginine and L-lysine and L-methionine and L-tyrosine plus	500 mg each twice daily, on an empty stomach. Take with water or juice. Do not take with milk. Take with 50 mg vitamin B6 and 100 mg vitamin C for better absorption. It is best to take a complex containing all the amino acids as well (but separately).	See AMINO ACIDS in Part One for the benefits of amino acids.
L-carnitine	500 mg twice daily, on an empty stomach.	Protects the heart and liver; decreases blood triglycerides; enhances the effectiveness of antioxidants; improves muscle strength.
and N-acetylcysteine	500 mg twice daily, on an empty stomach.	Used by the body to produce glutathione, a powerful antioxidant and detoxifier.
Multivitamin and mineral complex with		Needed for brain function and to protect the heart. Use a high-potency formula with chelated trace minerals.
vitamin A and	25,000 IU daily.	Important antioxidants. Protect the lungs, needed for growth and repair of body tissues and smooth skin.
natural beta-carotene and	15,000 IU daily.	
potassium and	99 mg daily.	Plays a role in cellular integrity and water balance.
selenium and	300 mcg daily.	Prevents premature aging, boosts immunity, protects against cancer.
zinc	50 mg daily. Do not exceed a total of 100 mg daily from all supplements.	Needed for wound healing and healthy skin; enhances immune function.
Omega-3 essential fatty acids (flaxseed oil, primrose oil, and salmon oil are good sources)	As directed on label 3 times daily, with meals.	Plays an important role in cell formation; essential for proper brain function; protects the heart and helps to keep plaque from sticking to the arteries.
Pycnogenol or grape seed extract	50 mg twice daily. As directed on label.	Possibly the most powerful free radical scavengers. They can pass the blood-brain barrier to protect brain cells.
Superoxide dismutase (SOD) or Cell Guard from Biotec Foods	As directed on label. As directed on label.	A potent antioxidant that destroys free radicals, which damage body cells and cause premature aging. Consider injections (under a doctor's supervision). An antioxidant complex that contains SOD.
Vitamin B complex injections plus extra pantothenic acid (vitamin B5) and	As prescribed by physician. As prescribed by physician.	The B vitamins fight depression; aid in transforming proteins, fats, and carbohydrates into energy; are necessary for the formation of certain proteins and for the functioning of the
choline and inositol and para-aminobenzoic acid (PABA)	As prescribed by physician. As prescribed by physician.	nervous system; and are essential for healthy red blood cells and the absorption of nutrients, including iron. Injections (under a doctor's supervision) are best. If injections are not available, use a sublingual form.
Vitamin E	Start with 200 IU daily and slowly increase to 800 IU daily.	A potent antioxidant that fights cellular aging by protecting cell membranes. Also improves circulation and prolongs the life of red blood cells.
Vitamin C with bioflavonoids	4,000–10,000 mg daily, in divided doses.	Powerful antioxidant and immune system enhancer that reduces allergies, protects the brain and spinal cord, keeps white blood cells healthy, fights fatigue, and increases energy.
Taurine Plus from American Biologics	As directed on label.	A building block for all amino acids that improves white blood cell function. Use the sublingual form.

Very Important

Supplement	Suggested Dosage	Comments
Boron	3 mg daily. Do not exceed this amount.	Aids calcium absorption and brain function.
Calcium and	1,500 mg daily.	Necessary to prevent bone loss and for normal heart function. Use calcium chelate or calcium asporotate form.
magnesium and	750 mg daily.	Needed to balance with calcium.
vitamin D or	600–1,000 mg daily.	Enhances calcium absorption.
Bone Defense from KAL	As directed on label.	Contains calcium, magnesium, phosphorus and other valuable bone-reinforcing nutrients.
Chromium picolinate	400–1,000 mcg daily.	Improves insulin efficiency, which maintains the health of the glands that control aging.
Free-form amino acid complex	As directed on label 3 times daily. Take with 50 mg vitamin B6 and 100 mg vitamin C for better absorption.	To supply needed protein. Elderly people often have difficulty assimilating dietary protein, and so are likely to have amino acid deficiencies.
Lecithin granules or capsules	1 tbsp 3 times daily, with meals. 1,200 mg 3 times daily, with meals.	Improves brain function and memory. Protects nervous system cells. A fat emulsifier.
Phosphatidyl serine	1,000 mg 3 times daily.	Improves brain function.
RNA and DNA	As directed on label.	Good for healthy cell reproduction. Use a sublingual form. Caution: Do not take this supplement if you have gout.

Helpful

Supplement	Suggested Dosage	Comments
Bio-Bifidus from American Biologics or Kyo-Dophilus from Wakunaga	As directed on label. As directed on label.	To improve liver function and aid in digestion by replacing bowel flora.
Brewer's yeast	Start with ½ tsp daily and work up slowly to 1 tbsp daily.	A natural source of the B vitamins.
Glucosamine sulfate or N-Acetylglucos-amine (N-A-G from Source Naturals)	As directed on label. As directed on label.	Important for the formation of bones, skin, nails, connective tissues, and heart valves; also plays a role in the mucous secretions of the digestive, respiratory, and urinary tracts.
Melatonin or Chronoset from Allergy Research Group	1.5–5 mg daily, taken 2 hours or less before bedtime. As directed on label.	Delays the aging process and improves sleep. Good for many disorders associated with aging. Contains melatonin.
Raw thymus glandular	500 mg daily.	Stimulates the immune system.

Multienzyme complex with pancreatin	As directed on label, after meals.	To aid digestion. Most elderly people lack sufficient digestive enzymes. *Caution:* If you have a history of ulcers, do not use a formula containing HCl.
Silica or horsetail	As directed on label.	Protects connective tissues and cells; keeps skin, bones, hair, nails, and other tissues youthful. *See under* Herbs, below.
Smart Longevity from E'Ola Products	As directed on label.	A liquid supplement containing antioxidants and nutrients to enhance brain function.
Zinc plus copper	50 mg daily. Do not exceed a total of 100 mg daily from all supplements. 3 mg daily.	Increases antibodies and protects the eyes against macular degeneration and vision loss. Very important for the prostate. Needed to balance with zinc.

HERBS

❑ Burdock root and red clover cleanse the bloodstream. They can be used separately or in combination.

❑ Echinacea helps to boost the immune system.

❑ Garlic helps immune function and protects the heart.

❑ Ginseng and ginkgo biloba extract are good for giving extra energy, improving brain function, and increasing circulation.

Caution: Do not use ginseng if you have high blood pressure.

❑ Horsetail, taken in tea or extract form, is an excellent source of silica, a form of the trace mineral silicon. Silicon is important for maintaining the strength of bones and connective tissue, and possibly the walls of blood vessels.

❑ Licorice root is an effective anti-inflammatory and anti-allergenic agent that supports the organ systems.

Caution: Do not use this herb on a daily basis for more than seven days in a row. Avoid it completely if you have high blood pressure.

❑ Milk thistle promotes good liver function.

❑ Nettle is full of vital minerals and is good for hypoglycemia, allergies, depression, prostate and urinary tract disorders, and a host of other problems.

❑ Valerian root is valuable as a sleep aid and tranquilizer.

❑ Wild yam contains natural steroids that have a rejuvenating effect. Steroids are what help exercise to melt off more weight and build muscle. This hormone is found in the human body as dehydroepiandrosterone (DHEA). Take larger amounts—2,400 mg daily, dropping to 1,600 mg daily—for two weeks, then stop for two weeks.

RECOMMENDATIONS

❑ Eat a balanced diet that includes raw vegetables, fruits, grains, seeds, nuts, and quality protein. Decrease your over-all food consumption, but increase your intake of raw foods. Include in the diet broccoli, cabbage, cauliflower, fish, fruits, whole grains, nuts, oats, seeds, and soybeans.

❑ Consume steam-distilled water. Drink even when you don't feel thirsty—your body needs plenty of water.

❑ Include in the diet garlic, onions, shiitake mushrooms, and pearl barley. These foods are good sources of germanium, which lessens free radical damage and is involved as a catalyst in the supply of oxygen to oxygen-poor tissue.

❑ Avoid alcohol, caffeine, red meat, salt, tobacco, white flour, white sugar, chemical food additives, drugs, pesticides, and tap water.

❑ Get regular exercise. Exercise is most important in slowing the aging process because it increases the amount of oxygen available to body tissues, a key determinant of energy and stamina. Brisk walking is good. Swimming is even better. It is the original low-impact whole-body aerobic exercise, a terrific torso toner, and even a meditative mind-relaxer.

❑ Improve your blood's oxygenation and circulation with deep breathing exercises. Try holding your breath for thirty seconds every half hour. Inhale and hold for thirty seconds, then place your tongue on the roof of your mouth where your teeth meet your gums and release the air slowly. Repeat this exercise every day for one month.

❑ Keep the colon clean. This is crucial for warding off degenerative diseases and slowing the aging process. Eat a high-fiber diet and use a cleansing enema once weekly. Get extra fiber by eating plenty of fresh vegetables, whole grains, bran, and oats. Consider retention enemas, a potent way to assure your body will assimilate and use needed nutrients (*see* ENEMAS and COLON CLEANSING in Part Three.)

❑ Eat only when you are hungry, and cut your total caloric intake. Laboratory experiments suggest that life span may increase if caloric intake is decreased.

❑ Learn how to relax. Keep active and be enthusiastic about life. By keeping up your appearance, exercising every day, and being involved in hobbies and other activities, you can keep your mind active. This is most important.

❑ Allow yourself sufficient sleep. Proper rest is important.

❑ Do not use harsh soaps on your skin. Use olive, avocado, or almond oil to cleanse the skin. Pat the oil on, then wash it off with warm water and a soft cloth. Use a facial loofah occasionally with the oil and warm water to remove dead skin. Use liquid creams and lotions (not solid creams) that contain nutrients and natural ingredients to keep your skin from becoming too dry. Do not use cold creams, cleansing creams, or solid moisturizing creams. These are hardened saturated fats that become rancid rapidly and then create free radicals, which can cause premature wrinkles. Free radicals can cause the brownish spots on the skin known as age spots. (*See* AGE SPOTS in Part Two.) Exposing the skin to the sun also promotes free radicals. To halt wrinkles, stay out of the sun.

CONSIDERATIONS

❑ Many elderly people complain of sleep difficulties. One common cause is the consumption of sugar after dinner. Complex carbohydrates have a relaxing effect. A good night-time snack is popcorn, or nut butter and crackers. Protein, on the other hand, promotes alertness, so it should be consumed earlier in the day.

❑ A burning sensation, mainly on the bottom of the feet, is not unusual among elderly people. A deficiency of the B vitamins, especially vitamin B_{12}, is often the cause. Since many older people have problems with absorption of the B vitamins, it is best to take supplements of these nutrients in a way that bypasses the digestive tract. Injections are best. Sublingual administration is also effective.

❑ The *American Journal of Clinical Nutrition* reported that up to 30 percent of people over the age of sixty-five are unable to absorb vitamin B_{12} and folic acid properly because they do not produce enough hydrochloric acid and/or they suffer from an overgrowth of bacteria in the intestinal tract.

❑ GH3 (formerly known as Gerovital H-3) is a formula based on the anesthetic procaine that has been shown to slow the aging process and rejuvenate the body. Procaine acts like and enhances the action of vitamin B_6 and para-aminobenzoic acid (PABA, one of the B vitamins). GH3, marketed by Gero Vita International, has helped many people with arthritis and other diseases of aging.

Caution: This product should not be used by individuals who are allergic to sulfites.

❑ In laboratory experiments, the drug selegiline (Eldepryl [also known as Deprenyl]) has been shown to increase the life expectancy of adult rats by an astounding 210 percent. Researchers suggest that tiny doses of selegiline may rescue brain cells from death in the event of trauma or disease. Depending on the outcome of future research, selegiline may have a wide range of uses beyond the treatment of Parkinson's disease, the only condition for which it is now officially approved. There are other drugs currently under research as potential anti-aging treatments as well. These include substances known as alphaphenyltertiarybulylnitrone (PBN), which appears to improve memory and block free radical damage; centrophenoxine, which blocks the accumulation of waste products and toxic substances in the cells; growth hormone-releasing hormone (GRH) and insulin, two hormones that stimulate the production of human growth hormone (*see* GROWTH HORMONE THERAPY in Part Three); isoprinosine, an immune booster and nerve growth factor that shows some promise against Alzheimer's disease; and thymosins, hormones from the thymus gland that boost immune function and play a role in the endocrine system.

❑ There are a number of substances available that have properties that make them "natural life extenders":

• Coenzyme Q_{10} protects the heart, increases tissue oxygenation, and is vital for many bodily functions. The liver has the highest level of coenzyme Q_{10} of any tissue. Since the liver is the main detoxifying organ of the body, optimal liver function is vital for minimizing damage to all the body's tissues.

• Dehydroepiandrosterone (DHEA) is an adrenal hormone that enhances immune function. It has been found to help prevent and treat many of the disorders associated with aging. (*See* DHEA THERAPY in Part Three.)

• Dimethylglycine (DMG) is a derivative of the amino acid glycine. It boosts immune function and improves tissue oxygenation.

• Ginkgo biloba is an herb that has powerful antioxidant properties and that supplies oxygen to the brain cells, enhancing brain function.

• Glutathione is an amino acid compound that is a valuable antioxidant and detoxifier. Cellular glutathione levels tend to drop by 30 to 35 percent with age; increasing glutathione, particularly in the liver, lungs, kidneys, and bone marrow, may have an anti-aging effect. Glutathione can be taken in supplement form. Glutathione levels can also be increased by taking supplements of N-acetylcysteine, which is converted into glutathione in the body.

• Human growth hormone (HGH or GH), also known as somatotropin, is the hormone that regulates growth. Administered to older adults, it rebuilds muscle mass and reduces the amount of fat tissue, reversing changes that occur with aging. It is available only under the supervision of a physician. (*See* GROWTH HORMONE THERAPY in Part Three.)

• L-Carnitine, L-glutamine, L-methionine, L-phenylalanine, L-tyrosine, N-acetylcysteine, and taurine are amino acids and related compounds that have various important anti-aging actions (*see* AMINO ACIDS in Part One).

• Lipoic acid is critical in glycolysis and in the Kreb's cycle, two complex biochemical processes essential for the generation of cellular energy. The liver relies on these processes to meet its large energy demands. Lipoic acid is used extensively in Germany to enhance liver function.

• Melatonin is a natural hormone that acts as an antioxidant. Early in life, the body produces an abundant supply, but as we age, production steadily declines. In one laboratory experiment, mice given melatonin lived almost one-third beyond normal life expectancy. Melatonin may also help prevent cancer, counteract insomnia, and boost immunity.

• Morel, reishi, shiitake, and maitake are mushrooms that were touted by the ancient Chinese as superior medicines that give eternal youth and longevity. They prevent high blood pressure and heart disease, lower cholesterol, prevent fatigue and viral infections, and much more. They are found in supplement form as well as fresh.

• Pantothenic acid (vitamin B_5) keeps hair healthy, with little graying, and prevents premature hair loss. It is also very important for normal adrenal and immune function.

• Para-aminobenzoic acid (PABA) is one of the B vitamins. It keeps skin healthy and delays wrinkles. In addition, the a combination of PABA and dimethylaminoethanol (DMAE) has been found to enhance brain function, immunity, and cellular regeneration.

• Pycnogenol is a powerful bioflavonoid and antioxidant.

• Superoxide dismutase (SOD) is an enzyme that is a powerful free radical scavenger that protects the cells.

❑ Aging is not an illness, but it does increase one's chances of developing certain health problems. Constipation, depression, diarrhea, dizziness, heart palpitations, heartburn and indigestion, and weight gain are some of the more common complaints that accompany aging. Detailed information on the causes of and treatments for many problems that commonly afflict older people may be found in the relevant sections of this book. See AGE SPOTS; ALZHEIMER'S DISEASE; APPETITE, POOR; ARTERIOSCLEROSIS/ATHEROSCLEROSIS; ARTHRITIS; BEDSORES; CANCER; CARDIOVASCULAR DISEASE; CIRCULATORY PROBLEMS; CONSTIPATION; DEPRESSION; DIABETES; EYE PROBLEMS; GLAUCOMA; HAIR LOSS; HEARING LOSS; HEART ATTACK; HIGH BLOOD PRESSURE; HIGH CHOLESTEROL; INDIGESTION; INSOMNIA; MEMORY PROBLEMS; MUSCLE CRAMPS; OBESITY; OSTEOPOROSIS; PROSTATITIS/ENLARGED PROSTATE; SENILITY; WEAKENED IMMUNE SYSTEM; and/or WRINKLING OF SKIN, all in Part Two.

❑ If you follow the suggestions in this section and do not feel a positive change in your energy level, see COLITIS; DIVERTICULITIS; and/or MALABSORPTION SYNDROME in Part Two.

AIDS (Acquired Immune Deficiency Syndrome)

AIDS is an immune system disorder in which the body's ability to defend itself is greatly diminished. When human immunodeficiency virus (HIV, the virus that causes AIDS) invades key immune cells called T lymphocytes and multiplies, it causes a breakdown in the body's immune system, eventually leading to overwhelming infection and/or cancer—and, ultimately, to death. Most deaths among people with AIDS are not caused by AIDS itself, but by one of the many infections or cancers to which the syndrome makes the body vulnerable.

The origin of HIV is unknown. The earliest documented case of AIDS appeared in 1981, but researchers acknowledge that there may have been unidentified cases in the 1970s. Some investigators have wondered if HIV might be a genetically engineered virus gone awry. Whatever its origin, HIV is a type of virus known as a retrovirus that is spread primarily through sexual or blood-to-blood contact, such as occurs with the sharing of needles by intravenous drug users. It can also be spread by blood transfusion or the use of blood products such as clotting factors, if the blood used for these purposes is infected. Hemophiliacs, who require a specific coagulation factor from blood concentrates, have historically been especially vulnerable to

HIV. In the United States, as well as in many other parts of the world, blood is now screened for the presence of antibodies to HIV—a sign of HIV infection—and is discarded if found to contain them. It is possible, however, that HIV-infected blood may occasionally pass through the screening process. HIV antibodies may not show up in the blood for as much as three to six months after a person is infected, so their presence in blood taken from a person who contracted the virus recently may not be detectable. Blood products are now subjected to heat to destroy the virus, although some AIDS advocates have raised concerns that this process may not be 100-percent effective.

It is possible for dentists and medical workers who come into close contact with the bodily fluids of infected persons to become infected under certain circumstances. This is why paramedics, emergency medical technicians, dentists and dental hygienists, and hospital, clinic, and emergency room personnel—even police officers—now routinely use rubber gloves to prevent contact with blood products or saliva. The practice of wearing gloves also protects patients.

Babies of mothers with HIV can contract the virus during pregnancy or birth, or through breastfeeding, although this is not inevitable. In fact, statistics show that most such babies do not contract the virus themselves. According to the 1993 Surgeon General's report on HIV and AIDS, about 25 percent of these babies do become infected, either before or during birth. Scientists do not know what factors influence whether or not a child will become infected but are working diligently to find the answers. It is known that the use of drug therapy during pregnancy plus bottle-feeding after birth may dramatically decrease the likelihood of mother-to-baby transmission.

Many people who are infected with HIV are not even aware that they have it. While some people experience a mild flulike illness within two to four weeks of exposure to the virus, it generally takes at least two to five years before any symptoms of HIV infection appear. In many cases, the first symptoms are nonspecific and variable. They include diarrhea, fever, fatigue, inflamed gums, loss of appetite and weight, mouth sores, night sweats, skin disorders, swollen lymph nodes, and an enlarged liver and/or spleen. If such symptoms become chronic, an individual may be said to have AIDS-related complex (ARC).

In other cases, the first sign of HIV is the development of one or more of the opportunistic infections or cancers associated with AIDS. One of the most common is a tongue that is coated with white bumps. This is oral thrush, or candidiasis. Candidiasis indicates a compromised immune system. Intestinal parasites are another common problem. Other common AIDS-related illnesses include *Pneumocystis carinii* pneumonia (PCP), which is caused by a parasite found in about 60 percent of people with AIDS; an otherwise rare skin cancer called Kaposi's sarcoma; Epstein-Barr virus (EBV); cytomegalovirus (CMV); herpes simplex virus (HSV); *Mycobacterium aviumintracellulare*; salmonellosis; toxoplasmosis; and tuberculosis.

Women and AIDS

The majority of people with HIV and/or AIDS in the United States are men, but the incidence of AIDS in women is rising nearly six times as fast as that in men. The AIDS epidemic disproportionately affects women who are members of racial and ethnic minorities. According to the U.S. Centers for Disease Control, 1 in 98 black women and 1 in 222 Hispanic women between the ages of twenty-seven and thirty-nine are infected, compared with only 1 in 1,667 white women. Being a member of a particular racial or ethnic group does not mean a woman is any more susceptible to AIDS, however. Instead, it reflects the fact that members of minority groups are more likely to live in places with a high incidence of HIV infection. In the early years of the epidemic, most women with AIDS contracted the disease through intravenous drug use, but sexual contact has now surpassed intravenous drug use as the leading means of transmission among women.

Most women remain undiagnosed as HIV-positive until after the onset of AIDS or until they give birth to a child with HIV who becomes ill. This delay in diagnosis can have grave consequences for survival, and has contributed to the continuing myth that women's expected survival time is shorter than that for men. Experts say that if women were diagnosed at the same point in the disease as men are, their average length of survival would be essentially the same. Compounding the problems women with HIV face is the fact that the majority of them come from economically disadvantaged backgrounds, and their access to quality health care is often limited. In contrast, the gay men with HIV who were the primary ones affected in the early days of the epidemic were generally more affluent and lived in areas with better medical resources. This factor alone has helped to distort the figures kept by various advocacy groups and medical researchers. Moreover, until relatively recently, the list of opportunistic infections considered in diagnosing AIDS did not include diseases that are unique to women, such as chronic vaginal candidiasis (yeast infection). Thus, even a woman who was HIV-positive and had one or more opportunistic infection might not have qualified for an official diagnosis of AIDS.

Because recurrent vaginal candidiasis is the most common early indicator of HIV infection in women, the FDA mandated in 1992 that manufacturers of certain over-the-counter medications include a new warning label on their products. The warning states that frequent vaginal yeast infections, especially when persistent or recurrent, can be the result of a serious medical condition, such as HIV infection. The label advises women with these symptoms to consult their physicians.

Other infections and illnesses in women that should raise concern about possible HIV infection are pelvic inflammatory disease, cervical dysplasia (precancerous changes in the cervix), yeast infections of the mouth and throat, and any sexually transmitted disease, such as genital ulcers and warts, and herpesvirus infection.

The medical criteria for a diagnosis of full-blown AIDS are quite specific, requiring the presence of one or more opportunistic infections or cancers known to be associated with HIV infection. Testing HIV-positive does *not* mean that one has AIDS. Rather, it means that one has been exposed to HIV, as demonstrated by the presence in the blood of antibodies to the virus. However, a confirmed positive HIV test result is often the earliest indication that the person may eventually develop AIDS.

Some authorities believe that, although strongly linked to HIV, AIDS must be considered a disease caused by many factors. It may be that HIV is necessary but not sufficient to cause the onset of AIDS—that is, the virus needs help in bringing about immune deficiency. For example, epidemiologists have observed that those infected with both HIV and another retrovirus, such as the less frequently seen but similarly transmitted human T cell lymphoma virus (HTLV), develop the disease far more quickly than those infected with HIV alone. Conversely, some people with signs of full-blown generalized immune deficiency, consistent with a diagnosis of AIDS, actually test *negative* for HIV antibodies.

To date, only 50 to 60 percent of individuals exposed to HIV, as documented by an antibody test, have actually developed AIDS. This is probably due in part to the dis-ease's long incubation period, but there are some people who have tested positive for HIV for many years and have never developed any symptoms of immune deficiency. We believe that a person who becomes infected with HIV is more likely to go on to develop AIDS if his or her immune system is severely suppressed by other factors at the time of exposure and later. The risk of developing AIDS is proportional to the degree of immune suppression and the amount and duration of exposure to HIV. If the immune system is functioning well, it may be possible to avoid developing AIDS, even if one is a member of a high-risk group. Studies have repeatedly shown that immune-compromised persons are at greatest risk of contracting AIDS.

HIV is highly adaptable and capable of changing its form. According to scientists at Oxford University in England, this may be the key to its survival. They say that through subtle mutations, or changes in its genetic structure, HIV evades and ultimately defuses the body's mechanisms for the elimination of infected cells. As a result, it continues to survive despite the immune system's aggressive attacks.

Meanwhile, studies conducted at the Pasteur Institute indicate that the virus may be more hardy and virulent than we have ever been told. Health authorities have long maintained that the AIDS virus cannot survive without a host, but the Pasteur Institute researchers demonstrated that HIV can survive outside the body, and that it can live for up to eleven days in untreated sewage. Apparently, HIV is not as fragile as has been thought. While there are varying points of view, we believe it is possible that the virus may live for many days outside the body, even in a dried, inactive state, and then become infectious again.

At this time, there is no cure for AIDS. According to the U.S. Centers for Disease Control and Prevention, over half a million Americans have been diagnosed with AIDS since 1981, and approximately 62 percent of that number have died. AIDS is now a leading cause of premature death among Americans. In this country, it tends to disportionately affect members of minority communities, especially African-Americans and Hispanics, and men who have sex with other men. Those who abuse drugs and those who engage in sexual intercourse (anal, oral, or vaginal) with persons whose sexual or drug history places them at risk of HIV, with persons whose sex or drug history is unknown, or who have had multiple partners, are likewise considered to be at risk for the disease. In all population groups, young males are more likely than others to have contracted HIV. AIDS education seems to have had some impact on the spread of the virus in the United States, but in recent years the number of new cases among young people has been rising again, even though they grew up in an atmosphere of widespread concern and awareness about AIDS.

Anyone with HIV or AIDS can make a major contribution to his or her survival and quality of life by getting into an early treatment program, especially a program in which immune enhancement is encouraged. The person with AIDS needs higher amounts of all nutrients than normal because malabsorption is a common problem. Those at risk of becoming infected with HIV or of developing AIDS can also be helped through the following program. For all nutritional supplements, we strongly recommend the use of sublingual and injectable forms, as well as rectal suppositories, if available, for improved absorption.

Unless otherwise specified, the dosages recommended here are for adults. For a child between the ages of twelve and seventeen, reduce the dose to three-quarters the recommended amount. For a child between six and twelve, use one-half the recommended dose, and for a child under the age of six, use one-quarter the recommended amount.

NUTRIENTS

SUPPLEMENT	SUGGESTED DOSAGE	COMMENTS
Very Important		
Aerobic 07 from Aerobic Life Industries	9 drops in water 3 times daily.	For tissue oxygenation. Kills harmful bacteria and viruses.
or		
Dioxychlor from American Biologics	As directed on label 3 times daily.	
Acetyl-L-carnitine	As directed on label.	An energy carrier, metabolic facilitator, and cell membrane protector. Also protects the heart.
Acidophilus	As directed on label 3 times daily.	To supply essential "friendly" bacteria for the intestinal tract and liver function. Fights candida infection, often associated with HIV. Use a high-potency, nondairy formula. For adults.
plus Bifido Factor from Natren	As directed on label.	
or Lifestart from Natren	As directed on label.	For infants and children.
or Kyo-Dophilus from Wakunaga	As directed on label.	
AE Mulsion Forte from American Biologics	As directed on label. Reduce the dosage if you have liver disease.	To supply vitamins A and E, which destroy free radicals and enhance immune function. Avoid capsule forms of these vitamins.
Body Language Super Antioxidant from OxyFresh	As directed on label.	Protects the body from free radical damage, environmental stresses, and pollutants.
Bone Support from Synergy Plus	As directed on label.	Contains minerals needed for better absorption of calcium.
Bovine colostrum	As directed on label.	Enhances immune function and controls AIDS-related diarrhea.
Coenzyme Q10	100 mg daily.	Increases circulation and energy, and protects the heart. A powerful antioxidant and significant immune stimulant.
Colloidal silver	As directed on label.	A broad-spectrum antiseptic that subdues inflammation and promotes healing of skin lesions.
Dimethylglycine (DMG) (Aangamik DMG from FoodScience Labs)	As directed on label.	Good for breathing difficulties. Enhances oxygen transport, increases interferon production, and has antiviral and anticancer properties.
Dimethylsulfoxide (DMSO)	As directed on label.	Acts as a "second immune system" and promotes healing of keloids. Use only DMSO from a health food store.
Egg lecithin	20 g daily, in divided doses. Take on an empty stomach.	For cellular protection.
Germanium	200 mg daily.	Improves tissue oxygenation and interferon production.
Free-form amino acid complex	As directed on label. Take on an empty stomach with water or juice. Do not take with milk. Take with 50 mg vitamin B6 and 100 mg vitamin C for better absorption.	To supply protein for repair and rebuilding of body tissues. Use a formula containing all of the essential amino acids.
plus extra L-arginine and	As directed on label, on an empty stomach.	Enhances the immune system and retards the growth of tumors.
L-ornithine plus	As directed on label, on an empty stomach.	Necessary for the immune system.
L-cysteine and	As directed on label, on an empty stomach.	Protects against cancer; destroys free radicals.
L-histidine and	As directed on label, on an empty stomach.	Aids in healing. May help in the prevention of AIDS.
L-methionine	As directed on label, on an empty stomach.	An antioxidant and free radical scavenger.

Garlic (Kyolic)	2 capsules 3 times daily, with meals. Or place 1 dropperful of Kyolic liquid in a 6- to 8-ounce glass of distilled water, add 5 drops of Concentrace mineral drops from Trace Mineral Research, and gradually sip the mixture. Do this 2 or 3 times daily.	A powerful immunostimulant that also aids in digestion, endurance, and strength. It is a natural antibiotic and is good for candida infections.
Glutathione	As directed on label, on an empty stomach.	Inhibits the formation of free radicals. Aids in red blood cell integrity and protects immune cells.
Hydrochloric acid (HCl)	As directed on label.	Replenishes stomach acid to aid digestion. *Caution:* Do not take this supplement if you have a history of ulcers.
Infla-Zyme Forte from American Biologics	4 tablets 3 times daily, with meals.	Supplies proteolytic enzymes to aid in proper breakdown and absorption of nutrients.
Kyo-Green from Wakunaga	As directed on label.	Supplies nutrients and chlorophyll needed for repair. Important in immune response.
L-Lysine	As directed on label, on an empty stomach.	To aid in preventing mouth sores and herpes outbreaks. *Caution:* Do not take lysine longer than 6 months at a time.
Malic Acid and magnesium	As directed on label.	Involved in energy production in many cells of the body, including muscle cells. Needed for sugar metabolism. Reduces pain.
Multimineral complex with copper and zinc	3 mg daily. 80 mg daily. Do not exceed a total of 100 mg daily from all supplements.	All nutrients are needed because of malabsorption. Use a high-potency, hypoallergenic form. Use a formula without iron if fever is present.
Natural carotenoid complex (Betatene)	As directed on label.	Powerful antioxidant, free radical scavenger, potential cancer fighter, and immune enhancer. Also protects against heart disease.
Pycnogenol and/or grape seed extract or OPC-85 from Primary Source	As directed on label 3 times daily. As directed on label. As directed on label.	A unique bioflavonoid. A potent antioxidant and immune enhancer. One of the most potent antioxidants known. Protects the cells. A combination of grape seed and pine bark extracts.
Quercetin plus bromelain or Activated Quercetin from Source Naturals	As directed on label. As directed on label. As directed on label.	Aids in preventing allergic reactions and increases immunity. Increases absorption of quercetin. Contains quercetin plus bromelain and vitamin C.
Raw thymus glandular plus multiglandular complex with raw spleen	As directed on label. As directed on label.	Enhances T-cell production. *See* GLANDULAR THERAPY in Part Three. Glandulars from lamb source are best.
Selenium	400 mcg daily.	Free radical scavenger and powerful immune enhancer.

Shark cartilage (BeneFin)	As directed on label. Take on an empty stomach.	Inhibits tumor growth. Be sure to use 100% pure dried shark cartilage.
Superoxide dismutase (SOD)	As directed on label.	Free radical scavenger needed for cell protection.
Taurine Plus from American Biologics	As directed on label.	An important antioxidant and immune regulator necessary for white blood cell activation and neurological function. Use the sublingual form.
Vitamin B complex injections plus extra vitamin B6 (pyridoxine) and vitamin B12	As prescribed by physician. As prescribed by physician. As prescribed by physician.	Anti-stress vitamins, especially important for normal brain function. Injections (under a doctor's supervision) are most effective. If injections are not available, use a sublingual form.
Vitamin C with bioflavonoids	10,000–20,000 mg daily, in divided doses. *See* ASCORBIC ACID FLUSH in Part Three.	Strengthens the immune system. Use buffered powdered ascorbic acid or Ester-C with minerals.
Wobenzym N from Marlyn Nutraceuticals	3–6 tablets 2–3 times daily, between meals.	Destroys free radicals and aids in proper breakdown and absorption of foods. Also good for inflammation.

Helpful		
Acid-Ease from Prevail	As directed on label. Take with meals. Take between meals also if excess acid is a problem.	Contains pure plant enzymes that function in the breakdown and assimilation of foods.
Aloe vera		*See under* Herbs, below.
Chromium picolinate	At least 600 mcg daily.	Helps to build and maintain muscle mass. Stabilizes blood sugar.
Maitake	As directed on label.	Enhances the activity of T-helper cells in people with AIDS. Has been shown to kill HIV in the laboratory.
Shark liver oil	As directed on label.	Aids in rebuilding and functioning of all cells, and has anticancer properties.
Shiitake or reishi	As directed on label. As directed on label.	Boosts immunity, fights fatigue and viral infection, and has anticancer properties.
Ultimate Oil from Nature's Secret	As directed on label.	Supplies essential fatty acids, a most important element of the diet.

HERBS

❑ Aloe vera contains carrisyn, which appears to inhibit the growth and spread of HIV. Use a pure, food-grade product. Take 2 cups twice daily. If diarrhea occurs, reduce the dosage.

❑ Astragalus boosts the immune system.
Caution: Do not use this herb in the presence of a fever.

❑ Black radish, dandelion root, and silymarin (milk thistle extract) protect and aid in repairing the liver, and also cleanse the bloodstream. The liver is *the* organ of detoxification and must function optimally. Use these extracts as directed on the product label.

❑ Burdock root, echinacea, goldenseal, mullein, red clover, and suma are good for cleansing the blood and lymphatic systems, for viral and bacterial infections, and for boosting the immune system. Cayenne (capsicum) may also be helpful.

Caution: Do not take goldenseal on a daily basis for more than one week at a time, and do not use it during pregnancy. If you have a history of cardiovascular disease, diabetes, or glaucoma, use it only under a doctor's supervision.

❑ Cat's claw enhances immune function, and has been shown to be helpful for people with AIDS and AIDS-related cancers. Cat's Claw Defense Complex from Source Naturals is a combination of cat's claw and other herbs, plus antioxidants such as beta-carotene, N-acetylcysteine, vitamin C, and zinc.

Caution: Do not use cat's claw during pregnancy.

❑ The seeds and peels of the Chinese cucumber inhibit cancer. The root is currently being used in AIDS research.

❑ ClearLungs from Natural Alternatives is a Chinese herbal formula that is good for all lung disorders.

❑ Essiac is a combination herbal tea that has been used in cancer treatment with good results. Essiac teas are available in health food stores.

❑ Ginkgo biloba extract is good for the brain cells and circulation.

❑ For mouth sores, place alcohol-free goldenseal extract on a pure cotton ball or piece of gauze and apply the cotton to the gums or mouth sores before going to bed. Leave it on overnight; sores and inflammation should heal in a few days with this treatment.

❑ Licorice and wild yam root are good for endocrine gland function.

Caution: Do not use this herb on a daily basis for more than seven days in a row. Avoid it completely if you have high blood pressure.

❑ Magnolia vine berries increase oxygen absorption and boost the immune system. They coordinate the activities of the internal organs and help control the balance of the body's physiological processes.

❑ Pau d'arco is a natural antibiotic, and potentiates immune function. It is also a powerful antioxidant and is good for destroying candida in the colon.

❑ St. Johnswort contains two substances, hypericin and pseudohypericin, that inhibit retroviral infections, and could be useful in the treatment of AIDS.

❑ Siberian ginseng helps bronchial disorders and boosts energy.

Caution: Do not use this herb if you have hypoglycemia, high blood pressure, or a heart disorder.

RECOMMENDATIONS

❑ If you test positive for HIV, arrange for repeat testing as soon as you can to rule out the possibility of a false-positive result. If this is ruled out, *immediately* begin taking

measures to boost your immune system. This is the single most important factor in disease prevention, and it is the best defense for the person with HIV. Correct diet, appropriate supplements, exercise, stress reduction, a proper environment, and a healthy mental outlook all play significant roles in keeping the immune system working adequately.

❑ Pay special attention to meeting your nutritional needs and requirements, and keep in mind that a higher than normal intake of nutrients will probably be necessary.

❑ Increase your intake of fresh fruits and vegetables. Eat a diet consisting of 75 percent raw foods, organically grown if possible (avoid foods that have been treated with pesticides and other sprays), plus lentils, beans, seeds, nuts and whole grains, including brown rice and millet. Raw foods are particularly important because cooking depletes foods of their vital enzymes.

❑ Eat plenty of cruciferous vegetables, such as broccoli, Brussels sprouts, cabbage, and cauliflower. Also consume yellow and deep-orange vegetables such as carrots, pumpkin, squash, and yams.

❑ Consume plenty of fresh live juices. Juicing is extremely beneficial for supplying nutrients. (*See* JUICING in Part Three.) "Green drinks" made from leafy greens such as kale, spinach, and beet greens, and carrot and beet root juice, should be consumed on a daily basis, with garlic and onion added. Kyo-Green from Wakunaga is an excellent "green drink" product that contains chlorophyll, protein, vitamins, minerals, and enzymes. Take this drink three times a day.

❑ Drink steam-distilled water only (not tap water), and lots of it—eight or more 8-ounce glasses daily—to flush out toxins from the body. All cells and organ systems need water. Drink plenty of water even if you are not thirsty. The organs, and especially the brain, become dehydrated long before thirst develops.

❑ Eat unripened papaya (including a few of the seeds), fresh pineapple, and *Aspergillus oryzae* (a type of fungus) frequently. These foods are good sources of proteolytic enzymes, which are crucial for proper digestion of foods and assimilation of nutrients. Without enzymes, the body cannot be supplied with the energy it needs for its activities. Enzymes can also be taken in supplement form. These help in digestion in the lower stomach and intestinal tract.

❑ Eat onions and garlic, or take garlic in supplement form (*see under* Nutrients, above).

❑ Add shiitake, reishi, and maitake mushrooms to the diet, or take them in supplement form (*see under* Nutrients).

❑ Limit your intake of soybeans and soy products, which contain enzyme inhibitors, but do not completely eliminate them from your diet, as they are valuable sources of protein.

❑ Eliminate from the diet colas, foods with additives and colorings, junk foods, peanuts, processed refined foods, saturated fats, salt, sugar and sugar products, white flour, *all* animal protein, and anything that contains caffeine.

❑ Take supplemental fiber daily. Alternate between psyllium husks and freshly ground flaxseeds. Take psyllium with a glass of water and drink it quickly before it thickens.

Note: Always take supplemental fiber separately from other supplements and medications.

❑ Exercise caution in your choice of foods so as to avoid exposure to foodborne illness. Food poisoning can be very dangerous for people with AIDS or HIV infection. (*See* FOOD POISONING in Part Two.)

❑ Do not smoke, and stay away from those who do.

❑ Avoid alcohol, noxious chemicals, and everything else that can damage the liver.

❑ Try using bee propolis and royal jelly to fight bacterial infections invading the lungs, mouth, throat, and mucous membranes.

❑ Obtain as much fresh air and rest as possible, and moderate amounts of sunshine.

❑ Use coffee retention enemas to eliminate toxins and supply nutrients. *See* ENEMAS in Part Three.

❑ Determine what food sensitivities or allergies may be present. The best way to do this is to have yourself tested by a health care professional. (*See* ALLERGIES in Part Two.) It is important to eliminate allergenic foods from the diet because they wreak havoc in the body, causing damage to the immune system.

❑ *Always* use a condom (latex, not sheepskin) and spermicide (spermicide kills HIV) for any sexual contact. If you use a lubricant with a latex condom, use only a water-based lubricant such as K-Y jelly; *do not* use petroleum jelly (Vaseline), vegetable shortening (Crisco), hand lotion, or baby oil, as these substances can break down latex in a matter of minutes. Be aware, however, that even the proper use of a condom is not a guarantee against the transmission of HIV.

❑ Seek out the care of a qualified health care provider—if possible, one who has a great deal of experience, in treating people with HIV. Research has found that the length of survival of a person with AIDS is closely linked to how much his or her physician knows about treating the condition. The median length of survival after diagnosis is twenty-six months for those whose doctors have the most experience with AIDS, compared with fourteen months for those whose doctors have the least experience with AIDS.

❑ Educate yourself. HIV and AIDS are complicated conditions, and treatment options are constantly changing and expanding. In order to stay well, it is vital to be as informed as possible.

CONSIDERATIONS

❑ Ever since the AIDS epidemic began, researchers have been looking for a "silver bullet"—a single miracle drug to combat the virus, or a vaccine to seek out and destroy the virus in the bloodstream. If there is such a cure, scientists say it is still years away. The best answer is prevention, through avoidance of high-risk behavior and enhancement of the immune system. For persons already infected with HIV, the most logical approach to staying well is to eliminate all known causes of immune suppression and to implement the use of therapies that inhibit viral activity and stimulate immune function.

❑ The most destructive immunosuppressive factors in life are excessive alcohol and drug use, especially recreational drug use; poor diet; and sexual excess, especially in non-monogamous relationships.

❑ Research has shown that dehydroepiandrosterone (DHEA), a hormone, may enhance the functioning of the immune system. (*See* DHEA THERAPY in Part Three.)

❑ Human growth hormone (HGH) therapy has been shown to help prevent and/or reverse wasting syndrome. This treatment must be given under a doctor's supervision. (*See* GROWTH HORMONE THERAPY in Part Three.)

❑ Hyperbaric oxygen therapy is sometimes used, together with medications and other treatments, to help overcome opportunistic infections associated with AIDS. (*See* HYPERBARIC OXYGEN THERAPY in Part Three.)

❑ N-acetylcysteine and L-carnitine have both shown some promise in the ability to prevent and counteract the extreme weight loss common in people with AIDS.

❑ Maitake mushroom polysaccharide has shown anti-HIV activity in test tubes and under laboratory conditions. Whether it would be useful in combating the disease in infected people has not yet been determined, however.

❑ People with AIDS are almost always underweight, and often have malabsorption problems that contribute to malnutrition, which is common in people with AIDS. A lack of quality protein and adequate calories is a common reason for immune deficiency.

❑ The only *truly* safe sex is sex between life partners who are HIV-free. Other than that, abstinence is the only way to avoid any chance of infection with a sexually transmitted disease (STD). Changing partners particularly puts one at risk.

❑ There are thousands of AIDS survivors (epidemiologists call them "long-term non-progressors") who are free from all symptoms and lead absolutely normal lives years after being identified as HIV-positive. As reported at the World AIDS Conference in Japan in 1994, there are at least 10,000 such people worldwide, and they are being studied intensively. A key to the AIDS cure may reside in these people, some of whom have had HIV for over ten years and who have nevertheless remained healthy. Many thousands will continue to be HIV-positive but *not* manifest full-blown AIDS. And unknown to the general public and many in the medical establishment, there are also people who are now "antibody-negative"—once diagnosed as HIV-positive, they apparently no longer have the virus present in their bodies. The medical community is amazed by this, and doctors continue to monitor the blood of such people frequently, as if in disbelief. For more information about this, read *They Conquered AIDS! True Life Adventures* by Scott Gregory and Bianca Leonardo (True Life Publications, 1989).

❑ Standard medical approaches to treatment of HIV focus on using drugs to try to block replication of the virus and thus slow the progression of disease, plus taking aggressive measures as needed to fight opportunistic infections and cancers. Medical science has probably had more success finding ways to defeat opportunistic infections than in combating the virus directly, but research continues on both fronts and progress is being made. One currently accepted element of anti-HIV drug treatment is that combination therapy—the use of two or more drugs that act in different ways—is often more effective than the use of any single medication or type of medication.

❑ Most of the agents now widely used to target HIV fall into one of two categories:

• Nucleoside analogues. These drugs work by taking the place of one of the building blocks of the virus as it attempts to replicate, in effect blocking the virus's attempts to reproduce. Most of these drugs are commonly known by initials or combinations of letters and numbers derived from their original chemical names. Examples include zidovudine (Retrovir), better known as AZT; zalcitabine (HIVID), better known as ddC; didanosine (Videx), better known as ddI; stavudine (Zerit), better known as d4T; and lamivudine (Epivir), better known as 3TC. AZT was the first drug to be approved for use against HIV and has been the primary drug used to treat HIV infection ever since. It also has shown considerable effectiveness in preventing the transmission of the virus from an infected woman to a fetus during pregnancy and birth. The other nucleoside analogues were originally conceived as alternatives to AZT, but have since been found to work well with AZT in many cases. These drugs appear to prolong survival and delay the progression from the asymptomatic stage of HIV infection to full-blown AIDS, at least in some individuals. They can be used singly or in combination with each other (usually AZT plus one or more other drugs). Drawbacks include potential toxicity (especially in the case of AZT) and unpleasant side effects. In addition, the virus eventually develops resistance to these drugs, usually after a year or more of therapy.

• Protease inhibitors. These are drugs that bind to and block the action of a viral enzyme, protease, that plays a central role in the replication of HIV. If protease is prevented from exerting its normal action, the virus cannot reproduce. This class of drugs has shown great promise, at least in some studies, as a treatment for HIV infection. They are often used as an adjunct to treatment with AZT or another of the nucleoside analogues. Examples of protease inhibitors include indinavir (Crixivan), ritonavir (Norvir), and saquinivir (Invirase).

❑ There are different theories and some conflicting evidence about when to initiate treatment with nucleoside analogues and/or protease inhibitors, as well as about which agents are most effective (and for whom). Individual practitioners differ in their views on these issues. In addition, because of the tremendous amount of research being done on AIDS and its potential treatments, new possibilities for drugs and approaches to different aspects of the disease are emerging all the time. It is vital to work with a health care professional whose experience and judgment you trust.

❑ Some directions of antiviral drug research now being pursued include the following:

• Antisense compounds. By locking onto strands of viral DNA or RNA, these drugs act a bit like chewing gum stuck in the teeth of a zipper—they "gum up" the zipper so that the virus's genetic instructions are blocked.

• Cellular targets. These compounds inhibit factors inside the immune cells that HIV needs for replication, and have shown promise in interfering with the virus's ability to reproduce. One such compound is the cancer chemotherapy drug hydroxyurea (Hydrea), which appears to be particularly effective when used in combination with ddI.

• Cyclophilin inhibitors. These inhibit the fusion of infected and uninfected cells.

• Glucosidase inhibitors. These substances disrupt the structural integrity of sugars in the viral coat.

• Reverse transcriptase inhibitors. Reverse transcriptase is an enzyme used by retroviruses such as HIV to create copies of its genetic material, which then are incorporated into infected cells. By this mechanism the virus in effect turns normal immune cells into "factories" that continue to produce copies of viral DNA. In theory, by inhibiting reverse transcriptase, you suppress the virus.

❑ It is hoped that as scientists develop newer and more effective means of attacking the virus at various points in its life cycle, it will become possible to combine them in such a way that long-term suppression of the virus can be achieved—in effect, turning AIDS into a chronic but manageable illness rather than a terminal one. The principal unanswered question is whether, if near-perfect viral suppression does become reality, the immune system will be capable of restoring itself. The data are not yet clear on this point, though evidence from protease inhibitor studies has been encouraging. At the very least, it is fair to say that the new generation of antiviral drugs and their combinations is bringing a new era of new hope in the fight against AIDS.

❑ At an international conference on AIDS in Vancouver, British Columbia, Canada, in 1996, researchers reported that in some test subjects given "AIDS cocktails" containing mixtures of two, three, or more anti-AIDS drugs, the amount of HIV present in the body was dramatically reduced. They theorize that if given early enough, potent combination treatments might even be able to eliminate the virus and allow the immune system to recover.

❑ It is *not* possible to contract HIV by donating blood. Blood donors *do not* come in contact with the blood of other and only sterile materials, including single-use, disposable needles, are used to collect blood donations.

❑ *See also* SEXUALLY TRANSMITTED DISEASES in Part Two.

SOURCES OF FURTHER ASSISTANCE

❑ The following organizations and groups provide information and help for people with HIV and AIDS:

AIDS Hot Line
English: 800–342–AIDS
   (seven days a week, twenty-four hours a day)
Spanish: 800–344–7432
   (seven days a week, 8:00 a.m.–2:00 p.m. Eastern time)
TTY: 800–243–7889
   (Monday–Friday, 10:00 a.m.–10:00 p.m. Eastern time)
Sponsored by the Centers for Disease Control, the AIDS Hot Line offers information and educational services on HIV- and AIDS-related topics. Also provides medical and support-group referrals.

AIDS Action Committee
131 Clarendon Street
Boston, MA 02116
617–437–6200

American Foundation for AIDS Research (AMFAR)
733 Third Avenue, 12th Floor
New York, NY 10017
212–682–7440

Gay Men's Health Crisis (GMHC)
129 West 20th Street
New York, NY 10011–3629
212–807–6655   TTY 212–645–7470

National Association of People With AIDS (NAPWA)
1413 K Street NW, Suite 700
Washington, DC 20005
202–898–0414

Project Inform
1965 Market Street, Suite 220
San Francisco, CA 94103
800–822–7422

Alcoholism

Alcoholism is a chronic condition marked by a dependence on ethanol (ethyl alcohol). This dependence can be physiological, psychological, or a combination of the two. Of the estimated 75 percent of the American population that consumes alcohol, one in ten people can be expected to have a problem with alcohol consumption. Alcoholism currently affects approximately four times as many men as women, but the incidence of alcoholism among women is on the rise, as is the use of alcohol by children, adolescents, and college students.

Alcohol affects everyone differently. Some become intoxicated with the first drink; others may be able to consume four or five drinks before showing any effects. In alcoholics, each drink triggers a craving for another. Alcoholism is a progressive disease that usually starts with acceptable social drinking. This leads to a drink for every mood: one to calm down, one to perk up, one to celebrate, one to "drown one's sorrows," and so on. The alcoholic soon needs no excuse to drink. In time, the alcoholic is completely controlled by his or her dependence on alcohol. Alcoholics often become ashamed and angry at their compulsive behavior, and harbor deep feelings of inadequacy inside. This usually only leads to further alcohol abuse, however, as they use alcohol to numb the pain. They may also begin taking out their frustrations on those closest to them.

Alcoholism is unique to each individual; no two cases are alike. Some people drink moderate to heavy amounts of alcohol for years before becoming clinically dependent on it; others may become addicted to alcohol the very first time they ever take a drink. There is considerable debate as to whether alcoholism is a result of genetics or environment. While there are sizable bodies of evidence to support both sides, the truth probably lies somewhere in between; alcoholism is probably the result of a combination of the two.

As far as the body is concerned, alcohol is a poison. Some of the effects of chronic alcohol consumption include damage to the brain, liver, pancreas, duodenum, and central nervous system. Alcoholism causes metabolic damage to every cell in the body and depresses the immune system. It may take years before the consequences of excessive drinking become evident, but if an alcoholic continues to drink, his or her life span may be shortened by ten to fifteen years or more.

Alcohol is broken down in the liver. The repeated consumption of alcohol inhibits the liver's production of digestive enzymes, impairing the body's ability to absorb proteins, fats, and the fat-soluble vitamins (vitamins A, D, E, and K), as well as B-complex vitamins (especially thiamine and folic acid) and other water-soluble vitamins. Many essential nutrients are not retained for use by the body; they are rapidly eliminated through the urine. The toxic effect of alcohol on the liver is very serious. First, excessive amounts of fat accumulate in the liver, a result of alcohol's effect on the body's ability to digest fats properly. Next, the alcoholic may develop hepatitis, a condition in which liver cells become inflamed and may die. The final, usually fatal, stage of alcoholic liver damage is cirrhosis of the liver, a disease characterized by inflammation, hardening, and scarring of the liver. This prevents the normal passage of blood through the liver, inhibiting the organ's ability to filter out toxins and foreign substances.

The liver is one of the most robust organs of the body. It is the only organ that has the ability to regenerate itself after certain types of damage. Up to 25 percent of the liver can be removed, and within a short period of time, it will grow back to its original shape and size. It continually takes abuse, but if cared for properly, it will function more than adequately for decades. Alcohol is one of the toxins that the liver doesn't handle as well as others. The liver cannot regenerate after being severely damaged by alcohol.

There are many other health consequences of alcoholism as well. Alcoholics often experience damage to their peripheral nervous systems. This damage may show up initially as a loss of sensation in the hands or feet, with an accompanying difficulty in walking. Chronic drinking also causes inflammation of the pancreas. This further hampers the body's ability to digest fats and other nutrients, and can lead to diabetes. Alcoholics face an increased risk of mouth and throat cancer due to the direct toxicity of the alcohol. They may also experience high blood pressure, reduced testosterone production, visible dilation of blood vessels just beneath the skin's surface, and pathological enlargement of the heart that can progress to congestive heart failure. The social consequences of alcoholism can be very destructive as well. Alcohol abuse takes a tremendous toll on society through traffic and other accidents, poor job performance, and emotional damage to entire families.

Drinking during pregnancy is particularly dangerous. The consumption of alcohol during pregnancy can cause birth defects and increases the chance of miscarriage. Alcohol passes through the mother's placenta and into the fetal circulation. This toxic substance depresses the central nervous system of the fetus. Further, the fetal liver must try to metabolize the alcohol, but since the fetus's liver is not fully developed, the alcohol remains in the fetal circulation. Women who drink during pregnancy generally give birth to babies with lower birth weights. Their growth may be retarded or stunted; their brains may be smaller than normal, and there may be mental retardation as well. Limbs, joints, fingers, and facial features may be deformed. Heart and kidney defects may occur. Some children exposed to alcohol *in utero* become hyperactive at adolescence and exhibit learning disabilities. Every drink a pregnant woman consumes increases her child's risk of being born with fetal alcohol syndrome, and also increases her chances of miscarriage. Even moderate amounts of alcohol may be harmful, especially in the first three to four months of pregnancy.

Alcoholics who stop drinking often experience withdrawal symptoms, especially during the first week or so that they abstain from alcohol. Insomnia, visual and auditory hallucinations, convulsions, acute anxiety, a rapid pulse, profuse perspiration, and fever can occur. With time, however, and with appropriate supervision if necessary, these symptoms pass and the alcoholic is set free to begin the lifelong work of recovery.

Dietary supplements, while important for everyone, are especially vital for alcoholics. Alcoholics need to supplement *all* the known vitamins and minerals. The program outlined below is designed to help recovering alcoholics to improve their nutritional condition. There are also some supplements that help with the psychological aspects of recovery by decreasing the desire for alcohol.

NUTRIENTS

SUPPLEMENT	SUGGESTED DOSAGE	COMMENTS
Essential		
Free-form amino acid complex	500 mg each 3 times daily, on an empty stomach.	Aids in withdrawal; needed for brain and liver function; necessary for regeneration of liver cells. See AMINO ACIDS in Part One.
plus extra L-cysteine or N-acetylcysteine	Start with 500 mg daily and slowly work up to 1,000 mg daily.	
Gamma-aminobutyric acid (GABA)	750 mg once or twice daily, as needed.	To calm the body and prevent anxiety and stress.
plus inositol	As directed on label.	
and niacinamide	500 mg once or twice daily, as needed.	
Glutathione	3,000 mg daily, on an empty stomach.	Protects the liver and reduces craving for alcohol. *Note:* Do not take substitute glutamic acid for glutathione.
and L-methionine	1,000 mg daily, on an empty stomach. Take with water or juice. Do not take with milk. Take with 25 mg vitamin B$_6$ and 100 mg vitamin C for better absorption.	Protects glutathione, making it available to the liver. *See* AMINO ACIDS in Part One.
Pantothenic acid (vitamin B$_5$)	100 mg 3 times daily.	Aids the body in alcohol detoxification. Needed to counteract stress.
Vitamin B complex injections	As prescribed by physician.	To correct deficiencies. Injections (under a doctor's supervision) are best.
plus vitamin B$_{12}$	25 mg 3 times daily.	If injections are not available, use a sublingual form.
Vitamin B$_1$ (thiamine)	200 mg 3 times daily.	Alcoholics often are deficient in B vitamins, especially B$_1$.
Very Important		
Multienzyme complex	As directed on label. Take with meals.	To aid digestion.
plus proteolytic enzymes	As directed on label. Take between meals.	Essential for assimilation of protein. *Caution:* Do not give these supplements to a child.
Calcium and magnesium	2,000 mg daily, at bedtime. 1,000 mg daily, at bedtime.	A vital mineral that has a sedative effect. Works with calcium. Magnesium is depleted from the body with alcohol use.
Primrose oil	1,000 mg 3 times daily, with meals.	Used successfully in Europe, this supplement is a good source of essential fatty acids.
Vitamin C with bioflavonoids	3,000–10,000 mg daily, in divided doses.	Acts as a powerful antioxidant with healing potential, and promotes production of interferon, which helps the body resist infection, to which alcoholics are generally more susceptible.
Important		
Lecithin granules or capsules	1 tbsp 3 times daily, before meals. 1,200 mg 3 times daily, before meals.	Good for brain function. Helps correct fatty liver degeneration. May protect against cirrhosis.

Multivitamin and mineral complex with	As directed on label.	All nutrients are needed because of malabsorption problems.
manganese and	200 mcg daily. Take separately from calcium.	Important trace minerals that enhance immune function.
selenium	200 mcg daily.	

Helpful		
Acidophilus or	As directed on label. Take on an empty stomach.	Needed for proper digestion. Helps the damaged liver.
Bifido Factor from Natren	As directed on label.	Helps prevent candidiasis from developing.
Choline complex or	As directed on label.	Effective combinations that reduce fatty liver changes, improving liver function.
acetylcholine complex or	As directed on label.	
phosphatidyl choline	As directed on label.	
Dimethylglycine (DMG) (Aangamik DMG from FoodScience Labs)	125 mg 3 times daily.	Carries oxygen to the cells.
Lithium	As prescribed by physician.	A trace mineral that may help depression. Available by prescription only.
Raw liver extract	As directed on label.	A rich source of vitamins and minerals that aids in repairing the liver and in preventing anemia. See GLANDULAR THERAPY in Part Three.
and raw pancreas glandular	As directed on label.	Helps prevent pancreatic damage; beneficial for people with diabetes associated with alcoholism.
Vitamin A	25,000 IU daily. If you are pregnant, do not exceed 10,000 IU daily.	To counteract deficiencies. These vitamins are poorly absorbed if the liver is damaged. Use emulsion forms for easier assimilation and greater safety at higher doses. Avoid capsule or tablet forms.
and vitamin D and	400 IU daily.	
vitamin E	400–1,200 IU daily.	
Zinc	50 mg daily. Do not exceed a total of 100 mg daily from all supplements.	Deficiency can cause pathological changes in the stomach similar to those caused by alcohol.

HERBS

❑ Alfalfa is a good source of needed minerals.

❑ Burdock root and red clover cleanse the bloodstream.

❑ Dandelion root and silymarin (milk thistle extract) help to repair damage done to the liver.

❑ Valerian root has a calming effect. It is best taken at bedtime.

RECOMMENDATIONS

❑ Avoid *all* alcohol. Total abstinence is an absolute requirement for regaining control over your life and your health. Even after years of sobriety, you cannot begin drinking again and expect to maintain control over it. As little as one sip of something containing alcohol can renew the drinking pattern. You must choose *not* to drink.

❑ Seek help from a person or persons knowledgeable about this disorder. Alcoholics Anonymous has been doing wonderful work for many years in helping alcoholics achieve and maintain sobriety. Al-Anon is a similar group that provides support for the friends and families of alcoholics. The assistance and counseling services of these groups are available in nearly every city and town nationwide. Look in your local telephone directory for the group nearest you, or call your local mental health association for information.

❑ If possible, consult a nutritionally oriented physician to determine your specific nutritional needs.

❑ Go on a ten-day live juice and cleansing fast to remove toxins from the body quickly. *See* FASTING in Part Three.

❑ Eat a nutrient-dense diet of fresh whole foods, organically grown if possible, and follow the nutritional supplement program outlined above. Your primary foods should be raw fruits and vegetables, whole grains, and legumes.

❑ Avoid saturated fats and fried foods, which put stress on the liver. For essential fatty acids, use primrose oil supplements plus small amounts of cold-pressed organic vegetable oils.

❑ Do not consume refined sugar or anything that contains it. Alcoholics often have disorders of sugar metabolism.

❑ Get plenty of rest, especially in the early weeks of recovery, to allow your body to cleanse and repair itself.

❑ Avoid people, things, and places that are associated with drinking. Make new friendships with people who do not drink. Taking up a hobby, becoming involved in sports, and exercising promote self-esteem and provide a productive outlet for energy.

❑ As much as possible, avoid stress. Cultivate patience; this will be needed for the long, slow road to recovery.

❑ Do not take any drugs except for those prescribed by your physician.

❑ If you suspect that someone you know may be abusing alcohol, encourage the person to seek professional care.

CONSIDERATIONS

❑ Alcoholics are at much greater risk of malnutrition than other people, since as much as 50 percent of their caloric intake may come from ethanol at the expense of other nutritious foods. Alcoholics are commonly deficient in folic acid, and malabsorption due to pancreatic insufficiency is often a major problem.

❑ Long-term alcohol abuse can promote a zinc-deficient state, most likely because of increased fecal and urinary losses. Zinc plays a vital role in a variety of enzyme systems in the body, as well as in DNA and RNA production. A deficiency of zinc can result in anorexia, impaired senses of smell and taste, growth retardation, disorders of the reproductive system, and impaired wound healing and immune function. Pathological changes in the stomach occur due to zinc deficiency as well. Alcohol-related zinc deficiency accelerates the poisoning of cells that come into contact with alcohol by altering the metabolism of fats, carbohydrates, and nutrients. This leads to malabsorption problems and other nutritional deficiencies. Chronic alcohol intake often results in a depressed metabolism caused by zinc deficiency.

❑ A Department of Health and Human Services study showed that tobacco smokers and alcohol drinkers who regularly use high-alcohol mouthwash may be more likely than other people to get oral and pharyngeal cancers.

❑ Alcohol is one of the most damaging substances to the stomach and the small intestine. It is one of the few substances that can penetrate the lining of the stomach and cause damage. Gastric secretions increase with alcohol consumption, causing excess acidity and diluting digestive enzymes. This can lead to gastritis.

❑ Chronic alcohol consumption alters red blood cell membranes and causes various other types of cells, including gastrointestinal cells, to lose their normal flexibility.

❑ A recovering alcoholic who resumes drinking, even after years of sobriety, will damage his or her liver as though the drinking had never stopped in the first place.

❑ The drug naltrexone (Trexan) blocks the pleasurable effects of endogenous opioids, opiate-like substances released by the brain in response to alcohol, and may help problem drinkers remain sober. In two separate studies conducted at the University of Pennsylvania and the Yale University School of Medicine, people who took this drug were three times likelier than other patients to stick with their recovery programs. This drug is not suitable for people with liver disease, however.

❑ Some physicians prescribe the drug disulfram (Antabuse) to help alcoholics stay sober. Those on this drug experience nausea, vomiting, severe headaches, blurred vision, and sometimes an impending feeling of death if they take even a small sip of alcohol. Abstinence from alcohol often results with use of this drug.

❑ In some countries, hyperbaric oxygen has been used successfully in the treatment of alcoholism (see HYPERBARIC OXYGEN THERAPY in Part Three).

❑ Alcoholism and substance abuse specialists sometimes recommend a supervised "intervention" to force an alcoholic into admitting the problem and entering treatment. Psychological techniques have been developed and refined over the past few years, which seems to have increased the success rate among alcoholics seeking to recover and remain sober. Such interventions are delicate matters, however, and should be undertaken only under the supervision of a trained professional.

❑ Research has shown that college students today are getting drunk more often, and are drinking in order to become drunk. The number of students who drink to become intoxicated was two to three times as high today as it was two decades ago.

❑ Binge drinking is a sign of severe alcoholism. The binge drinker will drink to the point of intoxication and stay that way for a couple of days. The binge may end in vomiting and passing out. Frequently the person does not remember the events that happened during the binge. Binge drinkers consume larger quantities of alcohol on a regular basis and also experience more intoxication and alcohol-related problems than non-binge drinkers do.

❑ Some research has indicated that the children of teetotalers are actually at higher risk of becoming alcohol abusers even than children of alcoholics. This has been taken to mean that children reared in homes where alcohol is accepted as a social norm and not abused are less likely than others to become alcoholics. However, the latest research has found that children of alcoholics are more inclined than children of nonalcoholics to use drugs, including cocaine. These children are 400 times more likely to use drugs than those who do not have a family history of alcohol addiction. Studies conducted in Sweden revealed that the majority of babies of alcoholics who were adopted by nonalcoholic families eventually grew up to become alcoholics, indicating a correlation between chemical dependency and genetics.

❑ Limiting one's drinking to beer or wine does not protect against alcoholism or damage from alcohol. Twelve ounces of beer or 5 ounces of wine is comparable in alcohol content to 1¼ ounces of whiskey.

❑ Medications such as tranquilizers, phenobarbital, and even over-the-counter pain remedies such as acetaminophen (found in Tylenol, Datril, and many other products) can form toxic combinations with alcohol. Combining alcohol with antihistamines can enhance depression of the central nervous system.

❑ In recovery, it is best to avoid tranquilizers, as there is a danger of substituting one drug addiction for another. Sobriety should be drug-free.

❑ Pregnant women should avoid all alcohol.

❑ See also CIRRHOSIS OF THE LIVER and DRUG ADDICTION, both in Part Two.

Alkalosis

Alkalosis is the inverse of acidosis—it is a condition in which the body is too alkaline. Alkalosis is less common than acidosis, and produces overexcitability of the nervous system. The peripheral nerves are affected first. The symptoms may be manifested as a highly nervous condition, including hyperventilation and even seizures. Other symptoms can include sore muscles, creaking joints, bursitis, drowsiness, protruding eyes, hypertension, hypothermia, seizures, edema, allergies, night cramps, asthma, chronic indigestion, night coughs, vomiting, too-rapid blood clotting and thick blood, menstrual problems, hard dry stools, prostatitis, and thickening of the skin, with burning, itching sensations. Alkalosis may cause calcium to build up in the body, as in bone or heel spurs.

Acidity and alkalinity are measured according to the pH (potential of hydrogen) scale. Water, with a pH of 7.0, is considered neutral—neither acid nor alkaline. Any substance with a pH above 7.0 is alkaline, while anything with a pH below 7.0 is acid. The ideal pH range for the human body is between 6.0 and 6.8 (the human body is naturally mildly acidic). For the body, values above pH 6.8 are considered to be on the alkaline side; values below pH 6.3 are on the acidic side.

Alkalosis is often the result of excessive intake of alkaline drugs, such as sodium bicarbonate for the treatment of gastritis or peptic ulcers. It can also result from excessive vomiting, high cholesterol, endocrine imbalance, poor diet, diarrhea, and osteoarthritis.

ACID AND ALKALINE SELF-TEST

This test will determine whether your body fluids are either too acidic or too alkaline. An imbalance can cause illnesses such as acidosis or alkalosis.

Purchase nitrazine paper, available at any drugstore, and apply saliva and/or urine to the paper. The paper will change color to indicate if your system is overly acidic or alkaline. Red litmus paper turns blue in an alkaline medium and blue litmus paper turns red in an acid medium. Always perform the test either before eating or at least one hour after eating.

Depending on the results of your test, you should alter your diet to help bring your body back into the normal range. If your test indicates that your body is too alkaline, eat more acid-forming foods and omit alkaline-forming foods from your diet until another pH test shows that you have returned to normal. Conversely, if your body is too acidic, eat more alkaline-forming foods and omit acid-forming foods. Use the list below as a guide to which foods are acid-forming and which are alkaline-forming. Low-level acid-forming and low-level alkaline-forming foods are almost neutral.

Acid-Forming Foods

Alcohol	Legumes
Asparagus	Lentils
Beans	Meat
Brussels sprouts	Milk
Catsup	Mustard
Chickpeas	Noodles
Cocoa	Nuts and seeds (most)
Coffee	Oatmeal
Cornstarch	Olives
Cranberries	Organ meats
Eggs	Pasta
Fish	Pepper
Flour; flour-based products	Plums
Poultry	Sugar; all foods with
Prunes	sugar added
Sauerkraut	Tea
Shellfish	Vinegar
Soft drinks	

Aspirin, tobacco, and most drugs are also acid forming.

Low-Level Acid-Forming Foods

Butter	Grains (most)
Canned or glazed fruit	Ice cream
Cheeses	Ice milk
Dried coconut	Lamb's quarters
Dried or sulfured fruit (most)	Seeds and nuts (most)

Alkaline-Forming Foods

Avocados	Honey
Corn	Maple syrup
Dates	Molasses
Fresh coconut	Raisins
Fresh fruits (most)	Soy products
Fresh vegetables (most)	Umeboshi plums

Although it might seem that citrus fruits would have an acidifying effect on the body, the citric acid they contain actually has an alkalinizing effect in the system.

Low-Level Alkaline-Forming Foods

Almonds	Chestnuts
Blackstrap molasses	Lima beans
Brazil nuts	Millet
Buckwheat	Soured dairy products

NUTRIENTS

SUPPLEMENT	SUGGESTED DOSAGE	COMMENTS
Helpful		
Alfalfa		*See under* Herbs, below.
Betaine hydrochloride (HCl)	As directed on label.	A digestive enzyme that releases acid in the digestive tract.
L-Cysteine	500 mg twice daily, on an empty stomach. Take with water or juice. Do not take with milk. Take with 50 mg vitamin B_6 and 100 mg vitamin C for better absorption.	Needed to produce glutathione, a major detoxifying chemical. Also aids in making the tissues more acid. *See* AMINO ACIDS in Part One.
Raw kidney glandular	500 mg daily.	Stimulates kidney function.
Selenium	200 mcg daily.	Protects against free radicals produced in alkalosis.
Sulfur	500 mg daily.	An acid-forming mineral; helps to correct pH balance.

Vitamin B complex	100 mg daily.	Essential for stable and normal pH.
plus extra vitamin B6 (pyridoxine)	50 mg 3 times daily.	Needed for hydrochloric acid (HCl) production. Also relieves fluid retention.
Vitamin C with rose hips and citrus bioflavonoids	3,000–6,000 mg daily, in divided doses.	A potent antioxidant and free radical scavenger.

HERBS

❑ Alfalfa is beneficial for the digestive tract. It is a good source of vitamin K and other nutrients. Use supplements plus natural sources, such as alfalfa sprouts.

RECOMMENDATIONS

❑ Adopt a diet consisting of 80 percent grains and including beans, breads, brown rice, crackers, lentils, macaroni, nuts, soy sauce, and whole-grain cereals. The other 20 percent of the diet should include fresh fruits and vegetables and fish, chicken, eggs, and natural cheese.

❑ Do not use antacids or mineral supplements, except those mentioned above, for two weeks.

❑ Avoid sodium.

❑ Cut back on megadoses of vitamins and minerals for two weeks.

❑ Check your urine pH daily using nitrazine paper. See the self-testing section for a list of alkaline-forming foods to avoid until your pH is corrected.

CONSIDERATIONS

❑ Your breathing can affect the acid-alkali balance of your body. Prolonged hyperventilation may cause temporary alkalosis, resulting in anxiety and a feeling that one cannot get enough air, despite the fact that breathing itself is not actually restricted in any way. If this happens, breathe into a *paper* bag and rebreathe the air from the bag. This often helps to correct the chemical imbalance.

Allergic Rhinitis

See HAY FEVER.

Allergies

An allergy is an inappropriate response by the body's immune system to a substance that is not normally harmful. The immune system is the highly complex defense mecha-

nism that helps us to combat infection. It does this by identifying "foreign invaders" and mobilizing the body's white blood cells to fight them. In some people, the immune system wrongly identifies a nontoxic substance as an invader, and the white blood cells overreact and do more damage to the body than the invader. Thus, the allergic response becomes a disease in itself. Common responses are nasal congestion, coughing, wheezing, itching, hives and other skin rashes, headache, and fatigue.

The substances that provoke allergic responses are called allergens. Almost any substance can cause an allergic reaction in someone somewhere in the world, but the most common allergens include pollen, dust, certain metals (especially nickel), some cosmetics, lanolin, animal hair, insect venom, some common drugs (such as penicillin and aspirin), some food additives (such as benzoic acid and sulfur dioxide), and chemicals found in soap and washing powder.

Many people are allergic to mold. Molds are microcospic living organisms, neither animal nor insect, that thrive where no other life form can. Molds live throughout the house—under the sink and in the bathroom, basement, refrigerator, and any other damp, dark place. They also flourish in the air, in the soil, on dead leaves, and on other organic material. They may be destructive, but they are also beneficial. They help to make cheese, fertilize gardens, and speed decaying of garbage and fallen leaves. Penicillin is made from molds.

Mold spores are carried by the wind and predominate in the summer and early fall. In warm climates they thrive year round. Cutting grass, harvesting crops, or walking through tall vegetation can provoke a reaction. People who repair old furniture are also at risk.

Foods also can provoke allergic reactions. Some of the most common allergenic foods include chocolate, dairy products, eggs, shellfish, strawberries, and wheat. Food allergies and food intolerances are not the same thing. A person with a food intolerance is unable to digest and process that food correctly, usually due to a lack of a certain enzyme or enzymes. A food allergy, on the other hand, occurs when a person's immune system generates an antibody response to the ingested food. Food intolerance can lead to allergy, however, if particles of undigested food manage to enter the bloodstream and cause a reaction.

Some allergic reactions to food occur as soon as one starts chewing. Foods that are highly allergenic are easy to identify and eliminate from the diet. A delayed reaction is harder to detect. An irritating cough or tickle in the throat may be a sign of food allergy.

No one knows why some people are allergic to certain substances. However, allergies do run in families, and it is also believed that babies that are not breastfed are more likely to develop allergies. There may be an emotional cause to the problem as well; stress and anger, especially if the immune system is not functioning properly, are frequently contributing factors.

FOOD ALLERGY SELF-TEST

If you suspect that you are allergic to a specific food, a simple test can help you determine if you are correct. By recording your pulse rate after consuming the food in question, you can reveal if you are having an allergic reaction. Using a watch with a second hand, sit down and relax for a few minutes. When completely relaxed, take your pulse at the wrist. Count the number of beats in a sixty-second period. A normal pulse reading is between 52 and 70 beats per minute. After taking your pulse, consume the food that you are testing for an allergic reaction. Wait fifteen to twenty minutes and take your pulse again. If your pulse rate has increased more than ten beats per minute, omit this food from your diet for one month, and then retest yourself.

For the purposes of this test, it is best to use the purest form of the suspect food available. For example, if you are testing yourself for an allergy to wheat, it is better to use a bit of plain cream of wheat cereal than to use wheat bread, which contains other ingredients besides wheat. This way you will know that whatever reaction you observe (or fail to observe), it is the wheat that is responsible.

NUTRIENTS

SUPPLEMENT	SUGGESTED DOSAGE	COMMENTS
Very Important		
AntiAllergy formula from Freeda Vitamins	As directed on label.	A combination of quercetin, calcium pantothenate, and calcium ascorbate (vitamin C).
Bee pollen	Start with a few granules at a time and work up to 2 tsp daily.	Strengthens the immune system. Use raw crude pollen, preferably produced within 10 miles of your home. *Caution:* Bee pollen may cause an allergic reaction in some individuals. Discontinue use if a rash, wheezing, discomfort, or other symptom occurs.
Calcium and	1,500–2,000 mg daily.	Needed to help reduce stress. Use calcium chelate form.
magnesium	750 mg daily.	Needed to balance with calcium.
Multienzyme complex or pancreatin	As directed on label. Take with meals.	For improved digestion. *Caution:* If you have a history of ulcers, do not use a formula containing HCl.
Raw adrenal and raw spleen and raw thymus glandulars	500 mg each twice daily.	To stimulate proper immune function.
Vitamin B complex	100 mg daily.	Needed for proper digestion and nerve function. Use a high-stress formula. Consider injections.
plus extra pantothenic acid (vitamin B5) and	100 mg 3 times daily.	The anti-stress vitamin. Use a lozenge or sublingual form.
vitamin B12	300 mcg 3 times daily.	Needed for proper assimilation of nutrients. Use a lozenge or sublingual form.
Vitamin C with with bioflavonoids	5,000–20,000 mg daily, in divided doses. *See* ASCORBIC ACID FLUSH in Part Three.	Protects the body from allergens and moderates the inflammatory response.
Important		
Natural carotenoid complex (Betatene)	As directed on label.	Free radical scavengers that stimulate immune response.
Quercetin (Quercitin-C from Ecological Formulas is a good source) plus	500 mg twice daily.	Increases immunity and decreases reactions to certain foods, pollens, and other allergens.
bromelain or	100 mg twice daily.	Enhances absorption of quercetin.
Activated Quercetin from Source Naturals	As directed on label.	Contains quercetin plus bromelain and vitamin C.
Helpful		
Acidophilus	As directed on label. Take on an empty stomach for easier access into the small intestine.	Helps to maintain healthy intestinal flora. Use a nondairy formula.
Aller Bee-Gone from CC Pollen	As directed on label.	A combination of herbs, enzymes, and nutrients designed to fight acute allergy attacks.
Coenzyme Q10	100 mg daily.	Improves cellular oxygenation and immune function.
Free-form amino acid complex	As directed on label.	Supplies protein in a form that is rapidly absorbed and assimilated. Use a sublingual form.
Germanium	60 mg daily.	Stimulates immune response.
Glucosamine sulfate or N-Acetylglucosamine (N-A-G from Source Naturals)	As directed on label. As directed on label.	Important for regulating the mucous secretions of respiratory system.
L-Cysteine and L-tyrosine	500 mg each daily, on empty stomach. Take with water or juice, not milk. Take with 50 mg vitamin B6 and 100 mg vitamin C for better absorption.	Promotes healing from respiratory disorders. Helpful for stress and allergic disorders. *See* AMINO ACIDS in Part One.
Manganese	4 mg daily for 3 months. Take separately from calcium.	An important component in many of the body's enzyme systems. Use manganese chelate form.
Multivitamin and mineral complex	As directed on label.	All nutrients are needed in balance. Use a hypoallergenic formula.
Potassium	99 mg daily.	Necessary for adrenal gland function. Use potassium protinate or potassium chelate form.
Proteolytic enzymes or Infla-Zyme Forte from American Biologics	As directed on label. Take between meals, on an empty stomach. As directed on label.	To aid digestion and destroy free radicals. *Caution:* Do not give these supplements to a child.
Vitamin A and	10,000 IU daily.	Three nutrients necessary for proper immune function.
vitamin E and	600 IU daily.	
zinc	50 mg daily.	Do not exceed a total of 100 mg daily from all supplements.
Vitamin D	600 IU daily.	Essential in calcium metabolism.

HERBS

❑ Ephedra (ma huang) is good for relieving nasal and chest congestion.

Caution: Do not use this herb if you suffer from anxiety, glaucoma, heart disease, high blood pressure, or insomnia, or if you are taking a monoamine oxidase (MAO) inhibitor drug for depression.

❑ Goldenseal root aids absorption of nutrients.

Caution: Do not take goldenseal on a daily basis for more than one week at a time, and do not use it during pregnancy. If you have a history of cardiovascular disease, diabetes, or glaucoma, use it only under a doctor's supervision.

❑ Other herbs that can be beneficial for allergies include burdock, dandelion, and echinacea.

❑ For relief of allergic symptoms, take 2 to 3 teaspoons of yerba maté in 16 ounces of hot water on an empty stomach.

RECOMMENDATIONS

❑ Rotate your foods. (*See* Rotating Foods: Sample Daily Menus, at the end of this section.) Eat a different group of foods for each of four days and then repeat the cycle. You can select as many of the foods allowed on a specific day as you like, but it is essential that no type of food be ingested more often than every four days.

❑ *See* Detecting Your Hidden Food Allergies on page 114 and fill out the Food Sensitivity Questionnaire. Then omit from your diet for thirty days any food you have listed as consumed four times per week or more.

❑ Avoid the following foods until it is determined you are not allergic to them: bananas, beef products, caffeine, chocolate, citrus fruits, corn, dairy products, eggs, oats, oysters, peanuts, processed and refined foods, salmon, strawberries, tomatoes, wheat, and white rice.

❑ Follow a fasting program. *See* FASTING in Part Three. After a fast, you can try adding back the "foods to avoid" (listed above) in very small amounts, such as 1 teaspoon at a time. Record your reactions after eating. If you feel bloated or have a slight headache, an upset stomach, gas, diarrhea, a rapid pulse, or heart palpitations after eating certain foods, eliminate them from your diet for sixty days, then try introducing them again in small amounts. If you experience a reaction again, eliminate them from your diet permanently.

❑ Avoid any food products that contain artificial color, especially FD&C Yellow No. 5 dye. Many people are allergic to food colorings. Other food additives to avoid include vanillin, benzyldehyde, eucayptol, monosodium glutamate, BHT-BHA, benzoates, and annatto. Read labels carefully.

❑ Take the underarm temperature test to determine if you have an underactive thyroid. *See* HYPERTHYROIDISM in Part Two.

❑ Be sure to take only hypoallergenic supplements, as these do not contain potentially irritating substances.

❑ Keep rooms free from dust and use a dehumidifier in the basement. Use mold-proof paint and a disinfectant on walls and furniture.

❑ Do not smoke, and avoid secondhand smoke.

❑ Avoid taking aspirin within three hours of eating.

❑ For airborne allergies, try using an air purification device. The Air Supply personal air purifier from Wein Products is a miniature unit that is worn around the neck. It sets up an invisible pure air shield against microorganisms (such as viruses, bacteria, and mold) and microparticles (including dust, pollen, and pollutants) in the air. It also eliminates vapors, smells, and harmful volatile compounds in the air. The Living Air XL-15 unit from Alpine Air of America is an ionizing unit that is good for purifying the air in the home or workplace.

CONSIDERATIONS

❑ IgE is an antibody formed by the body as part of an allergic response to a food substance. If IgE is present in your lung tissue, it frequently causes symptoms such as shortness of breath or asthma. If present in the skin, it can cause hives. If IgE is present in the wall of the intestinal tract, it can result in severe pain, gas, or bloating. IgE can be present anywhere in the body, causing severe problems. Even healthy natural foods can have an adverse effect if you are allergic to them.

❑ Cerebral allergies cause swelling of the lining of the brain. Entire food families can cause such allergic reactions in susceptible individuals. Recurrent headaches, or schizophrenic, violent, or aggressive reactions, can be an indicator of cerebral allergy. Foods such as corn, wheat, rice, milk, and chocolate, and certain food additives, are the most common offenders.

❑ The *British Medical Journal* reported that taking aspirin before consuming an allergenic food makes it possible for more of the allergy-provoking food to be absorbed. In contrast, taking Aerobic Bulk Cleanse from Aerobic Life Industries combined with aloe vera juice may slow the absorption of foods that cause a reaction. Taking oat bran or guar gum in the morning works in the same way. Wheat bran is not recommended as a source of fiber for allergy-prone individuals because wheat is highly allergenic. (*See* NATURAL FOOD SUPPLEMENTS in Part One for a discussion of fiber.)

❑ Research is being conducted on the ability of coenzyme Q_{10} to counter histamine for asthma and allergy sufferers.

❑ *See also* CHEMICAL ALLERGIES in Part Two and FASTING in Part Three.

Sulfite Allergies

Sulfites are common food additives used as sanitary agents and preservatives to prevent discoloration of foods. They are commonly used in restaurant salad bars and are also present in many supermarket foods, including frozen foods, dried fruits, and certain fresh fruits and vegetables.

Many people are allergic to sulfites. The types and severity of reactions to sulfites in sensitive individuals vary, and may include breathing difficulties, anaphylactic shock, severe headaches, abdominal pain, stuffy and/or runny nose, flushing of the face and a "hot flash" feeling, diarrhea, irritability, and/or feelings of anger. These symptoms tend to occur quickly, usually within twenty to thirty minutes after consuming sulfites.

Sulfites pose a greater danger to some people than to others. People with asthma, a history of allergies, or a deficiency of the liver enzyme sulfite oxidase can suffer great harm. Sulfites have been implicated in at least thirteen deaths in the United States.

It is not always easy to tell if a food product contains sulfites. Sulfiting agents appear in food ingredient lists in a variety of ways, including "sodium sulfite," "sodium bisulfite," "sodium metabisulfite," "potassium bisulfite," "potassium metabisulfite," and "sulfur dioxide." Any ingredient ending in "-sulfite" should be assumed to be a sulfiting agent. If you have ever suffered a reaction after ingesting a food you believe contained sulfites, you should beware of the foods and beverages listed below, which often contain these substances. Sulfite-free forms of some of these foods may be found in health food stores.

FOODS AND BEVERAGES THAT OFTEN CONTAIN SULFITES

Fresh Fruits and Beverages

Avocado dip (guacamole)	Grapes	Potatoes	Prepared cut fruit or
Cole slaw	Mushrooms		vegetable salads

Fish and Shellfish

Canned seafood soups	Dried fish	Frozen, canned, or dried	Oysters
Clams	Fresh shellfish, especially	shellfish	Scallops
Crabs	shrimp	Lobster	Shrimp

Prepared Processed Foods

Beet sugars	Cornstarch	Horseradish	Sauerkraut
Breading mixes	Dietetic processed foods	Jams and jellies	Shredded coconut
Breakfast cereals	Dried or canned soups	Maraschino cherries	Trail mixes
Brown sugar	Dry salad dressing mixes	Noodle and rice mixes	Wine vinegar
Canned fruit pie fillings	Glacéed fruits	Olives	
Canned mushrooms	Frozen, canned, or dried	Onion relish	
Caramels	fruits and vegetables	Pickles	
Corn, maple, and	Frozen French fries	Potato chips	
pancake syrups	Hard candies	Sauces and gravies	

Miscellaneous

Apple cider	Bottled, canned, or frozen	Cordials	Gelatin
Baked goods	vegetable juices	Cornmeal	Instant tea mixes
Beer	Cocktail mixes	Frozen doughs	Wines
Bottled, canned, or frozen	Colas	Fruit drinks	
fruit juices			

Detecting Your Hidden Food Allergies

The first step in discovering hidden food allergies is to develop a list of suspect foods. Using the form below, keep track of how often you consume different foods. Be careful to note each time you consume each of the foods listed below, then add up your weekly total for each food. Do this for a four-week period.

FOOD SENSITIVITY QUESTIONNAIRE

Type of Food	First Week	Second Week	Third Week	Fourth Week
Beans and Legumes				
Kidney beans	_____	_____	_____	_____
Lentils	_____	_____	_____	_____
Lima beans	_____	_____	_____	_____
Mung beans	_____	_____	_____	_____
Pinto beans	_____	_____	_____	_____
Soybeans	_____	_____	_____	_____
Soymilk	_____	_____	_____	_____
White beans	_____	_____	_____	_____
Tofu and tofu products	_____	_____	_____	_____
Condiments				
Catsup	_____	_____	_____	_____
Gravy	_____	_____	_____	_____
Jams and jellies	_____	_____	_____	_____
Mustard	_____	_____	_____	_____
Pepper	_____	_____	_____	_____
Pickles	_____	_____	_____	_____
Salsa	_____	_____	_____	_____
Salt	_____	_____	_____	_____
Soy sauce	_____	_____	_____	_____
Dairy Products				
Butter	_____	_____	_____	_____
Buttermilk	_____	_____	_____	_____
Cheese	_____	_____	_____	_____
Cottage cheese	_____	_____	_____	_____
Cow's milk	_____	_____	_____	_____
Cream cheese	_____	_____	_____	_____
Eggs	_____	_____	_____	_____
Goat's milk	_____	_____	_____	_____
Ice cream	_____	_____	_____	_____
Margarine	_____	_____	_____	_____
Milk shake	_____	_____	_____	_____
Sour cream	_____	_____	_____	_____
Yogurt	_____	_____	_____	_____

Type of Food	First Week	Second Week	Third Week	Fourth Week
Fruits and Their Juices				
Apples	_____	_____	_____	_____
Apricots	_____	_____	_____	_____
Bananas	_____	_____	_____	_____
Blackberries	_____	_____	_____	_____
Blueberries	_____	_____	_____	_____
Cherries	_____	_____	_____	_____
Coconut	_____	_____	_____	_____
Cranberries	_____	_____	_____	_____
Dates	_____	_____	_____	_____
Dried fruits (most)	_____	_____	_____	_____
Figs	_____	_____	_____	_____
Grapefruit	_____	_____	_____	_____
Grapes	_____	_____	_____	_____
Lemons	_____	_____	_____	_____
Melons	_____	_____	_____	_____
Oranges	_____	_____	_____	_____
Nectarines	_____	_____	_____	_____
Papayas	_____	_____	_____	_____
Peaches	_____	_____	_____	_____
Pears	_____	_____	_____	_____
Pineapple	_____	_____	_____	_____
Plums	_____	_____	_____	_____
Prunes	_____	_____	_____	_____
Raisins	_____	_____	_____	_____
Raspberries	_____	_____	_____	_____
Strawberrles	_____	_____	_____	_____
Tangerines	_____	_____	_____	_____
Grains and Grain Products				
Brown rice	_____	_____	_____	_____
Buckwheat	_____	_____	_____	_____
Cold cereal	_____	_____	_____	_____
Cornmeal	_____	_____	_____	_____
Millet	_____	_____	_____	_____
Oats	_____	_____	_____	_____
Quinoa	_____	_____	_____	_____
Pancakes	_____	_____	_____	_____
Pasta	_____	_____	_____	_____
Rye	_____	_____	_____	_____
Spelt	_____	_____	_____	_____
Tapioca	_____	_____	_____	_____
White flour products	_____	_____	_____	_____
White rice	_____	_____	_____	_____
Wheat and whole-wheat products	_____	_____	_____	_____

Type of Food	First Week	Second Week	Third Week	Fourth Week
Meats, Poultry, and Fish				
Bacon	_____	_____	_____	_____
Beef	_____	_____	_____	_____
Bologna	_____	_____	_____	_____
Chicken	_____	_____	_____	_____
Fish	_____	_____	_____	_____
Ham	_____	_____	_____	_____
Lamb	_____	_____	_____	_____
Liver	_____	_____	_____	_____
Luncheon meat	_____	_____	_____	_____
Pork	_____	_____	_____	_____
Sausage	_____	_____	_____	_____
Shellfish	_____	_____	_____	_____
Turkey	_____	_____	_____	_____
Veal	_____	_____	_____	_____
Nuts and Seeds				
Almonds	_____	_____	_____	_____
Brazil nuts	_____	_____	_____	_____
Cashews	_____	_____	_____	_____
Chestnuts	_____	_____	_____	_____
Hazelnuts	_____	_____	_____	_____
Nut butter (other than peanut)	_____	_____	_____	_____
Nut milk	_____	_____	_____	_____
Peanut butter	_____	_____	_____	_____
Peanuts	_____	_____	_____	_____
Pecans	_____	_____	_____	_____
Pistachios	_____	_____	_____	_____
Sesame seeds	_____	_____	_____	_____
Sunflower seeds	_____	_____	_____	_____
Walnuts	_____	_____	_____	_____
Oils				
Canola oil	_____	_____	_____	_____
Corn oil	_____	_____	_____	_____
Cottonseed oil	_____	_____	_____	_____
Olive oil	_____	_____	_____	_____
Peanut oil	_____	_____	_____	_____
Safflower oil	_____	_____	_____	_____
Sesame oil	_____	_____	_____	_____
Soy oil	_____	_____	_____	_____

Type of Food	First Week	Second Week	Third Week	Fourth Week
Sweeteners				
Aspartame (NutraSweet)	_____	_____	_____	_____
Brown sugar	_____	_____	_____	_____
Corn syrup	_____	_____	_____	_____
Fructose	_____	_____	_____	_____
Honey	_____	_____	_____	_____
Maple syrup	_____	_____	_____	_____
Saccharin	_____	_____	_____	_____
White sugar	_____	_____	_____	_____
Vegetables				
Alfalfa sprouts	_____	_____	_____	_____
Artichokes	_____	_____	_____	_____
Asparagus	_____	_____	_____	_____
Avocado	_____	_____	_____	_____
Beets	_____	_____	_____	_____
Broccoli	_____	_____	_____	_____
Brussels sprouts	_____	_____	_____	_____
Cabbage	_____	_____	_____	_____
Carrots	_____	_____	_____	_____
Cauliflower	_____	_____	_____	_____
Celery	_____	_____	_____	_____
Corn	_____	_____	_____	_____
Cucumbers	_____	_____	_____	_____
Eggplant	_____	_____	_____	_____
Garlic	_____	_____	_____	_____
Green beans	_____	_____	_____	_____
Kale	_____	_____	_____	_____
Lettuce	_____	_____	_____	_____
Mushrooms	_____	_____	_____	_____
Okra	_____	_____	_____	_____
Olives	_____	_____	_____	_____
Onions	_____	_____	_____	_____
Parsley	_____	_____	_____	_____
Peas	_____	_____	_____	_____
Peppers	_____	_____	_____	_____
Potatoes	_____	_____	_____	_____
Radishes	_____	_____	_____	_____
Spinach	_____	_____	_____	_____
Summer squash	_____	_____	_____	_____
Sweet potatoes	_____	_____	_____	_____
Swiss chard	_____	_____	_____	_____
Tomatoes	_____	_____	_____	_____
Turnips	_____	_____	_____	_____
Winter squash	_____	_____	_____	_____
Zucchini	_____	_____	_____	_____

Type of Food	First Week	Second Week	Third Week	Fourth Week
Miscellaneous and Junk Foods				
Alcoholic beverages	_____	_____	_____	_____
Candy	_____	_____	_____	_____
Cheeseburger	_____	_____	_____	_____
Chewing gum	_____	_____	_____	_____
Chocolate	_____	_____	_____	_____
Coffee	_____	_____	_____	_____
Cola	_____	_____	_____	_____
Corn chips	_____	_____	_____	_____
Flavored gelatin	_____	_____	_____	_____
French fries	_____	_____	_____	_____
Fried foods	_____	_____	_____	_____
Hamburger	_____	_____	_____	_____
Pastry	_____	_____	_____	_____
Peppermint	_____	_____	_____	_____
Pizza	_____	_____	_____	_____
Popcorn	_____	_____	_____	_____
Potato chips	_____	_____	_____	_____
Pudding	_____	_____	_____	_____
Tea	_____	_____	_____	_____

Note any other snacks or other foods not listed above that you eat regularly. _____

_____

After the one-month recording period, go through the form and compile a list of all the foods you ate four times a week or more. This is your list of suspect foods.

KEEPING A FOOD DIARY

Once you have your list of suspect foods, omit these foods from your diet for a period of thirty days to give your body a rest from them. Then reintroduce the suspect foods, one at a time. Add only one new food a day.

As you add foods back to your diet, keep a diary of any symptoms you experience and monitor your reaction with the Food Allergy Self-Test (see page 111), as in the following sample:

Sample Food Diary

Date	Meal	Time	Foods Consumed	Symptoms
4/12	Breakfast	8:39 a.m.	milk, toast	gas, bloating
	Lunch	12:30 p.m.	pea soup, salad	no symptoms

If you note a reaction to any of the reintroduced foods, omit that food from your diet for another two months, then try a small amount of it again. If you have a reaction after the second reintroduction, eliminate that food from your diet permanently.

Use the form that follows to record your experiences as you reintroduce the banished foods into your diet. By first eliminating foods, then slowly adding them back into your diet, you will be able to pinpoint exactly which foods are giving you trouble.

Food Diary

Date	Meal	Time	Foods Consumed	Symptoms
_____	Breakfast			
_____	Lunch			
_____	Dinner			
_____	Snack			
_____	Breakfast			
_____	Lunch			
_____	Dinner			
_____	Snack			
_____	Breakfast			
_____	Lunch			
_____	Dinner			
_____	Snack			
_____	Breakfast			
_____	Lunch			
_____	Dinner			
_____	Snack			
_____	Breakfast			
_____	Lunch			
_____	Dinner			
_____	Snack			
_____	Breakfast			
_____	Lunch			
_____	Dinner			
_____	Snack			
_____	Breakfast			
_____	Lunch			
_____	Dinner			
_____	Snack			

Medications: _____

_____

_____

Herbs: _____

_____

Miscellaneous: _____

_____

When monitoring your reactions to different foods, it is important to be aware that food allergies can manifest themselves in many ways, not all of them obvious. The following symptoms are the most common manifestations of food allergies:

- Acne, especially pimples on the chin or around the mouth.
- Arthritis.
- Asthma.
- Chest and shoulder pains.
- Colitis.
- Depression.
- Fatigue.
- Food cravings.
- Headaches.
- Hemorrhoids.
- Insomnia.
- Intestinal problems.
- Muscle disorders.
- Obesity.
- Sinus problems.
- Ulcers.
- Unexplained dramatic weight gain or loss.

Your health care provider may look also for the following signs and symptoms when trying to determine if you have an allergy:

- Acid/alkaline imbalance.
- Anemia.

- Bed-wetting.
- Conjunctivitis.
- Diarrhea.
- Dizzy spells and floating sensations.
- Excessive drooling.
- Dark circles under the eyes or puffy eyes.
- Eye pain, tearing.
- Fluid retention.
- Hearing loss.
- Hyperactivity.
- Learning disabilities.
- Nasal congestion or chronic runny nose.
- Noises in the ear.
- Periods of blurred vision.
- Phobias.
- Poor memory and concentration.
- Poor muscle coordination.
- Red circles on the cheeks (as if wearing rouge, even in children).
- Repeated colds or ear infections, especially in children.
- Sensitivity to light.
- Severe menstrual symptoms.
- Swollen fingers and cold hands.
- Unusual body odor.
- Watery, itchy, red eyes.
- Recurrence of any illness despite treatment.

THE ROTATION DIET

Although some people have a reaction soon after ingesting a particular food for the first time, food allergies often develop slowly. The reason for this is that if you consume the same foods daily, your body eventually develops an intolerance to them. Then, rather than nourishing the body, these foods provoke harmful reactions.

Once you have identified and avoided an allergenic food for sixty to ninety days, you can usually reintroduce it without any adverse reactions, as long as you maintain a rotation diet. The basic principle behind the rotation diet is that each type of food is to be consumed only on one out of every four days. For example, if you eat beans on Monday, you wouldn't eat beans again on Tuesday, Wednesday, or Thursday. If you eat salmon on Friday, you would wait at least until Tuesday before consuming any other fish. Rotating foods in this way will not only make you feel better, it will also help to stabilize your weight.

Before starting the rotation diet, follow a fasting program to cleanse your system of offending foods and toxins. (*See* FASTING in Part Two.) After you have finished the program, consume only the following foods for the next two weeks:

- Baked or broiled chicken or turkey.
- Broiled, boiled, or baked fish.
- Brown rice.
- Fresh, unsweetened fruit and vegetable juices.
- Fresh fruits (except oranges).
- Herbal teas.
- Raw, steamed, or broiled vegetables.

Although you may feel that this list of foods does not offer much variety, there are numerous fruits and vegetables available, in addition to a variety of fish. After two weeks on this cleansing diet, you can once again begin to eat a greater number of different foods, but on a rotating basis—eating each type of food on no more than one out of four days. Use the sample menus below as a guide to help you put together daily menus rotating among different foods. Of course, if you are sensitive to any of the foods listed, substitute a food that agrees with you. Once you start following this program, you should start seeing an increase in your energy level in a week or less.

Rotating Foods: Sample Daily Menus

Breakfast	Lunch	Dinner	Snacks
Day 1			

Glass of distilled water
Papaya juice with vitamin C
Fresh papaya or peach
Oatmeal or oat bran cereal
  with 1 tbsp raw honey
Skim milk
Rose hip tea
	Tomato stuffed with tuna
	  salad or tuna burger on
	  wheat-free bread with
	  tomato, onion, alfalfa
	  sprouts, and eggless
	  mayonnaise
	Fresh lemonade
		Broiled whitefish or salmon
		  with dill
		Cole slaw or sprout salad
		  with tomato, onion, celery,
		  and eggless mayonnaise
		Steamed asparagus
		Herbal tea or lemonade
		
		Substitutions: Cauliflower,
		  Brussels sprouts, or
		  sauerkraut can be
		  substituted for asparagus.
			Celery sticks
			Pecans
			Fresh papaya or peach

Day 2			

Glass of distilled water
Apple juice with vitamin C
Fresh apple
Cream of wheat cereal with
  pure maple syrup and
  soymilk
Herbal tea
	Home-cooked sliced turkey
	  or chicken on whole
	  wheat bread with lettuce
	  and mustard
	Potato soup and wheat
	  crackers (make soup
	  with soymilk)
	Herbal tea or apple juice
	
	Substitutions: Soy burger
	  or eggless egg salad
	  with eggless mayonnaise
	  for turkey or chicken;
	  tofu soup for potato soup.
		Baked skinless turkey or
		  chicken with lemon juice,
		  garlic, and onion powder
		Baked potato with 2 tsp
		  sesame oil, chopped
		  chives, and a dash of
		  onion powder
		Tossed salad with radishes,
		  zucchini, yellow squash,
		  kale, and soy oil dressing
		Herbal tea
		
		Substitutions: Cornish game
		  hens for turkey or chicken;
		  vinaigrette dressing for
		  soy oil dressing.
			Apple
			Walnuts
			
			Substitutions: Baked apple
			  with pure maple syrup;
			  wheat crackers; sugar-
			  free applesauce topped
			  with walnuts.

Day 3			

Glass of distilled water
Cranberry juice with
  vitamin C
Sliced banana with almond
  milk
Cream of rice or puffed rice
  cereal
Herbal tea
	½ avocado filled with
	  cooked brown rice and
	  fresh peas, water
	  chestnuts, and a dash of
	  herbal seasoning and
	  lemon juice, topped with
	  slivered almonds
	Split pea soup with rice
	  crackers (make soup
	  with rice milk)
		Stir-fried vegetables with
		  broccoli, green peppers,
		  leeks, pea pods, sweet
		  red peppers, bean
		  sprouts, bamboo shoots,
		  and grated fresh ginger,
		  served over cooked
		  brown rice
		Rice cakes with almond butter
		Coffee substitute (from a
		  health food store) or
		  herbal tea
			Raw almonds
			Rice crackers with almond
			  butter
			Sliced bananas

Breakfast	Lunch	Dinner	Snacks
Day 4			
Glass of distilled water	Egg salad with chopped	Spinach mushroom quiche	RyKrisp crackers with
Grape juice with vitamin C	cucumber, green onions,	Fresh spinach salad with	sugar-free grape jam or
2 poached or soft-boiled	black olives, and low-fat	hard-boiled eggs,	sesame butter and
eggs or corn cereal	cottage cheese, topped	artichoke, shredded raw	sesame seeds
Rye toast with sugar-free	with raisins	beets, raisins, and olive	Fresh grapes
grape jam	RyKrisp crackers with	oil and lemon dressing	Raisins
Herbal tea	sugar-free grape jelly or	Iced herbal tea flavored	Hard-boiled eggs
	jam	with grape juice	
	Lentil soup or cool lentil		
	salad		

Alopecia

See HAIR LOSS.

Aluminum Toxicity

Aluminum is not a heavy metal, but it can be toxic if present in excessive amounts—even in small amounts, if it is deposited in the brain. Many of the symptoms of aluminum toxicity are similar to those of Alzheimer's disease and osteoporosis. Aluminum toxicity can lead to colic, rickets, gastrointestinal disturbances, poor calcium metabolism, extreme nervousness, anemia, headaches, decreased liver and kidney function, forgetfulness, speech disturbances, memory loss, softening of the bones, and weak, aching muscles.

Because aluminum is excreted through the kidneys, toxic amounts of aluminum may impair kidney function. The accumulation of aluminum salts in the brain has been implicated in seizures and reduced mental faculties. To reach the brain, aluminum must pass the blood-brain barrier, an elaborate structure that filters the blood before it reaches this vital organ. Elemental aluminum does not readily pass through this barrier, but certain aluminum compounds, such as aluminum fluoride, do. Many municipal water supplies are treated with both alum (aluminum sulfate) and fluoride, and these two chemicals readily combine with each other in the blood. Moreover, aluminum fluoride, once formed, is very poorly excreted in the urine.

Intestinal absorption of high levels of aluminum and silicon can result in the formation of compounds that accumulate in the cerebral cortex and prevent nerve impulses from being carried to and from the brain in the proper manner. Chronic calcium deficiency can aggravate the situation. People who have worked in aluminum smelting plants for long periods have been known to experience dizziness, impaired coordination, and a loss of balance and energy. The accumulation of aluminum in the brain has been cited as a possible cause for these symptoms. Perhaps most alarming, there is evidence to suggest that long-term accumulation of aluminum in the brain may contribute to the development of Alzheimer's disease (*see* The Alzheimer's/Aluminum Connection, page 124).

It has been estimated that the average person ingests between 3 and 10 milligrams of aluminum a day. Aluminum is the most abundant metallic element in the earth's crust. It is absorbed into the body primarily through the digestive tract, but also through the lungs and skin, and is absorbed by and accumulates in body tissues. Because aluminum permeates our air, water, and soil, it is found naturally in varying amounts in nearly all food and water. Aluminum is also used to make cookware, cooking utensils, and foil. Many other everyday products contain aluminum as well, including over-the-counter painkillers, anti-inflammatories, and douche preparations. Aluminum is an additive in most baking powders, is used in food processing, and is present in products ranging from antiperspirants and toothpaste to dental amalgams to bleached flour, grated cheese, table salt, and beer (especially when packaged in aluminum cans). One prominent source of aluminum is our municipal water supplies.

The excessive use of antacids is probably the most common cause of aluminum toxicity in this country, especially in people who have kidney problems. Many over-the-counter antacids contain amounts of aluminum hydroxide that may be too much for the kidneys to excrete successfully. Even antacids that contain a mixture of aluminum and other ingredients may pose a problem; in some people, such products may cause the same reaction as products composed entirely of aluminum compounds.

NUTRIENTS

SUPPLEMENT	SUGGESTED DOSAGE	COMMENTS
Helpful		
Apple pectin	2 tbsp twice daily.	Binds with metals in the colon and excretes them from the body.
Calcium and magnesium	1,500 mg daily. 750 mg daily.	Minerals that bind with aluminum and eliminate it from the body. Use chelate forms.
Garlic (Kyolic)	2 capsules 3 times daily.	Acts as a detoxifier.
Kelp	2,000–3,000 mg daily.	Has a balanced mineral content. Acts as a detoxifier of excess metals.
Lecithin granules or capsules	1 tbsp 3 times daily, before meals. 1,200 mg 3 times daily, before meals.	Aids in healing of the brain and cell membranes.
Multivitamin and mineral complex	As directed on label.	Basic for stabilizing vitamin and mineral imbalances in toxic conditions. Use a hypoallergenic high-potency formula.
Vitamin B complex plus extra vitamin B$_6$ and vitamin B$_{12}$	100 mg 3 times daily. 50 mg 3 times daily. 300 mcg 3 times daily.	The B vitamins, especially B$_6$, are important in ridding the intestinal tract of excess metals and in removing them from the body. Sublingual forms are recommended for better absorption. Injections (under a doctor's supervision) may be necessary.

RECOMMENDATIONS

❑ Eat a diet that is high in fiber and includes apple pectin.

❑ Use only stainless steel, glass, or iron cookware. Stainless steel is best.

❑ Beware of products containing aluminum. Read labels and avoid those that contain aluminum, or dihydroxyaluminum. *See* The Alzheimer's/Aluminum Connection on page 124 for additional suggestions.

CONSIDERATIONS

❑ A hair analysis can be used to determine levels of aluminum in the body. (*See* HAIR ANALYSIS in Part Three.)

❑ If you use chelation therapy, use oral chelating agents only (*see* CHELATION THERAPY in Part Three). Many researchers believe that aluminum cannot be chelated out of the body, as some metals can, but that it can be displaced or moved.

❑ Some research indicates that the longer you cook food in aluminum pots, the more they corrode, and the more aluminum compounds migrate into food and are absorbed by the body. Aluminum is more readily dissolved by acid-forming foods, such as coffee, cheeses, meats, black and green tea, cabbage, cucumbers, tomatoes, turnips, spinach, and radishes.

❑ Acid rain leeches aluminum out of the soil and into drinking water.

❑ *See also* ALZHEIMER'S DISEASE in Part Two.

Alzheimer's Disease

Alzheimer's disease is a common type of dementia, or decline in intellectual function. There are currently more than 4 million people in the United States who suffer from Alzheimer's disease. It afflicts 10 percent of Americans over the age of sixty-five and as many as 50 percent of those over eighty-five. Dementia is the fourth leading cause of death in those over sixty, while Alzheimer's alone kills 100,000 people per year in the United States. However, Alzheimer's disease does not affect elderly people only, but may strike when a person is in his or her forties.

This disorder was first identified in 1907 by a German neurologist named Alois Alzheimer. It is characterized by progressive mental deterioration, to such a degree that it interferes with the ability to function socially and at work. Memory and abstract thought processes are impaired. Symptoms include depression, disoriented perceptions of space and time, an inability to concentrate or communicate, loss of bladder and bowel control, memory loss, personality changes, and severe mood swings. Health and functioning progressively deteriorate, until the individual is totally incapacitated. Death usually occurs within five to ten years.

Once considered a psychological phenomenon, Alzheimer's disease is now known to be a degenerative disorder that is characterized by a specific set of physiological changes in the brain. Nerve fibers surrounding the hippocampus, the brain's memory center, become tangled, and information is no longer carried properly to or from the brain. New memories cannot be formed, and memories formed earlier cannot be retrieved. Characteristic plaques accumulate in the brain as well. These plaques are composed largely of a protein-containing substance called beta-amyloid. Scientists believe that the plaques build up in and damage nerve cells.

Many people worry that their forgetfulness is a sign of Alzheimer's disease. Most of us forget where we have put our keys or other everyday objects at one time or another, but this is not an indication of Alzheimer's disease. A good example of the difference between forgetfulness and dementia is the following: If you do not remember where you put your glasses, that is forgetfulness; if you do not remember that you wear glasses, that may be sign of dementia.

Other disorders can cause symptoms similar to those of Alzheimer's disease. Dementia may result from arteriosclerosis (hardening of the arteries) that slowly cuts off the supply of blood to the brain. The death of brain tissue from a series of minor strokes, or from pressure exerted by an accumulation of fluid in the brain, may cause dementia.

The Alzheimer's/Aluminum Connection

Autopsies performed on persons who have died of Alzheimer's disease have revealed accumulations of up to four times the normal amount of aluminum in the nerve cells in the brain. Especially high concentrations have been found in the region of the hippocampus, which plays a central role in memory.

Early in 1989, the British medical journal *The Lancet* reported conclusions of a British government study: The risk of contracting Alzheimer's disease was 50 percent higher in areas of Great Britain where drinking water contained elevated levels of aluminum. The threat from aluminum may be increased by chronic calcium deficiency, which may change the way in which the body uses minerals and result in greater accumulations of aluminum.

While our British cousins must contend with the threat of aluminum-tainted water, Americans can ingest aluminum through a wide variety of products. While there is still much controversy as to whether the accumulation of aluminum in the neurons is the cause or a result of neuronal dysfunction, we believe it is best to avoid aluminum as much as possible. Why not check the following guide, and then prune your pantry or medicine cabinet of items that contain potentially hazardous aluminum derivatives?

ALUMINUM COOKWARE

Aluminum cookware contributes significantly to the amount of aluminum in the diet. According to a study by the University of Cincinnati Medical Center, using aluminum pots to cook tomatoes doubled the aluminum content of those tomatoes, from 2 milligrams to 4 milligrams per serving.

ANTACIDS

Several dozen antacids contain aluminum hydroxide, an aluminum salt. Included in this list are such nationally advertised products as Di-Gel liquid, Gaviscon tablets, Gelusil liquid and tablets, Extra Strength Maalox, Mylanta and Mylanta Double Strength liquid and tablets, and Tempo Soft Antacid. Concentrations of aluminum vary. If you use antacids, always read product labels carefully. Antacids that contain aluminum must state this in their list of ingredients. There are more than twenty aluminum-free antacid compounds available, including Alka-Seltzer and Alka-Mints, Di-Gel tablets, Maalox caplets, Mylanta gelcaps, Rolaids tablets, Titralac, and Tums E-X.

ANTIDIARRHEAL PREPARATIONS

More than a dozen nonprescription antidiarrheal drugs contain aluminum salts, including kaolin, aluminum magnesium silicate, and attapulgite, in doses of 100 mg/ml to 600 milligrams per tablet. Familiar preparations containing these substances include Donnagel, Kaopectate, Pepto-Bismol liquid, and Rheaban. Products containing the newer antidiarrheal loperamide (Imodium AD and others) do not usually contain aluminum.

BUFFERED ASPIRIN

With concentrations of 14.4 milligrams to 88 milligrams per dose, buffered aspirin can be a source of aluminum. One of two compounds, aluminum hydroxide or aluminum glycinate, is found in brands such as Arthritis Pain Formula, Arthritis Strength Bufferin, Ascriptin, Bufferin, Cope, and Vanquish. Ordinary aspirin is aluminum-free, as are many other painkillers.

CONTAINERS

Aluminum-coated waxed containers, used especially for orange and pineapple juices, cause juices inside to absorb aluminum. Beer and soft drinks stored in aluminum cans absorb small quantities of the metal as well. Bottled beverages are a better choice.

DEODORANTS

Many deodorants and antiperspirants and some skin powders contain aluminum chlorhydrate. Aluminum in this form is readily absorbed into the brain through the nasal passages.

DOUCHES

Many popular douche preparations contain aluminum salts. These include such nationally advertised products as Massengil powder. Research has not yet shown how much of these solutions the body absorbs. A homemade solution of vinegar and water can be substituted for over-the-counter products.

FOOD ADDITIVES

Manufacturers add aluminum to many of the food products Americans eat every day. Cake mixes, frozen doughs, self-rising flour, and sliced processed cheese food all contain from 5 to 50 milligrams of sodium aluminum phosphate per average serving. Baking powder contains from 5 to 70 milligrams of sodium aluminum sulfate per teaspoonful. Varying amounts of other aluminum compounds are contained in food starch modifiers and anti-caking agents. Pickling salts can contain one of two aluminum compounds: aluminum ammonium sulfate or aluminum potassium sulfate. If you eat fast food, you should be aware that the processed cheeses used on cheese-burgers contain aluminum, which is is added to give the cheese product its melting quality.

SHAMPOOS

A number of anti-dandruff preparations, such as Selsun Blue, contain magnesium aluminum silicate. Aluminum lauryl sulfate is a common ingredient in many nationally advertised shampoos. As with other products, always read the label before you buy.

The presence of small blood clots in vessels that supply the brain, a brain tumor, hypothyroidism, and advanced syphilis all can cause symptoms similar to those of Alzheimer's. In addition, the average person over the age of sixty-five is likely to be taking between eight and ten different prescription and over-the-counter drugs. Drug reactions, coupled with a nutrient-poor diet, often adversely affect people not only physically, but mentally as well.

The precise cause or causes of Alzheimer's disease are unknown, but research has revealed a number of interesting clues. Many of them point to nutritional deficiencies. For example, people with Alzheimer's tend to have low levels of vitamin B_{12} and zinc in their bodies. The B vitamins are important in cognitive functioning, and it is well known that the processed foods that make up so much of the modern diet have been stripped of these essential nutrients. The development of the neurofibrillary tangles and amyloid plaques in the brain that are characteristic of the disease have been associated with zinc deficiency. Malabsorption problems, which are common among elderly people, make them more prone than others to nutritional deficiencies, and alcohol and many medications further deplete crucial vitamins and minerals.

Levels of the antioxidant vitamins A and E and the carotenoids (including beta-carotene) also are low in people with Alzheimer's disease. These nutrients act as free radical scavengers; deficiencies may expose the brain cells to increased oxidative damage. In addition, deficiencies of boron, potassium, and selenium have been found in people with Alzheimer's disease.

Research has also revealed a connection between Alzheimer's disease and high concentrations of aluminum in the brain. Autopsies of people who have died of Alzheimer's disease reveal excessive amounts of aluminum in the hippocampus area and in the cerebral cortex, the external layer of gray matter responsible for higher brain functions. It may be that exposure to excessive amounts of aluminum, especially if combined with a lack of essential vitamins and minerals, may directly or indirectly predispose one to developing Alzheimer's disease.

Aluminum is not the only metal that has been linked to Alzheimer's disease. The brains of people with Alzheimer's disease have been found to have higher than normal concentrations of the toxic metal mercury. For most people, the release of mercury from dental amalgams is the main means of mercury exposure, and a direct correlation has been demonstrated between the amount of inorganic mercury in the brain and the number of amalgam surfaces in the mouth. Mercury from dental amalgam passes into body tissues, and it accumulates in the body over time. Mercury exposure, especially from dental amalgams, cannot be excluded as a major contributor to Alzheimer's disease.

Many researchers believe that beta-amyloid is a key player in this memory-destroying disease. This substance is not unique to the brain, but is produced in virtually every cell in the body as a result of the degeneration of tissue.

Amyloid itself is not highly toxic, but it is possible it may trigger dementia if a critical mass accumulates in the brain.

Yet another possible culprit in the death of brain cells is the immune system. Many illnesses result from immune system malfunction causing it to attack the body's own tissues. Powerful immune system proteins called *complement proteins* have been found around the plaques and tangles in the brains of deceased Alzheimer's victims. In animals, brain injury is known to result in an alteration in the genetic "instructions" for two kinds of complement proteins. Some experts theorize that complement proteins normally help clear away dead cells, but that in Alzheimer's disease, they begin to attack healthy cells as well, and the degeneration of the cells results in accumulations of amyloid. There is also evidence that the presence of amyloid may trigger the release of a cascade of complement proteins, perhaps sparking a vicious cycle of inflammation and further plaque deposits. However, an immune system attack on brain cells may be a result, or merely one element, of Alzheimer's disease, rather than its cause.

Although all of these findings offer hope that Alzheimer's disease may one day be more fully understood, and thereby prevented, science does not yet know what can be done to arrest the mental deterioration. Even diagnosis of the disease is not a precise science. There are tests that can suggest a diagnosis of Alzheimer's and that can rule out other problems as the cause of symptoms, but there currently is no single laboratory procedure or biochemical marker that can definitively confirm the disorder in a living person. Because dementia can be a symptom of many disorders, a diagnosis of Alzheimer's disease is usually made when all other possibilities have been eliminated.

NUTRIENTS

SUPPLEMENT	SUGGESTED DOSAGE	COMMENTS
Essential		
Acetylcholine	500 mg 3 times daily, on an empty stomach.	Deficiency has been implicated as possibly causing dementia.
Boron	3 mg daily. Do not exceed this amount.	Improves brain function.
Coenzyme Q$_{10}$	100–200 mg daily.	Increases oxygenation of cells and is involved in the generation of cellular energy.
Ginkgo biloba		*See under* Herbs, below.
Lecithin granules or capsules	1 tbsp 3 times daily, before meals. 1,200 mg 3 times daily, before meals.	Needed for improved memory. Contains choline.
Multivitamin and mineral complex with potassium	99 mg daily.	All nutrients are necessary in balance. Use a high-potency formula. Needed for proper electrolyte balance.
Pycnogenol or grape seed extract	60 mg three times daily. As directed on label.	Potent antioxidants that readily pass the blood-brain barrier to protect brain cells from free radical damage.

Selenium	200 mcg daily.	Powerful antioxidant for brain cell protection.
Vitamin B complex injections plus extra	2 cc 3 times weekly or as prescribed by physician.	Needed for brain function; aids in the digestion of food.
vitamin B$_6$ (pyridoxine) and	½ cc once weekly or as prescribed by physician.	Deficiency can cause depression and mental difficulties.
vitamin B$_{12}$	1 cc 3 times weekly or as prescribed by physician.	Important for brain function. Deficient in people with Alzheimer's. Injections (under a doctor's supervision) are fast and give good results.
or		
Vitamin B complex plus extra	100 mg 3 times daily.	If injections are not available, use a sublingual form.
vitamin B$_6$ (pyridoxine) and	50 mg daily.	
vitamin B$_{12}$ plus	2,000 mcg daily.	Use a lozenge or sublingual form.
pantothenic acid (vitamin B$_5$)	100 mg 3 times daily.	Plays a role in converting choline into acetylcholine, needed for memory.
Zinc	50–100 mg daily. Do not exceed this amount.	Helps stop amyloid plaque formation induced by zinc deficiency.

Important		
Acetyl-l-carnitine	500 mg twice daily.	Believed to enhance brain metabolism. Slows deterioration of memory.
Apple pectin	As directed on label.	Aids in removing toxic metals such as mercury, which can contribute to dementia.
Calcium and magnesium	1,600 mg daily, at bedtime. 800 mg daily.	Has a calming effect and works with magnesium. Acts as a natural calcium channel blocker.
Free-form amino acid complex	1,000–2,500 mg daily, before meals. Take with 8 oz fluid.	Needed for improved brain function and tissue repair. Use free-form amino acids for best absorption.
Kelp	1,000–1,500 mg daily.	Supplies needed minerals.
Melatonin	2–3 mg daily, taken 2 hours or less before bedtime.	Improves brain function and aids sleep.
RNA and DNA	As directed on label.	These are the brain's cellular building blocks. Use a formula containing 200 mg RNA and 100 mg DNA per tablet. *Caution:* Do not take this supplement if you have gout.
Superoxide dismutase (SOD) plus	As directed on label.	A potent antioxidant that improves utilization of oxygen.
copper	3 mg daily.	SOD needs copper to function properly as an antioxidant.
Vitamin C with bioflavonoids	6,000–10,000 mg daily, in divided doses.	Enhances immune function and increases energy level; a powerful antioxidant. Use a buffered form.
Vitamin E	Start at 400 IU daily and increase slowly to 800 IU daily.	An antioxidant that helps transport oxygen to the brain cells and protects them from free radical damage.

HERBS

❑ Butcher's broom promotes healthy circulation.

❑ Ginkgo biloba extract, taken in liquid or capsule form, acts as an antioxidant and increases blood flow to the brain. Studies have shown that it can improve brain function. Take 100 to 200 mg of ginkgo biloba extract three times daily.

RECOMMENDATIONS

❑ Eat a well-balanced diet of natural foods and follow the supplementation program recommended above.

❑ Consume steam-distilled water only.

❑ Include plenty of fiber in your diet. Try oat bran or rice bran.

❑ Avoid alcohol, cigarette smoke, processed foods, and environmental toxins, especially metals such as aluminum and mercury. (*See* The Alzheimer's-Aluminum Connection on page 124.)

❑ Have a hair analysis to rule out the possibility of heavy metal intoxication as the cause of symptoms. *See* HAIR ANALYSIS in Part Three.

❑ Have allergy testing peformed to rule out environmental and/or food allergies. *See* ALLERGIES in Part Two.

CONSIDERATIONS

❑ Some experts distinguish between a rapidly progressing form of Alzheimer's disease that begins earlier in life (usually between the ages of thirty-six and forty-five) and a more gradual form that develops in people around the ages of sixty-five or seventy. For more information, consult *Complete Guide to Symptoms, Illness and Surgery for People Over 50* by H. Winter Griffith, M.D. (The Body Press/Perigee Books, 1992).

❑ The signs of alcohol abuse and the symptoms of Alzheimer's can be very similar. The actress Rita Hayworth, who was afflicted with Alzheimer's disease, was at first thought to be an alcoholic.

❑ No one should accept a diagnosis of Alzheimer's disease without first undergoing a trial of intensive nutritional therapy, particularly vitamin B$_{12}$ injections. Vitamin B$_{12}$ functions in numerous metabolic processes that affect nerve tissue, including the synthesis of neurotransmitters and the formation of the insulating sheath that surrounds many nerves, and it may have a role to play in the fight against Alzheimer's disease. Strange prickly or tingling sensations, loss of coordination, and dementia can be caused by B$_{12}$ deficiency even if the person does not have pernicious anemia, the classic sign of that deficiency. If an individual responds to B$_{12}$ treatment, Alzheimer's can be ruled out.

❑ Beta-amyloid, the protein-containing substance that makes up the characteristic senile plaques in the brain, has also been found in the spinal fluid of people with Alzheimer's disease. This finding may lead to the development of methods for earlier diagnosis of the condition.

❑ A test that measures electrical activity in the brain and stores the information on a computer disk for analysis can be used to help diagnose Alzheimer's disease. A skin test is also under development, and may allow for earlier and more rapid diagnosis.

❑ A decline in the ability to smell often occurs as much as two years prior to the beginning of mental decline in people with Alzheimer's. Scientists at the University of California—San Diego Medical Center found that people with this disorder need to be exposed to very strong concentrations of a substance before they can detect its odor. The rate at which the ability to distinguish smells is lost is a useful predictor of how rapidly an individual will lose cognitive functioning. Smoking can damage cells involved in the sense of smell, however, making this less useful as an indicator of disease in smokers.

❑ Researchers at the University of California–Davis questioned the caregivers of eighty-eight elderly people, half of whom had either Alzheimer's or a related form of dementia, about their eating habits. Half of the people with Alzheimer's disease had such a strong desire for sweets that their access to these foods had to be restricted.

❑ The hormone dehydroepiandrosterone (DHEA) may help to prevent Alzheimer's disease. (*See* DHEA THERAPY in Part Three.)

❑ High doses of lecithin may be helpful for people with Alzheimer's disease. However, a double-blind controlled trial of high doses of lecithin reported in the *Journal of Neurology, Neurosurgery, & Psychiatry* found that there may be a "therapeutic window" for the effects of lecithin on people with Alzheimer's disease, and that this may be more evident in older people.

❑ In his book *Beating Alzheimer's* (Avery Publishing Group, 1991), Tom Warren cites evidence that diet and chemical allergies may play an important role in Alzheimer's disease. Reactions to allergens can cause swelling in the brain. Recurring headaches are a common symptom of cerebral (brain-related) allergies. (*See* ALLERGIES in Part Two.)

❑ Research done at the University of Kentucky found that the brains of a group of individuals with Alzheimer's disease contained higher levels of mercury than the brains of a comparable control group, particularly in areas of the brain responsible for cognitive functioning, movement, and expression. The Alzheimer's group also had higher ratios of mercury to the trace minerals selenium and zinc, which help to protect the body against the toxic effects of mercury.

❑ Women with Alzheimer's disease have been found to have lower estrogen levels than their healthy counterparts.

❑ Researchers at the Massachusetts Institute of Technology discovered that levels of choline and ethanolamine are significantly lower than normal in people suffering from Alzheimer's disease. Both choline and ethanolamine are used for the synthesis of phospholipids that are major components of the cell membranes of neurons in the brain.

❑ Scientists at the University of Kentucky found that levels of glutamine synthetase, an enzyme that controls the production of ammonia and glutamate, were higher in a group of people with Alzheimer's disease than in a healthy control group. Glutamate is vital to the brain in small amounts, but can be poisonous in high concentrations. Abnormally high levels of glutamate have recently been associated with amyotrophic lateral sclerosis (ALS, also known as Lou Gehrig's disease) and glaucoma as well.

❑ An estimated 2 percent of Americans have two copies of a gene for the production of a substance called apolipoprotein E4, or APO-E4. APO-E4 transports cholesterol through the bloodstream and also changes the form of amyloid in the brain. Those with two copies of the gene have a 50-percent chance of getting Alzheimer's before the age of seventy. In contrast, for those with no copies of the gene, the risk of developing the disease does not rise to 50 percent until the after age of ninety.

❑ Hopes for the drug tacrine (Cognex) as a treatment for Alzheimer's disease have been deflated. Trials of tacrine yielded ambiguous results. It resulted in at best a modest decline in the progression of some cases of the disease, while at the same time raising concerns about liver damage.

❑ Experts say that it is in an individual's best interest to be told as soon as there is reason to suspect a diagnosis of Alzheimer's disease. Early warning cannot prevent the disease, but it gives people time to settle their affairs and make informed judgments about future care and other matters.

❑ Anyone who takes care of a person with Alzheimer's disease will eventually find the job overwhelming and need some help. For many, adult day-care centers are a godsend. A good day-care center should be clean, safe (without glass doors, uneven or slippery floors, furniture with sharp corners, and so on), and have barriers at entrances and exits to protect wanderers without making them feel trapped. The food should be nutritious and appetizing. Staff members should be warm and friendly, and professionally trained to work with people with Alzheimer's. There should be psychologists or social workers on hand to help people work through the ordinary frustrations of daily life and to assist them in coping with anger and depression. A quiet room should be available where an agitated or ill person can be separated from others, since some people find an active, stimulating environment upsetting. The availability of other specific services, such as physical therapy, help with hygiene, family counseling, or support groups for caregivers, as well as the usual activities of the center, should be suited to particular needs of the individual and his or her family.

❑ Further information about this disorder is available from the Alzheimer's Association, located at 919 North Michigan Avenue, Suite 1000, Chicago, IL 60611; telephone 800–272–3900 or 312–335–8700.

❑ *See also* ALUMINUM TOXICITY in Part Two.

Amblyopia

See Dimness or Loss of Vision *under* EYE PROBLEMS.

Anemia

Millions of Americans suffer from anemia, a reduction in either the number of red blood cells or the amount of hemoglobin in the blood. This results in a decrease in the amount of oxygen that the blood is able to carry. Anemia reduces the amount of oxygen available to the cells of the body. As a result, they have less energy available to perform their normal functions. Important processes, such as muscular activity and cell building and repair, slow down and become less efficient. When the brain lacks oxygen, dizziness may result, and mental faculties are less sharp.

Anything that causes a deficiency in the formation or production of red blood cells, or that leads to the too-rapid destruction of red blood cells, can result in anemia. Drug use, hormonal disorders, chronic inflammation in the body, surgery, infections, peptic ulcers, hemorrhoids, diverticular disease, heavy menstrual bleeding, repeated pregnancies, liver damage, thyroid disorders, rheumatoid arthritis, bone marrow disease, and dietary deficiencies (especially deficiencies of iron, folic acid, and vitamins B_6 and B_{12}) can all lead to anemia. There are also a number of hereditary disorders, such as sickle cell disease and thalassemia, that cause anemia. *Pernicious anemia* is a severe form of anemia that is due to vitamin B_{12} deficiency. Persons with this disorder cannot absorb any form of vitamin B_{12} from the gastrointestinal tract.

The most common cause of anemia is iron deficiency. Iron is an important factor in anemia because this mineral is used to make hemoglobin, the component of red blood cells that attaches to oxygen and transports it. Red blood cells exist only to oxygenate the body, and have a life span of about 120 days. If a person lacks sufficient iron, the formation of red blood cells is impaired. Iron-deficiency anemia can be caused by insufficient iron intake and/or absorption, or by significant blood loss. The latter is commonly seen in women who suffer from menorrhagia (heavy or prolonged menstrual bleeding), which in turn may be caused by a hormonal imbalance, fibroid tumors, or uterine cancer. Women who use intrauterine devices for contraception are also at a higher risk of blood loss, as are those who overuse anti-inflammatory medications such as aspirin or ibuprofen, which can cause blood loss through irritation of the digestive tract. Excessive aspirin usage, particularly by elderly people, may cause internal bleeding.

Of those suffering from anemia, 20 percent are women and 50 percent are children. It is often a hidden disease, because the symptoms can easily go unrecognized. The first

signs of developing anemia may be loss of appetite, constipation, headaches, irritability, and/or difficulty in concentrating. Established anemia can produce such symptoms as weakness; fatigue; coldness of the extremities; depression; dizziness; overall pallor, most noticeable in pale and brittle nails; pale lips and eyelids; soreness in the mouth; and in women, cessation of menstruation.

Anemia is significant not so much as a health problem in its own right, but as a sign of an underlying disorder. It is sometimes the first detectable sign of arthritis, infection, or certain major illnesses, including cancer. Anemia should therefore always be investigated and the cause determined. If you are anemic and your diet is ironclad, your physician can run a simple test called ESR (erythrocyte sedimentation rate) to detect any inflammation lurking in the body.

NUTRIENTS

SUPPLEMENT	SUGGESTED DOSAGE	COMMENTS
Essential		
Raw liver extract	500 mg twice daily.	Contains all the elements needed for red blood cell production. Use liver from organically raised beef Consider injections (under a doctor's supervision).
Very Important		
Blackstrap molasses		*See under* Recommendations, on next page.
Folic acid plus	800 mcg twice daily.	Needed for red blood cell formation.
biotin	300 mcg twice daily.	
Iron or Floradix Iron + Herbs from Salus Haus	As prescribed by physician. Take with 100 mg vitamin C for better absorption. 2 tsp twice daily.	To restore iron. Use ferrous gluconate form. *Caution:* Do not take iron unless anemia is diagnosed. Contains a readily absorbable form of iron that is nontoxic and from a natural source.
Vitamin B_{12} injections or vitamin B_{12}	2 cc once weekly or as prescribed by physician. 2,000 mcg 3 times daily.	Essential in red blood cell production and to break down and prepare protein for cellular use. Injections (under a doctor's supervision) are best. If injections are not available, use a lozenge or sublingual form for best absorption.
Important		
Vitamin B complex plus extra	50 mg 3 times daily.	B vitamins work best when taken together. A sublingual form is recommended.
pantothenic acid (vitamin B_5) and	50 mg 3 times daily.	Important in red blood cell production.
vitamin B_6 (pyridoxine)	100 mg daily.	Involved in cellular reproduction. Aids absorption of vitamin B_{12}.
Vitamin C	3,000–10,000 mg daily.	Important in iron absorption.
Helpful		
Brewer's yeast	As directed on label.	Rich in basic nutrients and a good source of B vitamins.

Copper	2 mg daily.	Needed in red blood cell production. *Note:* If more zinc is used, increase copper proportionately.
and zinc	30 mg daily. Do not exceed this amount.	Needed to balance with copper.
Raw spleen glandular	As directed on label.	*See* GLANDULAR THERAPY in Part Three for its benefits.
Vitamin A plus	10,000 IU daily.	Important antioxidants.
natural beta-carotene or	15,000 IU daily.	
carotenoid complex (Betatene)	As directed on label.	
Vitamin E	600 IU daily. Take separately from iron supplements.	Important for red blood cell survival; prolongs the life span of these cells. Use emulsion form for easier assimilation.

HERBS

❑ Alfalfa, bilberry, cherry, dandelion, goldenseal, grape skins, hawthorn berry, mullein, nettle, Oregon grape root, pau d'arco, red raspberry, shepherd's purse, and yellow dock are good for anemia.

Caution: Do not take goldenseal or Oregon grape root during pregnancy. Do not take goldenseal for more than one week at a time, and use it only under a doctor's supervision if you have a history of cardiovascular disease, diabetes, or glaucoma.

RECOMMENDATIONS

❑ Include the following in your diet: apples, apricots, asparagus, bananas, broccoli, egg yolks, kelp, leafy greens, okra, parsley, peas, plums, prunes, purple grapes, raisins, rice bran, squash, turnip greens, whole grains, and yams. Also eat foods high in vitamin C to enhance iron absorption.

❑ Consume at least 1 tablespoon of blackstrap molasses twice daily (for a child, use 1 teaspoon in a glass of milk or formula twice daily). Blackstrap molasses is a good source of iron and essential B vitamins.

❑ Eat foods containing oxalic acid in moderation or omit them from the diet. Oxalic acid interferes with iron absorption. Foods high in oxalic acid include almonds, cashews, chocolate, cocoa, kale, rhubarb, soda, sorrel, spinach, Swiss chard, and most nuts and beans.

❑ Avoid beer, candy bars, dairy products, ice cream, and soft drinks. Additives in these foods interfere with iron absorption. For the same reason, avoid coffee (which contains polyphenols) and tea (which contains tannins).

❑ Have a complete blood test to determine if you have an iron deficiency before taking iron supplements. Excess iron can damage the liver, heart, pancreas, and immune cell activity, and has been linked to cancer. Use iron supplements only under the supervision of a qualified health care provider.

❑ Because iron is removed through the stool, do not eat foods high in iron and/or iron supplements at the same time as fiber. Avoid using bran as a source of fiber.

❑ If you are a strict vegetarian, watch your diet closely. Taking supplemental vitamin B12 is advised (*see* VITAMINS in Part One).

❑ Do not smoke. Avoid secondhand smoke.

❑ Minimize your exposure to lead and other toxic metals. *See* ALUMINUM TOXICITY; CADMIUM TOXICITY; LEAD POISONING; and/or MERCURY TOXICITY for suggestions.

❑ Do not take calcium, vitamin E, zinc, or antacids at the same time as iron supplements. These can interfere with iron absorption.

CONSIDERATIONS

❑ Eating fish at the same time as vegetables containing iron increases iron absorption. Omitting all sugar from the diet increases iron absorption as well.

❑ Iron-deficiency anemia should disappear when the underlying cause is corrected.

❑ Persons with pernicious anemia must take vitamin B12 sublingually (dissolved under the tongue), by retention enema, or by injection. This treatment must be maintained for life, unless the underlying cause of the deficiency can be corrected.

Angina

See under CARDIOVASCULAR DISEASE.

Ankylosing Spondylitis

See under ARTHRITIS.

Anorexia Nervosa

The term *anorexia nervosa* was first coined in 1988. A doctor writing in the British medical journal *The Lancet* used the term to describe people who, although thin and weak, insisted that they needed to lose weight and would not eat a sufficient amount of food to remain alive.

Anorexia nervosa is an eating disorder characterized by a refusal to eat, even to the point of starvation. Other symptoms include an intense fear of becoming fat that never goes away, no matter how thin the individual becomes; extreme overactivity and an obsession with working out; negative feelings about the way the body looks; deep feelings of shame; and problems with drug and/or alcohol abuse. Ninety-five percent of the people who suffer from this disorder are female. Anorexia typically appears during adolescence; 1 to 2 percent of the female population between the ages of twelve and eighteen is affected.

Some people with anorexia just quit eating; some make themselves vomit immediately after eating; some take laxatives after eating; and some do all three. While most people with anorexia have normal feelings of hunger at the onset of the disease, they teach themselves to ignore them. Despite their refusal to eat, people with anorexia often become obsessed with food, and may spend hours fantasizing about it, reading recipes, or even preparing elaborate meals for others. Another characteristic feature of the disorder is that people with anorexia usually deny that there is anything wrong, but say that they simply "aren't hungry" and even insist that they need to lose more weight.

Many females who are anorexic are also bulimic. *Bulimia nervosa* is defined as the consumption of extremely large quantities of food in short periods of time (binging), followed by self-induced vomiting or the use of either diuretics or cathartics (purging). If anorexia and bulimia occur in the same individual, the disorder is called *bulimarexia.*

Anorexia can lead to underweight, extreme weakness, dizziness, cessation of menstruation, swelling of the neck, ulcers and erosion of the esophagus, erosion of the enamel of the back teeth from repeated vomiting, broken blood vessels in the face, and a low pulse rate and blood pressure. In some extreme cases, spoons or sticks used to induce vomiting have become stuck in the digestive tract and have had to be surgically removed. Systemic physiological changes in those suffering from anorexia include thyroid dysfunction, disturbances in the heartbeat, and irregularity in the secretion of growth hormone and the hormones cortisol, gonadotropin, and vasopressin.

Eventually, if anorexic behavior goes on long enough, classic complications associated with starvation appear. Electrolyte imbalances brought on by insufficient potassium and sodium levels cause dehydration, muscle spasms, and, ultimately, cardiac arrest. If laxatives are used, these further deplete the body of potassium. Hypokalemia (potassium deficiency) is a major problem for people with anorexia. Chronic hypokalemia can cause an irregular heartbeat, which can lead to heart failure and death.

Initially, anorexia nervosa was thought to be strictly a psychological problem. However, in the last few years, medical scientists and nutritionists have identified several physical components as well. For example, people with eating disorders have been found to have chemical imbalances similar to those found in individuals with clinical depression. Some cases of anorexia have been found to be caused by severe zinc deficiency.

As researchers have become increasingly aware of the physiological elements of anorexia, the psychological ones continue to be important. Teasing by peers or parents can play a role in making individuals obsessed with the idea that they are fat. In addition, many people who suffer from anorexia display great fear at the prospect of growing up, and girls often have difficult mother/daughter relationships. Some may try to live up to images their parents set for them, but feel inadequate—that they are not as beautiful or intelligent as their parents want them to be. A girl with anorexia may then develop an inferiority complex, seeing herself as fat and/or ugly, and no amount of common sense or persuasion can alter her distorted mental image.

About 30 percent of all people with anorexia struggle with the disorder all their lives. Another 30 percent have at least one life-threatening bout with it, while the remaining 40 percent outgrow it. Even if an individual recovers fully from the acute phase of the disorder, serious damage may have been done to the body.

NUTRIENTS

SUPPLEMENT	SUGGESTED DOSAGE	COMMENTS
Very Important		
Multivitamin and mineral complex with natural beta-carotene and	25,000 IU daily.	All nutrients are needed and must be taken in extremely high doses because they are passed through the gastrointestinal tract rapidly and are poorly assimilated.
vitamin A and	10,000 IU daily.	
calcium and	1,500 mg daily.	
magnesium and	1,000 mg daily.	
potassium and	99 mg daily.	
selenium	200 mcg daily.	
Zinc	80 mg daily. Do not exceed a total of 100 mg daily from all supplements.	All enzymes important for increased appetite and taste require zinc and copper. Zinc and copper work together to prevent copper deficiency.
plus copper	3 mg daily.	
Important		
Acidophilus	As directed on label. Take on an empty stomach so that it passes quickly to the small intestine.	Needed to replace the "friendly" bacteria lost from use of laxatives and/or from vomiting.
Free-form amino acid complex	As directed on label.	To supply easily assimilable protein, needed for tissue repair.
Multimineral complex	As directed on label.	Needed to replace lost minerals.
Vitamin B complex	100 mg 3 times daily.	Helps to prevent anemia and replaces lost B vitamins.
Vitamin B_{12} injections	1 cc 3 times weekly or as prescribed by physician.	Increases appetite; prevents loss of hair and damage to many bodily functions. If injections are not available, use a lozenge or sublingual form.
plus liver extract injections	2 cc 3 times weekly or as prescribed by physician.	To supply B vitamins and other valuable nutrients.
Vitamin C	5,000 mg daily, in divided doses.	Needed for the impaired immune system and to alleviate stress on the adrenal glands.
Helpful		
Bio-Strath from Bioforce or	3 times daily.	An herbal and yeast-based tonic.
Floradix Iron + Herbs from Salus Haus	As directed on label 3 times daily.	A natural source of iron.

Brewer's yeast	Start with 1 tsp daily and work up to 1 tbsp daily.	Contains balanced amounts of the B vitamins.
Kelp	2,000–3,000 mg daily.	Needed for mineral replacement.
Proteolytic enzymes	As directed on label. Take between meals and with meals.	To aid in digestion and in rebuilding of tissue.
Vitamin D	600 IU daily.	Needed for calcium uptake and to prevent bone loss.
Vitamin E	600 IU daily.	Increases oxygen uptake in the body for healing.

HERBS

❑ To rebuild the liver and cleanse the bloodstream, use dandelion, milk thistle, red clover, and wild yam.

❑ The following herbs are appetite stimulants: ginger root, ginseng, gotu kola, and peppermint.

Caution: Do not use ginseng if you have high blood pressure.

RECOMMENDATIONS

❑ While a normal eating pattern is being established, eat a well-balanced diet that is high in fiber. Eat plenty of fresh raw fruits and vegetables. These foods are cleansing to the system. When the body is cleansed, the appetite tends to return to normal.

❑ Consume no sugar, and avoid white flour products.

❑ Avoid processed and junk foods. The additives these foods contain tend to add to the aversion to eating.

❑ Seek out a practitioner or practitioners who specialize in the treatment of eating disorders and who can address the complex of physical and psychological elements involved. Some type of specialized counseling, in addition to nutritional counseling, is usually necessary for recovery.

❑ Look at your level of self-esteem. Women with low self-esteem tend to engage in self-destructive behaviors such as entering into abusive relationships, compulsive sexual behavior, and eating disorders. Cultivate relationships with people who make you feel important—people who are admiring and encouraging of your accomplishments and interests. As much as possible, remove from your life anything and anyone who makes you feel put-down, and consider counseling to help you learn to cope with those negative situations you cannot avoid.

CONSIDERATIONS

❑ If an individual shows any of the signs of anorexia, he or she should be seen by a physician.

❑ In many cases, a person with anorexia must be hospitalized and given intravenous nutrient feedings of potassium and multivitamins.

❑ Starvation tends to increase feelings of depression, anxiety, irritability, and anger. It may take up to a year or more for a person recovering from anorexia to improve his or her body

image, to reestablish normal eating patterns, and to reverse the effects of starvation on mood and behavior.

❑ Some researchers believe that neurotransmitters—such as dopamine, serotonin, norepinephrine, and the endogenous opioids—play a role in anorexia.

❑ Zinc, whether as part of the diet or in supplemental form, has been successful in helping many individuals with anorexia to regain their normal appetite and weight.

❑ The self-esteem problems typical of those with anorexia often begin at an early age. A child who is told that she is stupid, worthless, and/or unlovable is likely to come to believe it. In addition, recent research has shown that many (if not most) American girls undergo a severe loss of self-esteem in early adolescence, the very time that eating disorders are most likely to occur.

ADDITIONAL SOURCES OF INFORMATION

To learn more about eating disorders and treatments, contact any of the following organizations:

American Anorexia/Bulimia Association (AABA)
293 Central Park West, Suite 1R
New York, NY 10024
212–501–8351

Anorexia Nervosa and Related Eating Disorders (ANRED)
P.O. Box 5102
Eugene, OR 97405
503–344–1144

Institute for the Study of Anorexia and Bulimia
1 West 91st Street
New York, NY 10024
212–595–3449

National Eating Disorders Organization (NEDO)
445 East Granville Road
Worthington, OH 43085-3195
614–436–1112

Anxiety Disorder

Anxiety disorder is a far more common problem than was once thought. It can affect people in their teenage years through middle age and later. Anxiety disorder appears to affect twice as many women as men, though there may not actually be that wide a disparity between the sexes; psychologists believe that men are far less prone to report or even acknowledge having a problem of this nature.

Anxiety disorder can be either acute or chronic. Acute anxiety disorder manifests itself in episodes commonly known as panic attacks. A panic attack is an instance in which the body's natural "fight or flight" reaction occurs at the wrong time. This is a complex, involuntary physiological response in which the body prepares itself to deal with an emergency situation. Stress causes the body to produce more adrenal hormones, especially adrenaline. The increased production of adrenaline causes the body to step up its metabolism of proteins, fats, and carbohydrates to quickly produce energy for the body to use. In addition, the muscles tense, and heartbeat and breathing become more rapid. Even the composition of the blood changes slightly, to make it more prone to clotting.

In the face of a threat such as an assault, an accident, or a natural disaster, this type of reaction is perfectly normal and helpful for survival. At other times, the symptoms caused by a surge in adrenaline can be distressing and frightening. A person having a panic attack often is overwhelmed by a sense of impending disaster or death, which makes it impossible to think clearly. Other feelings that can accompany a panic attack include shortness of breath; a smothering, claustrophic sensation; heart palpitations; chest pain; dizziness; hot flashes and/or chills; trembling; numbness or tingling sensations in the extremities; sweating; nausea; a feeling of unreality; and a distorted perception of the passage of time. Eventually, the disorder can have other, cumulative effects, such as generalized aches and pains, muscular twitching and stiffness, depression, insomnia, nightmares and early waking, decreased libido, and abnormal feelings of tension with an accompanying inability to relax. Women may experience changes in the menstrual cycle and increased premenstrual symptoms.

Panic attacks are usually abrupt and intense. They can occur at any time of the day or night, and can last from a few seconds up to half an hour. To the panic sufferer, it often feels as though they are much longer. A person having a panic attacks often believes that he or she is experiencing a heart attack or a stroke. The attacks themselves are very unpredictable; some people experience one every few weeks, while others may have several a day. They are often triggered by stress (conscious or unconscious) or certain emotions, but may also occur in response to certain foods, drugs, or illness. Food allergies and hypoglycemia are both common among people with this disorder, and can promote panic attacks. An attack may follow ingestion or overindulgence in caffeine-based stimulants such as tea or coffee. Some attacks occur with no apparent cause. The unpredictability of the attacks makes them even more distressing.

Many people with acute anxiety disorder become fearful of being alone and of visiting public places because they fear having a panic attack. Of course, this only adds to the level of anxiety and leads to their lives being abnormally restricted. Many psychologists believe that at least in some cases, panic attacks are self-induced; that is, the fear of a panic attack is the very thing that brings one about.

For years, panic attacks were dismissed as a psychosomatic phenomenon. However, repeated studies have shown that this disorder has a real, physical basis. Many experts believe that panic attacks are caused principally by a malfunction in brain chemistry, wherein the brain sends and receives false "emergency signals." Hyperactivity in certain areas of the brain causes the release of norepinephrine, which causes the pulse, blood pressure, and breathing to become more rapid—the classic symptoms of a panic attack.

Chronic anxiety is a milder, more generalized form of this disorder. Many people feel a vague sense of anxiety much of the time, but the intensity of the feeling does not reach the levels of those in an actual panic attack. They may feel chronically uneasy, especially in the presence of other people, and tend to startle easily. Headaches and chronic fatigue are common among people with this form of the disorder. Generalized anxiety disorder can begin at any age, but the onset typically occurs in one's twenties or thirties. Some people with chronic anxiety disorder also suffer from occasional panic attacks.

Anxiety disorder may be hereditary to some extent, as it seems to run in families. Some cases may be linked to a relatively harmless abnormality of heart function called mitral valve prolapse. Anxiety disorder manifests itself in different ways, but doctors agree that conflict, whether internal or interpersonal, promotes a state of anxiety.

NUTRIENTS

SUPPLEMENT	SUGGESTED DOSAGE	COMMENTS
Very Important		
Calcium and	2,000 mg daily.	A natural tranquilizer.
magnesium	600–1,000 mg daily.	Helps to relieve anxiety, tension, nervousness, muscular spasms, and tics. Best taken in combination with calcium.
Floradix Iron + Herbs from Salus Haus	As directed on label.	Check for iron deficiency; this can increase the risk of panic attacks. Floradix is a natural source of iron.
Multivitamin and mineral complex with		To provide all needed nutrients in balance.
potassium	99 mg daily.	Essential for proper functioning of the adrenal glands.
Vitamin B complex plus extra	As directed on label.	Helps maintain normal nervous system function.
vitamin B$_1$ (thiamine) and	50 mg 3 times daily, with meals.	Helps reduce anxiety and has a calming effect on the nerves.
vitamin B$_6$ (pyridoxine)	50 mg 3 times daily, with meals.	A known energizer that also exerts a calming effect. Important in the production of certain brain chemicals.
and niacinamide	1,000 mg daily.	In large doses, has a calming effect. *Caution:* Do not substitute niacin for niacinamide. Niacin can be toxic in such high doses.
Vitamin C	5,000–10,000 mg daily, in divided doses.	Necessary for proper function of adrenal glands and brain chemistry. In large doses, can have a powerful tranquilizing effect and is known to decrease anxiety. Vital for dealing with stress.
Zinc	50–80 mg daily. Do not exceed a total of 100 mg daily from all supplements.	Can have a calming effect on the central nervous system.

Important		
Chromium picolinate	200 mcg daily.	Chromium deficiency can produce symptoms of anxiety.
DL-Phenylalanine (DLPA)	600–1,200 mg daily. Discontinue use if no improvement is seen in 1 week.	For chronic anxiety. Increases the brain's production of endorphins, which help relieve anxiety and stress. *Caution:* Do not take this supplement if you are pregnant or nursing, or suffer from panic attacks, diabetes, high blood pressure, or PKU.
L-Glutamine	500 mg 3 times daily, on an empty stomach. Take with water or juice. Do not take with milk. Take with 50 mg vitamin B$_6$ and 100 mg vitamin C for better absorption.	Has a mild tranquilizing effect. *See* AMINO ACIDS in Part One.
and L-tyrosine	500 mg 3 times daily, on an empty stomach.	Important for anxiety and depression. *Caution:* Do not take this supplement if you are taking an MAO inhibitor drug.
plus L-glycine	500 mg 3 times daily, on an empty stomach.	Necessary for central nervous system function.
Helpful		
Gamma-aminobutyric acid (GABA) plus inositol	750 mg twice daily.

As directed on label. | Necessary for proper brain function. *See* AMINO ACIDS in Part One. Combined with inositol, has a tranquilizing effect. |
| Melatonin | Start with 2–3 mg daily, taken 2 hours or less before bedtime. If necessary, gradually increase the dosage until an effective level is reached. | A natural sleep aid. Helpful if symptoms include insomnia. |

HERBS

❑ When the body is under stress, it is more vulnerable to free radical damage. Bilberry, ginkgo biloba, and milk thistle are rich in flavonoids that neutralize free radicals.

❑ Catnip, chamomile, cramp bark, kava kava, hops, linden flower, motherwort, and passionflower promote relaxation and aid in preventing panic attacks.

Caution: Do not use chamomile on an ongoing basis, as ragweed allergy may result. Avoid it completely if you are allergic to ragweed. Kava kava can cause drowsiness. If this occurs, discontinue use or reduce the dosage.

❑ Skullcap and valerian root can be taken at bedtime to promote sleep and aid in preventing panic attacks at night.

❑ *Avoid* ephedra (ma huang), as it can aggravate anxiety.

RECOMMENDATIONS

❑ Include in the diet apricots, asparagus, avocados, bananas, broccoli, blackstrap molasses, brewer's yeast, brown rice, dried fruits, dulse, figs, fish (especially salmon), garlic, green leafy vegetables, legumes, raw nuts and seeds, soy products, whole grains, and yogurt. These foods supply valuable minerals such as calcium, magnesium, phosphorus, and potassium, which are depleted by stress.

❑ Try eating small, frequent meals rather than the traditional three meals a day.

❑ Limit your intake of animal protein. Concentrate on meals high in complex carbohydrates and vegetable protein.

❑ Avoid foods containing refined sugar or other simple carbohydrates. For a nutritional treatment plan to have maximum benefits, the diet should contain *no* simple sugars, carbonated soft drinks, or alcohol.

❑ Do not consume coffee, black tea, cola, chocolate, or anything else that contains caffeine.

❑ Keep a food diary to detect correlations between your attacks and the foods you eat. Food allergies and sensitivities may trigger panic or anxiety attacks.

❑ Learn relaxation techniques. Biofeedback and meditation can be very helpful.

❑ Get regular exercise. Any type of exercise will work—a brisk walk, bicycle riding, swimming, aerobics, or whatever fits your individual lifestyle. After a few weeks of regular exercise, most people notice an improvement in anxiety symptoms.

❑ Be sure to get adequate rest. If sleep is a problem, consult INSOMNIA in Part Two for suggestions.

❑ To help manage an acute attack, use breathing techniques. Inhale slowly to a count of four, hold your breath for a count of four, exhale slowly to a count of four, and then do nothing for a count of four. Repeat this sequence until the attack subsides. Remind yourself that panic attacks last for a limited amount of time, and that the attack *will* pass.

❑ Call a trusted friend or family member. Talking things over can diffuse anxiety.

❑ If the self-help recommendations in this section do not help, and particularly if panic or anxiety is interfering with your life, consult your health care provider. If an underlying physical problem is ruled out, expect to be referred to a mental health professional for evaluation and treatment.

CONSIDERATIONS

❑ People with anxiety disorder, especially those who experience acute attacks, often seek medical assistance in hospital emergency rooms, only to be told they are just suffering from stress and that everything will be fine with rest. In one study, up to 70 percent of people who had panic attacks were found to have seen ten or more different physicians before being correctly diagnosed.

❑ Taking tricyclic antidepressants such as imipramine hydrochloride (Janimine, Tofranil) or imipramine pamoate (Tofranil-PM) in the presence of low serum levels of iron may increase the risk of developing anxiety and jitteriness.

❑ Chromium deficiency can produce nervousness, shakiness, and other general symptoms of anxiety. Chromium deficiency is common among alcoholics and people who consume large amounts of refined sugars. Brewer's yeast is a rich source of this essential trace element.

❑ There have been numerous reports on the benefits of DL-phenylalanine (DLPA) in treating anxiety and depression. DLPA is a supplement consisting of both D-phenylalanine and L-phenylalanine, and is much more potent than either of these amino acids taken alone. This should be used under the supervision of a nutritionally oriented physician.

❑ Selenium has been shown to elevate mood and decrease anxiety. These effects were more noticeable in people who had lower levels of selenium in their diets to begin with.

❑ Biofeedback can aid in managing anxiety symptoms. *See under* PAIN CONTROL in Part Three.

❑ Music can be effective in reducing anxiety. (*See* MUSIC AND SOUND THERAPY in Part Three.) Color also can be used to induce relaxation and calm. (*See* COLOR THERAPY in Part Three).

❑ A number of different drugs are used to block panic attacks. Their use must be carefully monitored by a physician. The effectiveness of any given drug varies from individual to individual, and all drugs used for this disorder can cause unpleasant side effects. Alprazolam (Xanax), one of the drugs most commonly used for this illness, has varying effectiveness and can cause drowsiness and lightheadedness. It also can be very addictive. The risk of dependence and its severity seem to be higher if this drug is taken in relatively high doses (more than 4 milligrams per day) and for more than eight weeks.

❑ A healthy diet plus appropriate nutritional supplementation can be of considerable benefit, reducing overall anxiety and even decreasing the frequency and intensity of panic attacks. If you are taking antianxiety medication, following the plan outlined in this section may make it possible to stop taking the medication, or at least to reduce the dosage. You should always consult with your physician before making any change in a prescription regimen, however.

❑ *See also* STRESS in Part Two.

Appetite, Poor

A poor appetite is not a disorder in itself, but usually a symptom of some other problem. Emotional factors such as depression, illness, stress, and trauma may cause a person's appetite to diminish noticeably. Certain controllable factors, such as the use of alcohol, tobacco, or other drugs, can also result in poor appetite. An undetected underlying illness, heavy metal poisoning, and/or nutritional deficiencies may also be involved.

NUTRIENTS

SUPPLEMENT	SUGGESTED DOSAGE	COMMENTS
Very Important		
Bio-Strath from Bioforce	As directed on label.	A yeast and herb formula that aids in gaining back strength and energy.
Floradix Iron+ Herbs from Salus Haus	As directed on label.	Helps digestion and stimulates appetite.
Multivitamin and mineral complex with		All nutrients are needed in large amounts. Use a high-potency formula.
vitamin A	25,000 IU daily. If you are pregnant, do not exceed 10,000 IU daily.	
and calcium	1,500 mg daily.	
and magnesium	750 mg daily.	
Vitamin B complex	100 mg or more daily, before meals.	Increases the appetite. Use a high-stress formula. A sublingual form is recommended. Injections (under a doctor's supervision) may be necessary.
Zinc	80 mg daily. Do not exceed a total of 100 mg daily from all supplements.	Enhances the sense of taste.
plus copper	3 mg daily.	Needed to balance with zinc.
Helpful		
Brewer's yeast	Start with ½ tsp daily and work up to 1 tbsp daily.	Rich in nutrients, especially the B vitamins. Improves the appetite.
Spiru-tein from Nature's Plus	As directed on label. Take between meals.	To supply protein, needed to build and repair tissue. Also acts as an appetite stimulant.

HERBS

❑ To stimulate a poor appetite, try using catnip, fennel seed, ginger root, ginseng, gotu kola, papaya leaves, peppermint leaves, and/or saw palmetto berries.

Caution: Do not use ginseng if you have high blood pressure.

RECOMMENDATIONS

❑ To obtain needed protein and calories, drink 3 or more cups a day of skim milk, soymilk, Rice Dream, or almond milk. Use a soy carob drink and yogurt fruit shakes. Eat only whole-grain bread, rolls, macaroni, crackers, and hot and cold cereals. Use cream soups (made with soymilk) as desired. These are usually higher in protein than broth soups.

❑ Between meals, snack on foods such as avocados, banana soy pudding, buttermilk, cheese, chicken or tuna, custard, fruit shakes, nuts and nut butters, whole-grain breads and cereals, turkey, and yogurt. In addition to promoting weight gain, these snacks are easy to digest, are high in protein and essential fatty acids, and contain "friendly" bacteria.

❑ Do not drink liquids before or during meals.

❑ Take supplemental B vitamins as outlined under Nutrients, above. The B-complex vitamins increase appetite.

❑ Try eating small quantities of food at frequent intervals throughout the day rather than two or three large meals. The sight of large amounts of food can cause a person to lose his or her appetite. Frequent small meals may be better tolerated, with a gradual increase in the volume of food.

❑ Exercise if possible, but avoid strenuous exercise. Walking and/or moderate exercise can increase the appetite. Exercise also helps the body to assimilate nutrients better.

❑ If you smoke, quit. Smoking decreases the appetite. It is one of the main causes of loss of appetite.

❑ When trying to stimulate a poor appetite, consider whether the appearance and aroma of the foods are appealing, and whether the environment is conducive to eating.

❑ If you experience a significant loss of appetite, see your physician to rule out an underlying physical problem.

CONSIDERATIONS

❑ To stimulate a poor appetite, the diet must be individualized according to the person's tolerances and tastes.

❑ There are many products on the market that can be helpful for people with appetite and weight problems. They are often found in the "sports" sections of health food stores, but they are not only for those who are into sports.

❑ See also ANOREXIA NERVOSA and BULIMIA in Part Two. See also HYPOTHYROIDISM in Part Two for the self-test.

Arsenic Poisoning

Arsenic is a highly poisonous metallic element that can be found in some amount in a wide variety of sources, including pesticides, laundry aids, smog, tobacco smoke, bone meal, dolomite, kelp, table salt, beer, seafood, and even drinking water. When ingested, inorganic arsenic is deposited in the hair, skin, and nails. Once it makes its way into the hair follicles, its presence can be detected in the hair shaft for years.

Headaches, confusion, drowsiness, convulsions, and changes in fingernail pigmentation may occur with chronic arsenic poisoning. Symptoms of acute arsenic poisoning include vomiting, diarrhea, bloody urine, muscle cramps and/or weakness, fatigue, hair loss, dermatitis, gastrointestinal pain, and convulsions. Arsenic poisoning primarily affects the lungs, skin, kidneys, and liver. The accumulation of toxic levels of arsenic can result in coma and death.

Exposure to arsenic has been implicated in the development of certain types of cancer as well. Workers involved in pesticide production, copper smelting, making and spraying insecticides, mining, sheep dipping, and metallurgical industries are at a high risk for skin cancer, scrotal cancer, a type of liver cancer, cancer of the lymphatic system, and lung cancer due to arsenic exposure. The toxic effects of arsenic are cumulative.

NUTRIENTS

SUPPLEMENT	SUGGESTED DOSAGE	COMMENTS
Very Important		
Garlic (Kyolic)	2 tablets 3 times daily, with meals.	A potent detoxifier.
Superoxide dismutase (SOD) or	As directed on label.	A powerful detoxifying agent.
Cell Guard from Biotec Foods	As directed on label.	An antioxidant complex that contains SOD.
Vitamin C with bioflavonoids	5,000–20,000 mg daily, in divided doses. *See* ASCORBIC ACID FLUSH in Part Three.	A potent detoxifier. Use a buffered form.
Helpful		
L-Cysteine and L-methionine	500 mg each daily, on an empty stomach. Take with water or juice. Do not take with milk. Take with 50 mg vitamin B_6 and 100 mg vitamin C for better absorption.	Potent detoxifiers of the liver. Cysteine contains sulfur, which eliminates arsenic. *See* AMINO ACIDS in Part One.
Pectin plus	As directed on label.	Aids in removing arsenic from the body.
antioxidant complex (ACES + Zinc from Carlson Labs)	As directed on label.	To protect against free radical damage.
Selenium	200 mcg daily.	Helps to rid the body of arsenic.

RECOMMENDATIONS

❑ Eat eggs, onions, beans, legumes, and garlic to obtain sulfur. You can also obtain sulfur from garlic supplements. Sulfur helps eliminate arsenic from the body. The amino acid cysteine also provides sulfur. Sulfur can be purchased in tablet form as well.

❑ Supplement your diet with plenty of fiber daily.
Note: Always take supplemental fiber separately from other supplements and medications.

❑ If you have symptoms of chronic arsenic poisoning, have a hair analysis done to determine the level of toxic metals in your body. *See* HAIR ANALYSIS in Part Three.

❑ In case of accidental arsenic ingestion, *immediately* take 5 charcoal tablets, and take 5 more every fifteen minutes until you reach your health care provider or the emergency room of the nearest hospital. Charcoal tablets should be kept on hand in every household in case of accidental overdose of drugs.

CONSIDERATIONS

❑ Chelation therapy removes toxic metals from the body. (*See* CHELATION THERAPY in Part Three.)

❑ *See also* CHEMICAL POISONING and ENVIRONMENTAL TOXICITY in Part Two.

Arteriosclerosis/ Atherosclerosis

Arteriosclerosis and atherosclerosis involve the buildup of deposits on the insides of the artery walls, which causes thickening and hardening of the arteries. In arteriosclerosis, the deposits are composed largely of calcium; in atherosclerosis, the deposits consist of fatty substances. Both conditions have about the same effect on circulation, causing high blood pressure and ultimately leading to angina (chest pain brought on by exertion), heart attack, stroke, and/or sudden cardiac death.

Although arteriosclerosis causes high blood pressure, high blood pressure can also *cause* arteriosclerosis. Calcium-based and fatty deposits typically form in areas of the arteries that have been weakened by high blood pressure or strain. The consequent narrowing of the arteries then makes blood pressure that is already high even higher. As the arteries become less pliable and less permeable, cells may experience ischemia (oxygen starvation) due to insufficient circulation. If one of the coronary arteries becomes obstructed by accumulated deposits, or by a blood clot that has either formed or snagged on the deposit, the heart muscle will be starved for oxygen and an individual will suffer a heart attack, also referred to as a myocardial infarction (MI) or coronary occlusion (a coronary). Older people are at a greater risk for this kind of heart trouble. When arteriosclerosis occludes the arterial supply of blood to the brain, a cerebrovascular accident, or stroke, occurs.

An estimated 1 million Americans are disabled by peripheral vascular disease (diseases involving the blood vessels in the extremities) each year. Most of those affected have at least one of the major risk factors for atherosclerosis: smoking, family history of the disease, hypertension, diabetes, or abnormal cholesterol levels. Advancing age increases the likelihood of developing these diseases, as does atherosclerosis of the coronary or cerebral arteries.

Peripheral atherosclerosis, also called *arteriosclerosis obliterans*, is a type of peripheral vascular disease in which the lower limbs are affected. In the early stages, the major arteries that carry blood to the legs and the feet become narrowed by fatty deposits. Atherosclerosis of the leg or foot not only can limit a person's mobility, but can also lead to loss of a limb. People who have diseased arteries in the leg or foot are likely to have them elsewhere, mainly in the heart and brain. Early signs of peripheral atherosclerosis are aching muscles, fatigue, and cramplike pains in the ankles and legs. Depending on which arteries are blocked, there may also be pain in the hips and thighs.

Pain in the legs (most often in the calf, but sometimes in the foot, thigh, hip or buttocks) that is brought on by walking and is promptly relieved by rest is called *intermittent claudication*. This is often the first symptom of developing peripheral atherosclerosis. Additional symptoms include numbness, weakness, and a heavy feeling in the legs. These symptoms occur because the amount of oxygenated blood that makes it through the plaque-clogged arteries is insufficient to meet the needs of the exercising leg muscles. The closer the problem lies to the abdominal aorta—the central artery that branches into the legs—the more tissue is affected and the more dangerous the condition.

PERIPHERAL ARTERY FUNCTION SELF-TEST

A simple test can determine how well the blood is flowing through the arteries of the legs. There are three places on the lower leg where a pulsating artery can be felt by lightly touching the skin covering the artery. One spot is the top of the foot; the second spot is the inner aspect of the ankle; and the third spot is behind the knee.

Apply pressure lightly to the skin on these spots. If you cannot find a pulse, this is an indication that the artery supplying the leg may be narrowed. Special studies may be needed. Consult your health care provider.

NUTRIENTS

SUPPLEMENT	SUGGESTED DOSAGE	COMMENTS
Very Important		
Calcium and	1,500 mg daily, taken at bedtime.	Needed to maintain proper muscle tone in the blood
magnesium plus	750 mg daily, taken at bedtime.	vessels. Use chelate forms.
vitamin D	400 mg daily.	Aids calcium uptake.
Coenzyme Q10	100 mg daily.	Improves tissue oxygenation.
Essential fatty acids (flaxseed oil and MaxEPA are good sources)	As directed on label.	Reduces blood pressure, lowers cholesterol levels, and helps to maintain proper elasticity of blood vessels. Be sure to use a product that contains vitamin E to keep the essential fatty acids from becoming rancid.
Garlic (Kyolic)	As directed on label.	Has a lipid (fat) regulating effect.
Multivitamin and mineral complex	As directed on label.	All nutrients are needed for protection.
Selenium	200 mcg daily.	Promotes the action of vitamin E.
Vitamin A	25,000 IU daily. If you are pregnant, do not exceed 10,000 IU daily.	A potent antioxidant and free radical scavenger. Use emulsion form for easier assimilation.
plus natural beta-carotene or	15,000 IU daily.	An antioxidant and precursor of vitamin A.
carotenoid complex (Betatene) and	As directed on label.	
vitamin E	Start with 200 IU daily and increase by 200 IU each week until you reach 1,000 IU daily.	Helps to block the first steps leading to the disease. Use emulsion form for easier assimilation.
Vitamin C with bioflavonoids	5,000–20,000 mg daily, in divided doses. *See* ASCORBIC ACID FLUSH in Part Three.	Antioxidant that acts as a free radical scavenger. Works with vitamin E. Use a buffered form.

Important		
Choline or lecithin granules or capsules	As directed on label. 1 tbsp 3 times daily, with meals. 2,400 mg 3 times daily, with meals.	Aids in breaking down fat and expelling it from the body. Phosphatidyl choline is best. A good source of choline.
Citrin		*See under* Herbs, below.
Dimethylglycine (DMG) (Aangamik DMG from FoodScience Labs)	125 mg 3 times daily.	Improves tissue oxygenation.
Germanium	200 mg daily.	Lowers cholesterol and improves cellular oxygenation.
Heart Science from Source Naturals	As directed on label.	Contains antioxidants, herbs, vitamins, and other nutrients that promote cardiovascular function.
Melatonin	2–3 mg daily, taken 2 hours or less before bedtime.	A powerful antioxidant that also improves sleep.
Multienzyme complex	As directed on label. Take with meals.	Important for proper digestion.
Proteolytic enzymes	As directed on label. Take with meals.	Aids in destroying free radicals. Improves digestive function.
Pycnogenol or grape seed extract	50 mg twice daily. As directed on label.	Possibly the most powerful free radical scavengers. Also enhance the action of vitamin C and strengthen connective tissue, including that of the cardiovascular system.

Helpful		
L-cysteine and L-methionine plus L-carnitine	500 mg daily, on an empty stomach. Take with water or juice. Do not take with milk. Take with 50 mg vitamin B_6 and 100 mg vitamin C for better absorption. 500 mg daily, on an empty stomach. 500 mg daily, on an empty stomach.	Promotes the burning of fat and the building of muscle. Helps to prevent fatty buildup in the arteries. Protects the heart and lowers blood triglyceride levels.
Vitamin B complex plus extra niacinamide	100 mg 3 times daily. 100 mg 3 times daily.	The B vitamins work together as a complex. Dilates small arteries. *Caution:* Do not substitute niacin for niacinamide.
Zinc plus copper	50 mg daily. Do not exceed a total of 100 mg daily from all supplements. 3 mg daily.	Aids in cleansing and in the healing process. Use chelate forms. *See also* CHELATION THERAPY in Part Three. Needed to balance with zinc.

HERBS

❑ The following herbs are helpful if you suffer from arteriosclerosis: cayenne (capsicum), chickweed, ginkgo biloba extract, and hawthorn berries.

❑ Citrin is an herbal extract that inhibits the synthesis of potentially dangerous fats in the body.

RECOMMENDATIONS

❑ Eat high-fiber foods that are low in fat and cholesterol. Fruits, vegetables, and grains should be your main foods.

❑ Eat plenty of foods rich in vitamin E to improve circulation. Good choices include dark green leafy vegetables, legumes, nuts, seeds, soybeans, wheat germ, and whole grains.

❑ Use only pure cold-pressed olive oil or unrefined canola oil (in moderate amounts) as fats in the diet. These may aid in lowering cholesterol. Do not heat these oils.

❑ Drink steam-distilled water only.

❑ Do not eat any candies, chips, fried foods, gravies, high-cholesterol foods, junk foods, pies, processed foods, red meat, or saturated fats. Avoid egg yolks, ice cream, salt, and all foods containing white flour and/or sugar. Do not use stimulants such as coffee, colas, and tobacco; also eliminate alcohol and highly spiced foods.

❑ Maintain a healthy weight for your height. Obesity causes unfavorable changes in serum lipoprotein levels.

❑ Reduce stress and learn techniques to help you handle stress that cannot be avoided. *See* STRESS in Part Two.

❑ Get regular moderate exercise. A daily walk is good. *Caution:* If you are over thirty-five and/or have been sedentary for some time, consult your health care provider before beginning any type of exercise program.

❑ Periodically monitor your blood pressure, and take steps to lower it if necessary. *See* HIGH BLOOD PRESSURE in Part Two. Control of high blood pressure is important.

❑ Do not smoke. Avoid exposure to secondhand smoke. Cigarette smoke contains large quantities of free radicals, many of which are known to oxidize low-density lipoproteins (LDL, the so-called "bad cholesterol"), making them more likely to be deposited on the walls of blood vessels. The free radical is one of the primary factors in the development of atherosclerosis. The effect of cigarette smoke may be due to the direct oxidation of lipids and proteins, and it may also have indirect effects, such as the depletion of various antioxidant defenses, which then allows other cellular processes (inflammation, for example) to modify LDL. In addition, smoking increases levels of LDL, lowers levels of high-density lipoproteins (HDL, or "good cholesterol"), and increases the blood's tendency to form clots.

❑ Do not take any preparations containing shark cartilage unless specifically directed to do so by your health care provider. Shark cartilage may inhibit the formation of new blood vessels, the mechanism by which the body can increase circulatory capacity.

CONSIDERATIONS

❑ In the Lifestyle Heart Trial study, eighteen of twenty-two people (82 percent) who adopted a vegetarian diet that restricted fat intake to 10 percent of total calories showed a significant regression of advanced coronary artery disease after one year. The diet also limited dietary cholesterol to no more than 5 milligrams per day. In contrast, most Americans consume 37 percent of their total calories as fats, and 300 to 500 milligrams of dietary cholesterol each day.

❑ Kombucha tea may help prevent and treat arteriosclerosis. (*See under* NATURAL FOOD SUPPLEMENTS in Part One.)

❑ Dehydroepiandrosterone (DHEA) is a natural hormone that has been shown to help prevent hardening of the arteries. (*See* DHEA Therapy in Part Three.)

❑ Chelation therapy can break up arterial plaque and improve circulation. (*See* CHELATION THERAPY in Part Three.)

❑ Hyperbaric oxygen is used in some countries to treat arteriosclerosis. (*See* HYPERBARIC OXYGEN THERAPY in Part Three.)

❑ Many doctors recommend angioplasty or bypass surgery for people with hardening of the arteries, particularly for those with disabling angina. Angioplasty is a procedure in which blocked vessels are reopened by flattening cholesterol and debris against artery walls. Bypass surgery involves taking healthy blood vessels from elsewhere in the body (usually the leg) and inserting them to detour around a diseased coronary artery. Unless people undergoing these procedures make significant nutritional and lifestyle changes, however, the disease process (atherosclerosis) will continue, and it is only a matter of time before the fatty deposits begin to build up again.

❑ Anticoagulants such as aspirin are often prescribed to make the blood less prone to clotting. For this to be effective, supplemental vitamin K and foods rich in vitamin K must be avoided. (*See* CARDIOVASCULAR DISEASE in Part Two.)

❑ Impotence can result from this disease. (*See* IMPOTENCE in Part Two.)

Arthritis

Arthritis is the inflammation one or more joints. It is characterized by pain, swelling, stiffness, deformity, and/or a diminished range of motion. More than 50 million Americans suffer from osteoarthritis, rheumatoid arthritis, and related conditions, such as fibromyalgia, gout, lupus, Lyme disease, psoriatic arthritis, Reiter's syndrome, Sjögren's syndrome, and ankylosing spondylitis.

These conditions affect the body's movable, or *synovial*, joints. Joints of the body are found at the knees, wrists, elbows, fingers, toes, hips, and shoulders. The neck and back also have joints between the bones of the spine. There are six different types of synovial joints (hinge, ball-and-socket, and so on), but although the types of motion they allow are different, their underlying physiological structure is essentially the same: Two or more adjoining movable bones, whose adjacent surfaces are covered with a layer of cartilage, are surrounded by a fluid-filled capsule made up of ligaments (tough, fibrous tissue). The fluid is secreted by a thin membrane, the synovial

membrane, that lines the inside of the joint capsule. Thanks to this viscous fluid, and to the smooth, rubbery, blue-white cartilage that covers the ends of the bones, the bones within the joint normally glide smoothly past one another.

In healthy joints, the synovial membrane is thin, the cartilage that covers the bones is smooth, and a thin layer of synovial fluid covers the bone surfaces. If anything goes wrong with any of these factors, arthritis can result. Arthritis may appear suddenly or come on gradually. Some people feel a sharp burning or grinding pain. Others compare the pain to that of a toothache. Moving the joint usually hurts, although sometimes there is only stiffness. The swelling and deformity that takes place in arthritic joints can result from a thickening of the synovial membrane, an increase in the secretion of synovial fluid, enlargement of the bones, or some combination of these factors. There are many different types of arthritis. Here we primarily discuss the most common forms: osteoarthritis and rheumatoid arthritis.

Osteoarthritis involves deterioration of the cartilage that covers the ends of the bones. It is a degenerative joint disease sometimes caused by injury or a defect in the protein that makes up cartilage. More commonly, it is related to the wear and tear of aging. The once-smooth surface of cartilage becomes rough, resulting in friction. The cartilage begins to break down, and the normally smooth sliding surfaces of the bones become pitted and irregular. The tendons, ligaments, and muscles holding the joint together become weaker, and the joint itself becomes deformed, painful, and stiff. There is usually some pain, but little or no swelling. Any resulting disability is usually minor. However, fractures become an increasing risk because osteoarthritis makes the bones brittle. As osteoarthritis advances, bony outgrowths called osteophytes tend to develop. These spurs, which can be detected by x-ray, develop near degenerated cartilage in the neck or lower back. This condition does not change a person's appearance.

Osteoarthritis rarely develops before the age of forty, but it affects nearly everyone past the age of sixty. However, it may be so mild that a person is unaware of it until it shows up on an x-ray. It typically runs in families, and afflicts almost three times as many women as men.

Rheumatoid arthritis (RA) and juvenile rheumatoid arthritis are types of inflammatory arthritis. RA is an autoimmune disorder—a "self-attacking-self" disease—in which the body's immune system improperly identifies the synovial membranes that secrete the lubricating fluid in the joints as *foreign*. Inflammation results, and the cartilage and tissues in and around the joints are damaged or destroyed. Often the bone surfaces are destroyed as well. The body replaces this damaged tissue with scar tissue, causing the normal spaces within the joints to become narrow and the bones to fuse together. Rheumatoid arthritis creates stiffness, swelling, fatigue, anemia, weight loss, fever, and, often, crippling pain.

RA frequently occurs in people under forty years of age, including young children. Currently, 2.1 million Americans are afflicted with rheumatoid arthritis, two thirds of them

Types of Arthritis

Swollen, painful joints can have a variety of causes. The particular symptoms involved make different arthritic conditions distinguishable from one another. The following table gives an overview of different types of arthritic disorders, their relative incidence, and characteristic features.

Cause of Arthritis	Incidence in U.S.	Typical Age at Onset	Symptoms
Osteoarthritis	15.8 million.	Over 40.	Stiffness and pain on joint motion. Most often comes on gradually, over a period of years. Inflammation is not usually present at first, but in the later stages, inflammation, enlargement of the joint, and muscle contractures may occur. Joint mobility may become limited, and movement may be accompanied by a grating sensation.
Rheumatoid arthritis	2.9 million.	25–50.	Joint stiffness upon awakening that lasts an hour or longer; swelling in specific finger or wrist joints; swelling in the soft tissue around the joints; swelling on both sides of the joint. Swelling can occur without or without pain, and can worsen progressively or remain the same for years before progressing.
Spondyloarthropathies (including psoriatic arthritis, ankylosing spondylitis, Reiter's syndrome)	2.5 million.	20–40.	A group of disorders that tend to affect the spine, causing pain, stiffness, inflammation, and changes in posture.
Gout	1.6 million (85 percent male).	40.	Sudden onset of extreme pain and swelling of a large joint (usually a big toe, but occasionally other joints).
Systemic lupus erythematosus	300,000 (90 percent female).	18–50.	Fever, weakness, upper body and facial pain, joint pain.
Juvenile rheumatoid arthritis	250,000.	Under 18.	Joint stiffness, often in knee, wrist, and hand. Can also involve kidneys, heart, lungs, and nervous system.
Infectious arthritis	100,000.	Any age.	Body aches, chills, and fever; confusion, dizziness, low blood pressure, pneumonia, and shock; redness, swelling, tenderness, and throbbing pain in the affected joint. Pain sometimes spreads to other joints and worsens with movement.
Kawasaki syndrome	Hundreds of cases in local outbreaks.	6 months–11 years.	Fever, joint pain, red rash on palms and soles, heart complications.

women. Juvenile rheumatoid arthritis affects 71,000 young Americans (aged eighteen and under), six times as many girls as boys. The onset of rheumatoid arthritis is often associated with physical or emotional stress; however, poor nutrition or bacterial infection may also be involved. Rheumatologists have discovered that the blood of many people with RA contains antibodies called rheumatoid factors, a finding that can aid in diagnosis of the condition.

While osteoarthritis affects individual joints, rheumatoid arthritis affects all of the body's synovial joints. Joints afflicted with rheumatoid arthritis tend to make a sound like crinkling cellophane, whereas osteoarthritic joints make popping, clicking, and banging noises.

Arthritis can also be caused by bacterial, viral, or fungal infection of a joint. The microorganisms most commonly involved in this type of the disorder, termed *infectious arthritis*, are streptococci, staphylococci, gonococci, hemophilus or tubercle bacilli, and fungi such as *Candida albicans*. Usually the infecting organism travels to the joint through the bloodstream from an infection elsewhere in the body, but injury or even surgery can result in joint infection as well. Symptoms of infectious arthritis include redness, swelling, pain, and tenderness in the affected joint, often accompanied by systemic symptoms of infection such as fever, chills, and body aches.

The *spondyloarthropathies* are a group of rheumatic disorders that tend to affect the spine. *Ankylosing spondylitis* (AS) is the most common of these. In this disorder, certain joints of the spine become inflamed, stiffen, become rigid, and then fuse together. If confined to the lower back, AS causes virtually no limitation of movement. In some cases, however, the entire spine may become rigid and bent. If the joints between the ribs and spine are affected, breathing problems may result as the chest wall's ability to expand becomes limited. Postural deformities are common. More than 400,000 Americans suffer from AS. Two and a half times as many men as women have this disorder.

Gout, an acute form of inflammatory arthritis, occurs most often in people who are overweight and/or who indulge regularly in rich foods and alcohol. It typically attacks the smaller joints of the feet and hands, especially the big toe. Deposits of crystallized uric acid salt in the joint cause swelling, redness, and a sensation of heat and extreme pain. Some 1 million Americans suffer from gout. Unlike most forms of arthritis, gout overwhelmingly affects men— 90 percent of those who suffer from gout are male.

NUTRIENTS

SUPPLEMENT	SUGGESTED DOSAGE	COMMENTS
Essential		
Boron	3 mg daily. Do not exceed this amount.	A trace mineral required for healthy bones.
Bromelain	As directed on label 3 times daily, with meals.	An enzyme that helps to stimulate production of prostaglandins. Also helps digestion of protein.
Glucosamine sulfate or N-Acetylglucosamine (N-A-G from Source Naturals)	As directed on label. / As directed on label.	Important for the formation of bones, tendons, ligaments, cartilage, and synovial (joint) fluid.
Pantothenic acid (vitamin B5)	500–1,000 mg daily.	Especially for rheumatoid arthritis; vital for the production of steroids in the adrenal gland.
Primrose oil or salmon oil	As directed on label twice daily. Take before meals.	To supply essential fatty acids that increase production of anti-inflammatory prostaglandins. Helps to control arthritis pain and inflammation.
Sea cucumber (bêche-de-mer)	As directed on label.	A rich source of specific lubricating compounds found abundantly in all connective tissues, especially the joints and joint fluid. It may take 3 to 6 weeks to note an improvement.
Silica	As directed on label.	Supplies silicon, important for rebuilding of the connective tissues and formation of bones.
Superoxide dismutase (SOD) or Cell Guard from Biotec Foods	As directed on label. / As directed on label.	An antioxidant that protects the fluid in the joints from destruction by free radicals. A sublingual form is recommended. Consider injections (under a doctor's supervision). / An antioxidant complex that contains SOD.
Vitamin E	400 IU daily.	A powerful antioxidant that protects the joints from damage by free radicals. Increases joint mobility.
Very Important		
Calcium and magnesium plus copper and zinc	2,000 mg daily. / 1,000 mg daily. / 3 mg daily. / 50 mg daily. Do not exceed a total of 100 mg daily from all supplements.	Needed to prevent bone loss. Use calcium chelate form. / Needed to balance with calcium. / A cofactor for lysyl oxidase, which strengthens connective tissue. / Needed for bone growth. Often deficient in those with arthritis. Use zinc picolinate form.
Coenzyme Q10	60 mg daily.	Increases tissue oxygenation to aid in repair of connective tissues.
Dimethylglycine (DMG) (Aangamik DMG from FoodScience Labs)	125 mg 3 times daily.	Helps to prevent further damage to joints.
Free-form amino acid complex	As directed on label.	To supply protein, needed for tissue repair.
Kelp or alfalfa	As directed on label.	A rich source of minerals needed for good skeletal health. See under Herbs, below.
Manganese	2 mg daily.	Needed for normal bone growth. Note: Do not take manganese and calcium at the same time, as they compete for absorption.
Multienzyme complex	As directed on label. Take with meals.	To aid digestion. Caution: If you have a history of ulcers, do not use a product containing HCl.
Selenium	200 mcg daily.	A powerful antioxidant.

Vitamin B complex with para-aminobenzoic acid (PABA) plus extra	50 mg 3 times daily.	B vitamins work best when taken together. Use a hypoallergenic formula. Good for swelling.
vitamin B$_3$ (niacin) or niacinamide	100 mg 3 times daily. Do not exceed this amount.	Increases blood flow by dilating small arteries. *Caution:* Do not take niacin if you have a liver disorder, gout, or high blood pressure. Reduces swelling in tissue.
plus vitamin B$_6$ (pyridoxine)	50 mg daily.	
Vitamin B$_{12}$ and folic acid	1,000 mcg daily. 400 mcg daily.	Needed for proper digestion, the formation of cells, and the production of myelin, the protective coating surrounding the nerves. Prevents nerve damage.
Vitamin C plus bioflavonoids	3,000–10,000 mg daily, in divided doses. 500 mg daily.	Powerful free radical destroyer that also aids in pain relief because of its anti-inflammatory effect. Use a buffered form. Boosts the activity of vitamin C.
Vitamin K	As directed on label.	Helps deposit minerals into the bone matrix.

Important		
Germanium (GE-132 from American Biologics	150 mg with each meal.	A powerful antioxidant that also relieves pain.

Helpful		
Bone Defense from KAL or	As directed on label.	Contains calcium, magnesium, phosphorus and other valuable bone-reinforcing nutrients.
Joint Support from Now Foods	As directed on label.	A combination of vitamins, minerals, herbs, and other nutrients that is excellent for joint problems.
DL-Phenylalanine (DLPA)	500 mg daily every other week.	Good for pain relief. *Caution:* Do not take this supplement if you are pregnant or nursing, or if you suffer from panic attacks, diabetes, high blood pressure, or PKU.
Garlic (Kyolic)	2 capsules 3 times daily, with meals.	Inhibits the formation of free radicals, which can damage the joints.
L-Cysteine	500 mg twice daily, on an empty stomach. Take with water or juice. Do not take with milk. Take with 50 mg vitamin B$_6$ and 100 mg vitamin C for better absorption.	A detoxifier essential for immune function; a source of sulfur and component of collagenous tissue. See AMINO ACIDS in Part One.
Multivitamin complex with vitamin A and natural beta-carotene	10,000 IU daily. 15,000 IU daily.	All nutrients are needed to aid in repairing tissues and cartilage.
Proteolytic enzymes or Infla-Zyme Forte from American Biologics	As directed on label. Take between meals. As directed on label.	To protect the joints from free radical damage.
Pycnogenol or grape seed extract	As directed on label. As directed on label.	Powerful free radical scavengers that also act as anti-inflammatories and strengthen connective tissue.
Shark cartilage (BeneFin)	Start with 1 gram per 15 lbs of body weight daily, divided into 3 doses. When relief is achieved, reduce the dosage to 1 gm per 40 lbs of body weight daily.	Treats pain and inflammation.
VitaCarte from Phoenix BioLabs	As directed on label.	Contains bovine cartilage, which has been shown to be effective in improving rheumatoid arthritis.

HERBS

❑ Alfalfa contains all the minerals essential for bone formation, and may be helpful for arthritis. It can be taken in capsules or in whole, natural form.

❑ Cat's claw is helpful for relieving arthritis pain. Feverfew and ginger also are good for pain and soreness.

Caution: Do not use cat's claw or feverfew during pregnancy.

❑ The hot peppers known as cayenne (capsicum) contain a compound called capsaicin that relieves pain, apparently by inhibiting the release of substance P, a neurotransmitter responsible for communicating pain sensations. Capsaicin can be absorbed through the skin; mix cayenne powder with enough wintergreen oil to make a paste and apply it to painful joints, or use cayenne peppers in a poultice (*see* USING A POULTICE in Part Three). This may cause a stinging sensation at first, but with repeated use, pain should diminish markedly. Cayenne can also be taken in capsule form.

❑ Other herbs that can be beneficial for arthritis include brigham tea, buchu leaves, burdock root, celery seed, corn silk, devil's claw tea, horsetail, nettle, and parsley tea, and yucca.

RECOMMENDATIONS

❑ Eat more sulfur-containing foods, such as asparagus, eggs, garlic, and onions. Sulfur is needed for the repair and rebuilding of bone, cartilage, and connective tissue, and aids in the absorption of calcium. Other good foods include green leafy vegetables, which supply vitamin K; fresh vegetables; nonacidic fresh fruits; whole grains; oatmeal; brown rice; and fish.

❑ Consume foods containing the amino acid histidine, including rice, wheat, and rye. Histidine is good for removing excess metals from the body. Many people with arthritis have high levels of copper and iron in their bodies.

❑ Eat fresh pineapple frequently. Bromelain, an enzyme found in pineapple, is excellent for reducing inflammation. To be effective, the pineapple must be fresh, as freezing and canning destroy enzymes.

❑ Eat some form of fiber, such as ground flaxseeds, oat bran, or rice bran, daily.

❑ Reduce the amount of fat in your diet. Do not consume milk, dairy products, or red meat. Also avoid caffeine, citrus fruits, paprika, salt, tobacco, and everything that contains sugar.

❑ Avoid the nightshade vegetables (peppers, eggplant, tomatoes, white potatoes). These foods contain a substance called solanine, to which some people, particularly those suffering from arthritis, are highly sensitive. Solanine interferes with enzymes in the muscles, and may cause pain and discomfort.

❑ If you use ibuprofen or other nonsteroidal anti-inflammatory drugs (NSAIDs), avoid sodium (salt), which causes water retention. Spread doses of these medications out through the day, take them only after eating, and take an antacid an hour after taking the drug. Ask your health care provider about a protective agent to take along with the NSAID, especially if you are over sixty-five or have had previous gastrointestinal bleeding.

❑ Do not take iron supplements, or a multivitamin containing iron. Iron is suspected of being involved in pain, swelling, and joint destruction. Consume iron in foods instead. Good sources include blackstrap molasses, broccoli, Brussels sprouts, cauliflower, fish, lima beans, and peas.

❑ For relief of pain, try using cold gel packs. These retain cold for long periods when frozen. Place them on inflamed joints. Alternate with applications of heat.

❑ Hot tubs and baths may provide relief. Raw lemon rubs and hot castor oil packs are also extremely beneficial. To make a hot castor oil pack, place castor oil in a pan and heat but do not boil it. Dip a piece of cheesecloth or other white cotton material into the oil until the cloth is saturated. Apply the cloth to the affected area and cover it with a piece of plastic that is larger in size than the cotton cloth. Place a heating pad over the plastic and use it to keep the pack warm. Keep the pack in place for one-half to two hours, as needed.

❑ In the morning, take a hot shower or a bath to help relieve morning stiffness.

❑ Take a free-form amino acid complex regularly to help repair tissue.

❑ Check for possible food allergies. Many sufferers of neck and shoulder pain have found relief when they eliminate certain foods.

❑ Consider having a hair analysis to determine the levels of toxic metals in your body. Lead levels have been found to be higher than normal in some arthritis sufferers. (See HAIR ANALYSIS in Part Three.)

❑ Spend time outdoors for fresh air and sunshine. Exposure to the sun prompts the synthesis of vitamin D, which is needed for proper bone formation.

❑ Get regular moderate exercise. Exercise is essential for reducing pain and retarding joint deterioration. Regular activity that does not put stress on affected joints, but that strengthens surrounding bones, muscles, and ligaments, is valuable for many types of arthritis. Bicycle riding, walking, and water exercises are good choices. Avoid weight-bearing or impact exercises.

❑ If you are overweight, lose the excess pounds. Being overweight can cause and aggravate osteoarthritis.

CONSIDERATIONS

❑ If the blood is too acidic, this may cause the cartilage in the joints to dissolve. The joints lose their normal smooth sliding motion, the bones rub together, and the joints become inflamed. This causes pain.

❑ Researchers at Jefferson Medical College in Philadelphia have identified a possible genetic component of osteoarthritis. They found that in some individuals, there is a defect in the gene that instructs cartilage cells to manufacture collagen, an important protein in connective tissue. As a result, the collagen in these individuals' joints is more prone to wear down, depriving the bones of their protective cushion.

❑ In one study, people with rheumatoid arthritis were found to have lower blood levels of folic acid, protein, and zinc than healthy persons. The researchers concluded that drugs prescribed for arthritis had brought about biochemical changes in the subjects' bodies, increasing their a need for certain nutrients.

❑ Eating deep-sea fish, which are rich in eicosapentaenoic acid (EPA) and docosahexaenoic acid (DHA), was found to help relieve the symptoms of rheumatoid arthritis in a study conducted by Charles Dinarello, M.D., of the Tufts University School of Medicine. Albany Medical College researcher Joel M. Kremer conducted a study in which 20 people with rheumatoid arthritis were given daily doses of 15 capsules of MaxEPA, a fish oil concentrate, and 20 were given a placebo. After 14 weeks, the groups were switched. The people taking the fish oil reported only about half as many tender joints as the placebo group. The fish oil also slowed the onset of fatigue.

❑ Researchers are currently looking at an ointment containing the immunosuppressant drug cyclosporine, which is used in transplant patients to prevent rejection of the transplanted organ, as a treatment for a variety of autoimmune diseases, including rheumatoid arthritis. Using the ointment form of cyclosporine apparently lessens the potentially hazardous side effects this drug has when administered by mouth or by injection, such as kidney damage and reduced resistance to infection.

❑ Chlamydia, the organism responsible for many cases of urethritis, has been linked to a form of arthritis that affects young women. In nearly half of the women with unexplained arthritis tested in one study, chlamydia was found in the joints. Seventy-five percent had elevated levels of antibodies to chlamydia in their blood.

❑ Silicone gel breast implants and other silicone prostheses may cause arthritis-like symptoms, such as swelling of joints, contractures, fever, chronic fatigue, and pain. Silicone has also been known to trigger such severe autoimmune diseases as scleroderma and lupus. In a study at the University of California in Davis, sixteen of forty-six women with implants had antibodies that attacked collagen, whereas in a group of forty-five women without implants, only four had the antibodies. Some women have seen arthritic symptoms disappear after having the implants removed, but this is not true in all cases.

❑ In one laboratory study, injections of a protein called anti-TGF-B banished painful joint swelling in 75 percent of the subjects, according to Dr. David Pisetsky of the National Arthritis Foundation. This protein destroys TGF-B, a chemical produced by the body in response to infection that causes inflammation and triggers swelling in the hands and feet.

❑ Mobility from Parametric Associates and Cosamin from Nutramax Laboratories are two formulas that may help the joints and ligaments. They are not generally available in health food stores, however, so they may have to be ordered directly from the manufacturers. (*See* MANUFACTURER AND DISTRIBUTOR INFORMATION in the Appendix.)

❑ Kombucha tea, which contains many vital nutrients as well as compounds that are essential components of connective tissue, has been reported to increase energy, relieve pain, and improve mobility in people with arthritis. (*See* MAKING KOMBUCHA TEA in Part Three.)

❑ Dimethylsulfoxide (DMSO), a byproduct of wood processing, is a liquid that can be applied topically to relieve pain, reduce swelling, and promote healing.

Note: Only DMSO from a health food store should be used for the treatment of arthritis. Commercial-grade DMSO such as that found in hardware stores is not suitable for healing purposes. The use of DMSO may result in a garlicky body odor. This is temporary, and is not a cause for concern.

❑ Arthritis pain and inflammation may respond to treatment with honeybee venom. The venom contains a powerful anti-inflammatory substance and also acts as an immune system stimulant. It is administered by injection, either with a hypodermic needle or by the bees themselves. It is believed to be effective for both osteoarthritis and rheumatoid arthritis, although the latter generally takes longer to respond. Further information is available from the American Apitherapy Society in Hartland Four Corners, Vermont; telephone 802–436–2708.

❑ Nonsteroidal anti-inflammatory drugs (NSAIDs) such as ibuprofen (found in Advil, Nuprin, and numerous other products), indomethacin (Indocin), and piroxicam (Feldene) are commonly prescribed for relief of arthritis pain. Unfortunately, these drugs also can have side effects. At least 1 in 100 people who take NSAIDs on a regular basis for arthritis develops stomach ulcers or experiences severe gastrointestinal bleeding—effects that are potentially very dangerous. The U.S. Food and Drug Administration recently estimated that as many as 200,000 cases of gastrointestinal bleeding, including 10,000 to 20,000 deaths, occur each year in the United States as a result of nonsteroidal anti-inflammatory drugs prescribed for arthritis. These drugs also can cause kidney or liver damage. According to a study reported in *Annals of Internal Medicine*, the use of NSAIDs can lead to serious health problems if you have even mild kidney dysfunction.

❑ Misoprostol (Cytotec) and ulcer drugs like ranitidine (Zantac) and sucralfate (Carafate) can prevent the development of ulcers associated with NSAIDs. However, these drugs have their own side effects, and they double the cost of treatment.

❑ Diclofenac sodium (Voltaren), a drug often prescribed for arthritis, may cause serious liver problems in some cases. People who take it should be monitored very carefully. If this medication is prescribed, the physician should perform a blood liver enzyme study to determine whether there is a risk of side effects. This test should be done within eight weeks after the beginning of treatment.

❑ For some forms of arthritis, drugs such as hydroxychloroquine (Plaquenil) and gold compound (Ridaura) may be prescribed.

❑ For some individuals, the ulcer drug sucralfate (Carafate) may give the same relief as aspirin and other anti-inflammatory drugs without damaging the stomach lining.

❑ Acetaminophen (sold as Tylenol, Datril, and others) may be a better medication for osteoarthritis than NSAIDs. In many cases, it may be able to relieve the pain of osteoarthritis as well as ibuprofen. Acetaminophen is relatively safe and inexpensive. However, it is important not to exceed the recommended dose of acetaminophen, and it should not be used by persons who consume alcohol. If taken in excessive amounts or in combination with alcohol, this drug can cause liver damage.

❑ Drugs do not always help everyone. Some people who use drugs obtain only partial relief.

❑ Kawasaki syndrome is an infectious disease that can cause symptoms of arthritis in children, accompanied by conjunctivitis; fever; a red rash on the body; a swollen, red tongue; and/or red or purplish-red discoloration and swelling of the palms of the hands and the soles of the feet. The cause of this disorder is not known. It primarily affects children under five years of age. Most children recover, but in some cases it causes permanent heart damage.

❑ Sjögren's (pronounced SHOW-grens) syndrome is a chronic illness that sometimes accompanies rheumatic diseases, including rheumatoid arthritis and lupus. It is characterized by changes in the immune system that result in the destruction of moisture-producing glands. The lack of moisture can affect many parts of the body, including the eyes, joints, lungs, mouth, and kidneys. Symptoms include coughing; dental cavities; difficulty chewing and/or swallowing; dry eyes, sometimes leading to damage to the cornea; dryness of the mouth, skin, throat, and all the mucous membranes; fatigue; hair loss; muscle weakness; and swollen salivary glands. Information on this condition may be obtained from the National Sjögren's Syndrome Association, P.O. Box 42207, Phoenix, AZ 85023, telephone 800–395–NSSA; or the Sjögren's Syndrome Foundation, 333 North Broadway, Suite 2000, Jericho, NY 11753, telephone 516–933–6365.

❑ Lyme disease can mimic arthritis, causing many of the same symptoms. (*See* LYME DISEASE in Part Two.)

❑ Systemic lupus erythematosus (SLE) is an autoimmune disease that often manifests itself as arthritis. For reasons unknown, the body produces antibodies that act against its own tissues. (*See* LUPUS in Part Two.)

❑ In its early stages, ulcerative colitis can cause symptoms like those of arthritis. Because this may occur before there are any abdominal symptoms, it can lead to misdiagnosis and delayed treatment. (*See* COLITIS in Part Two.)

❑ More information about arthritis is available from the Arthritis Foundation, telephone 800–283–7800.

❑ *See also* GOUT in Part Two and PAIN CONTROL in Part Three.

Asthma

Asthma is a lung disease that causes obstruction of the airways. During an asthma attack, spasms in the muscles surrounding the bronchi (small airways in the lungs) constrict, impeding the outward passage of stale air. Sufferers often describe this plight as "starving for air." Typical symptoms of an asthma attack are coughing, wheezing, a feeling of tightness in the chest, and difficulty in breathing.

The spasms that characterize the acute attack are not the cause of the disorder, but a result of chronic inflammation and hypersensitivity of the airways to certain stimuli. An attack may be triggered if a susceptible individual is exposed to an allergen or irritants. Common asthma-provoking allergens include animal dander, chemicals, drugs, dust mites, environmental pollutants, feathers, food additives such as sulfites, fumes, mold, and tobacco smoke, but any kind of allergen can precipitate an asthma attack in a susceptible individual. Other things that can bring on asthma attacks include adrenal disorders, anxiety, changes in temperature, exercise, extremes of dryness or humidity, fear, laughing, low blood sugar, and stress. A respiratory infection such as bronchitis may also be involved.

Whatever the particular instigator, it causes the bronchial tubes to swell and become plugged with mucus. This inflammation further irritates the airways, resulting in even greater sensitivity; the attacks become more frequent and the inflammation more severe.

Asthma specialists speculate that rising levels of environmental pollution lead to a higher incidence of asthma. Asthma epidemics related to atmospheric contamination—situations in which dust and chemical particulate matter are abundant, especially in enclosed environments—are well known. Occupational exposure to certain substances—chemicals such urethane and polyurethane, used in the adhesives and plastics industry; rubber epoxy resins from paint; welders' cloth cleaners; fumes in auto body shops; dry cleaning chemicals; and others—may also be a major risk factor. A predisposition to asthma may be hereditary.

In the last decade, the number of Americans with asthma has increased by one third. Today, asthma affects over 10 million people (3 million children and 7 million adults), or 4 percent of the U.S. population. Children under sixteen and adults over sixty-five are more likely than other people to suffer from asthma. Among children, the incidence of hospitalization for asthma has increased fivefold in the last twenty-nine years; the rate for adults has doubled.

Asthma can be difficult to diagnose conclusively. Its symptoms may resemble those of other diseases, including emphysema, bronchitis, and lower respiratory infections. To distinguish asthma from other conditions, a physician may recommend blood tests, chest x-rays, and spirometry (a procedure that measures air taken into and out of the lungs). With prompt diagnosis and appropriate treatment, serious danger from asthma should be preventable.

Cardiac asthma is a condition that causes the same symptoms as other types of asthma, but is caused by heart failure. Intrinsic asthma, a less common form of the disease, generally appears during adulthood, is often associated with other respiratory diseases such as bronchitis or sinusitis, and tends to appear during upper respiratory viral infections. People who suffer from intrinsic asthma are usually vulnerable to changes in weather, exercise, emotional stress, and other factors related to inner feelings.

NUTRIENTS

SUPPLEMENT	SUGGESTED DOSAGE	COMMENTS
Essential		
Quercitin-C from Ecological Formulas plus	500 mg 3 times daily.	Powerful immunostimulants. Quercetin-C has an antihistaminic effect. Also stabilizes cells to stop inflammation. Take these supplements together for best results.
bromelain	100 mg 3 times daily.	
or		
Activated Quercetin from Source Naturals	As directed on label.	Contains quercetin plus bromelain and vitamin C.
Flaxseed oil or primrose oil	1,000 mg twice daily, before meals.	Sources of essential fatty acids needed for production of anti-inflammatory prostaglandins.
Pantothenic acid (vitamin B5)	50 mg 3 times daily.	The anti-stress vitamin.
Vitamin A plus	15,000 IU daily. If you are pregnant, do not exceed 10,000 IU daily.	Needed for tissue repair and immunity.
natural beta-carotene or	10,000 IU daily.	An antioxidant and precursor of vitamin A.
carotenoid complex (Betatene)	As directed on label.	
Vitamin B complex plus extra	50 mg 4 times daily.	Stimulates the immune system.
vitamin B6 (pyridoxine) injections	½ cc weekly or as prescribed by physician.	Helpful in the treatment of allergies and asthma. Injections (under a doctor's supervision) are best.
or		
capsules plus	50 mg 3 times daily.	
vitamin B12	1,000 mcg twice daily, between meals.	Decreases inflammation that occurs in the lungs during an attack. Use a lozenge or sublingual form.
Vitamin E	600 IU and up daily.	A potent antioxidant.

Supplement	Suggested Dosage	Comments
Vitamin C with bioflavonoids	1,500 mg 3 times daily.	Needed to protect lung tissue and keep down infection. Also increases air flow and fights inflammation.
Very Important		
ClearLungs from Natural Alternatives		*See under* Herbs, below.
Coenzyme Q$_{10}$	100 mg daily.	Has the ability to counter histamine.
Magnesium plus calcium	750 mg daily. 1,500 mg daily.	May stop the acute asthmatic episode by increasing the vital capacity of the lungs. Has a dilating effect on the bronchial muscles. Use chelate or asporotate forms.
Multivitamin and mineral complex with selenium	200 mcg daily.	Necessary for enhanced immune function. Use a high-potency formula. A powerful destroyer of free radicals created from air pollutants.
Helpful		
Bee pollen	Start with a few granules at a time and slowly work up to 2 tsp daily.	Strengthens the immune system. Use raw crude pollen, preferably produced within 10 miles of your home. *Caution:* Bee pollen may cause an allergic reaction in some individuals. Discontinue use if a rash, wheezing, discomfort, or other symptom occurs.
Dimethylglycine (DMG) (Aangamik DMG from FoodScience Labs)	As directed on label twice daily.	Improves oxygenation in lung tissue.
Glucosamine sulfate or N-Acetylglucosamine (N-A-G from Source Naturals)	As directed on label. As directed on label.	Important for regulation of mucous secretions of the respiratory tract.
Kelp	2,000–3,000 mg daily for 21 days, then reduce to 1,000–1,500 mg daily.	For minerals in balanced amounts.
L-Cysteine and L-methionine	500 mg twice daily, on an empty stomach. Take with water or juice. Do not take with milk. Take with 50 mg vitamin B$_6$ and 100 mg vitamin C for better absorption. 500 mg twice daily, on an empty stomach.	Repairs lung tissue and reduces inflammation. *See* AMINO ACIDS in Part One. An important antioxidant.
Pycnogenol or grape seed extract	As directed on label. As directed on label.	Powerful antioxidants and anti-inflammatories.
Urban Air Defense from Source Naturals	2 tablets daily.	Contains many of the necessary nutrients listed in this table.
Vitamin D	600 IU daily.	Needed for repair of tissues.

HERBS

❑ Ginkgo biloba, an herb containing the active ingredient ginkgolide B, has shown good results in many studies.

❑ Lobelia extract is helpful during an asthma attack; it is a bronchial smooth muscle relaxant and expectorant.
   Caution: Do not take lobelia internally on an ongoing basis.

❑ ClearLungs from RidgeCrest Herbals is a Chinese herbal formula designed to reduce inflammation and mucus, opening up the airways to the lungs and promoting free breathing. Take 2 capsules twice daily.

❑ Mullein oil is said to be a powerful remedy for bronchial congestion. The oil stops coughs, unclogs bronchial tubes, and helps clear up asthma attacks. Users say that when they take it in tea or fruit juice, the effect is almost immediate.

❑ Pau d'arco acts as a natural antibiotic and reduces inflammation. Drink 3 cups of pau d'arco tea daily.

❑ Other herbs beneficial for asthma include echinacea, ephedra (ma huang), goldenseal, horsetail, juniper berries, licorice root, and slippery elm bark tablets.
   Caution: Do not use ephedra if you suffer from anxiety, glaucoma, heart disease, high blood pressure, or insomnia, or if you are taking a monoamine oxidase (MAO) inhibitor drug for depression. Do not take goldenseal on a daily basis for more than one week at a time and do not use it during pregnancy; if you have a history of cardiovascular disease, diabetes, or glaucoma, use it only under supervision. Do not use licorice on a daily basis for more than seven days in a row, and avoid it completely if you have high blood pressure.

RECOMMENDATIONS

❑ Eat a diet consisting primarily of fresh fruits and vegetables, nuts and seeds, oatmeal, brown rice, and whole grains. The diet should be relatively high in protein, low in carbohydrates, and contain no sugar. *See* HYPOGLYCEMIA in Part Two for suggestions.

❑ Include garlic and onions in your diet. These foods contain quercetin and mustard oils, which have been shown to inhibit an enzyme that aids in releasing inflammatory chemicals.

❑ Include "green drinks" in your program. Kyo-Green from Wakunaga is excellent. Take it three times a day, one-half hour before meals.

❑ Avoid gas-producing foods, such as beans, brassicas (broccoli, cauliflower, and cabbage) and large amounts of bran, or take an enzyme complex such as Be Sure from Wakunaga of America. Gas can irritate an asthmatic condition by putting pressure on the diaphragm.

❑ Do not eat ice cream or drink extremely cold liquids. Cold can shock the bronchial tubes into spasms.

❑ Use a juice fast, a fast using distilled water and lemon juice, or a combination of both for three days each month to help rid the body of toxins and mucus. *See* FASTING in Part Three.

❑ Try using bee propolis, which is soothing to the mucous membranes.

❑ Eat lightly—a large meal can cause shortness of breath by making the stomach put pressure on the diaphragm.

❑ Use an elimination diet to see if certain foods aggravate the asthmatic condition. Common culprits include alfalfa, corn, peanuts, soy, eggs, beets, carrots, colas, cold beverages (which may cause bronchial spasm), dairy products (including milk and ice cream), fish, red meat (especially pork), processed foods, salt, spinach, chicken and turkey, white flour, and white sugar. (See ALLERGIES in Part Two.)

❑ If you use aspirin or other nonsteroidal anti-inflammatory drugs (NSAIDs), do so with caution. Painkillers such as aspirin, ibuprofen (Advil, Nuprin, and others), naproxen (Naprosyn), and piroxicam (Feldene) account for over two thirds of drug-related asthmatic reactions, with aspirin causing over half of these. Chemotherapeutic agents and antibiotics also can induce asthma reactions.

❑ Use Urban Air Defense from Source Naturals two to three times daily. Also apply castor oil packs on the back and around the lung and kidney areas. To make a castor oil pack, place castor oil in a pan and heat but do not boil it. Dip a piece of cheesecloth or other white cotton material into the oil until the cloth is saturated. Apply the cloth to the affected area and cover it with a piece of plastic that is larger in size than the cotton cloth. Place a heating pad over the plastic and use it to keep the pack warm. Keep the pack in place for one-half to two hours, as needed.

❑ Practice methods to relieve stress. Stress and strong emotions like worry and fear can trigger an asthma attack. See STRESS in Part Two.

❑ Avoid furry animals; the food additives BHA and BHT; FD&C Yellow No. 5 food dye; tobacco and other types of smoke; and the amino acid tryptophan.

❑ If you suspect that dust mites are causing your asthma symptoms, try to get rid of the bugs. There are vacuum cleaners on the market that destroy these mites. An application of benzyl benzoate powder (such as X-MITE from Allersearch) will eliminate mites for two to three months. One pound of this powder treats approximately 150 square feet of carpeting or fabric. If local pharmacies don't carry the powder, you can order it from Aller-Guard Corporation of Ocean, New Jersey; telephone 800–234–0816.

CONSIDERATIONS

❑ People with asthma may be deficient in certain nutrients, such as vitamin B6 (pyridoxine), vitamin C, magnesium, manganese, and selenium, as well as in the enzyme glutathione peroxidase. People with asthma often have lower than normal levels of gastric hydrochloric acid, which is needed for proper digestion. Dr. Jonathan Wright, a noted nutritionist, claims excellent results using a combination of gastric acid replacement therapy (usually in the form of betaine hydrochloride) and supplementation with vitamin B6, vitamin B12, and magnesium for treatment of asthma.

❑ According to Nutrition Health Review, strong feelings of anger, anxiety, and depression may be an important cause of asthma attacks. Unfortunately, many of the drugs used to control and alleviate asthma themselves cause jittery nerves, mood swings, and insomnia.

❑ Many people with asthma are sensitive to food additives known as sulfites. Some people have had severe attacks after consuming foods containing sulfites. Many restaurants use sulfiting agents—including sodium bisulfite, potassium metabisulfite, potassium bisulfite, and sulfur dioxide—to prevent discoloration and bacterial growth in green salads, cut and sliced fruit, frozen shellfish, and other foods. Although most common in these foods, sulfites can be found in any type of food. (See Sulfite Allergies on page 113 for additional information.)

❑ Goose feathers may cause lung ailments.

❑ Beta-blocking medications, used to treat high blood pressure, can constrict the bronchial muscles and cause life-threatening problems for a person with asthma.

❑ Ozone, sulfur dioxide, nitrogen dioxide, cigarette smoke, carbon monoxide, hydrocarbons, nitrogen oxide, and photochemical substances are air pollutants that can trigger asthma attacks.

❑ Inhaling a muscle-relaxing medication such as albuterol (Proventil, Ventolin) from a bronchodilator can relieve an acute asthma attack immediately by opening the bronchial tubes. Bronchodilators do not treat the underlying problem, however.

❑ A sustained-release form of the drug theophylline, sold under the brand name Theo-Dur Sprinkle, has been used with good results. For children, this medication can be administered by opening a capsule and sprinkling the contents on a soft food such as applesauce.

❑ Researchers at Harvard and the U.S. Environmental Protection Agency (EPA) have shown that people with asthma who drink coffee and other caffeine-containing drinks generally have one-third fewer symptoms than those who do not. This is most likely due to the action of the caffeine, which has a dilating effect on the bronchial airways.

❑ A study reported in the Journal of Allergy and Clinical Immunology suggested that taking 2 salmon oil capsules before each meal and eating fish three times weekly may be beneficial for asthma.

❑ The Air Supply personal air purifier from Wein Products is a miniature unit that is worn around the neck. It sets up an invisible pure air shield against microorganisms (such as viruses, bacteria, and mold) and microparticles (including dust, pollen, and pollutants) in the air. It also eliminates vapors, smells, and harmful volatile compounds in the air. The Living Air XL-15 unit from Alpine Air of America is an ionizing unit that is good for purifying the air in the home or workplace.

❑ Regular exercise is beneficial, but exercise can also trigger an acute attack in some individuals. No one is sure why this is, but it has been speculated that inhaling lots of cool, dry air while working out aggravates the respiratory system. Running, for example, induces many more asthma attacks than swimming. One way to control exercise-induced asthma is to wear a mask that retains heat and moisture and limits the effects of breathing cold, dry air.

Atherosclerosis

See ARTERIOSCLEROSIS / ATHEROSCLEROSIS.

Athlete's Foot

Athlete's foot (tinea pedis) is a fungal infection that thrives in an environment of warmth and dampness. It is the most common fungal infection of the skin and affects about 4 percent of Americans, mostly men. The fungi live off the dead skin cells and calluses of the feet, especially on the skin between the toes. Symptoms include inflammation, burning, itching, scaling, cracking, and blisters.

The fungus that causes athlete's foot spreads rapidly when beneficial bacteria are destroyed by antibiotics, drugs, or radiation. It is especially prevalent and highly contagious in warm, damp places such as gyms and swimming pool locker rooms.

NUTRIENTS

SUPPLEMENT	SUGGESTED DOSAGE	COMMENTS
Essential		
Acidophilus	1 tsp in water twice daily, on an empty stomach.	Replenishes the "friendly" bacteria that inhibit pathogenic organisms. Use a nondairy formula.
Colloidal silver	Apply topically as directed on label.	A natural antibiotic and disinfectant. Destroys fungi, viruses, and bacteria. Promotes healing.
Very Important		
Garlic (Kyolic)	2 capsules 3 times daily.	Aids in destroying fungus.
Important		
Kyo-Dophilus from Wakunaga	As directed on label.	Contains acidophilus and aged garlic extract, both beneficial in treating fungal disease.
Vitamin B complex	As directed on label.	Needed for healthy skin. Use a yeast-free, high-potency formula. A sublingual form is best.
Vitamin C	3,000–10,000 mg 3 times daily, in divided doses.	Reduces stress and promotes immune function. Use a buffered form.
Zinc	50 mg daily. Do not exceed a total of 100 mg daily from all supplements.	Inhibits fungus and stimulates the immune system.

Helpful		
Aerobic 07 from Aerobic Life Industries	9 drops in a glass of water twice daily. Also apply a few drops directly on affected areas and let dry.	Supplies oxygen to the cells, which kills germs and harmful bacteria.
Essential fatty acids (fish oil from Omega-Life and Ultimate Oil from Nature's Secret are good sources)	As directed on label.	Promotes healing of skin disorders.
Vitamin A	50,000 IU daily for 1 month, then reduce to 25,000 IU. If you are pregnant, do not exceed 10,000 IU daily.	Needed for healing of tissues and to stimulate the immune system.
Vitamin E	Start with 400 IU daily and increase slowly to 1,000 IU daily.	An antioxidant that promotes healthy skin.

HERBS

❑ Drink 3 cups of pau d'arco tea daily. Pau d'arco tea can also be used topically. Prepare a strong pau d'arco tea, using 6 teabags to 2 quarts of warm water. Add 20 drops of Aerobic 07 from Aerobic Life Industries. Soak your feet in this mixture for fifteen minutes three times daily for quick relief.

❑ As an alternative footbath, add 20 drops of tea tree oil to a small tub of water, and use this to soak your feet for fifteen minutes three times daily. After soaking your feet, dry them thoroughly and dab a few drops of undiluted tea tree oil on the affected area. Tea tree oil is a powerful natural antifungal.

RECOMMENDATIONS

❑ Eat a balanced diet that includes plenty of raw fruits and vegetables, broiled fish, broiled skinless chicken, whole grains, and yogurt and other acidophilus-containing foods.

❑ Avoid cola drinks, processed foods, refined grains, and all forms of sugar. Do not eat fried or greasy foods.

❑ Take supplements of vitamins A, B, and C as outlined under Nutrients, above.

❑ Keep your feet dry. After bathing, dry carefully between your toes. Make sure to use each towel only once before laundering. Wear absorbent socks made of cotton. Air your shoes out and change socks daily. Wash socks, towels, and anything that comes into contact with the infected area in very hot water, with chlorine bleach added if possible.

❑ Cut raw garlic into tiny pieces and wear them in your shoes for a few days. The garlic will be absorbed into the skin. Also dust your feet with garlic powder. Though there are nonprescription antifungal drugs available, we believe garlic works better.

❑ Bathe your feet daily in a half-and-half mixture of vinegar and water. Dry them thoroughly and apply pure, unprocessed oil, such as olive oil, to the infected area. Or soak your feet in a solution of 2 teaspoons of salt in a pint of warm water for ten minutes. Repeat this treatment daily until the condition clears up.

❑ To ease pain and itching, use cold compresses. Soak a white cotton cloth in Burow's solution (available in drugstores) dissolved in 1 pint of cold water. Apply compresses several times a day for fifteen to twenty minutes at a time.

❑ Take care to protect your feet from direct contact with floors in communal areas such as locker rooms. Wear shoes or slippers in such places. Do not share shoes, socks, towels, or anything else that comes into contact with the feet.

❑ If the condition doesn't clear up in four weeks, if there is pus in the blisters or in the cracked skin, if a fever develops, or if there is swelling in the foot or leg, see your health care provider. Severe cases may require medical attention.

CONSIDERATIONS

❑ Athlete's foot can become complicated by a fungal toenail infection (*see* NAIL PROBLEMS in Part Two). Keep the toenails clean, but do not use a metal file that can damage the nail and give the fungus a place to grow. If the toenails become thick and discolored, see a podiatrist.

❑ Those with recurrent fungal infections of the feet often have a fungal infection in the groin area. Both areas must be treated simultaneously. To prevent transmission of the foot fungus to the groin area, put clean socks on before putting on your underwear when dressing.

❑ *See also* CANDIDIASIS and FUNGAL INFECTION in Part Two.

Attention Deficit Disorder

See HYPERACTIVITY.

Autism

Autism is a little-understood brain disorder that affects approximately 4 out of every 10,000 people. There are well over 100,000 autistic individuals in the United States. Autism is usually diagnosed in early childhood (before the age of three) and is characterized by a marked unresponsiveness to other people and to the surrounding environment. Physically, autistic individuals do not appear different from others, but they exhibit marked differences in behavior from a very early age. While most babies love to be held and cuddled, autistic infants appear indifferent to love and affection. As they grow older, they fail to form attachments to others in the way most children do, and instead seem to withdraw into themselves. Many autistic children also exhibit unpredictable and unusual behaviors that can range from constant rocking, to pounding their

feet while sitting, to sitting for long periods of time in total silence. Some experience bursts of hyperactivity that include biting and pounding on their bodies.

Autistic children have learning disabilities, and are often mentally disabled. Speech development is usually delayed, and in many cases is absent or limited to nonsensical rhyming or babbling. Some autistic children seem to have lower than normal intelligence, while others seem to fall into the normal range. Still others have low intelligence in most areas but almost supernatural abilities in others, such as mathematics or music. Most develop a strong resistance to any changes in familiar environments or routines.

The cause of autism is unknown. Studies comparing twins suggest that there may be a hereditary component to this disorder. Some experts believe that it is a result of some neurological imbalance or malfunction that renders the autistic individual painfully oversensitive to external stimuli. It is known that autism is not caused by parental neglect or actions, as was once believed.

Unless otherwise specified, the following recommended dosages are for persons over the age of eighteen. For a child between twelve and seventeen years old, reduce the dose to three-quarters the recommended amount. For a child between six and twelve, use one-half the recommended dose, and for a child under six years old, use one-quarter the recommended amount.

NUTRIENTS

SUPPLEMENT	SUGGESTED DOSAGE	COMMENTS
Very Important		
Calcium and	1,500 mg daily.	Essential for normal brain and nervous system function.
magnesium	1,000 mg daily.	
Choline	500–2,000 mg daily.	Improves brain function and circulation to the brain. Use under professional supervision.
Coenzyme Q$_{10}$	As directed on label.	Improves brain function.
Dimethylglycine (DMG) (Aangamik DMG from FoodScience Labs)	100 mg daily.	An oxygen carrier to the brain. Important for normal brain and nervous system function.
Ginkgo biloba		*See under* Herbs, below.
Vitamin B complex	50 mg 3 times daily, with meals.	Essential for normal brain and nervous system function. A sublingual form is recommended.
plus extra vitamin B$_3$ (niacin)	50 mg 3 times daily. Do not exceed this amount.	Improves circulation. Helpful for many psychological disorders. *Caution:* Do not take niacin if you have a liver disorder, gout, or high blood pressure.
and niacinamide and	300 mg daily.	Aids circulation.
pantothenic acid (vitamin B$_5$) and	500 mg daily.	Helps reduce stress.
vitamin B$_6$ (pyridoxine)	50 mg 3 times daily. Do not exceed this amount except at the direction of a physician.	Deficiencies have been linked to autism.

Vitamin C with bioflavonoids	5,000–20,000 mg daily, in divided doses. *See* ASCORBIC ACID FLUSH in Part Three.	A powerful free radical scavenger.
Helpful		
Multivitamin and mineral complex with	As directed on label.	All nutrients are needed in balance. Use a high-potency formula.
vitamin A	15,000 IU daily. If you are pregnant, do not exceed 10,000 IU daily.	
and natural beta-carotene	25,000 IU daily.	
and selenium	200 mcg daily.	
and zinc	50 mg daily. Do not exceed a total of 100 mg daily from all supplements.	
L-Glutamine and L-phenylalanine and L-tyrosine and taurine	500 mg each daily, on an empty stomach. Take with water or juice. Do not take with milk. Take with 50 mg vitamin B6 and 100 mg vitamin C for better absorption.	Amino acids needed for normal brain function. *See* AMINO ACIDS in Part One. *Caution:* Do not take phenylalanine if you are pregnant or nursing, or suffer from panic attacks, diabetes, high blood pressure, or PKU.
Melatonin	2–3 mg daily for adults, 1 mg or less daily for children, taken 2 hours or less before bedtime. If this is not effective, gradually increase the dosage until an effective level is reached.	Helpful if symptoms include insomnia.
RNA and DNA	200 mg daily. 100 mg daily.	To aid in repairing and building of new brain tissues. *Caution:* Do not take this supplement if you have gout.
Vitamin E	200–600 IU daily.	Improves circulation and brain function.

HERBS

❑ Ginkgo biloba is a powerful free radical destroyer that protects the brain. It also improves brain function by increasing circulation to the brain. Take it in capsule or extract form as directed on the product label, three times daily.

RECOMMENDATIONS

❑ Eat a high-fiber diet consisting of 50 to 75 percent raw foods, including large amounts of fruits and vegetables plus brown rice, lentils, and potatoes. For protein, eat beans and legumes, fish, raw nuts and seeds, skinless white turkey or white chicken breast, tofu, and low-fat yogurt.

❑ Eliminate alcohol, caffeine, canned and packaged foods, carbonated beverages, chocolate, all junk foods, refined and processed foods, salt, sugar, sweets, saturated fats, soft drinks, and white flour from the diet . Avoid foods that contain artificial colors or preservatives. Avoid fatty foods such as bacon, cold cuts, fried foods, gravies, ham, luncheon meats, sausage, and all dairy products except for low-fat soured products.

❑ Omit wheat and wheat products from the diet.

❑ Drink steam-distilled water.

❑ Get regular moderate exercise.

❑ Use an elimination diet to test for food allergies, which can aggravate the condition. *See* ALLERGIES in Part Two.

❑ Have a hair analysis done to rule out heavy metal poisoning. *See* HAIR ANALYSIS in Part Three.

❑ Try to improve blood oxygen supply to the brain with deep breathing exercises. Hold your breath for thirty seconds every half hour for a thirty-day period. This stimulates deeper breathing and helps to increase oxygen levels in the tissues of the brain.

❑ Do not go without food. Eating frequent small meals daily is better than eating two or three large meals.

CONSIDERATIONS

❑ Studies have shown that supplementation with vitamin B6 (pyridoxine) and magnesium can produce good results in autistic children and adults. In addition, there is often dramatic improvement after chemical additives and allergenic foods are eliminated from the diet.

❑ In studies of autistic children, a significant number have been found to have gastrointestinal disorders, including celiac disease and other food intolerances.

❑ Elevated serum and tissue copper levels may be a factor in autism and other mental problems, as may excessive exposure to lead and mercury. Excessive copper also seem to contribute to autism. Even low-level lead exposure in young children has been associated with impaired intellectual development and behavior problems.

❑ Infants and toddlers whose diets consist largely of processed baby foods need supplemental vitamins and minerals to ensure that all of their nutritional needs are met. Nutritional deficiencies are a factor in many psychological disorders.

❑ The prognosis for autistic children is difficult to predict. There have been documented cases of apparent recovery from autism, usually after adolescence. Some children seem to progress well only to inexplicably regress. Many become marginally self-sufficient and independent. However, most autistic individuals ultimately need lifelong care of some type.

❑ *See also* HYPOGLYCEMIA and HYPERACTIVITY in Part Two.

Backache

Nearly 80 percent of adults are affected by back pain at some point in their lives. It is one of the most common reasons for hospitalization in the United States. A variety of problems in the muscles, tendons, bones, ligaments, or an underlying organ, such as the kidneys, may cause backaches. Aches and pain in the lower back can be a chronic problem. Lumbago is a folk term for muscle pain in the lower back, near the pelvis.

For many years, it was assumed that back pain was usually the result of spinal degeneration or injury, especially damage to the intervertebral disks. These are structures located between the vertebrae that act as cushions. Each disk consists of a tough, fibrous outer layer surrounding a soft interior, which is what provides the cushioning. With the ordinary wear and tear of living, the disks show signs of aging and may be injured. When a disk begins to degenerate, a strain—even something as small as a sneeze—can cause the disk to rupture, or herniate, allowing the soft interior material to protrude out of the disk and press against the spinal cord. This situation is sometimes erroneously referred to as a "slipped disk." A herniated disk can indeed cause severe intermittent or constant back pain. However, it is difficult to pinpoint disk disease as the cause of most cases of back pain. That is because most adults past the age of forty—whether they experience back pain or not—can be shown to have some degree of disk degeneration. Further, in most instances, disk degeneration and even herniation do not produce any symptoms.

It is now believed that the leading cause of back pain is simple muscle strain. Although symptoms may come on suddenly and can be acutely painful, this is actually a problem that develops over a long period of time. When muscles contract, lactic acid and pyruvic acid are produced as byproducts of muscular activity. It is the presence of lactic acid in the muscles that produces the familiar sensation of muscle fatigue following strenuous activity. If high levels of these acidic byproducts accumulate in the muscles, they cause irritation that can eventually turn into pain and interfere with the normal conduction of electrical impulses in the muscle tissue. This results in a phenomenon called *delayed-onset muscle soreness* (DOMS). Problems with acidic buildup are often made worse by dehydration.

Most cases of back pain also have an important psychological component, usually a deep-seated emotional or stress-related problem. Other contributors to back pain can include poor posture, improper footwear and walking habits, improper lifting, straining, calcium deficiency, slouching when sitting, and sleeping on a mattress that is too soft. Kidney, bladder, and prostate problems, female pelvic disorders, and even constipation may produce back pain. Chronic conditions that can cause back pain include arthritis, rheumatism, bone disease, and abnormal curvature of the spine. Fractures are rarely the cause of back pain.

NUTRIENTS

SUPPLEMENT	SUGGESTED DOSAGE	COMMENTS
Very Important		
DL-Phenylalanine (DLPA)	Take daily every other week, as directed on label.	Helps to alleviate pain. *Caution:* Do not take this supplement if you are pregnant or nursing, or suffer from panic attacks, diabetes, high blood pressure, or PKU.
Calcium	1,500–2,000 mg daily.	Needed for strong bones. To assure absorption, use a mixture of 3 different forms: calcium carbonate, calcium chelate, and calcium asporotate.
and magnesium and	700–1,000 mg daily.	Works with calcium. Use magnesium chelate form.
vitamin D	400 IU daily.	Aids absorption of calcium and magnesium.
Multivitamin and mineral complex with		To supply a balance of nutrients important in formation and metabolism of bone and connective tissue and needed for healing.
vitamin A	15,000 IU daily. If you are pregnant, do not exceed 10,000 IU daily.	
and natural beta-carotene	15,000 IU daily.	
and vitamin E	400–800 IU daily.	
Silica or horsetail	3 times daily, as directed on label.	Supplies silicon, which improves calcium uptake. *See under* Herbs, below.
Vitamin B12	2,000 mg daily.	Aids in calcium absorption and digestion. Use a lozenge or sublingual form.
Zinc	50 mg daily. Do not exceed a total of 100 mg daily from all supplements.	Required for protein synthesis and collagen formation. Promotes a healthy immune system.
plus copper	3 mg daily.	Works in balance with zinc and vitamin C to form elastin, and is needed for healthy nerves.
Important		
Boron	3 mg daily. Do not exceed this amount.	Improves calcium uptake. Take boron only until healed, unless you are over age 50.
Free-form amino acid complex	As directed on label.	Essential in bone and tissue repair.
L-Proline	500 mg daily, on an empty stomach. Take with water or juice. Do not take with milk. Take with 50 mg vitamin B6 and 100 mg vitamin C for better absorption.	Heals cartilage and strengthens muscles and tissues. *See* AMINO ACIDS in Part One.
Manganese	2–5 mg daily. Take separately from calcium.	Aids in healing cartilage and tissue in the neck and back. Use manganese gluconate form.
Helpful		
Essential fatty acids (flaxseed oil is a good source)	As directed on label. Take with meals.	Needed for repair and flexibility of muscles.
GlucosaMend from Source Naturals	As directed on label.	To supply glucosamine, an important component of many body tissues, including bones and connective tissue.
Multienzyme complex with bromelain and pancreatin	As directed on label. Take with meals.	To aid digestion and relieve muscle tension and inflammation.
Vitamin B complex	As directed on label 3 times daily.	Needed for repair and to relieve stress in the back muscles. Use a high-stress formula high in vitamin B6 (pyridoxine) and vitamin B12.

Vitamin C with bioflavonoids	3,000–10,000 mg daily.	Essential for formation of collagen, which holds the tissues together. Needed for repair of tissues. Relieves tension in the back area.

HERBS

❑ Arth-X from Trace Minerals Research is a formula containing herbs, sea minerals, calcium, and other nutrients for the bones and joints.

❑ Horsetail is a good source of silica, which is necessary for bones and connective tissue.

❑ Other herbs recommended for backache include alfalfa, burdock, oat straw, slippery elm, and white willow bark. They can be taken in capsule, extract, or tea form.

RECOMMENDATIONS

❑ Avoid all meats and animal protein products until you are healed. Animal foods contain uric acid, which puts undue strain on the kidneys that can contribute to back pain. Eat no gravies, oils, fats, sugar, or rich or highly processed foods.

❑ Follow a fasting program. See FASTING in Part Three.

❑ When pain hits, immediately drink two large glasses of quality water. This often gives relief within minutes. Muscle aches and back pain are frequently connected to dehydration. The body needs a minimum of eight 8-ounce glasses of water daily to keep acidic wastes from building up in muscles and other tissues.

❑ If pain follows an injury or sudden movement, apply ice for the first forty-eight hours, then apply heat. Rest on a firm bed. When getting up, roll to your side, draw your knees up, push up to a sitting position, and stand by pushing up with your legs.

❑ To relieve back muscle pain, soak in a very warm bath or apply a heating pad directly to your back.

❑ Once the acute pain has subsided, doing exercises to strengthen the abdominal muscles may help to prevent recurrences; these muscles help to support the back. Sit-ups are good for this purpose. Always do sit-ups with your knees bent, not with your legs flat on the floor.

❑ When sitting, keep your knees a little higher than your hips and keep your feet flat on the floor.

❑ When carrying things on your shoulder, switch the weight to the other side from time to time. Carrying heavy shoulder bags may produce neck, back, and shoulder pain.

❑ Learn to recognize and reduce stress. Relaxation techniques can be very helpful.

❑ Always push large objects; never pull them.

❑ Wear comfortable, well-made shoes. The higher the heels of your shoes, the greater the risk of backache.

❑ Move around. Do not sit in the same position for long periods of time.

❑ Never lean forward without bending your knees. Lift with your legs, arms, and abdomen—not with the muscles of the small of your back. Avoid lifting anything heavier than twenty pounds. If you must work close to the ground, squat down so that you avoid bending at the waist.

❑ Do not sleep on your stomach with your head raised on a pillow. Instead, rest your back by lying on your side with your legs bent, so that your knees are about an inch higher than your hips. Sleep on a firm mattress with your head supported on a pillow. If your mattress is not firm enough, place a board between the box spring and the mattress.

❑ Maintain a healthy weight and get regular moderate exercise. A lack of exercise can cause back pain. Activities that are good for the back include swimming, cycling, walking, and rowing. *Avoid* the following activities:

• *Baseball, basketball, football.* The quick responses needed for these sports involve sudden twisting and jumping motions.

• *Bowling.* Lifting a heavy weight while bending and twisting puts strain on the back.

• *Golf.* The twisting motion involved in the swing, and the body's tendency to bend forward at the waist, are stressful to the lower back.

• *Tennis.* Playing tennis puts strain on the back due to the quick "stop-and-go action of the game.

• *Weightlifting.* This sport is potentially the most damaging because it places great strain on the lower portion of the spine and back.

❑ If pain lasts longer than seventy-two hours, if the pain radiates into the legs, or if other symptoms such as unexplained weight loss occur, consult your health care provider. If your backaches are chronic, look for a physician who specializes in backs—and who does not rush to recommend surgery.

❑ If you have pain in one side of the small of your back, feel sick, and have a fever, see your physician immediately. You may have a kidney infection.

❑ If pain follows an injury and is accompanied by sudden loss of bladder or bowel control, if you have difficulty moving any limb, or if you feel numbness, pain, or tingling in a limb, do not move, but call for medical help immediately. You may have hurt your spinal cord.

CONSIDERATIONS

❑ People seeking professional advice about back pain face a bewildering array of generalists and specialists to choose from. Complex back problems are rapidly becoming a subspecialty. True specialists now focus on people with back problems only. For treatment of back pain, you can consult any of the following types of practitioners:

• *Chiropractors* are licensed to perform spinal manipulation and may recommend nutritional and/or lifestyle changes. They primarily use high-velocity manipulations of the neck and back to correct problems. According to a 1994 report issued by the U.S. Agency for Health Care Policy and Research, spinal manipulation may be the most effective treatment for acute back pain. Chiropractors are not medical doctors, and therefore cannot prescribe drugs or perform surgery. A good chiropractor should be willing to recommend a medical doctor if necessary.

• *Massage therapists* work with muscles and tendons, using different techniques like muscle kneading and compression to lessen tension in the muscles. This increases circulation and helps the body flush out cellular debris, which speeds tissue repair and aids in healing back problems.

• *Orthopedic surgeons* are medical doctors who prescribe medication (painkillers, muscle relaxers, anti-inflammatory drugs), bed rest, and physical therapy for some cases of back pain. Since these doctors can perform surgery, they may be more likely to recommend it than other practitioners.

• *Osteopaths* can prescribe drugs and perform surgery, but because of their philosophy of treatment, they often try manipulation or physical therapy first.

• *Physiatrists*, also known as doctors of physical rehabilitation medicine, are medical doctors who treat back pain by the use of various physical therapies, lifestyle changes, and back braces, which promote healing by reducing the load on the spine. Physiatrists are not licensed to perform surgery, and are less likely than other M.D.s to hospitalize their patients. They have a good record for treating back problems, including low back pain and herniated disks.

• *Physical therapists* specialize in improving joint and spine mobility and muscle strength. They are not medical doctors, and are strictly limited to physical therapy.

❑ With signs of rapidly progressive nerve damage (increasing weakness in a leg, or loss of bladder or bowel function), back surgery moves high on the list of options. It must also be considered when pain is unremitting or getting worse. Surgery always entails a degree of risk; there is always the chance of permanent damage and impaired mobility. According to U.S. government data, only 1 percent of those who suffer from back pain appear to benefit from surgery. Back surgery is useful only for problems in four broad categories:

1. Disk displacement (a protruded or "slipped" disk).
2. Painful (and abnormal) motion of one vertebra in relation to another.
3. Narrowing of the spine around the spinal cord itself from overgrowth of bone (spinal stenosis).
4. Some cases in which misalignment of one vertebra with another (spondylolisthesis) leads to pain.

❑ X-rays are often considered a routine part of back pain diagnosis, yet only a few back conditions show up on x-rays. If the pain is caused by muscle strain or a herniated disk, an x-ray will do little to aid the diagnosis, since disks, muscles, and ligaments are all soft tissues. X-ray exposure bears special hazards for pregnant women.

❑ With the new imaging procedures such as computerized tomography (CT) and magnetic resonance imaging (MRI), disks can be seen. However, Dr. Richard A. Deyo, a professor of medicine and health services at the University of Washington School of Medicine and School of Public Health, notes that 20 to 30 percent of people with back pain have herniated disks that are not the source of their discomfort. If these disks show up during imaging procedures, a person may end up having surgery for a condition that, while present, is not really the cause of his or her pain.

❑ If pain comes after lifting something heavy, after coughing, or after unusually heavy exercise, and the pain prevents you from moving or shoots down one leg, you may have a herniated disk.

❑ Epidemiological studies in the United States, as well as studies of smoking and nonsmoking pairs of twins in Scandinavia, have shown that smoking aggravates problems in the disks.

❑ Numerous studies have shown that people with lower back pain who are treated at chiropractic clinics recover faster, and at less cost, and end up with less pain and more mobility than those treated in hospitals.

❑ *See also under* PREGNANCY-RELATED PROBLEMS in Part Two.

❑ *See also* PAIN CONTROL in Part Three.

Bad Breath

See HALITOSIS.

Baldness

See HAIR LOSS.

Bedsores

Bedsores, also known as pressure sores, are deep ulcers that form when pressure is exerted over bony areas of the body, restricting circulation and leading to the death of cells in the overlying tissue. They are most commonly found on the heels, buttocks, hips, sacrum, and shoulder blades. As their name implies, they tend to occur during periods of prolonged bed rest. However, wheelchair users also may develop bedsores. People who suffer from bedsores are usually seriously deficient in many nutrients, especially zinc and vitamins A, E, B_2 (riboflavin), and C, and often have a high bodily pH.

NUTRIENTS

SUPPLEMENT	SUGGESTED DOSAGE	COMMENTS
Very Important		
Vitamin E	400 IU daily and up.	Improves circulation.
Zinc	50–80 mg daily. Do not exceed a total of 100 mg daily from all supplements.	Important in healing of tissues.
plus copper	3 mg daily.	Needed to balance with zinc.
Important		
Free-form amino acid complex	As directed on label.	To supply protein needed for healing.
Natural beta-carotene or	15,000 IU daily.	Protects the lungs, improving breathing. Repairs bedsores by improving skin tissue.
carotenoid complex	As directed on label.	
Vitamin B complex plus extra vitamin B$_{12}$	100 mg twice daily, with meals. 2,000 mcg twice daily.	Needed to reduce stress and for healing. Use a lozenge or sublingual form.
Vitamin C	3,000–10,000 mg daily, in divided doses.	Aids in healing, improves circulation, and enhances immune function.
Vitamin D	400–1,000 IU daily.	Essential for healing. Lack of exposure to sunshine increases the need for this nutrient.
Helpful		
All-Purpose Bactericide Spray from Aerobic Life Industries or	Apply topically to irritated areas as directed on label.	Destroys harmful bacteria.
colloidal silver	Apply topically as directed on label.	A natural antibiotic. Destroys bacteria, viruses, and fungi. Protects against infection and promotes healing.
Calcium and	2,000 mg daily.	Needed for the central nervous system and to keep bones from softening through disuse.
magnesium	1,000 mg daily.	
Garlic (Kyolic)	2 capsules 3 times daily, with meals.	Has a natural antibiotic effect; protects against infection.
Kelp	500–1,000 mg daily.	Provides necessary minerals.
Panoderm I from American Biologics	Apply topically as directed on label.	A natural antioxidant skin moisturizer and cleanser that contains squalene.
Vitamin A	50,000 IU daily for 1 month, then reduce to 15,000 IU daily. If you are pregnant, do not exceed 10,000 IU daily.	Needed for healing of skin tissue. Use emulsion form for easier assimilation.

HERBS

❑ Comfrey ointment or Natureworks Marigold Ointment from Abkit can be used externally.

Note: Comfrey is recommended for external use only.

❑ Goldenseal, myrrh gum, pau d'arco, and suma, taken in tea or extract form, are beneficial for bedsores. Buckwheat tea and lime flower tea are also helpful.

Caution: Do not take goldenseal for more than one week at a

time; do not use it during pregnancy; and use it under supervision if you have heart disease, diabetes, or glaucoma.

❑ Mix equal amounts of goldenseal powder or extract and vitamin E oil with a small amount of honey to make paste, and apply the mixture to the sores often. This mixture gives fast relief and helps the healing process. Alternate this with raw honey, vitamin E cream, and aloe vera gel.

RECOMMENDATIONS

❑ Eat a well-balanced diet with 70 percent raw fruits and vegetables.

❑ Consume liquids around the clock, even if you are not thirsty. Use steam-distilled water, herbal teas, and sugar-free juices. Liquids are important in keeping the colon clean and the bladder functioning properly.

❑ Eliminate animal fats, fried foods, junk foods, processed foods, and sugar from the diet.

❑ Use oat bran, psyllium husks, ground flaxseeds, or Aerobic Bulk Cleanse (ABC) from Aerobic Life Industries to provide fiber. Fiber absorbs dangerous toxins and helps prevent constipation.

Note: Always take supplemental fiber separately from other supplements and medications.

❑ Make sure that the bowels move every day. On days when the bowels do not move, use an enema. *See* ENEMAS in Part Three.

❑ Give immediate attention to lowering the body's pH level, to 5.5 or lower, to prevent bacteria in the sores from multiplying. Place 2 to 3 teaspoons of apple cider vinegar in glass of water, add a little honey, and sip this with meals. *See* ALKALOSIS in Part Two for additional suggestions.

❑ Try applying essential oils and/or aloe vera with a little tea tree oil added to the affected area. This is very good for the skin, and helps existing bedsores to heal as well as preventing new ones from forming. (Keep these oils away from the eyes, however, because they burn.)

❑ Take measures to prevent bedsores from developing:

• Do not let an immobilized individual stay in one position for too long—move him or her to alternate positions every two hours.

• Keep the skin dry; include thorough drying after bathing.

• Inspect pressure points daily for reddening or other signs that a sore may be developing.

• If the person can sit up, have him or her do so three to four times daily, or use pillows as a prop.

• Give a sponge bath daily using warm water and a mild herbal or vitamin E soap. Do not use harsh soaps.

• Gently but firmly massage pressure points and other affected areas once daily to increase circulation.

• Give frequent alcohol rubs to stimulate circulation and prevent blood vessels from closing up. Use isopropyl (rubbing) alcohol and cotton balls or sterile gauze to apply the alcohol. As an alternative, witch hazel can be used instead.

• Allow as much light and fresh air into the bedridden person's room as he or she can tolerate.

• Have the individual wear loose-fitting clothing made from all-natural materials. Cotton is best because it allows air to penetrate to the skin. Pay attention to clothing construction as well. Avoid items with seams, gathers, or other features that may press on sensitive areas.

• Keep the bed clean, dry, and tidy. Lying on wrinkled bed linens can lead to bedsores.

CONSIDERATIONS

❑ People who suffer from bedsores are usually seriously deficient in many nutrients, especially zinc and vitamins A, E, B2 (riboflavin), and C. Vitamins A and E are useful in healing bedsores.

❑ There is a special mattress designed for people who are bedridden. It has pockets of air connected by small tubes. When placed between the sheet and the standard mattress, it decreases the pressure on sensitive areas when a person has to lie in one position for long periods of time.

❑ Dimethylsulfoxide (DMSO) is helpful for promoting healing. It is applied topically directly to the affected area.

Note: Only DMSO from a health food store should be used for therapeutic purposes. Commercial-grade DMSO found in hardware stores is not suitable. The use of DMSO may result in a garlicky body odor. This is temporary, and is not a cause for concern.

Bed-Wetting

Bed-wetting, known in the medical community as *enuresis*, is the act of urinating in bed habitually and, especially, involuntarily. Bed-wetting is common in early childhood. It also occurs sometimes in early adulthood and frequently among the aging. The causes are often unknown. The most popular theories center on the roles of behavioral disturbances, very sound sleeping, the consumption of too much liquid before bedtime, dreaming about using the rest room, food allergies, heredity, stress, nutritional deficiencies, and psychological problems (one of the most common factors in young adults).

In children under the age of five or so, the most common cause of bed-wetting is simply the size of the bladder; it is often too small to hold enough urine to last through the night every single night. This type of bed-wetting is usually outgrown. Occasional bed-wetting by older children usually stops spontaneously by the teenage years. An underlying illness such as a urinary tract infection or diabetes may also result in bed-wetting.

Unless otherwise specified, the following recommended doses are for persons over the age of eighteen. For a child between twelve and seventeen years old, reduce the dose to three-quarters the recommended amount. For a child between six and twelve, use one-half the recommended dose, and for a child under six years old, use one-quarter the recommended amount.

NUTRIENTS

SUPPLEMENT	SUGGESTED DOSAGE	COMMENTS
Very Important		
Free-form amino acid complex	As directed on label.	Helps to strengthen bladder muscle. Use a product made from a vegetable source.
Important		
Calcium and magnesium	1,500 mg daily. 350 mg daily.	To aid in controlling bladder spasms.
Helpful		
Multivitamin and mineral complex with vitamin B complex	As directed on label.	Aids in relieving stress and supplies all needed nutrients.
Potassium	99 mg daily.	Aids in balancing sodium and potassium in the body.
Vitamin A or cod liver oil and vitamin E	As directed on label. If you are pregnant, do not exceed 10,000 IU daily. As directed on label. 600 IU daily.	To aid in normalizing bladder muscle function.
Zinc	10 mg daily for children; 80 mg daily for adults. Do not exceed these amounts.	For improved bladder function. Also enhances the immune system.

HERBS

❑ For bed-wetting, try using buchu, corn silk, oat straw, parsley, and/or plantain. Take these herbs before 3:00 p.m.

RECOMMENDATIONS

❑ Consume more foods that are high in vitamin B2 (riboflavin) and pantothenic acid (vitamin B5), including bee pollen, brewer's yeast, soaked nuts, spirulina, and all kinds of sprouts.

Caution: Both bee pollen and brewer's yeast can cause an allergic reaction in some individuals. Start with a small amount at first, and discontinue use if any allergic symptoms occur.

❑ Do not drink liquids within thirty minutes of bedtime.

❑ See your health care provider for food allergy testing. Bed-wetting is often caused by food allergies. Omit cow's milk, which is highly allergenic, from your diet. Also eliminate from the diet carbonated beverages, chocolate, refined carbohydrates (including junk food), and products containing food coloring.

□ Do not spank or scold a child for bed-wetting. This only complicates the problem. Instead, give rewards for *not* wetting the bed.

CONSIDERATIONS

□ We know of several cases of bed-wetting (among children and adults) that were relieved within a matter of days when supplements of certain nutrients were supplied. Among these were magnesium, vitamin B$_2$, and pantothenic acid. In addition, all allergy-causing foods were removed from the diet, and a protein supplement was added. Spirulina, brewer's yeast, and bee pollen are all excellent sources of protein.

□ Supplemental magnesium is especially helpful for certain people. Magnesium citrate is one of the better forms to use, since the body can readily assimilate it.

□ Behavior modification techniques have proved useful in some cases, especially with children. One technique involves the use of an alarm that goes off as soon as the individual starts to wet the bed. Over time, this is believed to help a child respond to the body's cues and wake up when he or she needs to urinate during the night.

Bee Sting

There are a number of common stinging insects in the United States. While not all of them are bees—certain hornets, yellow jackets, wasps, spiders, and ants can also inflict stings—stings are most commonly associated with bees.

When an insect stings, it injects venom through its stinger into the victim. Bees generally leave their stingers behind at the sting site; wasps most often do not. Usually, a stinging insect attacks because it is trying to protect itself from danger or what it perceives as its territory from invasion. This is why a person who stumbles on a beehive may end up receiving multiple stings from the hive's residents.

Most stings cause localized swelling, redness, and acute pain that may feel throbbing and/or burning, a reaction to the insect's venom. However, some people are highly allergic to insect venom, and if they are stung, a very severe reaction can occur. Symptoms of such a reaction can include difficulty swallowing, hoarseness, labored breathing, weakness, confusion, severe swelling, and a feeling of impending disaster. A more severe reaction can result in closing of the airway and/or shock.

Unless otherwise indicated, the following recommended dosages are for persons over the age of eighteen. For a child between twelve and seventeen years old, reduce the dose to three-quarters the recommended amount. For a child between six and twelve, use one-half the recommended dose, and for a child under six years old, use one-quarter the recommended amount.

NUTRIENTS

SUPPLEMENT	SUGGESTED DOSAGE	COMMENTS
Helpful		
Calcium	1,500 mg daily.	Helps relieve pain. Use calcium gluconate form.
Pantothenic acid (vitamin B$_5$)	500 mg daily.	Acts to inhibit allergic reponse.
Vitamin C with bioflavonoids	10,000 mg within the first hour. Then 5,000–25,000 mg daily in divided doses. *See* ASCORBIC ACID FLUSH in Part Three.	Protects the body from allergens and moderates the inflammatory response.
Vitamin E	Cut open a capsule or use vitamin E oil and apply topically to the sting site.	Aids in healing.

HERBS

□ Poultices made from comfrey, slippery elm, and white oak bark and leaves ease pain and promote healing. Also good are lobelia poultices and plantain poultices or salve.
Note: Comfrey is recommended for external use only.

□ Take echinacea and/or goldenseal in tea or capsule form to boost immune function. Goldenseal is a natural antibiotic.

□ Drink as much yellow dock tea as you can, or take 2 capsules of yellow dock every hour until symptoms are relieved.

RECOMMENDATIONS

□ If you are stung, *immediately and carefully* remove any stinger left in the skin. Do not pull out the stinger with your fingers or tweezers. Instead, gently scrape it out. A sterilized knife is best for this purpose, but you can use your fingernail or the edge of a credit card if nothing else is available. Take care not to squeeze the stinger or the attached venom sac, as this may inject more poison into the skin. Then wash the area and rinse thoroughly. If you have ever had an allergic reaction to a sting in the past, seek emergency medical attention *immediately*. Life-threatening allergic reactions can come on suddenly and progress very quickly, so you do not want to waste time. If you have no history of insect allergy, no medical treatment is needed, but do remain alert for symptoms of a developing allergic reaction. Reactions can occur within minutes or hours, and they can happen the first time or the thousandth time you are stung by a bee. If you notice any allergic symptoms, or if you are not sure, seek professional attention.

□ Once any stinger has been removed and the area cleansed, try one or more of the following home remedies to ease pain and swelling:

• Make a paste by adding a bit of cool water to baking soda, a crushed aspirin, or a crushed papaya enzyme tablet, and apply the mixture to the sting. If none of these items is available, a bit of meat tenderizer containing the enzyme papain may be substituted.

• Open a charcoal capsule or crush a charcoal tablet and place it on a cotton ball. Place the cotton ball on the affected area and cover it with an adhesive bandage.

• Apply a cold pack or an ice cube directly on the sting.

• Place a drop of plain ammonia on the site of the sting.

CONSIDERATIONS

❑ Anyone who has had an allergic reaction to an insect sting should keep an emergency insect sting kit containing epinephrine, such as EpiPen, available at all times. These kits are available by prescription only.

❑ A venom extractor called Lil Sucker fits inside a pocket or purse. If you get stung, it produces a vacuum that sucks the venom out within two minutes. The end of the extractor can also be used to remove a honeybee stinger. For more information on this, call International Reforestation Suppliers at 800–321–1037.

❑ Taking large doses of vitamin C has been known to reduce the severity of bee stings.

❑ To avoid bee stings, wear plain, light-colored clothing. Also avoid wearing clothing that is flowered or dark-colored; perfume, suntan lotion, hair spray, or anything scented; shiny jewelry; and open sandals or loose-fitting clothes.

❑ When a yellow jacket is squashed, its body releases a chemical that causes other yellow jackets in the area to attack. It is better to leave the area than to swat at these insects.

❑ *See also* INSECT ALLERGY and INSECT BITE in Part Two.

Benign Prostatic Hypertrophy

See under PROSTATITIS / ENLARGED PROSTATE.

Beriberi

Beriberi is a disease caused by a deficiency of the B vitamins, particularly vitamin B_1 (thiamine). This disease occurs mainly in the Far East, where the diet consists principally of polished rice, which does not supply sufficient thiamine. Cases of beriberi that occur in the United States are usually associated with alcoholism, hypothyroidism, infections, pregnancy, and/or stress.

Symptoms of beriberi in children can include impaired growth, muscle wasting, mental confusion, convulsions, gastrointestinal problems, nausea, vomiting, constipation, and diarrhea. In adults, the symptoms are diarrhea, edema, fatigue, and weight loss, as well as heart failure and nerve damage that can lead to paralysis.

NUTRIENTS

SUPPLEMENT	SUGGESTED DOSAGE	COMMENTS
Important		
Multivitamin and mineral complex	As directed on label.	For essential balanced vitamins and minerals.
Vitamin B complex	100 mg daily.	B vitamins work best when taken together. A sublingual form is recommended. Injections (under a doctor's supervision) may be necessary.
plus extra vitamin B_1 (thiamine)	50 mg 3 times daily.	To counteract deficiency.
Helpful		
Brewer's yeast	Start with 1 tsp twice weekly and slowly increase to 1 tbsp twice weekly.	Supplies the B vitamins.
Vitamin C	2,000–5,000 mg daily, in divided doses.	Important for immune function, improved circulation, and healing. Needed for proper uptake of the B vitamins.

RECOMMENDATIONS

❑ Include brown rice, legumes, raw fruits and vegetables, seeds and nuts, whole grains, and yogurt in your daily diet. These foods are rich in B vitamins, particularly thiamine.

❑ Do not drink liquids with meals. This dilutes digestive juices and leads to many of the B vitamins being washed away.

Bite

See BEE STING; DOG BITE; INSECT ALLERGY; SNAKEBITE; SPIDER BITE.

Bitot's Spots

See under EYE PROBLEMS.

Bladder Infection (Cystitis)

Infection of the bladder, usually caused by some type of bacteria, results in cystitis, an inflammation of the bladder. Nearly 85 percent of urinary tract infections are caused by *Escherichia coli*, a bacterium that is normally found in the intestines. Chlamydia may also cause bladder problems. In women, bacteria introduced by means of fecal contamination or from vaginal secretions can gain access to the bladder by traveling up through the urethra. Cystitis occurs much more frequently in women than in men because of the close proximity of the anus, vagina, and urethra in females, and also because of the short length of the female urethra. This allows for relatively easy transmission of bacteria from the anus to the vagina and urethra, and thus to the bladder. In males, bacteria can reach the bladder either by ascending through the urethra or by migrating from an infected prostate gland. While bladder infections are relatively common in women, bladder infections in men may signal a more serious problem, such as prostatitis.

Bladder infections are characterized by an urgent desire to empty the bladder. Urination is typically frequent and painful; even after the bladder has been emptied, there may be a desire to urinate again. The urine often has a strong, unpleasant odor, and may appear cloudy. Children suffering from bladder infections often complain of lower abdominal pain and a painful burning sensation while urinating. There may be blood in the urine. While cystitis itself is usually more of an annoyance than a serious health problem, it can lead to kidney infection if left untreated.

The possibility of developing a bladder infection can be increased by many factors, including pregnancy, sexual intercourse, the use of a diaphragm, and systemic disorders such as diabetes. The risk of cystitis is also increased if there is a structural abnormality or obstruction of the urinary tract resulting in restriction of the free flow of urine, or if past infections have resulted in a narrowing of the urethra.

URINARY TRACT INFECTION SELF-TEST

A home testing kit is available to help determine if you have a urinary infection. Ames N-Multistix reagent strips, manufactured by Miles Inc. Diagnostics Division of Elkhart, Indiana, are available in drugstores.

NUTRIENTS

SUPPLEMENT	SUGGESTED DOSAGE	COMMENTS
Very Important		
Cranberry		*See under* Herbs, below.
Colloidal silver	As directed on label.	A natural antibiotic. Destroys bacteria, viruses, and fungi. Promotes healing.
Garlic (Kyolic)	2 capsules 3 times daily.	A natural antibiotic and immune enhancer.
SP-6 Cornsilk Blend from Solaray or KB formula from Nature's Way		*See under* Herbs, below.
Vitamin C plus bioflavonoids	4,000–5,000 mg daily, in divided doses. 1,000 mg daily.	Produces antibacterial effect through acidification of urine. Important in immune function.
Important		
Acidophilus	As directed on label. Take on an empty stomach. Also use 1 tbsp in 1 qt warm water as a douche.	Needed to restore "friendly" bacteria. Especially important if antibiotics are prescribed.
Calcium and magnesium	1,500 mg daily. 750–1,000 mg daily.	Reduces bladder irritability. Aids in the stress response and works best when balanced with calcium. Use magnesium chelate form.
Dioxychlor from American Biologics	10 drops twice daily. Also use 30 drops in 1 qt warm water as a douche.	An important antibacterial, antifungal, and antiviral agent.
Multivitamin and mineral complex with vitamin A and natural beta-carotene	10,000 IU daily. 15,000 IU daily.	Needed for essential balanced vitamins and minerals. Use a high-potency, hypoallergenic form.
N-Acetylcysteine	500 mg twice daily, on an empty stomach.	A potent detoxifier that neutralizes free radicals.
Potassium	99 mg daily.	Replaces potassium lost as a result of frequent urination.
Vitamin B complex	50–100 mg twice daily, with meals.	Necessary for proper digestion. High doses are necessary if antibiotics are used.
Vitamin E	600 IU daily.	Combats infecting bacteria.
Zinc plus copper	50 mg daily. Do not exceed a total of 100 mg daily from all supplements. 3 mg daily.	Important in tissue repair and immunity. Needed to balance with zinc.

HERBS

❑ Cranberry is the best herbal remedy for bladder infections. Quality cranberry juice produces hippuric acid in the urine, which acidifies the urine and inhibits bacterial growth. Other components in cranberry juice prevent bacteria from adhering to the lining of the bladder. Drink 1 quart of cranberry juice daily. Purchase pure, unsweetened juice. If pure cranberry juice is not available, cranberry capsules can be substituted. Always take these with a large glass of water. Avoid commercial cranberry juice cocktail products. These contain relatively little pure cranberry juice (less than 30 percent in some cases) and have high-fructose corn syrup or other sweeteners added.

❑ Birch leaves are a natural diuretic and reduce some of the pain associated with bladder infections; dandelion tea or extract acts as a diuretic and liver cleanser, and aids in relieving bladder discomfort; hydrangea is good for stimulating the kidneys and flushing them clean. Diuretics help to cleanse the system. By promoting the release of fluids from the tissues, diuretics also help to relieve the false sensations of urgency that are characteristic of cystitis. Combinations of these herbs are often most effective in flushing the kidneys and aiding in reducing the urgent need to urinate.

❑ Goldenseal is good for bladder infections if there is bleeding, and is most effective as an herbal antimicrobial agent.

Caution: Do not take goldenseal on a daily basis for more than one week at a time, and do not use it during pregnancy. If you have a history of cardiovascular disease, diabetes, or glaucoma, use it only under a doctor's supervision.

❑ Buchu is good for a bladder infection with a burning sensation upon urination.

❑ KB formula from Nature's Way and SP-6 Cornsilk Blend from Solaray are herbal formulas that have a diuretic effect and reduce bladder spasms. Take 2 capsules twice daily.

❑ Marshmallow root increases the acidity of urine, inhibiting bacterial growth. Drink 1 quart of marshmallow root tea daily. It helps to strengthen and cleanse the bladder.

❑ Uva ursi (bearberry, a type of cranberry), used in small amounts and diluted with other herbal teas, acts as a mild diuretic and antiseptic. It is effective against *E. coli.*

❑ Other beneficial herbs include burdock root, juniper berries, kava kava, and rose hips.

Caution: Kava kava may cause drowsiness. If this occurs, discontinue use or decrease the dosage.

RECOMMENDATIONS

❑ Drink plenty of liquids, especially cranberry juice (*see under* Herbs, above). Drink at least one 8-ounce glass of quality water every hour. This is extremely beneficial for urinary tract infections. Steam-distilled water is preferable to tap water.

❑ Include celery, parsley, and watermelon in your diet. These foods act as natural diuretics and cleansers. Celery and parsley juice or extract can be purchased at a health food store or made fresh at home if you have a juicer.

❑ Avoid citrus fruits; these produce alkaline urine that encourages bacterial growth. Increasing the acid content in urine inhibits the growth of bacteria. *See* ACIDOSIS in Part Two for a list of acid-forming foods.

❑ Stay away from alcohol, caffeine, carbonated beverages, coffee, chocolate, refined or processed foods, and simple sugars. Chemicals in food, drugs, and impure water have an adverse effect on the bladder.

❑ Perform a one- to three-day cleansing fast.

❑ Take 2 teaspoonfuls of whey powder or 2 acidophilus tablets or capsules with each meal. This is especially important if antibiotic therapy is required.

❑ Take a twenty-minute hot sitz bath twice daily. Hot sitz baths help to relieve the pain associated with cystitis. Batherapy, a product that can be found in health food stores, is excellent. Or you can add one cup of vinegar to a sitz bath (or to shallow bath water) once a day. A woman should position her knees up and apart so that the water can enter the vagina. Alternate this with a bath made with two cloves of crushed garlic or an equivalent amount of garlic juice. *See* SITZ BATH in Part Three.

❑ Use acidophilus douches as recommended under Nutrients, above. If cystitis is associated with vaginitis, alternate this with apple cider vinegar douches.

❑ Avoid taking excess zinc and iron supplements until healed. Taking over 100 mg of zinc daily can depress the immune system; bacteria require iron for growth. If a bacterial infection is present, the body stores iron in the liver, spleen, and bone marrow in order to prevent further growth of the bacteria.

❑ Do not delay emptying the bladder. Making sure that you urinate every two to three waking hours—"voiding by the clock"—can help.

❑ Keep the genital and anal areas clean and dry. Women should wipe from front to back after emptying the bladder or bowels, should empty the bladder before and after exercise and sexual intercourse, and wash the vagina after intercourse.

❑ Wear white cotton underwear; nylon underwear should be avoided.

❑ Change into dry clothes as soon as possible after swimming; avoid sitting around in a wet bathing suit.

❑ Do not use "feminine hygiene sprays," packaged douches, bubble baths, or tampons, sanitary pads, or toilet paper containing fragrance. The chemicals these products contain are potentially irritating.

❑ If you suffer from frequent urinary tract infections, use sanitary pads rather than tampons.

❑ If urination is painful but bacteria cannot be cultured by the laboratory, discontinue use of all types of soaps and use only water to cleanse the vaginal area. Some people are sensitive to soap; an all-natural soap from a health food store is recommended.

❑ If there is blood in the urine, consult your health care provider. This can be a sign of a more serious problem that warrants medical attention.

CONSIDERATIONS

❑ Optimal immune function is important in both fighting and preventing all bacterial disorders.

❑ Caffeine causes the muscles around the bladder neck to contract, and can produce painful bladder spasms.

❑ Habitually retaining the urine in the bladder for long periods increases a woman's risk of urinary tract infection, and may increase the risk of bladder cancer.

❑ Shrinkage of urethral and vaginal membranes, which most commonly occurs after menopause as as result of a reduction in the amount of estrogen in the body, can increase the tendency to develop bladder infections. Urethral dilation helps stretch a contracted urethra.

❑ Food allergies often cause symptoms that mimic bladder infections. Food allergy testing can determine which foods are causing the allergic reaction. (*See* ALLERGIES in Part Two.)

❑ Using aluminum cookware may cause cystitis symptoms. Cadmium, a toxic metal, may cause urinary problems as well.

❑ Colloidal silver is a natural broad-spectrum antiseptic that fights infection, subdues inflammation, and promotes healing. It is a clear golden liquid composed of 99.9-percent pure silver particles approximately 0.001 to 0.01 micron ($\frac{1}{1,000,000}$ to $\frac{1}{100,000}$ millimeter) in diameter that are suspended in pure water. It can be taken by mouth, administered intravenously, or applied topically. Colloidal silver is available in health food stores.

❑ Antibiotics and analgesics may be necessary treatments for cystitis, especially for persistent and/or painful infections. Beware of resorting to them too often, however. Antibiotics disturb the normal internal flora and may actually promote recurrent infections by promoting the development of antibiotic-resistant strains of bacteria. In fact, because antibiotics have been widely overprescribed over the years, many of the bacteria in our bodies (estimates run from 50 to 80 percent) are now resistant to common antibiotics, such as sulfa drugs and tetracycline. This forces doctors to resort to more powerful and potentially more dangerous antibiotics that pose a greater risk of adverse reactions and side effects. For most bladder infections, a natural approach to treatment appears to be best.

❑ Recurrent cystitis may be a sign of a more serious problem, such as bladder cancer, an anatomical anomaly, or immune deficiency. Cystoscopy, a simple visual examination of the bladder, is indicated.

❑ *See also* PROSTATITIS and KIDNEY DISEASE in Part Two.

Blepharitis

See under EYE PROBLEMS.

Blood Pressure Problems

See HIGH BLOOD PRESSURE.

Blood Sugar Problems

See DIABETES; HYPOGLYCEMIA.

Boil

Boils, referred to as *furuncles* by medical professionals, are round pus-filled nodules on the skin that result from infection with *Staphylococcus aureus* bacteria. The infection begins in the deepest portion of a hair follicle, and then the bacteria bore into the skin's deeper layers and the inflammation spreads. Poor nutrition, illness that has depressed

immune function, diabetes mellitus, and the use of immunosuppressive drugs are common contributing factors.

This disorder is common, especially among children and adolescents. Boils often appear on the scalp, buttocks, face, or underarms. They are tender, red, and painful, and they appear suddenly. Symptoms that a boil may be forming include itching, mild pain, and localized swelling. Within twenty-four hours, the boil becomes red and filled with pus. Fever and swelling of the lymph glands nearest the boil may occur.

Boils are contagious. The pus that drains when a boil opens can contaminate nearby skin, causing new boils, or can enter the bloodstream and spread to other body parts. A *carbuncle* is a cluster of boils that occurs when the infection spreads and other boils are formed. The formation of a carbuncle may be an indication of immune depression.

Without treatment, a boil usually comes to a head, opens, drains, and heals in ten to twenty-five days. With treatment, symptoms are less severe and new boils should not appear.

Unless otherwise specified, the following recommended doses are for persons over the age of eighteen. For a child between twelve and seventeen years old, reduce the dose to three-quarters the recommended amount. For a child between six and twelve, use one-half the recommended dose, and for a child under six years old, use one-quarter the recommended amount.

NUTRIENTS

SUPPLEMENT	SUGGESTED DOSAGE	COMMENTS
Essential		
Chlorophyll liquid	1 tbsp 3 times daily.	To cleanse the bloodstream.
Colloidal silver	Apply topically as directed on label.	A natural antibiotic and disinfectant. Destroys bacteria, viruses, and fungi. Promotes healing.
Garlic (Kyolic)	2 capsules 3 times daily.	A natural antibiotic that potentiates immune function.
Very Important		
Proteolytic enzymes	As directed on label. Take on an empty stomach.	Speeds up cleansing process at infection sites.
Vitamin A and vitamin E	75,000 IU daily for 1 month, then reduce to 25,000 IU daily. If you are pregnant, do not exceed 10,000 IU daily. 600 IU daily.	Antioxidants necessary for proper immune system function. Use emulsion forms for easier assimilation and greater safety at high doses.
Vitamin C	3,000–8,000 mg daily, in divided doses.	Powerful anti-inflammatory and immune system stimulant.
Helpful		
Coenzyme Q10	60 mg daily.	Important for oxygen utilization and immune function.
Kelp plus multimineral complex	2,000–3,000 mg daily, in divided doses. As directed on label.	To supply balanced minerals. Use a high-potency formula.
Raw thymus glandular	500 mg daily.	Stimulates the immune system. *See* GLANDULAR THERAPY in Part Three.

Silica or oat straw	As directed on label.	Supplies silicon, which reduces inflammatory reaction. *See under* Herbs, below.

HERBS

❑ Burdock root and pau d'arco are natural antibiotics that help rid the body of infections and toxins.

❑ Dandelion and milk thistle are liver cleansers.

❑ Echinacea and goldenseal help to cleanse the lymph glands.

Caution: Do not take goldenseal on a daily basis for more than one week at a time, and do not use it during pregnancy. If you have a history of cardiovascular disease, diabetes, or glaucoma, use it only under a doctor's supervision.

❑ Oat straw, taken in tea form, supplies silica, which has an anti-inflammatory effect.

❑ Onion poultices are good for boils. Apply pieces of onion wrapped in a piece of cloth—not directly to the area. *See* USING A POULTICE in Part Three.

❑ Red clover acts as an antibiotic and blood purifier, and is good for bacterial infections.

❑ Suma boosts the immune system.

RECOMMENDATIONS

❑ Use a cleansing fast to clear the system and rid the body of toxins that may cause boils. *See* FASTING in Part Three.

❑ To relieve pain and help to bring the boil to a head, apply moist heat three or four times a day. Wet a clean towel or sterile gauze pad with warm water and apply it to the boil. Place a heating pad or a hot water bottle on top. Do this for twenty minutes three or four times a day. Use a clean towel or fresh piece of gauze each time to prevent spreading the infection. Warm Epsom salts baths are also good.

❑ Do not cover a boil with an adhesive bandage, but do avoid irritation, injury, or trauma to the affected area. To avoid sweating, do not exercise or engage in strenuous activity until the boil heals.

❑ Keep the skin clean. Wash the infected area several times a day and swab it with antiseptic. You can also apply honey directly to the boil. Vitamin A and E emulsion, applied directly on boils, is helpful. Clay packs and/or chlorophyll are also good. Both of these can be found in health food stores. Apply them directly to the boil with a sterile gauze pad.

❑ If a boil is very large, persistent, or recurrent, consult your physician. Surgical incision and drainage may be necessary. Severe cases may require bed rest.

CONSIDERATIONS

❑ A doctor may prescribe an oral antibiotic. These drugs have side effects, however. It is best not to use them unless other measures fail.

❑ Over-the-counter antibiotic ointments are ineffective for boils and should be avoided.

Bone, Broken

See FRACTURE.

Bone Spur

See HEEL OR BONE SPUR.

Breast Cancer

Cancer of the breast is the leading cause of cancer death for women in the United States. Every year, about 180,000 people are diagnosed as having breast cancer. According to the American Cancer Society, one in nine women will get breast cancer before she is eighty-five.

The human breast is a gland that contains milk ducts, lobes, fatty tissue, and a network of lymphatic vessels. Cancerous tumors can arise in virtually any part of the breast, and are most often detected when a woman feels a lump. In general, cancerous lumps are firm, never go away, and are usually (though not always) pain-free. The vast majority of breast lumps are not cancerous (many are cysts or fibroid masses), but there is no way to tell without a professional's examination. A lump that seems to be growing or does not move when pushed may be cancerous, or may simply be caused by normal fibrocystic changes during the menstrual cycle. A biopsy is required to identify the lump. Breast cancer can also cause a yellow, bloody, or clear discharge from the nipple.

People tend to think of breast cancer as a single entity, but there are actually different types of the disease. Some types of breast cancer include the following:

• *Adenoid cystic carcinoma, malignant cytosarcoma phylliodes, medullary carcinoma, and tubular carcinoma.* These and several other relatively uncommon types of breast cancer tend to be less aggressive than the other forms.

• *Infiltrating ductal carcinoma.* This is a cancer that arises in the lining of the milk ducts and infiltrates (invades) the surrounding breast tissue. Approximately 80 percent of all cases of breast cancer are infiltrating ductal carcinomas.

• *Inflammatory carcinoma.* In this type of cancer, a tumor arises in the lining of the milk ducts and, as it grows, it plugs the lymphatic and blood vessels. The skin thickens and turns red, and the breast becomes extremely tender and looks infected. This type of cancer spreads very quickly due to the rich blood and lymph vessel supply associated with the inflammatory reaction.

• *Intraductal carcinoma in situ*. This is a localized type of cancer in which cancerous cells grow within the ducts. This type of cancer may not invade other tissues.

• *Lobular carcinoma*. A less common form of breast cancer, lobular carcinoma—breast cancer that arises in the lobes—accounts for about 9 percent of breast cancers. Lobular carcinomas occasionally occur in both breasts simultaneously.

• *Paget's disease of the nipple*. This form of cancer occurs when cells from an underlying cancerous tumor migrate to the nipple. The symptoms are itching, redness, and soreness of the nipple. Paget's disease always signals the presence of primary ductal carcinoma elsewhere in the breast tissue.

There is probably no single answer as to what causes breast cancer, but the female sex hormone estrogen is the most likely culprit in many cases. Estrogen promotes cellular growth in the tissues of the breasts and reproductive organs, and cancer is a disorder of unrestrained cellular growth. Moreover, some of the known risk factors for breast cancer include onset of menstruation before age nine, menopause after age fifty-five, having a first child after age forty, and having no or few children. One thing all of these risk factors have in common is that they result in the breasts being exposed to more estrogen for longer periods. Obesity also increases a woman's risk of developing breast cancer, and obese women tend to have higher levels of estrogen in their bodies than thin women. Similarly, eating a high-fat diet has been associated with an increased risk of breast cancer, and when a woman eats a diet high in fat and low in fiber, her body produces more estrogen.

Environmental factors may be involved in the development of breast cancer as well, among them exposure to such hazards as radiation and pesticides and the use of breast implants. Although the use of silicone/polyurethane implants—silicone-filled implants coated with polyurethane—has been banned since 1992 because of concerns about their safety, an estimated 200,000 American women still have these implants in their bodies. Polyurethane releases a human carcinogen known as toluene diisocyanate, or TDA, which was banned for use in hair dye long before the controversy over breast implants arose. Silicone has been shown to cause malignant tumors in test animals. Further, even if there were no potential danger from the implants themselves, breast implants can make it harder to detect breast cancer in the earlier stages because they may hide some breast tissue, interfering with the ability to take and interpret mammograms properly. Heredity is a factor in breast cancer as well; there are certain types of the disease that clearly run in families.

Although it is possible for a woman to get breast cancer at any age, the disease is most common in women over forty, especially postmenopausal women. Men also can get breast cancer, but they account for fewer than 1 percent of breast cancer cases. However, while it occurs less frequently, breast cancer in men usually is diagnosed at a later, and therefore more serious, stage because neither physicians nor their patients tend to suspect it.

It is important to detect breast cancer in its earliest and most curable stage. Making healthy changes in diet and lifestyle, examining your breasts regularly (*see* Breast Self-Examiniation, below), and having regular mammograms can increase your chances of avoiding or, if need be, overcoming, breast cancer.

BREAST SELF-EXAMINATION

It is important to examine your breasts each month, at the same point in your menstrual cycle. Do not examine them during your menstrual period. Before the period, a woman's breasts may swell and become tender or lumpy. This usually decreases after the period. The breasts also become larger and firmer during pregnancy, in preparation for breastfeeding. Familiarize yourself with the normal feel of your breasts so that you can detect any changes such as enlargement of a lump. A women who is accustomed to the way her breasts feel is better able to notice subtle changes. Any changes in your breasts should be reported to your health care provider, and you should be rechecked by a professional if you have any doubt concerning your examination. Since men also can get breast cancer, they can benefit from self-examination as well. The following is the recommended procedure for breast self-examination:

1. While standing and looking in the mirror, raise your hands over your head and press them together. Notice the shape of your breasts. Place your hands on your hips, apply pressure, and look for dimpling of the skin, nipples that seem to be out of position, one breast that looks different from the other, or red scaling or thickening of the skin and nipples.

2. Raise one arm above your head. With the other hand, firmly explore your breast. Beginning at the outer edge, using a circular motion, gradually work toward the nipple. Take your time when examining the area between the nipple and the armpit, and feel the armpit as well. You have lymph nodes in the armpit; they move freely and feel soft, and are not painful to the touch. Look for lumps that are hard and not mobile. Cancers are often attached to underlying muscle or the skin. When you have finished examining one breast, repeat this on the other side.

3. Lie down on your back and repeat step 2. Lumps may be more easily detected in this position. Also, squeeze each nipple gently to check for blood or a watery yellow or pink discharge.

In addition to monthly self-examination, the American Cancer Society recommends that women between the ages of twenty and forty have their breasts examined by a physician every one to three years. After age forty, the exam should be performed every year. Women should get their first mammogram by age forty, then have one every one to two years until the age of fifty. After age fifty, a mammogram should be performed annually.

The program recommended below is designed for women who have been diagnosed with breast cancer as well as for women who want to increase their odds of avoiding breast cancer.

NUTRIENTS

SUPPLEMENT	SUGGESTED DOSAGE	COMMENTS
Essential		
Natural beta-carotene	10,000 IU daily.	A powerful antioxidant that destroys free radicals.
or carotenoid complex (Betatene)	As directed on label.	
Coenzyme Q10	100 mg daily.	Improves cellular oxygenation.
Dimethylglycine (DMG) (Aangamik DMG from FoodScience Labs)	As directed on label.	Improves cellular oxygenation.
Essential fatty acids (black currant seed oil, borage oil, and flaxseed oil are good sources)	As directed on label.	Needed for proper cell reproduction.
Garlic (Kyolic)	2 capsules 3 times daily.	Enhances immune function.
Germanium	200 mg daily.	A powerful immunostimulant that improves cellular oxygenation, deterring cancer growth.
Proteolytic enzymes	As directed on label. Take with meals.	Powerful free radical scavengers.
Selenium	200–400 mcg daily.	Powerful free radical scavenger.
Shark cartilage (BeneFin)	For cancer treatment, 1 gm per 2 lbs of body weight daily, divided into 3 doses. If you cannot tolerate taking it orally, it can be administered in a retention enema. For cancer prevention, 2,000–4,500 mg 3 times daily.	Inhibits tumor growth and stimulates the immune system.
Superoxide dismutase (SOD)	As directed on label.	Destroys free radicals. Consider injections (under a doctor's supervision).
Vitamin A	50,000 IU daily. If you are pregnant, do not exceed 10,000 IU daily.	Vital to immunity.
Vitamin B complex	100 mg 3 times daily.	To improve circulation, build red blood cells, and aid liver function; necessary for normal cell division and function. Involved in the regulation of enzyme and hormone production. *Caution:* Do not take niacin if you have a liver disorder, gout, or high blood pressure.
plus extra vitamin B3 (niacin)	100 mg daily. Do not exceed this amount.	
and choline	100 mg 3 times daily.	Aids in reducing estrogen production.
plus brewer's yeast	As directed on label.	A source of B vitamins.
Vitamin C with bioflavonoids	5,000–20,000 mg daily, in divided doses.	Powerful anticancer agent. *See* ASCORBIC ACID FLUSH in Part Three.
Vitamin E	Start with 400 IU daily and increase slowly to 1,000 IU daily.	Deficiency has been linked to breast cancer. Also aids in hormone production and immune function. Use emulsion form for easier assimilation and greater safety at higher doses.
Important		
Maitake	4,000–8,000 mg daily.	Inhibits the growth and spread of cancerous tumors. Also boosts immune response.
Helpful		
Acidophilus	As directed on label. Take on an empty stomach.	To replenish "friendly" bacteria in the colon. Use nondairy formula.
Aerobic 07 from Aerobic Life Industries	As directed on label.	Antimicrobial agents.
or Dioxychlor from American Biologics	As directed on label.	
Kelp	1,000–1,500 mg daily.	For mineral balance.
or seaweed	As directed on label.	
L-Carnitine	As directed on label.	Protects the skin after mastectomy and/or radiation treatment. Use a form derived from fish liver (squalene).
L-Cysteine and L-methionine	As directed on label. Take with water or juice. Do not take with milk. Take with 50 mg vitamin B6 and 100 mg vitamin C for better absorption.	To detoxify harmful substances. *See* AMINO ACIDS in Part One.
Multienzyme complex	As directed on label. Take with meals.	To aid digestion.
Multimineral complex with calcium and magnesium and potassium	2,000 mg daily. / 1,000 mg daily. / 99 mg daily.	Essential for normal cell division and function. Use a comprehensive formula that contains all major minerals and trace elements but that is iron-free.
Multivitamin complex	As directed on label. Take with meals.	All nutrients are needed in balance. Do not use a sustained-release formula or a formula that contains iron.
Raw glandular complex plus raw thymus and raw adrenal glandulars	As directed on label.	To stimulate glandular function, especially the thymus, the site of T lymphocyte production. *See* GLANDULAR THERAPY in Part Three.
Taurine Plus from American Biologics	As directed on label.	Functions as foundation for tissue and organ repair. Use the sublingual form.
Vitamin B12 and folic acid	2,000 mcg daily. / 400 mcg daily.	To prevent anemia and aid in proper digestion and absorption of nutrients. Consider injections (under a doctor's supervision). If injections are not available, a sublingual form is best.

162

HERBS

❑ Astragalus root and echinacea enhance immune function. These herbs are best used in a rotating fashion, for no more than seven to ten days in a row.

Caution: Do not use astragalus in the presence of a fever.

❑ Burdock root, dandelion root, milk thistle, and red clover all protect the liver and aid in cleansing the bloodstream.

❑ Ginkgo biloba enhances circulation and brain function.

❑ Licorice root aids in maintaining proper organ function.

Caution: If overused, licorice can elevate blood pressure. Do not use this herb on a daily basis for more than seven days in a row. Avoid it completely if you have high blood pressure.

RECOMMENDATIONS

❑ Eat a diet based on fresh fruits and vegetables, plus grains, legumes, raw nuts (except peanuts) and seeds, and soured products such as low-fat yogurt. Very important are the cruciferous vegetables, such as broccoli, Brussels sprouts, cabbage, and cauliflower, and yellow/orange vegetables, such as carrots, pumpkin, squash, sweet potatoes, and yams. Eat vegetables raw or lightly steamed. For grains, use unpolished brown rice, millet, oats, and wheat. Eat whole grains only. If at all possible, consume only organically grown foods. Pesticides and other chemicals have been linked to breast cancer (they may mimic the effect of estrogen on the body).

❑ Include in the diet fresh apples, cherries, grapes, plums, and all types of berries.

❑ Eat onions and garlic, or take garlic in supplement form.

❑ Drink spring or steam-distilled water only, never tap water. Also drink fresh homemade vegetable and fruit juices. Drink fruit juices in the morning, vegetable juices in the afternoon.

❑ Do not eat meat or other animal products. Many animals are treated with hormones to hasten growth. Meat also contains saturated fat. Avoid all dairy products except for unsweetened low-fat yogurt.

❑ Do not consume any alcohol, caffeine, junk foods, processed refined foods, saturated fats, salt, sugar, or white flour. Limit your intake of soy products, which contain enzyme inhibitors. It is not necessary to eliminate soy foods completely, however.

❑ Take extra fiber daily. Fiber keeps toxic wastes from being absorbed into the bloodstream. Psyllium husks are a recommended source. The colon must be kept clean and the bowels must move daily for healing. *See* COLON CLEANSING, ENEMAS, and FASTING in Part Three.

Note: Always take supplemental fiber separately from other supplements and medications.

❑ Do not take supplements containing iron. Iron may be used by tumors to promote their growth.

❑ If you experience itching, redness, and soreness of the nipples, especially if you are not currently breastfeeding a baby, seek evaluation by a physician. These can be symptoms of Paget's disease.

❑ If you are undergoing treatment for breast cancer and find yourself feeling depressed or frightened, try to keep in mind that when medications (especially chemotherapy drugs) are stopped, you will probably start to feel better and to look at things in a different light. Think about all the women, including many celebrities and public figures, who have had breast cancer, and have gone on to have fulfilling lives and careers. Thousands of women who have had breast cancer are living happy, normal lives.

CONSIDERATIONS

❑ A study done by the American Health Foundation found that consuming wheat bran can reduce blood estrogen levels.

❑ People with breast cancer have been found to have lower than normal levels of vitamin E and the mineral selenium, two important antioxidants that work together to neutralize free radicals. Research has shown that people with cancer of the lung, bladder, breast, colon, and skin all have levels of vitamin A that are lower than normal.

❑ Being physically fit appears to help protect against breast cancer.

❑ Evidence is strong for a link between breast cancer and lifestyle. *The New England Journal of Medicine* has stated that consuming as few as three alcoholic drinks a week increases the potential for breast cancer by 50 percent. The National Women's Health Network urges all women to cut their total fat intake to 20 percent of total calories. Saturated fats should account for no more than 5 percent of calories.

❑ A study reported in the journal *Cancer* showed that women who gained more than 22 pounds since their teenage years doubled their chances of getting breast cancer.

❑ Treatment for breast cancer may include surgery or radiation therapy, or both, to control the breast tumor. Hormone therapy may be added in the form of drugs such as tamoxifen (Nolvadex).

❑ Options for the surgical treatment of breast cancer have expanded greatly in the past couple of decades. Surgical treatment now emphasizes breast conservation—preserving the breast when possible. Some of the treatment options in breast surgery include:

• Lumpectomy, also known as *segmental mastectomy* or *tylectomy*. The tumor and a small amount of surrounding tissue are removed. This is the least extensive type of breast cancer surgery.

• Quadrantectomy, also known as *partial mastectomy*. The quadrant of the breast in which the tumor was found is removed, including some skin and the lining of the chest muscle below the tumor.

• Simple mastectomy. The entire breast is removed and a sample of the underarm lymph nodes is taken.

• Modified radical mastectomy, also known as *total mastectomy*. The entire breast and all underarm lymph nodes are removed. The lining over the chest muscles may also be removed.

• Radical mastectomy, also known as the *Halsted radical mastectomy*. The entire breast, all the axillary (underarm) lymph nodes, and the underlying chest muscle are removed. This procedure was once the standard in breast cancer surgery, but today, fewer than 5 percent of women with breast cancer undergo this type of surgery.

No single procedure can be recommended as ideal for all individuals. A woman and her surgeon must base their decision on the patient's medical status and her particular concerns. Her choice may be influenced by emotional considerations, finances, access to care, body image, and personal beliefs. Depending on the type of surgery that is done, there is the option of having breast reconstruction later.

❑ After surgery, analysis of the tumor is done to determine the type of cancer and to test for the presence of a substance called estrogen-receptor protein, to determine whether the cancer is estrogen-dependent. If the tumor is found to be estrogen-dependent, an alternative to conventional chemotherapy may be the drug tamoxifen (Nolvadex). This drug blocks estrogen from binding with receptors on any developing breast cancer cells in the early stages, thus "starving" the cancer cells of the estrogen that promotes their growth. It can cause adverse side effects, however. In premenopausal women, hormonal treatment may be accomplished by removing the hormone-producing ovaries.

❑ In any type of breast cancer surgery, some or all of the underarm lymph nodes may be removed. This is done to check for possible spread of the cancer. If the cancer has spread to the lymph nodes, postoperative therapy may include radiation, chemotherapy, or hormonal therapy. Radiation is always required after a lumpectomy or quadrantectomy to ensure that no more cancer cells remain.

❑ After surgery, women are usually advised to avoid moving or carrying heavy objects, to wear loose-fitting clothes and gloves, and to avoid overexposure to the sun. Some women whose lymph nodes are removed during breast cancer surgery have a problem with swelling of the arm on that side due to an accumulation of lymphatic fluid. This is not unusual. Certain arm exercises are usually prescribed to keep the arm from becoming stiff and to assist in healing. If there is any unusual swelling, redness, or pain in the hand or arm, this should be evaluated by a physician.

❑ When breast cancer is caught in the very early stages—when it has not invaded nearby tissues—the cure rate is near 100 percent with surgery alone. Tumors of 1 centimeter or less in size carry a particularly good prognosis—less than a 10-percent likelihood of recurrence within 10 years. In general, the risk of recurrence rises with increasing tumor size and lymph node involvement.

❑ A relatively new approach to breast cancer treatment involves a combination of high-dose chemotherapy and a bone marrow transplant. Doctors first extract and freeze a small amount of marrow, then administer extremely high doses of chemotherapy to eradicate the cancer cells. The marrow is then reinjected into the patient to replace the marrow destroyed by chemotherapy. This treatment was tested at Duke University on women with advanced breast cancer that had spread to the lymph nodes in the armpits. After two years, 72 percent of the treated women were free of cancer, compared with 38 percent of those who received standard chemotherapy treatment. This treatment is very expensive, however; it can cost more than $100,000, and many insurance companies are reluctant to pay for it because they consider it "experimental." It is also extremely difficult physically for the woman who undergoes it.

❑ Once treatment has been completed and a woman is declared free of cancer, her physician will usually want to follow her progress for at least five years.

❑ Family support is necessary for the person with breast cancer. Depression, anxiety, and fear are not uncommon.

❑ *See also* CANCER in Part Two.

Breastfeeding-Related Problems

Breastfeeding, or lactation, is the natural way in which the mother of a newborn can feed her child instead of relying on cow's milk or artificial formula preparations. A woman's breasts are ideally suited for the task of feeding a baby, and nursing provides many benefits to both mother and baby that bottles and formulas do not. For example, mother's milk is much easier to digest, prevents constipation, lowers the incidence of food allergies, and protects the baby from many infectious diseases. Nursing also promotes healthy oral development, satisfies suckling needs, and enhances bonding and skin-to-skin contact between mother and child. Breastfeeding is beneficial to the mother in that it reduces the chance of hemorrhaging from the placental site, gives the mother an opportunity to rest, and encourages the uterus to contract, returning it to its prepregnant size.

In breastfeeding, as with anything else that is new and unfamiliar, problems may occur. This section offers explanations and solutions to the most common breastfeeding problems.

ENGORGEMENT

This is a temporary problem that most commonly occurs between two to five days after childbirth. It is caused by a combination of the increased blood supply to the breast and the pressure of the newly produced milk, resulting in the swelling of the tissues in the breast. A low-grade fever may be present; the breasts feel full, hard, tender, and tight; and the skin of the breasts is hot, shiny, and distended. This condition does not have to be present in order to allow nursing.

Recommendations

❑ Give your baby short, frequent feedings. A feeding schedule of every one and a half to two hours day and night should be maintained while engorgement lasts.

❑ Express milk between feedings to relieve pressure.

❑ Apply moist heat for thirty minutes preceding each feeding, and massage the breast during feedings to help get the milk flowing.

❑ Do not use nipple shields, as they can confuse the baby's sucking pattern, damage nipples, reduce stimulation of the breast, and decrease the milk supply.

❑ To prevent engorgement, feed your baby on demand and without delay, and allowing unrestricted suckling time. Do not skip or delay feedings during the day or night. Do not give your baby any formula or sugar water, and allow the baby to empty each breast completely at each feeding. This should take about seven minutes on each side.

MASTITIS (BREAST INFECTION)

If a plugged duct is not taken care of, mastitis can result. Soreness and redness in the breast, fever, and flulike symptoms are indicators of this problem. In fact, in a nursing mother all flulike symptoms should be considered a breast infection until proven otherwise.

Recommendations

❑ Drink plenty of fluids.

❑ Get plenty of rest.

❑ Apply heat with a hot water bottle or heating pad.

❑ Do not stop nursing your baby; if you do, the ducts will remain full, and overfilled ducts can worsen the problem.

Considerations

❑ Your health care provider may prescribe antibiotics that can be taken by a nursing mother.

❑ In rare cases, a breast infection results in a breast abscess, in which the sore breast fills with pus. An abscess may have to be incised to allow drainage. This procedure is performed in a physician's office. If an abscess develops, milk should be hand-expressed (massaged) from the infected breast and discarded. Breastfeeding should continue on the uninfected breast until the abscess is healed.

PLUGGED DUCT

Incomplete emptying of the milk ducts by the baby, or the wearing of a tight bra, can cause a plugged duct. Soreness and a lump in one area of a breast is an indication of this problem.

Recommendations

❑ Check the nipple very carefully for any tiny dots of dried milk, and remove them by gentle cleansing. Together with frequent nursing on the affected breast, this should allow the duct to clear itself within twenty-four hours.

❑ Massage the breasts with firm pressure, from the chest wall toward the nipple, to stimulate milk flow.

❑ Alter the position of the baby on the nipple so all the ducts are drained.

❑ Make sure you offer the affected breast first, when the baby's sucking is strongest.

SORE NIPPLES

Sore nipples are usually caused by improper nursing positions and nursing schedules, or incorrect sucking by the baby. They can also be caused by infection, most commonly with the fungus *Candida albicans*.

Recommendations

❑ Nurse on the least sore side first. However, if both breasts are sore, hand-express (massage the breast) until letdown occurs and milk is readily available to the baby.

❑ Make sure that the baby's jaws exert pressure on the least tender spots. Do not pull away when the baby is about to begin feeding. Learn to relax.

❑ Use dry heat such as a low-wattage electric bulb placed twelve to eighteen inches from the breast for ten to fifteen minutes following each feeding.

❑ If cracked nipples accompany soreness, apply aloe vera gel to the nipples to alleviate pain and promote healing.

❑ To prevent sore nipples, feed your baby frequently to avoid having a baby who is overly hungry bite down roughly on the nipple. Change nursing positions often to rotate the pressure of the baby's mouth on the breast, and learn to break suction correctly. Between feedings, keep the nipples dry. Expose them to sunlight and air. Do not wash them with soap, alcohol, or petroleum-based products, which can wash away their natural protection.

❑ If the pain is severe and persists despite these measures, it may be a sign of a candida infection (*see* FUNGAL INFECTION in Part Two). Consult your health care provider.

NUTRITIONAL HEALTH WHILE NURSING

The following supplements are beneficial for nursing mothers. After discussion with your health care provider, you may decide to supplement your diet with these vitamins and minerals.

NUTRIENTS

SUPPLEMENT	SUGGESTED DOSAGE	COMMENTS
Essential		
Free-form amino acid complex	As directed on label.	To supply needed protein. Soy protein and free-form amino acids are better sources than animal protein.
Helpful		
Calcium and	1,000–1,500 mg daily.	Needed by both mother and baby. Use chelate forms. Do not use bone meal or dolomite, as these may contain lead.
magnesium	500–750 mg daily.	
Bifido Factor from Natren	½ tsp daily, between meals.	For mother. Boosts immune system and provides necessary "friendly" bacteria. Use only unchilled water in preparation.
and LifeStart from Natren	¼ tsp daily, added to water or juice.	For infant. Use only unchilled water in preparation.
Multivitamin and mineral complex with vitamin B complex plus extra	As directed on label.	All nutrients are needed by both mother and baby. Use a high-potency formula.
folic acid and	400 mcg daily.	
vitamin C and	3,000 mg daily.	
vitamin D and	400 IU daily.	
iron and	As directed by physician.	
manganese	2 mg daily. Note: Do not take calcium and manganese together, as they compete for absorption.	
Vitamin B complex or	50 mg twice daily.	Needed for production of milk and to relieve stress.
brewer's yeast	Start with 1 tsp and work up to 1 tbsp 3 times daily, taken in juice.	

Herbs

❑ Any of the following herbs can be beneficial for the nursing mother: alfalfa, blessed thistle, dandelion, fennel, horsetail, and raspberry.

❑ Nettle leaf has a tonic effect and contains iron in addition to many other nutrients.

❑ The following herbs *decrease* milk supply, and should be avoided until a woman is no longer nursing: black walnut, sage, and yarrow.

Recommendations

❑ Eat plenty of brewer's yeast, eggs, nuts and seeds, and whole grains. Raw foods should be plentiful in the diet.

❑ Discuss the need for supplements for your baby with your health care provider. Mother's milk is nearly a perfect food. However, it is low in vitamins C and D and iron.

❑ If you need to supplement mother's milk, try almond milk, Rice Dream (made from brown rice), or a soymilk formula with a small amount of papaya (put through a blender). This resembles mother's milk. You can add a small amount of blackstrap molasses and brewer's yeast after the baby is a few months old. Always consult your health care provider before making any changes in your baby's diet.

Considerations

❑ The UCLA Medical School reported that mother's milk kills a tiny parasite (*Giardia lamblia*) that can cause intestinal disease in children.

❑ In recent studies, mothers who consumed garlic increased their babies' desire for milk, and the babies nursed longer. Garlic is good for both the mother and the infant. Kyolic from Wakunaga is an ideal way to consume garlic since it is odorless and therefore more "sociable."

❑ Almost all drugs have been found to enter a nursing mother's milk, including acetaminophen (Tylenol and others), alcohol, amphetamines, antibiotics, antihistamines, aspirin, barbiturates, caffeine, cimetidine (Tagamet), cocaine, decongestants, diazepam (Valium), ergotamine, chlordiazepoxide (Librium), marijuana, nicotine, and opiates (codeine, meperidine [Demerol], morphine). Some of the effects these drugs can have on an infant include diarrhea, rapid heart rate, restlessness, irritability, crying, poor sleeping, vomiting, and convulsions. In addition, some of these drugs may accumulate in an infant's body and cause addiction.

❑ In a study of new mothers, those who were trained and sent home from the hospital with a breast pump were found to breastfeed their infants longer than those who were given formula but no pumps.

❑ Breastfed babies run a very low risk of ever developing meningitis or severe blood infections. They also have a 500- to 600-percent lower risk of developing childhood lymphoma and suffer from 50 percent fewer middle ear infections than bottlefed babies.

❑ Breast milk contains high amounts of inositol, a B vitamin that plays a crucial role in survival and infant development.

❑ Women who undergo reduction mammoplasty (breast reduction surgery) and subsequently become pregnant can retain the ability to lactate and nurse. However, in one study, only 35 percent of such women breastfed successfully, whereas 65 percent either did not breastfeed or discontinued nursing for various reasons. It was not disclosed whether any of these women were actually unable to secrete sufficient amounts of milk to nurse their babies. Women who are considering breast reduction surgery should nevertheless consider this if they wish to have children later on and hope to breastfeed.

❑ There are resources available to help women learn to breastfeed successfully and to overcome any problems that arise. Certified lactation consultants are practitioners who specialize in this area. Your health care provider or the facility where you give birth should be able to give you a referral. La Leche League is another valuable resource for the breastfeeding mother. This is an organization of nursing women that can serve as both an educational resource and a support group. Consult your local telephone directory for the chapter nearest you, or contact La Leche League International at 1400 North Meacham Road, Schaumburg, IL 60173; telephone 708–455–7730.

Bright's Disease

See under KIDNEY DISEASE.

Bronchitis

Bronchitis is the inflammation or obstruction of the bronchi, the breathing tubes that lead to the lungs. The inflammation results in a buildup of mucus plus coughing, fever, pain in the chest and/or back, fatigue, sore throat, difficulty breathing, and, often, sudden chills and shaking. Bronchospasm may also occur. Swelling of the mucous membranes and hypersecretion by the bronchial glands frequently accompany bronchospasm.

Bronchitis can be either acute or chronic. Acute bronchitis is usually caused by an infection, which can be bacterial, viral, chlamydial, mycoplasmal, or caused by a combination of agents. It typically follows an upper respiratory tract infection, such as a cold or influenza. In acute bronchitis, bronchospasm is more often associated with viral (rather than bacterial) infection. Most cases of acute bronchitis are self-limiting, with full recovery in a matter of weeks. In some cases, however, the condition can lead to pneumonia. This is more likely to occur in persons who also have a chronic respiratory disease or other debilitating health problem.

Chronic bronchitis results from frequent irritation of the lungs, such as from exposure to cigarette smoke or other noxious fumes, rather than from infection. Allergies also may be the cause of chronic bronchitis. As chronic bronchitis diminishes the exchange of oxygen and carbon dioxide in the lungs, the heart works harder in an attempt to compensate. Over time, this can lead to pulmonary hypertension, enlargement of the heart, and, ultimately, heart failure.

Chronic bronchitis is one of the most common diseases seen by otolaryngolosits, allergists, and primary care physicians. Specialists in occupational medicine have long known that an adverse environment produces a vulnerability to respiratory infections. Climatic factors and epidemics of viral infections also increase the risk. Among people who live or work in unhealthy environments, shortness of breath is frequently aggravated by dampness and cold, exposure to dust, or even minor respiratory infections.

NUTRIENTS

SUPPLEMENT	SUGGESTED DOSAGE	COMMENTS
Essential		
Colloidal silver	As directed on label.	A natural antibiotic that destroys bacteria, viruses, and fungi. Promotes healing.
Natural beta-carotene or	50,000 IU daily.	Needed for protection and repair of lung tissue.
carotenoid complex (Betatene)	As directed on label.	
Quercitin-C from Ecological Formulas or	500 mg 3 times daily.	For allergic bronchitis. Has an antihistiminic effect.
Activated Quercetin from Source Naturals	As directed on label.	Contains quercetin plus bromelain and vitamin C for increased absorption.
Vitamin A	20,000 IU twice daily for 1 month; then reduce to 15,000 IU daily. If you are pregnant, do not exceed 10,000 IU daily.	For healing and protection of all tissues.
Vitamin C with bioflavonoids	3,000–10,000 mg daily, in divided doses.	Enhances immune function and reduces histamine levels. Use a buffered powder form.
Very Important		
Coenzyme Q$_{10}$	60 mg daily.	For improved circulation and breathing.
Proteolytic enzymes with bromelain	As directed on label. Take between meals.	Helps reduce inflammation.
Vitamin E	400 IU and up twice daily. Take with 50–100 mg vitamin C.	Powerful free radical scavenger and oxygen carrier. Needed for healing of tissues and improved breathing.
Zinc lozenges (Ultimate Zinc-C Lozenges from Now Foods)	1 15-mg lozenge 5 times daily. Do not exceed a total of 100 mg daily from all supplements.	Needed for repair of all tissues.
Important		
Chlorophyll or	As directed on label, 3 times daily.	To improve circulation, and to keep tissues free of toxic substances. Use liquid or tablet form.
"green drinks" (fresh wheatgrass juice, Kyo-Green from Wakunaga)	As directed on label.	To supply chlorophyll and important nutrients.
ClearLungs from Natural Alternatives		*See under* Herbs, below.
Garlic (Kyolic)	2 tablets 3 times daily, with meals.	A natural antibiotic that reduces infection and detoxifies the body.
Vitamin B complex	100 mg 3 times daily.	Activates many enzymes needed for healing.
Helpful		
Calcium and	1,000 mg daily.	Necessary for healing. Use in chelate or asporotate form.
magnesium	500 mg daily.	Needed to balance with calcium.
Maitake or	As directed on label.	To boost immunity and fight viral infection.
shiitake or	As directed on label.	
reishi	As directed on label.	

Multivitamin complex	As directed on label.	All nutrients are needed in balance for healing.
N-Acetylcysteine	500 mg twice daily, on an empty stomach. Take with water or juice. Do not take with milk. Take with 50 mg vitamin B_6 and 100 mg vitamin C for better absorption.	Protects and preserves the cells and contains sulfur, needed to lessen viscosity of bronchial mucus. *See* AMINO ACIDS in Part One.
plus L-arginine and	500 mg twice daily, on an empty stomach.	Aids in liver detoxification.
L-lysine and	500 mg twice daily, on an empty stomach.	Needed for protein synthesis to aid in healing.
L-ornithine	500 mg twice daily, on an empty stomach.	Lowers blood ammonia levels, which can be increased by respiratory illness.
Silica or horsetail	As directed on label.	Acts as an anti-inflammatory, reduces mucus flow, and reduces coughing. *See under* Herbs, below.
Raw thymus glandular	500 mg twice daily.	Needed to protect and enhance immune function. *See* GLANDULAR THERAPY in Part Three.

HERBS

Rather than using only one of the herbs listed here, alternate among several to get all of their healing benefits.

❑ Astragalus, myrrh, and pau d'arco are natural antibiotics.
Caution: Do not use astragalus in the presence of a fever.

❑ Black radish, chickweed, ginkgo biloba, lobelia, and mullein improve lung and bronchial congestion and circulation.

❑ Boneset contains immunostimulatory polysaccharides that are good for inflammation of the mucous membranes.
Caution: Do not use boneset on a daily basis for more than one week, as long-term use can lead to toxicity.

❑ Bronc-Ease from Nature's Herbs is an excellent herbal formula. It relieves congestion, coughing, and irritation.

❑ ClearLungs from Natural Alternatives is a Chinese herbal formula that helps provide relief from shortness of breath, tightness in the chest, and wheezing due to bronchial congestion. It is available in two formulas: one with ephedra and the other without. Both have been found to be equally effective. Take 2 capsules three times daily.

❑ Coltsfoot, slippery elm bark, and wild cherry bark soothe the throat and are good for a cough.

❑ Alcohol-free echinacea and goldenseal extract helps to fight viruses and bacteria and boost the immune system. At the first sign of illness, put ½ dropperful in your mouth. Hold it there for ten minutes, then swallow. Do this every three hours until symptoms are relieved (but not for longer than one week at a time).

❑ Ephedra (ma huang) is good for relieving nasal and chest congestion, as well as bronchial spasms.
Caution: Do not use this herb if you suffer from anxiety, glaucoma, heart disease, high blood pressure, or insomnia, or if you are taking a monoamine oxidase (MAO) inhibitor drug for depression.

❑ Inhaling the vapors of eucalyptus leaves helps to relieve respiratory problems.

❑ Fenugreek is good for reducing the flow of mucus.

❑ Goldenseal has antibiotic properties and is good for all conditions involving inflammation of the mucous membranes of the bronchial tubes, throat, nasal passages, and sinuses. In addition to taking goldenseal orally, you can place a cloth soaked with a strong goldenseal tea under a hot water bottle. Place 3 wet goldenseal tea bags on each lung under the soaked cloth.
Caution: Do not take goldenseal on a daily basis for more than one week at a time, and do not use it during pregnancy. If you have a history of cardiovascular disease, diabetes, or glaucoma, use it only under a doctor's supervision.

❑ Horsetail, taken in extract form, is a good source of silica, which has anti-inflammatory and expectorant properties, and also reduces coughing.

❑ Iceland moss is good for mucous congestion.

❑ Siberian ginseng is especially good for the lungs. It clears bronchial passages and reduces inflammation.
Caution: Do not use this herb if you have hypoglycemia, high blood pressure, or a heart disorder.

RECOMMENDATIONS

❑ Include garlic and onions in your diet. These foods contain quercetin and mustard oils, which have been shown to inhibit lipoxygenase, an enzyme that aids in releasing an inflammatory chemical in the body. Garlic is also a natural antibiotic.

❑ Drink plenty of fluids. Pure water, herbal teas, and soups are all good choices.

❑ Avoid mucus-forming foods such as dairy products, processed foods, sugar, sweet fruits, and white flour; also avoid gas-producing foods such as beans, cabbage, cauliflower, and so on. A vegetarian diet is best.

❑ Do not smoke, and avoid secondhand smoke. Cigarette smoke is very harmful. If you have chronic bronchitis, little improvement can be expected unless the irritating substances that cause the mucus to clog the air passages are eliminated.

❑ Add moisture to the air. Use a humidifier, a vaporizer, or even a pan of water placed on a radiator. Clean the equipment frequently to prevent the growth of bacteria.

❑ Rest in bed in the early stages, when fever is present. Once fever subsides and you are feeling better, alternate periods of rest with periods of moderate activity to prevent secretions from settling in the lungs.

❑ Apply warm, moist heat, or a hot water bottle over the chest and back before bedtime to aid in sleeping and reduce inflammation.

❑ To aid recovery, blow up a balloon a few times daily. One research study showed that after eight weeks of this therapy, people with bronchitis were much less breathless.

❑ Supplement your diet with vitamin C. Vitamin C is essential for all infectious disorders because the white blood cells use up large amounts in fighting infection.

❑ Do not use a cough suppressant if you have bronchitis. Coughing is essential for eliminating mucous secretions.

❑ If persistent and/or severe coughing, high fever, wheezing sounds, weakness and lethargy, difficulty breathing, and/or chest pain develop, consult your health care provider. These may be signs of developing pneumonia (*see* PNEUMONIA in Part Two).

CONSIDERATIONS

❑ If bacteria are the cause of acute bronchitis, treatment with antibiotics may be necessary to cure the infection and to prevent pneumonia from developing.

❑ Diet, nutrition, and environment all play important roles in any respiratory disease. A healthy household environment can make respiratory problems easier to control.

❑ For people who are unable to cough up sputum, bronchoscopy may be recommended. This is a procedure in which a flexible tube is inserted to examine the bronchial tree. It can be done simply for the sake of a visual examination, to suction out congestion, to remove foreign bodies, or even to biopsy (sample) tissue from the bronchial tubes for the purpose of identifying the infecting organism.

❑ If bronchitis does not clear up in a reasonable amount of time, a chest x-ray may be recommended to rule out lung cancer, tuberculosis, or other conditions that can cause similar symptoms.

❑ It is not unusual for persons with chronic respiratory disorders to be taking a variety of medications—inhalers, antianxiety medications, even diuretics—to help them breathe. Exercise is important; it helps one to breathe more efficiently and to tolerate daily activities.

❑ In recent years a new type of bronchitis, probably viral in origin, has afflicted many women. It is very difficult to treat, and often lasts three weeks to five months. Antibiotics, especially doxycycline hyclate (Doryx, Vibramycin), sometimes help, although we believe that the herb goldenseal works as well or better.

❑ A common treatment for bronchitis is a bronchodilator. If you use a bronchodilator, do not inhale more than the prescribed dose, as larger doses may cause side effects, including nervousness, restlessness, and trembling. Before using an inhaler, discuss with your doctor possible side effects and warning signs of dangerous reactions, plus any personal health concerns you have, such as possible pregnancy; a medical problem such as diabetes, hypothyroidism, or a seizure disorder; a history of drug use or adverse reactions to drugs; and current use of other over-the-counter or prescription drugs.

❑ The Air Supply personal air purifier from Wein Products is a small unit worn around the neck. It sets up an invisible pure air shield against microorganisms (such as viruses, bacteria, and mold) and microparticles (including dust, pollen, and pollutants) in the air. It also eliminates vapors, smells, and harmful volatile compounds in the air. The Living Air XL-15 unit from Alpine Air of America is an ionizing unit that is good for purifying the air in the home or workplace.

❑ *See also* ASTHMA; HAY FEVER; SINUSITIS; EMPHYSEMA; and PNEUMONIA in Part Two.

Bruising

A bruise occurs when the tissues underlying the skin are injured. The skin is not broken, but blood collects under the skin, resulting in pain, swelling, and "black-and-blue marks"—discoloration that starts out red, then turns dark and bluish, and finally may become a yellowish color as the blood under the skin is absorbed. Body parts often become bruised after banging into hard objects; this is normal. However, there are several factors that predispose people to bruising more easily than they should. People who do not eat enough fresh, uncooked foods to supply the body with needed nutrients are prone to easy bruising. Anemia, overweight, vitamin C deficiency, malnutrition, heavy smoking, leukemia, menstruation, and the use of anticlotting drugs are other factors that can result in a tendency to bruise. Bruising easily without a known cause can be an early sign of cancer.

NUTRIENTS

SUPPLEMENT	SUGGESTED DOSAGE	COMMENTS
Very Important		
Vitamin C with bioflavonoids	3,000–10,000 mg daily, in divided doses.	Helps to prevent bruising by supplying oxygen to the injured cells and strengthening capillary walls.
Important		
Vitamin K or alfalfa	As directed on label.	Necessary for blood clotting and healing. *See under* Herbs, below.
Helpful		
Coenzyme Q10	60 mg daily.	Essential for construction and reconstruction of body cells.
Dimethylglycine (DMG) (Aangamik DMG from FoodScience Labs)	100 mg daily.	Improves oxygen metabolism in the cells and tissues.
Iron (ferrous fumarate from Freeda Vitamins) or	As directed by physician. Take with 100 mg vitamin C for better absorption.	To correct deficiencies. *Caution:* Do not take iron unless anemia is diagnosed.
Floradix Iron + Herbs from Salus Haus	As directed on label.	A natural iron supplement.

Multienzyme complex	As directed on label. Take with meals.	To prevent inflammation in bruised areas.
plus proteolytic enzymes	As directed on label. Take between meals.	
Pycnogenol or grape seed extract	As directed on label. As directed on label.	Potent antioxidants for protecting skin tissue.
Vitamin B complex plus extra folic acid	100 mg twice daily. 400 mcg daily.	Aids in protecting the tissues.
Vitamin D plus calcium and magnesium	400–800 IU daily. 2,000 mg daily. 1,000 mg daily.	To help protect the skin. Needed for blood cell formation.
Vitamin E	Start with 400 IU daily and increase slowly to 800 IU daily. Do not exceed 400 IU daily if you take anticoagulant medication.	Improves circulation in body tissues.

HERBS

❑ Alfalfa supplies beneficial minerals and vitamin K, which is needed for healing. Take it in tablet form as directed on the product label.

❑ Dandelion and yellow dock are good sources of iron.

❑ Other beneficial herbs include black walnut, horsetail, and rose hips.

RECOMMENDATIONS

❑ To minimize bruising, as soon as possible after an injury, place an ice pack on the bruised area and keep it in place for thirty minutes.

❑ Eat a diet including an abundance of dark green leafy vegetables, buckwheat, and fresh fruits. These foods are high in vitamin C and bioflavonoids, which help to prevent bruising. Leafy greens such as kale are also good sources of vitamin K, which is necessary for blood clotting and healing.

❑ Do not take aspirin, ibuprofen (Advil, Nuprin, and others), or other nonsteroidal anti-inflammatory drugs (NSAIDs).

❑ If bruising is frequent, consult your health care provider.

CONSIDERATIONS

❑ Studies show that people with vitamin C deficiencies bruise more easily than others, probably because their blood vessels are generally weaker.

Bruxism

Bruxism is the medical term for tooth-grinding. This usually occurs during sleep, often without the person being aware of it (although family members may be). Over time, chronic tooth-grinding can result in loosened teeth and receding gums. The teeth may be pushed out of line, and the bite may need adjusting. Eventually, tooth loss can occur.

Bruxism can develop if the teeth are sensitive to heat and cold. Fluctuations in blood sugar levels may be involved. Stress and anxiety are often the cause of tooth-grinding.

NUTRIENTS

SUPPLEMENT	SUGGESTED DOSAGE	COMMENTS
Essential		
Calcium and magnesium	1,500–2,000 mg daily. 750 mg daily.	Deficiencies have been linked to tooth-grinding.
Pantothenic acid (vitamin B5)	500 mg twice daily.	Reduces stress.
Very Important		
Vitamin C	3,000–5,000 mg daily.	Potentiates adrenal function; acts as an anti-stress vitamin.
Helpful		
Chromium	200 mcg daily.	Helps to normalize blood sugar levels. Hypoglycemia is often linked to this disorder. Use chromium picolinate form.
Multivitamin and mineral complex plus raw adrenal glandular	As directed on label. As directed on label.	All nutrients are needed to reduce stress. To support adrenal function. *See* GLANDULAR THERAPY in Part Three.
Vitamin B complex	100 mg twice daily.	Necessary for proper nerve function. Use a high-stress formula.
Zinc	50 mg daily. Do not exceed a total of 100 mg daily from all supplements.	Helps to support the immune system and reduce stress.

RECOMMENDATIONS

❑ Adopt a hypoglycemic diet that is high in fiber and protein and includes plenty of fresh vegetables and high-fiber fruits, plus legumes, raw nuts and seeds, skinless white turkey or chicken, broiled fish, and whole grains. Consume starchy vegetables and very sweet fruits in moderation only. Eat six to eight small meals spread evenly throughout the day rather than two or three large meals. Hypoglycemia, related to low adrenal function, is often the cause of bruxism. (*See* HYPOGLYCEMIA in Part Two.)

❑ Do not consume alcoholic beverages. Alcohol often makes the problem worse.

❑ Avoid fast foods, fried foods, processed foods, red meat, refined sugar, saturated fats, and all dairy products except for yogurt, kefir, and raw cheese. Also avoid all foods with artificial flavors, colors, preservatives, and other chemicals.

❑ Do not eat anything sweet within six hours of going to bed. If you are hungry, have a light protein-and-fiber snack.

❑ As much as possible, avoid stress. Learn stress management and relaxation techniques. *See* STRESS in Part Two.

❑ Take supplemental calcium and pantothenic acid as directed under Nutrients, above. Calcium is often effective for treating involuntary movement of muscles.

❑ Consider having a hair analysis done to determine if you have any mineral imbalances, such as abnormal levels of sodium and potassium. *See* HAIR ANALYSIS in Part Three.

CONSIDERATIONS

❑ Dentists sometimes recommend a type of splint that is worn over the teeth for people with bruxism. This does not cure the problem, but it can help to prevent tooth damage.

❑ Biofeedback is helpful for overcoming bruxism in some cases. (*See* Biofeedback *under* PAIN CONTROL in Part Three.)

Bulimia

Bulimia nervosa is an eating disorder characterized by episodes of uncontrolled binge eating, often involving extremely large amounts of high-calorie foods, followed by induced vomiting or the use of laxatives to "purge" the body of the food eaten during the binge. The binge eating and purging are carried out in secret. This is a serious medical and psychological problem with potentially dangerous complications. Bulimia can lead to serious medical problems, including ulcers, internal bleeding, hypoglycemia, a ruptured stomach, kidney damage, erratic heartbeat, cessation of menstrual cycles, and a low pulse rate and blood pressure.

The causes of bulimia are most often psychological in nature, and episodes of binging are often stress related. Binging may be a means by which an individual with bulimia attempts to manage emotions; they allow the person to focus attention away from unpleasant or uncomfortable emotional problems. People with bulimia may also be obsessed with exercise as a means of controlling weight.

This disorder affects many more women than men, especially those in professions that stress appearance, such as modeling, acting, or dance. Obsession with weight can also result from social factors. In today's society, we are constantly bombarded with the message that "thin is in"— and the thinner the better. As many as one in eight girls between the ages of thirteen and nineteen, including many college students, may have an eating disorder.

Many individuals who suffer from this disorder come from families in which they were subjected to physical or sexual abuse. In some families, substance abuse is also a factor. Many women started their first binge because of real or imagined male rejection. Others are perfectionists and overachievers with high standards but low self-esteem. Particularly if a woman's basic emotional needs were not met in childhood, she may come to believe that her problems would be resolved if only she were attractive (that is, thin) enough, and this obsession leads to bulimia.

There are indications of possible physiological elements in this disorder as well. For example, people with eating disorders tend to have a type of chemical imbalance similar to one found in persons with clinical depression. Both have high levels of adrenocorticotropic hormone (ACTH), a hormone produced by the pituitary gland that inhibits T cell function and thereby depresses immunity. People who suffer from bulimia may also have low levels of the neurotransmitter serotonin, which can lead to cravings for simple carbohydrates—common binge foods.

Unlike people with anorexia, whose self-starvation eventually becomes obvious, those with bulimia can hide the disorder for long periods, even years, because their weight is usually in the normal range (some are even overweight) and the binging and purging are done in secret. Physical signs of bulimia may be swollen glands in the face and neck; erosion of the enamel of back teeth; broken blood vessels in the face; swollen salivary glands, resulting in a "chipmunk" appearance; constant sore throat; inflammation of the esophagus; and hiatal hernia. All of these are the consequences of induced vomiting. Sometimes emboweled spoons or sticks used to induce vomiting have to be surgically removed. If laxative abuse is part of the picture, damage to the bowel, rectal bleeding, and perpetual diarrhea may result. Laxative use also washes potassium and sodium from the body, which can result in electrolyte imbalances that may lead to dehydration, muscle spasms, and, eventually, cardiac arrest. Other signs of bulimia can include hair loss, yellow skin, premature wrinkles, bad breath, extreme weakness, muscle fatigue, and dizziness.

People with bulimia often feel extremely guilty about their behavior, which is why they may successfully hide the disorder for years, even from their spouses and children. Trips to the bathroom after meals, the sudden disappearance of large quantities of food, frequent dental visits, and mood changes may be hints that something is wrong.

NUTRIENTS

SUPPLEMENT	SUGGESTED DOSAGE	COMMENTS
Very Important		
Multivitamin and mineral complex with vitamin A and natural beta-carotene and potassium and selenium	As recommended by physician. Take with meals. 15,000 IU daily. If you are pregnant, do not exceed 10,000 IU daily. 25,000 IU daily. 99 mg daily. 200 mcg daily.	The bulimic syndrome results in extreme vitamin and mineral deficiencies. Extremely high doses are needed because nutrients pass rapidly through the gastrointestinal system and are poorly assimilated. Do not use a sustained-release formula.
Zinc plus copper	50–100 mg daily. Do not exceed a total of 100 mg daily from all supplements. 3 mg daily.	Necessary in protein metabolism; aids the sense of taste and increases the appetite. Deficiencies are common in people with this disorder. Needed to balance with zinc.

171

Important		
Acidophilus	As directed on label. Take on an empty stomach so it can pass quickly to the small intestine.	Stabilizes intestinal bacteria. Protects the liver.
Calcium and magnesium	1,500 mg daily, at bedtime. 750 mg daily.	Has a calming effect and replaces lost calcium stores. Relaxes smooth muscle and has a bronchodilating effect.
Free-form amino acid complex	As directed on label.	To counteract protein deficiency, a serious problem in bulimia. Free-form amino acids are more readily available for use by the body than other protein forms.
Vitamin B complex	100 mg 3 times daily.	Essential for all cellular functions.
Vitamin B_{12} injections	1 cc 3 times weekly or as prescribed by physician.	Needed for the digestion of foods and the assimilation of all nutrients, including iron. Injections (under a doctor's supervision) are best. If injections are not available, use a lozenge or sublingual form.
plus liver extract injections	2 cc 3 times weekly or as prescribed by physician.	A good source of B vitamins and other valuable nutrients.
Vitamin C	5,000 mg daily, in divided doses.	Necessary for all cellular and glandular functions.

Helpful		
Bio-Strath from Bioforce	As directed on label 3 times daily.	For increased strength and energy. Aids in tissue repair and increases the appetite. Contains the B vitamins and other necessary nutrients.
or brewer's yeast	Start with 1 tsp daily and work up to the amount recommended on label.	A good source of B vitamins.
Iron (ferrous fumarate from Freeda Vitamins) or	As directed by physician. Take with 100 mg vitamin C for better absorption.	To correct deficiencies and increase appetite. Caution: Do not take iron unless anemia is diagnosed.
Floradix Iron + Herbs from Salus Haus	As directed on label, 3 times daily.	A natural source of iron that is easily assimilated.
Kelp	2,000–3,000 mg daily.	Supplies essential minerals, especially iodine.
Proteolytic enzymes or Infla-Zyme Forte from American Biologics	As directed on label. Take with meals and between meals.	Important for proper digestion and absorption of nutrients.
Vitamin D	600 IU daily.	Needed to aid in calcium uptake and prevent bone loss, which can lead to tooth loss.
Vitamin E or	600 IU daily.	Necessary for tissue repair and a powerful antioxidant.
ACES + Zinc from Carlson Labs	As directed on label.	To supply a combination of antioxidants.

RECOMMENDATIONS

❑ While healthier eating behaviors are being established, try to eat a well-balanced, high-fiber diet.

❑ Consume no sugar in any form. Avoid junk foods and white flour products. Be aware that you may experience withdrawal symptoms such as anxiety, depression, fatigue, headache, insomnia, and/or irritability for a time after you eliminate sugar from the diet.

CONSIDERATIONS

❑ Psychiatric consultation is frequently necessary to overcome bulimia, as the cause is most often psychological. Long-term treatment may be needed to improve self-esteem.

❑ According to researchers at the National Institute of Mental Health (NIMH) and Duke University, lack of a hormone that controls appetite may be the reason bulimics fail to feel full. In such persons, eating a meal apparently does not stimulate adequate production of the hormone cholecystokinin-pancreozymin (CCK), which is found in the small intestine and the brain. They have to keep eating, and binging, in order to feel satisfied. However, more research is needed to determine whether this is the cause behind the majority of cases of binge eating.

❑ A study conducted at the University of Iowa College of Medicine and the University of Wisconsin found that reducing weight as part of athletic training may lead to bulimia. A survey of 700 high school wrestlers found that 2 percent were involved with binge eating followed by vomiting, fasting, excessive exercise, or the use of laxatives to avoid weight gain.

ADDITIONAL SOURCES OF INFORMATION

❑ To obtain more information about eating disorders and treatments, contact any of the following:

American Anorexia/Bulimia Association (AABA)
293 Central Park West, Suite 1R
New York, NY 10024
212–501–8351

Anorexia Nervosa and Related Eating Disorders (ANRED)
P.O. Box 5102
Eugene, OR 97405
503–344–1144

Institute for the Study of Anorexia and Bulimia
1 West 91st Street
New York, NY 10024
212–595–3449

National Eating Disorders Organization (NEDO)
445 East Granville Road
Worthington, OH 43085-3195
614–436–1112

Burns

There are three basic classifications of burns, depending on severity. First-degree burns affect only the outer layer of the skin, causing redness and sensitivity to the touch. Sunburn is usually a first-degree burn. Second-degree burns extend somewhat into underlying skin layers, and are characterized by redness, blistering, and acute pain. In third-degree burns, the entire thickness of the skin and possibly underlying tissues such as muscle are destroyed. The skin may be red, or it may be white or yellowish, or leathery and black. There is usually little or no pain because the nerves in the skin are severely damaged.

The following nutrients are important for healing once appropriate local treatment has been administered.

NUTRIENTS

SUPPLEMENT	SUGGESTED DOSAGE	COMMENTS
Very Important		
Colloidal silver	Apply topically as directed on label.	A natural antibiotic and disinfectant. Promotes healing.
Free-form amino acid complex	As directed on label.	Important in the healing of tissues.
Potassium	99 mg daily.	Needed to replace potassium lost from burns.
Vitamin A	100,000 IU daily for 1 month, then reduce to 50,000 IU daily. If you are pregnant, do not exceed 10,000 IU daily.	Needed for tissue repair. Use emulsion form for easier assimilation and greater safety at high doses.
plus natural beta-carotene or	25,000 IU daily.	An antioxidant and precursor of vitamin A.
carotenoid complex (Betatene)	As directed on label.	
Vitamin B complex plus extra	100 mg daily, with meals.	Important in the healing of skin tissue.
vitamin B12	1,000 mcg twice daily.	Needed for protein synthesis and cell formation. Use a lozenge or sublingual form.
Vitamin C with bioflavonoids	10,000 mg immediately after a burn; 2,000 mg 3 times a day thereafter until healed.	An antioxidant that is essential in the formation of collagen; promotes the healing of burns.
Vitamin E	Start with 600 IU daily and increase slowly to 1,600 IU daily. Also open a capsule and apply the oil directly to the scar once healing has begun.	Needed for healing and to prevent scarring.
Zinc	30 mg 3 times daily. Do not exceed a total of 100 mg daily from all supplements.	Needed for healing of tissues.
Important		
Essential fatty acids (flaxseed oil and primrose oil are good sources)	As directed on label.	Speeds healing.
Selenium	200 mcg daily.	Needed for tissue elasticity. Provides antioxidant protection at the cellular level.
Helpful		
Calcium and	1,500 mg daily.	Promotes healthy skin.
magnesium and	750 mg daily.	Loss of body fluids increases the need for magnesium.
vitamin D	400 IU daily.	Needed for calcium uptake.
All-Purpose Bactericide Spray from Aerobic Life Industries	Apply topically as directed on label.	Kills bacteria and prevents infection.
Coenzyme Q10	100 mg daily.	Helps circulation and healing of tissue.
Germanium	200 mg daily.	Enhances circulation and healing of tissue.
Infla-Zyme Forte from American Biologics	As directed on label. Take between meals.	Reduces inflammation.

HERBS

❑ Aloe vera pulp, gel, or liquid can be applied to the burn as needed to relieve pain and speed healing.

❑ Goldenseal is a natural antibiotic that helps to prevent infection.

Caution: Do not take goldenseal on a daily basis for more than one week at a time, and do not use it during pregnancy. If you have a history of cardiovascular disease, diabetes, or glaucoma, use it only under a doctor's supervision.

❑ Bayberry, black or green tea, blackberry leaves, sumac leaves, sweet gum, and white oak bark contain tannic acid, which has been used in clinics for surface burns that have begun to heal. These herbs can be used as teas and as wet compresses.

❑ Horsetail and slippery elm help skin tissues to heal.

RECOMMENDATIONS

❑ If you suspect a third-degree burn, see your physician at once or go to the emergency room of the nearest hospital. Do not attempt to treat the injury, do not remove clothing that is stuck to the burned area, and do not put ice or water on the burn. A third-degree burn requires professional treatment.

❑ Cool a first- or second-degree burn at once to reduce pain and swelling. Immerse the area in cool running water, or use cool compresses for a minimum of ten minutes. *Do not* use ice water, and do not stop prematurely. While cooling the burn, remove rings, wristwatches, belts, or anything else that could constrict the injured area once it begins to swell.

❑ To remove hot tar, wax, or melted plastic from the skin, use ice water to harden the heated substance.

❑ After the burn has been cooled, apply aloe vera gel or a product such as Burn Gel from Aerobic Life Industries, which contains aloe vera, to ease pain and promote healing. Do not put oils, greasy ointments, or butter on burns. Do not break blisters.

❑ While your body is recovering from a burn—especially a second- or third-degree burn—change your diet to provide a high protein intake and up to 5,000 or 6,000 calories per day. This is needed for tissue repair and healing.

❑ Watch for signs of infection, odor, pus, or extreme redness in the area of the burn. Protect the injury from exposure to sun.

❑ Drink plenty of fluids throughout the healing phase.

❑ Keep burn injuries elevated to minimize swelling and promote healing. This is especially important for burns on the hands, legs, or feet.

❑ Keep the burn *lightly* covered to minimize the chance of bacterial infection.

❑ Try adding 1 tablespoon of powdered vitamin C to 1 quart of cold water and spraying it on the burn site. This has been found to enhance healing. Or try using cold clay poultices. *See* USING A POULTICE in Part Three.

❑ If infection starts to set in, apply honey three times a day after gently washing the area with hydrogen peroxide.

CONSIDERATIONS

❑ For third-degree burns, your doctor may prescribe silver sulfadiazine cream (Silvadene). Reactions to silver sulfadiazine are rare, but they can occur.

❑ A medically supervised program for a more serious burn, or a burn in a sensitive location, may include the use of antibiotics, debridement to remove dead tissue, hydrotherapy to loosen dead skin, and physical therapy or splinting to prevent contractures.

❑ In cases of severe burns, hyperbaric oxygen therapy may be employed to reduce edema, scarring, and contracture. This treatment also improves the chances that a skin graft will take. (*See* HYPERBARIC OXYGEN THERAPY in Part Three.)

❑ A study on the effects of high-dose vitamin C therapy for third-degree burns that was reported in the *Journal of Burn Care and Rehabilitation* concluded that persons with serious burns should immediately begin taking vitamin C (*see under* Nutrients, above).

❑ Applied topically to burned skin, dimethylsulfoxide (DMSO), a byproduct of wood processing, has been reported to have a remarkable ability to relieve pain and promote healing.

Note: Only DMSO from a health food store should be used for healing purposes. Commercial-grade DMSO found in hardware stores is not suitable. The use of DMSO may result in a garlicky body odor. This is temporary, and is not a cause for concern.

❑ *See also* SUNBURN in Part Two.

❑ *See also* PAIN CONTROL in Part Three.

Bursitis

Bursitis is an inflammation of a bursa. The bursae are small fluid-filled sacs located between tendons and bone in various places in the body. They help to promote muscular movement by cushioning against friction between bones and other tissues. An inflamed bursa causes pain, tenderness to the touch of the affected body part, and limitation of motion. There may be redness and swelling as well.

Bursitis can be caused by injury, chronic overuse, reactions to certain foods, airborne allergies, or calcium deposits. Tight muscles also may lead to bursitis. The bursae in the hip and shoulder joints are most often affected. Bursitis affecting the arm is often called "tennis elbow" or "frozen shoulder." Occupational bursitis is not uncommon, and is known by old, familiar names such as "housemaid's knee," "policeman's heel," or the "beat knee" or "beat shoulder" of coal miners. One of the most common foot ailments, the bunion, is actually a form of bursitis caused by friction; a tight-fitting shoe causes a sac on the joint of the big toe to become inflamed.

Bursitis can affect anyone, at any age. However, older people, especially athletes, are more likely than others to get bursitis. It can sometimes be difficult to differentiate between bursitis and tendinitis, the inflammation of a tendon. Bursitis is usually characterized by a dull, persistent ache that increases with movement, whereas tendinitis typically causes sharp pain on movement. Tendinitis often afflicts people who routinely have to reach to perform certain activities, such as domestic workers and painters. Tendon inflammation may also result from calcium deposits that press against a tendon. Unlike tendinitis, bursitis is often accompanied by swelling and fluid accumulation.

NUTRIENTS

SUPPLEMENT	SUGGESTED DOSAGE	COMMENTS
Very Important		
Calcium and	1,500 mg daily.	Needed for repair of connective tissue.
magnesium	750 mg daily.	Needed to balance with calcium and for proper muscular function. Use magnesium chelate form.
Free-form amino acid complex	As directed on label. Take on an empty stomach.	Needed for healing.
Multienzyme complex with pancreatin	As directed on label. Take with meals.	To aid digestion. Use a formula with high amounts of pancreatin.
Proteolytic enzymes or Infla-Zyme Forte from American Biologics	As directed on label. Take between meals. 2 tablets 2–3 times daily, between meals.	Contains a powerful anti-inflammatory substance.
Vitamin A plus	15,000 IU daily. If you are pregnant, do not exceed 10,000 IU daily.	Needed for tissue repair and immune function.
natural beta-carotene or	25,000 IU daily.	Potent antioxidant and precursor of vitamin A.
carotenoid complex (Betatene)	As directed on label.	
plus selenium	200 mcg daily.	
Vitamin E	Start with 400 IU daily and increase slowly to 1,000 IU daily.	An anti-inflammatory free radical scavenger.

Vitamin C with bioflavonoids	3,000–8,000 mg daily, in divided doses.	Reduces inflammation and potentiates immune function. Essential for the formation of collagen, a protein in connective tissue.
Zinc plus copper	50 mg daily. Do not exceed a total of 100 mg daily from all supplements. 3 mg daily.	Important in all enzyme systems and tissue repair. Needed to balance with zinc.
Helpful		
Boron	3 mg daily. Do not exceed this amount.	For better calcium absorption.
Coenzyme Q₁₀	60 mg daily.	Good for circulation.
Glucosamine sulfate or N-Acetylglucosamine (N-A-G from Source Naturals)	As directed on label. As directed on label.	Important for the formation of connective tissues.
Multivitamin and mineral complex	As directed on label.	Needed for tissue repair.
Pycnogenol or grape seed extract (Vitrenol)	As directed on label. As directed on label.	Powerful antioxidants and anti-inflammatories.
Silica or horsetail	As directed on label.	Supplies silicon, necessary for repair of connective tissues. *See under* Herbs, below.
Vitamin B complex	100 mg twice daily.	Important in cellular repair.
Vitamin B₁₂ injections	As prescribed by physician.	Needed for proper digestion and absorption of foods and for the repair of nerve damage. Injections (under a doctor's supervision) are best. If injections are not available, use a lozenge or sublingual form.

HERBS

❑ Horsetail extract supplies silica, a form of the trace mineral silicon, which is necessary for tissue repair and healing.

RECOMMENDATIONS

❑ Go on a seven-day raw food diet, followed by a three-day cleansing fast. *See* FASTING in Part Three.

❑ Eat no processed foods or any form of sugar.

❑ To relieve pain, use hot castor oil packs. Place castor oil in a pan and heat but do not boil it. Dip a piece of cheesecloth or other white cotton material into the oil until the cloth is saturated. Apply the cloth to the affected area and cover it with a piece of plastic that is larger in size than the cotton cloth. Place a heating pad over the plastic and use it to keep the pack warm. Keep the pack in place for one-half to two hours, as needed. Some physicians recommend ice packs.

❑ You may need to abstain from activity and get plenty of rest. When engaging in physical activity, do not push yourself too hard or too long. If you are in pain, stop.

CONSIDERATIONS

❑ Treatment for bursitis involves removing the cause of the injury (this usually means rest and/or immobilization of the affected area), clearing up any underlying infection, and possibly surgically removing calcium deposits.

❑ Applied topically, dimethylsulfoxide (DMSO), a byproduct of wood processing, can relieve pain and reduce swelling.

Note: Only DMSO from a health food store should be used for healing purposes. Commercial-grade DMSO found in hardware stores is not suitable. The use of DMSO may result in a garlicky body odor. This is temporary, and is not a cause for concern.

❑ A new, still experimental, treatment for bursitis involves injecting honeybee venom directly at the site. The venom contains a powerful anti-inflammatory and can provide rapid relief. It can be injected either with a hypodermic needle or by the bees themselves. Further information is available from the American Apitherapy Society in Hartland Four Corners, Vermont; telephone 802–436–2708.

❑ *See also* PAIN CONTROL in Part Three.

Cadmium Toxicity

A toxic trace metal, cadmium can be detrimental to your health. Like lead, cadmium accumulates in the body and has varying degrees of toxicity. Cadmium replaces the body's stores of the essential mineral zinc in the liver and kidneys. Not surprisingly, therefore, cadmium levels rise in people who have zinc deficiencies.

Elevated levels of cadmium may result in hypertension (high blood pressure); a dulled sense of smell; anemia; joint soreness; hair loss; dry, scaly skin; and loss of appetite. Cadmium toxicity threatens the health of the body by weakening the immune system. It causes a decreased production of T lymphocytes (T cells), key white blood cells that protect the body by destroying foreign invaders and cancer cells. Because cadmium is retained in the kidneys and liver, excessive exposure can lead to kidney disease and serious liver damage. Possible effects of intense cadmium exposure include emphysema, cancer, and a shortened life span.

Tobacco smoke—whether cigarette, cigar, or pipe smoke—contains cadmium, and studies have shown that cigarette smokers have higher levels of cadmium in their bodies than nonsmokers. You can also accumulate cadmium from secondhand smoke. Cadmium is used in plastics and in the production of nickel-cadmium batteries. In addition to cigarette smoke and plastics, common sources of cadmium exposure include drinking water, fertilizer, fungicides, pesticides, soil, air pollution, refined grains, rice, coffee, tea, and soft drinks.

NUTRIENTS

SUPPLEMENT	SUGGESTED DOSAGE	COMMENTS
Important		
Alfalfa		*See under* Herbs, below.
Calcium and magnesium	2,000 mg daily. 1,000 mg daily.	Minerals that help rid the body of cadmium.
Garlic (Kyolic)	2 capsules 3 times daily.	Helps to rid the body of cadmium. A potent detoxifier.
Lecithin granules or capsules	2 tbsp 3 times daily, with meals. 2,400 mg 3 times daily, with meals. Take with vitamin E (see below) for better assimilation.	Protects all cells.
L-cysteine and L-lysine and L-methionine	500 mg each daily, on an empty stomach. Take with water or juice. Do not take with milk. Take with 50 mg vitamin B$_6$ and 100 mg vitamin C for better absorption.	These amino acids act as antioxidants; they protect the organs, especially the liver. *See* AMINO ACIDS in Part One.
Rutin	200 mg 3 times daily. Take with 100 mg vitamin C.	Aids in removing high amounts of metals from the body.
Vitamin E	600–1,000 IU daily.	An antioxidant. Use emulsion form for easier assimilation.
Zinc	50–80 mg daily. Do not exceed a total of 100 mg daily from all supplements.	Needed to restore zinc displaced by cadmium, and to prevent cadmium levels from rising.
Helpful		
Copper	3 mg daily.	Works with zinc to remove cadmium deposits.
Iron or Floradix Iron + Herbs from Salus Haus	As directed by physician. Take with 100 mg vitamin C for better absorption. As directed on label.	To correct deficiency. Use ferrous fumarate form. *Caution:* Do not take iron unless anemia is diagnosed. Contains nontoxic, natural iron from food sources that is easily assimilated into the body.

HERBS

❑ Alfalfa contains chlorophyll and vitamin K, and helps to remove cadmium from the body. Take 2,000 to 3,000 milligrams in tablet form daily.

RECOMMENDATIONS

❑ If you suspect cadmium toxicity, have a hair analysis done to determine the level of toxic metals in your system. *See* HAIR ANALYSIS in Part Three.

❑ Make sure that you include plenty of fiber and apple pectin in your diet. Also eat pumpkin seeds and other foods that are high in zinc.

CONSIDERATIONS

❑ Chelation removes toxic metals from the body. (*See* CHELATION THERAPY in Part Three.)

❑ *See also* ENVIRONMENTAL TOXICITY in Part Two.

Cancer

When your body is injured—for example, if you have a cut—the cells surrounding the cut reproduce to replace the ones that have been harmed. These cells "know" to stop reproducing once they have filled in the injured area.

Sometimes, however, a cell begins to reproduce for no obvious reason. The "daughter" cells that it produces form a lump. This is cancer. Often, a cell from this lump, or tumor, spreads to another part of the body and begins reproduction there. These cells are not receptive to the normal signal to stop reproducing. Eventually, this abnormal tissue interferes with the ability of the body and its cells, organs, and other structures to perform their appointed functions, and illness or death results.

No one knows exactly why some cells behave in this way. We do know, however, that certain things increase the likelihood of certain types of cancer. Environmental factors and diet are widely believed to be two of the major causes of cancer. Persons exposed to cigarette smoke have significantly higher rates of lung cancer than other people. Regular alcohol consumption increases the risk of mouth and throat cancers. A diet that is high in fat and low in fiber is associated with a greater risk of colorectal cancer, and is a factor in breast and prostate cancer as well. Many experts believe that what these apparently different risk factors have in common is that they increase the body's exposure to free radicals. They theorize that damage from free radicals is an important factor in causing the uncontrolled cellular growth that is characteristic of cancer (*see* Free Radicals on page 44). Others believe that factors such as cigarette smoking and poor dietary habits increase the risk of cancer because they impair the immune system. In addition to blaming diet and environmental pollutants, many experts link cancer to stress.

In the United States, one person dies from cancer every minute. Another 3 million have cancer, and one out of three will eventually die of some form of this disease. There are more than 100 different varieties of cancer. They have different causes, cause different symptoms, and vary in aggressiveness (the speed at which they spread). However, most types of cancer fall into one of four broad categories:

1. Carcinomas affect the skin, mucous membranes, glands, and internal organs.

2. Leukemias are cancers of blood-forming tissues.

3. Sarcomas affect muscles, connective tissue, and bones.

4. Lymphomas affect the lymphatic system.

The nutritional program and other recommendations outlined in this section are designed for persons who have been diagnosed with cancer, as well as for those who wish

The Warning Signs and Possible Causes of Certain Cancers

Knowing early warning signs and factors that increase the risk of developing different forms of cancer can save your life. The American Cancer Society estimates that there are 170,000 or more deaths from cancer in the United States each year that could have been prevented. The table below indicates the risks and signs that have been associated with various types of cancer. If you experience one or more of the symptoms described, that does not necessarily mean you have cancer (many can be caused by other, less serious disorders as well), but you should consult your health care provider for an evaluation.

Type of Cancer	Risk Factors	Symptoms
Bladder and kidney	Exposure to certain chemicals, such as benzidines, aniline dyes, naphthalenes; smoking; excessive consumption of caffeine and/or artificial sweeteners; a history of schistosomiasis (a tropical disease); frequent urinary tract infections.	Blood in the urine; pain and burning with urination; increased frequency of urination.
Breast	First childbirth after age 35; having no children; family history of cancer; high alcohol and/or caffeine intake; high-fat diet; diabetes. There is a link between sugar intake in older women and breast cancer. Estrogens and oral contraceptives have also been linked to breast and uterine cancer.	Lump(s), thickening, and other physical changes in the breast; itching, redness, and/or soreness of the nipples not associated with breastfeeding.
Cervical and uterine	More than 5 complete pregnancies; first intercourse before age 18; a history of gonorrhea or genital warts; multiple sex partners; infertility.	Bleeding between menstrual periods; unusual discharge; painful menstrual periods; heavy periods.
Colon	Lack of dietary fiber and calcium; polyps; family history of colon cancer; continued constipation and/or diarrhea; a buildup of toxins in the colon; a high-fat diet.	Rectal bleeding; blood in the stool; changes in bowel habits (persistent diarrhea and/or constipation).
Endometrial	Never having been pregnant; being past menopause; family history of cancer; diabetes; obesity; hypertension.	Bleeding between menstrual periods; unusual discharge; painful menstrual periods; heavy periods.
Laryngeal	Heavy smoking; alcohol consumption.	Persistent cough; hoarse throat.
Leukemia	Hereditary factors; radiation exposure; chronic viral infections.	Paleness; fatigue; weight loss; repeated infections; easy bruising; bone and joint pain; nosebleeds.
Lung	Smoking; exposure to asbestos, nickel, chromates, or radioactive materials; chronic bronchitis; history of tuberculosis; exposure to certain chemicals, such as pesticides and herbicides.	A persistent cough; sputum with blood; chest pain.
Lymphoma	Hereditary factors; immune system dysfunction. At least some cases are linked to a viral cause.	Enlarged, rubbery lymph nodes; itching; night sweats; unexplained fever and/or weight loss.
Mouth and Throat	Irritants inside the mouth, such as a broken tooth, or ill-fitting or broken dentures; excessive alcohol intake; smoking; use of chewing tobacco.	A chronic ulcer of the mouth, tongue, or throat that does not heal.

Type of Cancer	Risk Factors	Symptoms
Ovarian	Not having had children; high-fat diet.	Often no obvious symptoms until it is in its later stages of development.
Prostate	Recurring prostate infection; history of venereal disease; diet high in animal fat; high intake of milk, meat, and/or coffee; use of male hormone testosterone in treatment of impotence; vasectomy; being over age 50.	Weak or interrupted urine flow; continuous pain in the lower back, pelvis, and/or upper thighs.
Skin	Exposure to the sun, especially for those who have fair skin; history of moles (malignant or otherwise); moles on the feet or in areas irritated by clothing; scars from severe burns and scars or sores that won't heal; family history of skin cancer.	Tumor or lump under the skin, resembling a wart or an ulceration that never heals; moles that change color or size; flat sores; lesions that look like moles.
Stomach	Pernicious anemia; lack of hydrochloric acid and dietary fiber; high-fat diet; chronic gastritis; stomach polyps.	Indigestion and pain after eating; weight loss.
Testicular	Undescended testicle.	Lump(s); enlargement of a testicle; thickening of the scrotum; sudden collection of fluid in the scrotum; pain or discomfort in a testicle or in the scrotum; mild ache in the lower abdomen or groin; enlargement or tenderness of the breasts.

Projected U.S. Cancer Rates by State

Information regarding the projected incidence (cases per 1,000 individuals) of new cases of cancer of all types by state was developed from data provided by the American Cancer Society and the U.S. Bureau of the Census. The states below are listed from highest to lowest projected incidence of cancer.

1. Florida
2. West Virginia
3. Pennsylvania
4. Arkansas
5. Maine
6. Kentucky
7. District of Columbia
8. Delaware
9. Rhode Island
10. New Jersey
11. Missouri
12. Oregon
13. Tennessee
14. Massachusetts
15. Nevada
16. North Dakota
17. Ohio
18. Alabama
19. Iowa
20. Mississippi
21. Montana
22. Oklahoma
23. Tennessee
24. Wisconsin
25. Kansas
26. Indiana
27. Illinois
28. South Carolina
29. Arizona
30. Maryland
31. Louisiana
32. Michigan
33. Connecticut
34. New York
35. South Dakota
36. Nebraska
37. Vermont
38. Washington
39. Virginia
40. New Hampshire
41. Minnesota
42. Texas
43. Georgia
44. Idaho
45. Wyoming
46. Colorado
47. California
48. New Mexico
49. Hawaii
50. Utah
51. Alaska

to enhance their chances of avoiding this disease. Vitamins should be taken in injection form whenever possible. If you must use oral supplements, take them daily with meals (except for vitamin E, which should be taken before meals). Use only *natural* vitamin supplements.

SELF-TESTS

Breast Cancer Self-Test

See under BREAST CANCER in Part Two.

Colon Cancer Self-Test

A test kit can be purchased at most drugstores for detecting blood in the stool (an early sign of colon cancer). In one test, you simply drop a strip of chemically treated paper into the commode after a bowel movement. The paper will change to the color blue if blood is present in the stool.

If your test result is positive, take a second test in three days. If the second test is also positive, see your physician immediately. The presence of blood in the stool does *not* necessarily mean that you have cancer. The consumption of red meat or the presence of diverticulitis, hemorrhoids, polyps, ulcers, or an inflamed colon can all cause a positive test result. About 10 percent of those who test positive for blood in the stool have cancer.

Testicular Cancer Self-Test

With the fingers of both hands, gently roll each testicle between the thumb and the fingers, checking for hard lumps or nodules. If you find a suspicious lump, see your physician. You will be better able to feel for lumps if you check for them after a warm bath or shower, when the scrotal skin is relaxed.

NUTRIENTS

SUPPLEMENT	SUGGESTED DOSAGE	COMMENTS
Essential		
Coenzyme Q10	90 mg daily.	Improves cellular oxygenation.
Dimethylglycine (DMG) (Aangamik DMG from FoodScience Labs)	As directed on label.	Enhances oxygen utilization.
Garlic (Kyolic)	2 capsules 3 times daily.	Enhances immune function.
Melatonin	2–3 mg daily, taken 2 hours or less before bedtime.	A powerful antioxidant that also aids sleep.
Natural beta-carotene or	25,000 IU daily.	Needed by all cells for repair and rebuilding.
carotenoid complex	As directed on label.	
Omega-3 Forte and	As directed on label.	For repair and production of new cells.
Omega-Plex, both from American Biologics	As directed on label.	

Proteolytic enzymes or Wobenzym N from Marlyn Nutraceuticals	As directed on label. Take with meals. 2–6 tablets 2–3 times daily, between meals.	Powerful free radical scavengers.
Selenium	200 mcg daily.	Powerful free radical scavenger. Aids in protein digestion.
Shark cartilage (BeneFin)	For cancer treatment, 1 gm per 2 lbs of body weight daily, divided into 3 doses. If you cannot tolerate taking it orally, it can be administered in a retention enema. For cancer prevention, 2,000–4,500 mg 3 times daily.	Has been shown to inhibit and even reverse the growth of some types of tumors. Also stimulates the immune system.
Superoxide dismutase (SOD)	As directed on label.	Destroys free radicals. Consider injections (under a doctor's supervision).
Vitamin A and	50,000–100,000 IU daily for 10 days, then 50,000 IU daily for 30 days, then reduce to 25,000 IU daily. If you are pregnant, do not exceed 10,000 IU daily.	People with cancer require higher than normal amounts of this antioxidant. Use emulsion form for easier assimilation and greater safety at higher doses. Capsule forms put more stress on the liver.
vitamin E	Up to 1,000 IU daily.	A powerful antioxidant and cancer-fighter. Use emulsion form for easier assimilation and greater safety at high doses.
Vitamin B complex plus	100 mg daily.	Necessary for normal cell division and function.
brewer's yeast	1 tsp daily for 1 week, then gradually increase to 1 tbsp 3 times daily.	A good source of B vitamins.
Vitamin C with bioflavonoids	5,000–20,000 mg daily, in divided doses. *See* ASCORBIC ACID FLUSH in Part Three.	Powerful anticancer agent that promotes the production of interferon in the body.
Important		
Maitake	As directed on label.	Contains a substance that prevents carcinogenesis and inhibits the growth of cancerous tumors. Also helps the body adapt to the stress of cancer treatments such as chemotherpy.
Shiitake or	As directed on label.	Has valuable immune-boosting and anti-tumor properties.
reishi	As directed on label.	
Helpful		
Acidophilus	As directed on label. Take on an empty stomach.	Has an antibacterial effect on the body. Use a nondairy formula.
Aerobic 07 from Aerobic Life Industries or	As directed on label.	Antimicrobial agents.
Dioxychlor from American Biologics	As directed on label.	
Chromium picolinate	At least 600 mcg daily.	Helps to build and maintain muscle mass. Useful if muscle atrophy exists.
Grape seed extract	As directed on label.	A powerful antioxidant.

Kelp or seaweed	1,000–1,500 mg daily. As directed on label.	For mineral balance and to help the body avoid damage resulting from radiation therapy.
L-Carnitine	As directed on label.	Protects against damage from free radicals and toxins. Use a form derived from fish liver (squalene).
Multienzyme complex	As directed on label, with meals.	To aid digestion. Caution: Do not give this supplement to a child.
Multimineral complex with		Essential for normal cell division and function. Use a comprehensive formula that contains all major minerals and trace elements except iron.
calcium and	2,000 mg daily.	
magnesium and	1,000 mg daily.	
potassium	99 mg daily.	
Multivitamin complex	As directed on label, with meals.	Do not use a sustained-release formula. Use a formula without iron.
N-Acetylcysteine plus L-methionine	As directed on label, on an empty stomach. Take with water or juice. Do not take with milk. Take with 50 mg vitamin B_6 and 100 mg vitamin C for better absorption.	To detoxify harmful substances and protect the liver and other organs. See AMINO ACIDS in Part One.
Taurine	As directed on label.	Functions as foundation for tissue and organ repair.
Vitamin B_3 (niacin) and choline	100 mg daily. Do not exceed this amount. 500–1,000 mg daily.	B vitamins that improve circulation, build red blood cells, and aid liver function. Caution: Do not take niacin if you have a liver disorder, gout, or high blood pressure.
plus vitamin B_{12}	2,000 mcg daily.	To prevent anemia. Use a lozenge or sublingual form.
Raw glandular complex plus	As directed on label.	Stimulates glandular function, especially the thymus (site of T lymphocyte production).
raw thymus and	As directed on label.	See GLANDULAR THERAPY in Part Three.
raw spleen glandulars	As directed on label.	

HERBS

❑ Include some of the following in your cancer prevention or cancer therapy program: dandelion, echinacea, green tea, pau d'arco, red clover, and suma.

❑ Many people with external cancers, such as skin cancers, have responded well to poultices made from comfrey, pau d'arco, ragwort, and wood sage. See USING A POULTICE in Part Three.

Note: Comfrey is recommended for external use only.

❑ Cat's claw enhances immune function and has anti-tumor properties. Cat's Claw Defense Complex from Source Naturals is a combination of cat's claw and other herbs, plus antioxidant nutrients such as beta-carotene, N-acetylcysteine, vitamin C, and zinc.

Caution: Do not use cat's claw during pregnancy.

❑ Essiac from Resperin Corporation is an herbal remedy

that activates the body's natural defenses, helps relieve pain, and has anti-tumor properties. Many people with cancer have credited it with extending and improving the quality of their lives. Jason Winters Tea from Tri-Sun International is a combination herbal tea that is good as well.

RECOMMENDATIONS

❑ Eat a diet that includes grains, nuts, seeds, and unpolished brown rice. Millet cereal is a good source of protein. Eat wheat, oat, and bran.

❑ Eat plenty of cruciferous vegetables, such as broccoli, Brussels sprouts, cabbage, and cauliflower. Also consume yellow and deep-orange vegetables such as carrots, pumpkin, squash, and yams. Apples, berries, Brazil nuts, cantaloupes, cherries, grapes, legumes (including chickpeas, lentils, and red beans), and plums all help to fight cancer. Berries protect DNA from damage.

❑ Cook all sprouts slightly (except for alfalfa sprouts, which should be eaten raw).

❑ Eat onions and garlic, or take garlic in supplement form.

❑ Eat ten raw almonds every day. They contain laetrile, which has anticancer properties.

❑ Drink beet juice (from roots and greens), carrot juice (a source of beta-carotene), fresh cabbage juice, and asparagus juice often. Grape, black cherry, and all dark-colored juices are good, as are black currants. Also beneficial is apple juice, if it is fresh. Fruit juices are best taken in the morning, vegetable juices in the afternoon.

❑ Drink spring or steam-distilled water only, not tap water.

❑ Do not consume any of the following: peanuts, junk foods, processed refined foods, saturated fats, salt, sugar, or white flour. Instead of salt, use kelp or a potassium substitute. If necessary, a small amount of blackstrap molasses or pure maple syrup can be used as a natural sweetener in place of sugar. Use whole wheat or rye instead of white flour. Do not consume anything containing alcohol or caffeine. Avoid all teas except for herbal teas.

❑ Do not eat any animal protein—never eat luncheon meat, hot dogs, or smoked or cured meats. As your condition improves, eat broiled fish three times a week.

❑ Limit your consumption of dairy products; a little yogurt, kefir, or raw cheese occasionally is enough.

❑ Limit, but do not eliminate altogether, your intake of soybean products; they contain enzyme inhibitors.

❑ See FASTING in Part Three, and follow the program.

❑ Take coffee enemas daily to help the body eliminate toxins. Use cleansing enemas with lemon and water or garlic and water two or three times weekly. See ENEMAS in Part Three.

❑ Do not take supplemental iron. The body naturally withholds iron from cancer cells to inhibit their growth.

❑ Use only glass cookware and wooden cooking utensils.

❑ Get regular exercise. Cancer is less prevalent in physically active people. Exercise also helps to stave off depression and promotes oxygenation of the tissues.

❑ Because of potential low-level radiation leakage, avoid microwave ovens. Do not sit close to television sets—sit at least eight feet away. Also avoid x-rays.

❑ Avoid chemicals such as hair sprays, cleaning compounds, waxes, fresh paints, and garden pesticides. Do not use any products in aerosol cans. Many chemicals promote the formation of free radicals in the body, which may lead to cancer. People with cancer can further weaken their immune systems by coming into contact with chemicals. The body then must expend energy trying to protect itself from the damaging chemicals instead of fighting the cancer.

❑ Remove known and suspected carcinogens from your life and from your home. *The Safe Shoppers Bible* by David Steinman and Samuel S. Epstein, M.D. (Macmillan, 1995) provides information on the safety of many different types of products, including cleaning products, paints, pesticides, pet supplies, auto products, art and craft supplies, cosmetics, personal care products, as well as foods and beverages. Another good source of information is Mary Kerney Levenstein's *Everyday Cancer Risks and How to Avoid Them* (Avery Publishing Group, 1992).

❑ Do not take any drugs except for those prescribed by your physician.

❑ As much as possible, avoid stress. Learn relaxation and stress management techniques to help you deal with those stresses you cannot avoid. *See* STRESS in Part Two.

CONSIDERATIONS

❑ The amount of data linking diet and nutrition to the development of cancer is massive, and is continuing to grow. Some of these connections include:

• A lack of the nutrients beta-carotene, vitamin E, and the B vitamins in lung tissue may be related to lung cancer.

• Calcium may prevent precancerous cells from becoming cancerous.

• People in Japan and Iceland have low rates of both goiter and breast cancer. In fact, breast cancer is almost nonexistent in Japanese women. Colon cancer rates in Japan are also low. Breast cancer has been linked to iodine deficiency, and the soil in both Japan and Iceland is rich in both iodine and selenium. Japanese people also consume large amounts of fish, which may be a factor. The Cancer Control Convention in Japan has reported that germanium may be important in the prevention and cure of cancer.

• Obesity in men may cause or contribute to colon and rectal cancer; in women, it has been linked to gallbladder, cervical, uterine, and breast cancer. Overweight women are more likely to develop cancer of the uterine lining than other women and

tend to do poorly if they develop breast cancer. Fat affects the level of sex hormones in the body. Hormones produced by the adrenal glands are converted into estrogen in fat tissue, so the greater the amount of fat present, the higher a woman's estrogen levels are likely to be. Estrogen stimulates cells in the breast and reproductive system to divide.

• People with excess iron levels in their blood tend to have an increased risk of developing cancer. Excess iron may suppress the cancer-killing function of macrophages (cells that engulf and devour bacteria and other foreign invaders) and interfere with the activity of lymphocytes.

• Niacin has been discovered to play a major role in the prevention and treatment of cancer.

• A high-fat diet dramatically increases the incidence of colon and breast cancer, as compared to a low-fat diet. High dietary fat is a promoter of cancer.

• The incidence of leukemia among children who were breastfed has been found to be significantly lower than that among bottlefed children.

❑ Surveys indicate that 40 percent of the U.S. population rarely consume any fruit or fruit juices, and 20 percent never eat vegetables. In addition, 80 percent of Americans do not consume quality high-fiber cereals or whole-grain bread. Meanwhile, more than 85,000 Americans are diagnosed as having colon cancer each year, and that number is growing.

❑ A group of seventy-five Environmental Protection Agency (EPA) experts ranked pesticide residues among the top three environmental cancer risks.

❑ People whose mothers smoked during pregnancy are 50 percent more likely than children of nonsmoking mothers to develop cancer later in life. These findings confirm the harmful effects smoking has on the developing fetus.

❑ The risk of prostate cancer for males who have undergone vasectomies may be as much as three times greater than that of males who have not had vasectomies.

❑ The single most *avoidable* cancer risk is smoking. Lung cancer was a rare disease until the twentieth century, when cigarette smoking became widespread. Today lung cancer is the leading cause of cancer death in the United States.

❑ It is now thought that intestinal cancer takes about twenty years to develop.

❑ Some types of cancer are treated with chemotherapy and can apparently be cured with this treatment. Cancer chemotherapy is the administration of highly toxic medications meant to kill cancer cells. Side effects of chemotherapy can include hair loss, extreme nausea, vomiting, fatigue, weakness, sterility, and damage to the kidneys and heart. Certain nutrients may help the body avoid some of the damage done by this treatment, among them vitamin B_6 (pyridoxine) and coenzyme Q_{10}.

❑ Many people with cancer have achieved good results with a macrobiotic diet.

Alternative Cancer Therapies

A growing number of people with cancer are now benefiting from alternative means of cancer treatment. Some of the available alternative therapies provide help by strengthening the body and controlling the side effects of conventional treatments. Other approaches, because of their gentle, noninvasive nature, may in some cases be preferred over more orthodox treatments.

Although there are a large number of different alternative therapies, most of them do have common themes. For instance, many of them are based on the belief that a truly healthy body is less vulnerable to cancer. They emphasize that cancer develops as the result of a problem with the immune system or an imbalance in the body, either or both of which may allow the cancer to develop. Thus, they try to reduce or eliminate the underlying problem that allowed the cancer to take hold, and to activate the body's own inherent healing processes so that the body can heal itself.

Usually, alternative treatments are holistic in approach. This means that the goal is to treat the whole body, rather than just the area seemingly affected by the cancer. Many also aim to treat the individual on a number of different levels, including physical, mental, spiritual, and emotional.

TYPES OF ALTERNATIVE TREATMENTS

Most of the alternative treatments used in cancer therapy fall into one of the following categories: biologic and pharmacologic therapies, immunologic therapies, herbal therapies, metabolic therapies, mind-body therapies, and nutritional therapies. Although there is a certain amount of overlapping between categories—an immunologic therapy, for instance, may have nutritional components—these categories do serve to highlight the central focus of the many treatments and regimens that fall within them. Be aware though, that the following discussion by no means mentions all of the individual therapies available. It is meant to familiarize you with the various approaches that may be used.

Biologic and Pharmacologic Therapies

These therapies use biologic substances or nontoxic pharmacologic agents—nontoxic medications usually derived from biological sources, such as plants or human cells. Each of these treatments works in a different way. Antineoplaston therapy, for instance, uses amino acid derivatives to inhibit the growth of cancer cells. Another such treatment, shark cartilage therapy, is thought to work by blocking angiogenesis, the creation of new blood vessels required for tumor growth, and thus starve the tumor of needed nourishment.

Immunologic Therapies

Immunologic therapies are based on the belief that cancer develops because of a breakdown of the immune system. The aim of these therapies is to bolster those parts of the immune system that combat and destroy cancer cells. Examples of the treatments in this category include the

therapy of Dr. Virginia Livingston, which uses vaccines, diet, nutritional supplements, and gamma globulin; and Dr. Josef Issels' whole-body program, which uses vaccines, diet, and fever therapy.

Herbal Therapies

In these therapies, herbal remedies—probably the oldest form of treatment in the world—are used to strengthen the body's ability to eliminate cancer cells. Hoxsey therapy, for instance, employs internal and external herbal preparations, along with diet, vitamin and mineral supplements, and psychological counseling, to strengthen the body and fight the cancer.

Metabolic Therapies

These therapies are based on the idea that many factors cause the occurrence of cancer, and that a multifaceted healing approach is required to eliminate the disorder. The therapies use detoxification, including colon cleansing, to flush out toxins; anticancer diets based on whole foods; and vitamins, minerals, and enzymes, which further cleanse the body, repair damaged tissues, and stimulate immune function. Dr. Max Gerson's therapy—which is based on a diet of organically grown fresh fruits and vegetables, as well as nutritional supplements—is one such regimen.

Mind-Body Therapies

These treatments focus on the role that emotions, behavior, and faith play in recovery from illness. In the case of some therapies, counseling, hypnosis, biofeedback, or other techniques are used to promote greater emotional and spiritual well-being. In other therapies, the aim is to use mind-body techniques to actually change the course of the illness, possibly bringing the person into remission. For instance, Dr. O. Carl Simonton and Stephanie Matthews-Simonton have developed a visualization technique to help patients increase the effectiveness of their immune systems.

Nutritional Therapies

Therapies that focus on nutrition are perhaps the most popular alternative approach to cancer, especially since research began showing the link between diet and health. For instance, studies have indicated that a high-fat diet increases the risk of cancer, while a low-fat diet that is rich in fiber, fresh fruits and vegetables, and whole grains actually helps the body to fight cancer. Three of the therapies that fall into this category are wheatgrass therapy, a diet based on wheatgrass and other raw foods; the macrobiotic diet, a traditional Japanese diet high in whole grains and vegetables; and the Moerman regimen, a meatless high-fiber diet that includes nutritional supplements.

CHOOSING AN ALTERNATIVE THERAPY

Unless you already have a specific therapy in mind, the first step in choosing one is to learn more about those that are available. By visiting libraries and bookstores and contacting health organizations that focus on cancer, you should be able to find a number of comprehensive, up-to-date books that provide additional information about alternative treatments. Richard Walters' *Options: The Alternative Cancer Therapy Book* (Avery Publishing Group, 1993) can help you evaluate and compare a number of alternative cancer therapies, as can Ralph Moss's *Cancer Therapy: The Independent Consumer's Guide to Non-Toxic Treatment & Prevention* (Equinox Press, 1995).

Once you have a better idea of the therapy or therapies that would best serve your needs, contact educational organizations and patient-referral services that provide information on these treatments. *Options*, mentioned above, provides a list of these groups. Another good source of information is John Fink's *Third Opinion: An International Directory to Alternative Therapy Centers for the Treatment and Prevention of Cancer and Other Degenerative Diseases* (Avery Publishing Group, 1992).

When researching a particular therapy, try to get information from other people who have used that treatment. Some information organizations and some alternative clinics will provide lists of recovered patients whom you can call or write to. Focus on those people who have the same kind of cancer you have, and ask them what specific treatments they found helpful.

When screening alternative practitioners and clinics, ask what their success has been in treating your specific form of cancer. Keep in mind that a therapy that is effective against one type of cancer will not necessarily be effective against another. Ask to see supportive studies, documented cases, and patients' testimonials, and view all information with a healthy dose of skepticism. As much as possible, pin the practitioner down regarding what you can expect from the treatment—short-term improvement or long-term survival, for instance. Finally, consider whether the therapy fits in with your lifestyle, personality, and belief system. Be honest with yourself. Some therapies may require a degree of commitment that you are not willing to make. Others may require too much time, too much travel, or too much money to truly be feasible.

❑ In some cases, radiation therapy may be recommended. This involves aiming concentrated x-rays directly at a tumor to kill the cancerous cells. Radiation therapy too has unpleasant side effects, including fever, headache, nausea and vomiting, and loss of appetite.

❑ Shark cartilage has been shown to be helpful for certain types of cancer, including cancer of the breast, cervix, pancreas, and prostate, as well as Kaposi's sarcoma, a type of skin cancer. It suppresses angiogenesis (the development of new blood vessels), depriving cancerous tumors of nourishment and, often, causing them to shrink and die.

❑ Hyperbaric oxygen therapy has been effective in reducing the death of healthy tissue due to radiation treatment for cancer (*see* HYPERBARIC OXYGEN THERAPY in Part Three).

❑ German physician Dr. Hans Nieper has been using fresh raw cabbage and carrot juice with excellent results. Dr. Nieper also uses Carnivora, a substance derived from a South American plant, to fight cancer.

❑ Some physicians use dimethylsulfoxide (DMSO), either alone or in combination with other therapies, to treat certain forms of cancer.

❑ The hormone dehydroepiandrosterone (DHEA) is believed to help prevent cancer by blocking an enzyme that promotes cancer cell growth. (*See* DHEA THERAPY in Part Three.)

❑ Kombucha tea has energizing and immune-boosting properties, and may be valuable in fighting cancer. (*See* MAKING KOMBUCHA TEA in Part Three.)

❑ Dr. Virginia Livingston of the Livingston-Wheeler Clinic in San Diego developed a vaccine against an organism called *Progenitor cryptocides*. According to Dr. Livingston, if the immune system is weakened through poor diet, the consumption of "infected" foods, or old age, this microbe can gain a foothold and initiate cancer cell growth. She claimed that nine out of ten people who are treated with her vaccine, plus dietary and vitamin therapy, experience improvement.

❑ *See also* BREAST CANCER; PROSTATE CANCER; SKIN CANCER; and TUMORS, all in Part Two.

❑ *See also* PAIN CONTROL in Part Three.

Candidiasis

Candida albicans is a type of parasitic yeastlike fungus that inhabits the intestines, genital tract, mouth, esophagus, and throat. Normally this fungus lives in healthy balance with the other bacteria and yeasts in the body; however, certain conditions can cause it to multiply, weakening the immune system and causing an infection known as candidiasis. The fungus can travel through the bloodstream to many parts of the body.

Because candidiasis can affect various parts of the body—the most common being the mouth, ears, nose, gastrointestinal tract, and vagina—it can be characterized by many symptoms. These include constipation, diarrhea, colitis, abdominal pain, headaches, bad breath, rectal itching, impotence, memory loss, mood swings, prostatitis, canker sores, persistent heartburn, muscle and joint pain, sore throat, congestion, nagging cough, numbness in the face or extremities, tingling sensations, acne, night sweats, severe itching, clogged sinuses, PMS, burning tongue, white spots on the tongue and in the mouth, extreme fatigue, vaginitis, kidney and bladder infections, arthritis, depression, hyperactivity, hypothyroidism, adrenal problems, and even diabetes. Symptoms often worsen in damp and/or moldy places, and after consumption of foods containing sugar and/or yeast. Because of its many and varied symptoms, this disorder is often misdiagnosed.

When candida infects the vagina, it results in vaginitis characterized by a large amount of white, cheesy discharge and intense itching and burning. When the fungus infects the oral cavity, it is called thrush. White sores may form on the tongue, gums, and inside the cheeks. In a baby, the white spots of oral thrush may resemble milk spots. Oral thrush in an infant can spread to the mother's nipples by breastfeeding, and can lead to a situation in which mother and baby continually reinfect each other. Thrush may also infect a baby's buttocks, appearing as a diaper rash. Candida infection may also take the form of athlete's foot or jock itch. *Systemic candidiasis* is an overgrowth of candida everywhere, throughout the body. In the most severe cases, candida can travel through the bloodstream to invade every organ system in the body, causing a type of blood poisoning called *candida septicemia*. This condition almost always occurs in persons with serious underlying illnesses, such as advanced cancer or AIDS.

Candidiasis may affect both men and women; however, it is rarely transmitted sexually. It is most common in babies (an infected mother may pass the fungal infection to her newborn) and in persons with compromised immune systems. Virtually all people with AIDS have some type of fungal infection. Anyone who has been on long-term antibiotic therapy, or has taken antibiotics often, probably has an overgrowth of candida somewhere in his or her body. Antibiotics weaken the immune system and also destroy the "friendly" bacteria that normally keep candida under control. As it proliferates, the fungus releases toxins that weaken the immune system further. Other factors that increase the chances of contracting a yeast infection include pregnancy and the use of corticosteroid drugs.

Very often, allergies to foods are present in people with candida infections. Oral thrush, athlete's foot, ringworm, jock itch, fingernail or toenail fungus, and even diaper rash can develop as a result of the combination of food allergies and *C. albicans*. The symptoms of a food allergy or environmental sensitivity can also mimic those of candidiasis. To further complicate matters, some people with candidiasis go on to develop environmental sensitivities as well. Many cannot tolerate contact with rubber, petroleum products, tobacco, exhaust fumes, and chemical odors.

NUTRIENTS

SUPPLEMENT	SUGGESTED DOSAGE	COMMENTS
Very Important		
Essential fatty acids (black currant seed oil and flaxseed oil are good sources)	As directed on label.	Important in healing and preventing the fungus from destroying cells.
Acidophilus or Bio-Bifidus from American Biologics	As directed on label. Take on an empty stomach. As directed on label.	Fights candida infection. Use a nondairy formula.
or Eugalan Forte from Bio Nutritional	As directed on label.	
or Kyo-Dophilus from Wakunaga	As directed on label.	
Caprylic acid (Caprystatin from Ecological Formulas, Capralin from Synergy Plus)	As directed on label.	An antifungal agent that destroys the candida organism.
Dioxychlor from American Biologics	5 drops in water twice daily.	A stabilized oxygen product that destroys the fungus while preserving the "good" bacteria.
Garlic (Kyolic)	2 capsules 3 times daily. For candida vaginitis, use Kyolic vaginal suppositories as directed on label.	Inhibits the infecting organism.
Quercetin plus bromelain	500 mg twice daily, 30 minutes before meals. 100 mg twice daily, 30 minutes before meals.	Speeds healing and reduces the effects of food allergies and inflammation. Improves absorption of quercetin.
or Activated Quercetin from Source Naturals	As directed on label.	Contains quercetin plus bromelain and vitamin C for increased absorption.
Vitamin B complex	100 mg 3 times daily.	B vitamins are required for all bodily functions, resistance to infection, and all enzyme systems. Important for brain function. Use a yeast-free formula. Consider injections (under a doctor's supervision).
plus extra biotin	50 mg 3 times daily.	Needed for healthy skin.
plus vitamin B12	2,000 mcg 3 times daily.	Important for digestion. Needed for metabolism of carbohydrates, fats, and proteins. Use a lozenge or sublingual form.
Important		
Calcium	1,500 mg daily.	Often deficient in people with this disorder. Use calcium citrate form.
and magnesium	750–1,000 mg daily.	Needed to balance with calcium.
and vitamin D	400 IU daily.	Enhances calcium absorption.
Helpful		
Coenzyme Q10	100 mg daily.	Improves tissue oxygenation.
Free-form amino acid complex	As directed on label. Take between meals, on an empty stomach.	Rebuilds damaged tissue. Use a sublingual form for best absorption.
Glutathione	500 mg twice daily.	Needed for brain function. Candida impairs brain function.
Multivitamin and mineral complex with vitamin A	25,000 IU daily. If you are pregnant, do not exceed 10,000 IU daily.	All nutrients are needed for proper immune function and for repair of intestinal lining and all tissues; build resistance to infection. Choose a yeast-free formula that includes zinc and iron.
and natural beta-carotene	15,000 IU daily.	
and selenium	200 mcg daily.	

184

Grapefruit seed extract	As directed on label. Always dilute before use.	Rids the body of potentially harmful microorganisms.
L-Cysteine	500 mg twice daily, on an empty stomach. Take with water or juice. Do not take with milk. Take with 50 mg vitamin B$_6$ and 100 mg vitamin C for better absorption.	A potent antioxidant and free radical destroyer. *See* AMINO ACIDS in Part One.
Orithrush from Ecological Formulas	Use as a mouth rinse or as a douche.	Destroys candida.
Vitamin C	1,000 mg 3 times daily.	Builds up immunity and protects the body tissues from damage by the toxins released from candida. Use an esterified form.

HERBS

❑ Pau d'arco (also known as lapacho or taheebo) contains an antibacterial and antifungal agent, although it does have an alkaloid base and a small percentage of people may not benefit from its use. If you do not benefit from this tea, try clove tea instead. It is a good idea to alternate between the two, because clove tea has some benefits that pau d'arco does not have and vice versa. To make pau d'arco tea, boil 1 quart of distilled water with 2 tablespoons of herb for five minutes. Cool and store it in the refrigerator with the tea leaves in. Strain before drinking, if needed. Drink 3 to 6 cups daily.

❑ Some people who no longer respond to pau d'arco can benefit from maitake tea. It is a good alternative. While pau d'arco must be boiled, maitake is prepared as a regular tea. Resistant strains of candida develop rapidly due to genetic mutation. Rotating treatment programs is beneficial.

RECOMMENDATIONS

❑ Eat vegetables, fish, and gluten-free grains such as brown rice and millet.

❑ Eat plain yogurt that contains live yogurt cultures. For vaginal candidiasis, apply yogurt directly to the vagina. This helps to inhibit the growth of the fungus.

❑ Take supplemental acidophilus or bifidus to help to restore the normal balance of flora in the bowel and vagina.

❑ Take some type of fiber daily. Oat bran is a good source.

❑ Drink distilled water only.

❑ Make sure the diet is fruit-free, sugar-free, and yeast-free. Candida thrives in a sugary environment, so your diet should be low in carbohydrates and contain no yeast products or sugar in any form.

❑ Avoid aged cheeses, alcohol, baked goods, chocolate, dried fruits, fermented foods, all grains containing gluten (wheat, oats, rye, and barley), ham, honey, nut butters, pickles, potatoes, raw mushrooms, soy sauce, sprouts, and vinegar.

❑ Eliminate citrus and acidic fruits such as oranges, grapefruit, lemons, tomatoes, pineapple, and limes from your diet for one month; then add back only a few twice weekly.

Although they seem acidic, these fruits are actually alkaline-forming in the body and candida thrives on them.

❑ To replace "friendly" intestinal bacteria, use an *L. bifidus* retention enema. *See* ENEMAS in Part Three.

❑ Take only hypoallergenic supplements.

❑ To prevent reinfection, replace your toothbrush every thirty days. This is a good preventive measure against both fungal and bacterial infections of the mouth.

❑ Wear white cotton underwear. Synthetic fibers lead to increased perspiration, which creates a hospitable environment for candida, and also traps bacteria, which can cause a secondary infection. Change underclothing daily.

❑ Do not use corticosteroids or oral contraceptives until your condition improves. Oral contraceptives can upset the balance of microorganisms in the body, leading to proliferation of *C. albicans*.

❑ Avoid household chemical products and cleaners, chlorinated water, mothballs, synthetic textiles, and damp and moldy places, such as basements.

❑ If you have chronic and/or unusually persistent candida infections, consult your health care provider. This may be a sign of an underlying illness such as diabetes or immune system dysfunction, which makes for an environment more conducive to the growth of yeast.

CONSIDERATIONS

❑ All persons on long-term antibiotics or chemotherapy are at high risk for severe cases of candidiasis. Taking antibiotics also can cause a deficiency of vitamin K, which is manufactured by the "good bacteria" in the intestines. Eating plenty of leafy greens, alafalfa, strawberries, whole grains, and yogurt can restore the vitamin K balance.

❑ If a breastfed baby develops oral thrush or a nursing mother develops a thrush infection of the nipples, both mother and baby should be treated to eradicate the infection, even if only one of them seems to be affected.

❑ Because there is no simple, accurate test for candida, it is difficult to determine if it is the cause of a baby's diaper rash.

❑ Allergy testing is advised for anyone with symptoms of candida infection. (*See* ALLERGIES in Part Two.)

❑ Medical treatment for candidiasis may involve the use of antifungal medications such as nystatin (sold under the brand names Mycolog, Mycostatin, Mytrex, Nilstat, and Nystex), ketoconazole (Nizoral), and amphotericin (Fungizone). Unfortunately, the use of these agents, especially if chronic or repeated, can lead to the development of stronger strains of yeast that are drug resistant. Higher dosages are then required, which in turn further weaken the immune system. Many doctors no longer use nystatin or antibiotics because they weaken the immune system and can damage certain organs. Others prescribe them for short-term treatment only.

❑ Colloidal silver is a natural broad-spectrum antiseptic that fights infection, subdues inflammation, and promotes healing. It is a clear golden liquid composed of 99.9-percent pure silver particles approximately 0.001 to 0.01 microns ($\frac{1}{1,000,000}$ to $\frac{1}{100,000}$ millimeter) in diameter that are suspended in pure water. Colloidal silver can be taken by mouth, administered intravenously, or applied topically.

❑ High levels of mercury in the body can result in candidiasis. Mercury salts inhibit the growth of the necessary "friendly" bacteria in the intestines. You may want to have a hair analysis done to determine the levels of toxic metals. (*See* HAIR ANALYSIS in Part Three.)

❑ Systemic yeast infection (candidiasis) and AIDS both cause immunosuppressive symptoms. Because they can mimic each other, misdiagnosis is common. Severe yeast infections are common in people with AIDS.

❑ Candida Forte from Nature's Plus is good for mild cases.

❑ Kombucha tea may be helpful. It contains many of the B vitamins, boosts energy, and improves the immune response. (*See* MAKING KOMBUCHA TEA in Part Three.)

❑ Candidiasis may be related to hypoglycemia. (*See* HYPOGLYCEMIA in Part Two.)

❑ *See also* FUNGAL INFECTION and YEAST INFECTION in Part Two.

Canker Sores (Aphthous Ulcers)

Canker sores are small, painful ulcers that can appear on the tongue, the lips, the gums, or the insides of the cheeks. A canker sore begins as a red, ulcerated spot with a yellowish border. The ulcer then becomes covered by a coagulated yellowish mixture of fluids, bacteria, and white blood cells. The development of the sore may be preceded by a burning and tingling sensation. Canker sores do not form blisters as cold sores (fever blisters) do.

Canker sores range in size from as small as a pinhead to as large as a quarter. They appear suddenly and often leave suddenly, usually lasting from four to twenty days. Some experts believe that these painful mouth ulcerations are contagious, but others disagree. Canker sores occur most often in females. They can be triggered by any of a number of factors, including poor dental hygiene, irritation from dental work, food allergies, nutritional deficiencies, hormonal imbalances, viral infection, an underlying immunologic disease, trauma (such as that caused by biting the inside of the cheek or using a hard-bristled toothbrush), stress, and/or fatigue. They may result from an abnormal immune response to normal bacteria in the mouth. Canker sores are occasionally associated with Crohn's disease, which affects the bowels. Deficiencies of iron, lysine, vitamin B12, and folic acid have been linked to this disorder in some people.

NUTRIENTS

SUPPLEMENT	SUGGESTED DOSAGE	COMMENTS
Very Important		
Acidophilus	As directed on label. Take on an empty stomach.	Aids in maintaining healthy balance of intestinal flora ("friendly" bacteria). Use a high-potency powdered form.
L-Lysine	500 mg 3 times daily, on an empty stomach. Take with water or juice. Do not take with milk. Take with 50 mg vitamin B_6 and 100 mg vitamin C for better absorption.	A deficiency may cause an outbreak of sores in and around the mouth. *See* AMINO ACIDS in Part One. *Caution:* Do not take lysine for longer than 6 months at a time.
Vitamin B complex plus extra	50 mg 3 times daily.	B vitamins are basic for immune function and healing. Deficiencies have been linked to mouth sores.
vitamin B_3 (niacin)	50–100 mg 3 times daily. Do not exceed this amount.	*Caution:* Do not take niacin if you have a liver disorder, gout, or high blood pressure.
and pantothenic acid (vitamin B_5)	50–100 mg 3 times daily.	An anti-stress vitamin necessary for adrenal function.
and vitamin B_{12}	2,000 mcg 3 times daily, on an empty stomach.	Use a lozenge or sublingual form.
and folic acid	400 mcg daily.	Use a lozenge or sublingual form.
Vitamin C with bioflavonoids	3,000–8,000 mg daily, in divided doses.	Fights infection and boosts the immune system. Use a buffered form.
Important		
Zinc lozenges (Ultimate Zinc-C Lozenges from Now Foods)	1 15-mg lozenge every 3 waking hours for 2 days. Do not exceed a total of 100 mg daily.	Enhances immune function and aids healing.
Helpful		
Garlic (Kyolic)	3 capsules 3 times daily.	Acts as a natural antibiotic and immunostimulant.
Multivitamin and mineral complex	As directed on label.	A balance of minerals is always important.
Vitamin A	50,000 IU daily for 2 weeks, then reduce to 25,000 IU daily. If you are pregnant, do not exceed 10,000 IU daily. Also put a few drops of vitamin A oil directly on the affected area.	Speeds healing, especially of the mucous membranes. Use emulsion form for easier assimilation.

HERBS

❑ Use burdock, goldenseal, pau d'arco tea, and red clover to cleanse the bloodstream and decrease infection.

Caution: Do not take goldenseal on a daily basis for more than one week at a time, and do not use it during pregnancy. If you have a history of cardiovascular disease, diabetes, or glaucoma, use it only under a doctor's supervision.

❑ Goldenseal extract or tea tree oil, applied gently on the sore twice during the day and again at bedtime, helps to speed healing. To use these as mouthwashes, add three drops to 4 ounces of water. Add a drop or two to your toothpaste before brushing. Use alcohol-free goldenseal extract.

❑ Red raspberry tea contains valuable flavonoids and is very helpful.

RECOMMENDATIONS

❑ Eat plenty of salad with raw onions. Onions contain sulfur and have healing properties.

❑ Include in the diet yogurt and other soured products, such as kefir, cottage cheese, and buttermilk.

❑ Avoid sugar, citrus fruits, and processed and refined foods.

❑ Do not eat fish or meat of any kind for two weeks. The consumption of animal protein increases the body's acidity, which slows healing.

❑ Avoid chewing gum, lozenges, mouthwashes, tobacco, coffee, citrus fruits, and any other foods that you know trigger these sores.

❑ If you have repeated attacks of canker sores, check for nutritional deficiencies.

❑ To avoid getting canker sores, it is important to maintain a proper balance of minerals, acidity, and alkalinity in the body. *See* ACIDOSIS in Part Two for the acid and alkaline self-test. Have a hair analysis done to test for mineral levels. *See* HAIR ANALYSIS in Part Three.

❑ Do not take iron supplements unless your doctor prescribes them. Obtain iron from natural food sources.

❑ Consult your dentist if you have a mouth sore that does not heal.

CONSIDERATIONS

❑ Stress and allergies are probably the most common cause of open sores in the mouth.

❑ Some doctors prescribe mouthwashes that contain tetracycline, an antibiotic, for canker sores.

❑ The drug Zilactin is a gel-like ointment that is applied directly to the ulcer. It sticks to the canker sore and gives relief from irritating foods.

❑ *See also* COLD SORES in Part Two.

Cardiovascular Disease

The cardiovascular system is made up of the heart and blood vessels. Blood is pumped by the heart and circulated throughout the body through the blood vessels. Cardiovascular disease is the leading health problem in the Western world. It is the number one cause of death in the United States, claiming more than 1 million lives annually. An estimated 50 million Americans are afflicted with heart and blood vessel disease, although many do not know it because they have no symptoms.

The arteries that supply blood to the heart are called the *coronary arteries*. If the heart's blood vessels narrow, the amount of blood they supply to the heart may be insufficient to provide the oxygen the heart needs. This oxygen deprivation is what causes a type of chest pain known as *angina pectoris*. Angina is characterized by a heavy, tight pain in the chest area, usually after some type of exertion. The pain usually recedes with rest.

If the coronary arteries that carry oxygen and nutrients to the heart muscle become obstructed, the flow of blood is cut off completely, and a *heart attack*, or *myocardial infarction*, can occur, resulting in damage to the heart muscle. Arteriosclerosis, or hardening of the arteries, and the presence of a thrombus, or clot, in a blood vessel are the most common causes of obstruction. Arteriosclerosis is responsible for most of the deaths resulting from heart attacks. Spasms of the coronary arteries can also result in a heart attack. A heart attack may feel as if someone is applying intense pressure to the chest. This pain may last for several minutes, often extending to the shoulder, arm, neck, or jaw. Other signs of heart attack include sweating, nausea, vomiting, shortness of breath, dizziness, fainting, feelings of anxiety, difficulty swallowing, sudden ringing in the ears, and loss of speech. The amount and type of chest pain vary from one person to another. Some people have intense pain, while others feel only mild discomfort. Many mistake the signs of a heart attack for indigestion. Some have no symptoms at all, a situation referred to as a "silent" heart attack.

Hypertension (high blood pressure) is often a precursor to heart problems. Hypertension is an extremely common form of cardiovascular disease. It usually results from a decrease in the elasticity or a reduction in the interior diameter of the arteries (or both), which may be caused by arteriosclerosis, defects in sodium metabolism, stress, nutritional deficiencies, and enzyme imbalances. Kidney disease, hyperthyroidism, disorders of the pituitary or adrenal glands, and the use of oral contraceptives can also lead to hypertension, and heredity may be a factor. Because it is essentially painless, especially in the early stages, many people don't even know they have it—hence the term "silent killer." By the time hypertension causes complications that result in symptoms (such as rapid pulse, shortness of breath, dizziness, headaches, and sweating), the disorder is more difficult to treat. Untreated hypertension is the leading cause of stroke, and also greatly increases the risk of heart attack, heart failure, and kidney failure.

Other types of cardiovascular disease include heart failure, arrhythmias, and valvular disease. While a heart attack occurs because of an interruption in blood flow *to* the heart, *heart failure* is characterized by inadequate blood flow *from* the heart—the heart fails to pump enough blood to meet the body's needs. Symptoms include fatigue, poor color, shortness of breath, and edema (swelling due to the accu-

Common Heart Problems and Procedures

If either you or a loved one has heart trouble, you can better understand and participate in treatment if you familiarize yourself with the following medical terms that may be used by your physician:

• **Aneurysm.** An aneurysm is a spot in a blood vessel where the wall becomes thin and bulges outward as blood presses against it. If it ruptures, circulation is disrupted. Depending on the location of the aneurysm, the consequences of this can be grave. If detected in time, aneurysms can be repaired surgically in many cases.

• **Angina pectoris.** Angina refers to pain or heavy pressure in the chest that is caused by an insufficient supply of oxygen to the heart tissue. This chest pain may be severe or mild and is usually associated with physical exertion and relieved by rest. It can be a warning sign of impending heart attack.

• **Angiogram.** This is a diagnostic picture produced by injecting into the heart and/or blood vessels a type of dye that is visible on x-ray. It may be done to diagnose valvular disease, blood vessel blockage, and other conditions.

• **Arrhythmia.** Cardiac arrhythmias are disruptions in the natural rhythm of the heartbeat that are caused by improper functioning of electrical system cells in the heart. There are different kinds of arrhythmias. *Palpitations* is a term that refers to the feeling of a pounding heartbeat, whether regular or irregular. *Tachycardia* is an abnormal increase in the resting heart rate; *bradycardia* is the opposite, an abnormally slow heart rate. *Ectopic beats* are premature beats (often felt as "skipped" beats). *Flutter* and *fibrillation* are situations in which the normal steady beating of the heart are converted by electrical error into a rapid twitching of the heart muscle. This ineffective functioning results in an insufficient supply of blood being carried to the body's tissues.

• **Cardiac arrest.** Cardiac arrest occurs when the heart stops beating. When this happens, the blood supply to the brain is cut off and the person loses consciousness. A person in apparent good health who experiences cardiac arrest usually has unsuspected coronary artery disease.

• **Cardiomegaly.** This is the medical term for enlargement of the heart. If the heart is unable to function effectively, as in heart failure, or if there is too much resistance to the normal pumping of blood through the blood vessels, as in high blood pressure, the body attempts to increase the strength of the heart by increasing its size. Cardiomegaly is characteristic of a number of different heart disorders. It is also known as *cardiac hypertrophy*.

• **Cardiomyopathy.** Any of a group of diseases of the heart muscle that result in impaired heart function and, ultimately, heart failure. Cardiomyopathies are classified according to characteristic physical changes in the heart, such as enlargement of the heart, dilation of one or more of the heart's chambers, or rigidity of the heart muscle. These disorders may be related to inherited defects or may be caused by any of a number of different diseases. Often, the cause is unknown.

• **Carditis.** Carditis is an inflammation of the heart muscle. This can result from infection or from an inflammatory response, as in rheumatic fever, and it can lead to permanent heart damage if not treated.

• **Catheterization.** This is a procedure sometimes used to diagnose the condition of the heart and/or circulatory system and, in some cases, to treat cardiovascular disease. A hollow, flexible tube called a catheter is inserted by means of a very fine flexible wire into a blood vessel somewhere in the body (usually the arm, neck, or leg), and from there is threaded through the blood vessel to the heart or other location being investigated. Catheterization can be used to detect (and in some cases to treat) arterial blockage, to discover malformations of the heart, and to study electrical conduction in the heart, among other things.

• **Congestive heart failure.** This is a condition of chronic heart failure that results in fluid accumulation in the lungs, labored breathing after even mild exertion, and edema (swelling) in the ankles and feet.

• **Echocardiogram.** An echocardiogram is a procedure in which ultrasound technology is used to form an image of the heart. It is used to detect structural and functional abnormalities, enlargement or inflammation of the heart, and other conditions.

• **Endocarditis.** This is an inflammation of the endocardium, the membrane surrounding the heart muscle, usually as a result of bacterial infection. Endocarditis is not uncommon in persons with compromised immune systems, such as those with HIV and AIDS. It also can occur as a complication of surgery to replace defective heart valves. This disorder can result in permanent heart damage.

• **Heart attack.** The medical term for a heart attack is *myocardial infarction (MI)*. This refers to the formation of *infarcts* (areas of local tissue death or decay) in the *myocardium* (heart muscle). Infarction occurs when the blood supply to an area of the heart is cut off, usually as a result of a blood clot that blocks a narrowed coronary artery. Depending on the size and location of the areas affected, a heart attack may be described as mild or severe, but it always involves some irreparable damage to the heart.

• **Heart failure.** This disorder occurs when a damaged heart becomes unable to pump effectively, depriving the body's tissues of adequte oxygen and nutrients to function properly. Heart failure can be either acute (short-term) or chronic, and has a variety of different causes.

• **Ischemic heart disease.** Ischemic heart disease is caused by obstruction of the blood flow to the heart, usually as a result of atherosclerosis. Ischemia (lack of sufficient oxygen) can lead to angina, cardiac arrhythmias, congestive heart failure, or a heart attack.

mulation of fluid in the body's tissues), especially around the ankles. *Arrhythmias* are disturbances in the normal rhythm of the heartbeat. There are different kinds of arrhythmias. Some are quite dangerous—even immediately life threatening—while others may be merely annoying (or scarcely noticeable), and pose no particular danger. *Valvular disease* is a term for disorders that impair the functioning of one or more of the heart's valves. It may be caused by congenital defect, or it may be the consequence of illness such as rheumatic fever or endocarditis (infection of the heart muscle).

Unfortunately, despite remarkable new technology for both diagnosis and treatment of heart conditions, the first sign of cardiovascular disease may be a life-threatening calamity. Disorders of the cardiovascular system are often far advanced before they become symptomatic. An estimated 25 percent of people who have heart attacks have no previous symptoms of heart trouble. Every minute, someone in the United States dies of a heart attack.

Cardiovascular disease is not an inevitable result of aging. Many preventive measures can be taken to avoid heart disease. Controllable factors that can contribute to heart disease include smoking, high blood pressure, elevated serum cholesterol, a type-A personality, stress, obesity, a sedentary lifestyle, and diabetes. You *can* alter your lifestyle to keep your heart healthy.

HEART FUNCTION SELF-TEST

Your heart is the most important muscle in your body. A simple pulse test can help you determine how well your heart is functioning. The best time to check your pulse is first thing in the morning. If your pulse is under 60, your heart is functioning at a good pace. If your pulse is above 80, you may need to change your diet and lifestyle. If your pulse remains rapid, consult your health care provider to rule out problems. A chronically high pulse rate is often a precursor of hypertension. Taken daily, this pulse test can forewarn you of oncoming illness.

NUTRIENTS

SUPPLEMENT	SUGGESTED DOSAGE	COMMENTS
Essential		
Coenzyme Q10	50–100 mg 3 times daily.	Increases oxygenation of heart tissue. Has been shown to prevent recurrences in individuals who have had a heart attack.
Very Important		
Bio-Cardiozyme Forte from Biotics Research	1 tablet 3 times daily, on an empty stomach.	A complex that strengthens the heart muscle.
or Heart Science from Source Naturals	As directed on label.	Contains antioxidants, cholesterol-fighters, herbs, and vitamins that work together to protect the heart and promote cardiovascular function.
Calcium and magnesium	1,500–2,000 mg daily, in divided doses, after meals and at bedtime. 750–1,000 mg daily, in divided doses, after meals and at bedtime.	Important in the proper functioning of the cardiac muscle. Use chelate forms.
Garlic (Kyolic) and Kyo-Green from Wakunaga	2 capsules 3 times daily. As directed on label.	Lowers blood pressure and thins the blood. Concentrated barley and wheatgrass juice; contains nutrients needed for healing and prevention of heart disease.
L-Carnitine	500 mg twice daily, on an empty stomach. Take with 50 mg vitamin B6 and 100 mg vitamin C for better absorption.	Reduces fat and triglyceride levels in the blood. Increases oxygen uptake and stress tolerance.
Lecithin granules or capsules	1 tbsp 3 times daily, before meals. 2,400 mg 3 times daily, with meals. Take with vitamin E (see below).	Acts as a fat emulsifier.
Phosphatidyl choline or lipotropic factors	As directed on label. As directed on label.	Reduces fat and triglyceride levels in the blood.
Important		
Citrin		*See under* Herbs, below.
Dimethylglycine (DMG) (Aangamik DMG from FoodScience Labs)	50 mg 4 times daily.	Promotes the utilization of oxygen.
Essential fatty acids (black currant seed oil, flaxseed oil, MaxEPA, primrose oil, and salmon oil are good sources)	As directed on label.	Helps prevent hardening of the arteries. If you use a fish oil, use a product with vitamin E added to prevent rancidity.
Potassium	99 mg daily.	Needed for electrolyte balance, especially if taking cortisone or blood pressure medication.
Selenium	200 mcg daily.	Deficiency has been linked with heart disease.
Superoxide dismutase (SOD)	As directed on label.	A powerful antioxidant.
Taurine Plus from American Biologics	1,000 mg daily. Take with 50 mg vitamin B6 and 100 mg vitamin C for better absorption.	Helps stabilize the heartbeat and correct cardiac arrhythmias. An important antioxidant and immune regulator, necessary for white blood cell activation and neurological function. Use the sublingual form.
Vitamin E	Start with 100–200 IU daily and increase slowly, adding 100 IU each week until daily dosage is 800–1,000 IU. If you take an anticoagulant drug, do not exceed 400 IU daily.	Strengthens the immune system and heart muscle, improves circulation, and destroys free radicals. *Caution:* Use this supplement only under the supervision of a physician.
Helpful		
Kelp	1,000–1,500 mg daily, with meals.	A rich source of important vitamins, minerals, and trace elements.
Copper	As directed by physician.	Deficiency may be linked to some heart problems.

Melatonin	2–3 mg daily, taken 2 hours or less before bedtime.	A powerful antioxidant that may help prevent stroke and also aids sleep.
Multienzyme complex (Infla-Zyme Forte from American Biologics) plus	As directed on label. Take between meals.	To aid digestion.
bromelain	300 mg daily.	
Octacosanol and/or	As directed on label.	Improves endurance; relieves muscle pain.
wheat germ	As directed on label.	
Sea mussel	As directed on label.	A source of protein that aids in the functioning of the cardiovascular system.
Vitamin B complex plus extra	50 mg 3 times daily, with meals.	B vitamins work best when taken together.
vitamin B$_1$ (thiamine) and	50 mg daily.	Deficiency in the heart muscle leads to heart disease.
vitamin B$_3$ (niacin)	50 mg daily. Do not exceed a total of 200 mg daily if you have a history of rheumatic heart disease or other valvular heart problem.	Lowers cholesterol and improves circulation. Caution: Do not take niacin if you have a liver disorder, gout, or high blood pressure.
and vitamin B$_6$ (pyridoxine) and	50 mg daily.	Deficiency has been linked to heart disease.
folic acid	400 mcg daily.	
Vitamin C with bioflavonoids	1,000 mg 3 times daily.	Extremely important in treating cardiovascular disease.

HERBS

❑ Citrin, an extract from the plant *Garcinia cambogia*, inhibits the synthesis of fatty acids in the liver, thus helping to prevent the accumulation of potentially dangerous fats in the body.

❑ Sanhelio's Circu Caps from Health From the Sun is an herbal combination formula that has given good results.

❑ People with cardiovascular disease may benefit from suma tea. Take 3 cups of this herbal tea daily with ginkgo biloba extract as directed on the product label.

❑ Other herbs beneficial for cardiovascular disorders include barberry, black cohosh, butcher's broom, cayenne (capsicum), dandelion, ginseng, hawthorn berries, SP-8 Hawthorn Motherwort Blend from Solaray, and valerian root.

Caution: Do not use barberry or black cohosh during pregnancy. Do not use ginseng if you have high blood pressure.

❑ *Avoid* the herbs ephedra (ma huang) and licorice; they can cause a rise in blood pressure.

RECOMMENDATIONS

❑ If you experience any of the symptoms of a heart attack, contact your doctor or go *immediately* to the emergency room of the nearest hospital, even if symptoms last only a few minutes. Half of all heart attack deaths occur within three to four hours of the onset of the attack, so a person suffering from a heart attack requires immediate medical attention.

❑ Make sure your diet is well balanced and contains plenty of fiber. Eat plenty of raw foods. For protein, eat broiled fish and skinless turkey and chicken, which are low in fat.

❑ Include in the diet garlic, onions, and lecithin. They effectively reduce serum cholesterol levels.

❑ Add raw nuts (except peanuts), olive oil, pink salmon, trout, tuna, Atlantic herring, and mackerel to your diet. These foods contain essential fatty acids.

❑ Do not consume stimulants, such as coffee and black tea, that contain caffeine. Also avoid tobacco, alcohol, chocolate, sugar, butter, red meat, fats (particularly animal fats and hydrogenated oils), fried foods, processed and refined foods, soft drinks, spicy foods, and white flour products, such as white bread.

❑ Drink steam-distilled water only.

❑ Eliminate *all* sources of sodium from your diet. Read all labels and avoid those food products that have "soda," "sodium," or the symbol "Na" on the label. These indicate that the product contains sodium. Some foods and food additives that should be avoided on a salt-free diet include:

• Monosodium glutamate or MSG (Accent flavor enhancer).

• Baking soda.

• Canned vegetables.

• Commercially prepared foods.

• Diet soft drinks.

• Foods with mold inhibitors.

• Foods with preservatives.

• Meat tenderizers.

• Saccharin (found in Sweet'n Low), and products containing saccharin.

• Some medicines and dentifrices.

• Softened water.

❑ If you take an anticoagulant (blood thinner) such as warfarin (Coumadin) or heparin, or even aspirin, limit your intake of foods high in vitamin K. Eating foods containing vitamin K increases the blood's tendency to clot, so they should be eaten only in small quantities. Foods that are rich in vitamin K include alfalfa, broccoli, cauliflower, egg yolks, liver, spinach, and all dark green vegetables. To enhance the effect of anticoagulants, eat more of the following: wheat germ, vitamin E, soybeans, and sunflower seeds.

❑ Learn all about the drugs that have been prescribed for you. Know what to do in case of an emergency. Keep emergency and ambulance numbers easily accessible. If you have a heart condition, someone close to you should know what to do if cardiac arrest occurs. Make sure your loved one knows how to do cardiac massage and mouth-to-mouth breathing. The American Red Cross and many local hospitals offer training in these techniques.

❑ Keep your weight down. Obesity is a risk factor for heart

attacks and high blood pressure. Get regular moderate exercise.

Caution: If you are over thirty-five and/or have been sedentary for some time, consult with your health care provider before beginning an exercise program.

❑ Avoid stress, and learn stress-management techniques. *See* STRESS in Part Two.

CONSIDERATIONS

❑ Studies suggest that the hormone dehydroepiandrosterone (DHEA) may help to prevent cardiovascular disease. DHEA therapy has been linked with a 48-percent reduction in death from heart disease in research populations. (*See* DHEA THERAPY in Part Three.)

❑ Being exposed to excessive noise for more than thirty minutes can increase blood pressure and can affect the heart for up to thirty minutes *after* the noise subsides.

❑ Controlling high blood pressure, either with drugs or lifestyle changes (or a combination of the two), can prevent, or at least delay, dangerous complications.

❑ According to some studies, magnesium supplementation can correct some types of irregular heartbeat, and could save the lives of many people with heart trouble.

❑ The use of a test called cardiokymography (CKG) together with electrocardiograms (ECGs) may help to detect "silent" heart disease. A comparison study revealed that electrocardiograms alone missed 39 percent of heart disease cases. When CKG was used with ECGs, only 8 percent of cases were undetected.

❑ Nitroglycerin, which is sold in sublingual tablet, patch, and lingual spray form, is commonly prescribed to relieve chest pain and to improve the oxygen supply to the heart. This drug is taken at the first sign of chest pain. If dry mouth prevents sublingual nitroglycerin tablets from dissolving, the spray form may be a better choice. Nitroglycerin has some side effects, including headache, weakness, and dizziness. These usually disappear with continued use.

❑ Substances known as thrombolytic agents, including streptokinase and alteplase (also known as TPA [Tissue Plasminogen Activator] and sold under the brand name Activase) have the ability to break up clots. When injected intravenously, they circulate through the arteries, locating and disintegrating blood clots. Studies have shown that thrombolytic therapy within the first six hours of the onset of a heart attack increases the chances of survival. However, this treatment may be contraindicated in people who have peptic ulcers, extremely high blood pressure, a history of stroke, or recent head injury or abdominal surgery.

❑ The FDA asserts that taking one baby aspirin a day can reduce the risk of heart attack without side effects, although a Harvard Medical School newsletter states that there is insufficient evidence to support this. If you do use aspirin, keep in mind that it can cause internal bleeding and stomach ulceration.

❑ Allergies may be linked to some heart attacks. When a reaction in the walls of the arteries triggers a spasm in the coronary arteries, a heart attack may result. Allergy tests are recommended to determine food sensitivities. (*See* ALLERGIES in Part Two.)

❑ Certain viruses may infect blood vessels, causing changes that eventually lead to heart disease. According to an article in *Circulation* magazine, researchers have discovered traces of herpesviruses in blood vessels from people undergoing coronary bypass surgery. Researchers theorize that viruses may injure blood vessels.

❑ *See also* ARTERIOSCLEROSIS; CIRCULATORY PROBLEMS; HEART ATTACK; and HIGH BLOOD PRESSURE, all in Part Two, and CHELATION THERAPY in Part Three.

Carpal Tunnel Syndrome

Almost unheard of only a generation ago, carpal tunnel syndrome (CTS) has rapidly become a bane of modern existence. CTS is the term used to describe a set of symptoms that occur when the median nerve in the wrist is compressed or damaged. The median nerve controls the thumb muscles, and is also responsible for sensation felt in the thumb, the palm, and the first three fingers of the hand. The carpal tunnel is a very small opening about one-quarter inch below the surface of the wrist through which the median nerve passes. The median nerve is vulnerable to compression or injury from a number of sources—swelling due to pregnancy or water retention, pressure from bone spurs, inflammatory arthritis, or even tendinitis.

CTS is associated with repetitive wrist motion injury, which is linked to continuous rapid use of the fingers. Once considered an occupational hazard affecting only supermarket checkout clerks and bookkeepers, CTS did not become widely known until the 1980s, when personal computers came to dominate the workplace. Today, CTS is commonplace among people who earn a living using word processors or other computerized keyboards. Carpal tunnel syndrome can also be caused by strong, steady vibrations that shake the wrist for long periods (such as using a jackhammer or chain saw). Other people whose occupations have been linked to CTS include assembly line workers, athletes, drivers, hairstylists, musicians, restaurant servers, and writers. Although CTS affects both sexes, women between the ages of twenty-nine and sixty-two seem to be affected more than any other segment of the population. Factors that increase the risk of CTS include menopause, Raynaud's disease, pregnancy, hypothyroidism, and diabetes mellitus.

Symptoms of CTS can range from mild numbness and faint tingling to excruciating pain accompanied by a crippling atrophy of the muscles in the thumb. Most commonly, it is experienced as burning, tingling, or numbness in the thumb and the first three fingers. (The little finger is spared because it receives its nerve impulses from outside the carpal tunnel.) The tingling is often referred to as feeling similar to the "pins and needles" associated with a limb "falling asleep," and it also involves a gradual weakening of the thumb. In the beginning, symptoms are often intermittent, but they become persistent as the condition worsens. CTS can affect one or both hands. Symptoms are often worse at night or in the morning, when circulation slows down. Pain may spread to the forearm and, in severe cases, to the shoulder.

Not all nerve entrapment problems are in the carpal tunnel area. Though far less common, entrapment of the ulnar nerve, located in the elbow, produces symptoms almost identical to those of CTS. This condition can be very painful and disabling.

CTS SELF-TEST

The symptoms of CTS are often similar to those of other disorders, particularly arthritis in the neck. A simple self-test can help you determine whether you have carpal tunnel syndrome.

Place the backs of your hands together, with the fingers pointing straight down and the wrists at a 90-degree angle, so that your elbows point straight out to the sides. If holding this position for over a minute brings on symptoms, you probably have CTS. If your job or hobby causes you to develop a burning sensation, numbness, or clumsiness affecting the first three fingers of one or both hands, chances are that CTS is the culprit.

This self-test is not foolproof, however. The only truly conclusive tests for CTS is *electromyography* (EMG), which involves transmitting elecrical impulses through the arm. The nerve impulses that direct motion are nothing more than a very low voltage current. Normal nerve impulse transmission occurs at a speed of approximately 136 meters per second, which is fast enough to appear instantanous to us. If nerves are damaged or entrapped by swollen tissue, however, they cannot transmit electrical neural impulses at the normal rate of speed. If you are found to have a neurotransmission speed of only 90 to 95 meters per second, nerve damage or compression is strongly suggested.

NUTRIENTS

SUPPLEMENT	SUGGESTED DOSAGE	COMMENTS
Essential		
Coenzyme Q$_{10}$	30–90 mg daily.	Improves tissue oxygenation.
Lecithin granules or capsules	1 tbsp 3 times daily, before meals. 1,200 mg 3 times daily, before meals.	Supplies choline and inositol for nerve function. A fat emulsifier.
Vitamin B complex plus extra vitamin B$_1$ (thiamine) and vitamin B$_6$ (pyridoxine)	100 mg 3 times daily. 50 mg 3 times daily for 12 weeks. 100 mg twice daily for 12 weeks. Do not exceed this amount, or nerve damage may result.	B vitamins are essential in nerve function. Increases the uptake of vitamin B$_6$ and improves tissue oxygenation. A potent diuretic.
Zinc	50 mg daily. Do not exceed a total of 100 mg daily from all supplements.	Enhances healing. Use zinc gluconate lozenges or OptiZinc for best absorption.
Helpful		
Grape seed extract	As directed on label.	A powerful antioxidant and anti-inflammatory.
Kelp	As directed on label.	Beneficial to nerves.
Manganese	As directed on label. Take separately from calcium.	Helpful for nerve problems.
Multivitamin and mineral complex	As directed on label.	For general nutritional supplementation.
Primrose oil	As directed on label.	Contains essential fatty acids necessary for nerve function.
Vitamin A	25,000 IU daily. If you are pregnant, do not exceed 10,000 IU daily.	An important antioxidant.
Vitamin C	1,000 mg 4 times daily.	Important in healing and a potent antioxidant.
Vitamin E	400 IU daily.	An important antioxidant.

HERBS

❑ Aloe vera, devil's claw, yarrow, and yucca are helpful for restoring flexibility and reducing inflammation.

❑ Butcher's broom helps to relieve inflammation.

❑ Capsicum relieves pain and is a catalyst for other herbs.

❑ Corn silk and parsley are natural diuretics.

❑ Ginkgo biloba, taken in either tea or capsule form, is beneficial for improving circulation and also aids nerve function.

❑ Gravel root tightens and soothes tissues and acts as an antiseptic.

❑ Marshmallow root soothes and softens tissues and promotes healing.

❑ St. Johnswort stimulates circulation and helps to restore local nerve impulse transmission.

❑ Skullcap relieves muscle spasms and pain.

❑ Wintergreen oil aids in pain relief and circulation to the muscles.

RECOMMENDATIONS

❑ Consume foods that contain or lead to the production of oxalic acid in moderation only. These include asparagus, beets, beet greens, eggs, fish, parsley, rhubarb, sorrel, spinach, Swiss chard, and vegetables of the cabbage family. Large amounts of oxalic acid can promote joint problems.

Minimizing the Risk of Carpal Tunnel Syndrome

Carpal tunnel syndrome is an occupational hazard for anyone whose job involves making repetitive movements with the hands and/or fingers. In this age of computers, that means virtually anyone who works in an office, as well as assembly line workers, bookkeepers, cashiers, jackhammer operators, musicians, and many others. Spending a great deal of time engaging in a hobby such as knitting and needlework can also cause problems. No matter what your occupation, the following measures are recommended to help you reduce the risk of developing this painful and disabling condition:

• Use your whole hand and all of your fingers when you grip an object.

• Whenever possible, use a tool instead of flexing your wrists forcibly.

• Make sure your posture is correct. For keyboard tasks, sit straight in your chair with your body tilted slightly back. Raise or lower your chair so that your knees are bent at a right angle and your feet are flat on the floor. Your wrists and hands should be straight and your forearms parallel to the floor. Keep your wrists and hands consistently in a straight line.

• Keep your elbows bent. This lessens the load close to your body and reduces the amount of force required to do your job. Give yourself elbow room to allow you to use as much of your arm as you can while keeping your wrist straight. Use your whole arm while performing tasks in order to minimize the stress on your elbow.

• Adjust your computer screen so that it is about two feet away from you and just below your line of sight.

• Use arm rests that attach to the chair to keep your wrists from flexing too much.

• If the relative positions of your desk, chair, and keyboard do not allow you to keep your wrists straight while keyboarding, the use of a "wrist rest" pad in front of the keyboard is highly recommended to alleviate pressure on the carpal tunnel.

• Slow your rhythm while varying wrist and hand movements.

• Take a break from handwork for a few minutes every hour.

• Shake out your hands periodically throughout the day.

• Perform simple stretching exercises before your daily tasks to improve overall circulation and aid in warming up the muscles. The American Physical Therapy Association recommends these exercises:

1. Resting one forearm on a table, grasp the fingertips of that hand and pull back gently.
   Hold this position for five seconds, then repeat the exercise with the other hand.

2. Press the palms flat on a table, as if doing a push-up. Lean forward to stretch the forearm muscles and the wrists.

• Another recommended gentle exercise is done by rotating the wrist. Move your hands around in a circle for about two minutes, thoroughly stretching the muscles of the hand. This helps to restore circulation and improve the posture of the wrist.

• Do strengthening exercises by placing a rubber band around the fingers to provide resistance, and opening and closing the fingers. Three times a day, do a set of ten repetitions with each hand.

❑ Eat half of a fresh pineapple daily for one to three weeks, until relief is achieved. Pineapple contains bromelain, which reduces pain and swelling. Only fresh pineapple is effective.

❑ Avoid salt and all foods containing sodium. They promote water retention and may aggravate carpal tunnel syndrome. They will also counteract any diuretics that your physician may prescribe.

❑ If you engage in repetitive mechanical tasks, try to reduce the impact on your wrists and hands. *See* Minimizing the Risk of Carpal Tunnel Syndrome, above.

❑ If possible, stop all repetitive finger movements for several days and see if any improvement occurs. If it does, try to rearrange your schedule so that you spend less time in CTS-stimulating activities. If possible, alternate tasks rather than performing a single task for long periods. Fortunately, employers have become more mindful of the possibility of repetitive motion injuries and are often more understanding than they might have been only a few years ago. Many now try to have their employees rotate the tasks they perform so that the risk of injury is reduced.

❑ Maintain ideal weight, and lose weight if necessary. Excess weight results in extra pressure on the carpal tunnel. Losing weight has brought relief to many people with CTS.

❑ Try homeopathic *Rhus toxicodendron* for relief of acute swelling and pain. Zhen Gu Shi, a potent Chinese liniment for inflamed joints, is also good. It is sold in many Asian markets,

❑ Use a splint to help prevent flare-ups. Splints are cloth-covered metal or plastic braces that attach to the forearm with an elastic bandage (an Ace bandage or the equivalent) or hook and loop fasteners (Velcro). These devices are available at medical supply houses and many pharmacies. If you cannot find one that fits properly, have one custom-made. Be sure to apply and wear the splint properly; if you don't, its effectiveness may be reduced or it may even aggravate the problem. Cock your wrist back slightly so that your thumb is parallel to your forearm. Your hand should be in approximately the same position as if it were holding a pen. This position keeps the carpal tunnel as open as possible. Wear the splint as much as possible for several days to see if your symptoms are reduced. Splinting is often very helpful for those who have suffered a repetitive motion injury that results in CTS.

❑ Keep your workplace warm and dry. Cool and/or damp conditions tend to aggravate CTS.

❑ Avoid taking supplements that contain iron. They are suspected of aggravating pain and swelling in joints.

CONSIDERATIONS

❑ If CTS develops as a result of the edema of pregnancy, it usually clears up of its own accord once the baby arrives and the excess fluid of pregnancy disappears.

❑ Physicians treat CTS in a variety of ways, most often with a combination of anti-inflammatory medications, splints, and the recommendation that you avoid any aggravating activity. Sometimes corticosteroid injections in the wrist are used. This treatment is controversial, however, and should not be used unless the pain from CTS is debilitating, since the injections themselves are a source of considerable discomfort.

❑ If weakness develops in the thumb, it is an indication that the median nerve has sustained some amount of damage, and surgical treatment may be recommended. This surgery involves cutting the transverse carpal ligament, a thick, fibrous band that covers part of the carpal tunnel. The surgeon can make either a small incision or a relatively large one. A small incision causes minimal scarring, but it affords the surgeon a very limited area view, which increases the risk of damage to other important structures in the wrist. A larger incision reduces the risk of peripheral damage, but a more prominent scar is usually the result, and the scarring itself may cause some pain and disability. A splint or cast must be worn for two to four weeks following surgery.

❑ Many doctors maintain that surgery for CTS is too often performed unnecessarily. A second opinion should always be obtained before surgery is agreed to. However, if the second doctor's opinion confirms that surgery is unavoidable, it is best not to put the operation off for too long, as delay may result in permanent nerve damage.

❑ The numbness, tingling, and pain of CTS usually subside within a few days after surgery, but some people find that it takes as much as two years for the symptoms to resolve. When this happens, it is often because the median nerve has sustained some damage and a long time is needed for any nerve regeneration to occur. If surgery is necessary and is put off for too long, the thumb may be left permanently weakened and the mobility of the affected hand may be diminished.

❑ A new treatment for CTS involves the use of a low-energy ("cold") laser to penetrate tissues, stimulate nerves, and increase microcirculation in the affected area.

❑ *See also* PAIN CONTROL in Part Three.

Cataracts

See under EYE PROBLEMS.

Cavities

See TOOTH DECAY.

Celiac Disease

Celiac disease (also called celiac sprue) is a rare disorder caused by an intolerance to gluten, a component of wheat, rye, barley, and oats. An estimated 1 in 5,000 persons in the United States is affected. Gluten contains a protein called alpha-gliadin. In persons with celiac disease, this protein causes a reaction in the mucous lining of the intestine. The villi lining the small intestine suffer damage and destruction, which impairs the body's ability to absorb vital nutrients. Malabsorption becomes a serious problem, and the loss of vitamins, minerals, and calories results in malnutrition despite an adequate diet. Diarrhea compounds the problem. Because celiac disease impairs digestion, food allergies may also appear.

Celiac disease affects both adults and children, and can appear at any age. It often appears when a child is first introduced to cereal foods, at around three or four months of age. The first signs are usually diarrhea, weight loss, and nutritional deficiencies such as anemia. Other symptoms include nausea; abdominal swelling; large, and frequently pale and/or light-yellow-colored, foul-smelling stools that float; depression; fatigue; irritability; muscle cramps and wasting; and joint and/or bone pain. Infants and children may exhibit stunted growth, vomiting, an intense burning sensation in the skin, and a red, itchy skin rash called dermatitis herpetiformis. A baby with celiac disease may gain weight more slowly than normal or may lose weight. The infant may have a poor appetite, gas, and offensive-smelling bowel movements. The child is likely to have an anemic, undernourished appearance. Ulcers may develop in the mouth.

Since it is a rare condition and many physicians are not aware of the various symptoms associated with gluten intolerance, they may misdiagnose celiac disease. It is often misdiagnosed as irritable bowel syndrome or spastic colon, for example. There have been cases in which doctors unable to diagnose the illness have referred their patients to psychiatrists. Many people go a long time before being diagnosed correctly, and often the correct diagnosis is arrived at only because of something they have heard or read that enables them to identify the disease themselves. Yet if left untreated, celiac disease can be quite serious, even life-threatening. Bone disease, central and peripheral nervous system impairment, internal hemorrhaging, pancreatic disease, infertility, miscarriages, and gynecological disorders are just some of the long-term maladies that can complicate celiac disease. It also increases the risk of developing intestinal lymphoma and other intestinal malignancies. Certain autoimmune disorders can also be associated with celiac disease, including dermatitis herpetiformis, kidney disease (nephrosis), sarcoidosis (the formation of lesions in the lungs, bones, skin, and other places), insulin-dependent diabetes mellitus, systemic lupus erythematosus, thyroid disease, and, rarely, chronic active hepatitis, scleroderma, myasthenia gravis, Addison's disease, rheumatoid arthritis, and Sjögren's syndrome.

NUTRIENTS

SUPPLEMENT	SUGGESTED DOSAGE	COMMENTS
Essential		
Free-form amino acid complex	As directed on label.	To supply protein in a form readily available for use by the body.
Multivitamin and mineral complex with		All nutrients are necessary in balance. Use a wheat- and yeast-free product only.
vitamin A	15,000 IU daily. If you are pregnant, do not exceed 10,000 IU daily.	
and natural beta-carotene	10,000 IU daily.	
and vitamin E	400 IU daily.	
Vitamin B complex injections plus extra	2 cc weekly, or as prescribed by physician.	Necessary for proper digestion. Injections (under a doctor's supervision) are best because they bypass the digestive system.
vitamin B$_6$ (pyridoxine) or	½ cc weekly, or as prescribed by physician.	
vitamin B complex	100 mg 3 times daily.	If injections are not available, a sublingual form is recommended. Use a wheat- and yeast-free product.
Vitamin B$_{12}$ and	As directed on label.	Malabsorption of vitamin B$_{12}$ results from celiac disease. Injections may be necessary. If injections are not available, use a lozenge or sublingual form.
folic acid	As directed on label.	
Important		
N-acetylglucosamine (N-A-G from Source Naturals)	As directed on label.	Forms the basis of complex molecular structures of the mucous membranes of the intestinal lining.
Vitamin K or alfalfa	As directed on label.	Fat-soluble vitamins are not absorbed well in this disorder. *See under* Herbs, below.
Zinc lozenges (Ultimate Zinc-C Lozenges from Now Foods) plus	1 15-mg lozenge 5 times daily. Do not exceed a total of 100 mg daily from all supplements.	Needed for immunity and healing.
copper	3 mg daily.	Needed to balance with zinc.

Helpful		
Essential fatty acids (primrose oil and salmon oil are good sources)	As directed on label.	Needed for the villi in the intestines.
Magnesium plus	750 mg daily.	Helps maintain the body's normal pH balance. Deficiency is common in people with celiac disease.
calcium	1,500 mg daily.	Works with magnesium.
Proteolytic enzymes	As directed on label, 3 times daily. Take between meals, on an empty stomach.	Additional digestive enzymes may be needed to aid in breakdown and absorption of foods.
Psyllium seed or Aerobic Bulk Cleanse (ABC) from Aerobic Life Industries	As directed on label. Take separately from other supplements and medications.	A fiber product not absorbed by the intestines. Drink large amounts of water because the fiber expands to several times its dry volume.
Vitamin C	2,000–5,000 mg daily, in divided doses.	Boosts immune function.

HERBS

❑ Alfalfa supplies vitamin K, which is often deficient in those with celiac disease. Take 2,000 to 3,000 mg in tablet form daily.

RECOMMENDATIONS

❑ Eat fresh vegetables, legumes (such as lentils, beans, and peas), rice bran, nuts, sunflower seeds, raisins, figs, and "seedy" fruits, such as strawberries, raspberries, and blackberries. Include in the diet blackstrap molasses, which is high in iron and the B vitamins. People with celiac disease need fiber and foods rich in iron and the B vitamins.

❑ Do not eat sugary products, processed foods, dairy products, bouillon cubes, chocolate, and bottled salad dressings.

❑ Celiac disease causes malabsorption of the B vitamins and the fat-soluble vitamins (vitamins A, D, E, and K), so take these nutrients. Note that gluten is found in many nutritional supplements. Read labels carefully, and use supplements that are hypoallergenic, wheat-free, and yeast-free.

❑ If a child develops any of the symptoms of celiac disease, omit all gluten-containing foods from the child's diet and see if the problem clears up. Eliminate milk, as lactose intolerance can occur with celiac disease. The disease can begin in the first few months of life, depending on the child's diet.

❑ Avoid any and all foods that contain gluten. Do not eat any products that contain barley, oats, rye, or wheat. Rice and corn can be eaten. Substitute rice, potato, cornmeal, and soy flour for wheat flour. Read all labels carefully. Watch for "hidden" sources of gluten, such as hydrolyzed vegetable protein, textured vegetable protein, hydrolyzed plant protein, and all derivatives of wheat, rye, oats, and barley, including malt, modified food starch, some soy sauces, grain vinegars, binders, fillers, excipients, and "natural flavorings." Do not consume hot dogs, gravies, luncheon meat, beer, mustard, catsup, nondairy creamer, white vinegar, curry powder, or seasonings. Gluten-free products are available at health food stores.

CONSIDERATIONS

❑ If celiac disease is suspected, an intestinal biopsy should be performed to make a definitive diagnosis.

❑ A child who gets blisters and sores all over his or her body should be checked for celiac disease.

❑ Martin F. Kagnoff, M.D., of the University of California at San Diego says that heredity is a vital factor in the development of this disease. He also says that celiac sprue often develops in childhood but may trail off in adolescence; in some cases, reappearing in adults in their thirties and forties. Factors that may trigger the onset of celiac disease are emotional stress, physical trauma, a viral infection, pregnancy, or surgery.

❑ Vitamin K deficiency caused by celiac disease may lead to a hypoprothrombinemia (a lack of clotting factors in the blood). One form of vitamin K is manufactured by "friendly" bacteria in the intestines; another is present in certain foods, especially leafy greens, alfalfa, tomatoes, strawberries, whole grains, and yogurt. Bacteria such as those found in yogurt and acidophilus can also help to restore the intestinal flora necessary for vitamin K production.

❑ A report published in the British medical journal *The Lancet* pointed to a possible connection between celiac disease and epilepsy. Theories as to how the two might be linked include the possibility that endorphin-like substances may be created from wheat gluten and may affect brain metabolism; another possibility is that celiac disease increases intestinal permeability, which in turn allows the absorption of substances that may affect brain chemistry.

❑ It may be necessary to remove milk and milk products from the diet because of a secondary lactase deficiency (*see* LACTOSE INTOLERANCE in Part Two).

❑ Schizophrenia has been observed to occur more often in those with celiac disease. (*See* SCHIZOPHRENIA in Part Two.)

❑ For more information about celiac disease, you can contact the Celiac Disease Foundation at 13251 Ventura Boulevard, Suite 3, Studio City, CA 91604–1838; telephone 818–990–2354. There are also good books on this subject available in health food stores.

❑ *See also* MALABSORPTION SYNDROME in Part Two.

Chemical Allergies

When the body is exposed to certain foreign chemicals, it may respond by producing antibodies to defend itself against the foreign invaders. Virtually any substance can provoke a reaction in some individuals. Some of the environmental contaminants that most frequently cause problems include air pollution; gas, oil, or coal fumes; formaldehyde; chlorine; phenol; carbolic acid; insecticides; disinfectants; paint; hair sprays; household cleaning products; and metals such as nickel, mercury, chrome, and beryllium. Chemical allergies often manifest themselves as skin reactions. Other possible allergic responses to foreign chemicals include watery eyes, ringing in the ears, stuffy nose, diarrhea, nausea, upset stomach, asthma, bronchitis, arthritis, fatigue, eczema, intestinal disorders, depression, and headache. Some people may have a reaction immediately after encountering a chemical allergen; others may not develop a rash for twenty-four hours after coming in contact with the irritant.

The following supplement program is designed to protect you from, and help you cope with the effects of chemical allergies.

NUTRIENTS

SUPPLEMENT	SUGGESTED DOSAGE	COMMENTS
Very Important		
Vitamin A and vitamin E	50,000 IU daily for 30 days, then reduce to 25,000 IU daily. If you are pregnant, do not exceed 10,000 IU daily. 400–800 IU daily.	Powerful free radical scavengers and immune enhancers. Use emulsion forms for easier assimilation.
Vitamin B complex plus extra vitamin B6 (pyridoxine) plus niacinamide	100–200 mg daily. 100 mg 3 times daily. 500 mg 3 times daily.	Allergies hinder absorption of B vitamins. Consider injections (under a doctor's supervision). Natural antihistamine. Also aids in detoxifying foreign substances and eliminating them through the kidneys. Aids circulation. *Caution:* Do not substitute niacin for niacinamide, or toxicity may result.
Vitamin C with bioflavonoids	5,000–20,000 mg daily, in divided doses. *See* ASCORBIC ACID FLUSH in Part Three.	Protects the body from allergens and moderates the inflammatory response.
Important		
Coenzyme Q10	60 mg daily.	Helps to counter histamine, a body chemical involved in allergic reactions.
Selenium	200 mcg daily.	Essential in immune function and protection of cells.
Superoxide dismutase (SOD) or Cell Guard from Biotec Foods	As directed on label. As directed on label.	A potent free radical scavenger. An antioxidant complex that contains SOD.
Zinc plus copper	50 mg daily. Do not exceed a total of 100 mg daily from all supplements. 3 mg daily.	Important in proper immune function. Use zinc gluconate lozenges or OptiZinc for best absorption. Needed to balance with zinc. Copper is lost when high doses of vitamin C are taken.

Helpful		
Aller Bee-Gone from CC Pollen	As directed on label.	A combination of herbs, enzymes, and nutrients that fight allergic outbreaks.
Dioxychlor from American Biologics	5 drops in water twice daily.	A potent detoxifier.
Garlic (Kyolic)	2 capsules 3 times daily.	A powerful immunostimulant.
L-Cysteine and L-methionine plus L-glutamic acid	500 mg each daily. Take on an empty stomach with juice or water. Do not take with milk. Take with 50 mg vitamin B$_6$ and 100 mg vitamin C for better absorption.	Excellent detoxifiers, especially of the liver. See AMINO ACIDS in Part One.
Manganese	As directed on label. Take separately from calcium.	Interacts with zinc and copper. Use manganese chelate form.
Pancreatic enzymes and proteolytic enzymes	As directed on label 3 times daily, with meals. As directed on label 3 times daily, between meals.	Both pancreatic and proteolytic enzymes are needed for proper digestion and assimilation of necessary nutrients. Protelytic enzymes also control inflammation.
Taurine Plus from American Biologics	500 mg daily.	The most important antioxidant and immune regulator, necessary for white blood cell activitation and neurological function. Use the sublingual form.
Raw thymus glandular	As directed on label.	Important for immune function.

HERBS

❑ If you develop a skin rash from exposure to metal in watchbands, earrings, snaps, or other items that come in contact with the skin, try using Natureworks Marigold Ointment from Abkit. Calendula, chamomile, elder flower, and tea tree oil can also be used as a soothing wash on rashes.

RECOMMENDATIONS

❑ The first step in managing chemical allergies is to determine which chemicals are provoking the allergic reaction, then avoid coming in contact with these chemicals. If the source of the problem is not obvious, see an allergy specialist.

❑ Avoid foods that have been sprayed or that contain artificial colorings (found in some apples and oranges), ripening agents, or protective waxes (found on some apples, cucumbers, and other items). Avoid things containing FD&C Yellow No. 5 dye. Read all food product labels carefully.

❑ Supplement your diet with plenty of fiber. Oat bran is a good source of fiber. Apple pectin can also be a useful addition to your diet. It removes unwanted metals that may trigger allergic reactions.

Note: Always take supplemental fiber separately from other supplements and medications.

CONSIDERATIONS

❑ Mercury and silver in dental fillings can cause allergic reactions as well as heavy metal poisoning. See MERCURY TOXICITY in Part Two.

❑ See also CHEMICAL POISONING in Part Two.

Chemical Poisoning

Like toxic metals, poisonous chemicals such as chlorine, disinfectants, heavy metals, herbicides, insecticides, petroleum products, and solvents can enter the body and decrease the functioning capacity of its organs. This is chemical poisoning. Some chemicals are absorbed through the skin; others may be inhaled or ingested. The body's immune system is threatened by these chemicals, and tries to cleanse itself of the poisons. Damage to internal organs, especially the liver, may occur.

Chronic chemical poisoning occurs most often in people who use or who are exposed to chemicals in their work environments, or who use excessive amounts of chemical sprays. People who live near landfills or certain industrial installations may also be chronically exposed to toxic chemicals. Acute chemical poisoning can result from accidental ingestion of household chemicals (particularly among children) or taking improper or excessive medications.

NUTRIENTS

SUPPLEMENT	SUGGESTED DOSAGE	COMMENTS
Very Important		
Free-form amino acid complex	As directed on label twice daily, on an empty stomach.	Helps liver function. Use a sublingual form.
Raw liver extract	As directed on label or as prescribed by physician.	Supplies needed B vitamins and iron, and detoxifies chemicals. For severe chemical poisoning, injections (under a doctor's supervision) are best.
Superoxide dismutase (SOD) or	As directed on label.	A powerful free radical destroyer.
Cell Guard from Biotec Foods	As directed on label.	An antioxidant complex that contains SOD.
Vitamin B complex injections	As prescribed by physician.	Protects the liver and bodily functions. Injections (under a doctor's supervision) are best. If injections are not available, use a sublingual form.
plus choline and inositol	50 mg 3 times daily, with meals. 50 mg 3 times daily, with meals.	
Vitamin C with bioflavonoids	5,000–20,000 mg daily, in divided doses. See ASCORBIC ACID FLUSH in Part Three.	Protects the body from pollutants and aids in the elimination of toxic substances.

Important		
Grape seed extract	As directed on label.	A powerful antioxidant.
L-Cysteine and L-methionine	500 mg each daily, on an empty stomach. Take with water or juice. Do not take with milk. Take with 50 mg vitamin B$_6$ and 100 mg vitamin C for better absorption.	To remove toxins and rebuild the body. See AMINO ACIDS in Part One.
Selenium	200 mcg daily.	Works with vitamins C and E to detoxify the body.
Vitamin E	400–800 IU daily.	A powerful antioxidant.

Helpful		
Coenzyme Q$_{10}$	30–60 mg daily.	Aids in rebuilding the immune system and providing oxygen to the tissues.
Dioxychlor from American Biologics	5 drops in water twice daily.	Delivers oxygen to the tissues.
Garlic (Kyolic)	2 capsules 3 times daily.	Helps to detoxify and cleanse the bloodstream.
Multivitamin and mineral complex	As directed on label.	All nutrients are needed to aid in strengthening the immune system and lessening toxicity.

RECOMMENDATIONS

❑ To aid recovery, eat a well-balanced diet that is high in fiber. Fiber helps to cleanse the system. Recommended foods include almonds, apricots, bananas, barley, beans, beets, Brazil nuts, brown rice, carrots, dates, fish, garlic, grapes, hazelnuts, lemons, lentils, onions, spinach, oatmeal, and yogurt.

❑ If at all possible, eat only organically grown foods.

❑ Drink steam-distilled water only.

❑ Perform a cleansing fast for three days each month to help the body get rid of toxins. See FASTING in Part Three.

❑ Avoid chemicals whenever possible.

CONSIDERATIONS

❑ See also CHEMICAL ALLERGIES and POISONING in Part Two.

Chickenpox

Most children contract this childhood disease before age nine. It is caused by a virus and first manifests itself as a fever and headache, usually starting between seven and twenty-one days after exposure to the virus. Twenty-four to thirty-six hours later, small round "pimples" appear on the face and body. They are filled with fluid and look like water blisters. The fluid leaks from the swollen areas of the skin, forming a crust. These eruptions continue in cycles, lasting from three days to one week. The blisters and crusts are infectious and itchy, and scratching them can lead to

infection and scarring. Once the scabs are gone, the individual is no longer infectious. Chickenpox usually runs its course in two weeks, although the infection can be serious in newborns. Adults who contract the infection tend to have more severe cases than children do.

One bout with chickenpox generally affords lifetime immunity against the illness. Second attacks are possible, but rare. However, the virus that causes chickenpox, *Varicella-zoster*, is the same virus that causes shingles in adults. This virus can lie dormant for years, then resurface as shingles in adulthood. A person can contract chickenpox (but not shingles) from direct contact with a shingles rash.

Unless otherwise specified, the dosages recommended here are for adults. For a child between the ages of twelve and seventeen, reduce the dose to three-quarters the recommended amount. For a child between six and twelve, use one-half the recommended dose, and for a child under the age of six, use one-quarter the recommended amount.

NUTRIENTS

SUPPLEMENT	SUGGESTED DOSAGE	COMMENTS
Essential		
Natural beta-carotene or carotenoid complex	15,000 IU daily. As directed on label.	Heals tissues and stimulates the immune system.
Vitamin A capsules or emulsion	20,000 IU daily for 1 month, then 15,000 IU daily for 1 week. 100,000 IU daily for 1 week, then 75,000 IU daily for 1 week. If you are pregnant, do not exceed 10,000 IU daily.	An immunostimulant that aids healing of tissues. Emulsion form is recommended for easier assimilation and greater safety at higher doses.
Vitamin C	1,000 mg 4 times daily.	Powerful immune stimulant that aids in keeping down fever.
Very Important		
Potassium and zinc	99 mg daily. 80 mg daily. Do not exceed a total of 100 mg daily from all supplements.	Helps reduce fever and speed healing. Enhances immune function. Use zinc gluconate lozenges or OptiZinc for best absorption.
Vitamin E	400–600 IU daily.	A powerful free radical scavenger that increases oxygenation and promotes healing.
Helpful		
Maitake or shiitake or reishi	As directed on label. As directed on label. As directed on label.	Mushrooms with immune-stimulating and antiviral properties.
Multivitamin and mineral complex	As directed on label.	All nutrients help to speed the healing process.
Raw thymus glandular	As directed on label.	Stimulates the production of T lymphocytes by the thymus gland. Needed for immune function. See GLANDULAR THERAPY in Part Three.

HERBS

❑ Other recommended herbs include burdock root, echinacea, ginger, goldenseal, pau d'arco, and St. Johnswort.

❑ Catnip tea sweetened with molasses is good for fever, and can be given to infants and children as well as to adults. For a child over age two, catnip tea enemas can reduce fever.

RECOMMENDATIONS

❑ Drink freshly made juices with protein powder and brewer's yeast added. Also drink pure vegetable broth.

❑ When the fever drops and the appetite returns, use a "starter diet" consisting of only mashed bananas, avocados, fresh raw applesauce, and/or yogurt. Do not use cooked or processed foods.

❑ Do not give any cow's milk or formula to a feverish infant. Instead, use pure, freshly made juices that have been diluted with a combination of 4 ounces of steam-distilled water and 100 to 1,000 milligrams of vitamin C for each 4 ounces of juice. Infants who are six months old or older can have almond or soy milk, available in health food stores. Give a sick infant lots of water to prevent dehydration.

❑ Take care not to scratch the pocks. Keep a child's nails short and clean, and bathe the child often. Put mittens on a young child's hands if necessary. Use hot baths made with tea prepared with the recommended herbs, or ginger baths using cool water. Sponge the affected area with the tea. Wet compresses help to control the itching; use these often.

❑ Keep infected children separated, and keep an infected child away from elderly people, newborn babies, and pregnant women who have not had chickenpox.

❑ Never give aspirin to a child who has a fever. Studies have shown an increased risk of Reye's syndrome, a rare and potentially fatal disorder, in children given aspirin for fever. (See REYE'S SYNDROME in Part Two.)

❑ If you are unlucky enough to contract chickenpox in adulthood, contact your health care provider. Use a fasting program to help speed healing. See FASTING in Part Three.

CONSIDERATIONS

❑ Fetal exposure to chickenpox has been associated with an increased risk of birth defects.

❑ If the sores become infected, an antibiotic ointment is usually prescribed.

❑ See also SHINGLES in Part Two.

Chlamydia

According the U.S. Centers for Disease Control and Prevention (CDC), sexually transmitted chlamydia infection ac-

counts for the bulk of the sexually transmitted disease (STD) epidemic in the United States. Sexually transmitted chlamydia infection is believed to be twice as common as gonorrhea. Each year, some 4 million new cases are diagnosed and an estimated 50,000 women are rendered sterile by the disease. About 18 percent of American adolescents have had a chlamydial infection, and one recent study found that 50 percent of the women on one college campus had been infected.

Symptoms of chlamydia include genital inflammation, vaginal or urethral discharge, difficulty in urinating, painful intercourse, and itching around the inflamed area. These symptoms can appear in both men and women. However, as many as 10 percent of the men and 70 percent of the women who have chlamydia experience no symptoms at all. This is unfortunate, as untreated chlamydial infection in women leads to sterility in an estimated 30 percent of cases. Pelvic inflammatory disease and irreparable damage to the reproductive system can occur, and hysterectomy may be required.

In males, prostatitis and inflammation of the seminal vesicles may be caused by chlamydia. Symptoms of prostatitis include pain when urinating and a watery mucous urethral discharge.

Diagnosis of chlamydia infection is made on the basis of bacteriologic examination of urine or vaginal or urethral discharge.

NUTRIENTS

SUPPLEMENT	SUGGESTED DOSAGE	COMMENTS
Important		
Garlic (Kyolic)	2 capsules 3 times daily.	Acts as a natural antibiotic and aids in healing.
Vitamin B complex	50–100 mg 3 times daily, with meals.	Needed for proper functioning of the liver and gastrointestinal tract.
Vitamin C	1,500 mg 4 times daily.	Immunostimulant that aids healing. Use a buffered form.
Vitamin E	600 IU daily. Can also be used directly on the inflamed site; cut open a capsule and apply.	Needed to protect red blood cells. Immune enhancer.
Helpful		
Acidophilus	As directed on label. Take on an empty stomach.	Replenishes "friendly" bacteria destroyed by antibiotics.
Bio-Bifidus from American Biologics	Use as a vaginal douche as directed on label.	Replaces normal vaginal and bowel flora.
Coenzyme Q10	60 mg daily.	Aids in healing and is a powerful antioxidant and immune stimulant.
Dioxychlor from American Biologics	As directed on label.	An important antibacterial, antifungal, and antiviral agent.
Kelp	2,000–3,000 mg daily.	A rich source of minerals.
Multivitamin complex with natural beta-carotene	As directed on label.	Necessary for healing of all bodily tissues. Use a high-potency formula.

Zinc	50 mg daily. Do not exceed a total of 100 mg daily from all supplements.	Important for immune function and healing. Use zinc gluconate lozenges or OptiZinc for best absorption.
plus		
copper	3 mg daily.	Needed to balance with zinc.

HERBS

❑ Astragalus, echinacea, goldenseal, pau d'arco, and red clover aid in healing.

   Caution: Do not take goldenseal on a daily basis for more than one week at a time, and do not use it during pregnancy. If you have a history of cardiovascular disease, diabetes, or glaucoma, use it only under a doctor's supervision.

RECOMMENDATIONS

❑ Eat a diet consisting mainly of fresh vegetables and fruits, plus brown rice, raw seeds and nuts, turkey, white fish, and whole grains.

❑ Avoid highly processed, fried, and junk foods, as well as chicken. Approximately one third of all chickens sold in this country contain pathogenic bacteria such as salmonella. Turkey is acceptable; such bacteria are not found in turkey.

❑ Drink only steam-distilled water, sugar-free juices, and herbal teas.

❑ Take acidophilus to replenish the "friendly" bacteria destroyed by antibiotics.

❑ If you have symptoms of chlamydia infection, do not delay seeking treatment. Complications increase as time passes.

CONSIDERATIONS

❑ If you are under thirty-five and have more than one sexual partner, you should be tested for infection yearly.

❑ Both partners must be treated for this disorder so that the disease is not transmitted back and forth. (Both sexes have similar discharges, and it is through this discharge that the disease is transmitted during sexual contact.) Antibiotics such as tetracycline and doxycycline (Doryx, Vibramycin, and others) kill chlamydia. Alternatively, a single 1-gram oral dose of azithromycin (Zithromax) may be used. This is relatively expensive (a single dose costs as much as a one-week regimen of doxycycline), but the convenience of single-dose treatment may be worth it.

❑ Chlamydia has been linked to a form of arthritis in young women. In one study, the microorganism was found in the joints of nearly half those with unexplained arthritis.

❑ *See also* SEXUALLY TRANSMITTED DISEASES in Part Two.

Cholesterol Problems

See HIGH CHOLESTEROL.

Chronic Fatigue Syndrome

Chronic fatigue syndrome (CFS) is a condition that has become widespread in the United States. Symptoms associated with CFS include aching muscles and joints, anxiety, depression, difficulty concentrating, fever, headaches, intestinal problems, irritability, jaundice, loss of appetite, mood swings, muscle spasms, recurrent upper respiratory tract infections, sensitivity to light and heat, sleep disturbances, sore throat, swollen glands (lymph nodes), temporary memory loss—and most of all, extreme and often disabling fatigue.

The symptoms of this syndrome resemble those of flu and other viral infections, so it is often mistaken for other disorders. It is often misdiagnosed as hypochondria, psychosomatic illness, or depression, because routine medical tests do not detect any problems. The syndrome is three times more prevalent in women than in men, and primarily affects young adults between the ages of twenty and forty.

The major criteria used to distinguish chronic fatigue syndrome are:

1. Persistent fatigue that does not resolve with bed rest and that is severe enough to reduce average daily activity by at least 50 percent for at least six months.

2. The presence of other chronic clinical conditions, including psychiatric disorders, can be ruled out.

The cause or causes of chronic fatigue syndrome are not well understood. Some experts believe it is linked to infection with the Epstein-Barr virus (EBV), a member of the herpesvirus family that is also the cause of mononucleosis. This belief is based in large part on the fact that many people with chronic fatigue syndrome have been found to have high levels of EBV antibodies in their blood, and that many people date the onset of symptoms to a prolonged bout with a viral infection. However, no connection between EBV and chronic fatigue has ever been conclusively proved. Moreover, it is now known that many people have high EBV antibody levels without any apparent ill effects on their health, and that many cases of chronic fatigue occur without any known preceding infection. This has led researchers to look for other possible causes. Some suspect an as-yet-unidentified immune system problem, or a defect in the mechanisms that regulate blood pressure. Other proposed causes of chronic fatigue syndrome include anemia, chronic mercury poisoning from amalgam dental fillings, hypoglycemia, hypothyroidism, infection with the fungus *Candida albicans*, and sleep problems. Fibromyalgia, a muscle disorder that causes muscle weakness and fatigue, has been found in many people with chronic fatigue syndrome. Intestinal parasites are also comparatively common in people with this condition. It is likely that there are different combinations of factors that can result in chronic fatigue in susceptible individuals.

Even though chronic fatigue syndrome is not life-threatening, it cannot be cured, and it can result in serious damage to the immune system. Some people appear to recover spontaneously, but once you have had this condition, it can recur at any time, usually following a bout with another illness or during times of stress.

NUTRIENTS

SUPPLEMENT	SUGGESTED DOSAGE	COMMENTS
Essential		
Acidophilus or Bifido Factor from Natren	As directed on label. As directed on label.	To replace necessary "friendly" bacteria. Also fights candida infection. Chronic fatigue and candidiasis often occur together. Use a nondairy formula.
Coenzyme Q10	75 mg daily.	Enhances the effectiveness of the immune system and protects the heart.
Lecithin granules or capsules	1 tbsp 3 times daily, with meals. 1,200 mg 3 times daily, with meals.	Promotes energy and enhances immunity.
Malic acid and magnesium	As directed on label. 500–1,000 mg daily.	Involved in energy production in many cells of the body, including muscle cells. Needed for sugar metabolism. Deficiency has been linked to CFS.
Manganese	5 mg daily.	Influences the metabolic rate by its involvement in endocrine function.
Proteolytic enzymes or Infla-Zyme Forte from American Biologics or Wobenzym N from Marlyn Nutraceuticals	As directed on label, 6 times daily, on an empty stomach. Take with meals, between meals, and at bedtime.	Reduces inflammation and improves absorption of nutrients, especially protein, which is needed for tissue repair.
Vitamin A and vitamin E	25,000 IU daily for 1 month, then slowly reduce to 10,000 IU daily. If you are pregnant, do not exceed 10,000 IU daily. 800 IU daily for 1 month, then slowly reduce to 400 IU daily.	Powerful free radical scavengers that protect the cells and enhance immune function to fight viruses. Use emulsion forms for easier assimilation and greater safety at high doses.
Vitamin C with bioflavonoids	5,000–10,000 mg daily.	Has a powerful antiviral effect and increases the energy level. Use a buffered form.
Very Important		
Dimethylglycine (DMG) (Aangamik DMG from FoodScience Labs)	50 mg 3 times daily.	Enhances oxygen utilization and destroys free radicals.
Garlic (Kyolic) plus Kyo-Green from Wakunaga	2 capsules 3 times daily, with meals. As directed on label.	Promotes immune function and increases energy. Destroys common parasites. To improve digestion and cleanse the bloodstream.
Free-form amino acid complex	As directed on label.	For tissue and organ repair. Use a formula containing all the essential amino acids.
Vitamin B complex injections plus extra vitamin B6 (pyridoxine) and vitamin B12 plus liver extract injections or vitamin B complex plus extra vitamin B12	2 cc twice weekly or as prescribed by physician. ½ cc twice weekly or as prescribed by physician. 1 cc twice weekly or as prescribed by physician. 2 cc twice weekly or as prescribed by physician. 100 mg 3 times daily. 2,000 mcg daily.	B vitamins are essential for increased energy levels and normal brain function. Injections (under a doctor's supervision) are best. All injectables can be combined in a single syringe. Aids in absorption of vitamin B12. A natural energy booster needed to prevent anemia. A good source of B vitamins plus other valuable nutrients. If injections are not available, a sublingual form is recommended for best results. Use a lozenge or sublingual form.
Important		
Black currant seed oil or primrose oil	As directed on label. Take with meals.	To supply gamma-linolenic acid (GLA) and other essential fatty acids.
Gamma-aminobutyric acid (GABA)	As directed on label, on an empty stomach. Take with water or juice. Do not take with milk. Take with 50 mg vitamin B6 and 100 mg vitamin C for better absorption.	To maintain proper control of brain activity and to control anxiety. See AMINO ACIDS in Part One.
Maitake	As directed on label.	Normalizes immune function and helps the body adapt to stress.
Multivitamin and mineral complex with natural beta-carotene and calcium and magnesium and potassium and selenium and zinc	15,000 IU daily. 1,500 mg daily. 1,000 mg daily. 99 mg daily. 200 mcg daily. 50 mg daily.	All nutrients are necessary in balance. Use a high-potency, hypoallergenic product.
Raw thymus and spleen glandulars plus raw glandular complex	As directed on label. As directed on label. As directed on label.	To boost the immune system. See GLANDULAR THERAPY in Part Three.
Shiitake or reishi	As directed on label. As directed on label.	Helps to combat fatigue, boost immunity, and fight viral infection.

HERBS

❑ Astragalus and echinacea enhance immune function and are good for cold and flu symptoms.

Caution: Do not use astragalus in the presence of a fever.

❑ Ginkgo biloba improves circulation and brain function.

❑ Teas brewed from burdock root, dandelion, and red clover promote healing by cleansing the blood and enhancing immune function. Combine or alternate these herbal teas, and drink 4 to 6 cups daily.

❑ China Gold from Aerobic Life Industries is an herbal formula containing thirty-six different herbal extracts, including ten varieties of ginseng. It helps to enhance adrenal function and overcome fatigue.

❑ Use goldenseal to control infection. At the first signs of a sore throat, take a few drops of alcohol-free goldenseal extract, hold it in your mouth for a moment, then swallow.

Caution: Do not take goldenseal on a daily basis for more than one week at a time, and do not use it during pregnancy. If you have a history of cardiovascular disease, diabetes, or glaucoma, use it only under a doctor's supervision.

❑ Licorice root supports the endocrine system.

Caution: Do not use this herb on a daily basis for more than seven days in a row. Avoid it completely if you have high blood pressure.

❑ Milk thistle protects the liver.

❑ Pau d'arco, taken in capsule or tea form, is good for treating candida infection.

❑ St. Johnswort has antiviral properties.

❑ Skullcap and valerian root improve sleep.

RECOMMENDATIONS

❑ Eat a well-balanced diet of 50 percent raw foods and fresh "live" juices. The diet should consist mostly of fruits, vegetables, and whole grains, plus raw nuts, seeds, skinless turkey, and some deep-water fish. These quality foods supply nutrients that renew energy and build immunity.

❑ Add some form of acidophilus to your diet, and regularly consume soured products such as yogurt and kefir. Many people with chronic fatigue syndrome also are infected with candida. Acidophilus helps to keep candida under control.

❑ Consume plenty of water—at least eight 8-ounce glasses a day—plus juices, preferably freshly made vegetable juices. Drink a full glass of water every two to three waking hours. Water flushes out toxins and aids in reducing muscle pain.

❑ Do not eat shellfish, fried foods, junk foods, processed foods; stimulants such as coffee, tea, and soft drinks; sugar; and white flour products such as bread and pasta.

❑ Make sure that the bowels move daily, and add fiber to the diet. Give yourself occasional cleansing enemas. *See* ENEMAS in Part Three.

❑ Take chlorophyll in tablet form or obtain it from the liquid of vegetables, such as a "green drink" from leafy vegetables, wheatgrass, or Kyo-Green from Wakunaga. Take a protein supplement from a vegetable source—Spiru-tein from Nature's Plus is a good protein drink to take between meals.

❑ Get plenty of rest, and make sure that you do not overexert yourself. Melatonin is helpful for promoting sound, restful sleep. This natural sleep-regulating hormone is available in supplement form. Take it two hours or less before bedtime, not during the day, as it can cause drowsiness.

❑ Try using kombucha tea. Many people have reported new energy and feelings of well-being when using this supplement. *See* MAKING KOMBUCHA TEA in Part Three.

❑ Do not take aspirin. If a viral infection is present, Reye's syndrome may result.

CONSIDERATIONS

❑ There are other health problems that can cause symptoms of chronic fatigue, including anemia, depression, fibromyalgia, cardiovascular disease (especially in women), hepatitis, and Lyme disease, among others. Anyone who experiences extreme fatigue that persists for longer than a week or two should consult a health care provider. There may be an underlying medical disorder that requires treatment.

❑ If you are diagnosed as having chronic fatigue syndrome, it is wise to seek out a health care provider who has specific experience in the management and treatment of this complex condition.

❑ Taking regular cold showers may produce an improvement in CFS symptoms. However, people with heart or circulatory disorders or other serious health problems should not attempt cold water treatment without first consulting their health care providers.

❑ Certain of the amino acids may be beneficial to people with chronic fatigue. These include tyrosine, leucine, isoleucine, and valine, as well as lysine and taurine. (*See* AMINO ACIDS in Part One.)

❑ A recent study at Johns Hopkins University Hospital in Baltimore identified a link between chronic fatigue and a problem in the body's mechanisms for regulating blood pressure. In this study, twenty-two out of twenty-three subjects with chronic fatigue were found to have a syndrome in which the body responds inappropriately to periods of prolonged standing—the heart rate slows and blood pressure drops, resulting in lightheadedness, followed by a feeling of weakness and exhaustion that can persist for days afterward. A significant percentage of those in the study experienced an improvement when they were treated for the blood pressure problem.

❑ Some research points to chemical and/or food sensitivities as possible causes of chronic fatigue. People living in the past fifty years have been exposed to more different chemicals than all of the rest of humankind combined. It is no wonder that some people have become sensitive to chemicals. (*See* CHEMICAL ALLERGIES in Part Two.)

❑ Parasites are common in people with chronic fatigue.

☐ Family members, friends, and coworkers must understand the nature of the disorder, and realize that the person suffering from it is not exaggerating or faking symptoms.

☐ The National Institute of Allergy and Infectious Diseases (NIAID), a part of the National Institutes of Health, provides current information on chronic fatigue syndrome. You can write to them at Building 31, Room 7A50, 9000 Rockville Pike, Bethesda, MD 20892; or call 301–496–5717.

☐ *See also* CANDIDIASIS; FIBROMYALGIA; HYPOTHYROIDISM; and MONONUCLEOSIS, all in Part Two.

Circulatory Problems

There are many disorders associated with circulatory problems. When plaque or fatty deposits form along the walls of the arteries, it causes them to harden and constrict. *Hypertension,* or high blood pressure, results because the blood exerts greater force against the walls of the narrowed and/or more rigid blood vessels. Hypertension can lead to stroke, angina pectoris (chest pain), kidney damage, and heart attack.

A circulatory disease that is brought on by chronic inflammation of the blood vessels in the extremities is *thromboangiitis obliterans (Buerger's disease).* This disease is most prevalent among people who smoke. It usually affects the foot or lower leg, but it can occur in the hand, arm, or thigh as well. Early signs of Buerger's disease are a tingling sensation (commonly referred to as "pins and needles") and a burning sensation in the fingers and toes. It can lead to ulceration and gangrene; in severe cases, amputation may be required.

Another serious circulatory condition is *Raynaud's phenomenon,* which is characterized by constriction and spasm of the blood vessels in the extremities, such as in the fingers, toes, and tip of the nose. Cold, stress, smoking, and other factors may cause fingers and toes to become numb; extremities may appear colorless or bluish due to lack of circulation and arterial spasm. This disease most commonly affects women and occasionally leads to gangrene. Poor circulation can also result from *varicose veins,* which develop because of a loss of elasticity in the walls of the veins.

NUTRIENTS

SUPPLEMENT	SUGGESTED DOSAGE	COMMENTS
Essential		
L-Carnitine	500 mg twice daily.	Helps to strengthen the heart muscle and to promote circulation by transporting long fatty acid chains.
Very Important		
Garlic (Kyolic)	2 capsules 3 times daily, with meals.	Lowers blood pressure and helps to strengthen the heart muscle. Thins the blood.
Chlorophyll	As directed on label.	Enhances circulation and helps build healthy cells. Use liquid or tablet form. Also prepare fresh "green drinks" from green leafy vegetables.
Coenzyme Q_{10}	100 mg daily.	Improves tissue oxygenation.
Lecithin granules or capsules	1 tbsp 3 times daily, before meals. 2,400 mg 3 times daily, before meals.	Emulsifies (breaks up) fats.
Multienzyme complex	As directed on label. Take with meals.	To aid digestion and circulation and enhance oxygen use in all body tissues.
Vitamin B complex	50–100 mg 3 times daily.	Needed for metabolism of fat and cholesterol. Consider injections (under a doctor's supervision). If injections are not available, use a sublingual form. Enhances circulation and brain function.
plus extra vitamin B_1 (thiamine) and	50 mg daily.	
vitamin B_6 (pyridoxine) and	50 mg daily.	A natural diuretic that protects the heart.
vitamin B_{12} and	300 mcg daily.	Prevents anemia and acts as a natural energy booster.
folic acid and	400 mcg daily.	Needed for the formation of oxygen-carrying red blood cells.
para-aminobenzoic acid (PABA)	25 mg daily.	Assists in the formation of red blood cells.
Vitamin C with bioflavonoids	5,000–10,000 mg daily, in divided doses.	Helps prevent blood clotting.
Important		
Calcium and	1,500–2,000 mg daily, in divided doses, after meals and at bedtime.	Essential in normal blood viscosity.
magnesium	750–1,000 mg daily, in divided doses, after meals and at bedtime.	Strengthens the heartbeat. Calcium and magnesium work together.
Dimethylglycine (DMG) (Aangamik DMG from FoodScience Labs)	50 mg twice daily.	Enhances tissue oxygenation.
Multivitamin and mineral complex	As directed on label.	To provide a balance of nutrients basic to good circulatory function.
Vitamin A and	50,000 IU daily. If you are pregnant, do not exceed 10,000 IU daily.	Aids in storage of fat and acts as an antioxidant. Use emulsion form for easier assimilation and greater safety at high doses.
vitamin E	Start with 200 IU daily and increase slowly to 1,000 IU daily.	Inhibits the formation of free radicals. Use emulsion form.
Helpful		
Choline and inositol plus	100 mg each 3 times daily, with meals.	Helps to remove fat deposits and improve circulation. Helps to lower cholesterol.
vitamin B_3 (niacin)	50 mg 3 times daily. Do not exceed a total of 300 mg daily from all supplements.	Helps to lower cholesterol. *Caution:* Do not take niacin if you have a liver disorder, gout, or high blood pressure.
Pycnogenol or grape seed extract	As directed on label. As directed on label.	Neutralize free radicals, enhance the action of vitamin C, and strengthen connective tissue, including that of the cardiovascular system.

L-cysteine and L-methionine	500 mg each daily, on an empty stomach. Take with juice or water. Do not take with milk. Take with 50 mg vitamin B_6 and 100 mg vitamin C for better absorption.	Protects and preserves cells by detoxifying harmful toxins. Prevents accumulation of fat both in the liver and in the arteries, where it may obstruct blood flow. See AMINO ACIDS in Part One.
Proteolytic enzymes	As directed on label. Take between meals.	To combat "leaky gut syndrome."
Selenium	200 mcg daily.	Deficiency has been linked to heart disorders.
Shiitake or reishi	As directed on label. As directed on label.	Helps to prevent high blood pressure and heart disease; lowers cholesterol levels.
Zinc plus copper	50 mg daily. Do not exceed a total of 100 mg daily from all supplements. 3 mg daily.	Needed for immune function. Use zinc chelate form. Needed to balance with zinc.

HERBS

❑ The following herbs support the heart and cirulatory system: black cohosh, butcher's broom, cayenne (capsicum), chickweed, gentian root, ginkgo biloba, goldenseal, hawthorn berries, horseradish, horsetail, hyssop, licorice root, pleurisy root, rose hips, and wormwood. Cayenne increases the pulse rate, while black cohosh slows it. Ginkgo is being used for circulatory disorders in many clinics.

Caution: Do not use black cohosh if you are pregnant or have any type of chronic disease. Do not use licorice on a daily basis for more than seven days in a row, and avoid it completely if you have high blood pressure. Do not use wormwood during pregnancy. It is not recommended for long-term use, as it can be habit-forming.

❑ Sanhelio's Circu Caps from Health From the Sun is an herbal combination formula beneficial for circulatory disorders.

RECOMMENDATIONS

❑ Make sure that your diet is high in fiber. Oat bran can help lower cholesterol levels.

❑ Include the following in your diet: bananas, brown rice, endive, garlic, lima beans, onions, pears, peas, and spinach.

❑ Drink steam-distilled water only.

❑ Eliminate animal protein and fatty foods (such as red meat), sugar, and white flour from your diet. Do not use stimulants such as coffee, colas, or tobacco, or eat foods with a lot of spices.

❑ Get regular exercise to help blood flow and to keep the arteries soft and unclogged.

Caution: If you are over thirty-five and/or have been sedentary for some time, consult your health care provider before beginning any type of exercise program.

❑ Keep your weight down.

❑ To boost circulation, give yourself a dry massage over your entire body using a loofah sponge or natural bath brush. Also dip a towel in cold water and rub it briskly over parts of the body.

❑ If you have circulatory problems, *do not* take any preparations containing shark cartilage unless specifically directed to do so by your physician. Shark cartilage inhibits the formation of new blood vessels, the mechanism by which the body can increase circulatory capacity.

CONSIDERATIONS

❑ Because sluggish circulation can have a variety of different causes, you should see your health care provider if it is persistent.

❑ Chelation therapy is helpful for improving circulation. (*See* CHELATION THERAPY in Part Three.)

❑ *See also* ARTERIOSCLEROSIS/ATHEROSCLEROSIS; CARDIOVASCULAR DISEASE; HIGH BLOOD PRESSURE; HIGH CHOLESTEROL; HYPOTHYROIDISM; RAYNAUD'S PHENOMENON; and VARICOSE VEINS, all in Part Two.

Cirrhosis of the Liver

Cirrhosis of the liver is a degenerative inflammatory disease that results in hardening and scarring of liver cells. The liver becomes unable to function properly due to the scarred tissue, which prevents the normal passage of blood through the liver.

The most common cause of cirrhosis of the liver is excessive alcohol consumption; a less frequent cause is viral hepatitis. Malnutrition and chronic inflammation can also lead to liver malfunction.

In the early stages, symptoms of cirrhosis of the liver may include constipation or diarrhea, fever, upset stomach, fatigue, weakness, poor appetite, weight loss, enlarged liver, vomiting, red palms, and jaundice. Those in the later stages of the disease may develop anemia, bruising due to bleeding under the skin, and edema.

NUTRIENTS

SUPPLEMENT	SUGGESTED DOSAGE	COMMENTS
Essential		
Vitamin B complex	100 mg 3 times daily.	The B vitamins are necessary for proper digestion, absorption of nutrients, and formation of red blood cells. Use a high-potency formula. Injections (under a doctor's supervision) may be necessary.
plus extra vitamin B_{12}	1,000 mcg twice daily.	To prevent anemia and protect against nerve damage. Use a lozenge or sublingual form.
and folic acid	200 mcg daily.	To correct deficiencies.

Phosphatidyl choline plus	As directed on label.	For fatty liver.
choline and inositol	As directed on label.	
Primrose oil	500 mg twice daily, with meals.	To prevent an imbalance of fatty acids, found in cirrhosis of the liver.

Very Important

Garlic (Kyolic)	2 capsules 3 times daily, with meals.	Detoxifies the liver and bloodstream.
Infla-Zyme Forte from American Biologics	As directed on label.	Balanced potent enzymes that act to inhibit inflammation.
L-Arginine plus L-cysteine and L-methionine	500 mg each daily, on an empty stomach. Take with water or juice. Do not take with milk. Take with 50 mg vitamin B_6 and 100 mg vitamin C for better absorption.	Helps to detoxify ammonia, a byproduct of protein digestion that can accumulate when the liver isn't functioning properly. Helps detoxify harmful toxins.
plus L-carnitine	500 mg daily, on an empty stomach.	Helps prevent accumulation of fat in the liver.
plus glutathione	500 mg daily, on an empty stomach.	A powerful antioxidant that protects against liver cancer.
Lecithin granules or capsules	1 tbsp 3 times daily, with meals. 2,400 mg 3 times daily, with meals.	A powerful fat emulsifier.
Multienzyme complex with betaine and hydrochloric acid (HCl) plus ox bile extract	As directed on label. Take with each meal. As directed on label.	Needed for digestion to lessen the strain on the liver. Replaces the digestive enzymes normally produced by the gallbladder.
Raw liver extract	As directed on label.	Prevents anemia and aids in building the liver. See GLANDULAR THERAPY in Part Three.
Silymarin (milk thistle extract)		See under Herbs, below.
Taurine Plus from American Biologics	20 drops 3 times daily.	The most important antioxidant for health and stress from free radical damage. Use the sublingual form.

Important

Alfalfa		See under Herbs, below.
Bifido Factor from Natren or	As directed on label. Take on an empty stomach.	Repairs liver cells and aids in healing.
Kyo-Dophilus from Wakunaga	2–3 capsules 3 times daily.	Human-cultured flora from small intestine, primarily to improve assimilation of nutrients. Detoxifies ammonia.
Calcium and magnesium	1,500 mg daily, in divided doses, after meals and at bedtime. 750 mg daily.	To promote healing of tissue. Beneficial for the nervous system. Use chelate forms.
Vitamin C	3,000–8,000 mg daily, in divided doses.	An important antioxidant. Use a buffered form.

Dimethylglycine (DMG) (Aangamik DMG from FoodScience Labs)	As directed on label.	Supplies oxygen for healing.

Helpful

Aloe vera		See under Herbs, below.
Coenzyme Q_{10}	100 mg daily.	Promotes oxygenation.
Free-form amino acid complex	As directed on label.	A good source of protein that is easy on the liver.
Selenium	200 mcg daily.	A good detoxifier.
Spiru-tein from Nature's Plus	As directed on label. Take between meals.	A vegetable protein drink that supplies essential amino acids and stabilizes the blood sugar.
Vitamin A	As directed on label. Do not exceed 10,000 IU daily.	Needed for healing. Use emulsion form for easier assimilation and greater safety at higher doses. Caution: Do not substitute pill forms of vitamin A for emulsion. Pills put extra stress on liver.
plus vitamin D and	As directed on label.	To correct deficiencies.
vitamin E	As directed on label.	A potent antioxidant that aids circulation.
Zinc	50 mg daily. Do not exceed a total of 100 mg daily from all supplements.	Needed for the immune system and the healing process. Use zinc gluconate lozenges or OptiZinc for best absorption.

HERBS

❑ Alfalfa helps to build a healthy digestive tract and is a good source of vitamin K. It helps to prevent bleeding as a result of vitamin K deficiency, which is common with cirrhosis. It can be taken in tablet or liquid form.

❑ Aloe vera helps to cleanse and heal the digestive tract. Drink ¼ cup of aloe vera juice every morning and evening. George's Aloe Vera Juice from Warren Laboratories is a good product. It can be taken in a cup of herbal tea if you wish.

❑ Silymarin (milk thistle extract) has been shown in scientific studies to repair and rejuvenate the liver. Take 200 milligrams of silymarin three times daily.

❑ Other herbs that can be beneficial for people with cirrhosis include barberry, black radish, burdock, celandine, cheonanthus, dandelion, echinacea, fennel, goldenseal, hops, horsetail, Irish moss, red clover, rose hips, suma, thyme, and wild Oregon grape.

Caution: Do not use barberry, celandine, goldenseal, or wild Oregon grape during pregnancy. Do not take goldenseal on a daily basis for more than one week at a time, and use it only under supervision if you have a history of cardiovascular disease, diabetes, or glaucoma.

RECOMMENDATIONS

❑ Obtain protein from vegetable sources; do not eat foods containing animal protein.

The Liver

Weighing about four pounds, the liver is the largest gland of the body and the only internal organ that will regenerate itself if part of it is damaged. Up to 25 percent of the liver can be removed, and within a short period of time, it will grow back to its original shape and size.

The liver has many functions, perhaps the most important of which is the secretion of bile. This fluid is stored in the gallbladder and released as needed for digestion. Bile is necessary for the digestion of fats; it breaks fat down into small globules. Bile also assists in the absorption of the fat-soluble vitamins (A, D, E, and K), and helps to assimilate calcium. In addition, bile converts beta-carotene into vitamin A. It promotes intestinal peristalsis as well, which helps prevent constipation.

After nutrients have been absorbed into the bloodstream through the intestinal wall, they are transported by way of the hepatic portal system to the liver. In the liver, nutrients such as iron and vitamins A, B_{12}, and D are extracted from the bloodstream and stored for future use. These stored substances are utilized for everyday activities and in times of physical stress. The liver plays an important role in fat metabolism; in the synthesis of fatty acids from amino acids and sugars; in the production of lipoproteins, cholesterol, and phospholipids; and in the oxidation of fat to produce energy. The liver creates a substance called glucose tolerance factor (GTF) from chromium and glutathione. GTF acts with insulin to regulate blood sugar levels. Sugars not required for immediate energy production are converted into glycogen in the liver; the glycogen is stored in the liver and the muscles, and is converted back into sugar when needed for energy. Excess food is converted to fat in the liver, and the fat is then transported to the fatty tissues of the body for storage.

In addition to its important functions in digestion and energy production, the liver acts as a detoxifier. Protein digestion and bacterial fermentation of food in the intestines produce ammonia as a byproduct; this ammonia is detoxified by the liver. The liver combines toxic substances (including metabolic waste products, insecticide residues, drugs, alcohol, and other harmful chemicals) with substances that are less toxic. These substances are then excreted via the kidneys. Thus, in order for the liver to function properly, you must also have proper kidney function.

Finally, the liver is responsible for regulating thyroid function by converting thyroxine (T_4), a thyroid hormone, into its more active form, triiodothyronine (T_3). Inadequate conversion of T_4 into T_3 by the liver may lead to hypothyroidism. The liver also breaks down hormones like adrenaline, aldosterone, estrogen, and insulin after they have performed their needed functions.

The nutrients listed in the right column can help maintain proper liver function.

NUTRIENTS

SUPPLEMENT	SUGGESTED DOSAGE	COMMENTS
Coenzyme Q_{10}	60 mg daily.	Supplies oxygen to the liver. A potent liver protector.
Free-form amino acid complex	As directed on label. Take on an empty stomach.	A source of protein that is easy on the liver because it has already been broken down.
L-Cysteine and L-methionine	500 mg each daily, before meals. Take with water or juice, not with milk. Take with 50 mg vitamin B_6 and 100 mg vitamin C for better absorption.	To aid in liver detoxification and protect liver cells. *See* AMINO ACIDS in Part One.
plus glutathione	100 mg daily, before meals.	
Lecithin granules or capsules	1 tbsp 3 times daily, before meals. 1,200 mg 3 times daily, before meals.	Prevents fatty buildup in the liver.
Liver extract injections plus	As prescribed by physician.	To supply needed B vitamins, iron, and other nutrients that help to rebuild the liver cells.
vitamin B_{12} or	As prescribed by physician.	
desiccated liver	As directed on label.	Use liver from organically raised beef.
Liv-R-Actin from Nature's Plus		*See under* Herbs, below.
Multienzyme complex with ox bile	As directed on label.	Aids in digestion. Relieves the liver of some of its burden.
Multivitamin and mineral complex with		All nutrients are needed for repair of tissues.
vitamin B complex and	50 mg daily.	
selenium and	200 mcg daily.	
zinc	30 mg daily.	
Phosphatidyl choline	As directed on label.	Prevents fatty buildup and is important for energy production in the liver.
Vitamin C	5,000 mg daily, in divided doses.	An immune enhancer and powerful antioxidant. Neutralizes toxic substances.
Vitamin E	600 IU daily.	A powerful antioxidant. Protects the liver from damage.

HERBS

❑   Use celandine and silymarin (milk thistle extract) daily to help maintain liver function.

Caution: Do not use celandine during pregnancy.

❑   Liv-R-Actin from Nature's Plus is a good source of milk thistle. Take 2 capsules three times daily, before meals.

RECOMMENDATIONS

❑ Increase your consumption of foods high in potassium, such as almonds, bananas, blackstrap molasses, brewer's yeast, dulse, kelp, prunes, raisins, rice and wheat bran, and seeds.

❑ Drink plenty of water, especially steam-distilled water. When taking supplements, always take them with a full glass of water.

❑ Avoid constipating foods. The liver has to work twice as hard if you are constipated. Be sure your diet contains sufficient amounts of choline, inositol, and lecithin, as well as bulk and fiber.

❑ Do not smoke, and avoid alcohol, coffee, fish, fowl, meat, salt, soft drinks, sugar, tea, and spicy or fried foods.

❑ Perform a three-day juice fast once every thirty days. *See* FASTING in Part Three. To help cleanse the liver while fasting, drink beet juice, carrot juice, black radish extract, and dandelion extract. Chlorophyll and distilled water with lemon are excellent blood purifiers and liver cleansers. Regular cleansing of the body, especially the liver, is vital to maintaining good health.

❑ Do not take more than 10,000 international units of vitamin A daily on an ongoing basis, and avoid cod liver oil. Do not take more than 1,500 milligrams of niacin daily.

CONSIDERATIONS

❑ Animal studies indicate that the typical American diet is damaging to the liver. Improper diet results in allergies, digestive disorders, a low energy level, and an inability to detoxify harmful substances.

❑ The four basic reasons for poor liver function are:

1. *The presence of cumulative poisons.* Insecticides, preservatives, and other toxins can build up in and impair the liver. Even though a particular toxin may not accumulate in the liver, liver function may suffer if the functioning of other organs, especially the pancreas and/or kidneys, is adversely affected by the toxin.

2. *An improper diet.* A diet that is low in protein and high in carbohydrates and fats, especially saturated fats, fried foods, and hydrogenated fats, is hard on the liver and may not provide sufficient protein building blocks necessary for repair. Poor food choices include processed foods, junk foods, refined white flour products, white sugar products, and imitation foods that are designed to appear and taste like an original product but that have been robbed of natural vitamins, minerals, and enzymes.

3. *Overeating.* Overeating is probably the most common cause of liver malfunction. Overeating creates excess work for the liver, resulting in liver fatigue. In addition, the liver must detoxify all of the various chemicals present in our food supply today. When the liver is overworked, it may not detoxify harmful substances properly.

4. *Drugs.* Drugs put a great strain on the liver. Drugs are substances that are foreign and unnatural to the body. These foreign substances cause the liver to work overtime in excreting these toxins. The liver neutralizes the effects of drugs on the body. Alcohol is particularly toxic to the liver. When excessive amounts of alcohol enter the liver, the liver begins to lose its functioning capacity. Other substances that can contribute to liver malfunction include oral contraceptives and caffeine.

❑ Eat a diet consisting of 75 percent raw foods. If cirrhosis is severe, consume only fresh vegetables and fruits and their juices for two weeks.

❑ Include the following in your diet: almonds, brewer's yeast, grains and seeds, raw goat's milk, and products derived from goat's milk. Nuts must be raw and from tightly sealed packages.

❑ Eat plenty of foods high in vitamin K. Persons with cirrhosis of the liver are often deficient in vitamin K. Good sources of vitamin K include alfalfa sprouts and green leafy vegetables.

❑ Include legumes (kidney beans, peas, and soybeans) and seeds in your diet. These foods contain the amino acid arginine, which helps to detoxify ammonia, a byproduct of protein digestion.

❑ Drink fresh vegetable juices, such as beet, carrot, dandelion extract, and "green drinks."

❑ Drink steam-distilled or sip barley water throughout the day. *See* THERAPEUTIC LIQUIDS in Part Three for the recipe.

❑ Use only cold-pressed vegetable oils as sources of dietary fats. Consume oils in uncooked form only, such as in salad dressings.

❑ Limit your intake of fish—haddock, bluefish, salmon, and sardines—to a maximum of two servings a week, and *do not* eat raw or undercooked seafood. A damaged liver cannot handle the amount of vitamin A contained in these foods. Avoid cod liver oil.

❑ Keep the colon clean. Toxins accumulate in the liver and must be excreted via the colon and kidneys. *See* COLON CLEANSING in Part Three.

❑ Do not use harsh laxatives to cleanse the system. Lemon enemas are preferred; take these twice weekly. You can also alternate wheatgrass enemas with coffee enemas for two weeks. Both of these detoxify the system. *See* ENEMAS in Part Three.

❑ Do not take any drugs (over-the-counter or prescription) except for those prescribed by your doctor.

❑ Consume no alcohol in any form. Also eliminate the

following from your diet: animal products, candies, milk, pastries, pepper, salt, spices, stimulants of any kind (including caffeine and colas), white rice, and products containing sugar and/or white flour. Virtually all commercially prepared foods contain some of the above.

❑   Read all food labels carefully, and avoid most fats. Do not eat any of the following: butter, margarine, vegetable shortening, and any other hardened fats; fried or fatty foods; melted or hard cheeses; nuts or oils that have been subjected to heat (either in processing or in cooking); potato chips; and all refined and processed foods. These overwork and damage the liver.

CONSIDERATIONS

❑   In one study, people with cirrhosis of the liver were found to have an imbalance of essential fatty acids, which are needed for cell protection. After taking 10 capsules of primrose oil daily for three weeks, these individuals showed a marked improvement in the balance of their fatty acids.

❑   *See also* ALCOHOLISM and HEPATITIS, both in Part Two.

Cold

See COMMON COLD.

Cold Sores (Fever Blisters)

Cold sores, or fever blisters, are caused by herpes simplex virus I. They first appear three to ten days after exposure and may last up to three weeks. The virus then remains in the body, and repeated outbreaks may be triggered by fever, a cold or other viral infection, exposure to sun and wind, stress, menstruation, or depression of the immune system. These sores are very contagious.

The first sign of a developing cold sore is local tenderness with a small bump. The bump then turns into a blister, and there may be more tenderness in the area. The adjacent lymph nodes may become swollen and tender. In some cases, pus oozes from the blisters, which makes eating difficult. Fortunately, there is always less discomfort with recurrences of cold sores than with the initial outbreak.

NUTRIENTS

SUPPLEMENT	SUGGESTED DOSAGE	COMMENTS
Essential		
L-Lysine	500 mg twice daily.	Fights the virus that causes cold sores. *Caution:* Do not take lysine for longer than 6 months at a time.
L-Lysine cream	Apply topically as directed on label.	This amino acid fights herpes-viruses. *See* AMINO ACIDS in Part One.
Vitamin B complex	100–150 mg twice daily.	Important for healing and immune function. Use a high-stress formula.
Zinc lozenges (Ultimate Zinc-C Lozenges from Now Foods)	1 15-mg lozenge every 3 waking hours for 2 days, then 2 lozenges daily until healed. Do not exceed a total of 100 mg daily from all supplements.	Stimulates immune function to fight the virus. Zinc is absorbed quickly in lozenge form.
Very Important		
Acidophilus	As directed on label. Take on an empty stomach.	Inhibits pathogenic organisms.
Colloidal silver	Take orally or apply topically as directed on label.	An antiseptic and antibiotic that destroys bacteria, viruses, and fungi, and promotes healing.
Garlic (Kyolic)	2 capsules 3 times daily.	Acts as a natural antibiotic and immunity enhancer.
Vitamin C	3,000–6,000 mg daily, in divided doses.	Fights the virus and boosts immune function. Use a buffered form.
Important		
Calcium and	1,500 mg daily.	To help relieve stress.
magnesium	750–1,000 mg daily.	
Essential fatty acids	As directed on label.	Aids skin in healing.
Helpful		
Maitake or	As directed on label.	To fight viruses and build resistance to disease.
shiitake or	As directed on label.	
reishi	As directed on label.	
Multivitamin and mineral complex	As directed on label.	All nutrients are necessary in balance.
Vitamin A and vitamin E	50,000 IU daily. If you are pregnant, do not exceed 10,000 IU daily. 400 IU daily.	Needed for healing of tissue in mouth and lip area. Use emulsion forms for easier assimilation and greater safety at higher doses.

HERBS

❑   For cold sores, use echinacea, goldenseal, pau d'arco, and red clover.

Caution: Do not take goldenseal on a daily basis for more than one week at a time, and do not use it during pregnancy. If you have a history of cardiovascular disease, diabetes, or glaucoma, use it only under a doctor's supervision.

RECOMMENDATIONS

❑   Eat plenty of raw vegetables, as well as yogurt and other soured products.

❑   If cold sore outbreaks occur often, check for low thyroid function. *See* HYPOTHYROIDISM in Part Two.

CONSIDERATIONS

❑ The drug acyclovir (Zovirax), in oral or topical form, is sometimes prescribed for cold sores.

❑ If you are prone to allergies, you most likely have a malfunctioning immune system and may be susceptible to cold sores. *See* ALLERGIES in Part Two.

❑ *See also* HERPESVIRUS INFECTION in Part Two.

Colitis

See ULCERATIVE COLITIS.

Colorblindness

See under EYE PROBLEMS.

Common Cold

There are over 200 viruses that can cause the common cold, an infection of the upper respiratory tract. The well-known symptoms include head congestion, sore throat, coughing, headache, fever, restlessness, sneezing, watery eyes, and aches and pains. Most colds clear up on their own in a week to ten days, but occasionally a cold can lead to a more serious illness, such as bronchitis, pneumonia, or flu.

It is estimated that healthy adults get an average of two colds per year. Children generally get many more because their immune systems are immature, and because they have not yet developed immunity to many of the viruses that cause colds. If an adult gets colds often, it may be a sign that his or her immune system is not working properly.

NUTRIENTS

SUPPLEMENT	SUGGESTED DOSAGE	COMMENTS
Essential		
ACES + Zinc from Carlson Labs	As directed on label.	Contains vitamins A, C, and E, plus the minerals selenium and zinc.
Echinacea and goldenseal		*See under* Herbs, below.
Vitamin A	15,000 IU daily. If you are pregnant, do not exceed 10,000 IU daily.	Helps heal inflamed mucous membranes and strengthens the immune system.
plus natural beta-carotene	15,000 IU daily.	An antioxidant and precursor of vitamin A.
or carotenoid complex (Betatene)	As directed on label.	
Vitamin C	5,000–20,000 mg daily, in divided doses. *See* ASCORBIC ACID FLUSH in Part Three.	Fights cold viruses. For children, use buffered vitamin C or calcium ascorbate.
Zinc lozenges (Ultimate Zinc-C Lozenges from Now Foods)	For adults and children, 1 15-mg lozenge every 3 waking hours for 3 days, then 1 lozenge every 4 hours for 1 week. Do not exceed a total of 100 mg daily from all supplements.	Boosts the immune system. Keep these on hand and use them at the first sign of a cold.
Important		
Free-form amino acid complex	As directed on label.	To supply needed protein.
Garlic (Kyolic)	2 capsules 3 times daily.	A natural antibiotic and immune system enhancer.
L-Lysine	500 mg daily, on an empty stomach. Take with water or juice. Do not take with milk. Take with 50 mg vitamin B_6 and 100 mg vitamin C for better absorption.	Aids in destroying viruses and preventing cold sores in and around the mouth. *See* AMINO ACIDS in Part One. *Caution:* Do not take lysine for longer than 6 months at a time.
Helpful		
Acidophilus or	As directed on label. Take on an empty stomach.	To replace "friendly" bacteria.
Bifido Factor from Natren or	As directed on label.	For adults.
LifeStart from Natren	As directed on label.	For children.
Fenu-Thyme from Nature's Way		*See under* Herbs, below.
Maitake or	As directed on label.	Mushrooms with immune-boosting and antiviral properties.
shiitake or	As directed on label.	
reishi	As directed on label.	
Multimineral complex	As directed on label.	Minerals are needed for healing and for immune response.
or kelp	1,800–3,600 mg daily.	A rich source of necessary minerals.
Multivitamin complex with		For healing and to reduce stress.
vitamin B complex	50–100 mg 3 times daily.	

HERBS

❑ For fever, take catnip tea enemas and ¼ to ½ teaspoon of lobelia tincture every three to four hours until fever drops. This dosage can be used for children also.
Caution: Do not take lobelia internally on an ongoing basis.

❑ Ephedra (ma huang) is helpful for congestion and coughing.
Caution: Do not use this herb if you suffer from anxiety, glaucoma, heart disease, high blood pressure, or insomnia, or if you are taking a monoamine oxidase (MAO) inhibitor drug for depression.

❑ Ginger, pau d'arco, slippery elm, and yarrow tea can help the common cold.

Common Cold Remedies

Americans spend more than $1 billion every year on nonprescription treatments for coughs and colds. At best, these products can offer only temporary relief. The following is a list of some of the most common types of cold remedies, and what they can and cannot do:

• **Analgesics,** such as acetaminophen, aspirin, and ibuprofen, help to relieve aches and pains and reduce fever. By themselves, colds do not usually cause significant fever. Allowing a low-grade fever to run its course may actually be beneficial; an elevated temperature is one of the body's ways of fighting infection. If you have a fever that reaches 102°F or higher, chances are something other than the cold is causing it. It may be a sign of a developing bacterial infection somewhere in the body that requires treatment. By reducing fever, analgesics may mask this sign.

• **Antihistamines** decrease nasal secretions by blocking the action of histamine, a body chemical that causes swelling of small blood vessels, which results in sneezing and runny nose. These products may make you drowsy. In addition, it is better to allow the secretions that contain the virus to flow out of the body rather than trying to block them.

• **Cough medicines** come in two basic types: expectorants and antitussives. Expectorants make coughs more productive by increasing the amount of phlegm and decreasing its thickness. This helps remove irritants from respiratory airways. Guaifenesin, an expectorant found in many popular over-the-counter cough medicines, can be effective. The effectiveness of other over-the-counter expectorants is questionable. Antitussives reduce the frequency of coughing. An antitussive called dextromethorphan is generally considered reasonably safe and effective. It is often denoted by the initials "DM" on product labels. However, because coughing is the body's mechanism for clearing secretions from the lungs, it is probably best not to suppress it unless coughing is unusually severe or persistent, or it is interfering with sleep.

• **Decongestants** shrink nasal blood vessels to relieve swelling and congestion. These medications can cause side effects including jitteriness, insomnia, and fatigue.

Most over-the-counter cold remedies contain some combination of acetaminophen and various decongestants, antihistamines, and cough suppressants. Some experts believe that these ingredients may work against one another. For example, acetaminophen may increase nasal congestion, while the decongestant decreases it. If a cold is making you extremely uncomfortable and you feel you must take something for it, it is better to take a single-ingredient product appropriate for the particular symptom you are treating.

❑ Eucalyptus oil is helpful for relieving congestion. Put 5 drops in a hot bath, or put 6 drops in a cup of boiling water and inhale the steam.

❑ Fenu-Thyme from Nature's Way is an herbal formula that helps rid nasal passages of mucus. Take 2 capsules three times daily.

❑ For a sore throat, add 3 to 6 drops of pure tea tree oil to warm water and gargle. Repeat this up to three times daily. Take up to 2 tea tree oil lozenges and allow them to dissolve slowly in your mouth. Repeat this treatment as often as required, alternating it with goldenseal extract. These products can be found in most health food stores.

❑ At the first sign of a cold, use an alcohol-free echinacea and goldenseal combination extract to boost your immune system and keep the virus from multiplying. For adults, place 1 dropperful in the mouth, hold it for five minutes, then swallow. Do this every three hours for three days. For children, place 8 to 10 drops in the mouth, hold it for a few minutes (or as long as the child can manage), then swallow. Do this every two hours for three days. Then take 8 to 10 drops in liquid daily until symptoms are gone. Besides beating colds, flu, bronchitis, and other upper respiratory infections, echinacea is good for clearing up strep throat. *Caution:* Do not take goldenseal on a daily basis for more than one week at a time, and do not use it during pregnancy.

If you have a history of cardiovascular disease, diabetes, or glaucoma, use it only under a doctor's supervision.

RECOMMENDATIONS

❑ Sip hot liquids such as turkey or chicken broth.

❑ Drink Potato Peeling Broth twice a day—make it fresh daily. *See* THERAPEUTIC LIQUIDS in Part Three for the recipe. You can add a carrot or a stalk of celery to your drink.

❑ Remain as active as possible. Not only is staying in bed for ordinary sniffles unnecessary, but it will probably make you feel worse. Moving around helps to loosen built-up mucus and fluids. Unless you have a fever, a brisk walk or any other type of moderate exercise should make you feel better.

❑ Flush tissues after they have been used. Because they harbor the virus, tissues can pass on the virus or cause you to reinfect yourself.

❑ Wash your hands often. Cold viruses can survive for several hours on hands, tissues, or hard surfaces. A healthy person can contract the virus by touching a contaminated surface, then touching his or her own mouth or nose.

❑ Try not to spread the cold to your family or colleagues. Refrain from close contact with loved ones. Even shaking hands is out; hand contact can spread the virus.

❑ Do not give aspirin, or any product containing aspirin, to a child with symptoms of any viral infection, including a cold. (*See* REYE'S SYNDROME in Part Two).

CONSIDERATIONS

❑ Since there is no cure for the common cold, the best approach is prevention. Once a cold has a firm grip on you, it is hard to stop it.

❑ There are many over-the-counter cold medications available. None of them can actually cure a cold, although they may sometimes be helpful for alleviating symptoms. (*See* Common Cold Remedies on page 210.)

❑ It is unlikely that a vaccine will ever be developed to prevent the common cold because the viruses responsible have the ability to change in size and shape, and have hundreds of different forms.

❑ The possibility for real cold relief may lie in substances such as interferons, natural proteins that the body produces in response to viral infection. Interferons seem to improve the respiratory tract's ability to ward off viruses. Vitamin C promotes interferon production.

❑ Antibiotics are ineffective against viral infections, but many people still ask their doctors to prescribe them. It is important to understand that penicillin and most other antibiotics work only against bacterial infections, such as strep throat—not viral infections. Viruses and bacteria may produce similar symptoms, but they are very different kinds of microbes and do not respond to the same treatment. In fact, because antibiotics kill off "good" bacteria together with the bad, antibiotics actually inhibit the body's efforts to defend itself against viral invasion.

❑ You can, in a sense, catch a cold from yourself. When your immune system weakens from factors such as stress and/or a poor diet, viruses can take hold.

❑ A five-week study of seventy-nine young adults deliberately infected with a cold virus revealed that those given the drug naproxen (Naprosyn), which is commonly prescribed for arthritis, suffered almost a third fewer cold symptoms, such as headache and coughing, than those given a placebo.

❑ Medical researchers at Dartmouth College gave a group of thirty-five cold sufferers zinc lozenges, and told these individuals to take a lozenge as often as every two hours. Another thirty-five cold sufferers were given placebos. The zinc-takers' colds subsided in an average of four days, while the control group struggled with their colds for another nine days.

❑ Under experimental conditions, polysaccharides found in the herb echinacea have been shown to enhance the immune response.

❑ Allergies can cause symptoms that mimic those of colds and flu. Allergy testing is recommended. (*See* ALLERGIES in Part Two.)

❑ A child who has frequent colds or bouts with the flu should be checked for thyroid malfunction. When the child is well, perform the thyroid function self-test (*see under* HYPOTHYROIDISM in Part Two). If the child's temperature is low, consult your health care provider.

❑ Congestion, cough, and/or sore throat are signs of a cold, but if these symptoms occur together with fever or fatigue, you may have the flu. (*See* INFLUENZA in Part Two.)

❑ If congestion develops in the chest, it is best to consult a physician, as chest (lung) infections can be serious. Also contact your health care provider if your fever goes above 102°F for more than three days, if yellow or white spots appear in the throat, if the lymph nodes under the jaw and in the neck become enlarged, and/or if chills and shortness of breath occur.

Complexion Problems

See ACNE; DRY SKIN; OILY SKIN; PSORIASIS; ROSACEA; WRINKLING OF SKIN.

Conjunctivitis

See under EYE PROBLEMS.

Constipation

Constipation results when waste material moves too slowly through the large bowel, resulting in infrequent and/or painful elimination. Constipation can give rise to many different ailments, including appendicitis, bad breath, body odor, coated tongue, depression, diverticulitis, fatigue, gas, headaches, hemorrhoids (piles), hernia, indigestion, insomnia, malabsorption syndrome, obesity, and varicose veins. It may even be involved in the development of serious diseases such as bowel cancer.

It is important that the bowels move on a daily basis. The colon is a holding tank for waste matter that should be removed within eighteen to twenty-four hours. Harmful toxins can form after this period. Antigens and toxins from bowel bacteria and undigested food particles may play a role in the development of diabetes mellitus, meningitis, myasthenia gravis, thyroid disease, candidiasis, chronic gas and bloating, migraines, fatigue and ulcerative colitis.

In most cases, constipation arises from insufficient amounts of fiber and fluids in the diet. Other causative factors include inadequate exercise, advanced age, muscle disorders, structural abnormalities, bowel diseases, neurogenic disorders, and a poor diet, especially heavy consumption of junk food. Constipation may be a side effect of iron supplements and some drugs, such as painkillers and antidepressants. It is also common during pregnancy.

High levels of calcium and low levels of thyroid hormone are two metabolic disturbances that can lead to constipation. People with kidney failure or diabetes also tend to have problems with constipation. In older individuals, constipation is often caused by dehydration; in people of any age, depression can be a factor.

A small percentage of people, such as persons with spinal injuries, have problems with constipation because the nerves that usually regulate bowel movement have been damaged or destroyed. In a condition called Hirschsprung's disease, normal excretion of feces is impossible because the nerves inside the bowel are missing. The nerve cells in the wall of the colon can also be damaged by long-term, habitual use of laxatives. When this happens, constipation is inevitable. A thrombosed hemorrhoid, anal fissure, or a pocket of infection at the anus can create a spasm of pain strong enough to contract the muscles and hinder the evacuation of stools.

NUTRIENTS

SUPPLEMENT	SUGGESTED DOSAGE	COMMENTS
Important		
Aloe vera		*See under* Herbs, below.
Garlic (Kyolic)	2 capsules twice daily, with meals.	Destroys harmful bacteria in the colon.
Vitamin C	5,000–20,000 mg daily, in divided doses. *See* ASCORBIC ACID FLUSH in Part Three.	Has a cleansing and healing effect. Use a buffered form.
Helpful		
Acidophilus	1 tsp twice daily. Take on an empty stomach.	Allows survival and rapid passage of "friendly" bacteria through the stomach into the small intestine.
Apple pectin	500 mg daily. Take separately from other supplements and medications.	A source of fiber that aids in correcting constipation.
Bio-Bifidus from American Biologics	As directed on label. For fast results, use it in an enema.	For bowel flora replacement to improve assimilation of nutrients from foods.
Chlorophyll liquid or alfalfa	1 tbsp daily, before meals.	Eliminates toxins and bad breath. *See under* Herbs, below.
Essential fatty acids or freshly ground flaxseeds	As directed on label. 1 tbsp 3 times daily, with meals.	Needed for proper digestion and stool formation. Provides essential fatty acids plus many added added benefits, such as B vitamins and fiber.
Multienzyme complex	As directed on label. Take after meals.	To aid digestion.
Vitamin E	600 IU daily. Take before meals.	Aids in healing of the colon.
Multivitamin and mineral complex with vitamin A and natural beta-carotene	As directed on label. If you are pregnant, do not exceed 10,000 IU daily.	Constipation blocks proper absorption of nutrients, resulting in vitamin and mineral deficiencies.
Vitamin B complex plus extra vitamin B$_{12}$ and folic acid	50 mg 3 times daily, before meals. 1,000 mcg daily. 200 mcg daily.	Aids in proper digestion of fats, carbohydrates, and protein. Use a high-potency formula. A sublingual form is best. To aid in digestion and prevent anemia. Deficiency may result in constipation.
Vitamin D plus calcium and magnesium	400 mg daily. 1,500 mg daily. 750 mg daily.	Aids in preventing colon cancer. Needed for proper muscular contraction. May also help prevent colon cancer. Works with calcium to regulate muscle tone.

HERBS

❑ Alfalfa extract contains chlorophyll, which aids in detoxifying the body and cleansing the breath. Fennel seed tea also is good for freshening the breath.

❑ Aloe vera has a healing and cleansing effect on the digestive tract, and aids in forming soft stools. Drink ½ cup of aloe vera juice in the morning and at night. George's Aloe Vera Juice from Warren Laboratories is good. It can be mixed with a cup of herbal tea if you wish.

❑ Use milk thistle to aid liver function and to enhance bile output to soften stools.

❑ Other herbs that are helpful for constipation include cascara sagrada, goldenseal, rhubarb root, senna leaves, and yerba maté. If you take yerba maté, take 2 to 3 teaspoons in 16 ounces of hot water on an empty stomach.

Caution: Do not take goldenseal on a daily basis for more than one week at a time, and do not use it during pregnancy. If you have a history of cardiovascular disease, diabetes, or glaucoma, use it only under a doctor's supervision.

RECOMMENDATIONS

❑ Eat high-fiber foods such as fresh fruits, raw green leafy vegetables, and brown rice daily. Also eat asparagus, beans, Brussels sprouts, cabbage, carrots, garlic, kale, okra, peas, sweet potatoes, and whole grains.

❑ Drink more water. This is important when adding fiber to the diet. Drink at least eight 8-ounce glasses of water every day, whether you are thirsty or not.

❑ Consume plenty of foods that are high in pectin, such as apples, carrots, beets, bananas, cabbage, citrus fruits, dried peas, and okra. Pectin is also available in supplement form.

❑ Follow a low-fat diet. Eat no fried foods.

❑ Avoid foods that stimulate secretions by the mucous membranes, such as dairy products, fats, and spicy foods.

Types of Laxatives

Laxatives are substances that are used to promote bowel movement. There are four basic types of laxatives: bulk-forming agents, stool softeners, osmotic agents, and stimulants. The following are basic descriptions of the way the different laxatives work to achieve their effects:

• **Bulk-forming agents** increase the bulk and water content of the stools. They are the only type of laxatives that can be safe to take on a daily basis. Examples include bran (both in foods and in supplement form), psyllium, and methylcellulose.

• **Stool softeners,** such as mineral oil and docusate sodium, soften fecal matter so that it passes through the intestines more easily. They should not be used on a regular basis, because they can have other effects on the body. Mineral oil can damage the lungs if inhaled, and it reduces the absorption of fat-soluble vitamins. Docusate sodium (found in Colace and Dialose) may increase the toxicity of other drugs taken at the same time, and may cause liver damage to occur.

• **Osmotic agents** contain salts or carbohydrates that promote secretion of water into the colon, initiating bowel movement. They are among the safest laxatives for occasional use, but if they are used more than occasionally, dependency can result. Examples include lactulose (a prescription medication sold under the brand names Cephulac and Chronulac), sorbitol (which is cheaper than lactulose but just as effective), milk of magnesia, citrate of magnesia, and Epsom salts.

• **Stimulant laxatives** irritate the intestinal wall, stimulating peristalsis. They can damage the bowels with habitual use, and can lead to dependency. Examples include bisacodyl (found in Dulcolax), casanthranol (Peri-Colace), cascara sagrada, castor oil, phenolphthalein (Dialose Plus), and senna (Perdiem, Senokot).

❑ Do not consume dairy products, soft drinks, meat, white flour, highly processed foods, salt, coffee, alcohol, or sugar. These foods are difficult to digest and have little or no fiber.

❑ For quick relief of constipation, drink a large glass of quality water every ten minutes for half an hour. This can work wonders to flush out toxins and relieve constipation.

❑ Eat prunes or figs. These are the best natural laxatives.

❑ Eat smaller portions—no large, heavy meals.

❑ Consume barley juice, Green Magma from Green Foods Corporation, Kyo-Green from Wakunaga, or wheatgrass for chlorophyll.

❑ Get some exercise. Physical activity speeds the movement of waste through the intestines. A twenty-minute walk can often relieve constipation. Regular exercise is also important for preventing constipation in the first place.

❑ Go to the toilet at the same time each day, even if the urge does not exist, and relax. Stress tightens the muscles, and can cause constipation. Many people find reading helpful as a way to relax. Never repress the urge to defecate.

❑ Keep the bowel clean. See COLON CLEANSING in Part Three.

❑ If constipation is persistent, take cleansing enemas. See ENEMAS in Part Three.

❑ Do not consume products containing mineral oil, which can interfere with the absorption of fat-soluble vitamins. Also avoid taking Epsom salts, milk of magnesia, and citrate of magnesia, which draw volumes of fluid into the intestines and wash out minerals from the body.

❑ Heavy laxative users should take acidophilus to replace the "friendly" bacteria. The continued use of laxatives cleans out the intestinal bacteria and leads to chronic constipation.

CONSIDERATIONS

❑ Psyllium seed is helpful for constipation. If you take psyllium seed, be sure to take it with a full glass of water.

❑ Flaxseed oil or freshly ground flaxseeds help to soften stools. Freshly ground flaxseeds have a pleasant, nutty taste and can be sprinkled over cereals, salads, and other foods.

❑ Nutralax 2 from Nature's Way Products is good for constipation.

❑ Triphala from Planetary Formulas aids in the formation of odor-free, firm, and healthy stools.

❑ It can help to fast periodically. (See FASTING in Part Three.)

❑ Kombucha tea, which has detoxifying and immune-boosting properties, may be beneficial for relieving constipation and other digestive disorders. (See MAKING KOMBUCHA TEA in Part Three.)

❑ If added natural fiber and herbal laxatives do not improve constipation, you may have a problem with muscle coordination. Normally, the upper muscles in the bowel contract as the lower ones relax. Problems occur if the lower muscle tightens and goes into a spasm instead of relaxing.

❑ If constipation is more than an occasional problem, the possibility of a cancer or another obstruction in the lower bowel should not be dismissed unless a proctoscopic examination or a barium enema has shown that there is no blockage. Other symptoms of colon cancer include the presence of blood in the feces; severe cramping; a tender, distended abdomen; and markedly narrowed stools. However, cancer may be present even without these symptoms.

❑ Foul-smelling stools and a burning feeling in the anus may be signs of acidosis. (See ACIDOSIS in Part Two.)

❑   Alternating constipation and diarrhea may be a sign of irritable bowel syndrome. While this disorder is chronic and unpleasant, it is not dangerous. Other common symptoms are crampy pains, gassiness, and variation in the consistency of the stool. The cause of irritable bowel syndrome is not known, but many experts believe it is stress related. (*See* IRRITABLE BOWEL SYNDROME in Part Two.)

❑   *See also* DIVERTICULITIS and ULCERATIVE COLITIS, both in Part Two.

❑   *See also under* PREGNANCY-RELATED PROBLEMS in Part Two.

Copper Deficiency

Copper is an essential trace mineral. Even a mild copper deficiency impairs the ability of white blood cells to fight infection. Copper is necessary for proper absorption of iron in the body, and it is found primarily in foods containing iron. If the body does not get a sufficient amount of copper, hemoglobin production decreases and copper-deficiency anemia can result.

Various enzyme reactions require copper as well. Copper is needed as a cross-linking agent for elastin and collagen, as a catalyst for protein reactions, and for oxygen transport. It is also used for the metabolism of essential fatty acids. Copper deficiency can produce various symptoms, including diarrhea, inefficient utilization of iron and protein, and stunted growth. In babies, the development of nerve, bone, and lung tissue can be impaired, and the structure of these body parts may be altered.

For the body to work properly, it must have a proper balance of copper and zinc; an imbalance can lead to thyroid problems. In addition, low (or high) copper levels may contribute to mental and emotional problems. Copper deficiency may be a factor in anorexia nervosa, for example.

Copper deficiency is most likely to occur in babies who are fed only soymilk, persons suffering from sprue (a malabsorption syndrome) or kidney disease, and those who chronically take megadoses of zinc. Long-term use of oral contraceptives can upset the balance of copper in the body, causing either excessively high or excessively low copper levels. Copper levels can be determined through a blood test, urine samples, and hair analysis. Determining mineral levels and ratios is the basis for a nutritional program to balance body chemistry.

NUTRIENTS

SUPPLEMENT	SUGGESTED DOSAGE	COMMENTS
Important		
Copper	5 mg daily for 1 month, then reduce to 3 mg daily.	To restore copper in the body. Use copper amino acid chelate.
Zinc	30 mg daily. Do not exceed this amount.	Needed to balance with copper. Use zinc chelate form.

Helpful		
Iron	As directed by physician. Take with 100 mg vitamin C for better absorption.	Copper deficiency may cause anemia. Use a chelate form. *Caution:* Do not take iron unless anemia is diagnosed.
Multivitamin and mineral complex	As directed on label.	All nutrients are necessary in balance.

RECOMMENDATIONS

❑   If you suspect that you may have a copper deficiency, increase your intake of foods rich in copper, such as legumes (especially soybeans), nuts, cocoa, black pepper, seafood, raisins, molasses, avocados, whole grains, and cauliflower.

❑   Copper deficiency can be confirmed through hair analysis. (*See* HAIR ANALYSIS in Part Three.) If deficiency is confirmed, follow the supplementation plan above to restore proper mineral balance.

CONSIDERATIONS

❑   *Patent ductus arteriosus* is a congenital defect in which the ductus arteriosus, or fetal blood vessel, fails to close properly shortly after birth. It results in blood flow between the pulmonary artery, which goes to the lungs, and the aorta, which brings oxygenated blood to the rest of the heart. In a laboratory experiment reported in *Developmental Pharmacology and Therapy*, the ductus arteriosus remained open in 100 percent of offspring of a copper-deficient group of rats, but in only 20 percent of the offspring of a control group not suffering from copper deficiency.

Copper Toxicity

Small amounts of copper are essential for life. However, as with all trace minerals, excess amounts of copper in the body can be toxic. The liver and brain contain the largest amounts of copper in the body; other organs contain smaller amounts. Too much copper in the system can cause diarrhea, eczema, hemolytic anemia, high blood pressure, kidney disease, nausea, premenstrual syndrome, sickle cell anemia, stomach pain, weakness, and severe damage to the central nervous system. As with mercury and lead, high levels of copper are also associated with mental and emotional disorders, including autism, behavioral problems, childhood hyperactivity, clinical depression, hallucinatory and paranoid schizophrenia, insomnia, mood swings, stuttering, and senile dementia (senility).

Sources of copper include beer, copper cookware, copper plumbing, insecticides, pasteurized milk, tap water, and various foods, as well as swimming pool chemicals and permanent-wave solutions.

Copper levels can be determined through blood tests, urine samples, and hair analysis. Normal urine samples collected over a twenty-four-hour period contain 15 to 40 micrograms of copper. In people with diseases such as arthritis, heart disease, hypertension, schizophrenia, or cancer, serum copper levels tend to be high. During illness, copper is released from the tissues into the blood to promote tissue repair. High serum copper readings during illness should not be taken to mean that the copper is a cause of the illness; rather, it is an indication that the body's natural repair processes have been activated.

The use of oral contraceptives and/or tobacco can cause a rise in the amount of copper in the body. Excess serum copper is also characteristic of anemia, cirrhosis of the liver, leukemia, hypoproteinemia, and vitamin B_3 (niacin) deficiency. Serum copper levels during pregnancy tend to be higher than normal as well. Wilson's disease is a rare hereditary disorder in which the body is unable to metabolize copper properly, so the metal accumulates in the body.

With knowledge of how minerals interact in the body, it is possible to lower the amount of copper in the body and maintain a proper mineral balance.

NUTRIENTS

SUPPLEMENT	SUGGESTED DOSAGE	COMMENTS
Important		
Vitamin C with bioflavonoids plus	1,000 mg 4 times daily.	Copper chelators. Use ascorbic acid form.
rutin	60 mg daily.	A bioflavonoid that is a byproduct of buckwheat and lowers serum copper.
Zinc	50–80 mg daily. Do not exceed a total of 100 mg daily from all supplements.	Zinc deficiency predisposes one to excessive copper levels. Use zinc chelate form.
Helpful		
Calcium chelate or	1,500 mg daily.	Binds with metallic ions in the body.
calcium disodium edetate plus	As prescribed by physician.	Used by doctors to treat heavy metal poisoning. Available by prescription only.
magnesium	750 mg daily, at bedtime.	Works with calcium.
L-Cysteine and L-cystine and L-methionine	As directed on label, on an empty stomach. Take with water or juice. Do not take with milk. Take with 50 mg vitamin B_6 and 100 mg vitamin C for better absorption.	Aids in elimination of copper from the body and protects the liver. *See* AMINO ACIDS in Part One.
Manganese	2–4 mg daily. Take separately from calcium.	Aids in excretion of excess copper.
Molybdenum	30 mcg daily.	Prevents accumulation of excess copper in the body.

RECOMMENDATIONS

❑ Have your drinking water tested. Drinking water can be a source of copper. The level of copper and other minerals in household drinking water can be tested by special labs.

If there is more than 1 part per million of copper in your drinking water, an alternate source of water, such as bottled steam-distilled water, is advisable. If this is not feasible, always run the water for at least two minutes before using it to clear out some of the impurities.

❑ Increase your intake of sulfur, found in such foods as eggs, onions, and garlic. These help to rid the body of copper. In addition, supplement your diet with pectin, which can be found in apples.

❑ Do not take a multivitamin and/or mineral supplement that contains copper.

❑ Do not use copper pots or other cooking utensils.

CONSIDERATIONS

❑ Hair analysis has been shown to be a reliable test of the copper level in body tissues. (*See* HAIR ANALYSIS in Part Three.)

❑ If you have an extremely high level of copper, you may require medical treatment with chelation to remove the excess copper. Chelation therapy removes toxic metals from the body. (*See* CHELATION THERAPY in Part Three.) If the copper levels are higher than normal, but not extreme, this can often be managed with supplements.

❑ The trace minerals manganese, molybdenum, and zinc can prevent excess copper from accumulating in the body.

❑ Many people with schizophrenia have been found to have high levels of copper and iron, combined with deficiencies of zinc and manganese, probably as a result of lower than normal excretion of copper. Increasing the intake of zinc and manganese, whether through the diet or supplementation, increases elimination of copper and helps to return copper levels to normal.

❑ *See also* ENVIRONMENTAL TOXICITY and WILSON'S DISEASE, both in Part Two.

Corneal Ulcer

See under EYE PROBLEMS.

Corns and Calluses

Calluses are areas of *hyperkeratosis*, or overgrowth of skin tissue. The skin thickens and hardens. Calluses most commonly form on the feet and sometimes on the hands. Corns are small cone-shaped areas of skin overgrowth that most often form on or between the toes. They can be either soft or hard. If they form between the toes, the moisture of the area keeps them soft; corns that form on top of the toes are typically hard.

These growths can cause inflammation and pain. Corns especially may ache and be tender to the touch. Both corns and calluses usually form in response to repeated friction or pressure, such as from wearing ill-fitting shoes or performing certain tasks repeatedly. Other factors that may be involved include staphylococcus- or streptococcus-type infection, misalignment of the foot, and an acid/alkaline imbalance in the body. The heavy consumption of fats, sugars, and highly processed foods is the most common cause of imbalance in the acidity and alkalinity of the body.

HERBS

❑ Use alternate applications of alcohol-free goldenseal extract and tea tree oil to keep down infection and speed healing.

RECOMMENDATIONS

❑ Consume raw vegetables and juices for three days to aid in balancing the acidity/alkalinity of your system. Umeboshi (Japanese salt plum) can quickly balance the body's pH. These are available in health food stores and Asian markets. Take one every three hours for two days.

❑ Avoid fried foods, meats, caffeine, sugar, and highly processed foods.

❑ To treat corns and calluses, soften the thickened skin by adding 2 tablespoons of Dr. Bronner's liquid soap (available in health food stores) or a mild dish soap to ½ gallon of warm water. Soak your feet in this mixture for fifteen minutes. Afterwards, dry your feet with a soft towel and rub a couple of drops of vitamin E oil into the affected area. Then, using a pumice stone or a special callus file, *gently* file down the top layer of the corn or callus. Clean the area with mild soap and water, using a gauze pad or cotton ball. Do this twice a day. Wear clean white cotton socks after treatment.

❑ Apply a nonmedicated corn pad (a small round or oval-shaped foam pad with a hole in the center) around a corn to help to relieve the pressure. Stretch the pad so that it clears the corn by at least one-eighth inch on all sides. Then apply vitamin E oil to the corn, cover with a gauze square, and wrap the toe with adhesive tape. Alternate between using vitamin E oil and tea tree oil.

❑ For corns between the toes, dab on vitamin E oil and place a clean piece of cotton or a cotton ball over it. Make sure to use 100-percent cotton, not synthetic cosmetic puffs. Put on clean white cotton socks and leave them on overnight after treatment. Vitamin E oil mixed with a crushed garlic clove is good for softening corns or calluses.

❑ Never use a knife or any sharp instrument to cut the hardened area away, as infection can result.

CONSIDERATIONS

❑ Compresses made from hot Epsom salts or Footherapy solution from Para Laboratories/Queen Helene are good.

❑ Medicated pads are available that are supposed to treat corns and calluses. Most of these products are fairly aggressive, however, and may attack good tissue as well, provoking an allergic reaction.

❑ *See also* ACIDOSIS and/or ALKALOSIS, both in Part Two.

Cramps

See MUSCLE CRAMPS; PREMENSTRUAL SYNDROME.

Crohn's Disease

Crohn's disease is characterized by a chronic and long-lasting ulceration of a section or sections of the digestive tract. The ulceration extends through all layers of the intestinal wall and involves the entire digestive system, from the mouth to the anus, as well as the adjacent lymph nodes. The inflamed parts heal, leaving scar tissue that narrows the passageway. This disorder is not contagious. Its cause is still uncertain, although it known that a history of food allergies increases the risk of developing it; conversely, eliminating allergenic foods often relieves the symptoms. Studies also suggest that free radical damage may be involved, and that a lack of vitamins C and E may play a role.

Symptoms of Crohn's disease include chronic diarrhea, pain in the upper and lower abdomen, fever, headaches, malabsorption (and consequent malnutrition), steatorrhea (the presence of excess fat in the stool, which results in pale, bulky stools that float), and loss of energy, appetite, and weight. Chronic bleeding may cause iron-deficiency anemia. If the ulcerated intestinal wall leaks, peritonitis can result. Mouth and anal sores may be present when the disease is active. Because of pain, diarrhea, nausea, and sometimes severe headaches and even vomiting, the person with Crohn's disease may dread eating. Sometimes Crohn's disease is misdiagnosed as appendicitis because the pain it causes is centered in the same location.

In addition to the ulceration and inflammation, people with Crohn's disease may develop strictures that partially obstruct the bowel. They also may develop fistulas, abnormal passages that lead from one loop of intestine to another, or even to other organs.

The onset of Crohn's disease typically occurs between the ages of fourteen and thirty, although more and more cases are being reported in children. Attacks may occur every few months to every few years. In rare cases, it appears once or twice and does not return. If the disease continues for many years, bowel function gradually deteriorates. Left untreated, it can become extremely serious, even life threatening, and it may increase the risk of cancer by as much as twenty times.

Crohn's disease is similar to ulcerative colitis in many respects. Both involve loss of appetite, abdominal pain, general malaise, weight loss, diarrhea, and rectal bleeding. The primary difference between the two conditions is the degree of involvement of the wall of the intestinal tract. Ulcerative colitis is limited to the mucosa and submucosa, the first two layers of the lining of the bowel adjacent to the lumen (the central passageway); Crohn's disease also involves the next two layers, the muscular layer and the connective tissue layer below it.

NUTRIENTS

SUPPLEMENT	SUGGESTED DOSAGE	COMMENTS
Essential		
Duodenal glandular	As directed on label.	Aids in healing gastrointestinal ulcers.
Taurine Plus from American Biologics	500 mg daily, on an empty stomach. Take with 50 mg vitamin B_6 and 100 mg vitamin C for better absorption.	An important antioxidant and immune regulator. Use the sublingual form.
Liver extract injections plus	2 cc once weekly or as prescribed by physician.	Needed for proper digestion.
vitamin B complex and	1 cc once weekly or as prescribed by physician.	Helps to prevent anemia.
vitamin B_{12} and	1 cc twice weekly or as prescribed by physician.	Important for proper digestion and to prevent anemia. Deficiency aggravates malabsorption.
folic acid	¼ cc twice weekly or as prescribed by physician.	Needed for constant supply of new cells. Injections (under a doctor's supervision) are best.
or vitamin B complex plus extra	100 mg 3 times daily.	If injections are not available, use a sublingual form.
vitamin B_{12} and	200 mcg daily.	Use a lozenge or sublingual form.
folic acid	200 mcg daily.	
N-Acetylglucosamine (N-A-G from Source Naturals)	As directed on label.	A major constituent of the barrier layer that protects the intestinal lining from digestive enzymes and other potentially damaging intestinal contents.
Omega-3 essential fatty acids (flaxseed oil, primrose oil, and salmon oil are good sources)	As directed on label 3 times daily.	Needed for repair of the digestive tract; reduces inflammatory processes and is much needed in Crohn's disease.
Pancreatin plus bromelain	As directed on label. Take with meals. As directed on label.	To break down protein and assist digestion.
Vitamin C with bioflavonoids	1,000 mg 3 times daily.	Prevents inflammation and improves immunity. Use a buffered type.
Vitamin K	As directed on label.	Vital to colon health. Deficiency is common in people with this disorder due to malabsorption and diarrhea.
Zinc	50 mg daily. Do not exceed a total of 100 mg daily from all supplements.	Needed for the immune system and for healing. Use zinc gluconate lozenges or OptiZinc for best absorption.
Important		
Free-form amino acid complex	¼ tsp twice daily.	Protein is essential in the healing of the intestine. Use a sublingual form.
Garlic (Kyolic)	2 capsules 3 times daily, with meals.	Combats free radicals in Crohn's disease. Aids healing.
Lactobacilli or Capricin from Premier One Products	As directed on label, twice daily. Take on an empty stomach. As directed on label.	Aids in digestion. Use a nondairy formula. A product containing both *L. acidophilus* and *L. bifidus* organisms is best. Works in conjunction with butyric acid to reduce inflammation and seepage of undigested food particles.
L-Glutamine	500 mg twice daily, on an empty stomach. Take with water or juice. Do not take with milk. Take with 50 mg vitamin B_6 and 100 mg vitamin C for better absorption.	A major metabolic fuel for the intestinal cells; maintains the villi, the absorption surfaces of the gut. See AMINO ACIDS in Part One.
Spiru-tein from Nature's Plus	2 capsules 3 times daily.	Supplies necessary protein. Helps stabilize blood sugar between meals.
Helpful		
Aloe vera		See under Herbs, below.
Calcium and magnesium	2,000 mg daily. 1,500 mg daily.	Aids in preventing colon cancer.
Floradix Iron + Herbs from Salus Haus	2 tsp daily.	To prevent anemia. Floradix is a readily absorbable form of iron that is nontoxic and derived from food sources.
Multivitamin and mineral complex with copper and manganese and selenium plus extra	As directed on label.	Malabsorption is often a result of this disorder. Copper, selenium, and manganese are important for treating this disorder and are often deficient because of absorption problems. Use a liquid, powder, or capsule formula.
potassium	99 mg daily.	May reduce surgical complications and also the need for surgery.
Quercetin plus bromelain or Activated Quercetin from Source Naturals	500 mg twice daily, before meals. 100 mg twice daily, before meals. As directed on label.	Slows histamine release; helps control food allergies. Needed for a variety of enzyme functions. Improves absorption of quercetin. Contains quercetin plus bromelain and vitamin C.
Shark cartilage (BeneFin)	As directed on label. If you cannot tolerate taking it orally, it can be administered rectally in a retention enema.	Fights metastasis of cancerous tumors.
Vitamin A and vitamin E	50,000 IU daily. If you are pregnant, do not exceed 10,000 IU daily. Up to 800 IU daily.	Antioxidants that aid in controlling infection and in repair of the intestinal tract. Use emulsion forms for easier assimilation.
Vitamin D	400 IU daily.	Prevents metabolic bone disease from developing as a result of malabsorption.

217

HERBS

❑ Aloe vera is beneficial for Crohn's disease because it softens stools and has a healing effect on the digestive tract. Drink ½ cup of aloe vera juice three times daily.

❑ Other herbs that are good for this disorder include burdock root, echinacea, fenugreek, goldenseal, licorice, marshmallow root, pau d'arco, enteric-coated peppermint (do not use any other form), red clover, rose hips, silymarin (milk thistle extract), slippery elm, and yerba maté. These herbs support digestion, cleanse the bloodstream, and reduce inflammation and infection. For best results, use them on an alternating basis.

Caution: Do not use licorice on a daily basis for more than seven days in a row, and avoid it completely if you have high blood pressure. Do not take goldenseal on a daily basis for more than one week at a time, and do not use it during pregnancy. If you have a history of cardiovascular disease, diabetes, or glaucoma, use it only under a doctor's supervision.

RECOMMENDATIONS

❑ Eat a diet consisting mainly of nonacidic fresh or cooked vegetables such as broccoli, Brussels sprouts, cabbage, carrots, celery, garlic, kale, spinach, and turnips. Steam, broil, boil, or bake your food.

❑ Drink plenty of liquids, such as steam-distilled water, herbal teas, and fresh juices. Fresh cabbage juice is very beneficial.

❑ Add papaya to your diet. Chew a couple of the seeds to aid digestion.

❑ During an acute attack, eat organic baby foods, steamed vegetables, and well-cooked brown rice, millet, and oatmeal.

❑ Try eliminating all dairy foods (including cheese), fish, hard sausage, pickled cabbage, and yeast products from your diet, and see if symptoms improve. These foods are high in histamine. Many people with Crohn's disease are histamine-intolerant. Milk and other dairy products also contain carrageenan, a compound extracted from red seaweed. Carrageenan, which is widely used in the food industry for its ability to stabilize milk proteins, has been shown to induce ulcerative colitis in laboratory animals.

❑ Avoid alcohol, caffeine, carbonated beverages, chocolate, corn, eggs, foods with artificial additives or preservatives, fried and greasy foods, margarine, meat, pepper, spicy foods, tobacco, white flour, and all animal products, with the exception of white fish from clear waters. These foods are irritating to the digestive tract. Mucus-forming foods such as processed refined foods and dairy products should also be avoided. Limit your intake of barley, rye, and wheat.

❑ Avoid refined carbohydrates. Do not consume such foods as boxed dry cereals or anything containing any form of sugar. Diets high in refined carbohydrates have been

associated with Crohn's disease. These foods must be eliminated from the diet.

❑ Check stools daily for bleeding.

❑ As much as possible, avoid stress. Our thoughts, nervous systems, and bodily functions are deeply interconnected. Our bodies are affected by our thoughts and moods. During an attack, rest is important.

❑ Make sure the bowels move daily, but do not use harsh laxatives (*see* CONSTIPATION and/or DIARRHEA in Part Two). Gentle enemas made by adding a dropperful of alcohol-free herbal extract and 1 teaspoon of nondairy acidophilus powder to 2 quarts of lukewarm water are good. Accumulations of toxic body wastes often become breeding grounds for parasitic infestation. Toxins can also be absorbed into the bloodstream through the colon wall. Psyllium husks should be used daily for fiber; this aids in removing toxins before they are absorbed.

Note: Always take supplemental fiber separately from other supplements and medications.

❑ Do not use rectal suppositories that contain hydrogenated chemically prepared fats.

❑ If you are constipated, use a cleansing enema. *See* ENEMAS in Part Three. Use a heating pad to reduce abdominal pain.

CONSIDERATIONS

❑ It is important that nutritional deficiencies be corrected for healing. Persons with inflammatory bowel disorders require as much as 30 percent more protein than normal. If chronic diarrhea is present, electrolyte and trace mineral deficiencies should be considered. Chronic steatorrhea may result in deficiencies of calcium and magnesium.

❑ Drugs such as corticosteroids and sulfasalazine (Azulfidine), which are prescribed for inflammatory bowel diseases, and cholestyramine (Questran), which is prescribed to lower cholesterol levels, increase the need for nutritional supplements. Corticosteroids depress protein synthesis and inhibit normal calcium absorption by increasing excretion of vitamin C in the urine. Deficiencies of other nutrients, such as zinc, potassium, vitamin B_6 (pyridoxine), folic acid, and vitamin D, decrease bone formation and slow healing. Sulfasalazine inhibits the transport of folic acid and iron, causing anemia.

❑ Antioxidants have been shown to decrease the risk of developing Crohn's disease. The intestinal walls normally contain small amounts of the antioxidant enzymes superoxide dismutase (SOD), catalase, and glutathione peroxidase, but their ability to fight free radicals may be overwhelmed during periods of active inflammation, resulting in tissue damage.

❑ To reestablish a proper healing environment, it is necessary to maintain a generally alkaline bodily pH.

❑ Adhering to an allergen-free diet, replacing lost nutrients, and using selected herbs can speed healing and may prevent future disturbances. Studies have proven that when a person who has achieved remission goes back to his or her former diet, Crohn's returns. Other things that have been implicated in this disorder include prolonged stress, trauma, and psychosomatic and vascular factors.

❑ Nutritional deficiencies resulting from malabsorption may weaken the immune system, in turn prolonging the time required for the inflammation and ulcers to heal.

❑ Many microorganisms have been considered as possible causes of Crohn's disease, including fungi, bacteria, viruses, mycobacteria, pseudomonas-like organisms, and chlamydia. However, the cause of Crohn's disease has not yet been established. It is likely that multiple factors are involved.

❑ Antigenic reactions may result from "leaky gut syndrome," in which minute particles of undigested or partially digested food pass through the swollen and inflamed mucosal wall into the bloodstream, where they cause reactions. The mucosal wall must be repaired to avoid this. Avoiding foods that cause a reaction is important. (See ALLERGIES in Part Two.) Treatment with butyric acid, a monounsaturated fatty acid, reduces inflammatory conditions, reduces seepage of undigested food particles, and aids in repair of the mucosal wall. N-acetylglucosamine (NAG) prevents leaky gut syndrome.

❑ A study done in Italy found that people with Crohn's disease who took sustained-release fish oil supplements were less likely to suffer relapses than those who did not. Of the subjects in the one-year study who took fish oil, over half remained symptom-free, compared with only a quarter of those who took a placebo.

❑ Researchers have not been able to find a specific genetic marker for Crohn's disease, but they have found that the illness is four time more common in Caucasians and Jews than in people of other ethnic backgrounds. In 20 to 40 percent of reported cases, multiple family members have suffered either from Crohn's or ulcerative colitis.

❑ It is possible to have surgery for Crohn's disease. This involves removing the diseased segment of bowel. While this surgery doesn't cure the disease, it can relieve symptoms, and five years later at least 50 percent of people who undergo it are in good health, can work full time, and enjoy life without being restricted by diarrhea or pain.

Croup

Croup is a respiratory infection that causes the larynx or trachea to narrow due to swelling. The larynx goes into spasms, and the sufferer experiences difficulty breathing; a harsh, barking cough; hoarseness; tightness in the lungs; and feelings of suffocation. Mucus production may also increase, further clogging the airway. Croup most commonly occurs in young children, whose airways are much narrower than those of adults.

One of the trademarks of croup is a harsh, wheezing noise that is made when air is breathed in through the constricted windpipe and over inflamed vocal cords. Fits of coughing are another characteristic symptom. Croup is usually preceded by a cold, bronchitis, or allergy attack, but can also occur if a foreign body is inhaled. Attacks frequently occur at night.

NUTRIENTS

SUPPLEMENT	SUGGESTED DOSAGE	COMMENTS
Essential		
Vitamin C	60 mg 4 times daily for children 6–12 months old; 100 mg 4 times daily for ages 1–4; 500 mg 4 times daily for children over 4.	Helps control infection and fever by boosting the immune system.
Zinc lozenges (Ultimate Zinc-C Lozenges from Now Foods)	5 mg once daily for 3 days for children 6–12 months old; 5 mg twice daily for 3 days for ages 1–3; 5 mg 3 times daily for 3 days for children over 3.	Promotes immune function and is necessary in healing. Use lozenges for faster absorption.
Very Important		
Vitamin A	2,000 IU daily.	Needed for healing of the mucous membranes. Use an emulsion form.
Vitamin E	10 mg daily for children under 3; 20 mg daily for ages 3–6; 50 mg daily for children over 6.	Destroys free radicals and carries oxygen to all cells. Use an emulsion form.
Important		
Cod liver oil	1 tbsp twice daily in juice.	Can be used for children in place of vitamin A.

HERBS

❑ The following herbs are recommended for croup: echinacea, fenugreek, goldenseal, and thyme. Echinacea tincture should be taken if a fever is present. Take 15 drops in liquid every three to four hours.

Caution: Do not take goldenseal on a daily basis for more than one week at a time, and do not use it during pregnancy. If you have a history of cardiovascular disease, diabetes, or glaucoma, use it only under a doctor's supervision.

❑ Put a few drops of eucalyptus oil in a vaporizer and inhale the steam.

❑ Give a child with croup very warm ginger herb baths; then immediately wrap the child in a heavy towel or blanket, and put him or her to bed to perspire. This helps loosen mucus and rid the body of toxins.

❑ Fenu-Thyme combination from Nature's Way Products is good for congestion.

RECOMMENDATIONS

❑ Give a child with croup plenty of fluids to help to thin mucus. Steam-distilled water, herbal teas, and homemade soups are good choices.

❑ Apply hot onion packs over the chest and back three times a day. Slice onions and place them between cloths, and then apply the pack and cover it with a heating pad. Onion packs open the pores and relieve congestion.

❑ If a child with croup is having difficulty breathing, take him or her to the emergency room of the nearest hospital for treatment and for x-rays of the larynx. Antibiotics and oxygen may be needed. Milder cases of croup can be treated at home, but parents should be alert for signs of increasing breathing difficulty.

❑ If antibiotics are prescribed, use some form of acidophilus.

Cushing's Syndrome

See under ADRENAL DISORDERS.

Cystic Fibrosis

Cystic fibrosis (CF) is the most common inherited illness among Americans of northern and western European ancestry, affecting some 30,000 people. Although it occurs in people of all ethnic backgrounds, it is far more common in Caucasians (an estimated incidence of 1 in 2,400) than in African-Americans (1 in 17,000). It occurs with approximately equal frequency in men and women.

CF is caused by a defect in a gene that encodes instructions for a protein that regulates the passage of salt in and out of the cells of the body's exocrine glands. In most people with CF, the genetic instructions omit just one of the protein's 1,480 constituent amino acids—a tiny glitch, but a devastating one that affects many different glands in the body, including the pancreas, sweat glands, and glands of the digestive and respiratory systems.

Symptoms of CF begin early in life. Glands in the lungs and bronchial tubes secrete large quantities of thick, sticky mucus that blocks lung passages and traps harmful bacteria, resulting in chronic coughing and wheezing, difficulty breathing, and recurrent lung infections. Thick secretions also often obstruct the release of pancreatic enzymes, resulting in digestive difficulties and malabsorption problems, particularly problems with the metabolism of fats. Malnutrition may result because a lack of necessary digestive enzymes means that nutrients from foods are not properly absorbed. This in turn can cause pain after eating and, especially in young children, a failure to gain weight normally.

Persons with this disease also lose excessive amounts of salt through their sweat glands. Sweating may be profuse, and the sweat itself contains abnormally high concentrations of sodium, potassium, and chloride salts. Other signs suggestive of CF include clubbing of the fingers and toes (a result of poor circulation); infertility; greasy, bulky, foul-smelling stools; and salty-tasting skin. An individual may have any or all of thse symptoms.

The gene responsible for CF was identified in 1989. All human cells (except red blood cells, eggs, and sperm) contain two copies of this gene, one inherited from each parent. CF results when both copies of the the "CF gene" are abnormal. If one copy is abnormal and the other normal, an individual is said to be a carrier; he or she will show no signs of CF, but is capable of passing a defective gene on to offspring. A child of two carrier parents has a 1-in-4 chance of inheriting CF; a 1-in-4 chance of being completely free of the mutant gene; and a 1-in-2 chance of being a carrier, like the parents. About 8 million people in the US may be carriers.

The identification of the CF gene has enabled researchers to begin developing new approaches to diagnosis and treatment of the disease. A test is now available in which cells are swabbed from the inside of the cheek and then examined for the presence of defective genes. The presence of both normal and mutant CF genes indicates that the individual is a carrier. If only mutant genes are there, CF is indicated.

The most widely used test for CF is the electrolyte sweat test. It detects the excessive amounts of electrolytes (charged mineral salts) found on the skin of many people with CF. A physician would likely recommend that a sweat test be performed on a child who failed to gain weight despite adequate feeding, or who suffered from very frequent respiratory infections. CF testing is currently recommended only for those individuals with symptoms highly suggestive of the disease, or with a family history of the disorder.

Unless otherwise specified, the dosages recommended here are for adults. For a child between the ages of twelve and seventeen, reduce the dose to three-quarters the recommended amount. For a child between six and twelve, use one-half the recommended dose, and for a child under the age of six, use one-quarter the recommended amount.

NUTRIENTS

SUPPLEMENT	SUGGESTED DOSAGE	COMMENTS
Very Important		
Pancreatin	As directed on label. Take with meals.	Needed for protein digestion.
Proteolytic enzymes	As directed on label, on an empty stomach. Take between meals.	Aids in controlling infection, helps digestion, and thins the mucous secretions of the lungs.
Vitamin B complex plus extra vitamin B$_2$ (riboflavin)	100 mg 3 times daily, with meals. 50 mg 3 times daily.	Aids in digestion, healing, and tissue repair.
Vitamin B$_{12}$	1,000 mcg 3 times daily, on an empty stomach.	Needed for proper digestion and assimilation of nutrients, including iron. Use a lozenge, sublingual, or spray form.

Vitamin C	3,000–6,000 mg daily, in divided doses.	For tissue repair and immune function.
Vitamin K or alfalfa	100 mcg twice daily.	Deficiency is common in those with this disorder. Needed for proper digestion. *See under* Herbs, below.

Important		
Protein supplement	As directed on label.	Needed for healing. Use protein from a vegetable source or a free-form amino acid complex.
Essential fatty acids (primrose oil is a good source)	As directed on label.	Relieves inflammation.
Vitamin A	50,000 IU daily. If you are pregnant, do not exceed 10,000 IU daily.	For tissue repair. Also boosts the immune system. Use emulsion form for better absorption and greater safety at higher doses.
plus natural beta-carotene or	25,000 IU daily.	Precursor of vitamin A.
carotenoid complex (Betatene)	As directed on label.	
Vitamin E emulsion or	400–1,000 IU daily.	An antioxidant necessary for tissue repair. Emulsion form is recommended because it provides for easier assimilation and greater safety at high doses.
capsules	Start with 100–200 IU daily and slowly increase to 400–1,000 IU daily.	
Zinc	50 mg daily. Do not exceed a total of 100 mg daily from all supplements.	Important in immune function and healing of tissue. Use zinc gluconate lozenges or OptiZinc for best absorption.

Helpful		
Coenzyme Q10	100 mg daily.	Acts as an immunostimulant.
Copper and selenium	3 mg daily. 200 mcg daily.	Low levels of copper and selenium have been linked to cystic fibrosis.
Kyo-Green from Wakunaga or chloropyll	As directed on label. As directed on label.	To supply minerals and chlorophyll needed to control infection.
L-Cysteine and L-methionine	500 mg each twice daily, on an empty stomach. Take with water or juice. Do not take with milk. Take with 50 mg vitamin B6 and 100 mg vitamin C for better absorption.	Needed for repair of lung tissue and to protect the liver. *See* AMINO ACIDS in Part One.
Raw pancreas and raw spleen and raw thymus glandulars	As directed on label. As directed on label. As directed on label.	To relieve inflammation. *See* GLANDULAR THERAPY in Part Three.
Vitamin D	400 IU daily.	Aids in protecting the lungs.

HERBS

❑ ClearLungs from Natural Alternatives is a Chinese herbal formula that is highly recommended for this condition.

❑ Other herbs beneficial for cystic fibrosis include echinacea, ginger, goldenseal, and yarrow tea.

❑ Alfalfa extract supplies vitamin K and necessary minerals, which are often deficient in those with cystic fibrosis due to absorption problems. It is also a good source of chlorophyll.

RECOMMENDATIONS

❑ Eat a diet consisting of 75 percent raw fruits and vegetables, and raw nuts and seeds.

❑ Make sure your intake of calories, protein, and other nutrients is adequate. People with CF require as much as 50 percent more of many nutrients than normal. Take supplements to provide required enzymes, vitamins, and minerals.

❑ Include in the diet foods that are high in germanium, such as garlic, shiitake mushrooms, and onions. Germanium helps to improve tissue oxygenation at the cellular level.

❑ During hot weather, drink plenty of fluids and increase your salt intake.

❑ Do not eat foods that stimulate secretions by the mucous membranes. Cooked and processed foods cause excess mucus buildup and drain the body of energy. These foods are harder to digest. Do not eat animal products, dairy products, processed foods, sugar, or white flour products.

❑ When you must take antibiotics, take acidophilus to replace "friendly" bacteria.

CONSIDERATIONS

❑ The symptoms of cystic fibrosis are normally controlled with a number of different drugs. Antibiotics are used to combat the infections to which people with CF are prone, especially infection with *Pseudomonas aeruginosa*, a type of microbe that is attracted to the sticky mucus in the lungs. Pancrelipase (Viokase) is a prescription product containing a combination of digestive enzymes that is often prescribed for people with CF and other pancreatic insufficiencies. Many people also take anti-inflammatory drugs such as ibuprofen (Advil, Nuprin, and others), naproxen (Naprosyn), or prednisone (Deltasone and others).

❑ The future of CF treatment may lie in gene therapy. In the laboratory, normal CF genes have been successfully introduced into cells from people with CF. Experiments in rats have indicated that replacing the defective CF genes with normal ones in just 10 percent of the lung lining cells improves lung function. However, because the genes in the cells of the reproductive system are unaffected by this procedure, the defect can still be passed on to offspring.

❑ The drug amiloride (Midamor, Moduretic), which is used as an adjunct to treatment with some diuretic drugs, is being tested as a treatment for CF. It is believed to thin lung secretions by blocking sodium uptake by lung cells. Another substance undergoing testing as a potential treatment for CF is deoxyribonuclease (DNase), a protein administered in aerosol form to help thin secretions and clear the lungs. Studies suggest that its use may significantly reduce the risk of death and shorten hospital stays for people with CF.

☐ Low levels of selenium and vitamin E have been linked to cystic fibrosis and cancer.

☐ Further information about cystic fibrosis is available from the Cystic Fibrosis Foundation, 6931 Arlington Road, Bethesda, MD 20814; telephone 800–FIGHT–CF.

Cystitis

See BLADDER INFECTION.

Dandruff

Dandruff is a common scalp condition that occurs when dead skin is shed, producing irritating white flakes. The most common cause of dandruff is seborrhea, which is an inflammatory scaling skin disease caused by a disorder of the sebaceous (oil-secreting) glands. Dandruff can also be triggered by trauma, illness, hormonal imbalances, improper carbohydrate consumption, and the consumption of sugar. Deficiencies of nutrients such as the B-complex vitamins, essential fatty acids, and selenium have been linked to dandruff as well. Chronic dandruff may be associated with baldness and general hair loss.

NUTRIENTS

SUPPLEMENT	SUGGESTED DOSAGE	COMMENTS
Very Important		
Essential fatty acids (flaxseed oil, primrose oil, and salmon oil are good sources)	As directed on label.	Helps to relieve itching and inflammation; essential for healthy skin and scalp.
Kelp	1,000–1,500 mg daily.	Supplies needed minerals, especially iodine, for better hair growth and healing of the scalp.
Selenium	200 mcg daily.	An important antioxidant to aid in controlling dry scalp.
Vitamin B complex plus extra vitamin B$_6$ (pyridoxine) and vitamin B$_{12}$	100 mg twice daily, with meals. 50 mg twice daily. 200 mcg daily.	B vitamins are needed for healthy skin and hair. Use a high-stress formula. Sublingual forms are best for absorption.
Vitamin E	400 IU and up.	For improved circulation.
Zinc lozenges (Ultimate Zinc-C Lozenges from Now Foods)	1 15-mg lozenge 5 times daily for 1 week. Do not exceed a total of 100 mg daily from all supplements.	Protein metabolism depends on zinc. The skin is composed primarily of protein.

Important		
Free-form amino acid complex	As directed on label.	Needed for repair of all tissues and for proper hair growth. Use a formula containing both essential and nonessential amino acids.
L-Cystine	500 mg daily, on an empty stomach. Take with water or juice. Do not take with milk. Take with 50 mg vitamin B$_6$ and 100 mg vitamin C for better absorption.	Needed for flexibility of the skin and for hair texture. *See* AMINO ACIDS in Part One.
Vitamin A and natural beta-carotene or carotenoid complex (Betatene)	Up to 20,000 IU daily. If you are pregnant, do not exceed 10,000 IU daily. 15,000 IU daily. As directed on label.	Helps prevent dry skin. Aids in healing of tissue. An antioxidant and precursor of vitamin A.
Vitamin C with bioflavonoids	3,000–6,000 mg daily, in divided doses.	An important antioxidant to prevent tissue damage to the scalp and to aid in healing.
Helpful		
Lecithin granules or capsules	1 tbsp 3 times daily, before meals. 1,200 mg 3 times daily, before meals.	Protects the scalp and strengthens cell membranes of the scalp and hair.

HERBS

☐ An infusion of chaparral or thyme may be used as a hair rinse.

☐ Those with dandruff can benefit from taking dandelion, goldenseal, and red clover.

Caution: Do not take goldenseal on a daily basis for more than one week at a time, and do not use it during pregnancy. If you have a history of cardiovascular disease, diabetes, or glaucoma, use it only under a doctor's supervision.

RECOMMENDATIONS

☐ Eat a diet consisting of 50 to 75 percent raw foods. Eat soured products such as yogurt.

☐ Avoid fried foods, dairy products, sugar, flour, chocolate, nuts, and seafood.

☐ *See* FASTING in Part Three, and follow the program once a month.

☐ Before washing your hair, add about 8 tablespoons of pure organic peanut oil to the juice of half a lemon and rub the mixture into your scalp. Leave it on for five to ten minutes, then shampoo.

☐ Try rinsing your hair with vinegar and water instead of plain water after shampooing. Use ¼ cup vinegar to 1 quart of water.

☐ If antibiotics are prescribed, take extra B-complex vitamins. Also take an acidophilus supplement to replace the "friendly" bacteria that are destroyed by antibiotics.

❑ Do not pick or scratch the scalp. Make sure to wash your hair frequently, and use a non-oily shampoo. Use natural hair products that do not contain chemicals. Avoid using irritating soaps and greasy ointments and creams.

❑ Do not use a shampoo containing selenium on a daily basis, even if it aids in controlling dandruff.

❑ If dandruff is persistent or symptoms seem to be getting worse, consult your health care provider.

CONSIDERATIONS

❑ Some people have found that sun exposure helps clear up dandruff, but others find that it seems to make the problem worse.

❑ It is best not to use over-the-counter ointments for dandruff. They can often do more harm than good.

❑ Dermatologists usually prescribe a cleansing lotion containing a drying agent with sulfur and resorcinol, or a medicated product called Diprosone from Schering Laboratories, to clear up dandruff.

❑ *See also* SEBORRHEA in Part Two.

Deafness

See HEARING LOSS.

Depression

Depression is a whole-body illness—it involves the body, nervous system, moods, thoughts, and behavior. It affects the way you eat and sleep, the way you feel about yourself, and the way you react to and think about the people and things around you. Symptoms can last for weeks, months, or years. There are many types of depression, with variations in the number of symptoms, their severity, and persistence.

People with depression typically withdraw and hide from society. They lose interest in things around them and become incapable of experiencing pleasure. Symptoms of depression include chronic fatigue, sleep disturbances (either insomnia or excessive sleeping), changes in appetite, headaches, backaches, digestive disorders, restlessness, irritability, quickness to anger, loss of interest or pleasure in hobbies, and feelings of worthlessness and inadequacy. Many think of death and consider suicide. Things appear bleak and time seems to pass slowly. A person with depression may be chronically angry and irritable, sad and despairing, or display little or no emotion at all. Some try to "sleep off" depression, or do nothing but sit or lie around.

The two major classifications of depressive disorders are *unipolar* and *bipolar*. Unipolar disorders are characterized by depressive episodes that most often recur at least several times in the course of a person's life. Bipolar disorders usually begin as depression, but as they progress, they involve alternating episodes of depression and mania. As a result, bipolar depression is commonly known as *manic depression*. This section focuses primarily on various types of unipolar depression.

The causes of depression are not fully understood, but they are probably many and varied. Depression may be triggered by tension, stress, a traumatic life event, chemical imbalances in the brain, thyroid disorders, upset stomach, headache, nutritional deficiencies, poor diet, the consumption of sugar, mononucleosis, lack of exercise, endometriosis, any serious physical disorder, or allergies. One of the most common causes of depression is food allergies. Hypoglycemia (low blood sugar) is another common cause of depression.

Heredity is a significant factor in this disorder. In up to 50 percent of people suffering from recurrent episodes of depression, one or both of the parents also experienced depression.

Whatever the factors that trigger it, depression begins with a disturbance in the part of the brain that governs moods. Most people can handle everyday stresses; their bodies readjust to these pressures. When stress is too great for a person and his or her adjustment mechanism is unresponsive, depression may be triggered.

Perhaps the most common type of depression is a chronic low-grade depression called *dysthymia*. This condition involves long-term and/or recurring depressive symptoms that are not necessarily disabling but keep a person from functioning normally and interfere with social interactions and enjoyment of life. Research has found that this type of depression often results from (unconscious) negative thinking habits. *Double depression* is a variation of dysthymia in which a person with chronic, low-grade depression periodically experiences major depressive episodes, then returns to his or her "normal," mildly depressed state.

Some people become more depressed in the winter months, when the days are shorter and darker. This type of disorder is known as *seasonal affective disorder (SAD)*. Women are more likely to suffer from SAD than men are. People who suffer this type of depression in the winter months lose their energy, suffer anxiety attacks, gain weight as a result of craving the wrong foods, sleep too much, and have a reduced sex drive. Many people get depressed around the December holidays; while most of them probably just have the "holiday blues," some of them may be suffering from seasonal affective disorder. Suicides seem to be highest during this time of year.

Some researchers believe that depression can be "caught," like a cold or the flu. In his book *Contagious Emotions: Staying Well When Your Loved One Is Depressed* (Pocket Books, 1993), Dr. Ronald M. Podell says that in a marriage, if one partner is chronically depressed, both probably will be. Researchers have found that some people are powerful mood transmitters and others are mood receivers. Mood transmitters can control the mood of a family or group of coworkers just by being in the room. Mood receivers are very susceptible to the changing moods of those around them. This subconscious interaction is most dangerous when the mood transmitter is exhibiting depression through constant moodiness, anger, anxiety, or sadness; he or she can then "give" a case of depression to others.

Depression affects an estimated 11 million Americans every year and is on the rise. It is twice as common in women as in men. This disorder is the focus of a considerable amount of research, and as we learn more about this disease in all its complexity, perhaps we will abandon the catchall category called depression and diagnose people according to their particular chemical imbalances.

Foods greatly influence the brain's behavior. We believe that a poor diet, especially constant snacking on junk foods, is a common cause of depression. The levels of brain chemicals called neurotransmitters, which regulate our behavior, are controlled by what we eat, and neurotransmitters are closely linked to mood. The neurotransmitters most commonly associated with mood are dopamine, serotonin, and norepinephrine. When the brain produces serotonin, tension is eased. When it produces dopamine or norepinephrine, we tend to think and act more quickly and are generally more alert.

At the neurochemical and physiological level, neurotransmitters are extremely important. These substances carry impulses between nerve cells. The substance that processes the neurotransmitter called serotonin is the amino acid tryptophan. The consumption of tryptophan increases the amount of serotonin made by the brain. Thus, eating complex carbohydrates, which raise the level of tryptophan in the brain (thereby increasing serotonin production), has a calming effect. High-protein foods, on the other hand, promote the production of dopamine and norepinephrine, which promote alertness.

The following nutrients are helpful for those suffering from depression.

NUTRIENTS

SUPPLEMENT	SUGGESTED DOSAGE	COMMENTS
Essential		
L-Tyrosine	Up to 50 mg per pound of body weight daily. Take on an empty stomach with 50 mg vitamin B_6 and 100–500 mg vitamin C for better absorption. Best taken at bedtime.	Alleviates stress by boosting production of adrenaline. It also raises dopamine levels, which influence moods. See AMINO ACIDS in Part One. *Caution:* Do not take tyrosine if you are taking an MAO inhibitor drug.
Sub-Adrene from American Biologics	As directed on label.	A dietary supplement for adrenal support.
Zinc	50 mg daily. Do not exceed a total of 100 mg daily from all supplements.	Found to be deficient in people with depression. Use zinc gluconate lozenges or OptiZinc for best absorption.
Taurine Plus from American Biologics	As directed on label.	An important antioxidant and immune regulator, necessary for white blood cell activation and neurological function. Use the sublingual form.
Vitamin B complex injections	2 cc once weekly or as prescribed by physician.	B vitamins are necessary for the normal functioning of the brain and nervous system. If depression is severe, injections (under a doctor's supervision) are recommended. All injectables can be combined in a single shot.
plus extra vitamin B_6 (pyridoxine) and	½ cc once weekly or as prescribed by physician.	Needed for normal brain function. May help lift depression.
vitamin B_{12}	1 cc once weekly or as prescribed by physician.	Linked to the production of the neurotransmitter acetylcholine.
or liver extract injections	2 cc once weekly or as prescribed by physician.	A good source of B vitamins and other valuable nutrients.
plus vitamin B_{12}	1 cc once weekly or as prescribed by physician.	
or vitamin B complex	100 mg 3 times daily.	If injections are not available, a sublingual form of B complex is recommended.
plus extra pantothenic acid (vitamin B_5) and	500 mg daily.	The most potent anti-stress vitamin.
vitamin B_6 (pyridoxine) plus	50 mg 3 times daily.	
vitamin B_3 (niacin)	50 mg 3 times daily. Do not exceed this amount.	Improves celebral circulation. *Caution:* Do not take niacin if you have a liver disorder, gout, or high blood pressure.
and folic acid	400 mcg daily.	Found to be deficient in people with depression.
Important		
Choline and inositol	100 mg each twice daily.	Important in brain function and neurotransmission. *Caution:* Do not take these supplements if you suffer from manic (bipolar) depression.
or lecithin	As directed on label.	
GH3 from Gero Vita	As directed on label for those 35 years or older.	Aids in proper brain function; promotes alertness and increased energy. *Caution:* Do not use this product if you are allergic to sulfites.
Helpful		
Calcium and	1,500–2,000 mg daily.	Has a calming effect. Needed for the nervous system.
magnesium	1,000 mg daily.	Works with calcium. Use magnesium asporotate or magnesium chelate form.
Chromium	300 mcg daily.	Aids in mobilizing fats for energy.
Essential fatty acids (black currant seed oil and primrose oil are good sources)	As directed on label. Take with meals.	Aid in the transmission of nerve impulses; needed for normal brain function.
Gamma-aminobutyric acid (GABA)	750 mg daily. Take with 200 mg niacinamide for best results.	Has a tranquilizing effect, much as diazepam (Valium) and other tranquilizers do. See AMINO ACIDS in Part One.
Lithium	As prescribed by physician.	A trace mineral used to treat bipolar (manic) depression. Available by prescription only.

Megavital Forte from Futurebiotics or	As directed on label.	A balanced vitamin and mineral formula that increases energy and sense of well-being.
multivitamin and mineral complex	As directed on label.	To correct vitamin and mineral deficiencies, often associated with depression.
Vitamin C plus rutin	2,000–5,000 mg daily, in divided doses. 200–300 mg daily.	Needed for immune function. Aids in preventing depression. Buckwheat-derived bioflavonoid. Enhances vitamin C absorption.

HERBS

❑ Balm, also known as lemon balm, is good for the stomach and digestive organs during stressful situations.

❑ Ephedra (ma huang) may be helpful for lethargic depression.

Caution: Do not use this herb if you suffer from anxiety disorder, glaucoma, heart disease, high blood pressure, or insomnia, or if you are taking a monoamine oxidase (MAO) inhibitor drug.

❑ Ginger, ginkgo biloba, licorice root, oat straw, peppermint, and Siberian ginseng may be helpful.

Caution: Do not use licorice on a daily basis for more than seven days in a row. Avoid it completely if you have high blood pressure. Do not use Siberian ginseng if you have hypoglycemia, high blood pressure, or a heart disorder.

❑ Kava kava helps to induce calm and relieve depression.

Caution: This herb can cause drowsiness. If this occurs, discontinue use or reduce the dosage.

❑ St. Johnswort acts in the same way as monoamine oxidase (MAO) inhibitors do, but less harshly.

RECOMMENDATIONS

❑ Eat a diet that includes plenty of raw fruits and vegetables, with soybeans and soy products, brown rice, millet, and legumes. A diet too low in complex carbohydrates can cause serotonin depletion and depression.

❑ If you are nervous and wish to become more relaxed, consume more complex carbohydrates. For increased alertness, eat protein meals containing essential fatty acids. Salmon and white fish are good choices. If you need your spirits lifted, you will benefit from eating foods like turkey and salmon, which are high in tryptophan and protein.

❑ Omit wheat products from the diet. Wheat gluten has been linked to depressive disorders.

❑ Limit your intake of supplements that contain the amino acid phenylalanine. It contains the chemical phenol, which is highly allergenic. Most depressed people are allergic to certain substances. If you take a combination free-form amino acid supplement, look for a product that does not contain phenylalanine, such as that made by Ecological Formulas. For the same reason, avoid the artificial sweetener aspartame (Equal, NutraSweet); phenylalanine is one of the major components in this substance.

❑ Avoid foods high in saturated fats; the consumption of meat or fried foods, such as hamburgers and French fries, leads to sluggishness, slow thinking, and fatigue. They interfere with blood flow by causing the arteries and small blood vessels to become blocked and the blood cells to become sticky and tend to clump together, resulting in poor circulation, especially to the brain.

❑ Avoid all forms of sugar. The body reacts more quickly to the presence of sugar than it does to the presence of complex carbohydrates. The increase in energy supplied by the simple carbohydrates (sugars) is quickly followed by fatigue and depression.

❑ Avoid alcohol, caffeine, and processed foods.

❑ Investigate the possibility that food allergies are causing or contributing to depression. *See* ALLERGIES in Part Two.

❑ Have a hair analysis to rule out heavy metal intoxication as the cause of depression. *See* HAIR ANALYSIS in Part Three.

❑ Keep your mind active, and get plenty of rest and regular exercise. Studies have shown that exercise—walking, swimming, or any activity that you enjoy—is most important for all types of depression. Avoid stressful situations.

❑ Learn to recognize, and then to "reroute," negative thinking patterns. Working with a qualified professional to change ingrained habits can be rewarding (cognitive-behavioral therapists specialize in this type of work). Keeping a daily log also can help you to recognize disorted thoughts and develop a more positive way of thinking.

❑ If depression is seasonal, light therapy may help. Exposure to the sun and bright light seem to regulate the body's production of melatonin, a hormone produced by the pineal gland that is, in part, responsible for preventing the blues. Stay in brightly lit rooms on dark days. Keep all draperies, curtains, and blinds open and use full-spectrum fluorescent lights in your home. The normal room has about 500 to 800 lux of light. Choose one room and light it with about 10,000 lux of full-spectrum light and spend at least half an hour there each day. For information about devices for this type of light treatment, contact either The SunBox Company (telephone 301–869–5980 or 800–548–3968) or Apollo Light Systems, Inc. (telephone 801–226–2370 or 800–545–9667).

❑ *See* HYPOTHYROIDISM in Part Two and take the underarm test to detect an underactive thyroid. If your temperature is low, consult your physician. For people with hypothyroidism, we recommend Armour Thyroid Tablets. This product is produced by Forest Pharmaceuticals and is available by prescription only.

❑ Try using color to alleviate depression. *See* COLOR THERAPY in Part Three.

CONSIDERATIONS

❑ Tyrosine is needed for brain function. This amino acid is directly involved in the production of norepinephrine and dopamine, two vital neurotransmitters that are synthesized in the brain and the adrenal medulla. A lack of tyrosine can result in a deficiency of norepinephrine in certain sites in the brain, resulting in mood disorders such as depression. The effects of stress may be prevented or reversed if this essential amino acid is obtained in the diet or by means of supplements.

Caution: If you are taking an MAO inhibitor drug for depression, *do not* take tyrosine supplements, and avoid foods containing tyrosine, as drug and dietary interactions can cause a sudden, dangerous rise in blood pressure. Discuss food and medicine limitations thoroughly with your health care provider or a qualified dietitian.

❑ Selenium has been shown to elevate mood, and also to decrease anxiety. These effects were more noticeable in people who had lower levels of selenium in their diets to begin with.

❑ Vigorous exercise can be an effective antidote to bouts of depression. During exercise, the brain produces painkilling chemicals called endorphins and enkephalins. Certain endorphins and other brain chemicals released in response to exercise also produce a natural "high." Most of those who exercise regularly say that they feel really good afterward. This may explain why exercise is the best way to get rid of depression.

❑ Music can have powerful effects on mood and may be useful in alleviating depression. (*See* MUSIC AND SOUND THERAPY in Part Three.)

❑ In one study, people suffering from depression were found to have lower than normal levels of folic acid in their blood than nondepressed individuals. Other studies have shown that zinc levels tend to be significantly lower than normal when people suffer from depression.

❑ It may be possible to diagnose depression by using a computerized tomography (CT) scan to measure a person's adrenal glands. Researchers at Duke University found that people suffering from clinical depression have larger adrenal glands than nondepressed people.

❑ A variety of different drugs are commonly prescribed to treat depression. Antidepressant drugs fight depression by changing the balance of neurotransmitters in the body. These medications include:

• *Tricyclics.* These drugs work by inhibiting the uptake of the neurotransmitters serotonin, norepinephrine, and dopamine, making more of the mood-enhancing chemical messengers available to nerve cells. Examples include amitriptyline (Elavil, Endep), desipramine (Norpramin, Pertofrane), imipramine (Janimine, Tofranil), and nortriptyline (Aventyl, Pamelor). Possible side effects include blurred vision, constipation, dry mouth, irregular heartbeat, urine retention, and orthostatic hypotension, a severe drop in blood pressure upon sitting up or standing, which can lead to dizziness, falls, and fractures.

• *Tetracyclics.* These drugs have an action similar to that of the tricyclics, but have a slightly different chemical structure and appear to cause fewer side effects. Maprotiline (Ludiomil) is in this category.

• *Monoamine oxidase (MAO) inhibitors.* These drugs increase the amounts of mood-enhancing neurotransmitters in the brain by blocking the action of the enzyme monoamine oxidase, which normally breaks them down. Examples of MAO inhibitors include isocarboxazid (Marplan), phenelzine (Nardil), and tranylcypromine (Parnate). Possible side effects include agitation, elevated blood pressure, overstimulation, and changes in heart rate and rhythm. MAO inhibitors also have a high potential for dangerous interactions with other substances, including drugs and foods. Persons taking these drugs must adhere strictly to a diet that includes no foods containing the chemical tyramine, such as almonds, avocados, bananas, beef or chicken liver, beer, cheese (including cottage cheese), chocolate, coffee, fava beans, herring, meat tenderizer, peanuts, pickles, pineapples, pumpkin seeds, raisins, sausage, sesame seeds, sour cream, soy sauce, wine, yeast extracts (including brewer's yeast), yogurt, and other foods. In general, any high-protein food that has undergone aging, pickling, fermentation, or similar processes should be avoided. Over-the-counter cold and allergy remedies should also be avoided.

• *Other drugs.* Several drugs known as "second-generation" antidepressants have become available in the past few years. These new drugs have not been shown to be more effective than the others, but they tend to have fewer serious side effects. They include the newer tricyclic amoxapine (Asendin); fluoxetine (Prozac) and sertraline (Zoloft), which specifically block the uptake of the neurotransmitter serotonin but, unlike tricyclics, not that of norepinephrine or dopamine; buproprion (Wellbutrin), which is believed to act by inhibiting the uptake of dopamine but not serotonin or norepinephrine; and trazodone (Desyrel), an antidepressant with stimulant properties that also inhibits the uptake of dopamine.

❑ Steroid drugs and oral contraceptives may cause serotonin levels in the brain to drop.

❑ People who smoke are more likely than nonsmokers to be depressed.

❑ Allergies, hypoglycemia, hypothyroidism, and/or malabsorption problems can cause or contribute to depression. In people with these conditions, vitamin B$_{12}$ and folic acid are blocked from entering the system, which can lead to depression.

❑ Individuals with depression are more likely than other people to have various disturbances in calcium metabolism.

❑ There is no doubt that attitude affects health. Study after study has shown that optimistic people are not only happier but healthier. They suffer less illness, recover better from illness and surgery, and have stronger immune defenses.

Dermatitis

Dermatitis is an inflammation of the skin that produces scaling, flaking, thickening, color changes, and, often, itching. Many cases of dermatitis are the result of allergies. This type of condition is called *allergic* or *contact dermatitis*. It may be caused by contact with perfumes, cosmetics, rubber, medicated creams and ointments, plants such as poison ivy, and/or metals or metal alloys such as gold, silver, and nickel found in jewelry or zippers. Some people with dermatitis are sensitive to sunlight. Whatever the irritant, if the skin remains in constant contact with it, the dermatitis is likely to spread and become more severe. Stress, especially chronic tension, can cause or exacerbate dermatitis.

Atopic dermatitis is a hereditary form of the condition that usually becomes apparent in infancy. It typically appears on the face, in the bends of the elbows, and behind the knees. Often, other family members have histories of allergies or asthma. *Nummular* ("coin-shaped") *dermatitis* is a chronic condition in which round lesions appear on the limbs. It may be caused by an allergy to nickel, and is often associated with dry skin. *Dermatitis herpetiformis* is a very itchy type of dermatitis associated with intestinal and immune disorders. This form of dermatitis may be triggered by the consumption of dairy products and/or gluten. *Eczema* is a term sometimes used interchangeably with dermatitis, although some authorities define it as a specific type of dermatitis distinguished by the presence of fluid-filled blisters that weep, ooze, and crust over. *Seborrhea* is a form of dermatitis that most commonly affects the scalp and/or face.

NUTRIENTS

SUPPLEMENT	SUGGESTED DOSAGE	COMMENTS
Essential		
Vitamin B complex	50–100 mg 3 times daily, with meals.	Needed for healthy skin and proper circulation. Aids in reproduction of all cells. Use a high-stress, yeast-free formula. A sublingual form is recommended.
plus extra vitamin B$_3$ (niacin)	100 mg 3 times daily. Do not exceed this amount.	Important for proper circulation and healthy skin. *Caution:* Do not take niacin if you have a liver disorder, gout, or high blood pressure.
and vitamin B$_6$ (pyridoxine)	50 mg 3 times daily.	Deficiency has been linked to skin disorders.
and vitamin B$_{12}$	200 mcg daily.	Aids in cell formation and cellular longevity. Use a lozenge or sublingual form.
and biotin	300 mg daily.	Deficiency has been linked to dermatitis.
Important		
Kelp	1,000 mg daily or as directed on label.	Contains iodine and other minerals needed for healing of tissues.
Essential fatty acids (black currant seed oil, flaxseed oil, primrose oil, and salmon oil are good sources)	As directed on label.	Promotes lubrication of the skin.
Vitamin E	400 IU daily and up.	Relieves itching and dryness.
Zinc	100 mg daily. Do not exceed this amount.	Aids healing and enhances immune function. Use zinc gluconate lozenges or OptiZinc for best absorption.
Helpful		
Aller Bee-Gone from CC Pollen	As directed on label.	For allergic dermatitis. A combination of herbs, enzymes, and nutrients designed to fight allergic flare-ups.
Herpanacine from Diamond-Herpanacine Associates	As directed on label.	Contains antioxidants, amino acids, and herbs that promote overall skin health.
Free-form amino acid complex	As directed on label, on an empty stomach.	To supply protein, important for construction and repair of all tissues. Use a formula containing both essential and nonessential amino acids.
Shark cartilage (BeneFin)	1 gram per 15 lbs of body weight daily, divided into 3 doses.	Reduces inflammation in eczema.
Vitamin A emulsion or capsules and	100,000 IU daily for 1 month, then 50,000 IU daily for 2 weeks, then reduce to 25,000 IU daily. If you are pregnant, do not exceed 10,000 IU daily. 5,000 IU daily.	Needed for smooth skin. Aids in preventing dryness. Use emulsion form for easier assimilation and greater safety at high doses.
natural beta-carotene	25,000 IU daily.	Antioxidant and precursor of vitamin A.
Vitamin D	400–1,000 IU daily.	Aids in healing of tissues.

HERBS

❑ Poultices combining chaparral, dandelion, and yellow dock root can be helpful. *See* USING A POULTICE in Part Three.
Note: Chaparral is recommended for external use only.

❑ The following herbs can be used in tea or capsule form: dandelion, goldenseal, myrrh, pau d'arco, and red clover. Alternate among them for best results.
Caution: Do not take goldenseal on a daily basis for more than one week at a time, and do not use it during pregnancy. If you have a history of cardiovascular disease, diabetes, or glaucoma, use it only under a doctor's supervision.

❑ To relieve itching and promote healing, mix goldenseal root powder with vitamin E oil, then add a little honey until it is the consistency of a loose paste. Apply this mixture to the affected area.

RECOMMENDATIONS

❑ Add brown rice and millet to your diet.

❑ Avoid dairy products, sugar, white flour, fats, fried foods, and processed foods.

❑ Try a gluten-free diet for six weeks, then add gluten-containing foods back to the diet one at a time, and see if the condition changes. A gluten-free diet is often of therapeutic benefit in controlling dermatitis. *See* CELIAC DISEASE in Part Two for the recommended diet.

❑ Do not eat foods containing raw eggs, which contain avidin, a protein that binds biotin and prevents it from being absorbed. Biotin is needed for skin and scalp disorders.

❑ Keep the colon clean. Use a fiber supplement such as flaxseed, psyllium husk, or Aerobic Bulk Cleanse (ABC) from Aerobic Life Industries daily. Use occasional cleansing enemas for removing toxins for quicker healing. *See* COLON CLEANSING and/or ENEMAS in Part Three.

Note: Always take supplemental fiber separately from other supplements and medications.

CONSIDERATIONS

❑ Chemicals used in bubble bath products may cause dermatitis and may even irritate the tissues of the lower urinary tract sufficiently to cause bloody urine. This is most likely to occur if you soak in treated bathwater for too long.

❑ Primrose oil and vitamin B_6 (pyridoxine) have helped infants with dermatitis.

❑ Sensitivity to gluten is widespread, although it is often unrecognized. Research has shown that people suffering from virtually all skin disorders do better if they eliminate foods containing gluten and all dairy products from the diet.

❑ Food allergies can cause dermatitis. (*See* ALLERGIES in Part Two.)

❑ *See also* FUNGAL INFECTION; HIVES; INTERTRIGO; POISON IVY/POISON OAK; PSORIASIS; ROSACEA; SCABIES; and/or SEBORRHEA, all in Part Two.

Detached Retina

See Dimness or Loss of Vision *under* EYE PROBLEMS.

Diabetes

There are two basic types of diabetes: *diabetes insipidus* and *diabetes mellitus*. Diabetes insipidus is a rare metabolic disorder caused either by a deficiency of the pituitary hormone vasopressin or by the inability of the kidneys to respond properly to this hormone. Failure to produce adequate amounts of vasopressin is usually the result of damage to the pituitary gland. Diabetes insipidus is characterized by extreme thirst and by the production of enormous amounts of urine, regardless of how much liquid is consumed.

Diabetes mellitus results from a defect in the production of insulin by the pancreas. Without insulin, the body cannot utilize glucose (blood sugar), its principal energy source. As a result, the level of glucose circulating in the blood is high and the level of glucose absorbed by the body tissues is low. Perhaps more than most diseases, diabetes mellitus is associated with diet. It is a chronic disorder of carbohydrate metabolism that over time increases the risk of kidney disease, atherosclerosis, blindness, and neuropathy (loss of nerve function). It also creates a predisposition to infections such as candidiasis and can complicate pregnancy. Although genetics may make a person susceptible to diabetes, a diet high in refined, processed foods and low in fiber and complex carbohydrates is believed to be behind most cases of the disease. Those who are overweight face the greatest risk of developing diabetes.

Diabetes mellitus is generally divided into two categories: type I, called insulin-dependent or juvenile diabetes, and type II, or non-insulin-dependent diabetes. Type I diabetes is associated with destruction of the beta cells of the pancreas, which manufacture insulin. This type of diabetes occurs mostly in children and young adults. Recent evidence implicates a viral cause in some cases of this disorder. Autoimmune factors may also be involved.

Symptoms of type I diabetes include irritability, frequent urination, abnormal thirst, nausea or vomiting, weakness, fatigue, weight loss despite a normal (or even increased) intake of food, and unusual hunger. In children, frequent bedwetting—especially by a child who did not previously wet the bed—is another common sign.

People with type I diabetes are subject to episodes in which blood glucose levels are very high (hyperglycemia) and very low (hypoglycemia). Either of these conditions can lead to a serious medical emergency.

Episodes of hypoglycemia, which strike suddenly, can be caused by a missed meal, too much exercise, or a reaction to too much insulin. The initial signs of hypoglycemia are hunger, dizziness, sweating, confusion, palpitations, and numbness or tingling of the lips. If not treated, the individual may go on to experience double vision, trembling, and disorientation; may act strangely; and may eventually lapse into a coma.

In contrast, a hyperglycemic episode can come on over a period of several hours or even days. The risk for hyperglycemia is greatest during illness, when insulin requirements rise; blood sugar can creep up, ultimately resulting in coma, a reaction also known as *diabetic ketoacidosis*. One of the warning signs of developing hyperglycemia is the inability to keep down fluids. Possible long-term complications include stroke, blindness, heart disease, kidney failure, gangrene, and nerve damage.

The second category of diabetes mellitus, often referred to as maturity-onset diabetes, is most likely to occur in people with a family history of diabetes. In this type of the disorder, the pancreas does produce insulin, but the insulin is ineffective. Symptoms include blurred vision, itching, unusual thirst, drowsiness, fatigue, skin infections, slow wound healing, and tingling or numbness in the feet. The onset of type II diabetes typically occurs during adulthood and is linked to a poor diet. Other signs that may be associated with diabetes include lingering flulike symptoms, loss of hair on the legs, increased facial hair, and small yellow bumps known as xanthomas anywhere on the body. Balanoposthitis (inflammation of the penile glans and foreskin) often is the first sign of diabetes and is usually associated with frequent urination day and night.

Some individuals have impaired glucose tolerance (IGT), indicating an asymptomatic subclinical, or latent, form of diabetes. IGT describes those whose plasma glucose levels and responses to glucose are intermediate, somewhere between those of a diabetic and a healthy person.

An estimated 5.5 million Americans are being treated for diabetes. Studies indicate that there are 5 million adults with undetected type II diabetes, and another 20 million have impaired glucose tolerance that may lead to full-blown diabetes. The National Institutes of Health report that undiagnosed diabetes has caused millions of people to lose their vision. In addition, complications of diabetes are the third leading cause of death in the United States. Urinalysis can often detect unsuspected diabetes.

DIABETES SELF-TESTS

There are several ways to test yourself for diabetes. The tests for type I diabetes are also used for self-monitoring by persons diagnosed with the condition.

Type I Diabetes (Insulin-Dependent or Juvenile-Onset diabetes)

To test for type I diabetes:

1. Purchase chemically treated plastic strips at a drugstore.
2. Prick your finger and apply a drop of blood to the tip of the strip.
3. Wait one minute and compare the color on the strip to a color chart, which lists various glucose levels.

There are also electronic devices available that can analyze the test strip for you and give you a numerical readout of the glucose level. The Bayer Corporation of Elkhart, Indiana, manufactures two glucometer kits—Glucometer Elite and Glucometer Encore—for testing blood sugar in the convenience of your own home. You simply prick your finger with the spring-loaded needle, apply a drop of your blood to the test strip, and place it in the machine for analysis. This test gives you an immediate blood sugar result. It is a device that all people with diabetes should own.

Type II Diabetes (Maturity-Onset Diabetes)

Those with type II diabetes mellitus often cannot perceive sweet tastes. This abnormality may play an important role in how individuals with diabetes perceive the taste of their food, and also in how well they comply with the dietary aspects of treatment. Because our society as a whole is addicted to sugar, this distorted taste perception is very common among the population in general.

The following test can detect an impaired ability to taste sweets.

1. Do not consume stimulants (coffee, tea, soda) or sweets for one hour before the test.
2. Fill seven identical glasses with 8 ounces of water each and label the glasses as having no sugar, ¼ teaspoon sugar, ½ teaspoon sugar, 1 teaspoon sugar 1½ teaspoons sugar, 2 teaspoons sugar, and 3 teaspoons sugar. Add the appropriate amount of sugar to each glass, then ask someone else to rearrange the order of the glasses and hide the labels.
3. Take a straw and sip from each glass, then write down the amount of sugar you think it contains. Between sips, rinse your mouth with pure water.

Healthy people generally notice a sweet taste when a teaspoon or less of sugar is added to 8 ounces of water. By contrast, people with adult-onset diabetes usually do not notice sweetness until 1½ to 2 teaspoons of sugar have been added to the water.

NUTRIENTS

SUPPLEMENT	SUGGESTED DOSAGE	COMMENTS
Essential		
Chromium picolinate or	400-600 mcg daily.	Improves insulin's efficiency, which lowers blood sugar levels.
Diabetic Nutrition Rx from Progressive Research Labs or	As directed on label.	A combination of chromium picolinate, vanadyl sulfate, and other vitamins and minerals that work synergistically to
brewer's yeast with added chromium	As directed on label.	regulate blood sugar levels and correct deficiencies. *Caution:* If you have diabetes, consult with your physician before taking any supplement containing chromium.
L-Carnitine plus	500 mg twice daily, on an empty stomach. Take with water. Do not take with milk. Take with 50 mg vitamin B$_6$ and 100 mg vitamin C for better absorption.	Mobilizes fat.
L-glutamine plus	500 mg twice daily, on an empty stomach.	Reduces the craving for sugars.
taurine	500 mg twice daily, on an empty stomach.	Aids in the release of insulin.
Quercetin (Activated Quercetin from Source Naturals, Quercitin-C from Ecological Formulas)	100 mg 3 times daily.	Helps protect the membranes of the lens of the eye from accumulations of polyols as a result of high glucose levels.
Raw adrenal and	As directed on label.	Aids in rebuilding and nourishing these organs. *See* GLANDULAR THERAPY in Part Three.
raw pancreas and	As directed on label.	
thyroid glandulars	As directed on label.	

229

Supplement	Dosage	Comments
Vitamin B complex	50 mg 3 times daily. Do not exceed 300 mg daily from all supplements.	The B vitamins work best when taken together.
plus extra biotin and	50 mg daily.	Improves the metabolism of glucose.
inositol	50 mg daily.	Important for circulation and for prevention of atherosclerosis.
Vitamin B₁₂	As prescribed by physician or directed on label.	Needed to prevent diabetic neuropathy. Injections (under a doctor's supervision) are best. If injections are not available, use a lozenge or sublingual form.
Zinc	50–80 mg daily. Do not exceed a total of 100 mg daily from all supplements.	Deficiency has been associated with diabetes. Use zinc gluconate lozenges or OptiZinc for best absorption.

Very Important

Coenzyme Q₁₀	80 mg daily.	Improves circulation and stabilizes blood sugar.
Magnesium	750 mg daily.	Important for enzyme systems and pH balance. Protects against coronary artery spasm in arteriosclerosis.
Manganese	5–10 mg daily. Take separately from calcium.	Needed for repair of the pancreas. Also a cofactor in key enzymes of glucose metabolism. Deficiency is common in people with diabetes.
Psyllium husks or Aerobic Bulk Cleanse (ABC) from Aerobic Life Industries	As directed on label. Take with a large glass of water. Take separately from other supplements and medications.	Good fiber source and fat mobilizer.

Important

Vitamin A	15,000 IU daily. If you are pregnant, do not exceed 10,000 IU daily.	An important antioxidant needed to maintain the health of the eyes. Use emulsion form for best absorption.
Vitamin C	3,000–6,000 mg daily.	Deficiency may lead to vascular problems in people with diabetes.
Vitamin E	400 IU and up daily.	Improves circulation and prevents complications through its antioxidant properties.

Helpful

Calcium	1,500 mg daily.	Important for pH balance.
Copper complex	As directed on label.	Aids in protein metabolism and in many enzyme systems.
Garlic (Kyolic)	2 capsules each morning and evening.	Stabilizes blood sugar, enhances immunity, and improves circulation.
Maitake	1–4 gm daily.	May help to normalize blood sugar levels.
Multienzyme complex plus	As directed on label. Take with meals.	To aid digestion. Proper digestion is essential in management of diabetes.
proteolytic enzymes	As directed on label. Take between meals.	
Pycnogenol or grape seed extract	As directed on label. As directed on label.	A powerful antioxidant that also enhances the activity of vitamin C and strengthens connective tissue, including that of the cardiovascular system.

HERBS

❑ Cedar berries are excellent nourishment for the pancreas.

❑ Ginseng tea is believed to lower the blood sugar level. *Caution:* Do not use this herb if you have high blood pressure.

❑ Huckleberry helps to promote insulin production.

❑ Other herbs that may be beneficial for diabetes include bilberry, buchu, dandelion root, goldenseal, and uva ursi. *Caution:* Do not take goldenseal on a daily basis for more than one week at a time, and do not use it during pregnancy. If you have a history of cardiovascular disease, diabetes, or glaucoma, use it only under a doctor's supervision.

RECOMMENDATIONS

❑ Eat a high-complex-carbohydrate, low-fat, high-fiber diet including plenty of raw fruits and vegetables as well as fresh vegetable juices. This reduces the need for insulin and also lowers the level of fats in the blood. Fiber helps to reduce blood sugar surges. For snacks, eat oat or rice bran crackers with nut butter or cheese. Legumes, root vegetables, and whole grains are also good.

❑ Supplement your diet with spirulina. Spirulina helps to stabilize blood sugar levels. Other foods that help normalize blood sugar include berries, brewer's yeast, dairy products (especially cheese), egg yolks, fish, garlic, kelp, sauerkraut, soybeans, and vegetables.

❑ Get your protein from vegetable sources, such as grains and legumes. Fish and low-fat dairy products are also acceptable sources of protein.

❑ Avoid saturated fats and simple sugars (except when necessary to balance an insulin reaction).

❑ Eat more carbohydrates or reduce your insulin dosage before exercise. Exercise produces an insulinlike effect in the body. Talk to your doctor about the right approach for you.

❑ Do not take fish oil capsules or supplements containing large amounts of para-aminobenzoic acid (PABA), and avoid salt and white flour products. Consumption of these products results in an elevation of blood sugar.

❑ Do not take supplements containing the amino acid cysteine. It has the ability to break down the bonds of the hormone insulin and interferes with absorption of insulin by the cells.

❑ Do not take extremely large doses of vitamins B₁ (thiamine) and C. Excessive amounts may inactivate insulin. These vitamins may, however, be taken in normal amounts. Consult the Nutrients table, above, for recommendations.

❑ If symptoms of hyperglycemia develop, go to the emergency room of the nearest hospital. This is a potentially dangerous situation. Intravenous administration of proper fluids, electrolytes, and insulin may be required.

Chromium Picolinate:
A Complementary Nutritional Therapy for Diabetes

Chromium picolinate is a nutritional supplement that can help control diabetes. As the name implies, it is a combination of two different substances: chromium and picolinate. Chromium is a mineral that helps to increase the efficiency of insulin, the hormone that controls blood glucose (blood sugar) levels; picolinate is an amino acid derivative that allows the body to use chromium much more readily.

The shape of individual insulin molecules is important to the hormone's effectiveness. If the molecules maintain their proper shape, the insulin can effectively transport glucose into the cells, where it is needed. Without chromium, insulin molecules become misshapen, and can no longer serve as an effective transportation system for glucose. Without an effective transportation system, glucose builds up in the bloodstream, starting a chain reaction that eventually leads to diabetes.

Scientists have long known that chromium is a vital nutrient, but not until chromium was combined with picolinate was a truly effective means of providing supplemental chromium developed. In the body, chromium takes the form of an ion, a particle with an electrical charge. This charge is repelled by the body's cells, making it difficult for chromium to enter the cells. Picolinate is a chelator, a substance that can bind with an ion and neutralize its charge. Once chromium and picolinate join together, the chromium's repellent charge is done away with. The body's cells then are able to accept the chromium.

The effectiveness of chromium picolinate has been tested on individuals with a number of different health problems, including diabetes. Research shows that most people with diabetes experience a decline in blood glucose levels after they start taking daily chromium picolinate supplements. As a result, it is believed that chromium picolinate may be able to help many people with diabetes (especially type II diabetes) to control their blood sugar levels. This in turn would allow them to cut back on their intake of insulin and other drugs, likely resulting in fewer side effects. Furthermore, since improving the action of insulin also helps the body to use fat as a fuel, chromium picolinate can help reduce obesity. This means that it may enable some people with type II diabetes to lose enough weight to stop taking drugs entirely.

However, it is not recommended that people with diabetes simply go out and buy chromium picolinate supplements and start taking them. Anyone who has diabetes, especially type I diabetes, must exercise caution with this supplement. Its effects on insulin requirements are very real. Blood sugar levels must be monitored carefully and the appropriate dosages of insulin and/or other drugs adjusted as needed in response. Otherwise, a potentially dangerous insulin reaction may occur as a result of too little glucose in the blood.

Anyone interested in using chromium picolinate for the treatment of diabetes should first seek the advice of a qualified health care provider, preferably a nutritionally oriented physician who has experience in this area.

❑ Avoid taking large amounts of vitamin B3 (niacin). However, small amounts (50 to 100 milligrams daily), taken by mouth, may be beneficial.

❑ If you have a child with diabetes, be sure his or her teacher knows how to respond to the warning signs of hypoglycemia and hyperglycemia.

❑ If symptoms of hypoglycemia develop, *immediately* consume fruit juice, soda pop, or anything else that contains sugar. If that fails to help within twenty minutes, repeat this regimen. If the second treatment fails, or if you cannot ingest food, seek immediate medical attention and/or administer a glucagon injection. Anyone who has insulin-dependent diabetes should always carry a glucagon kit and know how to use it.

❑ Avoid tobacco in any form; it constricts the blood vessels and inhibits circulation. Keep your feet clean, dry, and warm, and wear only white cotton socks and well-fitting shoes. Lack of oxygen (because of poor circulation) and peripheral nerve damage (with loss of pain sensation) are major factors in the development of diabetic foot ulcers. Try to avoid injury, and take measures to improve the circulation in the feet and legs. *See* CIRCULATORY PROBLEMS in Part Two.

CONSIDERATIONS

❑ Because the management of type I diabetes is such a complex challenge, it is imperative that a person with this condition have a good relationship with the physician prescribing the insulin. There are more than thirty insulin formulations on the U.S. market, but all are variations of several basic types. The most commonly used are purified porcine (pork), purified bovine (beef), and recombinant DNA-origin (human) insulin. Purified porcine insulin is insulin derived from the pancreases of pigs that has undergone further purification; purified bovine insulin is cattle-pancreas-derived insulin that has undergone further purification. Recombinant DNA-origin insulin is genetically engineered by inserting the human gene for insulin production into a non-disease-producing laboratory strain of *Escherichea coli* bacteria or yeast.

❑ People with type II diabetes are less able than most people to perceive sweet tastes, and this may make it more difficult for them to lose weight. Because they do not recognize the sweet taste of substances, they often consume sugary products that they do not appreciate as sweet. If a person with type II diabetes attains a better understanding of food, exercises greater care in choosing foods, and reads food product labels carefully, he or she should be able to control the problem and avoid the need for treatment with drugs or insulin.

❑ Type II diabetes can usually be controlled by dietary modification and exercise; insulin treatment is not usually required. Obesity is a major factor in type II diabetes, and a weight reduction program is often all that is required to control it.

❑ Some people with diabetes may be able to abandon insulin injections for an inhaler in a few years. Researchers at Johns Hopkins School of Public Health in Baltimore reported that an experimental aerosol inhaler normalized blood glucose levels in six volunteers with type II diabetes, according to an article by Mike Snider in *USA Today*.

❑ Research indicates that supplementation with the hormone dehydroepiandrosterone (DHEA) may help prevent diabetes. (*See* DHEA THERAPY in Part Three.)

❑ Hypothyroidism may be a leading cause of diabetes. Well-known researcher and author Stephen Langer, M.D., has noticed that neuropathies, together with other diabetic complications, disappear when thyroid hormone is administered. Many complications of diabetes and hypothyroidism are a result of clogged arteries, which prevent the blood from delivering nutrients and oxygen and carrying off waste and debris.

❑ Glycosylation—the binding of glucose and other sugars onto proteins in the blood, nerve cells, and lenses of the eyes—may be responsible for many of the long-term effects of diabetes. Researchers at the University of Surrey's School of Biological Sciences and the Academic Unit of Diabetes and Endocrinology of London's Whittington Hospital have shown that vitamin C may inhibit this destructive process. They say that if glycosylation is part of the normal aging process, taking vitamin C supplements may slow it.

❑ A woman with diabetes who wants to become pregnant should watch her blood sugar levels long before she plans to conceive. The fetus has the greatest chance of developing birth defects during the first five to eight weeks of pregnancy, before most women know they are pregnant. It usually takes a few months to get the blood sugar under proper control; if a woman begins to monitor her blood sugar level the day she conceives, damage may already be done by the time it is under control.

❑ Damage to the retina from diabetes is the leading cause of blindness in the United States. One in twenty people with type I diabetes and one in fifteen people with type II diabetes develop retinopathy. However, the incidence of blindness from diabetic retinopathy will probably drop with the further development of laser surgery. Persons with diabetes should get annual retinal examinations to check on their condition.

❑ Diabetic nephropathy—damage to the kidneys from diabetes—is common and a leading cause of death among people with diabetes. It is important to monitor kidney function periodically. Controlling wide swings in blood sugar levels reduces the risks of these complications. A low-protein diet containing less than 40 grams of protein each day is recommended for prevention and treatment of diabetic nephropathy.

❑ Diabetic neuropathy (damage to the nerves caused by diabetes) usually affects the peripheral nerves, such as those in the feet, hands, and legs. Symptoms include numbness, tingling, and pain.

❑ In one study, large amounts of niacin raised blood sugar levels in people with non-insulin-dependent diabetes by as much as 16 percent. Over time, this could cause dependence on insulin or medication. Niacin can also cause the level of uric acid in the blood to rise, indicating probable kidney dysfunction and an increased risk of gout. However, niacinamide, a form of niacin, slows down the destruction and enhances the regeneration of the insulin-producing beta cells in the pancreas, and therefore may be helpful for those with type I diabetes.

❑ Elevated glucose levels in the lens of the eye can result in the accumulation of substances called polyols, whose presence can ultimately cause damage to the lens. High polyol concentrations resulting from high glucose levels can persist even if glucose levels subsequently return to normal. Flavonoids, such as quercetin, help to inhibit the accumulation of polyols.

❑ Diabetes and high blood pressure often go hand in hand, and both can lead to kidney disease. In one recent study, hypertensive diabetics who took drugs called angiotensin converting enzyme (ACE) inhibitors cut their risk of developing serious kidney disease in half.

❑ Researchers at the University of Colorado Health Sciences Center found that diabetics who smoke are two to three times more likely than nonsmoking diabetics to develop kidney damage, often leading to the need for dialysis or a transplant. Smoking constricts blood vessels. In people with diabetes, this helps to push large protein molecules out of the vessels and into the kidneys. That can eventually lead to kidney failure.

❑ For more information on diabetes and its potential complications, contact the following organizations:

American Diabetes Association
1660 Duke Street
Alexandria, VA 22314
703–549–1500
Also ask about state and local chapters.

American Heart Association
7272 Greenville Avenue
Dallas, TX 75231
800–AHA–USA1
214–373–6300
Also ask about state and local chapters.

International Diabetes Center
3800 Park Nicollet Boulevard
Minneapolis, MN 55416
612–927–3393

Joslin Diabetes Center
One Joslin Place
Boston, MA 02215
617–732–2415

Juvenile Diabetes Foundation (JDF)
120 Wall Street, 19th Floor
New York, NY 10005
800–533–2873 212–785–9500

National Diabetes Information Clearinghouse (NDIC)
1 Information Way
Bethesda, MD 20892–3560
301–654–3327

National Eye Institute (NEI)
National Institutes of Health
Building 31, Room 6A32
31 Center Drive, MSC 2510
Bethesda, MD 20892–2510
301–496–5248

National Institute of Diabetes and Digestive
   and Kidney Diseases (NIDDK)
National Institutes of Health
Building 31, Room 9A04
31 Center Drive, MSC 2560
Bethesda, MD 20892–2560
301–496–3583

Diabetic Retinopathy

See under EYE PROBLEMS.

Diarrhea

Diarrhea is characterized by frequent and loose, watery stools. Symptoms that may accompany diarrhea include vomiting, cramping, thirst, and abdominal pain. Some people run a fever as well. Diarrhea can exist alone or as a symptom of other problems. Among the many possible causes of diarrhea are incomplete digestion of food; food poisoning; stress; bacterial, viral, or other infection; consumption of contaminated water; pancreatic disease; cancer; the use of certain drugs; caffeine; intestinal parasites; inflammatory bowel disease such as ulcerative colitis or Crohn's disease; and the consumption of certain foods or chemicals, such as beans, caffeine, unripe fruits, spoiled or rancid foods, and foods the body cannot tolerate. Food

allergies are often the cause of diarrhea. Emotional stress also can cause diarrhea. Acute diarrhea accompanied by fever and mucus or blood in the stool can be a sign of infection or the presence of parasites.

NUTRIENTS

SUPPLEMENT	SUGGESTED DOSAGE	COMMENTS
Very Important		
Charcoal tablets	4 tablets every hour with water until the diarrhea subsides. Take separately from other supplements and medications.	Absorbs toxins from the colon and bloodstream.
Essential fatty acids	As directed on label.	Aids in forming stools.
Kelp	1,000 mg daily.	To replace minerals lost through diarrhea.
Potassium	99 mg daily.	To replace potassium lost in watery stools.
Aerobic Bulk Cleanse (ABC) from Aerobic Life Industries or	As directed on label.	To provide bulk that aids in forming stools.
psyllium seeds	4 capsules daily, at bedtime.	
Important		
Acidophilus	1 tsp in distilled water, twice daily, on an empty stomach.	Replaces lost "friendly" bacteria. Use a nondairy powder form.
Garlic (Kyolic)	2 capsules 3 times daily.	Kills bacteria and parasites. Enhances immunity.
Helpful		
Calcium and	1,500 mg daily.	To replace calcium depleted from the body. Also aids in forming stools.
magnesium and	1,000 mg daily.	Needed for calcium uptake. Promotes pH balance.
vitamin D	400 IU daily.	Needed for calcium uptake.
Multienzyme complex with pancreatin	As directed on label. Take with meals.	Needed for normal digestion.
Vitamin B complex plus extra	100 mg 3 times daily.	All B vitamins are necessary for digestion and absorption of nutrients. Sublingual forms are recommended for better absorption. Injections under a doctor's supervision) may be necessary.
vitamin B$_1$ (thiamine) and	200 mg daily for 2 weeks.	
vitamin B$_3$ (niacin) and	50 mg daily.	
folic acid	50 mg daily.	
Vitamin C	500 mg 3 times daily.	Needed for healing and immunity. Use a buffered form.
Vitamin E	400–1,000 IU daily.	Protects the cell membranes that line the colon wall.
Zinc	50 mg daily. Do not exceed a total of 100 mg daily from all supplements.	Aids in repair of damaged tissue of the digestive tract and enhances immune response. Use zinc gluconate lozenges or OptiZinc for best absorption.

HERBS

❑ If you suffer from occasional bouts of diarrhea, use blackberry root bark, chamomile, pau d'arco, and/or raspberry leaves. Herbs can be taken in tea form or added to applesauce, bananas, pineapple, or papaya juice.

Caution: Do not use chamomile on an ongoing basis, and avoid it completely if you are allergic to ragweed.

❑ Cayenne (capsicum) capsules, taken two to three times daily, may be beneficial.

❑ Ginger tea is good for cramps and abdominal pain.

❑ Slippery elm bark, taken in tea or extract form, is soothing to the digestive tract.

RECOMMENDATIONS

❑ Drink plenty of liquids, such as hot carob drink, carrot juice, and "green drinks," as well as plenty of quality water. The prolonged loss of fluids as a result of diarrhea can lead to dehydration and loss of necessary minerals, such as sodium, potassium, and magnesium.

❑ Eat oat bran, rice bran, raw foods, yogurt, and soured products daily. A high-fiber diet is important. When increasing fiber consumption, also increase your intake of liquids, especially steam-distilled water with a trace mineral concentrate added.

❑ Drink 3 cups of rice water daily. To make rice water, boil ½ cup of brown rice in 3 cups of water for forty-five minutes. Strain out the rice and drink the water. Eat the rice as well. Rice helps to form stools and supplies needed B vitamins.

❑ Do not consume any dairy products (except for low-fat soured products). They are highly allergenic. Moreover, diarrhea causes a temporary loss of the enzyme needed to digest lactose (milk sugar). Limit your intake of fats and foods containing gluten, including barley, oats, rye, and wheat. Avoid alcohol, caffeine, and spicy foods.

❑ Let a mild case of diarrhea run its course. It is the body's way of cleaning out toxins, bacteria, and other foreign invaders. Do not take any medication to stop diarrhea for at least two days. Stick to a liquid diet for twenty-four hours to give the bowel a rest.

❑ Consult your health care provider if any of the following conditions occur: the diarrhea lasts for more than two days, there is blood in the stool, the stool looks like black tar, you have a fever above 101°F, you have severe abdominal or rectal pain, you suffer from dehydration as evidenced by dry mouth or wrinkled skin, or urination is reduced or stops.

CONSIDERATIONS

❑ Carob powder is high in protein and helps halt diarrhea.

❑ Kombucha tea, which has detoxifying and immune-boosting properties, may be beneficial for diarrhea and other digestive disorders. (*See* MAKING KOMBUCHA TEA in Part Three.)

❑ Chronic diarrhea in very young children is evident if the child has five or more watery stools a day. A baby with diarrhea can become dehydrated very quickly, and should be evaluated by a health care provider.

❑ If diarrhea is chronic or recurrent, an underlying problem such as a food allergy, infection, or intestinal parasites may be the cause. Allergy testing can determine if you have any food allergies. A stool culture can be done to check for infection or the presence of parasites.

Diverticulitis

Diverticulitis is a condition in which the mucous membranes lining the colon become inflamed, resulting in the formation of small, pouchlike areas called diverticula in the large intestine. Once diverticula develop, they do not go away. The diverticula themselves cause no symptoms, but if waste matter becomes trapped in them, they can become infected or inflamed, causing fever, chills, and pain.

Diverticula typically form when an individual is constipated. Eating a low-fiber diet, as is typical in industrialized countries such as the United States, may contribute to the development of diverticulitis. Without fiber to soften and add bulk, stools are harder to pass. Greatly increased pressure is required to force small portions of hard, dry stool through the bowel. This rise in pressure can cause pouches to form at weak points in the wall of the colon.

Diverticulitis may be acute or chronic. Symptoms include cramping, bloating, tenderness on the left side of the abdomen that is relieved by passing gas or a bowel movement, constipation or diarrhea, nausea, and an almost continual need to eliminate. There may be blood in the stool. Diverticulitis usually strikes people between the ages of fifty and ninety. It affects millions of Americans, but many people do not even know they have the condition because they either experience no symptoms or accept their symptoms as simple indigestion.

Exactly why is not known, but it is known that smoking and stress make symptoms worse. In fact, this is a classic example of a stress-related disorder. Poor eating habits compound the problem. A poor diet, a family history of the disease, gallbladder disease, obesity, and coronary artery disease all increase the chances of developing diverticulitis.

There are several diagnostic tests available to help diagnose diverticulitis. A barium enema is a procedure in which the colon is filled with liquid barium and x-rays are taken to reveal pouches in the colon wall, narrowing of the colon, or other abnormalities. With sigmoidoscopy, a thin, flexible lighted tube is inserted into the rectum to give the physician a closer look at the lower colon. If necessary, tissue samples can be removed for examination. To see into other parts of the colon, a colonoscopy must be performed. This is similar to a sigmoidoscopy, but allows a view of the entire colon.

NUTRIENTS

SUPPLEMENT	SUGGESTED DOSAGE	COMMENTS
Essential		
Bio-Bifidus from American Biologics and	As directed on label.	To replace flora in the small intestine, primarily to improve assimilation.
Kyo-Dophilus from Wakunaga	As directed on label. Take on an empty stomach.	For bowel flora replacement to improve elimination and assimilation.
Fiber (oat bran, psyllium, ground flaxseeds, and Aerobic Bulk Cleanse (ABC) from Aerobic Life Industries are good sources)	As directed on label. Take 1 hour before meals with a large glass of liquid. Take separately from other supplements and medications.	Helps prevent constipation. Prevents infection by preventing accumulation of wastes in pouches in the colon walls.
Vitamin B complex	100 mg 3 times daily.	Needed for all enzyme systems in the body and for proper digestion. Use a hypoallergenic formula.
Very Important		
Multienzyme complex with pancreatin	As directed on label. Take with meals.	Needed to break down proteins. Use a formula high in pancreatin.
Proteolytic enzymes	As directed on label. Take between meals.	Aids in digestion and reduces inflammation of the colon.
Important		
Bio Rizin from American Biologics		*See under* Herbs, below.
Dioxychlor from American Biologics	As directed on label.	An important antibacterial, antifungal, and antiviral agent.
Essential fatty acids (flaxseed oil, primrose oil, salmon oil, and Ultimate Oil from Nature's Secret are good sources)	As directed on label 3 times daily, before meals.	Improves lymphatic function and aids in protecting the cells lining the wall of the colon.
Garlic (Kyolic)	2 capsules 3 times daily, with meals.	Aids in digestion and destroys unwanted bacteria and parasites. Use a yeast-free formula.
L-Glutamine	500 mg twice daily, on an empty stomach. Take with water or juice. Do not take with milk. Take with 50 mg vitamin B_6 and 100 mg vitamin C for better absorption.	A major metabolic fuel for the intestinal cells; maintains the villi, the absorption surfaces of the gut. *See* AMINO ACIDS in Part One.
Vitamin K or alfalfa	100 mcg daily.	Deficiency has been linked to intestinal disorders. *See under* Herbs, below.
Helpful		
Aloe vera		*See under* Herbs, below.
Free-form amino acid complex	As directed on label, on an empty stomach, ½ hour before meals.	To supply protein, needed for healing and repair of tissue.
Raw thymus glandular	As directed on label.	*See* GLANDULAR THERAPY in Part Three for its benefits. *Caution:* Do not give this supplement to a child.
Vitamin A	25,000 IU daily. If you are pregnant, do not exceed 10,000 IU daily.	Protects and heals the lining of the colon.
Vitamin C	3,000–8,000 mg daily, in divided doses.	Reduces inflammation and boosts immune response. Use a buffered form.
Vitamin E	Up to 800 IU daily.	A powerful antioxidant that protects the mucous membranes.

HERBS

❑ Alfalfa is a good natural source of vitamin K and valuable minerals, which are often deficient in people with intestinal disorders. It also contains chlorophyll, which aids healing. Take 2,000 milligrams daily in capsule or extract form.

❑ Aloe vera promotes the healing of inflamed areas. It also helps to prevent constipation. Drink ½ cup of aloe vera juice three times daily. George's Aloe Vera Juice from Warren Laboratories is good. It can be mixed with a cup of herbal tea if you wish.

❑ Bio Rizin from American Biologics is a licorice extract that improves glandular function and helps relieve allergy symptoms. Take 10 to 20 drops twice daily.

❑ Pau d'arco has an antibacterial, cleansing, and healing effect. Drink two cups of pau d'arco tea daily.

❑ Other herbs beneficial for diverticulitis include cayenne (capsicum), chamomile, goldenseal, papaya, red clover, and yarrow extract or tea.

Caution: Do not use chamomile on an ongoing basis, as ragweed allergy may result. Avoid it completely if you are allergic to ragweed. Do not take goldenseal for more than one week at a time, and do not use it during pregnancy. If you have a history of cardiovascular disease, diabetes, or glaucoma, use it only under a doctor's supervision.

RECOMMENDATIONS

❑ The key to controlling this disorder is to consume an adequate amount of fiber and lots of quality water. You need at least 30 grams of fiber each day. You may prefer to supplement your diet with a bulk product and/or a stool softener that contains methylcellulose or psyllium, since these do not promote as much gas formation in the colon as other sources of fiber, especially wheat bran. Drink at least eight 8-ounce glasses of water daily. Herbal teas, broth, and live juices can account for some of the liquid needed. Liquid aids in keeping the pouchlike areas clean of toxic wastes, preventing inflammation.

❑ Eat a low-carbohydrate diet with high levels of protein from vegetable sources and fish. Do not eat grains, seeds, or nuts, except for well-cooked brown rice. These foods are hard to digest and tend to get caught in the crevices of the colon wall, resulting in bloating and gas. Also eliminate from the diet dairy products, red meat, sugar products, fried foods, spices, and processed foods.

❑ Eat plenty of green leafy vegetables. These are good sources of vitamin K. Obtaining this vitamin through diet is especially important for people with intestinal disorders.

❑ Eat garlic for its healing and detoxifying properties.

❑ During an acute attack of diverticulitis, your health care provider may recommend a low-fiber diet temporarily. Once the inflammation clears you may slowly switch back to a high-fiber diet.

❑ When an attack or pain begins, give yourself a cleansing enema using 2 quarts of lukewarm water and the juice of a fresh lemon. *See* ENEMAS in Part Three. This helps to rid the colon of undigested and entrapped foods and to relieve pain.

❑ On the day of an acute attack, take 4 charcoal tablets or capsules with a large glass of water to absorb trapped gas. Charcoal tablets are available at health food stores. Always take charcoal separately from medications and other supplements, and do not take it for prolonged periods, as it absorbs beneficial nutrients as well as gas.

❑ During severe attacks, use liquid vitamin supplements for better assimilation and put all vegetables and fruits through a blender. Eat steamed vegetables only. Baby foods are good until healing is complete. Earth's Best produces organically grown baby foods that are available in health food stores and some supermarkets. Add supplemental fiber to the baby food. As healing progresses, gradually add raw fruits and vegetables to the diet. Drink carrot juice, cabbage juice, and "green drinks." Or take chlorophyll liquid or liquid alfalfa in juice.

❑ To relieve pain, massage the left side of the abdomen. Stand up and do stretching exercises.

❑ Clay tablets are beneficial. Take them as directed on the product label on an empty stomach upon arising.

❑ Check stools daily for blood. If the stool is black, take a portion of it to your physician for an analysis.

❑ Try to have a bowel movement at the same time each day. Take fiber and acidophilus first thing in the morning before breakfast to help the bowels move at this time.

Note: Always take supplemental fiber separately from other supplements and medications.

CONSIDERATIONS

❑ Food allergies are often a cause of intestinal disorders. Allergy testing is advised.

❑ If the diverticula are infected, your doctor may prescribe antibiotics. Be sure to consume plenty of soured products and some form of nondairy acidophilus if you are taking antibiotics.

❑ Do not overuse laxatives; they can irritate the colon wall.

❑ Fasting is beneficial. (*See* FASTING in Part Three.)

❑ *See also* CROHN'S DISEASE, IRRITABLE BOWEL SYNDROME, and ULCERATIVE COLITIS, all in Part Two.

Dizziness

See MÉNIÈRE'S DISEASE; VERTIGO. *See also under* PREGNANCY-RELATED PROBLEMS.

Dog Bite

A dog bite that breaks the skin poses the danger of infection, especially if the bite is deep. Any bite also carries the risk of rabies. Most household pets have been immunized against rabies, but the possibility of infection still exists. It is also possible to contract a tetanus infection from a dog bite.

NUTRIENTS

SUPPLEMENT	SUGGESTED DOSAGE	COMMENTS
Very Important		
Vitamin C	4,000–10,000 mg daily for 1 week, then reduce to 3,000 mg daily.	Fights infection. Important for repair of collagen and connective tissue.
Important		
Proteolytic enzymes or Infla-Zyme Forte from American Biologics	As directed on label. Take between meals.	Acts as an anti-inflammatory.
Helpful		
Garlic (Kyolic)	2 capsules 3 times daily.	Acts as a natural antibiotic.
L-Cysteine and L-methionine	500 mg each daily for 2 weeks. Take with water or juice on an empty stomach. Do not take with milk. Take with 50 mg vitamin B_6 and 100 mg vitamin C for better absorption.	Powerful detoxifying agents. *See* AMINO ACIDS in Part One.
Vira-Plex 135 from Enzymatic Therapy	As directed on label.	Aids in healing and fights infection.
Vitamin A or natural beta-carotene	25,000 IU daily. If you are pregnant, do not exceed 10,000 IU daily. 25,000 IU daily.	Powerful antioxidants that aid the immune system and assist healing of the skin.
plus vitamin E	400 IU daily.	
Vitamin B complex	50 mg 3 times daily.	Aids in tissue oxidation and antibody production.

HERBS

❑ Echinacea, goldenseal, pau d'arco, and red clover, taken in tea form, are good for dog bites. Goldenseal extract can also be applied directly on the affected area. This is a natural antibiotic that helps to fight infection.

Caution: Do not take goldenseal internally on a daily basis for more than one week at a time, and do not use it during pregnancy. If you have a history of cardiovascular disease, diabetes, or glaucoma, use it only under supervision.

RECOMMENDATIONS

❑ If you are bitten by a dog, the first thing you should do is remove the animal's saliva from the wound. Wash the area thoroughly with warm water, then add soap and wash for at least five minutes more. Rinse the wound for a few more minutes with plain water and cover it with a gauze dressing for twenty-four hours.

❑ See your health care provider to make sure that you do not need stitches or other professional treatment.

❑ If you know who the dog's owner is, inquire as to the animal's vaccination status. If the dog is unfamiliar, try to have someone confine it if possible so that its health can be checked and it can be placed under observation.

CONSIDERATIONS

❑ Your physician may prescribe an oral antibiotic to prevent infection. If so, make sure that you take acidophilus to replace the "friendly" bacteria that antibiotics destroy. Your doctor will also likely recommend that you have a tetanus booster shot if you haven't had one in six years or more.

❑ In most states, dog bite incidents must be reported to the local health department, and the dog must then be kept under observation for any signs of rabies—viciousness, paralysis, growling, foaming at the mouth, or agitation. If the animal cannot be located and rabies ruled out, a series of rabies injections will be necessary.

Down Syndrome

Down syndrome, also known as *trisomy 21*, is a congenital disorder—that is, it occurs during fetal development, but is not inherited. It is named for British physician John Langdon Haydon Down, who first described the condition in 1866. In 1959, Dr. Jerome LeJeune of France, discovered that Down syndrome was caused by a chromosomal anomaly, specifically the transmission of an extra 21st chromosome. The overall incidence of Down syndrome is about 1 in 700 live births. Almost half of the children with Down syndrome are born to mothers over the age of thirty-five.

Down syndrome is characterized by slow physical development, moderate to severe mental retardation, and skull and facial features that are somewhat flattened. Other physical characteristics include slanted eyes, a depressed nose bridge, low-set ears, and a large, furrowed tongue. The hands are broad and short, with a single crease, known as the simian crease, across the palm. Other common physical abnormalities include congenital heart disease, vision

problems, and susceptibility to acute leukemia. While females with Down syndrome may menstruate and be fertile, males are infertile.

Although the degree of mental retardation varies greatly among different individuals with Down syndrome, the average IQ falls within the range of 50 to 60. Generally, children with Down syndrome are able to learn everyday life skills and can be raised at home. Special education and training allow many individuals with Down syndrome to lead happy, useful, and love-filled lives. People with Down syndrome can live to middle or old age; however, as adults, they may be prone to developing pneumonia and other lung diseases.

The following nutrients are suggested for individuals with Down syndrome who are twelve years of age or older. Persons with malabsorption problems should consult a health care provider before starting any nutritional program.

NUTRIENTS

SUPPLEMENT	SUGGESTED DOSAGE	COMMENTS
Aangamik DMG from FoodScience Labs	50 mg 4 times daily.	Promotes the utilization of oxygen.
Coenzyme Q10	10 mg daily.	Prevents heart damage by improving oxygenation of cells.
Essential fatty acids	As directed on label.	Needed for proper brain and cardiovascular function.
Free-form amino acid complex	As directed on label.	To provide needed protein and bolster the immune system.
Garlic (Kyolic)	As directed on label.	Natural antibiotic that helps the body to eliminate toxins and strengthens the cardiovascular system.
Kelp	As directed on label.	To supply minerals helpful in establishing thyroid balance.
Lecithin granules or capsules	1 tsp 3 times daily. 2,400 mg 3 times daily.	Aids brain function.
Taurine Plus from American Biologics	500 mg daily, on an empty stomach. Take with water or juice. Do not take with milk. Take with 50 mg vitamin B6 and 100 mg vitamin C for better absorption.	Reduces stress and regulates nervous system.
Multivitamin and mineral complex with vitamin A and natural carotenoids and selenium	As directed on label. 10,000 IU daily. 15,000 IU daily. 200 mcg daily.	All nutrients are needed for proper immune function.
Potassium	200 mg daily.	Helps transmit nerve impulses.
Vitamin B complex with choline	As directed on label. 100 mg daily.	Prevents and/or treats memory loss and increases learning capacity. Also protects against cardiovascular disease.
Vitamin C	3,000 mg daily.	Enhances immune function and reduces cholesterol levels.

Alternative Approaches for Down Syndrome

There are a number of revolutionary treatments to maximize the learning potential and physical capabilities of those with Down syndrome that have shown significant success and have been gaining increasing scientific attention in recent years.

NUTRITIONAL APPROACH

The use of nutritional supplementation to help boost the metabolism of those with Down syndrome began with North American physician Dr. Henry Turkel in the 1950s. To address the unique biochemistry of those with Down syndrome, he began treating affected children with a combination of vitamins, minerals, and hormones. Although his program achieved some success, his work was generally rejected or ignored by mainstream scientists.

However, a growing population of parents of children with Down syndrome continued to use Dr. Turkel's nutritional program. Eventually, Kent MacLeod, a pharmaceutical biochemist and owner of Nutri-Chem Labs in Ottawa, Canada, learned of Dr. Turkel's formula after a number of parents asked him to evaluate the protocol. MacLeod and the biochemical team at Nutri-Chem joined with Dr. Turkel and other researchers in further developing and refining the original supplement. A nutritional formula known as MSBPlus was the eventual result.

MSBPlus is a formula of vitamins, minerals, amino acids, antioxidants, and enzymes that targets essential nutrients missing from the biochemical makeup of the person with Down syndrome. This supplement, which can be custom-formulated to meet individual age and metabolic needs, has met with marked success. Research is ongoing. The University of Miami School of Medicine is now collaborating with Nutri-Chem on clinical trials and studies on Down syndrome. One long-term, double-blind study will examine the cognitive development and language skills of children with Down syndrome who are taking MSBPlus.

Nutri-Chem is also working with Dr. Marie Peeters, a pediatrician and former member of the Institute de Progenese in Paris. Dr. Peeters was an associate of Dr. Jerome LeJeune, the scientist who discovered the cause of Down syndrome. In an effort to further study the effects of nutritional supplements (particularly amino acids) on those with this disorder, Dr. Peeters is involved in clinical trials.

For additional information on MSBPlus formula, or to receive information on the connection between nutrition and Down syndrome, you can write to Nutri-Chem Labs, 1303 Richmond Road, Ottawa, Ontario K2B 7Y4, Canada; or call them at 613–820–9065 or 613–829–2226.

The work of Dr. Turkel also influenced Jack Warner, M.D., F.A.A.P., founder of Warner House, Inc., a not-for-profit center for the clinical study and treatment of Down syndrome. Together with medical colleagues, biochemists, and other medical professionals, Dr. Warner developed a metabolic treatment called HAP CAPS for children with Down syndrome. This formula is a supplemental yet integral part of a multidisciplinary treatment approach that includes examination and evaluation by a physical therapist, a developmental optometrist, a clinical psychologist, a speech advisor, and a nutritionist, under the recommendation of a primary care pediatrician, plus a system of periodic reports, tests, and doctors' observations. In addition to seeing patients regularly at the clinic in Fullerton, California, the Warner House staff also travels across the United States to meet with patients in many cities.

Dr. Warner reports that data from over twelve years of research and treatment show the Warner House treatment protocol has resulted in changes in the physical features of children with Down syndrome, a reduction in the frequency of infections that typically affect these children, and an improvement in their cognitive ability.

More information about Warner House can be obtained by writing to The Warner House, 1023 East Chapman Avenue, Fullerton, CA 92631; or by calling 714–441–2600.

DEVELOPMENTAL STIMULATION APPROACH

The Institutes for the Achievement of Human Potential in Philadelphia, Pennsylvania, offers parents of children with Down syndrome a specialized program for helping their children develop and maximize their potential. In this program, parents are the key players in a home therapeutic approach that involves providing simple yet intensive neurological stimulation for their children. A carefully designed nutritional regimen is also an integral part of the program.

Before beginning the program, parents attend a five-day course of lectures and demonstrations at The Institutes. They learn about the Developmental Profile, a measuring instrument that clearly shows visual, auditory, tactile, mobility, language, and manual abilities a child should attain by certain ages, and they learn specific techniques to use in working on different skill areas with their children. Once home, the parents carry out an individualized brain-development program tailored to the needs of their child. Carried out properly, these techniques have produced most encouraging results, often leading children with Down syndrome to perform even above levels exhibited by most average children.

More information on this program can be obtained by writing to The Registrar, The Institutes for the Achievement of Human Potential, 8801 Stenton Avenue, Philadelphia, PA 19118; or by calling 800–736–4663.

Vitamin E	400 IU daily.	Boosts immune system and facilitates body's absorption of lecithin.
Zinc	50 mg daily.	Needed for proper brain function and a healthy immune system.

RECOMMENDATIONS

❑ Be patient when feeding a child with Down syndrome, and be sure to provide a balanced diet. Include fresh and whole foods that are rich in vegetable proteins, as well as foods that are high in magnesium, such as fresh green vegetables, figs, meat, fish and seafood, nuts and seeds, tofu, blackstrap molasses, apples, kelp, soybeans, cornmeal, rice, apricots, and brewer's yeast. Reduce consumption of foods high in gluten, such as wheat, rye, barley, and oats. Avoid refined foods, sugars, dairy products, and alcohol.

❑ Hold and nurture your child as much as possible.

❑ Provide plenty of exercise, including deep-breathing exercises, daily. This helps to oxygenate the brain.

❑ Provide environmental stimulation. Play music in your home, for example (studies suggest that classical music is best). Provide objects and toys that are safe to handle and that invite exploration. Talk to and interact with your child, and involve him or her as much as possible in whatever you happen to be doing (if you have other children, encourage them to do the same).

❑ Set realistic goals for your child, and remember the emotional needs of your other children.

❑ Use liquid or spray forms of supplements for a child with Down syndrome.

CONSIDERATIONS

❑ Care for the child with Down syndrome depends on the degree of mental and physical impairment. Carefully planned programs to promote development of motor and mental skills are important. Since learning potential is greatest during infancy, an *early* stimulation program of exercises based on the child's ability is necessary for teaching gross motor skills.

❑ The risk of giving birth to a Down syndrome child increases markedly after the age of thirty-four. Amniocentesis may be recommended if you become pregnant past this age. (For additional information on amniocentesis and other types of prenatal testing, *see under* PREGNANCY-RELATED PROBLEMS in Part Two.)

❑ Additional information on Down syndrome, parent support groups, and early intervention programs for children with Down syndrome is available from The National Down Syndrome Society, 666 Broadway, New York, NY 10012; telephone 800–221–4602 or 212–460–9330.

Drug Addiction (Substance Abuse)

In our drug-oriented society, it seems as if there is a pill available to soothe any possible discomfort. If you have a headache, you can reach into your medicine cabinet for some aspirin or acetaminophen to relieve the pain. If you are anxious or have trouble sleeping, you can take a couple of tranquilizers. If you are upset by work or marital problems, you can drown your sorrows in a stiff drink. It is not surprising, therefore, that many people have problems with drug addiction.

Addiction is said to exist when the body becomes so accustomed to the presence of a foreign substance that it can no longer function properly if the substance is withdrawn. This is why a person who is addicted to a drug experiences withdrawal symptoms if suddenly deprived of it. Drug withdrawal symptoms include headache, insomnia, sensitivity to light and noise, diarrhea, hot and cold flashes, sweating, deep depression, irritability, irrational thinking, and disorientation. Not surprisingly, individuals who are addicted to drugs can end up centering their lives on avoiding the excruciating pain of withdrawal—that is, on assuring a continuing supply of the drug. This need to obtain the drug at all costs leads ultimately to a disintegration of normal life, including broken personal relationships, loss of employment, and even criminal behavior.

Complicating the phenomenon of addiction is the problem of drug tolerance. With prolonged drug use, the body often ends up needing more and more of the substance to produce the desired effect and to prevent withdrawal symptoms. Some users end up increasing the dosage to the point that they die, or come close to dying, from overdose. In addition, addiction almost always has a powerful psychological as well as a physical component. In fact, with some types of drugs, addiction is entirely, or almost entirely, a matter of psychological dependence. While psychological dependence does not lead to physical withdrawal symptoms after the drug is discontinued, it does result in deep cravings that may persist long after any physical addiction has been overcome.

Drug use typically begins in adolescence. Although perceptions of alcohol and cigarette use have changed dramatically in recent years, these are still two of the most accessible drugs. Most young people who use drugs start with these, then move on to less accessible (that is, illegal) drugs such as marijuana. Many young drug users mistakenly believe that common drugs such as alcohol and marijuana are harmless. They also believe that they will never become dependent on drugs and that they can quit at any time. Unfortunately, instead of quitting, many end up turning to stronger drugs, including amphetamines, heroin, and cocaine. While the types of drugs most subject to abuse seem to vary from place to place and time to time, most experts agree that the potent form of cocaine popularly known as crack is a particular problem. It is less expensive than powdered cocaine, is easy to conceal, and offers a quick high.

It is also *extremely* addictive, and is associated with violent and criminal behavior. Newspaper reports have cited cases in which the use of this drug has filtered down even to the elementary school level.

Substances That Rob the Body of Nutrients

Different substances deplete the body of different nutrients. Use the list below to determine which supplements you may need as a result of the use of prescription or over-the-counter drugs, including alcohol and caffeine.

Substance	Depleted Nutrients	Substance	Depleted Nutrients
Allopurinol (Zyloprim)	Iron.	Hydralazine (Apresazide, Apresoline, and others)	Vitamin B_6 (pyridoxine).
Antacids	B-complex vitamins; calcium; phosphate; vitamins A and D.	Indomethacin (Indocin)	Iron.
Antibiotics, general (*see also* isoniazid, penicillin, sulfa drugs, and trimethoprim)	B-complex vitamins; vitamin K; "friendly" bacteria.	Isoniazid (INH and others)	Vitamins B_3 (niacin) and B_6 (pyridoxine).
Antihistamines	Vitamin C.	Laxatives (excluding herbs)	Potassium; vitamins A and K.
Aspirin	B-complex vitamins; calcium; folic acid; iron; potassium; vitamins A and C.	Lidocaine (Xylocaine)	Calcium; potassium.
		Nitrate/nitrite coronary vasodilators	Niacin; pangamic acid, selenium; vitamins C and E.
Barbiturates	Vitamin C.	Oral contraceptives	B-complex vitamins; vitamins C, D, and E.
Beta-blockers (Corgard, Inderal, Lopressor, and others)	Choline; chromium; pantothenic acid (vitamin B_5).	Penicillin preparations	Vitamin B_3 (niacin); niacinamide; vitamin B_6 (pyridoxine).
Caffeine	Biotin; inositol; potassium; vitamin B_1 (thiamine); zinc.	Phenobarbital preparations	Folic acid; vitamin B_6 (pyridoxine); vitamin B_{12}; vitamins D and K.
Carbamazepine (Atretol, Tegretol)	Dilutes blood sodium.	Phenylbutazone	Folic acid; iodine.
Chlorothiazide (Aldoclor, Diuril, and others)	Magnesium; potassium.	Phenytoin (Dilantin)	Calcium; folic acid; vitamins B_{12}, C, D, and K.
Cimetidine (Tagamet)	Iron.	Prednisone (Deltasone and others)	Potassium; vitamins B_6 (pyridoxine) and C; zinc.
Clonidine (Catapres, Combipres)	B-complex vitamins; calcium.	Quinidine preparations	Choline; pantothenic acid (vitamin B_5); potassium; vitamin K.
Corticosteroids, general (*see also* prednisone)	Calcium; potassium; vitamins A, B_6, C, and D; zinc.		
Digitalis preparations (Crystodigin, Digoxin, and others)	Vitamins B_1 (thiamine) and B_6 (pyridoxine); zinc.	Reserpine preparations	Phenylalanine; potassium; vitamins B_2 (riboflavin) and B_6 (pyridoxine).
Diuretics, general (see also chlorothiazide, spironolactone, thiazide diuretics, and triamterene)	Calcium; iodine; magnesium; potassium; vitamins B_2 (riboflavin) and C; zinc.	Spironolactone (Aldactone and others)	Calcium; folic acid.
		Sulfa drugs	Para-aminobenzoic acid (PABA); "friendly" bacteria.
Estrogen preparations	Folic acid; vitamin B_6 (pyridoxine).	Synthetic neurotransmitters	Magnesium; potassium; vitamins B_2 (riboflavin) and B_6 (pyridoxine).
Ethanol (alcohol)	B-complex vitamins; magnesium; vitamins C, D, E, and K.	Tobacco	Vitamins A, C, and E.
Fluoride	Vitamin C.	Thiazide diuretics	Magnesium; potassium; vitamin B_2 (riboflavin); zinc.
Glutethimide (Doriden)	Folic acid; vitamin B_6 (pyridoxine).	Triamterene (Dyrenium)	Calcium; folic acid.
Guanethidine (Esimil, Ismelin)	Magnesium; potassium; vitamins B_2 (riboflavin) and B_6 (pyridoxine).	Trimethoprim (Bactrim, Septra, and others)	Folic acid.

Signs of drug addiction can include a decreased desire to work and/or socialize, extreme drowsiness, inattentiveness, frequent mood swings, restlessness, personality changes, and a loss of appetite. Persons addicted to drugs want to be alone, and lose their tempers easily. They may experience crying spells and have slow, slurred speech. The pupils of the eyes may also change.

The nutrient program outlined below is designed to help those recovering from drug addiction. Unless otherwise specified, the dosages recommended here are for adults. For a child under the age of seventeen, use one-half to three-quarters of the recommended amount.

NUTRIENTS

SUPPLEMENT	SUGGESTED DOSAGE	COMMENTS
Very Important		
Vitamin B complex injections plus extra vitamin B$_{12}$	2 cc daily or as prescribed by physician. 1 cc daily or as prescribed by physician.	Needed when under stress to rebuild the liver. Injections (under a doctor's supervision) are most effective. If injections are not available, use a sublingual form.
Important		
Calcium and magnesium	1,500 mg at bedtime. 1,000 mg at bedtime.	Nourishes the central nervous system and helps control tremors by calming the body. Use chelate forms.
Free-form amino acid complex plus extra	As directed on label, on an empty stomach.	To supply needed protein in a readily assimilable form.
L-glutamine	500 mg 3 times daily, on an empty stomach.	Passes the blood-brain barrier to promote healthy mental functioning. Increases levels of gamma-aminobutyric acid (GABA), which has a calming effect.
and L-tyrosine	500 mg twice daily, on an empty stomach. Take these supplements with water or juice, not milk. Take with 50 mg vitamin B$_6$ and 100 mg vitamin C for better absorption.	Tyrosine and valerian root taken every 4 hours have given good results for cocaine withdrawal. *See* AMINO ACIDS in Part One. *Caution:* Do not take this supplement if you are taking an MAO inhibitor drug.
Gamma-aminobutyric acid (GABA)	As directed on label, on an empty stomach.	Acts as a relaxant and lessens cravings. *See* AMINO ACIDS in Part One.
Glutathione	As directed on label.	Aids in detoxifying drugs to reduce their harmful effects. Also reduces the desire for drugs or alcohol.
Lithium	As prescribed by physician.	A trace mineral that aids in relieving depression. Available by prescription only.
L-Phenylalanine	1,500 mg daily, taken upon arising.	Necessary as a brain fuel. Use for withdrawal symptoms. *Caution:* Do not take this supplement if you are pregnant or nursing, or suffer from panic attacks, diabetes, high blood pressure, or PKU.
Pantothenic acid (vitamin B$_5$)	500 mg 3 times daily.	Essential for the adrenal glands and for reducing stress.
Vitamin C	2,000 mg every 3 hours.	Detoxifies the system and lessens the craving for drugs. Use a buffered form such as sodium ascorbate. Intravenous administration (under a doctor's supervision) may be necessary.
Helpful		
Multivitamin and mineral complex	As directed on label.	All nutrients are needed in high amounts. Use a high-potency formula.
Niacinamide	500 mg 3 times daily.	Important for brain function. *Caution:* Do not substitute niacin for niacinamide. Niacin should not be taken in such high doses.

HERBS

❑ Siberian ginseng helps those experiencing cocaine withdrawal.

Caution: Do not use this herb if you have hypoglycemia, high blood pressure, or a heart disorder.

❑ Valerian root has a calming effect. Used with the amino acid tyrosine, it has been found to be helpful for those undergoing withdrawal from cocaine (*see under* Nutrients, above).

RECOMMENDATIONS

❑ Eat a well-balanced, nutrient-dense diet that emphasizes fresh, raw foods.

❑ Add high-protein drinks to the diet.

❑ Avoid heavily processed foods, all forms of sugar, and junk food. These foods are a quick source of energy, but are followed by a low feeling that may increase cravings for drugs.

❑ *See* FASTING in Part Three, and follow the instructions.

CONSIDERATIONS

❑ To minimize withdrawal symptoms, withdrawal from any drug should be done slowly. The dosage should be decreased gradually over a period of four weeks or longer. This task cannot be accomplished alone; most often hospitalization and/or professional help is required.

❑ Most people are aware that a drug overdose can kill, but many do not realize that these poisons kill in other ways as well. Angina, heart attack, coronary artery spasms, and life-threatening damage to the heart muscle may occur with the use of cocaine and heroin. All drugs weaken the immune system in one way or another. Chronic marijuana use can reduce the immune response by as much as 40 percent by damaging and destroying white blood cells. Without a strong immune system, the body is vulnerable to all kinds of infectious and degenerative diseases.

❑ Many drug users suffer from malnutrition. Because

drugs rob the body of necessary nutrients, those addicted to drugs need to take high doses of supplemental nutrients.

❑ Research has found that children of alcoholics are more inclined than others to use drugs, including cocaine. These individuals are 400 times more likely to use drugs than those who do not have a family history of alcohol addiction.

❑ An individual can be addicted to substances other than illegal drugs. Many are addicted to nicotine, caffeine, colas, alcohol, sugar, and even certain foods. Although these addictions may not pose as great a health risk, withdrawal may still be painful and difficult. Those who use these substances may also be more susceptible to illness and disease because these addictive substances deplete the body of needed nutrients. (*See* Substances that Rob the Body of Nutrients on page 240.)

❑ *See also* ALCOHOLISM and SMOKING DEPENDENCY in Part Two.

Dry Skin

A balance of oil and moisture is crucial for healthy, attractive skin. Oil is secreted by the sebaceous glands and lubricates the surface of the skin. Moisture is the water present inside the skin cells, and comes to the cells through the bloodstream. It is the water in the skin cells that keeps them plumped-up, healthy, and youthful-looking. Oil and moisture work together; there must be enough moisture in the skin cells, but there must also be enough oil to act as a shield, preventing excessive evaporation of moisture from the skin's top layers.

There are actually two types of dry skin: simple dry skin and complex dry skin. Simple dry skin results from a lack of natural oils. The reasons for this lack of oil vary. This condition most often affects women under the age of thirty-five. Complex dry skin lacks both oil and moisture, and is characterized by fine lines, brown spots, discolorations, enlarged pores, and sagging skin. It is usually associated with aging.

Dry skin tends to be dull-looking, even scaly and flaky, and readily develops wrinkles and fine lines. It usually feels "tight" and uncomfortable after washing unless some type of moisturizer or skin cream is applied. Chapping and cracking are signs of extremely dry, dehydrated skin.

Dry skin is most common on areas of the body that are exposed to the elements, such as the face and hands, but it can be a whole-body problem as well, especially in winter. It is probably primarily a genetic condition, but it may be caused (or aggravated) by a poor diet and by environmental factors such as exposure to sun, wind, cold, chemicals, or cosmetics, or excessive bathing with harsh soaps. Nutritional deficiencies, especially deficiencies of vitamin A and the B vitamins, can also contribute to dry skin. Fair-skinned people seem to be more likely than others to have dry skin, especially as they age; most people's skin tends to become thinner and drier as

they get older. Many people have skin that is dry in some areas and oily in others. In the classic case of "combination skin," the skin on the forehead, nose, and chin tends to be oily, while the skin on the rest of the face is dry.

NUTRIENTS

SUPPLEMENT	SUGGESTED DOSAGE	COMMENTS
Very Important		
Primrose oil	Up to 500 mg daily.	Contains linoleic acid, an essential fatty acid needed by the skin.
Vitamin A	25,000 IU daily for 3 months, then reduce to 15,000 IU daily. If you are pregnant, do not exceed 10,000 IU daily.	Strengthens and protects the skin tissue.
or ACES + Zinc from Carlson Labs	As directed on label.	Contains antioxidants that protect the skin by neutralizing free radicals.
Vitamin B complex plus extra vitamin B$_{12}$	As directed on label. 100 mg 3 times daily.	Anti-stress and anti-aging vitamins.
Important		
Kelp	1,000–1,500 mg daily.	Supplies balanced minerals. Needed for good skin tone.
Vitamin E	Start with 400 IU daily and increase slowly to 800 IU daily.	Protects against free radicals. Used topically, it can minimize wrinkling.
Zinc	50 mg daily. Do not exceed a total of 100 mg daily from all supplements.	Necessary for proper functioning of the oil-producing glands of the skin. Use zinc gluconate lozenges or OptiZinc for best absorption.
Helpful		
Ageless Beauty from Biotec Foods	As directed on label.	Protects the skin from free radical damage.
Aloe vera		*See under* Herbs, below.
Collagen	Apply topically as directed on label.	Good for very dry skin. A nourishing cream that can restore a healthy tone to damaged skin.
Elastin	Apply topically as directed on label.	Helps prevent and smooth wrinkles.
GH3 cream from Gero Vita International	Apply topically as directed on label.	Excellent for the prevention of wrinkles. Also good for any discoloration of the skin.
Glucosamine sulfate or N-Acetylglucosamine (N-A-G from Source Naturals)	As directed on label.	Important for healthy skin and connective tissue.
Herpanacine from Diamond-Herpanacine Associates	As directed on label.	Contains antioxidants, amino acids, and herbs that promote skin health.
L-Cysteine	500 mg daily, on an empty stomach. Take with water or juice. Do not take with milk. Take with 50 mg vitamin B$_6$ and 100 mg vitamin C for better absorption.	Contains sulfur, needed for healthy skin. *See* AMINO ACIDS in Part One.

Lecithin granules or capsules	1 tbsp 3 times daily, before meals. 1,200 mg 3 times daily, before meals.	Needed for better absorption of the essential fatty acids.
Pycnogenol or grape seed extract	As directed on label. As directed on label.	A free radical scavenger that also strengthens collagen.
Selenium	200 mcg daily.	Encourages tissue elasticity and is a powerful antioxidant. Protects against ultraviolet- induced damage.
Superoxide dismutase (SOD)	As directed on label.	A free radical destroyer. Also good for brown age spots.
Tretinoin (Retin-A)	As prescribed by physician.	Removes fine wrinkles; also excellent for age spots, precancerous lesions, and sun-damaged skin. Available by prescription only. Takes around 6 months to show results.
Vitamin C with bioflavonoids	3,000–5,000 mg daily, in divided doses.	Necessary for collagen production; strengthens the capillaries that feed the skin.

HERBS

❑ Used topically, aloe vera has excellent soothing, healing, and moisturizing properties. It also helps to slough off dead skin cells. Apply aloe vera gel topically on affected areas as directed on the product label.

❑ Calendula and comfrey have skin-softening properties. They can be used in a facial sauna or to make herbal or floral waters (see below). Comfrey also reduces redness and soothes irritated skin. Allantoin, an ingredient in many skin care products, is derived from comfrey.

Note: Comfrey is recommended for external use only.

❑ Spray an herbal or floral water mist on your skin throughout the day to replenish lost moisture. Almost all skin types, but particularly dry skin, benefit from lavender. You can purchase lavender water already made, or you can make your own by adding a few drops of essential oil to 4 ounces of distilled water, or by making an infusion of fresh lavender leaves and flowers.

❑ A weekly facial sauna using the herbs chamomile, lavender, and peppermint is good for dry skin. Using a glass or enameled pot, simmer a total of 2 to 4 tablespoons of dried or fresh herbs in 2 quarts of water. When the pot is steaming, place it on top of a trivet or thick potholder on a table, and sit with your face at a comfortable distance over the steam for fifteen minutes. You can use a towel to trap the steam if you wish. After fifteen minutes, splash your face with cold water and allow your skin to air dry or pat it dry with a towel. Then either apply a good natural moisturizer or facial oil, or apply a clay mask (*see under* Recommendations in this section). After the sauna, you can allow the herbal water to cool and save it for use as a toning lotion to be dabbed on your face with a cotton ball after cleansing.

RECOMMENDATIONS

❑ Eat a balanced diet that includes vegetables, fruits, grains, seeds, and nuts. Eat quality protein from vegetable sources. Increase your intake of raw foods.

❑ Eat foods high in sulfur, which helps to keep the skin smooth and youthful. Good sources include garlic, onions, eggs, and asparagus. Sulfur is also present in the amino acid L-cysteine, which can be purchased in pill form.

❑ Consume plenty of yellow and orange vegetables. These are high in beta-carotene, a precursor of vitamin A.

❑ Drink at least 2 quarts of quality water every day to keep the skin well hydrated.

❑ Avoid fried foods, animal fats, and heat-processed vegetable oils such as those sold in supermarkets. Use cold-pressed oils only. Beware of any oils that have been subjected to heat, whether in processing or cooking. Heating oils leads to the production of free radicals, which have a destructive effect on the skin. *Do* take supplemental essential fatty acids (*see under* Nutrients, above). This may be the best supplement available for dry skin, but be patient; it may take a month or more to see results.

❑ Do not drink soft drinks or eat sugar, chocolate, potato chips, or other junk foods.

❑ Avoid alcohol and caffeine. These substances have a diuretic effect, causing the body—including the skin cells—to lose fluids and essential minerals.

❑ Do not smoke, and avoid secondhand smoke. Smoking has a harmful effect on the skin for several reasons. First, nicotine constricts the blood vessels, including the tiny capillaries that serve the skin. This deprives the skin of the oxygen and nutrients it needs for good health. Second, smoking involves the frequent repetition of certain facial postures, which eventually become etched in the skin in the form of wrinkles. The characteristic "smoker's face" has wrinkles radiating in a circle outward from the mouth. Smoking also can make the skin dry and leathery.

❑ Do not use harsh soaps, cold cream, or cleansing creams on your skin. Cleansing creams are made from hydrogenated oils, which can cause free radical damage to the skin, resulting in dryness and wrinkles. Instead, use pure olive, avocado, or almond oil to cleanse the skin. Pat the oil on, then wash it off with warm water and a soft cloth.

❑ Twice weekly, use a loofah sponge for the face and warm water to boost circulation and remove dead skin cells. Avoid using the loofah around your eyes, however.

❑ Always moisturize your skin after cleansing, and at other times throughout the day, if necessary, to keep it from drying out. Use a liquid moisturizer or facial oil that contains nutrients and other natural ingredients. Do not use solid, waxy moisturizing creams. Wrinkle Treatment Oil and Vitamin A Moisturizing Gel from Derma-E Products are both good for dry age lines caused by the sun and the skin's natural aging. The Wrinkle Treatment Oil is also good for cleansing the skin. The moisturizing gel is non-oily and fast-absorbing.

❑ Look for skin care products that contain humectants. Humectants are substances that attract water to the skin to hold in moisture. Natural humectants include vegetable glycerine, vitamin E, and panthenol, a form of pantothenic acid (vitamin B5).

❑ Use a humidifier (or even a pan of water placed near a radiator) to humidify your environment, especially in winter. This helps to reduce the amount of moisture lost from the skin through evaporation.

❑ Once a week, use a facial mask to clarify the skin and remove dull, dry surface skin cells. (This can be done immediately after the facial sauna described under Herbs in this section.) Blend together well 1 teaspoon green clay powder (available in health food stores) and 1 teaspoon raw honey. Apply the mixture to your face, avoiding the eye area. Leave it on for fifteen minutes, then rinse well with lukewarm water. While your skin is still slightly damp, apply a natural skin oil or liquid moisturizer.

❑ If your skin is chapped or cracked, increase your consumption of water and essential fatty acids. Keep any chapped areas well lubricated and protected from the elements.

❑ For cracked, dry skin on the fingers, use calendula cream or oil with comfrey, vitamin E oil, and aloe vera. Apply the mixture to hands at bedtime, then wear plastic gloves overnight. Pure vitamin E oil can be found in health food stores.

❑ As much as possible, stay out of the sun. Sun is responsible for most of the damage done to the skin. It causes dryness, wrinkles, and even rashes and blisters. Always apply a good sunscreen to all exposed areas of skin if you must be in the sun.

❑ To care for combination skin, simply treat the dry areas as dry skin and the oily areas as oily skin. *See* OILY SKIN in Part Two.

CONSIDERATIONS

❑ Dry skin can be a sign of an underactive thyroid. (*See* HYPOTHYROIDISM in Part Two.)

❑ Certain drugs, including diuretics, antispasmodics, and antihistamines, can contribute to dry skin.

❑ Cocoa butter is a good skin cream and is not expensive. It also helps reduce skin wrinkling. Keep it in the refrigerator after opening.

❑ Balanced skin depends upon the production of natural moisturizing factors that help the skin attract and retain moisture. A group of acids known as alpha-hydroxy acids, applied topically, help to stimulate production of these naturally occurring substances. Alpha-hydroxy acids also encourage the formation of new skin cells. These acids occur naturally in apples, milk, sugar cane, citrus fruits, tomatoes, grapes, and blackberries. Of the alpha-hydroxy acids, lactic acid appears to be the best for improving moisturization, while glycolic acid is more effective at sloughing off dead skin cells and promoting cell renewal.

Dyspepsia

See INDIGESTION.

Dysthymia

See under DEPRESSION.

Ear Infection

It has been estimated that as many as 95 percent of all children have at least one ear infection by the age of six. There are several different types of ear infections. *External otitis*, or outer ear infection (also known as swimmer's ear), is an acute infection that is usually preceded by an upper respiratory infection or allergies. The ear canal, extending from the eardrum to the outside, becomes inflamed and swollen. Symptoms can include slight fever, discharge from the ear, and pain, often severe and throbbing, that worsens when the earlobe is touched or pulled. Impacted wax that traps water in the ear canal is often the culprit.

Middle ear infections (*otitis media*) are very common in infants and children. The site of this infection is behind the eardrum, where the small bones of the ear are located. Symptoms include earache; sharp, dull, or throbbing pain; a feeling of fullness and pressure in the ear; and a fever as high as 103°F or higher. Children often pull at their ears in an attempt to relieve the pressure. High altitudes and cold temperatures increase discomfort and can worsen an infection.

A severe middle ear infection can cause perforation of the eardrum. If this happens, it can actually cause a sudden *reduction* in pain. This is because the pain of an ear infection results when pressure builds up in restricted spaces; this pressure on sensitive nerve endings causes pain. A perforated eardrum results in hearing loss and a discharge of bloody fluid from the ear.

Frequent middle ear infections, or recurrent otitis media, affect 30 percent or more of children under the age of six. This is the most frequent diagnosis in clinical medical practice. A variety of different bacteria and viruses can cause middle ear infections. One of the leading causes of ear infection in children is a bacterium called *Branhamella catarrahalis* (B-cat). Another cause of frequent ear infections in children is food allergies.

Unless otherwise specified, the dosages recommended here are for adults. For a child between the ages of twelve and seventeen, reduce the dose to three-quarters the recommended amount. For a child between six and twelve, use one-half the recommended dose, and for a child under the age of six, use one-quarter the recommended amount.

NUTRIENTS

SUPPLEMENT	SUGGESTED DOSAGE	COMMENTS
Very Important		
AE Mulsion Forte from American Biologics or	As directed on label, to supply 50,000 IU vitamin A and 600 IU vitamin E daily.	For adults. Aids in controlling the infection.
natural beta-carotene or	20,000 IU daily.	
cod liver oil	1 tsp daily.	For children. A good source of vitamin A.
Manganese	10 mg daily. Take separately from calcium.	Deficiency has been linked to ear disorders.
Vitamin C with bioflavonoids	3,000–7,000 mg daily, in divided doses.	Boosts immunity and fights infection. Use an esterified or buffered form such as Ester-C or calcium or zinc ascorbate.
Zinc	10 mg in lozenge form 3 times daily for 5 days, then 50 mg daily in pill form. Do not exceed this amount.	Quickens immune response. Aids in reducing infection.
Important		
Dioxychlor from American Biologics	Add 3 drops to 10 drops distilled water to use as an earwash.	Important as an antibacterial, antifungal, and antiviral agent.
Vitamin B complex	50 mg 3 times daily.	Essential for healing and immune function. A sublingual form is recommended.
plus extra vitamin B6 (pyridoxine)	50 mg daily.	Important for immune function.
Primrose oil	1,000 mg daily for adults and children over 6; 500 mg daily for children under 6.	Reduces infection and inflammation.
Vitamin E	Start with 200 IU daily and increase weekly until you reach 800 IU daily.	Enhances immune function.
Helpful		
ThymuPlex #398 from Enzymatic Therapy	As directed on label.	Use if problem persists. Helps the immune system.

HERBS

❑ Take alcohol-free echinacea extract by mouth; this will generally end an ear infection if you catch it early.

❑ To alleviate pain, place a few drops of warm garlic oil or olive oil in the ear, then a drop or two of lobelia or mullein oil. You can plug the ear loosely with a cotton ball. You can also make a paste using onion powder or clay packs and apply it to the outside of the ear to relieve pain.

❑ Place ½ dropperful of alcohol-free goldenseal extract in your mouth and swish it around for a few minutes before swallowing. Do this every three hours for three days. Alternating echinacea with goldenseal works wonders. For an infant, put the extract in formula or expressed breast milk, or in fruit-flavored sugar-free yogurt.

Caution: Do not take goldenseal on a daily basis for more than one week at a time, and do not use it during pregnancy. If you have a history of cardiovascular disease, diabetes, or glaucoma, use it only under a doctor's supervision.

❑ Onion poultices are good for ear infections. *See* USING A POULTICE in Part Three.

RECOMMENDATIONS

❑ Avoid the most common allergenic foods: wheat, dairy products, corn, oranges, peanut butter, and all simple carbohydrates, including sugar, fruits, and fruit juices.

❑ To help reduce and prevent the development of food allergies, do not repeat foods frequently. A four-day rotation diet may be beneficial (*see* ALLERGIES in Part Two). With a young child, introduce new foods one at a time and watch carefully for any reaction.

❑ If a bottlefed baby has an ear infection, eliminate milk and dairy products from the child's diet for thirty days to see if any benefits result. Try feeding your baby soymilk, Rice Dream, or nut milk instead.

❑ Take garlic enemas if toxins accumulate to dangerous levels and cause the body to react. Signs of dangerous toxin levels include fever, chills, and general aches and pains. *See* ENEMAS in Part Three.

❑ For ringing in the ears, mix 1 teaspoonful of salt and 1 teaspoonful of glycerine (sold in drugstores) in 1 pint of warm water. Use a nasal spray bottle to spray each nostril with the solution until it begins to drain into the back of the throat. Spray the throat with the mixture as well. Do this several times a day.

❑ If you suffer from a chronic cough that lasts more than three weeks, see your health care provider. A chronic cough can be caused by impacted earwax that exerts pressure on a nerve in the ear canal, stimulating the coughing reflex. A physician can easily see if you have excessive earwax buildup and can remove it using careful suction or warm water with a slender blunt curette, plus a special microscope to aid in guiding the removal.

❑ Do not blow your nose if you have an ear infection. Keep the ear canal dry. Retained soap and water in the canal can be dangerous. Put cotton in the ear canal when showering or bathing. Do not go swimming until healing is complete.

❑ Avoid unsanitary conditions. An ear infection may result from lowered resistance due to a recent illness. Nonprescription ear drops may relieve the pain. A nasal spray may help open up the eustachian tube and relieve the pressure.

❑ If there are symptoms of dizziness, ringing in the ears, bleeding or a bloody discharge, sudden pain (or a sudden lessening of pain), and hearing loss in one or both ears, contact your health care provider immediately. These symptoms could indicte a ruptured eardrum.

CONSIDERATIONS

❑ Antibiotic therapy and/or surgical draining of the affected area may be necessary to heal an ear infection. However, some studies have shown that there is no significant overall difference in healing time or recurrence of ear infections between children treated with antibiotics and those not given antibiotics. In addition, many infants may also have reactions to the antibiotics used to treat ear infections, especially if they are used too frequently.

❑ In most cases, with proper treatment, a perforated eardrum heals naturally, with no permanent loss of hearing. An eardrum may rupture as a result of infection or due to sudden inward pressure to the ear from swimming, diving, a slap, a nearby explosion, or even a kiss over the ear.

❑ Breastfed babies are much less likely than bottlefed babies to suffer from ear infections.

❑ Ear problems are more common in the homes of smokers.

❑ *Branhamella catarrahalis* (B-cat), a common cause of ear infections, has developed strains that resist standard antibiotics. Fortunately, the antibiotic Augmentin (a combination of amoxicillin and clavulanate sodium) can still destroy the B-cat bacterium.

❑ Ear infection is not the only cause of ear pain. Rapid changes in air pressure, such as occur during air travel, often cause ear pain and can even result in damage to the eardrum. This is called *aerotitis* or *barotitis media*. If an infection is present, the effects of pressure changes are magnified.

❑ Children who have frequent ear infections should be tested for food allergies. The role of allergies as a major cause of chronic otitis media has been firmly established. (*See* ALLERGIES in Part Two.)

Eating Disorders

See ANOREXIA NERVOSA; APPETITE, POOR; BULIMIA; OBESITY; UNDERWEIGHT.

Eczema

See DERMATITIS.

Edema

Edema, formerly called dropsy, is the accumulation of fluid in body tissues. It most often occurs in the feet and ankles, but any part of the body may develop edema. The bloating and swelling of edema in turn can cause muscle aches and pains.

Fluid retention is often caused by allergies. Many women develop some degree of edema during pregnancy. Persistent edema may be caused by kidney, bladder, heart, or liver problems.

NUTRIENTS

SUPPLEMENT	SUGGESTED DOSAGE	COMMENTS
Very Important		
Free-form amino acid complex	As directed on label.	Sometimes edema is caused by inadequate protein assimilation. Protein deficiency has been linked to water retention.
SP-6 Cornsilk Blend from Solaray		*See under* Herbs, below.
Vitamin B complex plus extra vitamin B$_6$ (pyridoxine)	50–100 mg twice daily, with meals. 50 mg 3 times daily.	B vitamins work best when taken together. Reduces water retention.
Important		
Alfalfa		*See under* Herbs, below.
Calcium and magnesium	1,500 mg daily. 1,000 mg daily.	To replace minerals lost with correction of edema.
Silica	As directed on label.	A natural diuretic.
Helpful		
Bromelain	As directed on label, 3 times daily.	An enzyme derived from pineapples that helps digestion and allergies.
Garlic (Kyolic)	2 capsules 3 times daily, with meals.	A detoxifier.
Kelp	1,000–1,500 mg daily.	Supplies needed minerals.
Kidney-Liver Complex #406 from Enzymatic Therapy	As directed on label.	Improves kidney function.
Potassium	99 mg daily.	Very important if taking diuretics.
Pycnogenol	As directed on label.	A powerful antioxidant that also strengthens the tissues of the circulatory system.
Superoxide dismutase (SOD)	As directed on label.	Helpful in heart and liver disorders.
Taurine	As directed on label.	Aids heart function.
Vitamin C	3,000–5,000 mg daily, in divided doses.	Essential for adrenal function and production of adrenal hormones, which are vital for proper fluid balance and control of edema.
Vitamin E	400 IU and up daily.	Aids circulation.

HERBS

❑ Alfalfa is a good source of important minerals. It also contains chlorophyll, a potent detoxifier. Take 2,000 to 3,000 milligrams daily, in divided doses.

❑ SP-6 Cornsilk Blend from Solaray contains corn silk and other herbs that aid the body in expelling excess fluids. Take 2 capsules three times daily.

❑ Other herbs that can be beneficial if you are suffering from edema include butcher's broom, dandelion root, horsetail, juniper berries, lobelia, marshmallow, parsley, and pau d'arco tea.

Caution: Do not take lobelia internally on an ongoing basis.

RECOMMENDATIONS

❑ Increase your intake of raw foods. Eat plenty of apples, beets, garlic, grapes, and onions. A high-fiber diet is important.

❑ For protein, eat eggs, broiled white fish, and broiled skinless chicken or turkey. Consume small amounts of buttermilk, cottage cheese, kefir, and low-fat yogurt.

❑ Use kelp to supply needed minerals.

❑ Avoid alcohol, animal protein, beef, caffeine, chocolate, dairy products (except for those listed above), dried shellfish, fried foods, gravies, olives, pickles, salt, soy sauce, tobacco, white flour, and white sugar.

❑ Exercise daily and take hot baths or saunas twice a week.

❑ Avoid stress.

❑ *See* FASTING in Part Three and follow the program. Fasting flushes excess water from the tissues.

❑ If pressing with the fingers on your feet and ankles results in the formation of small "pits," consult your physician. This can be a sign of a serious health problem.

CONSIDERATIONS

❑ Food allergy testing is recommended. (*See* ALLERGIES in Part Two.)

❑ *See also under* PREGNANCY-RELATED PROBLEMS in Part Two.

Emphysema

Emphysema is a form of chronic obstructive pulmonary disease (COPD) caused by a loss of elasticity and dilatation of the lung tissue. A person with emphysema cannot exhale without great effort. Stale air remains trapped in the lungs, preventing the needed exchange of oxygen and carbon dioxide. The most common symptom of emphysema is breathlessness followed by coughing during exertion, no matter how slight.

Most people who are diagnosed with emphysema are long-term cigarette smokers. Symptoms may not occur until middle age, when the individual's ability to exercise or do heavy work begins to decline, and a productive cough begins. The symptoms may be subtle at first, but worsen with time.

In rare cases, emphysema is due to a deficiency of a blood protein called antitrypsin. The overwhelming majority of cases, however, are related to smoking. Smoking causes chronic low-level inflammation of the lungs, which increases the chance of developing this progressive disease.

NUTRIENTS

SUPPLEMENT	SUGGESTED DOSAGE	COMMENTS
Essential		
Chlorophyll (Kyo-Green from Wakunaga is a good source)	As directed on label 3 times daily.	Aids in clear breathing.
Dimethylglycine (DMG) Aangamik DMG from FoodScience Labs	250 mg 3 times daily.	Increases endurance. Use a sublingual form.
Very Important		
Coenzyme Q10	60 mg daily.	A powerful antioxidant; enhances oxygen in the lungs.
Free-form amino acid complex	As directed on label.	Important for repair of lung tissue.
Garlic (Kyolic)	2 capsules 3 times daily, with meals.	An immunity enhancer for protection against pneumonia.
L-Cysteine and L-methionine	500 mg each twice daily, on an empty stomach. Take with water or juice. Do not take with milk. Take with 50 mg vitamin B6 and 100 mg vitamin C for better absorption.	To aid in repairing damaged lung tissue and act as antioxidants protecting lung tissue. *See* AMINO ACIDS in Part One.
Vitamin A emulsion	100,000 IU daily for 1 month, then 50,000 IU daily until relief is achieved, then reduce	Needed for repair of lung tissues and for the immune system. Emulsion form is recommended for easier
or capsules	to 25,000 IU daily. If you are pregnant, do not exceed 10,000 IU daily.	assimilation and greater safety at higher doses.
plus natural beta-carotene	10,000 IU daily.	
or carotenoid complex	As directed on label.	
Vitamin E emulsion or	1,000 IU daily.	An oxygen carrier and potent antioxidant. A deficiency can lead to destruction of cell
capsules	Start with 400 IU daily and increase slowly to 1,600 IU daily. If you have heart problems, start with 200 daily and increase slowly to 800 IU daily.	membranes. Emulsion form is recommended for easier assimilation and greater safety at higher doses.
Vitamin C with bioflavonoids	5,000–10,000 mg daily, in divided doses.	Strengthens immune response and aids healing of inflamed tissue.
Important		
Licorice extract		*See under* Herbs, on next page.

Lung Complex #407 from Enzymatic Therapy	As directed on label.	See GLANDULAR THERAPY in Part Three for its benefits.
Helpful		
Aerobic 07 from Aerobic Life Industries	9 drops in water once daily.	Supplies oxygen and kills bacteria.
Calcium and magnesium	2,000 mg daily, at bedtime. 1,000 mg daily, at bedtime.	Act as a nerve tonic, protect nerve endings, and promote sound sleep. Use chelate forms.
Kelp	1,000–1,5000 mg daily.	Contains minerals needed for improved breathing and healing.
Multienzyme complex with pancreatin plus	As directed on label. Take with meals.	To keep infection in check by cleansing the lungs.
proteolytic enzymes or	As directed on label. Take between meals.	
Infla-Zyme Forte from American Biologics or	As directed on label.	A balance of potent enzymes and cofactors as a powerful inflammatory inhibitor.
Oxy-5000 Forte from American Biologics	As directed on label.	A potent nutritional antioxidant for health and stress that destroys free radicals.

HERBS

❑ ClearLungs from Natural Alternatives is an herbal combination that helps provide relief from shortness of breath, tightness in the chest, and wheezing due to bronchial congestion. It is available in two formulas, with ephedra and without. Both have been found to be equally effective.

❑ Ephedra (ma huang) is beneficial for respiratory disorders. Thyme is also very helpful.
Caution: Do not use ephedra if you suffer from anxiety, glaucoma, heart disease, high blood pressure, or insomnia, or if you are taking a monoamine oxidase (MAO) inhibitor drug for depression.

❑ Licorice extract increases energy levels and helps to improve organ function. Use an alcohol-free extract or Bio Rizin from American Biologics.
Caution: If overused, licorice can elevate blood pressure. Do not use this herb on a daily basis for more than seven days in a row. Avoid it completely if you have high blood pressure.

❑ Other beneficial herbs for emphysema include alfalfa, fenugreek, fresh horseradish, mullein tea, and rosemary.

RECOMMENDATIONS

❑ Avoid any and all contact with tobacco. Tobacco smoke is the single most dangerous thing anyone suffering from emphysema can encounter. If you have emphysema and smoke, you must quit. Avoid areas where people smoke and do not allow smoking in your home, your car, or anywhere near you.

❑ Eat a diet consisting of 50 percent raw foods. The other 50 percent should consist of soups, skinless chicken or turkey, fish, brown rice, millet, and whole grain cereals.

❑ Upon arising, take 1 teaspoonful of pure, cold-pressed olive oil mixed in apple juice. This will supply essential fatty acids while aiding in the elimination of toxic waste in the gallbladder and large intestine.

❑ Consume onions and garlic daily.

❑ Avoid fried and greasy foods, salt, and all foods that cause excess mucus to be formed in the gastrointestinal tract, lungs, sinuses, and nasal cavity. Foods that lead to the formation of mucus include meats, eggs, all dairy products and cheese, processed foods, tobacco, junk foods, and white flour products. Read labels carefully; these are sometimes "hidden" ingredients in food products.

❑ Avoid gas-forming foods such as legumes and cabbage. These foods cause abdominal distention that can interfere with breathing.

❑ Avoid foods that require a great deal of chewing, such as meats and nuts. Chronic lung disease can make it difficult to breathe while chewing. If necessary, vegetables can be steamed to make them easier to eat.

❑ Do not eat a typical American breakfast. Instead, sip hot, clear liquids (such as herbal teas) in the morning to help clear the mucus from the airways. Using a psyllium-based fiber product or Aerobic Bulk Cleanse (ABC) from Aerobic Life Industries (a colon cleanser available in health food stores) is helpful after consuming the liquids. Mix ABC with a glass of juice and drink it quickly. This will help rid the colon of excess mucus and reduce gas and distention.

❑ Use warm castor oil packs on the chest and back to help reduce mucus and enhance breathing. To make a castor oil pack, place a cup or so of castor oil in a pan and warm but do not boil it. Dip a piece of cheesecloth or other white cotton material into the oil until the cloth is saturated. Apply the cloth to the affected area and cover it with a piece of plastic that is larger in size than the cotton cloth, then place a warm cloth or a hot water bottle on top. Keep the pack in place for one-half to two hours, as needed.

❑ Because every extra chemical adds potential risk to the lungs, use only essential (and unscented) laundry products. Avoid perfume and anything containing fragrance. Avoid gas stoves as well; electric stoves are better for people with respiratory disorders. Choose flooring made from hardwood, ceramic tile, or stone rather than carpeting, which holds dust, mold, and many chemicals that get into the air and that can irritate the lungs. Avoid using window curtains and draperies, which also can harbor dust. Decorate with paint (new "odorless" formulas are now available) rather than wallpaper; the glues used to make the paper adhere to the wall can have volatile chemicals that may bother some people. Avoid plastic chairs, plastic dishes, and other plastic items in furnishing your home. Do not use aerosol products.

❏ Rest and avoid stress. Get plenty of fresh air.

❏ Go on a cleansing fast periodically, using carrot, celery, spinach, kale, and all dark green fresh juices. *See* FASTING in Part Three.

❏ Avoid air pollution. If your current working environment is dirty, dusty, or toxic to inhale, change jobs

❏ Leave the house during major housecleaning and other major household projects, and remain away for at least two hours afterward. Housecleaning stirs up dust and mold.

❏ Avoid hot, humid climates. If you must live in such a climate, continuous central air conditioning is essential. An air-conditioned car is also essential. Do not allow anyone to smoke or wear perfume in your car.

❏ Avoid letting furry or feathered animals into your home or car, as their hair and dander can irritate the lungs.

CONSIDERATIONS

❏ There is no known cure for emphysema, but the measures outlined in this section should ease discomfort and make breathing a bit easier.

❏ The Air Supply personal air purifier from Wein Products is a miniature unit that is worn around the neck. It sets up an invisible pure air shield against microorganisms (such as viruses, bacteria, and mold) and microparticles (including dust, pollen, and pollutants). It also eliminates vapors, smells, and harmful volatile compounds in the air. The Living Air XL-15 unit from Alpine Industries is an ionizing unit that purifies the air in the home or workplace.

❏ The University of Pennsylvania Hospital Department of Allergy reports that having an air conditioner and an electrostatic air cleaning machine in the bedroom of persons with respiratory disease is a major factor in the health of individuals with breathing trouble.

❏ *See also* ASCORBIC ACID FLUSH in Part Three and ENVIRONMENTAL TOXICITY in Part Two.

Endometriosis

Endometriosis is a condition in which the cells from the endometrium (the lining of the uterus) also grow elsewhere in the abdominal cavity. It can produce a host of different symptoms, including incapacitating pain in the uterus, lower back, and organs in the pelvic cavity prior to and during the menses; intermittent pain throughout the menstrual cycle; painful intercourse; excessive bleeding, including the passing of large clots and shreds of tissue during the menses; nausea, vomiting, and constipation during the menses; and infertility. Because menstruation is typically heavy, iron deficiency anemia is common. Women with cycles shorter than twenty-seven days and those with periods lasting over a week are at increased risk of anemia. Vulnerability to endometriosis seems to run in families; the condition often passes from mother to daughter.

Growths of endometrial tissue outside of the uterine cavity occur most often in or on the ovaries, the fallopian tubes, the urinary bladder, the bowel, the pelvic floor, and/or the peritoneum (the membrane that lines the walls of the abdominal cavity), and within the uterine musculature. The most common site of endometriosis is believed to be the deep pelvic peritoneal cavity, or the cul-de-sac. The presence of endometrial implants outside the pelvic area is uncommon.

During the normal menstrual cycle, a continually changing hormonal environment stimulates the endometrium to grow in preparation for a possible pregnancy. This same cycle causes a follicle within one of the ovaries to ripen, and an egg is released. Fingerlike tissues on the fallopian tube grasp the egg, and the tiny, hairlike cilia inside the tube transport it toward the uterus, the lining of which is now spongy and well supplied with blood. If the egg is not fertilized within twenty-four hours or so of being released, the uterine lining proceeds to "die," to be sloughed off, and to pass through the vagina during the menses.

Though not inside the uterus, the abnormal implants of endometriosis also respond to the hormonal changes controlling menstruation. Like the uterine lining, these fragments build tissue each month, then break down and bleed. Unlike blood from the uterine lining, however, blood from the implants has no way to leave the body. Instead, it must be absorbed by surrounding tissue, which is a comparatively slow process. In the meantime, the blood accumulates in body cavities. The entire sequence, from bleeding through absorption, can be painful.

As the menstrual cycle recurs month after month, the implants may get bigger. They may seed new implants and form localized scar tissue and adhesions—scar tissue that attaches to pelvic organs and binds them together. This contributes to the pain of endometriosis, and it can cause extreme pain in a subsequent pregnancy, as the uterus enlarges and the organs within the abdomen are pushed into different positions. Sometimes a collection of blood called a sac or cyst forms. Endometrial or "chocolate" cysts are common on the ovaries. These are usually found to contain moderate amounts of oxidized blood, which looks something like chocolate syrup. If a cyst ruptures, it can cause excruciating pain.

Because endometriosis depends on hormonal cycles, and pregnancy temporarily interrupts those cycles, many women find their symptoms improve during pregnancy. In some cases, the improvement may be permanent, presumably because the break from cycles of growth, bleeding, and scarring finally allows the implants to heal and be shed. In other cases, however, the relief is only temporary, and once the hormonal cycles return to normal, the symptoms of endometriosis recur.

No one knows what causes endometriosis, but several theories have been proposed. The *reflux menstruation* theory was developed by John Sampson, M.D., in 1920. According to this theory, menstrual fluid backs up into the fallopian tubes and drops into the peritoneal cavity, where endometrial cells implant themselves and grow. While this theory offers an answer to the question of what causes endometriosis, it has never been proved. Another popular theory states that

An Alternative Theory and Treatment for Endometriosis

An alternative theory of the origin of endometriosis has been developed by David Redwine, M.D., of St. Charles Medical Center in Bend, Oregon. Dr. Redwine disagrees with those obstetrician/gyecologists who accept reflux menstruation as the cause of endometriosis. Instead, he proposes that endometriosis is actually a type of birth defect. During fetal development, cells that are destined to become part of the female reproductive organs differentiate and migrate toward the appropriate locations. But if the mechanisms that control this process do not function properly, some endometrial cells may be "left behind" in places they do not belong, where they become embedded and grow.

Initially, these bits of misplaced tissue are colorless, but over time the tissue begins to change into the lesions known as endometriosis, probably at least in part in response to stimulation from sex hormones. The lesions begin to change color and gradually become darker until they appear as the classic dark-colored implants found primarily in women in their thirties. Before they reach that stage, however, they may appear white, yellow, red, or brown, and many colors in between. Thus, according to Dr. Redwine, endometrial growths only *appear* to spread progressively throughout the pelvis—that is, they are there all the time, even before birth, but they are not usually recognized for what they are until they take on a sufficiently dark color, a process that occurs over time.

Based on his understanding of the disease, Dr. Redwine developed a treatment for endometriosis in which the implants are physically removed through surgery. Using a laparoscope, the surgeon examines the entire pelvic cavity and the entire peritoneal surface at very close range to identify any possible endometrial lesions. Then all suspected endometrial growths are removed. Each lesion is biopsied and a tissue sample analyzed in a laboratory to determine whether or not it is endometrial in origin. With this identification method, Dr. Redwine says that he has been able to demonstrate that lesions other than the black "powder-burn" lesions normally considered characteristic of the condition have been endometrial in origin.

Many women who undergo surgery for endometriosis are diagnosed with recurrences later. This would seem to support the idea that this is a progressive disease that tends to come back despite treatment. However, Dr. Redwine maintains that the reason so many women have recurring problems with endometriosis is that only a portion of their endometrial implants are removed in surgery. Most surgeons remove only the "typical" black powder-burn lesions and chocolate cysts. Dr. Redwine estimates that a surgeon who excises only the black lesions may leave from 50 to 60 percent of the actual disease behind; he has found that only 40 percent of his patients have the typical lesions, while 60 percent have the multicolored, "atypical" type. He believes that endometriosis is indeed curable, as long as *all* the lesions—both typical and atypical, and not only within the pelvic cavity, but on the peritoneum as well—are removed. His follow-up studies indicate that after surgery, approximately 75 percent of his patients experience complete relief of symptoms, and approximately 20 percent experience an improvement in symptoms so that what was disabling pain becomes only minimal pain. Only about 5 percent report no relief. Dr. Redwine's treatment is now used also by several other gynecological surgeons in the United States.

The following table outlines some of the key differences between Dr. Redwine's theory and conventional medical theory.

ENDOMETRIOSIS THEORIES CONTRASTED

Conventional Theory	Dr. Redwine's Theory
Caused by retrograde menstruation.	Caused by a defect in embryonic cell differentiation.
A progressive disease primarily of women over 30.	A static disease affecting women of all ages.
Associated with menstruation.	Independent of menstruation.
Causes infertility.	May be associated with infertility, but is not the actual cause of it.
Lesions bleed monthly.	Lesions do not bleed.
Most lesions are black.	Lesions may be clear, white, pink, red, brown, black, or multicolored. Most are not black.
Peritoneal implants are not considered to be endometrial in origin.	Peritoneal implants have been proved to be endometrial in origin.
Recurrence following removal of lesions is common.	Recurrence following removal of lesions is rare if both typical and atypical lesions are removed.
Hysterectomy is recommended for severe cases. Surgery provides undependable levels of relief.	Surgical removal of all typical and atypical lesions is the treatment of choice for this disorder, and can provide complete relief in up to 75 percent of cases.

Further information on Dr. Redwine and his approach to endometriosis treatment can be obtained by writing to the Endometriosis Treatment Program, St. Charles Medical Center, 2500 NE Neff Road, Bend, OR 97701–6015, or by calling 503–382–4321.

endometriosis is caused when endometrial cells spread to other parts of the body through blood and lymphatic channels. Still another theory postulates that endometriosis is in effect a congenital condition (*see* An Alternative Theory and Treatment for Endometriosis on page 250).

Despite disagreement over the cause, more is known today about this condition than ever before. Once labeled the "working woman's disease," endometriosis is now known to affect 12 million American women—approximately 10 percent of the female adult population—from all walks of life. Many women fail to seek medical help because they mistake the symptoms of this disease for normal menstrual discomfort.

Most women who suffer from endometriosis have never been pregnant, and as many as 30 percent of women who report infertility problems actually have endometriosis. The exact relationship between infertility and endometriosis remains somewhat unclear, however. There is debate in the medical community over whether endometriosis causes infertility, or whether delaying childbearing results in endometriosis—or both.

Laparoscopy is the procedure most commonly used to diagnose endometriosis. This involves the insertion of a tiny lighted optical tube (a laparoscope) through a small incision in the navel. The surgeon can then see inside the abdominal cavity. Laparoscopic procedures are usually done on an outpatient basis.

The nutrient program and other recommendations outlined below may help to keep endometriosis under control if it is diagnosed in the early stages.

NUTRIENTS

SUPPLEMENT	SUGGESTED DOSAGE	COMMENTS
Very Important		
Vitamin E	Start with 400 IU daily and increase slowly to 1,000 IU daily.	Aids hormonal balance.
Vitamin K or alfalfa	200 mcg daily.	Needed for normal blood clotting. *See under* Herbs, below.
Important		
Essential fatty acids (primrose oil is a good source)	1,500 mg daily.	Provides essential fatty acids such as gamma-linolenic acid (GLA).
Iron or	As directed by physician.	Deficiency is common in those with this disorder. Use ferrous fumarate form. *Caution:* Do not take iron unless anemia is diagnosed. An easily assimilated and nontoxic source of iron.
Floradix Iron + Herbs from Salus Haus	As directed on label.	
Vitamin B complex plus extra	As directed on label.	Promotes blood cell productivity and proper hormone balance.
pantothenic acid (vitamin B$_5$) and	100 mg 3 times daily.	Relieves stress; needed for proper adrenal function.
vitamin B$_6$ (pyridoxine)	50 mg 3 times daily.	Aids the body in removing excess fluids.

Vitamin C with bioflavonoids	2,000 mg 3 times daily.	Important in the healing process. Use a buffered form.
Zinc	50 mg daily. Do not exceed a total of 100 mg daily from all supplements.	For tissue repair and immune function. Use zinc gluconate lozenges or OptiZinc for best absorption.
Helpful		
Calcium and	1,500 mg daily.	To supply needed minerals. Use chelate forms.
magnesium	1,000 mg daily, at bedtime.	
Kelp	1,000–1,500 mg daily.	To supply needed minerals.
Multivitamin and mineral complex	As directed on label.	All nutrients are required for repair and healing.

HERBS

❑ Alfalfa is a good source of vitamin K (necessary for blood clotting and healing) and needed minerals, including iron. Many women with endometriosis are iron-deficient.

❑ Astragalus, garlic, goldenseal, myrrh gum, pau d'arco, and red clover have antibiotic and antitumor properties.

❑ Burdock root, dong quai, and red raspberry leaf help to balance hormones.

❑ Nettle is rich in iron.

RECOMMENDATIONS

❑ Eat a diet consisting of 50 percent raw vegetables and fruits. In addition, eat only whole-grain products (no refined flour products) and raw nuts and seeds.

❑ Include "green drinks" made from dark green leafy vegetables in your diet.

❑ Use kelp to add iron to the diet. The heavy monthly bleeding that is common in women with endometriosis often leads to iron deficiency.

❑ Avoid alcohol, caffeine, animal fats, butter, dairy products, fried foods, foods that contain additives, all hardened fats, junk foods or fast foods, red meats, poultry (except organically raised and skinless), refined and processed foods, salt, shellfish, and sugar.

❑ Fast for three days each month before the anticipated beginning of the menstrual period. Use steam-distilled water and fresh live juices. *See* PREMENSTRUAL SYNDROME in Part Two and FASTING in Part Three.

❑ Use a heating pad, hot water bottle, or a hot bath to help relieve pain. The warmth relaxes the muscles that cramp and cause pain.

❑ If you are taking medication for endometriosis, report any new or worsened symptoms to your doctor immediately, especially problems such as difficulty breathing or chest or leg pain. These symptoms may indicate the presence of a blood clot. Frequent checkups are needed to monitor possible side effects such as thinning of the bones. Be aware,

251

however, that it is normal for endometriosis symptoms to worsen temporarily when a woman begins taking medicine.

❑ Use pads rather than tampons during menstruation. Tampons may make reflux menstruation more likely. They can also aggravate pain and cramping.

CONSIDERATIONS

❑ Diet is very important in managing endometriosis.

❑ Daily moderate exercise such as walking or stretching is beneficial.

❑ If you suspect you may have endometriosis, you should see a gynecologist promptly so that the condition can be controlled at the earliest possible stage of development.

❑ Medical treatment recommended for endometriosis depends on how far the condition has progressed.

❑ Doctors commonly prescribe a drug called danazol (Danocrine), which "shuts off" the normal hormonal cycles, in an attempt to control the blood flow and pain, and in hopes of keeping the abnormal tissue from spreading and inducing the growths to heal and shrink. Some doctors prescribe oral contraceptives (birth control pills) for essentially the same reason. Danazol has been shown to improve symptoms for 89 percent of women who take it and to reduce the size and number of implants. Weight gain and a deepened voice are possible side effects, but are usually reversible when the medication is stopped. However, symptoms may also reappear after medication is stopped.

❑ Nafarelin, available as a nasal spray called Synarel, relieves symptoms and helps shrink endometrial lesions. In a trial involving 247 women treated with nafarelin for six months, 85 percent had their implants shrink or disappear and their symptoms relieved. Six months after treatment, however, symptoms reappeared in half of those who had been helped. Possible side effects are similar to some of the discomforts of menopause, including hot flashes, vaginal dryness, and lighter, less frequent, or no menstruation. Other effects include headaches and nasal irritation.

❑ An injectable drug named leuprolide (Lupron) is similar to nafarelin. Treatment consists of one injection a month for six months. In clinical studies, the effectiveness of leuprolide has been found to be about the same as that of danazol, according to the manufacturer. Potential side effects are similar to those caused by nafarelin.

❑ A synthetic male hormone is sometimes used to temporarily stop menstrual cycles completely. This type of hormone causes excess facial hair growth and a deepening of the voice.

❑ If endometriosis is severe and disabling, or if drug therapy fails, and you do not wish to have any more children, hysterectomy may be recommended. However, hysterectomy does not always relieve all the symptoms, especially if there are implants of endometrial tissue throughout the pelvic region.

❑ An excision option less traumatic than hysterectomy that is used to treat milder cases is laparoscopy with laser surgery to identify and vaporize adhesions, cysts, and endometrial implants. The procedure has yet to be perfected; repeated laparoscopy may be necessary. Advances in this technique are being made at a rapid rate, however, and the need for repeat procedures may soon be a thing of the past.

❑ According to a report in the *Journal of the American Medical Association*, strenuous exercise lowers the level of estrogen in the body, and this may help suppress the symptoms of endometriosis. The more aerobic exercise a woman engages in and the earlier she starts, the lower her risk of developing the disease in the first place, according to a study of endometriosis led by Daniel W. Cramer of Brigham and Women's Hospital and Harvard Medical School. This study found that women who exercised more than seven hours a week had one-fifth the average risk of developing endometriosis. Unfortunately, this beneficial effect was limited to those who began exercising before the age of twenty-six.

❑ Some nutrition researchers have theorized that endometriosis is related to an inability to absorb calcium properly.

❑ For more information about endometriosis, you can contact the Endometriosis Association, P.O. Box 92187, Milwaukee, WI 53202. Or call 1–800–992–ENDO in the United States; 800–426–2END in Canada.

Enuresis

See BED-WETTING.

Enlarged Prostate

See PROSTATITIS/ENLARGED PROSTATE.

Environmental Toxicity

Today there is reason to be concerned about the quality of our water and food supply and about the effects of exposure to radiation and toxic metals, particularly on our immune systems. The body's immune system is a complex network that protects us from infectious agents (viruses, bacteria and other microorganisms), allergens (substances that induce allergic reactions), and other pathogens (substances that cause disease). When something foreign threatens the body, the body responds by forming antibodies and producing increased numbers of white blood cells to combat the intruder. The kidneys and liver work to rid the body of toxins. A properly functioning immune system is thus vital for good health.

Certain minerals, such as calcium and zinc, are necessary to sustain life. Other minerals, like copper, are essential in small amounts but are toxic in greater amounts. Some minerals not only have no nutritional value but also are toxic in any amount. These toxic metals—lead, aluminum, cadmium, and mercury—pervade our environment and threaten our health, impairing the function of our organs. Pesticides, herbicides, insecticides, fungicides, fumigants, and fertilizers containing these metals and other toxic substances seep into our soil and food. Food additives, preservatives, and artificial coloring pervade the products in our supermarkets. Fruits and vegetables are sprayed, treated with ripening agents, and waxed to make them appear more appetizing. Toxic chemicals and hazardous waste have contaminated our air and water.

Some of the common products and environmental factors that can have a detrimental effect on health include disinfectants, hair sprays, paint, solvents, bedding, animal hair, household cleaning products, dust, and mold. Some products used in the home emit volatile components into the air, such as styrene from plastics, benzene from solvents, and formaldehyde from manufactured wood products such as pressed wood furniture and kitchen cabinets. Permanent-press clothes and plastics emit traces of toxic vapors. Smoke from cigarettes, cigars, or pipes raises the level of toxic substances not only in the smoker, but also in those exposed to secondhand smoke.

When these and other pollutants in our environment invade our bodies, they can cause such reactions as watery eyes, diarrhea, nausea, upset stomach, and ringing in the ears. The symptoms of environmental toxicity are so varied that they also include asthma, bronchitis, stuffy nose, arthritis, fatigue, headache, eczema, and depression. If you suffer from chronic flulike symptoms, the culprit may not be a virus; you may be reacting to some material or item in your home or workplace. Exposure to environmental toxins has been linked to immune deficiency and cancer.

The symptoms of environmental toxicity and environmental allergies can be very similar, but the mechanisms that cause them are different. Allergies result from an overreaction by the immune system to some substance encountered in the environment. Environmental toxicity, on the other hand, is not a result of an immune system reaction, but a direct poisoning of tissues or cells, so that they can no longer function as they should. Allergic reactions usually begin to subside when contact with the offending allergen ceases, whereas toxicity-based problems can persist long afterwards, depending on the type and extent of the damage the toxins have caused.

NUTRIENTS

SUPPLEMENT	SUGGESTED DOSAGE	COMMENTS
Essential		
Coenzyme Q$_{10}$	30 mg 4 times daily.	Important in immune function.
Vitamin C with bioflavonoids and quercetin	3,000–10,000 mg daily, in divided doses.	Aids in removing toxins and heavy metals from the body.
Very Important		
Superoxide dismutase (SOD) (Cell Guard from Biotec Foods)	As directed on label.	A powerful antioxidant that protects against free radical formation and radiation.
Garlic (Kyolic)	2 capsules 3 times daily.	A potent immunostimulant.
L-Cysteine and L-methionine plus L-carnitine and glutathione	500 mg each 3 times daily, on an empty stomach. Take with water or juice. Do not take with milk. Take with 50 mg vitamin B$_6$ and 100 mg vitamin C for better absorption.	To protect the lungs, heart, and liver by destroying free radicals.
Proteolytic enzymes plus pancreatic enzymes	As directed on label. Take between meals. As directed on label. Take with meals.	Important for proper digestion and detoxification.
Taurine Plus from American Biologics	As directed on label.	An important antioxidant and immune regulator, necessary for white blood cell activation and neurological function. Use the sublingual form.
Important		
Apple pectin	As directed on label.	Binds with toxins and heavy metals to remove them from the body.
Grape seed extract	As directed on label.	A powerful antioxidant.
Vitamin A plus natural beta-carotene or carotenoid complex (Betatene) plus vitamin E	100,000 IU daily for 1 month, then reduce to 15,000 IU daily. If you are pregnant, do not exceed 10,000 IU daily. As directed on label. As directed on label. 400–800 IU daily.	Vitamins A and E both act as powerful antioxidants and detoxifiers. Use emulsion forms for easier assimilation and greater safety at high doses. Antioxidant and precursor of vitamin A.
Vitamin B complex plus extra pantothenic acid (vitamin B$_5$) and vitamin B$_6$ (pyridoxine) and niacinamide	100 mg 3 times daily, with meals. 100 mg 3 times daily. 50 mg 3 times daily. Up to 500 mg daily.	All B vitamins are vital for cellular function and repair; needed for proper digestion and to protect the lining of the digestive tract. Use a high-stress formula. Sublingual forms are recommended for best absorption.
Helpful		
Calcium plus copper and zinc	50 mg daily. 3 mg daily. 80 mg daily. Do not exceed a total of 100 mg daily from all supplements.	Minerals that aid the immune system. Use calcium pantothenate form. Use zinc gluconate lozenges or OptiZinc for best absorption.
Manganese	50 mg daily. Take separately from calcium.	Works with other trace minerals to aid the immune system. Use a chelate form.
Raw thymus glandular	500 mg daily.	Improves T cell production. *See* GLANDULAR THERAPY in Part Three for its benefits.

RECOMMENDATIONS

❑ Include in the diet fiber sources such as Aerobic Bulk Cleanse (ABC) from Aerobic Life Industries, oat bran, and wheat bran. Apple pectin also can be beneficial.

Note: Always take supplemental fiber separately from other supplements and medications.

❑ Drink only steam-distilled water.

❑ Use nontoxic cleaning products whenever possible.

❑ Try using an air cleaner or ionizer for symptomatic relief. These devices remove animal odors, bacteria, dust, pollen, smog, and smoke from the air. The Living Air XL-15 unit from Alpine Industries is an ionizing unit that is good for purifying the air in the home or workplace.

❑ To reduce your exposure to natural gas, pesticides, radon, smoke, and other chemicals in the household, ventilate your home well. Replace particleboard subflooring with exterior-grade plywood that does not contain formaldehyde. The wood should then be sealed with a nontoxic sealant.

❑ Scrape any peeling paint inside and outside your home, using appropriate protective devices. Older paints contain toxic lead residue. (*See* LEAD POISONING in Part Two.)

❑ Change vacuum cleaner bags frequently. Most vacuum cleaner bags do a poor job of filtering out dust, pollen, dust mites, and other potentially harmful particles. When shopping for a new vacuum, look for models that encase the bag in a hard, impermeable shell.

❑ Do not smoke, and do not let anyone else smoke in your home or car.

❑ Do not use insect sprays or bug bombs. If you need the services of an exterminator, make sure that anyone you hire is licensed.

CONSIDERATIONS

❑ It is advisable to see an allergy specialist to have a radioallergosorbent test (RAST) if you experience any of the symptoms listed above to rule out allergies as a cause of the problem. You may also want to have a hair analysis to determine the level of toxic substances in your system.

❑ Liver extract injections have produced good results for some people.

❑ Radon is a naturally occurring radioactive gas that can seep into buildings from the surrounding soil. It is most prevalent in certain areas of the country and is present in greater concentrations in newer, well-insulated homes. Exposure to radon is believed to be the number two cause of lung cancer in the United States. Home radon test kits are available in most hardware stores. If your home is found to have radon, you can probably correct the problem by sealing cracks and improving ventilation in the basement. Regional offices of the Environmental Protection Agency (EPA) can provide more information.

❑ One household item that can cause a lot of problems is carpeting. Some of the chemicals commonly used in carpeting have been shown to have an adverse effect on health. One suspect chemical is 4-phenylcyclohexene (4-PC), a byproduct of the production of styrene-butadiene. This substance is used for the backing of many carpets. Breakdown products from styrene-butadiene are also potentially toxic. Shampooing carpeting can be particularly bad for your health. When you shampoo a carpet, the bottom stays damp well after the surface you walk on is dry. This dampness becomes a breeding ground for thousands of microorganisms that can wreak havoc on your system. The moisture can also seep into the floor beneath, which in many buildings consists of particleboard made from formaldehyde-based glue and processed wood. When the particleboard gets wet, the formaldehyde can be released into the air in the home.

❑ *See also* ALUMINUM TOXICITY; ARSENIC POISONING; CADMIUM TOXICITY; CHEMICAL POISONING; COPPER TOXICITY; FOOD POISONING; LEAD POISONING; MERCURY TOXICITY; and NICKEL TOXICITY, all in Part Two.

Epilepsy

Epilepsy is a disorder characterized by recurring seizures, which are caused by electrical disturbances in the nerve cells in a section of the brain. In 75 percent of cases, the seizures begin in childhood and are characterized by staring spells and a few seconds of mental absence. In the remaining 25 percent of cases, seizures start later in life. The cause or causes of most cases of epilepsy are unknown. The condition is thought to be hereditary; however, a genetic predisposition alone probably does not cause most cases of the disorder. Other factors, such as oxygen deprivation at birth or a later head injury, are probably also present in most cases.

With epilepsy, seizures may occur for no apparent reason, or may be triggered by a wide range of things, including exposure to an allergen; drug or alcohol withdrawal; fever; flashing lights; hunger; hypoglycemia; infection; lack of sleep; metabolic or nutritional imbalances; or trauma, especially head injury. Epilepsy is the most common cause of seizures; it strikes 1 out of every 100 people in the U.S.

There are several types of seizures, including:

• *Absence (petit mal).* This type of seizure is most common in children. It is characterized by a blank stare lasting about half a minute; the person appears to be daydreaming. During this type of seizure, the individual is unaware of his or her surroundings.

• *Atonic (drop attack).* A childhood seizure in which the child loses consciousness for about ten seconds and usually falls to the ground because of a complete loss of muscle tone.

• *Complex partial (temporal lobe).* A blank stare, random activity, and a chewing motion are characteristic of this type of seizure. The person may be dazed and unaware of his or her surroundings, and may act oddly. There is no memory of this seizure. A person may experience a distinctive warning sign called an aura before this type of seizure. The aura is itself a form of partial seizure, but one in which the person retains awareness. The aura may be experienced as a peculiar odor, "butterflies" in the stomach, or a sound. One man with epilepsy, an ardent racetrack gambler, said he always heard the roar of a crowd, followed by the name of a favorite racehorse, just before he lost consciousness.

• *Generalized tonic-clonic (grand mal).* This type of seizure is characterized by sudden cries, a fall, rigidity and jerking of the muscles, shallow breathing, and bluish skin. Loss of bladder control is possible. The seizure usually lasts two to five minutes, and is followed by confusion, fatigue, and/or memory loss. It can be frightening to witness, especially for the first-time observer.

• *Myoclonic.* Brief, massive muscle jerks occur.

• *Simple partial (Jacksonian).* Jerking begins in the fingers and toes and progresses up through the body. The person remains conscious.

• *Simple partial (sensory).* The person may see, hear, or sense things that do not exist. This may occur as a preliminary symptom of a generalized seizure.

Nutritional supplementation is important for people with epilepsy. Unless otherwise specified, the dosages recommended here are for adults. For a child between twelve and seventeen, reduce the dose to three-quarters the recommended amount. For a child between six and twelve, use one-half the recommended dose, and for a child under the age of six, use one-quarter the recommended amount.

NUTRIENTS

SUPPLEMENT	SUGGESTED DOSAGE	COMMENTS
Essential		
Vitamin B complex	100 mg 3 times daily, with meals.	Extremely important in the functioning of the central nervous system. Injections (under a doctor's supervision) may be necessary.
plus extra vitamin B₃ (niacin)	50 mg daily.	Improves circulation and is helpful for many brain-related disorders.
and vitamin B₆ (pyridoxine)	100–600 mg 3 times daily, under the supervision of a health care professional.	Needed for normal brain function.
and vitamin B₁₂	200 mcg twice daily, on an empty stomach.	Involved in maintenance of the myelin sheaths that cover and protect nerve endings.
and folic acid	400 mcg daily.	A brain food vital for the health of the nervous system.
and pantothenic acid	500 mg daily.	The anti-stress vitamin.
Magnesium	700 mg daily, in divided doses. Take between meals, on an empty stomach, with apple cider vinegar or betaine HCl.	Needed to calm the nervous system and muscle spasms. Use magnesium chloride form.
L-Tyrosine and taurine	500 mg each 3 times daily, on an empty stomach. Take with water or juice. Do not take with milk. Take with 50 mg vitamin B₆ and 100 mg vitamin C for better absorption.	Important for proper brain function. *Caution:* Do not take tyrosine if you are taking an MAO inhibitor drug.
Taurine Plus from American Biologics	10–20 drops daily, in divided doses.	An important antioxidant and immune regulator, necessary for white blood cell activation and neurological function. Use the sublingual form.
Very Important		
Calcium	1,500 mg daily.	Important in normal nerve impulse transmission.
Zinc	50–80 mg daily. Do not exceed a total of 100 mg daily from all supplements.	Protects the brain cells. Use zinc gluconate lozenges or OptiZinc for best absorption.
Important		
Coenzyme Q₁₀	30 mg daily.	Improves brain oxygenation.
Dimethylglycine (DMG) (Aangamik DMG from FoodScience Labs)	50 mg twice daily, in the morning and at night.	Stimulates immune response and improves cellular oxygen levels. Use a sublingual form.
Oxy-5000 Forte from American Biologics	As directed on label.	A potent nutritional antioxidant for health and stress. Destroys free radicals.
Helpful		
Chromium picolinate	200 mcg daily.	Important in maintaining stable cerebral glucose metabolism.
Kelp or alfalfa	1,000–1,500 mg daily.	For necessary mineral balance. *See under* Herbs, below.
Melatonin	Start with 2–3 mg daily, taken 2 hours or less before bedtime. If necessary, gradually increase the dosage until an effective level is reached.	Helpful if symptoms include insomnia.
Proteolytic enzymes plus multienzyme complex	As directed on label. Take between meals. As directed on label. Take with meals.	Aids in healing if inflammation is the cause of seizures. Aids digestion, helping to make needed nutrients available.
Raw thymus and thyroid glandulars	As directed on label. As directed on label.	Both the thymus and thyroid are important in proper brain function. *See* GLANDULAR THERAPY in Part Three.
Vitamin A	25,000 IU daily. If you are pregnant, do not exceed 10,000 IU daily.	An important antioxidant that aids in protecting brain function.
Vitamin C with bioflavonoids	2,000–7,000 mg daily, in divided doses.	Vital to functioning of the adrenal glands, which are the anti-stress glands. A potent antioxidant.
Vitamin E	Start with 400 IU daily and gradually increase to 1,600 IU daily.	Aids circulation and immunity. Emulsion form is recommended for easier assimilation and greater safety at high doses.

HERBS

❑ Alfalfa is a good source of needed minerals. Take 2,000 milligrams daily in capsule or extract form.

❑ Black cohosh, hyssop, and lobelia are beneficial for people with epilepsy because they aid in controlling the central nervous system and have a calming effect. For best results, they should be used on an alternating basis.

Caution: Do not use black cohosh during pregnancy.

❑ *Avoid* the herb sage. This herb should not be used by anyone with a seizure disorder.

RECOMMENDATIONS

❑ Eat soured milk products like yogurt and kefir.

❑ Include beet greens, chard, eggs, green leafy vegetables, raw cheese, raw milk, raw nuts, seeds, and soybeans in the diet.

❑ Drink fresh "live" juices made from beets, carrots, green beans, green leafy vegetables, peas, red grapes, and seaweed for concentrated nutrients. *See* JUICING in Part Three.

❑ Eat small meals, do not drink large quantities of liquids at once, and take 2 tablespoons of olive oil daily.

❑ Avoid alcoholic beverages, animal protein, fried foods, artificial sweeteners such as aspartame (NutraSweet), caffeine, and nicotine. Avoid refined foods and sugar.

❑ If the bowels do not move each day, before going to bed, take a lemon enema using the juice of two lemons and 2 quarts of water. *See* ENEMAS in Part Three.

❑ Take an Epsom salts bath twice a week.

❑ Work toward self-care. Keep drug dosages as low as possible, and work toward becoming as free from drugs and seizures as possible. The correct diet and nutritional supplements are very important in the control of epilepsy.

❑ Get regular moderate exercise to improve circulation to the brain.

❑ As much as possible, avoid stress and tension. Learn stress management techniques. *See* STRESS in Part Two.

❑ Stay away from pesticides.

❑ Avoid using aluminum cookware. Use glass or stainless steel instead. Aluminum can leach into the food during cooking, and may contribute to seizures.

❑ Consider having a hair analysis to rule out metal toxicity as the cause of seizures.

CONSIDERATIONS

❑ Most people who have epilepsy are aware of their condition and take medication to control the seizures. Possible side effects of antiseizure medications include blood disorders, fatigue, liver problems, and mental fatigue and/or fogginess.

❑ Other types of drugs can interact with antiseizure medications, lessening or itensifying the effects of one drug or the other. Alcohol, birth control pills, the antibiotic erythromycin, and some types of asthma, ulcer, and heart medicines are known to interact with certain epilepsy drugs. Anyone who takes medication for epilepsy should always check with his or her doctor or pharmacist before taking other drugs, whether prescription or over-the-counter.

❑ Epilepsy is not the only cause of seizures. They can also be brought on by other factors, including alkalosis; excessive consumption of alcohol; arteriosclerosis; brain disorders such as a brain tumor, encephalitis, meningitis, or stroke; high fever (especially in children); the use of drugs; the formation of scar tissue as a result of an eye injury or a stroke; a lack of oxygen; and spasms of the blood vessels.

❑ High levels of aluminum have been found in the brains of people with epilepsy. Studies in animals have shown that trace amounts of aluminum in the brain may initiate the type of disordered electrical activity that causes seizures. (*See* ALUMINUM TOXICITY in Part Two.)

❑ According to research done by Arizona State University's Biochemical Department, the artificial sweetener aspartame (NutraSweet) has been associated with seizures in some people. Toxic agents such as aluminum and lead may contribute to the problem.

❑ Doses of folic acid in excess of 400 micrograms per day may increase seizure activity in people with epilepsy, especially if they are taking the commonly prescribed anticonvulsant phenytoin (Dilantin).

❑ A manganese deficiency in a pregnant woman may result in the birth of a child with epilepsy.

❑ Women taking epilepsy medication during pregnancy have about two to three times the standard risk of bearing a child with birth defects. Nevertheless, at least 90 percent of women who take epilepsy drugs during pregnancy give birth to normal, healthy infants. Because a seizure during pregnancy carries its own risks, most doctors advise pregnant women with epilepsy to continue taking their medication unless it is likely they will be seizure-free without it.

❑ Some good results have been reported using hyperbaric (high-pressure) oxygen therapy in treating people with epilepsy. (*See* HYPERBARIC OXYGEN THERAPY in Part Three.)

❑ In a Japanese study, the drug clorazepate dipotassium (Tranxene) helped twenty-one of twenty-nine people with epilepsy. The only side effect was a slight impairment in memory.

❑ Surgeons at the Mayo Clinic in Rochester, Minnesota, have pioneered a surgical technique that gives them access to the most remote and sensitive areas of the brain. Using a computer, a surgeon can view and vaporize the tiny tumors that cause some cases of epilepsy. This technique, called lesionectomy, can be performed with minimal damage to healthy tissue in the brain.

❑ A specialized dietary program called the *ketogenic diet* has been used with considerable success to control seizures in children. This is a rigidly controlled diet that is high in fats and extremely low in carbohydrates and proteins, which forces the body to use fats rather than the usual carbohydrates to generate cellular energy. When fats are burned, byproducts called *ketones* are formed. Normally, ketosis—the presence of high levels of ketones in the body—occurs only in cases of starvation or uncontrolled diabetes mellitus. Eating a diet containing virtually no carbohydrates, however, can produce essentially the same effect, and also causes biochemical changes that enable the body's tissues to burn these ketones for needed energy. Although it is not known exactly how, this process appears to control seizure activity. The majority of children who have been put on this diet benefit from it, and many have been able to stop taking, or reduce their dosage of, antiseizure medication. Using this dietary program can be challenging for parents, however; the child's foods, liquids, medications, and even personal hygiene products such as toothpaste must be strictly controlled, and the program must be followed to the letter (even slight deviations can negate its effects). It should be undertaken only under the direct supervision of a physician who is experienced in its use. Information about the ketogenic diet is available from the Pediatric Epilepsy Center at Johns Hopkins Hospital, 600 North Wolfe Street, Baltimore, MD 21287-7247; telephone 410–955–9100.

Epstein-Barr Virus

See CHRONIC FATIGUE SYNDROME; FIBROMYALGIA SYNDROME; MONONUCLEOSIS.

Eye Problems

We have all experienced eye trouble at one time or another—eyes that are tired, bloodshot, burning, dry, infected, irritated, itchy, sensitive to light, ulcerated, or watery, to name just a few. While some eye disorders—nearsightedness or cataracts, for example—are localized problems, eye disturbances are often a sign of disease elsewhere in the body. Watery eyes are a symptom of the common cold; a thyroid problem may be indicated by protruding or bulging eyes and reading difficulties; dark circles under the eyes and eyes that are red, swollen, and/or watery may indicate allergies; yellowing of the eyes from jaundice can be a sign of hepatitis, gallbladder disease, or gallstone blockage; droopy eyes are often an early sign of *myasthenia gravis,* a disorder in which the muscles of the eye weaken. A drastic difference in the sizes of the pupils can indicate a tumor somewhere in the body, whereas high blood pressure and diabetes may manifest themselves in periodic blurring of vision.

The eyeball is a sphere about an inch in diameter that is covered by a tough outer layer called the *sclera,* the "white of the eye." Underneath the sclera is the middle layer of the eye, the *choroid,* which contains the blood vessels that serve the eye. The front of the eye is covered by a transparent membrane called the *cornea.* Behind the cornea is a fluid-filled chamber called the *anterior chamber;* behind that—in the center of the sclera, on the front of the eyeball—is the highly pigmented *iris,* and in the center of the iris is the *pupil.* Behind the iris is the transparent *lens.* Inside, at the back of the eye, is the *retina,* a delicate light-sensitive membrane that is connected to the brain by the *optic nerve.*

The eye also contains two important fluids. The *ciliary body,* whose muscles are responsible for focusing the lens of the eye, also produces a waterlike substance called the *aqueous humor,* which fills the space between the cornea and the lens. The aqueous humor contains all of the constituents of blood except for red blood cells. The other fluid is the *vitreous humor,* a jellylike substance that fills the back of the eyeball, the space between the lens and the retina.

On the outside of the eyeball are six muscles that move the eyes. Under the upper eyelids are the lacrimal glands, which secrete tears. At the inner corners of the eyelids are the tear ducts, small openings through which the tears drain into the nose and the back of the throat. At the edges of the eyelids, where the eyelashes are, are glands that produce oils, sweat, and other secretions.

What we think of as the simple act of seeing is actually a complex, multistep process that goes on continuously and at breathtaking speed. Light enters the eye through the pupil, which changes size depending on the amount of light entering it. When there is very little light, the pupil dilates; in bright light, the pupil constricts. As light enters the eye, it is focused by the lens, which adjusts its shape by means of the action of the muscles and ligaments of the ciliary body. The lens becomes fatter or flatter depending upon the distance to the object being focused on. The lens projects light onto the retina, where special pigment absorbs the light and forms a corresponding image. Finally, this image is transmitted by means of the optic nerve to the brain, which interprets the image. Anything that interferes with any link in this chain of events can result in impaired vision.

Many cases of eye damage and vision loss are linked to underlying diseases of one type or another. Diabetes often leads to hemorrhages in the retina and the vitreous, eventually producing blindness. Early cataracts also may be related to diabetes. High blood pressure produces a gradual thickening of the blood vessels inside the eyes that can result in visual impairment and even blindness.

One major contributor to eye trouble is poor diet, specifically the denatured, chemical- and preservative-laden foods that most Americans consume daily. A deficiency of just one vitamin can lead to various eye problems. Supplementation with the correct vitamins and minerals can help

Maintaining Healthy Eyes

Like all other parts of the body, the eyes need to be nourished properly. In addition to making sure that the eyes are not strained by too much intense close work or inadequate light, proper eye care includes a healthy diet containing sufficient amounts of vitamins and minerals.

In order to promote good eyesight, you must make sure your diet contains the proper amounts of the B vitamins; vitamins A, C, and E; and the minerals selenium and zinc. Fresh fruits and vegetables are good sources of these vitamins and minerals; include plenty of these in your diet, especially yellow and yellow-orange foods such as carrots, yams, and cantaloupes. A well-balanced diet with plenty of fresh fruits and vegetables can help keep your eyes healthy.

NUTRIENTS

SUPPLEMENT	SUGGESTED DOSAGE	COMMENTS
Bilberry extract		*See under* Herbs, below.
Desiccated liver	As directed on label.	A good source of many important vitamins and minerals. Use only liver derived from organically raised beef.
Free-form amino acid complex plus	As directed on label.	For necessary protein. Free-form amino acids are assimilated best.
glutathione or	500 mg daily, on an empty stomach.	Powerful antioxidants that protect the lenses of the eyes.
N-acetylcysteine	500 mg daily, on an empty stomach. Take with water or juice. Do not take with milk. Take with 50 mg vitamin B_6 and 100 mg vitamin C for better absorption.	
Multivitamin and mineral complex with		All nutrients are needed in balance.
selenium	200 mcg daily.	Destroys free radicals that can damage the eyes.
Ocu-Care from Nature's Plus or	As directed on label.	These formulas provide many eye-strengthening nutrients, as well as protective and antioxidant substances, to support and nourish the eyes.
OcuGuard from Twinlab or	As directed on label.	
Vital Eyes from Source Naturals	As directed on label.	
Vitamin A emulsion or	75,000 IU daily. If you are pregnant, do not exceed 10,000 IU daily.	Absolutely necessary for proper eye function. Protects the eye from free radicals. Emulsion form is recommended for easier assimilation and greater safety at higher doses. Precursor of vitamin A.
capsules plus	15,000 IU daily. If you are pregnant, do not exceed 10,000 IU daily.	
natural beta-carotene or	15,000 IU daily.	
carotenoid complex (Betatene)	As directed on label.	

SUPPLEMENT	SUGGESTED DOSAGE	COMMENTS
Vitamin B complex	100 mg twice daily.	Needed for intracellular eye metabolism.
Vitamin C	2,000 mg 3 times daily.	An antioxidant that reduces intraocular pressure.
Vitamin E	400 IU daily.	Important in healing and immunity.
Zinc	50 mg daily. Do not exceed a total of 100 mg daily from all supplements.	Deficiency has been linked to retinal detachment. Use zinc gluconate lozenges or OptiZinc for best absorption.

HERBS

❑ Bayberry bark, cayenne (capsicum), and red raspberry leaves, taken by mouth, are beneficial.

❑ Bilberry extract has been shown to improve both normal and night vision.

❑ Eyebright is beneficial for the eyes. It can be taken orally in capsule or tea form. Eyebright tea can also be used as an eyewash.

❑ SP-23 Eyebright Blend from Solaray contains most of the herbs listed above.

RECOMMENDATIONS

❑ Include the following in your diet: broccoli, raw cabbage, carrots, cauliflower, green vegetables, squash, sunflower seeds, and watercress.

❑ Drink fresh carrot juice. This can help to prevent or alleviate some eye problems. Taking two tablespoons of cod liver oil daily can also be helpful.

❑ Eliminate sugar and white flour from your diet.

❑ If you wear glasses, wear clear spectacles that have been treated to keep out ultraviolet rays. This will help protect against damage from ultraviolet exposure. Avoid wearing tinted eyeglasses for this purpose, especially on a regular basis; dark glasses prevent needed light from entering the eyes. The functioning of the pineal gland, which plays an important role in the regulation of metabolism, behavior, and physiological functions, is largely governed by sunlight.

❑ Never use hair dyes containing coal tar on the eyelashes or eyebrows; doing so can cause injury or blindness. Although coal-tar dyes are legal, marketing them for the eyebrows and eyelashes is not.

❑ Be careful when using drugs, whether prescription or over-the-counter. Some may cause eye problems. Drugs that can cause damage to the optic nerve, retina, or other vital parts of the eye include:

- Adrenocorticotropic hormone, or ACTH (Acthar, Cortrosyn).

- Allopurinol (also sold under the brand name Zyloprim), which is used for gout.

- Anticoagulants such as heparin and warfarin (Coumadin).

- Aspirin.

- Corticosteroids, such as dexamethasone (Decadron), hydrocortisone (Cortenema, Hydrocortone, Solu-Cortef, VoSol HC), prednisolone (Blephamide, Hydeltra-T.B.A.), and prednisone (Deltasone).

- Chlorpropamide (Diabinese), which is used for non-insulin-dependent diabetes.

- Diuretics, antihistamines, and digitalis preparations. All of these can cause disturbances in color distinction.

- Indomethacin (Indocin), an arthritis medication.

- Marijuana.

- Nicotinic acid (niacin), if used for long periods.

- Streptomycin.

- Sulfa drugs.

- Tetracycline.

❑ Consult your health care provider if you develop any of the following conditions: change in pupil size; eye pain or pain on eye movement; impaired vision; intolerance to light; known exposure to gonorrhea or chlamydia; or swelling, tenderness, or redness around the eyes.

❑ If you have a baby or young child who exhibits any signs of eye infection, have the child evaluated by a professional.

CONSIDERATIONS

❑ There are three types of specialists who deal with the eyes:

1. Ophthalmologists are medical doctors who are eye specialists. They diagnose and treat eye disease, perform eye surgery, give eye tests, and prescribe corrective lenses.

2. Optometrists are not medical doctors, but they are licensed by the states to give eye tests and treat nonsurgical eye problems. They can prescribe corrective lenses, and in some states they can prescribe medication as well.

3. Opticians fill prescriptions for glasses and contact lenses. Only twenty-six states require opticians to be licensed.

❑ Because the light-absorbing retinal pigment is composed of vitamin A and protein, which are continually being used up as images are formed, adequate supplies of these nutrients are vital for proper eye function.

❑ The combination of nicotine, sugar, and caffeine may temporarily affect vision.

❑ Ophthalmologist and author Gary Price Todd, M.D., says that the use of margarine and vegetable shortening is dangerous for those with certain eye disorders. Butter and vegetable oils can be used as substitutes. For those who must undergo eye surgery, he suggests taking a multivitamin and mineral supplement the evening before the operation, preferably a formula including 10,000 international units of vitamin A, 1,000 milligrams of vitamin C, and 1,200 international units of vitamin E. He recommends continued use of these nutrients, plus 2 milligrams of copper and 20 milligrams of zinc daily, after surgery.

❑ Sea mussel is a source of protein that aids in the functioning of eye tissues and the secretion of eye fluids.

❑ Zinc may help reduce vision loss because it is a factor in the metabolic functioning of several enzymes in the chorioretinal complex (the vascular coating of the eye). Never take more than 100 milligrams daily, however.

❑ According to a report in *Ocular Diagnosis and Therapy,* ocular abnormalities can be hastened by anti-infective agents, diazepam (Valium), haloperidol (Haldol), some antidepressants, quinine, and sulfa drugs.

❑ People who work at computers every day are at risk for eyestrain, headaches, blurred vision, dry or irritated eyes, sensitivity to light, double vision, and after-images.

❑ People who wear contact lenses need to take precautions against eye damage because of the increased risk of injury and infection associated with them.

❑ Two recent studies have shown that leaving contact lenses in place for more than twenty-four consecutive hours can result in ulcerative keratitis, a condition in which the cells of the cornea are rubbed away by the contact lens, leading to infection and scarring. If not properly treated, this condition can cause blindness. Users of extended-wear lenses are ten to fifteen times more likely than other people to develop ulcerative keratitis, according to *The New England Journal of Medicine.* If ordinary daily-wear lenses are left in place overnight, the risk rises to the same level.

❑ Excise lasers, which break chemical bonds rather than produce heat, are used to shave dense superficial corneal scars so that people can see again. The scars must be no deeper than one-third the thickness of the cornea.

❑ Radial keratotomy is a surgical procedure in which a series of incisions is made in the cornea to alter its shape, in the hope of improving vision. It remains a controversial method of treating myopia (nearsightedness).

❑ Abnormalities in one or more of the six muscles that move the eyes, or a lack of coordination among these muscles, can result in a cross-eyed or walleyed condition. These muscles can be exercised and relaxed to improve their function. The internal muscles likewise can be exercised to improve the focusing ability of the eyes, both near and far.

prevent or correct eye trouble. Some of these supplements also protect against the formation of free radicals, which can damage the eyes. Specific eye problems that can be helped by supplementing the diet with vitamins and other nutrients are discussed in this section.

BAGS UNDER THE EYES

Skin loses some of its elasticity with age, and muscles within the eyelids lose tone, causing what is known as bags under the eyes. In addition, fat can gather in the eyelid, and fluids can accumulate and cause swelling. Puffiness around the eyes can also be caused by allergies or excessive consumption of salt. Smoking can aggravate the problem.

Recommendations

❑ Avoid drinking fluids before bed.

❑ Avoid salt.

❑ Do not smoke, and avoid secondhand smoke.

❑ Get plenty of sleep.

❑ Place a washcloth dipped in ice water over your eyes for fifteen minutes once or twice daily. You can also try using a wet tea bag or cold cucumber slices.

❑ *See* ALLERGIES in Part Two and take the self-test to determine allergens that may be causing the problem.

BITOT'S SPOTS

Bitot's spots are distinct elevated white patches on the conjunctiva, the membrane that covers most of the visible part of the eye. They may signify a severe deficiency of vitamin A.

NUTRIENTS

SUPPLEMENT	SUGGESTED DOSAGE	COMMENTS
Vitamin A	100,000 IU daily for two weeks, then 50,000 IU daily for 1 month, then reduce to 25,000 IU daily. If you are pregnant, do not exceed 10,000 IU daily.	Aids in dissolution of Bitot's spots, which may be caused by vitamin A deficiency. Use emulsion form for easier assimilation and greater safety at higher doses.

Recommendations

❑ Increase your intake of vitamin A.

❑ Avoid eyestrain and smoke-filled rooms.

BLEPHARITIS

Blepharitis is an inflammation of the outer edges of the eyelids that causes redness, itching, burning, and, often, a sensation of having something in one's eye. Other possible symptoms include swelling of the eyelids, loss of eyelashes, excessive tearing, and sensitivity to light. Secretions may form crusts that "glue" the eyes together during sleep.

This condition may be caused by an infection of the eyelash follicles or glands at the outer edges of the eyelids. Eyestrain, poor hygiene, poor living and sleeping habits, poor nutrition, and systemic disease with resulting immunodepression commonly contribute to the problem. Blepharitis may also be associated with seborrhea of the face or scalp.

NUTRIENTS

SUPPLEMENT	SUGGESTED DOSAGE	COMMENTS
Infla-Zyme Forte from American Biologics	As directed on label.	Aids in reducing inflammation.
Vitamin A plus	25,000 IU daily. If you are pregnant, do not exceed 10,000 IU daily.	Important in all eye disorders.
natural beta-carotene or	As directed on label.	Important antioxidants and precursor of vitamin A.
carotenoid complex (Betatene)	As directed on label.	
Vitamin C with bioflavonoids	6,000 mg daily, in divided doses.	A powerful antioxidant that protects the eyes and reduces inflammation.
Zinc	50 mg daily. Do not exceed a total of 100 mg daily from all supplements.	Needed for proper immune function. Use zinc gluconate lozenges or OptiZinc for best absorption.

Herbs

❑ Warm eyebright, goldenseal, or mullein compresses are soothing and help reduce inflammation. Prepare a tea using one of these herbs, cool it to a comfortably warm temperature, and soak a clean cloth or a piece of sterile cotton in it to make the compress. Apply the compress and relax for ten to fifteen minutes. Then make a fresh compress and gently wipe the edge of the eyelid and the area among the eyelashes to remove any scaly matter or dandruff-like debris. Do this twice a day or as needed. Use each compress only once before laundering or discarding it.

Recommendations

❑ Eat a well-balanced diet that emphasizes fresh, raw vegetables, plus grains, legumes, and fresh fruits.

❑ Keep the eyelids clean, especially along the edges (see the procedure described under Herbs, above), but do not touch or rub your eyes except when necessary. Always wash your hands before touching your eyes.

❑ Get sufficient sleep, and avoid eyestrain. Anything that increases eye fatigue makes the discomfort worse.

Considerations

❑ *See also* SEBORRHEA in Part Two.

BLOODSHOT EYES

Bloodshot eyes occur when the small blood vessels on the surface of the eye become inflamed and congested with blood, usually in response to an insufficient supply of oxygen in the cornea or tissues covering the eyes. They are a common consequence of eyestrain, fatigue, and improper diet, especially the consumption of alcohol.

A bloodshot appearance can also result from deficiencies in vitamins B_2 (riboflavin) and B_6 (pyridoxine), and the amino acids histidine, lysine, or phenylalanine. Once the body receives the nutrients it needs, the congestion in the blood vessels should disappear.

NUTRIENTS

SUPPLEMENT	SUGGESTED DOSAGE	COMMENTS
Vitamin A	50,000 IU daily. If you are pregnant, do not exceed 10,000 IU daily.	Needed for all eye disorders.
Vitamin B complex plus	100 mg 3 times daily.	Deficiencies have been linked to bloodshot eyes.
free-form amino acid complex	As directed on label.	Use a formula containing both essential and nonessential amino acids.

Herbs

❑ Use raspberry leaf to alleviate redness and irritation. Prepare a raspberry leaf tea, allow it to cool, and soak a clean cloth or piece of sterile cotton in the tea to make a compress. Apply the compress to the eyes with the lids closed for ten minutes or as needed.

BLURRED VISION

Vision may become blurred for any of a number of reasons. *Refractive error* (nearsightedness, farsightedness, and/or astigmatism) results in chronically blurry vision that can usually be overcome with corrective lenses. Eyestrain, fatigue, and excessive tearing can result in a temporary blurring of vision. A disturbance in the fluid balance in the body can also result in blurry vision.

A recurring tendency to periodic blurring can result from an inadequate supply of the light-sensitive pigment in the eye called rhodopsin, or visual purple, which is composed of vitamin A and protein. Any light that enters the eyes breaks down part of the visual purple, and the products of this purposeful breakdown set up nerve impulses that tell the brain what the eyes are seeing. If there is not enough pigment present, a time delay occurs between the time the eyes focus on an object and the time the brain forms an image of it. This is experienced as a blurring of vision.

NUTRIENTS

SUPPLEMENT	SUGGESTED DOSAGE	COMMENTS
Potassium	99 mg daily.	Needed to maintain proper fluid balance.
Vitamin A	25,000–50,000 IU daily. If you are pregnant, do not exceed 10,000 IU daily.	Necessary for pigment formation and proper balance of intraocular fluid.

CATARACTS

When the lens of the eye thickens, becoming clouded or opaque, it becomes unable to focus or admit light properly. This eye condition is referred to as a cataract. Some causes of cataracts include aging, diabetes, heavy metal poisoning, exposure to radiation, injury to the eye, and the use of certain drugs, such as steroids.

The main symptom of a developing cataract is a gradual, painless loss of vision. Cataracts are the number one cause of blindness in the world. Occasionally, a cataract may swell and cause secondary glaucoma.

The most common form of cataracts is senile cataracts, which affect people over sixty-five. This type of cataract is often caused by free radical damage. Exposure to ultraviolet rays and low-level radiation from x-rays leads to the formation of reactive chemical fragments in the eye. These free radicals attack the structural proteins, enzymes, and cell membranes of the lens. The free radicals in our food, water, and environment are probably a major factor in the increasing number of cataracts in our population.

NUTRIENTS

SUPPLEMENT	SUGGESTED DOSAGE	COMMENTS
Copper and	3 mg daily.	These minerals are important for proper healing and for
manganese	10 mg daily. Take separately from calcium.	retarding the growth of cataracts.
Grape seed extract	As directed on label.	A powerful antioxidant.
Glutathione	As directed on label.	A potent antioxidant that aids in maintaining a healthy lens and protects against toxins. Has been shown to slow the progression of cataracts.
L-Lysine	As directed on label, on an empty stomach. Take with water or juice. Do not take with milk. Take with 50 mg vitamin B_6 and 100 mg vitamin C for better absorption.	Important in collagen formation, which is necessary for lens repair. Also neutralizes viruses implicated in lens damage. *Caution:* Do not take lysine for longer than 6 months at a time.
Pantothenic acid (vitamin B_5)	500 mg daily.	An anti-stress vitamin.
Selenium	400 mcg daily.	An important free radical destroyer that works synergistically with vitamin E.
Vitamin A plus	25,000–50,000 IU daily. If you are pregnant, do not exceed 10,000 IU daily.	Vital for normal visual function.
natural beta-carotene or	As directed on label.	Precursor of vitamin A.
carotenoid complex (Betatene)	As directed on label.	
Vitamin B complex plus extra	As directed on label.	B vitamins work best when taken together.
vitamin B_1 (thiamine) and	50 mg each daily.	Important for intracellular eye metabolism.
vitamin B_2 (riboflavin)	50 mg each daily.	Deficiency has been linked to cataracts.
Vitamin C with bioflavonoids	3,000 mg 4 times daily.	A necessary free radical destroyer that also lowers intraocular pressure.

Vitamin E	400 IU daily.	An important free radical destroyer. Has been shown to arrest and reverse cataract formation in some cases.
Zinc	50 mg daily. Do not exceed a total of 100 mg daily from all supplements.	Protects against light-induced damage. Use zinc gluconate lozenges or OptiZinc for best absorption.

Herbs

❑ Bilberry extract, taken orally, supplies bioflavonoids that aid in removing toxic chemicals from the retina of the eye.

Recommendations

❑ Drink quality water, preferably steam-distilled. This is absolutely necessary in cataract prevention. Avoid fluoridated and chlorinated water. Even water from deeply driven wells may not be safe, since many aquifers (underground water sources), especially those located near or under farmland, are contaminated with toxic residue from farm runoff.

❑ Avoid dairy products, saturated fats, and any fats or oils that have been subjected to heat, whether by cooking or processing. These foods promote formation of free radicals, which can damage the lens. Use cold-pressed vegetable oils only.

❑ If you have cataracts, avoid antihistamines.

Considerations

❑ Taking vitamin C supplements for at least a decade and eating a diet rich in antioxidants can lower the risk of cataracts, according to researchers at the Harvard Medical School.

❑ In a study reported by the *British Medical Journal*, consumption of carotene and vitamin A was inversely related to the occurrence of cataracts. But only spinach—not carrots—appeared to protect against cataracts. Researchers theorize that a carotenoid other than beta-carotene is what exerts a protective effect.

❑ A number of heavy metals increase in concentration in the lenses of both aging people and people with cataracts. Cadmium, for instance, is found at levels two or three times higher than normal in lenses with cataracts. Concentrations of other metals, such as cobalt, nickel, iridium, and bromine, also are elevated.

❑ An article in *Science* magazine reported that the single greatest cause of cataracts is the body's inability to cope with food sugars. Lactose (milk sugar) was the worst offender, followed by refined white sugar. Many eye specialists note that most people with cataracts eat diets that include substantial amounts of dairy products and refined white sugar. Cataracts can also develop if the diet is inadequate and prolonged stress is endured.

❑ People who are deficient in the enzyme that converts galactose into glucose (ordinary blood sugar) develop cataracts much sooner than the rest of the population.

❑ Smoking is a risk factor for cataracts, probably because the free radicals it generates increase the oxidant stress on the body. A study of cigarette smoking and the risk of cataracts reported in the *Journal of the American Medical Association* found a significant association between smoking and the incidence of cataracts.

❑ The conventional treatment for cataracts is surgery. In cataract surgery, the eye's own dysfunctional lens is removed, and usually is replaced with a prosthetic lens implant. The lens may be removed whole, or a surgical procedure called phacoemulsification (often called the "phaco" technique) may be used. In this operation, the surgeon makes one minuscule incision, inserts the tip of a vibrating instrument into the cataract, and beats it until it turns liquid. The liquid is then sucked out and a new lens is implanted. With this type of surgery, the incision is only one-tenth of an inch long, compared to conventional one-third inch or one-half inch incisions.

❑ According to the National Eye Institute in Bethesda, Maryland, about 1.5 million Americans had cataract surgery in 1990, up from only 250,000 in 1980. Cataract surgery is among the most frequently performed operations in the United States. Yet a 1991 survey concluded that half of the people who had had cataract surgery were dissatisfied with the results. In some people, the capsules holding the lens implants become cloudy, diminishing vision. An ophthalmologist can correct this problem by using a laser to make a tiny hole in the capsule, clearing the passage to the retina. In 1991, this surgery was performed on more than 640,000 Medicare recipients, according to researchers at Georgetown University and Johns Hopkins Schools of Medicine. However, the *Wall Street Journal* has reported that people with cataracts who undergo this procedure are nearly four times more likely than others to suffer a detached retina or other difficulties, even vision loss. We believe that surgery should be resorted to only when absolutely necessary—when your natural lens becomes so opaque that you cannot read or drive.

COLORBLINDNESS

Colorblindness is a general term for the inability to see colors as most people see them. Specialized cells in the retina known as cones, which are vital for translating light waves into a perception of color, may be completely or partially lacking, or may not function properly, resulting in colorblindness. There are different types and varying severities of this condition. Most colorblind people confuse certain colors (they may not be able to tell red from green, for example); in rare cases, an individual may see no color at all. Some can distinguish colors only in certain lights.

There are also certain diseases, including pernicious anemia and sickle cell disease, as well as number of different medications, that can cause disturbances in color vision.

Because few people are tested for color vision, color-blindness is probably an underdiagnosed condition, especially among women. In most cases, colorblindness is present from birth, although the dimming of vision caused by cataracts can diminish a person's ability to distinguish colors later in life.

NUTRIENTS

SUPPLEMENT	SUGGESTED DOSAGE	COMMENTS
Vitamin A	50,000 IU daily. If you are pregnant, do not exceed 10,000 IU daily.	May be helpful because it is essential for proper functioning of the cones in the retina. Also improves night blindness. Use emulsion form, which is safe at higher doses than capsules.
Vitamin B12	2,000 mcg daily.	Deficiency can lead to yellow-blue colorblindness.

CONJUNCTIVITIS (PINKEYE)

Conjunctivitis is an inflammation of the conjunctiva, the membrane that lines the eyelid and wraps around to cover most of the white of the eye. The eyes may appear swollen and bloodshot; they are often itchy and irritated. Because the infected membrane is often filled with pus, the eyelids are apt to stick together after being closed for an extended period.

Factors that can contribute to conjunctivitis include bacterial infection, injury to the eye, allergies, and exposure to substances that are irritating to the eye, such as fumes, smoke, contact lens solutions, chlorine from swimming pools, chemicals, makeup, or any other foreign substance that enters the eye. Conjunctivitis is highly contagious if it is caused by a viral infection.

NUTRIENTS

SUPPLEMENT	SUGGESTED DOSAGE	COMMENTS
Vitamin A	100,000 IU daily for 1 month; then reduce to 25,000 IU daily. If you are pregnant, do not exceed 10,000 IU daily.	Vitamin A, vitamin C, and zinc all help to promote immunity, which is especially important in common viral conjunctivitis. Use an emulsion form for easier assimilation and greater safety at high doses.
Vitamin C	2,000–6,000 mg daily, in divided doses.	Protects the eye from further inflammation. Enhances healing.
Zinc	50 mg daily. Do not exceed a total of 100 mg daily from all supplements.	Enhances immune response. Use zinc gluconate lozenges or OptiZinc for best absorption.

Herbs

❑ Chamomile, fennel, and/or eyebright herbal teas can be used to make hot compresses. Eyebright can also be taken orally in capsule or tea form. It is good for any eye irritation or inflammation. The tea can also be used to rinse the eyes.

❑ Goldenseal, used as an alternative or in addition to eyebright, is very useful if conjunctivitis is caused by infection. *Caution:* Do not take goldenseal internally on a daily basis

for more than one week at a time. Do not use it during pregnancy.

Recommendations

❑ Apply hot compresses several times a day. Many of the microorganisms that cause conjunctivitis cannot tolerate heat. For greater benefit, use one of the herbal teas recommended above to make the compresses.

❑ If pain or blurred vision occurs, seek medical attention immediately. These can be signs of a more serious problem.

❑ If your eyelids are swollen, try peeling and grating a fresh potato, wrapping it with gauze, and placing it over your eyes. This acts as an astringent and has a healing effect.

Considerations

❑ Pinkeye associated with hay fever can be treated with prescription drops containing steroids.

❑ A bacterial infection is typically treated with antibiotics if the eye does not improve within four days of using compresses and taking supplements.

CORNEAL ULCER

If the cornea—the membrane covering the front of the eye—is damaged, the eye becomes inflamed and vulnerable to infection that can result in ulceration. Damage may occur as a result of injury, a foreign body in the eye, or excessive or inappropriate wearing of contact lenses. The infections that can result in ulceration of the cornea may be caused by viruses, bacteria, or fungi.

NUTRIENTS

SUPPLEMENT	SUGGESTED DOSAGE	COMMENTS
Vitamin A	50,000 IU daily. If you are pregnant, do not exceed 10,000 IU daily.	Needed for all eye disorders.
Vitamin C	6,000 mg daily, in divided doses.	A healing and antiviral substance.

Recommendation

❑ If you suspect that a corneal ulcer may be developing, consult a physician immediately.

DIABETIC RETINOPATHY

Diabetes can cause retinopathy, a disorder in which some of the tiny capillaries that nourish the retina leak fluid or blood that can damage the rod and cone cells. New capillaries then begin to form in the injured area, and these also interfere with vision. Diabetic retinopathy affects about 7 million Americans and causes blindness among about 7,000 each year. Unfortunately, there are few warning signs; the condition usually causes no symptoms until it is relatively advanced.

NUTRIENTS

SUPPLEMENT	SUGGESTED DOSAGE	COMMENTS
Vitamin A	50,000 IU daily. If you are pregnant, do not exceed 10,000 IU daily.	Needed for all eye disorders.
Shark cartilage (BeneFin)	1 gm per 15 lbs of body weight daily, divided into 3 doses. If you cannot tolerate taking it orally, it can be administered rectally in a retention enema.	To prevent or possibly halt the progression of the condition by inhibiting the growth of tiny blood vessels in the eye that contribute to vision loss.

Recommendations

❑ *See* DIABETES in Part Two and follow the dietary recommendations.

❑ If you have diabetes, make sure to have an annual eye examination to detect the onset of retinopathy. If the disorder is detected in time, laser surgery to seal leaking blood vessels can help stem vision loss.

Considerations

❑ A study reported that insulin-dependent (type I) diabetics who controlled their blood sugar levels tightly were able to slow the pace of retinopathy by about 60 percent.

❑ Researchers at the National Eye Institute induced a condition resembling diabetic retinopathy in dogs and then treated the animals with an experimental drug called sorbinil, which suppresses the action of an enzyme that converts excess sugar in the blood into an alcohol that seems to damage the retinal blood vessels. In this study, the sorbinil treatment totally blocked the progression of retinopathy.

DIMNESS OR LOSS OF VISION

Many different conditions can lead to a dimming or loss of vision. Among the most common are cataracts, glaucoma, and diabetic retinopathy. Macular degeneration and retinitis pigmentosa are less common, but do occur with some frequency. There are others as well. *Retinal detachment* causes a loss of vision often compared to having a curtain drawn across one's field of vision. Loss of vision may be preceded by a shower of "sparks" or lightning-like flashes of light, or by a dramatic increase in the number of black floaters in the field of vision. *Uveitis* is an inflammation in the middle layer of the eye, which consists of the iris, the ciliary body, and the choroid. In many cases it is caused by an underlying systemic disease such as rheumatoid arthritis or infection. Pain and redness may be present, but often symptoms consist primarily of diminished or hazy vision. Another condition that can lead to loss of vision is *blockage of a blood vessel serving the retina,* usually by a blood clot. Visual loss is generally sudden if the affected blood vessel is an artery, but it may be less rapid if the blocked vessel is a vein. Usually only one eye is affected.

Inflammation of the optic nerve is another possible cause of vision loss. Such inflammation may occur as a result of a systemic illness or infection, but in many cases the cause cannot be determined. This condition usually affects only one eye but it may affect both, causing varying degrees of vision loss over the course of a few days. *Toxic amblyopia* is a condition in which a toxic reaction damages the optic nerve, creating a small "hole" in the field of vision that enlarges over a period of time and may even lead to blindness. In most cases, both eyes are affected. This disorder is most common in people who smoke—in fact, it is sometimes referred to as *tobacco amblyopia*—and is seen most often in pipe smokers. It may also occur in those who consume excessive amounts of alcohol or who come into contact with lead, methanol, chloramphenicol, digitalis, ethambutol, and other chemicals.

Recommendations

❑ If any of the above symptoms develop, consult a physician. For most of these conditions, prompt treatment may help to preserve sight or at least slow vision loss.

❑ Do not smoke, and avoid those who do. Even people who have already developed toxic amblyopia as a result of smoking can have their vision improve if they quit.

Considerations

❑ The syndromes discussed here are usually painless. Physical discomfort is not a reliable indicator of visual health. Regular ophthalmic examinations are recommended for everyone over thirty-five.

❑ *See also* CATARACTS; DIABETIC RETINOPATHY; GLAUCOMA; MACULAR DEGENERATION; and RETINITIS PIGMENTOSA in this section.

DRY EYES

Dry eyes occur when the tear ducts do not produce enough fluid (tears) to keep the eyes moist, resulting in burning and irritation. This problem is more common in women than in men, and women's susceptibility increases after menopause. Contact lens wearers are particularly prone to develop dry eye problems. Dry eyes generally stem from a lack of vitamin A. This problem often comes with age, but it can also be caused by certain drugs, including the antidepressant imipramine (Tofranil), beta-blockers (used for treatment of high blood pressure and heart problems), and marijuana.

NUTRIENTS

SUPPLEMENT	SUGGESTED DOSAGE	COMMENTS
Primrose oil	1,000 mg 2–3 times daily.	A source of essential fatty acids.
Vitamin A ointment and/or	As directed on label.	Beneficial for eyes that seem dry and scratchy. Tears contain
vitamin A	25,000 IU daily. If you are pregnant, do not exceed 10,000 IU daily.	vitamin A.

Recommendations

❑ See your health care provider if you have dry eyes. It may be a symptom of a more serious condition, such as rheumatoid arthritis or lupus. Also, constant irritation to the eye as a result of dryness can result in injury and damage.

❑ If your tear ducts are swollen, add more calcium to your diet and avoid processed foods.

❑ Use a humidifier to add moisture to the air.

❑ Wear wraparound glasses on windy days.

❑ Avoid cigarette smoke and other types of smoke.

❑ Avoid products that claim they can "get the red out."

❑ Limit your use of hair dryers. Allow your hair to dry naturally.

Considerations

❑ In some cases, an ophthalmologist may perform a procedure to close the internal tear ducts, through which some tears drain from the eyes into the nose, to conserve tears and keep the eyes moist.

EYESTRAIN

Eyestrain causes a dull, aching sensation around and behind the eyes that can expand into a generalized headache. It may feel painful or fatiguing to focus the eyes. Eyestrain is commonly a result of overuse of the eyes for activities requiring close, precise focus, such as reading or computer work. People in certain occupations, such as jewelers, are particularly prone to eyestrain. Wearing improper lenses (whether the wrong prescription or an incorrectly made pair of glasses) can also cause eyestrain.

Acute closed-angle glaucoma can cause pain around the eyes as well, but the sensation is usually sharp and throbbing and accompanied by other symptoms. Most other eye disorders, even serious ones, cause little or no discomfort.

NUTRIENTS

SUPPLEMENT	SUGGESTED DOSAGE	COMMENTS
Vitamin A	50,000 IU daily. If you are pregnant, do not exceed 10,000 IU daily.	Needed for all eye disorders.
Vitamin B complex plus extra	50–100 mg daily.	Improves intraocular cellular metabolism.
vitamin B₂ (riboflavin)	25 mg 3 times daily.	Helps to alleviate eye fatigue.

Herbs

❑ Taking eyebright in capsule or tea form can be helpful. Eyebright tea can also be used to rinse the eyes.

❑ Goldenseal can be used as an alternative or in addition to eyebright.
Caution: Do not take goldenseal internally on a daily basis for more than one week at a time, do not use it during

pregnancy, and use it with caution if you are allergic to ragweed.

Recommendations

❑ Lie down, close your eyes, and place a cold compress over your eyes. Relax for ten minutes or longer, replacing the compress with a fresh one as necessary. This often helps to alleviate discomfort.

❑ Take measures to avoid eyestrain. Try to vary your tasks so that your eyes change focusing distance every so often. When doing close work for prolonged periods, take periodic "focus breaks." Every twenty minutes or so, look away from your work and focus your eyes on something in the distance for a minute or two.

❑ Get sufficient sleep. Fatigue promotes eyestrain.

❑ If pain is severe and comes on suddenly, and especially if vision is disturbed or the pain is accompanied by nausea and vomiting, seek professional help at once. This may be a sign of an acute glaucoma attack. *See* GLAUCOMA in Part Two.

FLOATERS

Bits of cellular debris floating within the eye are commonly referred to as floaters. Because these floaters cast shadows over the retina, the individual sees small specks that move slowly before the eyes, especially in certain lights and against certain backgrounds. Elderly and nearsighted people are most likely to complain of floaters. Most floaters eventually become less noticeable and are considered benign.

NUTRIENTS

SUPPLEMENT	SUGGESTED DOSAGE	COMMENTS
Apple pectin	As directed on label.	Chelates heavy metals that can circulate through the eyes.
L-Methionine	As directed on label, on an empty stomach. Take with water or juice. Do not take with milk. Take with 50 mg vitamin B₆ and 100 mg vitamin C for better absorption.	Chelates heavy metals. *See* AMINO ACIDS in Part One.
Oxy-5000 Forte from American Biologics	As directed on label.	A potent nutritional antioxidant for health and stress that destroys free radicals.
Vitamin A	50,000 IU daily. If you are pregnant, do not exceed 10,000 IU daily.	Needed for all eye disorders.

Recommendations

❑ It is normal to see a few floaters at times, but if you suddenly see a large number of them, consult an ophthalmologist. This may be a sign of developing retinal detachment. Delaying treatment can result in a detached retina requiring lengthy surgery.

GLAUCOMA

Glaucoma is a serious eye disease marked by an increase in the pressure that the fluids within the eyeball exert on other parts of the eye. If this pressure is unrelieved, it may harm the retina and ultimately damage the optic nerve, resulting in vision loss, even blindness. It is most common in people over thirty-five, in nearsighted people, and in people with high blood pressure. *See* GLAUCOMA in Part Two for a more complete discussion of this condition.

ITCHY OR TIRED EYES

Itchy or tired eyes can be the result of many different factors, including allergies, eyestrain, fatigue, infection (conjunctivitis), and an inadequate supply of oxygen to the cornea and outer eye tissues.

NUTRIENTS

SUPPLEMENT	SUGGESTED DOSAGE	COMMENTS
Vitamin A	50,000 IU daily. If you are pregnant, do not exceed 10,000 IU daily.	Needed for all eye disorders.
Vitamin B complex plus extra	50–100 mg daily.	Improves intraocular cellular metabolism.
vitamin B₂ (riboflavin)	50 mg daily.	Helps improve oxygenation of eye tissues.

Recommendations

❑ For quick relief of occasional itchy or tired eyes, close your eyes and apply a cold compress. Leave the compress in place for ten minutes. Compresses can be used as often as necessary.

Considerations

❑ If the problem is a recurrent one, allergies are a likely culprit. (*See* ALLERGIES in Part Two.)

❑ If itching and aching are accompanied by a bright pink or red color and thick secretions, you may have conjunctivitis. (*See* CONJUNCTIVITIS in this section.)

❑ If itchy and tired eyes persist over a long period of time, there may be an underlying nutritional cause. Supplement your diet with the B vitamins as described under Nutrients, above.

MACULAR DEGENERATION

This disorder causes a progressive visual loss due to degeneration of the macula, the portion of the retina responsible for fine vision. Macular degeneration is the leading cause of severe visual loss in the United States and Europe in people over fifty-five years old. This loss of vision may appear suddenly or it may progress slowly. Usually peripheral and color vision are unaffected.

There are two types of macular degeneration: atrophic (or "dry") and exudative ("wet"). In the latter type, the degeneration of the macula is accompanied by hemorrhaging or leaking of fluid from a network of tiny blood vessels that develop under the center of the retina. This results in scarring and loss of vision.

Macular degeneration is probably the result of free radical damage similar to the type of damage that induces cataracts. Factors that predispose a person to developing macular degeneration include aging, atherosclerosis, hypertension, annd environmental toxins. Heredity may play a role as well.

NUTRIENTS

SUPPLEMENT	SUGGESTED DOSAGE	COMMENTS
Natural beta-carotene or	2,000 IU daily.	Good for all eye disorders.
carotenoid complex (Betatene)	As directed on label.	
Bilberry		*See under* Herbs, below.
Grape seed extract	As directed on label.	A powerful antioxidant that protects against free radical damage.
Selenium	400 mcg daily.	An important antioxidant.
Shark cartilage (BeneFin)	1 gm per 15 lbs of body weight daily, divided into 3 doses. If you cannot tolerate taking it orally, it can be administered rectally in a retention enema.	To prevent and possibly halt the progression of exudative macular degeneration by inhibiting the growth of tiny blood vessels in the eye that contribute to vision loss.
Vitamin A	50,000–100,000 IU daily.	Potent antioxidant and important in eye function. Use emulsion form for easier assimilation and greater safety at high doses.
Vitamin C with bioflavonoids	1,000–2,500 mg 4 times daily.	An important antioxidant and a necessary free radical destroyer. Prevents eye damage; also relieves pressure from cataracts.
Vitamin E	600–800 IU daily.	An important antioxidant and free radical destroyer.
Zinc	45–80 mg daily. Do not exceed a total of 100 mg daily from all supplements.	Deficiency has been linked to eye disorders. Use zinc picolinate form.

Herbs

❑ Clinical studies have shown that taking bilberry extract (160 milligrams and up daily) and eating fresh blueberries (8 to 10 ounces per day), plus taking ginkgo biloba extract and zinc, can help halt the loss of vision. Blueberries are rich in valuable flavonoids. Treatment at an early stage is most effective.

Recommendations

❑ Increase your consumption of legumes; yellow vegetables; flavonoid-rich berries such as blueberries, blackberries, and cherries; and foods rich in vitamins E and C, such as raw fruits and vegetables.

❑ Avoid alcohol, cigarette smoke, all sugars, saturated fats, and foods containing fats and oils that have been subjected to heat and/or exposed to the air, such as fried foods, hamburgers, luncheon meats, and roasted nuts.

Considerations

❑ In a study reported in the *Archives of Ophthalmology*, ophthalmologists at Louisiana State University Medical School tested the effects of supplemental zinc on people suffering from macular degeneration. Half the group received a 100-milligram tablet of zinc twice a day; the other half received a placebo. After twelve to twenty-four months, the zinc group showed significantly less deterioration than the placebo group.

MUCUS IN THE EYES

❑ A number of different conditions can cause mucus to accumulate in the eyes, such as allergies, head colds, and infection (conjunctivitis).

Herbs

❑ Gently and carefully wash each eye with diluted alcohol-free goldenseal extract or cool goldenseal tea.

Caution: Do not use goldenseal during pregnancy, and use it with caution if you are allergic to ragweed.

PHOTOPHOBIA

Photophobia is an abnormal inability of the eyes to tolerate light; exposure to light hurts the eyes. It is more common in people with light-colored eyes, and usually is not a serious problem. In some cases, however, it may be associated with irritation or damage to the cornea, acute glaucoma, or uveitis. It can also be a symptom of developing measles.

NUTRIENTS

SUPPLEMENT	SUGGESTED DOSAGE	COMMENTS
Vitamin A	50,000 IU daily. If you are pregnant, do not exceed 10,000 IU daily.	Needed for all eye disorders.

Considerations

❑ *See also* GLAUCOMA and/or MEASLES, both in Part Two.

❑ *See also* the discussion of uveitis under Dimness or Loss of Vision in this section.

PINKEYE

See CONJUNCTIVITIS in this section.

RETINAL EDEMA

See VASCULAR RETINOPATHY in this section.

RETINAL HEMORRHAGE

See VASCULAR RETINOPATHY in this section.

RETINITIS PIGMENTOSA

Retinitis pigmentosa is an inherited disease that affects approximately 1 out of every 3,700 people. In this disorder, metabolic flaws slowly but progressively destroy retinal cells. The first symptom usually is loss of night vision, beginning in adolescence or young adulthood. This is followed by loss of peripheral vision and, ultimately, blindness, which sets in anywhere between the ages of thirty and eighty.

NUTRIENTS

SUPPLEMENT	SUGGESTED DOSAGE	COMMENTS
Vitamin A	75,000 IU daily. If you are pregnant, do not exceed 10,000 IU daily.	Helpful for all eye disorders. Use emulsion form for easier assimilation and greater safety at higher doses.

Considerations

❑ High doses of vitamin A can slow the loss of remaining eyesight by about 20 percent per year, according to Dr. Eliot Berson, professor of ophthalmology at Harvard Medical School.

❑ More information on this disorder can be obtained by calling the Retinitis Pigmentosa Foundation at 800–683–5555.

SHINGLES (HERPES ZOSTER)

Shingles is an infection caused by the varicella-zoster virus, a member of the herpes family and the same virus that causes chickenpox. The characteristic symptom is a rash of painful blisters. Shingles can appear anywhere on the body. If it occurs on the forehead near the eyes or on the tip of the nose, the eyes are likely to become involved, and damage to the cornea can occur. Taking the proper supplements when blisters first appear can make the blisters dry up quickly, and the discomfort may be alleviated.

NUTRIENTS

SUPPLEMENT	SUGGESTED DOSAGE	COMMENTS
Vitamin C with bioflavonoids	2,000–6,000 mg daily and up.	An antiviral and immune system enhancer.
Vitamin A	50,000 IU daily.	Needed for all eye disorders.
Vitamin B$_{12}$	2,000 mcg 3 times daily, on an empty stomach.	Prevents damage to the nerves in the eyes. Use a lozenge or sublingual form.
Vitamin E	1,000 IU daily. If you have high blood pressure and have not taken vitamin E previously, start with 400 IU daily and slowly increase to 800 IU daily.	Helps to prevent scarring and tissue damage.

| L-Lysine | 1,000 mg daily, on an empty stomach. Take with water or juice. Do not take with milk. Take with 50 mg vitamin B$_6$ and 100 mg vitamin C for better absorption. | Fights herpesviruses. *See* AMINO ACIDS in Part One. *Caution:* Do not take lysine longer than 6 months at a time. |

Recommendations

❑ If shingles appear on the forehead near the eyes or on the tip of the nose, seek treatment from an ophthalmologist.

❑ Apply zinc oxide cream to the blisters and the affected area. After the blisters have healed over, apply aloe gel and vitamin E to the area.

Considerations

❑ If zinc oxide, aloe gel, and/or vitamin E do not work to heal the blisters within three days, intravenous injections of 25 grams of vitamin C should provide relief almost immediately.

❑ *See also* SHINGLES in Part Two.

SCOTOMA

A scotoma is a blind spot in the visual field. Unless a scotoma is large or is located in the center of the field of vision, it may not be noticed. However, a professional can detect scotomas with a type of examination called a visual field test.

Scotomas are considered a symptom of disease, not a disease in themselves. They may be a sign of a problem with the retina or damage to the optic nerve, such as that caused by glaucoma.

NUTRIENTS

SUPPLEMENT	SUGGESTED DOSAGE	COMMENTS
Vitamin A emulsion or capsules	100,000 IU daily for 2 months. If you are pregnant, do not exceed 10,000 IU daily. 25,000 IU daily for 2 months. If you are pregnant, do not exceed 10,000 IU daily.	Essential for eye health. Use emulsion form for easier assimilation and greater safety at higher doses.

STYE

A stye is a bacterial infection within an oil gland on the edge of the eyelid. Because the tissues of the eye become inflamed from the infection, the stye takes on the appearance of a small pimple. This pimple gradually comes to a head, opens, and drains. Early treatment speeds the healing process and helps to avoid further complications.

Herbs

❑ Prepare raspberry leaf tea and use it as an eyewash to alleviate styes.

Recommendations

❑ Apply a hot compress to the affected area for ten minutes four to six times daily to help relieve discomfort and bring the stye to a head so that it can drain and healing can begin.

❑ If you suffer from styes frequently, supplement your diet with vitamin A. Recurring styes are often a sign of vitamin A deficiency.

Considerations

❑ If a stye does not heal promptly, it may need to be drained. This is a procedure that must be done by a health care professional. *Do not* squeeze the lump or attempt to drain it at home. This can cause the infection to spread into the bloodstream, leading to systemic illness.

❑ In severe and/or stubborn cases, treatment with antibiotics may be necessary.

THINNING EYELASHES

Many problems can lead to a thinning or even the total loss of the eyelashes. Among these are allergies, especially contact allergies to eye makeup; the use of certain drugs; exposure to environmental toxins; hypothyroidism; eye surgery; a poor diet and/or nutritional deficiencies; and trauma.

NUTRIENTS

SUPPLEMENT	SUGGESTED DOSAGE	COMMENTS
Vitamin A	50,000 IU daily. If you are pregnant, do not exceed 10,000 IU daily.	Promotes healthy skin and hair. Needed for all eye disorders.
Vitamin B complex plus extra	50–100 mg daily.	The B vitamins help prevent loss of eyelashes.
vitamin B$_2$ (riboflavin) and	As directed on label.	
vitamin B$_3$ (niacin) plus	As directed on label.	
brewer's yeast	2 tbsp daily.	A good source of B vitamins.

Recommendation

❑ Gently rub castor oil, linseed oil, or vitamin E oil on your eyelashes and into your eyelids at bedtime. This helps to thicken the lashes and promote normal growth.

ULCERATED EYE

See CORNEAL ULCER in this section.

ULCERATED EYELID

If an eyelid is scratched and the scratch becomes infected, an ulcerated area may develop. Ulcerated eyelids also can occur as a result of chronic blepharitis.

NUTRIENTS

SUPPLEMENT	SUGGESTED DOSAGE	COMMENTS
Vitamin A	50,000 IU daily. If you are pregnant, do not exceed 10,000 IU daily.	Promotes healing of skin.
Vitamin C with bioflavonoids	5,000–10,000 mg daily, in divided doses.	Improves circulation and aids in healing process. Also helps fight infection.
Vitamin E	400 IU daily.	Helps the body use oxygen efficiently and speeds healing.
Zinc	50 mg daily. Do not exceed a total of 100 mg daily from all supplements.	Promotes healing of tissues. Use zinc gluconate lozenges or OptiZinc for best absorption.

Herbs

❑ If an eye becomes inflamed due to an ulcerated eyelid, take yellow dock tea. Yellow dock tea can also be used to make a compress. Saturate a clean cotton cloth or piece of sterile cotton with the tea, and apply it to the inflamed eyelid. Leave the compress in place for ten to fifteen minutes. Repeat the procedure several times daily, as needed.

Considerations

❑ See also Blepharitis in this section.

VASCULAR RETINOPATHY

Vascular retinopathy is a general term for any of a group of disorders of the retina that arise from problems affecting the blood vessels, either locally (within the eye) or throughout the body. These problems can cause retinal hemorrhage (leakage from the vessels that transmit the fluids of the eye), microaneurysms (abnormally enlarged blood vessels in the eye), retinal edema (the accumulation of fluid in the eye), and, ultimately, loss of vision. Most cases are linked to diabetes or high blood pressure or both. Diabetic retinopathy is considered a form of vascular retinopathy.

NUTRIENTS

SUPPLEMENT	SUGGESTED DOSAGE	COMMENTS
Calcium and magnesium	1,000 mg daily. 500 mg daily.	A 2-to-1 ratio of calcium to magnesium helps microcirculation in the eye.
Selenium and superoxide dismutase (SOD) plus	100–200 mcg daily. As directed on label.	Potent free radical scavengers. Free radicals have been implicated in damage to the retina and microcirculation in the eye.
vitamin A and vitamin C and vitamin E	75,000 IU daily. If you are pregnant, do not exceed 10,000 IU daily. 2,000 mg 3 times daily. 400 IU daily.	Use emulsion form for easier assimilation and greater safety at higher doses.
Vitamin B complex	100 mg daily.	Improves intraocular cellular metabolism.

XEROPHTHALMIA

Xerophthalmia is an inflammation of the cornea that is associated with nutritional deficiency, especially a deficiency of vitamin A. The cornea becomes dry, and infection and/or ulceration may set in. Bitot's spots may appear, and night blindness may occur.

NUTRIENTS

SUPPLEMENT	SUGGESTED DOSAGE	COMMENTS
Vitamin A	25,000–50,000 IU daily. If you are pregnant, do not exceed 10,000 IU daily.	Specifically for dry eyes.
Vitamin B6 (pyridoxine) and	50 mg daily.	Nutrients that work well together to heal dry eyes.
vitamin C and	2,000–14,000 mg daily, in divided doses.	
zinc	50 mg daily. Do not exceed a total of 100 mg daily from all supplements.	Use zinc gluconate lozenges or OptiZinc for best absorption.

Considerations

❑ See also Bitot's Spots in this section.

Fatigue

Fatigue is not a disorder in itself; it is a symptom. Most illnesses, from the common cold to cancer, are accompanied by fatigue. Fatigue is often the earliest symptom of such health problems as diabetes, candidiasis, anemia, cancer, hypoglycemia, allergies, malabsorption, hypothyroidism, poor circulation, and mononucleosis. Extremely persistent and disabling fatigue is the chief symptom of chronic fatigue syndrome. Fatigue that is characterized by lack of energy only may be caused by boredom or depression. Persistent fatigue that is not caused by any underlying illness is usually the result of poor dietary lifestyle and habits, especially the combination of a high-fat and high-refined-carbohydrate diet and emotional stress. Alcohol, caffeine, drugs, tobacco, stress, and incorrect eating habits are all energy-robbers.

NUTRIENTS

SUPPLEMENT	SUGGESTED DOSAGE	COMMENTS
Very Important		
Bee pollen	A few granules daily for 3 days, then slowly increase to 2 tsp daily.	Often dramatically increases energy. *Caution:* Bee pollen may cause an allergic reaction in some individuals. Discontinue use if rash, wheezing, discomfort, or other symptom occurs.
Free-form amino acid complex	As directed on label.	Amino acids in free form are absorbed and assimilated quickly by the body.

Brewer's yeast or Bio-Strath from Bioforce	Start with 1 tsp daily and work up to 2 tbsp daily over a 2-week period. As directed on label.	A good source of B vitamins. A good tonic that contains B vitamins and herbs that increase energy levels.
Floradix Iron + Herbs from Salus Haus or desiccated liver	As directed on label. As directed on label.	A nontoxic form of iron from natural food sources.
Multivitamin and mineral complex with vitamin A and chromium and potassium and selenium and zinc	 25,000 IU daily. If you are pregnant, do not exceed 10,000 IU daily. 200 mcg daily. 99 mg daily. 100 mcg daily. 50 mg daily.	Vitamin and mineral deficiencies have been associated with a lack of energy. Use a high-potency formula.
Octacosanol	As directed on label.	Aids tissue oxygenation and increases endurance.
Vitamin B complex plus extra vitamin B$_{12}$ plus vitamin B$_1$ (thiamine) and pantothenic acid (vitamin B$_5$) and choline	100 mg 3 times daily, with meals. 2,000 mcg daily. 50 mg 3 times daily, with meals. 50–100 mg 3 times daily, with meals. 100 mg daily.	Deficiency can result in fatigue. Consider injections (under a doctor's supervision) if fatigue is severe. Fights fatigue and helps prevent anemia. Use a lozenge or sublingual form. Needed for normal brain function, hormone production, and conversion of fats, carbohydrates, and protein to energy.

Important		
Dimethylglycine (DMG) (Aangamik DMG from FoodScience Labs)	As directed on label.	Increases oxygen and energy levels in the body.
Vitamin C with bioflavonoids or E•mergen•C from Alacer	3,000–8,000 mg daily. As directed on label.	Increases energy levels. Increases energy levels quickly due to rapid assimilation into the body. Use between meals as a drink.

Helpful		
Energy Now from FoodScience Labs or PEP Formula from Pep Products	As directed on label. As directed on label.	Formulated to counteract fatigue.
Calcium and magnesium	1,500 mg daily. 750 mg daily.	Provides energy and plays an important role in protein structuring. Use calcium chelate or asporotate form. Needed to balance with calcium.
Kyo-Green from Wakunaga	As directed on label.	Supplies balanced nutrients for quick energy.
Pycnogenol or grape seed extract	As directed on label. As directed on label.	Powerful antioxidants that can pass the blood-brain barrier to protect brain cells.

L-Aspartic acid and L-citrulline plus L-phenylalanine	500 mg each twice daily, on an empty stomach. Take with water or juice. Do not take with milk. Take with 50 mg vitamin B$_6$ and 100 mg vitamin C for better absorption. 500 mg twice daily on an empty stomach.	Mood elevators that also increase stamina and endurance. Fatigue may result from low levels of aspartic acid. Elevates mood and helps overcome depression. *Caution:* Do not take phenylalanine if you are pregnant or nursing, or if you suffer from panic attacks, diabetes, high blood pressure, or PKU.
Royal Jelly from Montana Naturals	2 capsules 3 times daily.	Increases energy levels.
Shiitake or reishi	As directed on label. As directed on label.	To build immunity and boost energy levels.

HERBS

❑ Acacia, cayenne (capsicum), ginkgo biloba extract, gotu kola, guarana, and Siberian ginseng help combat fatigue.
   Caution: Do not use Siberian ginseng if you have hypoglycemia, high blood pressure, or a heart disorder.

❑ China Gold from Aerobic Life Industries is a liquid herbal combination formula that helps to boost energy.

RECOMMENDATIONS

❑ Include more fresh fruits and vegetables, grains, seeds, and nuts in your diet. Eat less red meat and more white fish.

❑ Avoid energy-robbers like sugar, alcohol, fats, caffeine, white flour products, and highly processed foods.

❑ Get regular exercise and adequate rest. If you are overweight, take measures to reduce your weight to normal. *See* OBESITY in Part Two.

❑ Use spirulina, an excellent protein source. Take 4 spirulina tablets three times a day with bee pollen, octacosanol, 3,000 milligrams of vitamin C, and free-form amino acids. This has been used for fatigue with good results.

❑ *See* FASTING in Part Three, and follow the program once monthly.

❑ If fatigue is persistent, consult your health care provider to determine whether some underlying health problem may be the cause.

CONSIDERATIONS

❑ Treatment with human growth hormone (available by a doctor's prescription only) can help to reduce fatigue. (*See* GROWTH HORMONE THERAPY in Part Three.)

❑ Allergies are often the cause of fatigue. Allergy testing, particularly testing for allergies to molds, is highly recommended.(*See* ALLERGIES and WEAKENED IMMUNE SYSTEM in Part Two.)

❑ Hypothyroidism can cause fatigue. (*See* HYPOTHYROID-ISM in Part Two for the underarm temperature test to determine if you have a low thyroid function.)

❑ Certain colors have energizing effects on the mind and body. (*See* COLOR THERAPY in Part Three.)

❑ If you find no physical reason for your fatigue, you should explore the possibility of a psychological basis and also seriously consider changing your lifestyle.

Fever

A fever is an elevation in body temperature. Fever is not a disease, but a symptom that may indicate the presence of disease.

Normal body temperature ranges from 98°F to 99°F. One should not have undue concern unless body temperature rises above 102°F in adults or 103°F in children. In fact, running a temperature is often helpful to the body. This defense mechanism of the body acts to destroy harmful microbes. A part of the brain called the hypothalamus regulates body temperature by regulating heat loss, mainly from the skin. When destructive microbes or tumor cells invade the body, the immune cells rushing to fight them release proteins that tell the hypothalamus to raise the temperature.

There are some situations, however, in which fever can cause problems. A moderately high fever may pose a risk for people with cardiac problems, since it makes the heart beat faster and work harder, and can cause irregular heart rhythms, chest pain, or a heart attack. Very high fever during the first trimester of pregnancy can cause birth defects. Fever over 105°F, especially for prolonged periods, can cause dehydration and brain injury. Fever can also cause discomfort.

Unless otherwise specified, the dosages recommended here are for adults. For a child between the ages of twelve and seventeen, reduce the dose to three-quarters the recommended amount. For a child between six and twelve, use one-half the recommended dose, and for a child under the age of six, use one-quarter the recommended amount.

NUTRIENTS

SUPPLEMENT	SUGGESTED DOSAGE	COMMENTS
Very Important		
Vitamin A emulsion or capsules	As directed on label. For adults: 50,000 IU daily for 1 week, then reduce to 25,000 IU daily. For children over 2 years: 1,000–10,000 IU daily. If you are pregnant, do not exceed 10,000 IU daily.	Essential in immune system function. Needed to fight infection and to strengthen the immune system. Emulsion form is recommended because it enters the system more quickly.
Dioxychlor from American Biologics	Take sublingually, as directed on label.	An important antibacterial, antifungal, and antiviral agent.
Infla-Zyme Forte from American Biologics	As directed on label.	A balanced, potent enzyme complex that moderates the inflammatory response.
Important		
Bio-Bifidus from American Biologics	As directed on label.	For bowel flora replacement to improve elimination and assimilation.
Free-form amino acid complex	As directed on label 3 times daily, on an empty stomach. Take with 50 mg each of vitamins B6 and C for better absorption.	A readily absorbed form of protein that helps repair tissue damaged by fever.
Taurine Plus from American Biologics	As directed on label.	An important antioxidant and immune regulator, necessary for white blood cell activation and neurological function. Use the sublingual form.
Vitamin C	5,000–20,000 daily, in divided doses. *See* ASCORBIC ACID FLUSH in Part Three.	To flush out toxins and reduce fever. For a child, use calcium ascorbate form—it does not produce heavy diarrhea.
Helpful		
Garlic (Kyolic)	2 capsules 3 times daily.	A natural antibiotic and powerful immunostimulant.
Royal jelly	As directed on label 3 times daily.	Has antifungal properties and improves adrenal function.
Spiru-tein from Nature's Plus	As directed on label, between meals.	A protein drink that contains all the amino acids, vitamins, and minerals needed for nourishment.

HERBS

❑ To bring a high fever down, use catnip tea enemas twice daily. These also relieve constipation and congestion, which keep fever up. *See* ENEMAS in Part Three.

❑ Catnip tea with dandelion and lobelia, taken in tea or extract form, is good for lowering fever. Lobelia can also be used on its own. Taking ½ teaspoon of lobelia extract or tincture every four hours helps to lower fever. If an upset stomach occurs, cut the dosage back to ¼ teaspoon.
Caution: Do not take lobelia internally on an ongoing basis.

❑ You can make a poultice from echinacea root to lower fever. *See* USING A POULTICE in Part Three.

❑ A combination of hyssop, licorice root, thyme, and yarrow tea can help a fever.
Caution: Do not use licorice on a daily basis for more than seven days in a row. Avoid it completely if you have high blood pressure.

❑ Other beneficial herbs include blackthorn, echinacea, fenugreek seed, feverfew, ginger, and poke root.
Caution: Do not use feverfew during pregnancy.

RECOMMENDATIONS

❑ Get plenty of rest while the temperature is elevated. Avoid rapid changes in temperature. Consume large quantities of liquids to prevent dehydration and flush out toxins.

❑ Drink plenty of distilled water and juices, but avoid solid food until the fever breaks.

❑ While feverish, avoid taking any supplements that contain iron or zinc. When an infection is present, the body attempts to "hide" iron in the tissues in an attempt to keep the infecting organism from using it for nourishment. Taking a supplement containing iron therefore causes undue strain on a body that is fighting an infection. Zinc is not properly absorbed while a fever is present.

❑ As long as a fever does not get too high (above 102°F), let it run its course. It helps to fight infection and eliminate toxins.

❑ If body temperature rises above 102°F (103°F in a child), take measures to reduce the fever, and consult your health care provider. This can be a sign of a worsening infection.

❑ Take cool sponge baths. Do not use rubbing alcohol to cool off; it gives off noxious fumes.

❑ See a health care professional immediately if you develop a fever associated with any of the following:

• Frequent urination, a burning sensation while urinating, or blood in the urine.

• Pain concentrated in one area of the abdomen.

• Shaking chills or alternating chills and sweats.

• Severe headache and vomiting.

• Profuse watery diarrhea lasting more than twenty-four hours.

• Swollen glands or rashes.

❑ Never give aspirin to a child with a fever. (*See* REYE'S SYNDROME in Part Two.)

CONSIDERATIONS

❑ Lingering or recurring flulike symptoms can be associated with diabetes (especially in children), hepatitis, Lyme disease, or mononucleosis (especially in adolescents). (*See* CHRONIC FATIGUE SYNDROME; DIABETES; HEPATITIS; LYME DISEASE; and/or MONONUCLEOSIS in Part Two.)

❑ Vigorous exercise, in which the muscles generate heat faster than the body can dissipate it, can cause a temporary rise in temperature.

Fibrocystic Disease of the Breast

It is estimated that more than 50 percent of adult females have fibrocystic disease of the breast. The condition is most common in women of childbearing age. It is characterized by the presence of round lumps in the breast that move freely and are either firm or soft. Symptoms include tenderness and lumpiness in the breasts. The discomfort is usually most pronounced before menstruation.

Normally, fluids from breast tissues are collected and transported out of the breasts by means of the lymphatic system. However, if there is more fluid than the system can cope with, small spaces in the breast may fill with fluid. Fibrous tissue surrounds them and thickens like a scar, forming cysts. Many breast cysts swell before and during menstruation, and the resulting pressure causes pain.

Cysts may even beget more cysts. A breast lump pressing against a milk gland can stimulate production of the pituitary hormone prolactin, which in turn results in milk secretion. The milk-producing glands may multiply and carry milk into the supporting fibrous tissue, causing further cyst formation.

Breast cysts may change in size, but they are benign. A cyst is tender and moves freely—it feels like an eyeball behind the lid. In contrast, a cancerous growth usually does not move freely, is most often not tender, and does not go away.

Most cysts are harmless. In fact, the normal structure of the breasts has a lumpy texture. However, this does not mean that any lumps should be disregarded. Each woman should be familiar with the normal feel of and cyclical changes in her breasts so that she can easily detect any new lumps. Ideally, she should check her breasts weekly, and if any new lumps become apparent between menstrual cycles, she should consult her health care provider promptly.

A physician can diagnose fibrocystic disease with a simple office procedure. Using a fine needle, he or she attempts to remove fluid from the lump. If fluid is present, the lump is a cyst. Usually a mammogram is recommended as well to rule out cancer.

NUTRIENTS

SUPPLEMENT	SUGGESTED DOSAGE	COMMENTS
Essential		
Coenzyme Q10	100 mg daily.	Similar to vitamin E in action, but more potent. A powerful antioxidant.
Kelp	1,500–2,000 mg daily, in divided doses.	A rich source of iodine. Iodine deficiency has been linked to this disease.
Primrose oil	1,500 mg daily.	May reduce the size of the lumps.
Vitamin E	400–600 IU daily.	Protects the breast tissue because of its antioxidant ability.
Very Important		
Vitamin A	15,000 IU daily. If you are pregnant, do not exceed 10,000 IU daily.	Needed for the ductal system of the breast.
plus natural beta-carotene or carotenoid complex (Betatene)	15,000 IU daily, with meals. As directed on label.	Antioxidant and precursor of vitamin A.
Vitamin B complex	50 mg 3 times daily, with meals.	B-complex vitamins are important for all enzyme systems in the body.
plus extra vitamin B6 (pyridoxine)	50 mg 3 times daily.	Needed for proper fluid balance and hormone regulation.

Important		
Vitamin C	2,000–4,000 mg daily, in divided doses.	Needed for proper immune function, tissue repair, and adrenal hormone balance.
Zinc	50 mg daily. Do not exceed a total of 100 mg daily from all supplements.	For repair of tissues and immune function. Use zinc gluconate lozenges or OptiZinc for best absorption.
Helpful		
Multimineral complex	As directed on label.	Balanced body minerals are important.
Proteolytic enzymes plus bromelain	As directed on label. Take with meals and between meals. As directed on label.	To reduce inflammation and soreness due to swelling.

HERBS

❑ The following herbs are good for fibrocystic disease of the breast: echinacea, goldenseal, mullein, pau d'arco, red clover, and squawvine.

Caution: Do not take goldenseal internally on a daily basis for more than one week at a time, as it may disturb normal intestinal flora. Do not use it during pregnancy, and use it with caution if you are allergic to ragweed.

❑ Use poke root or sage poultices to relieve breast inflammation and soreness. *See* USING A POULTICE in Part Three.

Note: Poke root is recommended for external use only.

RECOMMENDATIONS

❑ Eat a low-fat, high-fiber diet. Eat more raw foods, including seeds, nuts, and grains. Be sure nuts have not been subjected to heat. Include in your diet three or more servings daily of apples, bananas, grapes, grapefruit, raw nuts, seeds, fresh vegetables, and yogurt. Whole grains and beans should also be an important part of the diet.

❑ Include in the diet foods that are high in germanium, such as garlic, shiitake mushrooms, and onions. Germanium helps to improve tissue oxygenation at the cellular level.

❑ Do not consume any coffee, tea (except herbal teas), cola drinks, or chocolate. These foods contain caffeine, which has been implicated in fibrocystic disease. Also avoid alcohol, animal products (especially meats and animal fats), cooking oils from supermarket shelves, fried foods, salt, sugar, tobacco, and all white flour products.

CONSIDERATIONS

❑ Good results have been achieved using primrose oil to reduce the size of cysts.

❑ According to research done by Dr. John Peter Minton of the Department of Surgery at Ohio State University College of Medicine, Columbus, women who eliminate caffeine-containing substances from their diets have a high rate of success in eliminating cysts.

❑ The drug danocrine (Danazol), a hormone, acts through the pituitary gland, reducing the function of the ovaries. This in turn decreases the amount of estrogen in the breast, shrinking the lumps. Danocrine is not effective for all women, but about 60 percent notice results within a few weeks. Many report less pain or tenderness. The drug may have some unpleasant effects, however. It should be used only if the suggestions above fail to give the desired results.

❑ Thyroid function is important in fibrocystic disease; iodine deficiency can cause an underactive thyroid and has also been linked to fibrocystic disease. (*See* HYPOTHYROIDISM in Part Two.) Other factors include hormonal imbalance and abnormal production of breast milk brought about by high levels of the hormone estrogen.

Fibroids, Uterine

Uterine fibroids are benign growths that can form on the interior muscular wall as well as the exterior of the uterus. This disorder involves not only the uterus but sometimes the cervix also. The term "fibroid" may be somewhat misleading because the tumor cells are not fibrous. They are abnormal muscle cells.

It is estimated that 20 to 30 percent of all women develop fibroid tumors. For reasons not yet understood, they tend to form during the late thirties and early forties, and then to shrink after menopause. This would seem to suggest that estrogen is involved in the process, however, all women produce estrogen, but only some develop fibroid tumors. The presence of fibroid tumors does seem to have something to do with genetics, since they are known to run in families.

Most women who have fibroid tumors never even know it, unless they are discovered during the course of a routine pelvic examination. In roughly half of all cases, fibroid tumors cause no symptoms at all. In other cases, however, these growths cause abnormally heavy and frequent menstrual periods or even result in infertility. Other possible signs and symptoms include anemia, bleeding between periods, fatigue and weakness as a result of blood loss, increased vaginal discharge, and painful sexual intercourse or bleeding after intercourse. Depending upon their precise location, fibroids can cause pain and exert pressure upon the bowels or the bladder, or even block the urethra, producing kidney obstruction.

NUTRIENTS

SUPPLEMENT	SUGGESTED DOSAGE	COMMENTS
Coenzyme Q10	30 mg daily.	Promotes immune function and tissue oxygenation.
Floradix Iron + Herbs from Salus Haus	As directed on label. Do not take at the same time as vitamin E; iron depletes vitamin E in the body.	To supply iron in easily assimilable natural formula. Women with heavy menstrual flow as a result of fibroids are often anemic.

L-Arginine	500 mg daily, on an empty stomach. Take with water or juice. Do not take with milk. Take with 50 mg vitamin B$_6$ and 100 mg vitamin C for better absorption.	Enhances immune function and may retard tumor growth. *See* AMINO ACIDS in Part One.
and L-lysine	500 mg daily, on an empty stomach.	Needed to balance with arginine.
Maitake and/or shiitake	As directed on label. As directed on label.	To strengthen the body and improve overall health; have potent immunostimulant properties that inhibit tumor growth.
Multivitamin and mineral complex	As directed on label.	All nutrients are necessary in balance.
Vitamin A	25,000 IU daily.	Important in immune function and to promote tissue repair. Use emulsion form for easier assimilation and greater safety at higher doses.
Vitamin C	3,000–10,000 mg daily, in divided doses.	Promotes immune function and acts as an antioxidant.
Zinc	30–80 mg daily. Do not exceed a total of 100 mg daily from all supplements.	Needed for a healthy immune system.

RECOMMENDATIONS

❑ If you have unpleasant symptoms such as those outlined in this section, or if menstrual bleeding is so heavy that you saturate a pad or tampon more often than once an hour, consult your health care provider.

❑ If a fibroid is found, do not take oral contraceptives with a high estrogen content. High-estrogen birth control pills may stimulate the growth of fibroid tumors. Consider other forms of contraception, such as condoms and foam, a diaphragm, or a cervical cap.

CONSIDERATIONS

❑ Fibroids are almost never malignant, so treatment is not usually required as long as they remain relatively small and do not produce unpleasant symptoms.

❑ Women with fibroids may have higher levels of human growth hormone than other women.

❑ Uterine fibroids are five times more common in African-Americans than they are in Caucasians.

❑ A woman's chance of developing fibroids may be decreased if she avoids the use of oral contraceptives.

❑ In the past, it was a matter of general practice to perform surgery to remove fibroids if they grew to a point that the uterus was enlarged to the same extent it would be in a twelfth-week pregnancy. Increasingly, however, physicians are becoming more reluctant to remove these tumors based solely upon the "twelve-week rule" unless they are causing medical problems for the patient. Since these tumors usually shrink with the onset of menopause, the problem may well take care of itself over time.

❑ Over 30 percent of the hysterectomies performed in the U.S. are done to remove fibroid tumors. An alternative to hysterectomy is a procedure known as a myomectomy. This operation removes the fibroids, but leaves the uterus intact. This is an attractive alternative for a woman who wishes to bear children in the future, although it can be performed on any woman, regardless of age or childbearing desires. Myomectomy is more exacting surgery and places greater demands on the woman during recovery. There is also a slightly higher chance of complications with myomectomy than with hysterectomy, and the results are not always permanent. There is an estimated 50-percent chance that new tumors will form later, although they probably will not grow as large as the original fibroid tumors. If fibroids recur and cause symptoms, a repeat myomectomy can be performed.

❑ Any woman pondering a hysterectomy should give the matter close and careful consideration. (*See* HYSTERECTOMY-RELATED PROBLEMS in Part Two.)

Fibromyalgia Syndrome

Fibromyalgia is a rheumatic disorder characterized by chronic achy muscular pain that has no obvious physical cause. It most commonly affects the lower back, the neck, the shoulders, the back of the head, the upper chest, and/or the thighs, although any area or areas of the body may be involved. The pain is usually described as burning, throbbing, shooting, and stabbing. The pain and stiffness is often greater in the morning than at other times of day, and it may be accompanied by chronic headaches, strange sensations in the skin, insomnia, irritable bowel syndrome, and temporomandibular joint syndrome (TMJ). Other symptoms often experienced by people with fibromyalgia include premenstrual syndrome, painful periods, anxiety, palpitations, memory impairment, irritable bladder, skin sensitivities, dry eyes and mouth, a need for frequent changes in eyeglass prescription, dizziness, and impaired coordination. Such activities as lifting and climbing stairs are often very difficult and painful. Depression is frequently part of the picture as well. The most distinctive feature of fibromyalgia, however, is the existence of certain "tender points"—nine pairs of specific spots where the muscles are abnormally tender to the touch:

- Around the lower vertebra of the neck.
- At the insertion of the second rib.
- Around the upper part of the thigh bone.
- In the middle of the knee joint.
- In muscles connected to the base of the skull.
- In muscles of the neck and upper back.
- In muscles of the mid-back.
- On the side of the elbow.
- In the upper and outer muscles of the buttocks.

Most people with fibromyalgia also have an associated sleep disorder known as alpha-EEG anomaly. In this disorder, the individual's deep sleep periods are interrupted by bouts of waking-type brain activity, resulting in poor sleep. Some people with fibromyalgia are plagued by other sleep disorders as well, such as sleep apnea, restless leg syndrome, bruxism, and sleep myoclonus (a sudden rapid contraction of a muscle or a group of muscles during sleep or as one is falling asleep). Not surprisingly, given all these sleep difficulties, people with fibromyalgia often suffer from chronic fatigue that can range from mild to incapacitating.

This disorder is much more common in females than in males, and most often begins in young adulthood. In most cases, symptoms come on gradually and slowly increase in intensity. They can be triggered (or made worse) by a number of different factors, including overexertion, stress, lack of exercise, anxiety, depression, lack of sleep, trauma, extremes of temperature and/or humidity, and infectious illness. In the majority of cases, symptoms are severe enough to interfere with normal daily activities; a significant number of people with fibromyalgia are actually disabled by the condition. The course of the disorder is unpredictable. Some cases clear up on their own, some become chronic, and some go through cycles of flare-ups alternating with periods of apparent remission.

The cause or causes of fibromyalgia are not known. Some evidence points to a problem with the immune system; certain immunologic abnormalities are common among people with fibromyalgia. Their significance and relationship to the syndrome are not understood, however. A disturbance in brain chemistry may also be involved; many people who develop fibromyalgia have a history of clinical depression. Other possible causes that have been proposed include infection with the Epstein-Barr virus (EBV), the virus that causes infectious mononucleosis, or with the fungus *Candida albicans*; chronic mercury poisoning from amalgam dental fillings; anemia; parasites; hypoglycemia; and hypothyroidism. Some experts believe that fibromyalgia may be related to chronic fatigue syndrome (CFS), which causes similar symptoms, except that in fibromyalgia, muscle pain predominates over fatigue, whereas in CFS, fatigue predominates over pain.

Because malabsorption problems are common in people with this disorder, higher than normal doses of all supplemental nutrients are needed. Wherever possible, it is best to use sublingual vitamins and other supplements because they are more easily absorbed than tablets or capsules.

NUTRIENTS

SUPPLEMENT	SUGGESTED DOSAGE	COMMENTS
Essential		
Coenzyme Q10	75 mg daily.	Improves oxygenation of tissues, enhances the effectiveness of the immune system, and protects the heart.
Acidophilus (Kyo-Dophilus from Wakunaga, Bifido Factor from Natren)	As directed on label.	Candida infection is common in people with fibromyalgia. Acidophilus replaces "friendly" bacteria destroyed by candida. Use a nondairy formula.
Lecithin	As directed on label, with meals.	Promotes energy, enhances immunity, aids in brain function, and improves circulation.
Malic acid and magnesium	As directed on label.	Involved in energy production in many cells of the body, including the muscle cells. Needed for sugar metabolism.
Manganese	5 mg daily. Take separately from calcium.	Influences the metabolic rate by its involvement in the pituitary-hypothalamic-thyroid axis.
Proteolytic enzymes or Infla-Zyme Forte from American Biologics or Wobenzym N from Marlyn Nutraceuticals	As directed on label, 6 times daily, with meals, between meals, and at bedtime.	Reduces inflammation and improves absorption of foods, especially protein, which is needed for tissue repair.
Vitamin A and vitamin E or ACES + Zinc from Carlson Labs	25,000 IU daily for 1 month, then slowly reduce to 10,000 IU daily. 800 IU daily for 1 month, then slowly reduce to 400 IU daily. As directed on label.	Powerful free radical scavengers that protect the body's cells and enhance immune function. Use emulsion forms for easier assimilation. Contains vitamins A, C, and E plus the minerals selenium and zinc, to protect immune function.
Vitamin C with bioflavonoids	5,000–10,000 mg daily.	Has a powerful antiviral effect and increases the body's energy level. Use a buffered form.
Very Important		
Vitamin B complex injections plus extra vitamin B6 (pyridoxine) and vitamin B12 plus raw liver extract or	2 cc twice weekly for 1 month or as prescribed by physician. ¼ cc twice weekly for 1 month or as prescribed by physician. 1 cc twice weekly for 1 month or as prescribed by physician. 2 cc twice weekly for 1 month or as prescribed by physician.	Essential for increased energy and normal brain function. Injections (under doctor's supervision) are best. All injectables can be combined in a single syringe.
vitamin B complex	100 mg 3 times daily, with meals.	If injections are not available, or once the course of injections has been completed, use a sublingual form.
Dimethylglycine (DMG) (Aangamik DMG from FoodScience Labs)	50 mg 3 times daily.	Enhances oxygen utilization by the muscles and destroys free radicals that can damage cells.
Free-form amino acid complex	As directed on label.	To supply protein essential for repair and rebuilding of muscle tissue and for proper brain function. Use a formula containing all the essential amino acids.
Grape seed extract	As directed on label.	A powerful antioxidant that protects the muscles from free radical damage and enhances immunity.

Garlic (Kyolic) plus Kyo-Green from Wakunaga	2 capsules 3 times daily, with meals. As directed on label.	Promotes immune function and increases energy. Also destroys common parasites. To improve digestion and cleanse the bloodstream.

Important		
Calcium and magnesium or Bone Support from Synergy Plus plus potassium and selenium and zinc	2,000 mg daily. 1,000 mg daily. As directed on label. 99 mg daily. 200 mcg daily. 50 mg daily. Do not exceed a total of 100 mg daily from all supplements.	Needed to balance with magnesium. Needed for proper functioning of all muscles, including the heart; relieves muscle spasms and pain. Deficiency is common in people with this disorder. Contains calcium and magnesium plus other minerals to aid absorption. Involved in proper muscle function. An important antioxidant. Needed for proper functioning of the immune system.
Capricin from Probiologic	As directed on label.	To combat candida, which is associated with fibromyalgia.
DL-phenylalanine (DLPA)	500 mg daily every other week.	Can be very effective for controlling pain. Also increases mental alertness. Caution: Do not take this supplement if you are pregnant or nursing, or suffer from panic attacks, diabetes, high blood pressure, or PKU.
Essential fatty acids (black currant seed oil, flaxseed oil, and primrose oil are good sources)	As directed on label 3 times daily, with meals.	Protects against cell damage. Helps to reduce pain and fatigue.
Gamma-aminobutyric acid (GABA) or GABA Plus from Twinlab	As directed on label. As directed on label.	For proper control of brain function and to control anxiety. Contains a combination of GABA, inositol and niacinamide.
L-Leucine plus L-isoleucine and L-valine	500 mg each daily, on an empty stomach. Take with water or juice. Do not take with milk. Take with 50 mg vitamin B$_6$ and 100 mg vitamin C for better absorption.	These amino acids are found primarily in muscle tissue. They are available in combination formulas. See AMINO ACIDS in Part One.
L-Tyrosine	500–1,000 mg daily, at bedtime.	Helps to relieve depression and aids in relaxing the muscles. Caution: Do not take this supplement if you are taking an MAO inhibitor drug.
Melatonin	As directed on label, 2 hours or less before bedtime.	Promotes sound sleep. A sustained release formula is best.
Multivitamin and mineral complex plus natural carotenoids (Advanced Carotenoid Complex from Solgar)	As directed on label. 15,000 IU daily.	All nutrients are necessary in balance. Use a high-potency hypoallergenic formula.
Ocu-Care from Nature's Plus	As directed on label.	Contains essential nutrients to protect and nourish the eyes.

Raw thymus and raw spleen glandulars plus multiglandular complex	As directed on label. As directed on label. As directed on label.	To boost the immune system. See GLANDULAR THERAPY in Part Three.
Taurine	500 mg daily, on an empty stomach.	An important antioxidant and immune system regulator necessary for white blood cell activation and neurological function.
Vanadyl sulfate	As directed on label.	Protects the muscles and reduces overall body fatigue.

HERBS

❑ Astragalus and echinacea enhance immune function.

❑ Black walnut and garlic aid in removing parasites.

❑ Teas brewed from burdock root, dandelion, and red clover promote healing by cleansing the bloodstream and enhancing immune function. Combine or alternate these herbal teas, and drink 4 to 6 cups daily.

❑ Topical applications of cayenne (capsicum) powder mixed with wintergreen oil can help relieve muscle pain. Cayenne contains capsaicin, a substance that appears to inhibit the release of neurotransmitters responsible for communicating pain sensations. Use 1 part cayenne powder to 3 parts wintergreen oil. Cayenne can also be taken orally, in capsule form.

❑ Ginkgo biloba improves circulation and brain function.

❑ Licorice root supports the glandular system.
   Caution: If overused, licorice can elevate blood pressure. Do not use this herb on a daily basis for more than seven days in a row. Avoid it if you have high blood pressure.

❑ Milk thistle protects the liver.

❑ Pau d'arco, taken in tea or tablet form, is good for treating candida infection.

❑ Skullcap and valerian root improve sleep.

RECOMMENDATIONS

❑ Eat a well-balanced diet of 50 percent raw foods and fresh "live" juices. The diet should consist mostly of vegetables, fruits, whole grains (primarily millet and brown rice), raw nuts and seeds, skinless turkey or chicken, and deepwater fish. These quality foods supply nutrients that renew energy and build immunity.

❑ Eat four to five small meals daily to keep a steady supply of protein and carbohydrates available for proper muscle function. If the body does not have enough fuel for energy, it will rob the muscles of essential nutrients, causing muscle wasting and pain.

❑ Drink plenty of liquids to help flush out toxins. The best choices are steam-distilled water and herbal teas. Fresh vegetable juices supply necessary vitamins and minerals.

❑ Limit your consumption of green peppers, eggplant, tomatoes, and white potatoes. These foods contain solanine, which interferes with enzymes in the muscles, and may cause pain and discomfort.

❑ Do not eat meat, dairy products, or any other foods that are high in saturated fats. Saturated fats raise cholesterol levels and interfere with circulation. They also promote the inflammatory response and increase pain. Also avoid fried foods, processed foods, shellfish, and white flour products such as bread and pasta.

❑ Do not consume any caffeine, alcohol, or sugar. Eating sugar in any form—including fructose and honey—promotes fatigue, increases pain, and disturbs sleep. If these substances have been a regular part of your diet, your symptoms may actually get worse for a short period as a result of the "withdrawal" effect, but after that, you should experience a noticeable improvement in your condition.

❑ Avoid wheat and brewer's yeast until your symptoms improve.

❑ Maintain a regular program of moderate exercise. A daily walk followed by some gentle stretching exercises is good. If you have been sedentary before, start slowly and be careful not to overexert yourself; this can aggravate symptoms. Keep in mind that what you need is some amount of daily exercise, *not* a strenuous workout two or three times a week. Once your body is accustomed to regular exercise, symptoms are likely to improve.

❑ Be sure to give your body sufficient rest. Set aside at least eight hours for sleep each night.

❑ Take a hot shower or a bath upon arising to stimulate circulation and help relieve morning stiffness. Or alternate between hot water and cold water while showering. Recent studies have shown cold showers to be beneficial for relieving the pain of fibromyalgia.

❑ Take chlorophyll in tablet form or in "green drinks" such as Kyo-Green from Wakunaga of America. Spiru-tein from Nature's Plus is a good protein drink to use between meals to aid in maintaining energy levels and to reduce muscle pain.

CONSIDERATIONS

❑ Chronic pain sufferers, especially those with fibromyalgia and chronic fatigue syndrome, tend to be deficient in magnesium.

❑ Common painkillers such as aspirin, acetaminophen, and ibuprofen are not usually effective at relieving the pain of fibromyalgia. Other approaches, including attention to diet, exercise, and nutritional supplementation, are more likely to be of benefit.

❑ Many different disorders can cause symptoms similar to those of fibromyalgia, including anemia, depression, hepatitis, and Lyme disease, among others. Anyone who experiences muscular pain and/or fatigue that persists for longer than a week or two should consult a health care provider. There may be an underlying medical disorder that requires treatment.

❑ Recent research points to the possible involvement of chemical and/or food sensitivities in fibromyalgia, chronic fatigue syndrome, and the pain associated with these disorders. This would hardly be surprising, as humans have been exposed to more chemicals in the last fifty years than in all the rest of our history combined.

❑ Because malabsorption problems are common in this disorder, all nutrients are needed in greater than normal amounts, and a proper diet is essential. Colon cleansing is recommended to rid the gastrointestinal tract of mucus and debris, and so improve nutrient absorption. (*See* COLON CLEANSING in Part Three.)

❑ Many doctors prescribe low-dose antidepressants for fibromyalgia. These drugs can be beneficial in some cases, but can also cause a number of side effects, such as drowsiness. Other medical treatments that may or may not be of help to any given individual include muscle relaxants and/or local anesthetic sprays or injections for relief of pain. The antianxiety drug lorazepam (Ativan) is sometimes prescribed as well. This drug can cause a loss of equilibrium.

❑ Physical therapy, relaxation techniques, exercise therapy, massage therapy, deep heat therapy, and biofeedback are all helpful in some cases. Massage therapy is particularly beneficial for improved muscle function and pain relief. If you are diagnosed with fibromyalgia, it is wise to seek out a health care provider who has specific experience in the management and treatment of this condition.

❑ Food allergies can exacerbate the discomfort of many disorders. (*See* ALLERGIES in Part Two.)

❑ *See also* CHRONIC FATIGUE SYNDROME and DEPRESSION in Part Two.

❑ *See also* PAIN CONTROL in Part Three.

Flu

See INFLUENZA.

Food Poisoning

Food poisoning occurs when a person consumes food containing harmful toxins or microorganisms, usually bacteria. Each year more than 2 million Americans report illnesses that are traced to foods they have eaten. The actual number of food poisoning cases is almost certainly well above that number, however, because people often mistake the symptoms of food poisoning for those of intestinal flu.

Types of Food Poisoning

There are many different types of food poisoning, some more common than others. The following is a summary of some of these, together with the relative incidence and typical symptoms of each.

Type	Relative Incidence	Symptoms	Time Between Exposure and Onset of Symptoms
Botulism	Rare.	Double vision; difficulty speaking, breathing, and swallowing; nausea, vomiting, and abdominal pain; diarrhea; muscular weakness.	12–48 hours, but may be as long as 8 days.
Campylobacter infection	Common.	Muscular pain, nausea, vomiting, fever, abdominal cramps.	2–10 days.
Clostridium perfringens poisoning	Common.	Diarrhea, abdominal cramps.	9–15 hours.
Giardiasis	Common.	Nausea, gas, abdominal pain and/or cramping, diarrhea; in severe cases, malabsorption problems and weight loss.	1–3 weeks.
Listeriosis	Rare.	Flulike symptoms, including fever, chills; can cause spontaneous abortion or stillbirth; can cause severe illness in newborns and immune-depressed people.	2–4 weeks.
Norwalk virus infection	Common.	Nausea, vomiting, diarrhea, headache.	1–2 days.
Salmonellosis	Common.	Nausea, vomiting, diarrhea, abdominal cramps, fever, headache.	6–48 hours.
Scombroid poisoning	Uncommon.	Headache, dizziness, burning throat, hives, nausea, vomiting, abdominal pain.	5 minutes–1 hour.
Staphylococcal food poisoning	Common.	Vomiting, diarrhea; occasionally weakness, dizziness.	30 minutes–8 hours.
Trichinosis	Rare.	Fever, edema of eyelids, muscle pain.	1–2 days.

Symptoms of food poisoning may include nausea, vomiting, abdominal cramps and diarrhea, even chills, fever, severe headache, and worse, lasting from a few hours to a few days. Some types of food poisoning, such as botulism, are more serious, especially for elderly people and children. As many as 9,000 deaths occur annually from all types of food poisoning. In addition, many cases of food poisoning lead to chronic health disorders, such as reactive arthritis and chronic immune deficiency.

Pathogenic and toxigenic organisms—those that can cause disease and those that can produce harmful toxins—are silent killers because nothing about the taste, odor, or appearance of the food indicates their presence. All types of bacteria can potentially become toxigenic.

There are different types of food poisoning, depending on the agent that causes it (for a quick summary of some of these, see Types of Food Poisoning, above). The most common type is salmonellosis, or *Salmonella* infection. *Salmonella* bacteria are part of the natural intestinal flora of many animals. They are easily transmitted through the food supply, the hands of food preparers, and the surfaces of objects such as knives and tabletops. *Salmonella* thrive in livestock that have been given antibiotics. More than 50 percent of cattle, poultry, and swine in the United States are given antibiotics in their feed to make them grow faster and to prevent disease in crowded and unsanitary conditions. At least one-third of all chickens in the United States are infected with *Salmonella*. Salmonellosis is the leading cause of food poisoning death in America.

Symptoms of *Salmonella* infection can range from mild

abdominal pain to severe diarrhea and dehydration to typhoid-like fever. Symptoms usually develop within eight to thirty-six hours of eating contaminated foods. Diarrhea is often the first sign. *Salmonella* can also weaken the immune system and cause kidney and cardiovascular damage as well as arthritis.

Outbreaks of salmonellosis occur primarily in the warmer months. Most cases are the result of the consumption of contaminated foods, primarily chicken, eggs, beef, and pork products. People who eat raw or incompletely cooked meats are at greater risk of developing the disorder. Cooks who first handle raw meat or poultry and then handle other foods, without washing their hands in between, endanger others; cooks who lick their hands or fingers after handling raw meat or poultry put themselves at risk of *Salmonella* infection. People taking antibiotics are also at greater risk. Antibiotics can effectively treat bacterial infections, but, paradoxically, they can also promote infection by destroying good, competing bacteria and permitting the growth of bacteria that are antibiotic resistant.

In 1985, an outbreak of *Salmonella* from contaminated milk occurred in five Midwestern states. As a result, 17,000 people became ill and 2 died. Eggs were once thought to be free of *Salmonella*; however, there has been a dramatic increase in the number of reported cases of food poisoning from foods containing raw or only partly cooked eggs, particularly in the Northeast. These foods include ice cream, eggnog, Caesar salad dressing, and hollandaise sauce. Of thirty-five outbreaks of illness that were reported over a recent two-year period and determined to be food poisoning, twenty-four were caused by contaminated eggs or foods containing these infected eggs. Certain strains of bacteria found in eggs are not destroyed if the eggs are poached or prepared over easy or sunny-side up, in addition to other ways.

Salmonellosis as a result of the consumption of raw clams, oysters, and sushi made from raw fish has also been reported. Although this does not occur as often as *Salmonella* infection from eggs, meat, and poultry, it does happen.

After *Salmonella*, *Staphylococcus aureus* is the second most frequent cause of food-borne illness. Staphylococci are responsible for approximately 25 percent of all cases of food poisoning. This microorganism is commonly found in the nose and throat, but if a food product becomes contaminated with it (by being sneezed or coughed on, for example), the bacteria can grow and produce an enterotoxin, a toxin that specifically targets the cells of the intestines. It is this toxin, rather than the bacteria itself, that causes the food poisoning. Symptoms include diarrhea, nausea, vomiting, abdominal cramps, and prostration, usually beginning from two to eight hours after consumption of the contaminated food. Staphylococcal toxin is found most often in meat, poultry, egg products, tuna, potato and macaroni salads, and cream-filled pastries.

The bacterium *Clostridium botulinum*, which commonly inhabits the soil in the form of harmless spores, can cause a particularly dangerous type of food poisoning. Of the various types of food poisoning, botulism is the among the most severe. It affects the central nervous system. As with *Staphylococcus*, it is not the bacteria but rather toxins produced by the bacteria that cause the poisoning. The toxins produced by *C. botulinum* block the transmission of impulses from nerves to muscles, thus paralyzing the muscles. The paralysis often begins with the muscles that are responsible for eye movement, swallowing, and speech, and progresses to those in the torso and the extremities. Early symptoms of botulism include extreme weakness, double vision, droopy eyelids, and trouble swallowing. These symptoms typically appear twelve to forty-eight hours after ingestion of the contaminated food. Eventually, muscle weakness affecting the entire body, including the muscles required for breathing, can result. Paralysis and death may occur in severe cases.

Even though the U.S. Centers for Disease Control (CDC) reported only forty-two cases of botulism in the United States in 1994, it still remains a threat. Botulin toxin has been found in asparagus, beets, corn, stuffed eggplant, smoked and salted fish, green beans, ham, lobster, luncheon meats, mushrooms, peppers, sausage, soups, spinach, and tuna. Canned foods, especially those canned at home, are particularly prone to contamination with this potentially lethal organism. This is often due to improper canning techniques, usually the failure to use a pressure cooker to seal the jars adequately. A bulging lid or cracked jar can be a sign that the food within is contaminated, but botulism can occur even if a food container shows no signs of damage. Keeping food at room temperature for prolonged periods can also be a problem. In one reported case, a restaurant allowed a large batch of sautéed onions to be kept out throughout the day, instead of keeping them refrigerated, and small amounts were used as needed. Several people became very ill from botulin toxin in the onions.

Freezing, drying, and treatment with chemicals such as sodium nitrite prevent *C. botulinum* spores from growing and producing toxins. Although it does not kill the spores themselves, heating food to a temperature of at least 176°F for thirty minutes prevents food poisoning by destroying the lethal toxins.

A microorganism called *Campylobacter jejuni*, which has long been known to cause illness in cattle, has now been implicated in human illness as well. Many experts believe that the incidence of this infection is much higher than reported, because many people mistake it for a stomach virus. People tend not to associate their illness with food because it takes three to five days for these bacteria to produce symptoms, which include abdominal cramps, diarrhea, fever, and possibly blood in the stool. *C. jejuni* can be present in the intestinal tracts of apparently healthy cattle, turkeys, chickens, and sheep, and can be spread to all parts of the meat during the slaughtering process. Fortunately, heat destroys the bacteria, so it is possible to avoid this type of food poisoning by eating meat only if has been cooked thoroughly.

Another type of bacteria that can cause food poisoning

is *Clostridium perfringens*. *C. perfringens* often survives heat well, so it is not affected by normal cooking. The bacteria multiply, forming spores and generating toxins that proliferate as foods cool and while they are stored. The toxins also are often heat-resistant. The symptoms of *C. perfringens* poisoning usually are limited to mild nausea and vomiting that last a day or less, but that can be a very serious problem for elderly people. Contaminated meat and meat products are the most common sources of this type of food poisoning.

Not all food-borne illness is the result of bacterial contamination. *Giardia lamblia* is a protozoan that infects the small intestine. Giardiasis is associated with the consumption of contaminated water. It can also be transmitted to raw foods that have grown in contaminated water. Cool, moist environments are conducive to the growth of this microorganism. Symptoms generally occur within one to three weeks of infection and include diarrhea, constipation, abdominal pain, flatulence, loss of appetite, nausea, and vomiting. Norwalk virus is a very common virus that can be transmitted in food and water, and that causes many cases of diarrhea in both children and adults. *Trichinella spiralis* is a roundworm that causes the infection known as trichinosis. It is most often the result of eating raw or improperly cooked or processed pork or pork products. Scombroid poisoning (also called histamine poisoning) is a relatively rare type of food poisoning that can occur after the consumption of fish such as tuna and mackerel. After a fish is caught, decomposition by bacteria in the fish can trigger the production of high levels of a chemical called histamine. When the fish is eaten, in a matter of minutes the histamine can cause symptoms including facial flushing, nausea, vomiting, abdominal pain, and/or hives. Fortunately, symptoms usually subside in twenty-four hours.

Many people have the idea that food poisoning is a thing of the past. After all, the United States is among the wealthiest nations on earth. Our homes are equipped with the most modern appliances and conveniences, and most kitchens are kept reasonably clean. Thanks to our food safety, labeling, and inspection laws, our supermarket shelves are stocked with a nearly endless variety of foods that must meet strict government standards. Yet the truth is that food poisoning remains a major problem in this country, and strikes with a frequency that is both surprising and alarming.

The CDC offers several reasons for this. First, food animals are now raised in very close, confined quarters, a situation that is conducive to the spread of bacteria such as *Salmonella*. At the same time, food processing is becoming more and more centralized, so a single ingredient that is tainted with a contaminant can eventually show up in a multitude of different products. The United States now also imports record amounts of food from overseas, often from developing countries where proper hygiene in food production may not be as reliable as it is in this country.

Then there is the matter of food preparation. An increasing number of Americans are simply unaware of the prevalence of potentially dangerous microorganisms in the food supply, and lack knowledge of basic techniques for handling, preparing, and storing food safely. Most cases of food poisoning are easily preventable, provided you know how (*see* Tips for Preventing Food Poisoning on page 281). Also, more and more Americans, rather than eating meals prepared at home, purchase ready-made food at restaurants and from takeout establishments. One of the problems with this is that restaurants and food service companies may prepare large servings of turkey, chicken, beef, and other foods, and then leave them out at room temperature. Keeping food at room temperature encourages the growth of bacteria. *C. botulinum*, which is sometimes referred to as the "cafeteria germ," and *Salmonella* often breed in food that has not been cooked properly, or that has not been kept cold or hot enough.

If you contract food poisoning, the following supplements should be helpful.

NUTRIENTS

SUPPLEMENT	SUGGESTED DOSAGE	COMMENTS
Very Important		
Charcoal tablets	5 tablets at first signs of illness and again 6 hours later. Take separately from other medications and supplements.	Removes toxic substances from the colon and bloodstream.
Garlic (Kyolic)	2 capsules 3 times daily, with meals.	A powerful detoxifier that also destroys bacteria in the colon.
Potassium	99 mg daily.	To restore proper electrolyte balance.
Vitamin C with bioflavonoids	8,000 mg daily, in divided doses.	Detoxifies the body and aids in removing bacteria and toxins.
plus vitamin E	600 IU daily.	Reduces symptoms by enhancing immune function.
Important		
Acidophilus	As directed on label, twice daily, on an empty stomach.	Replaces essential intestinal bacteria.
Fiber (Aerobic Bulk Cleanse [ABC] from Aerobic Life Industries and oat bran are good sources)	As directed on label 6 hours after second dose of charcoal tablets and twice daily thereafter. Take separately from other supplements and medications.	Removes bacteria that have attached themselves to the colon walls, preventing them from entering the bloodstream; this reduces symptoms and speeds recovery.
Aerobic 07 from Aerobic Life Industries	20 drops in a glass of water every 3 hours.	Destroys harmful bacteria such as *Salmonella*.
Kelp	1,000–1,500 mg daily.	Contains needed minerals to restore electrolytes.
L-cysteine and L-methionine plus selenium and superoxide dismutase (SOD)	500 mg each daily, on an empty stomach. Take with 50 mg each of vitamins B6 and C for better absorption. 200 mcg daily. 5,000 mg daily.	All of these nutrients are essential in immune function.

Tips for Preventing Food Poisoning

Here are some fast, easy rules to help prevent food poisoning at home and while eating out:

• Keep food either hot or cold. Leaving food at room temperature encourages the growth of bacteria.

• Keep perishable products refrigerated.

• Refrigerate leftovers as soon as possible. Do not refrigerate foods in the same containers they were cooked or served in; transfer leftovers into clean containers so that they will cool more quickly.

• Cook meat, poultry, and seafood thoroughly. Meats should be cooked to an internal temperature of at least 165°F.

• Never use raw eggs that are cracked.

• Wash your hands before handling food, and after handling raw meat or poultry. Harmful bacteria can be transmitted if you handle food after diapering a baby or blowing your nose.

• Keep two cutting boards, one for meat and the other for vegetables. This will prevent the transfer of bacteria from meat to vegetables. At least three times a week, wash your cutting boards with a solution of ¼ cup of 3-percent hydrogen peroxide and 2 gallons of water. As an alternative, you can use a mixture of ½ cup of chlorine bleach and 1 quart of water, then rinse the board thoroughly with clean water.

• Go home directly after grocery shopping, especially in warm weather. Store foods immediately according to the instructions on the labels.

• Clean any utensil that has come in contact with raw hamburger, poultry, eggs, or seafood. Such utensils should not be allowed to come into contact with other foods until they have been disinfected.

• Wash out lunch boxes and Thermos bottles after every use.

• Beware of bulging cans, cracked jars, or loose lids on products. These can indicate botulism. Throw away cans that are bulging, rusted, bent, or sticky. Beware of cracks in jars and leaks in paper packaging, and exercise caution when consuming home-canned foods.

• When reheating food, bring it to a rapid boil, if possible, and cook it at that temperature for at least four minutes.

• Set your refrigerator temperature at 40°F or below. Freezers should be set at 0°F or below.

• Wash kitchen towels and sponges with a bleach-and-water solution (1 part bleach to 20 parts water) daily.

• Do not leave foods such as mayonnaise, salad dressing, and milk products at room temperature or, worse, out in the sun. Be especially careful at picnics and cookouts.

• Do not give honey to a young baby. This can lead to infant botulism, in which botulinal spores colonize the digestive tract and produce botulin toxin there. Honey is safe for babies after age one.

• Mold commonly grows on spoiled food products. The following foods should be avoided if mold is growing on them: bacon, bread, cured luncheon meats, soft dairy products, flour, canned ham, hot dogs, dried nuts, peanut butter, roast poultry, soft vegetables, and whole grains. Throw away any cooked or raw foods that are covered with mold.

• Thaw all frozen foods, especially meats and poultry, in the refrigerator.

• Eat hamburger and other meats only if they have been cooked at least until they turn brown. Meat or poultry that is even a little pink in color may still harbor bacteria. To ensure that all bacteria have been destroyed, it is best to cook meat until it is well done.

• When preparing a chicken or turkey with dressing, do not stuff the bird until you are ready to put it in the oven. Either cook the dressing separately or place it in the poultry *immediately* before putting it in the oven and then remove it as soon as the bird is done.

• Exercise caution when eating at restaurants and salad bars. Do not eat at salad bars that do not look fresh and clean or that do not have protective glass over them. Avoid the following foods when eating at salad bars: chicken, fish, creamed foods, foods containing mayonnaise, undercooked foods, and soups that are not kept at near-boiling temperatures.

• Before eating out, take 2 garlic tablets to help prevent food poisoning, as well as a product called ACES + Zinc from Carlson Labs to destroy any free radicals created by unknown toxins and oxidized fats in the food.

HERBS

❑ At the first sign of food poisoning, take a dropperful of alcohol-free goldenseal extract. Repeat this every four hours for one day. Goldenseal is a natural antibiotic that aids in destroying bacteria in the colon.

Caution: Do not take goldenseal internally on a daily basis for more than one week at a time, do not use it during pregnancy, and use it with caution if you are allergic to ragweed.

❑ Milk thistle and red clover aid in liver and blood cleansing.

❑ Use lobelia tea enemas to rid the body of the poison. Adding a dropperful of alcohol-free goldenseal extract to the enema is beneficial as well. *See* ENEMAS in Part Three.

RECOMMENDATIONS

❑ If you suspect food poisoning, call your regional poison control center immediately. Poison control centers can be reached twenty-four hours a day, and can provide you with up-to-date information regarding treatment. See page 432 for a list of poison control centers in the United States and

Canada. It is a good idea to keep the number of your local center posted by your telephone and/or entered into your telephone's automatic dialing program.

❑ At the first suspicion of food poisoning, protect your immune system by taking 6 charcoal tablets. These are available at most health food stores and should be kept on hand for emergencies. The agents in these tablets circulate through the bloodstream and help to neutralize and eliminate poisons. After six hours, take 6 more tablets. Consume a lot of quality water to aid in flushing toxins from the system.

❑ Use cleansing enemas to remove toxins from the colon and bloodstream. See ENEMAS in Part Three.

❑ If vomiting occurs, make sure that the individual does not choke. If vomiting does not subside in twenty-four hours, collect a sample of the vomit for analysis to aid in pinpointing the cause of the illness.

❑ If you suspect that you have been poisoned by food from a public restaurant or other eating place, contact your local health department right away. It may be possible to save others from food poisoning.

❑ For some cases of poisoning, it may be desirable to induce vomiting to help expel the toxin that is the cause of the problem. Keep syrup of ipecac (available in drugstores) on hand for this purpose.

Caution: Syrup of ipecac should be used only at the direction of a physician or poison control center.

❑ If symptoms of food poisoning are severe or prolonged, consult your health care provider.

CONSIDERATIONS

❑ David Hill, a microbiologist at England's University of Wolverhampton, monitored all the bacteria present in the intestines and found that in the presence of garlic, disease-causing microbes were eliminated. According to Hill, the sulfur compounds in garlic are the secret weapon that knocks out dangerous bacteria.

❑ It was once believed that nylon or plastic cutting boards were preferable to the wooden variety. Since then, research has indicated that wood is probably better after all. Researchers have discovered that when cutting boards are contaminated with organisms that can cause food poisoning, almost all the bacteria on the wooden boards die off within three minutes, while almost none die on the plastic ones. For added security, you can wash your wooden cutting board periodically with hydrogen peroxide and water or a bleach-and-water solution (*see* Tips for Preventing Food Poisoning on page 281).

❑ The overwhelming majority (an estimated 90 percent) of cases of botulism in the United States are attributable to improper home-canning techniques. The best safeguard against this illness is to avoid all home-canned meats, fruits, and vegetables unless they have been prepared in a pressure cooker in scrupulous accordance with the manufacturer's directions. The old "stovetop" method of home canning is *not* a reliable way to seal the jar lids properly.

❑ A person who experiences a severe headache and vomiting soon after eating may be suffering from food allergies. Charcoal tablets and a coffee retention enema can help rid the body of substances that cause allergic reactions. (*See* ALLERGIES in Part Three.)

❑ Interestingly, botulin toxin, one of the most potent toxins known to man, has been attracting attention from the medical community as a potential therapeutic tool. The U.S. Food and Drug Administration recently approved the use of a purified form of botulin toxin as a drug to treat two muscle disorders that affect the eyes, *blepharospasm* (uncontrollable muscle spasms of the eyelids) and *strabismus* (a tendency of one eye to deviate from parallelism with the other). A tiny amount of the toxin is injected directly into the muscles to paralyze them, reducing symptoms.

Fracture

A fracture is a break or a crack in a bone. If the skin over the bone remains intact, a fracture is referred to as *closed* or *simple*; if the bone breaks the skin, it is termed *open* or *compound*. A fracture may cause extreme pain and tenderness in the injured area; swelling; a protruding bone or blood under the skin; and numbness, tingling, or paralysis below the fracture. A major fracture, such as of an arm or leg, may also cause a loss of the pulse below the fracture, as well as weakness and an inability to bear weight. Broken arms, fingers, or legs may be bent out of alignment.

Fractures pose an increasing problem as we grow older and our bones become more brittle. An estimated 200,000 hip fractures occur in people over sixty-five years of age each year. Osteoporosis is a factor in the majority of these cases.

A broken bone calls for prompt professional help. After a bone has been set, the following supplements and other recommendations will aid in healing.

NUTRIENTS

SUPPLEMENT	SUGGESTED DOSAGE	COMMENTS
Very Important		
Bone Builder With Boron from Metagenics	As directed on label.	A microcrystalline hydroxy-apatite concentrate (MCHC) that contains the organic protein-calcium matrix of raw bone. Available only through health care professionals.
Bone Support from Synergy Plus or Bone Defense from KAL	As directed on label. Take with calcium and magnesium below. As directed on label.	To supply essential nutrients for bone health.

Boron	3 mg daily. Do not exceed this amount.	Important in bone health and healing. Studies show boron can increase calcium uptake by as much as 30 percent.
Calcium and magnesium	1,000–2,000 mg daily, in divided doses, after meals and at bedtime. 1,000 mg daily.	Vital for proper bone repair. Needed to balance with calcium.
Glucosamine sulfate	As directed on label.	Important for the repair of bones and connective tissue. Also relieves pain and inflammation.
Kelp	1,000–1,500 mg daily.	Rich in calcium and minerals in a natural balance.
Neonatal Multi-Gland from Biotics Research	As directed on label.	Promotes healing. See GLANDULAR THERAPY in Part Three for its benefits.
Proteolytic enzymes	As directed on label. Take between meals.	Reduces inflammation. Caution: Do not give this supplement to a child under 16 years of age.
Silica or horsetail	As directed on label.	Supplies silicon, needed for calcium uptake and connective tissue repair. See under Herbs, below.
Vitamin C with bioflavonoids	3,000–6,000 mg daily, in divided doses.	Important in repair of bones, connective tissue, and muscles.
Vitamin D	400–1,000 IU daily.	Needed for calcium absorption and bone repair.
Zinc	80 mg daily. Do not exceed a total of 100 mg daily from all supplements.	Important in tissue repair. Use zinc gluconate lozenges or zinc methionate (OptiZinc) for best absorption.
Helpful		
Free-form amino acid complex	As directed on label.	Speeds healing. Use a sublingual form.
Octacosanol	3,000 mg daily.	Improves tissue oxygenation.
Pantothenic acid (vitamin B5)	100 mg 3 times daily.	Anti-stress vitamin. Aids in vitamin utilization.
Potassium	99 mg daily.	Needed to keep swelling down and balance with sodium.
Raw liver extract	As directed on label.	Supplies balanced B vitamins and other needed vitamins and minerals. See GLANDULAR THERAPY in Part Three.
Vitamin A	50,000 IU daily for one month, then reduce to 25,000 IU daily until healed. If you are pregnant, do not exceed 10,000 IU daily.	Protein is not utilized without vitamin A. Use emulsion form for easier assimilation and greater safety at higher doses.

HERBS

❑ Horsetail extract is a good source of silica, which enhances the utilization of calcium and promotes healing and repair.

❑ Turmeric paste makes a good poultice. Combine turmeric with a little hot water and apply it to the site of the injury on a gauze dressing. This is also good for bruises and helps to reduce swelling. A poultice of fresh mullein leaves is also good. See USING A POULTICE in Part Three.

RECOMMENDATIONS

❑ Eat half of a fresh pineapple every day until the fracture is healed. Pineapple contains bromelain, an enzyme that acts to reduce swelling and inflammation. Use only fresh pineapple, not canned or processed.

❑ Avoid red meat, as well as colas and any other products containing caffeine. Foods with preservatives should also be avoided due to their phosphorus content. Phosphorus can lead to bone loss.

❑ Use clay poultices for bruises and swelling.

CONSIDERATIONS

❑ Glucosamine sulfate is a natural alternative to aspirin and other nonsteroidal anti-inflammatory drugs (NSAIDs). Glucosamine is found naturally in joint cartilage. It stimulates the production of the substances needed for joint repair.

❑ A study of senior citizens who took tranquilizers revealed that they suffered 70 percent more hip fractures than did other people their age.

❑ *See also* OSTEOPOROSIS and SPRAINS, STRAINS, AND OTHER INJURIES OF THE MUSCLES AND JOINTS in Part Two.

Frigidity

Frigidity is the inability of a woman to experience pleasure from sexual intercourse. Frigidity is usually of psychological origin, stemming from fear, guilt, depression, conflict with one's mate, and/or feelings of inferiority. Unpleasant childhood and adolescent experiences are often factors.

For some women, however, frigidity may be a result of physiological factors. Some women find intercourse painful due to insufficient lubrication, inadequate stimulation, underlying illness or infection, or some other physical cause. The pain causes them to fear and shrink from sexual contact. Vitamin deficiency can cause a deficiency in estrogen levels and result in improper lubrication. The supplement program outlined below will help.

NUTRIENTS

SUPPLEMENT	SUGGESTED DOSAGE	COMMENTS
Very Important		
Damiana		See under Herbs, below.
Kelp	2,000–2,500 mg daily.	A good source of iodine and other important minerals.
Vitamin B complex	100 mg twice daily.	Calms the nervous system and aids in reducing anxiety.
Vitamin E	Start with 200–400 IU daily and increase slowly to 1,600 IU daily.	Necessary for the functioning of the reproductive system and glands.

Helpful		
Fish liver oil	As directed on label. Take with meals.	Supplies vitamins A and D.
Lecithin granules or capsules	1 tbsp 3 times daily, with meals. 2,400 mg 3 times daily, with meals.	Contains essential fatty acids and aids in proper nerve function.
L-Phenylalanine and L-tyrosine	500 mg each daily, on an empty stomach. Take with water or juice. Do not take with milk. Take with 50 mg vitamin B$_6$ and 100 mg vitamin C for better absorption. Do not exceed the recommended dosage.	Amino acids needed for synthesis of crucial neurotransmitters involved in mood and nervous system function. *Caution:* Do not take phenylalanine if you are pregnant or nursing a baby, or if you suffer from panic attacks, diabetes, high blood pressure, or PKU. Do not take tyrosine if you are taking an MAO inhibitor drug.
Para-aminobenzoic acid (PABA)	100 mg daily.	A B vitamin that stimulates vital life functions.
Vitamin C with bioflavonoids	3,000–6,000 mg daily, in divided doses.	Important in glandular function and stress response.
Zinc	50–80 mg daily. Do not exceed a total of 100 mg daily from all supplements.	Zinc deficiency can result in impaired sexual function. Use zinc gluconate lozenges or OptiZinc for best absorption.

HERBS

❑ Damiana is the "woman's sexuality herb." It contains alkaloids that directly stimulate the nerves and organs and have a testosteronelike effect. Damiana is excellent for supporting the sexual organs and enhancing sexual pleasure. For best results, place a dropperful of damiana extract under your tongue an hour or two before sexual activity. It may take several days for the difference to become apparent.

❑ Wild yam contains a natural steroid called dehydroepiandrosterone (DHEA) that rejuvenates and gives vigor to lovemaking. Take it for two weeks, then stop for two weeks, and so on.

❑ Other herbs that are good for promoting energy and sexuality include fo-ti, gotu kola, sarsaparilla, saw palmetto, and Siberian ginseng.

Caution: Do not use Siberian ginseng if you have hypoglycemia, high blood pressure, or a heart disorder.

RECOMMENDATIONS

❑ Make sure to include the following in your diet: alfalfa sprouts; avocados; eggs that come fresh from hens (not those stored cold in the supermarket); olive oil; pumpkin seeds and other seeds and nuts; soy and sesame oil; and wheat.

❑ Try taking supplemental bee pollen to increase energy.

Caution: Bee pollen may cause an allergic reaction in some people. Start with a small amount at first, and discontinue use if a rash, wheezing, discomfort, or other symptom occurs.

❑ Avoid poultry, red meat, and sugar products.

❑ Avoid smoggy conditions. Smog is highly toxic and dangerous; it adversely affects immune function and hormonal activity, as well as a host of other body functions.

CONSIDERATIONS

❑ There are medical alternatives that can help some women by alleviating painful intercourse. Painful intercourse may also be a sign of certain gynecological diseases.

❑ If frigidity is due to interpersonal conflict or psychological causes, help from a couples counselor or other mental health professional is advised.

❑ Hypothyroidism or depression may be the underlying problem. (*See* HYPOTHYROIDISM and DEPRESSION in Part Two.)

Fungal Infection

Certain types of fungi (most commonly candida and tinea) can infect the skin and/or mucous membranes; they can also grow under the nails, between the toes, or on internal surfaces of the colon and other organs.

Fungal infection of the skin is most common in places where skin tends to be moist and one skin surface is in contact with another, such as the groin area ("*jock itch*") and between the toes ("*athlete's foot*"). However, moist, possibly itchy, red patches anywhere on the body can indicate fungal infection. In babies, a fungal infection can manifest itself as diaper rash that makes the skin bright red in light-skinned babies and darker brown in dark-skinned babies.

Fungal infection of the mouth is referred to as *oral thrush*, a condition in which creamy-looking white patches form on the tongue and the mucous membranes of the mouth. If the patches are scraped off, bleeding may result. This condition is most common in infants and in those with compromised immune systems.

Nursing mothers sometimes develop a *candida infection of the nipples* that causes severe pain while feeding. This can be further complicated if the baby develops oral thrush; it can lead to a "ping-pong" effect in which mother and baby continually reinfect each other.

Fungal infection under the nails (*paronychia*) or between the toes may cause discoloration and swelling, and the nails may become raised above the surface of the nail bed. In fungal infection of the vagina (*yeast infection*), a cheesy discharge is present, usually accompanied by intense itching.

Ringworm is a fungal infection of the skin or scalp characterized by the development of small red spots that grow to a size of about one-quarter inch in diameter. As the spots expand, the centers tend to heal and clear while the borders are raised, red, and scaly, giving them a ringlike appearance. Like other fungal infections, ringworm can be very itchy.

Recurrent fungal infections are a common sign of depressed immune function. The people most likely to be affected are those who have diseases such as diabetes or cancer, or who are infected with human immunodeficiency virus (HIV). Women who use oral contraceptives and people taking antibiotics are at higher risk as well, as are people who are obese and/or who perspire heavily.

NUTRIENTS

SUPPLEMENT	SUGGESTED DOSAGE	COMMENTS
Essential		
Acidophilus	As directed on label.	Supplies the "friendly" bacteria that are usually deficient in people with fungal infections.
Garlic (Kyolic)	2 capsules 3 times daily, with meals.	Neutralizes most fungi.
Important		
Aerobic 07 from Aerobic Life Industries	9 drops in 8 oz of water twice daily.	Increases tissue oxygenation, combats fungi, and destroys bacteria that can cause secondary infection.
Vitamin B complex plus extra pantothenic acid (vitamin B$_5$)	50 mg 3 times daily, with meals. 50 mg 3 times daily.	Needed for correctly balanced "friendly" bacteria in the body. Plays a role in the formation of antibodies and aids in the utilization of nutrients.
Vitamin C with bioflavonoids	5,000–20,000 mg daily, in divided doses. *See* ASCORBIC ACID FLUSH in Part Three.	Needed for proper immune function.
Vitamin E	400–800 IU daily.	Needed for proper immune function. Use emulsion for easier assimilation.
Zinc	50 mg daily. Do not exceed a total of 100 mg daily from all supplements.	Needed for proper immune function. Use zinc gluconate lozenges or OptiZinc for best absorption.
Helpful		
Essential fatty acids (black currant seed oil, primrose oil, and salmon oil are good sources)	As directed on label.	For relief of pain and inflammation.
Vitamin A	25,000 IU daily. If you are pregnant, do not exceed 10,000 IU daily.	Aids healing of skin and mucous membranes. Needed for proper immune function.

HERBS

❑ Tea tree oil is a natural antifungal for external use. It can be applied to the affected area several times a day, either full strength or diluted with distilled water or cold-pressed vegetable oil. You can also use black walnut extract.

❑ Drink 3 cups of pau d'arco tea daily.

❑ For toenail or fingernail fungus, soak nails in a mixture of pau d'arco and goldenseal. In a wide pan, make pau d'arco tea using 6 tea bags and a gallon of water. Bring to boil, then allow to cool to a very warm but tolerable temperature. Add the contents of 4 capsules of goldenseal. Soak your feet or hands in this mixture for fifteen minutes twice a day.

RECOMMENDATIONS

❑ Eat a diet of 60 to 70 percent raw foods. Eat plenty of fresh vegetables and moderate amounts of broiled fish and broiled skinless chicken.

❑ Do not eat any foods containing sugar or refined carbohydrates. Fungi thrive on sugar.

❑ Eliminate those foods from the diet that tend to promote secretion of mucus, especially meat and dairy products.

❑ Avoid cola drinks, grains, processed foods, and fried, greasy foods.

❑ *See* FASTING in Part Three and follow the program.

❑ Keep the skin clean and dry. Expose the affected area to the air as much as possible.

❑ Apply honey and crushed garlic, alternately, to the affected area.

❑ If the nails are affected, apply Aerobic 07 drops from Aerobic Life Industries directly on the area. Soak infected hands or feet in a solution of Aerobic 07 drops and pau d'arco tea daily for fifteen minutes. When not soaking them, keep the nails dry and clean.

❑ Wear clean cotton clothing and underwear. Do not wear clothing or use towels more than once without washing them, preferably in hot water with chlorine bleach added.

❑ To replace necessary "friendly" bacteria in the colon, use an *L. bifidus* retention enema. *See* ENEMAS in Part Three.

❑ Try not to allow an infected area of the body to come in contact with healthy skin. People who have fungal infections in one area often also have infections in other areas.

❑ If you are nursing a baby and your baby has thrush, *or* you develop sharp, shooting pains during feedings, *or* both, consult both your child's and your own health care provider. You may have a fungal infection. Both you and your baby should be treated to ensure a cure.

❑ For ringworm, put crushed raw garlic over the affected area and cover it with sterile gauze or a cotton cloth that allows air to penetrate. Do not cover it tightly with adhesive tape or a plastic bandage. These promote dampness.

❑ If you have been treating a fungal infection on your own and you develop symptoms of a worsening infection, such as increased redness and swelling or fever, consult your physician. You may have developed a bacterial infection on top of the fungal infection.

CONSIDERATIONS

❑ There are numerous topical antifungal preparations available in drug stores. However, we believe that garlic is safer and works just as well, if not better, than these drugs.

❑ *See also* ATHLETE'S FOOT; CANDIDIASIS; and/or YEAST INFECTION in Part Two.

Gallbladder Disorders

The gallbladder is a small organ located directly under the liver. It acts as a bile reservoir; it concentrates bile, which is secreted by the liver and is used by the body to digest fats. Bile contains cholesterol, bile salts, lecithin, and other substances.

If the gallbladder becomes inflamed, it causes severe pain in the upper right abdomen. This is accompanied by fever, nausea, and vomiting. This condition must be treated immediately. If left untreated, inflammation of the gallbladder, called *cholecystitis*, can be life threatening.

Sometimes cholesterol crystallizes and combines with bile in the gallbladder to form gallstones. Often persons with gallstones have no symptoms. If a stone blocks the bile passage, however, nausea, vomiting, and pain in the upper right abdominal region occur. These symptoms often arise after the individual has eaten fried or fatty foods.

NUTRIENTS

SUPPLEMENT	SUGGESTED DOSAGE	COMMENTS
Alfalfa		*See under* Herbs, below.
Essential fatty acids	As directed on label.	Important constituents of every living cell. Needed for repair and prevention of gallstones.
Lecithin granules or capsules	1 tbsp 3 times daily, before meals. 1,200 mg 3 times daily, before meals.	A fat emulsifier; aids digestion of fats.
L-Glycine	500 mg daily, on an empty stomach. Take with water or juice. Do not take with milk. Take with 50 mg vitamin B$_6$ and 100 mg vitamin C for better absorption.	Essential for the biosynthesis of nucleic and bile acids. *See* AMINO ACIDS in Part One.
Multienzyme complex with ox bile	As directed on label. Take before meals.	Aids in digestion if too little bile is secreted from the gallbladder. *Caution:* Do not give this supplement to a child. If you have a history of ulcers, *do not* use a formula containing HCl.
Vitamin A	25,000 IU daily. If you are pregnant, do not exceed 10,000 IU daily.	Needed for repair of tissues. Use emulsion form for easier assimilation.
Vitamin B complex plus extra vitamin B$_{12}$ and choline and inositol	50 mg 3 times daily, with meals. 2,000 mcg daily. 500 mg daily. 500 mg daily.	All B vitamins are necessary for proper digestion. Use a high-potency formula. Important in cholesterol metabolism and liver and gallbladder function.
Vitamin C	3,000 mg daily.	Deficiency can lead to gallstones.
Vitamin D	400 IU daily.	Gallbladder malfunction interferes with vitamin D absorption.
Vitamin E	600 IU daily.	Prevents fats from becoming rancid.

HERBS

❑ Alfalfa cleanses the liver and supplies necessary vitamins and minerals. Twice a day for two days, take 1,000 milligrams in tablet or capsule form with a glass of warm water.

❑ Peppermint oil capsules are used in Europe to cleanse the gallbladder.

❑ Other beneficial herbs include barberry root bark, catnip, cramp bark, dandelion, fennel, ginger root, horsetail, parsley, and wild yam.

Caution: Do not use barberry during pregnancy.

RECOMMENDATIONS

❑ For inflammation of the gallbladder, eat no solid food for a few days. Consume only distilled or spring water. Then drink juices such as pear, beet, and apple for three days. Then add solid foods: shredded raw beets with 2 tablespoons of olive oil, fresh lemon juice, and freshly made uncooked applesauce made in a blender or food processor.

❑ For gallstones, take 3 tablespoons of olive oil with the juice of a lemon before bed and upon awakening. Stones are often passed and eliminated in the stool with this technique—look for them. You can use grapefruit juice instead. To relieve pain, try using hot castor oil packs on the gallbladder area. Place castor oil in a pan and heat but do not boil it. Dip a piece of cheesecloth or other white cotton material into the oil until the cloth is saturated. Apply the cloth to the affected area and cover it with a piece of plastic that is larger in size than the cotton cloth. Place a heating pad over the plastic and use it to keep the pack warm. Keep the pack in place for one-half to two hours, as needed.

❑ Eat a diet consisting of 75 percent raw foods. Include in the diet applesauce, eggs, yogurt, cottage cheese, broiled fish, fresh apples, and beets.

❑ To cleanse the system, consume as much pure apple juice as possible for five days. Add pear juice occasionally. Beet juice also cleanses the liver.

❑ Avoid sugar and products containing sugar. Avoid all animal fat and meat, fried foods, spicy foods, margarine, soft drinks, commercial oils, coffee, chocolate, and refined carbohydrates.

❑ While you have pain, nausea and/or vomiting, and fever, follow a fasting program and use coffee enemas for a few days. The coffee enema is important. You can also use garlic in the enema. *See* FASTING and ENEMAS in Part Three.

❑ A detoxification program for the liver and colon is important for improved gallbladder function. Use cleansing enemas if you have chronic problems.

❑ Do not overeat. Obesity and gallbladder disease are related. Females age forty and over who are overweight and who have had children are more likely than most people to suffer from disorders of the gallbladder.

CONSIDERATIONS

❑ Kombucha tea may be beneficial for gallstones (*see* MAKING KOMBUCHA TEA in Part Three).

❑ Rapid weight changes can cause gallbladder problems.

❑ The recommended treatment for gallstones is usually surgical removal of the gallbladder. However, if gallstones show up on an x-ray but do not cause symptoms, there is no need for surgery. A gallstone may slip into a bile duct, one of the structures that drain the gallbladder and the liver. If this occurs, extraction or surgical removal may be necessary. Sometimes stones in the gallbladder can be fragmented or dissolved without surgery, using drugs or sound waves. Bile acid preparations used to dissolve stones work very slowly and can be used only on small stones.

Gangrene

Gangrene is a condition in which body tissues die, and ultimately decay, as a result of an inadequate oxygen supply. There are two types of gangrene: wet gangrene and dry gangrene.

Wet gangrene is the result of a wound or injury that becomes infected. The infection prevents adequate venous drainage, depriving the area of needed blood supply and oxygen. The disruption in oxygen supply in turn promotes the infection. Symptoms of wet gangrene include severe and rapidly worsening pain, swelling, and tenderness in the area. As the infection progresses, the affected tissue changes color, usually from pink to deep red to gray green or purple. Left untreated, wet gangrene can lead to shock and death in a matter of days. Fortunately, careful hygiene can usually prevent this type of gangrene.

Dry gangrene does not involve bacterial infection. It is caused by stopped or reduced blood flow, which results in oxygen-deprived tissue. Reduced blood flow may be caused by injury, hardening of the arteries, poor circulation, diabetes, or blockage in a blood vessel. The condition most often occurs in the feet and toes. Symptoms of the most common type of dry gangrene are a dull, aching pain and coldness in the area. Pain and pallor of the affected area are early signs.

Sometimes gangrene is caused by frostbite. In frostbite, the oxygen-deprived area dies, but the gangrene does not spread to any other area. As the flesh dies, it may be painful, but once the skin is dead, it becomes numb and slowly darkens.

NUTRIENTS

SUPPLEMENT	SUGGESTED DOSAGE	COMMENTS
Essential		
Dimethylglycine (DMG) (Aangamik DMG from FoodScience Labs)	100 mg 3 times daily.	Enhances oxygen utilization by affected tissue.
Very Important		
AE Mulsion Forte from American Biologics	As directed on label, to supply 50,000 IU vitamin A and 400–1,600 IU vitamin E daily. If you are pregnant, do not exceed 10,000 IU vitamin A daily.	Vitamin A is essential for tissue repair; vitamin E improves circulation. Both enhance immune function. Use this emulsion form for easier assimilation and safety at higher doses.
Chlorophyll	As directed on label 4 times daily.	A blood cleanser.
Coenzyme Q10	100 mg twice daily.	Improves circulation.
Potassium	99 mg daily.	Aids in reducing tissue swelling.
Proteolytic enzymes	As directed on label. Take with meals and between meals.	Aids in damaged tissue "cleanup" and repair. *Caution:* Do not give this supplement to a child under 16 years of age.
Vitamin C with bioflavonoids	5,000–20,000 mg daily. *See* ASCORBIC ACID FLUSH in Part Three.	For tissue repair and improved circulation.
Important		
Kelp	1,000–1,500 mg daily.	A rich source of chlorophyll and minerals good for circulation. A blood cleanser.
Helpful		
Aerobic 07 from Aerobic Life Industries	As directed on label. Also apply a few drops directly on the affected area.	A stabilized oxygen product. Kills infecting bacteria.
Calcium and magnesium	2,000 mg daily. 1,000 mg daily.	For connective tissue repair. Needed to balance with calcium.
Multivitamin and mineral complex	As directed on label.	All nutrients are necessary for healing.
Zinc	50–80 mg daily. Do not exceed a total of 100 mg daily from all supplements.	Speeds healing. Necessary for tissue repair and immune function. Use zinc gluconate lozenges or zinc methionate (OptiZinc) for best absorption.

HERBS

❑ Butcher's broom is important for circulation.

❑ Other beneficial herbs include bayberry, cayenne (capsicum), echinacea, ginkgo biloba, goldenseal, and red seal.

Caution: Do not take goldenseal internally on a daily basis for more than one week at a time, as it may disturb normal intestinal flora. Do not use it during pregnancy, and use it with caution if you are allergic to ragweed.

RECOMMENDATIONS

❑ Add "green drinks" made from vegetables to the diet. *See* JUICING in Part Three.

❑ Include in the diet foods that are high in germanium, such as garlic, shiitake mushrooms, and onions. Germanium helps to improve tissue oxygenation.

❑ If an injured area becomes red, swollen, and painful, or develops an odor, see your health care provider without delay.

CONSIDERATIONS

❑ For wet gangrene, treatment with antibiotics and surgical removal of the dead tissue are usually necessary. Hyperbaric oxygen therapy may be employed as well. (*See* HYPERBARIC OXYGEN THERAPY in Part Three.)

❑ Slowly developing dry gangrene may be reversed by arterial surgery. Chelation is an alternative. (*See* CHELATION THERAPY in Part Three.) If an acute arterial obstruction is involved, emergency surgery must be performed.

❑ *See also* ARTERIOSCLEROSIS and CIRCULATORY PROBLEMS in Part Two.

Gas

See HEARTBURN; INDIGESTION. *See also under* PREGNANCY-RELATED PROBLEMS.

Gastroenteritis

See FOOD POISONING. *See also under* INFLUENZA.

German Measles (Rubella)

German measles, also known as "three-day measles," is a mild but contagious viral infection that most often affects children. It affects the lymph glands in the neck and behind the ears. The first symptoms include coughing, fatigue, headache, mild fever, muscle aches, and stiffness, mainly in the neck. One to five days later, a pink rash often develops, usually starting on the face and neck and then spreading to the rest of the body. The virus usually runs its course in five to seven days.

German measles is a mild illness that does not usually cause anything more than slight discomfort and rarely leads to complications. However, if a woman contracts the disease in the first trimester of pregnancy, before the fetus's organs are formed, it can cause serious birth defects. The communicable period probably begins two to four days before the rash appears, and the virus most often disappears from the nose and throat by the time the rash on the body disappears, one to three days after the onset of symptoms. However, because of the danger it poses to pregnant women, German measles should be considered contagious from one week before the rash appears until one week after the rash fades.

Unless otherwise specified, the dosages recommended here are for adults. For a child between the ages of twelve and seventeen, reduce the dose to three-quarters the rec-ommended amount. For a child between six and twelve, use one-half the recommended dose, and for a child under the age of six, use one-quarter the recommended amount.

NUTRIENTS

SUPPLEMENT	SUGGESTED DOSAGE	COMMENTS
Helpful		
AE Mulsion Forte from American Biologics	As directed on label.	Supplies vitamins A and E, needed to reduce infection and repair tissues. For a child under 10, substitute cod liver oil.
Bio-Strath from Bioforce	As directed on label.	Acts as a tonic. Contains the vitamin B complex. Use the liquid form.
Calcium and magnesium	As directed on label. As directed on label.	Needed for tissue repair.
Proteolytic enzymes	As directed on label, on an empty stomach. Take between meals.	Reduces infection and aids digestion. *Caution:* Do not give this supplement to a child.
Raw thymus glandular	500 mg twice daily.	Stimulates the immune system. *Caution:* Do not give this supplement to a child.
Vitamin C with bioflavonoids	5,000–20,000 mg daily, in divided doses. *See* ASCORBIC ACID FLUSH in Part Three.	Very important for immune function. Controls fever and infection. Has antiviral properties. Use ascorbate or esterified form.
Zinc lozenges (Ultimate Zinc-C Lozenges from Now Foods)	1 15-mg lozenge 3 times daily for 4 days. Then reduce to 1 lozenge daily. Use this dosage for adults and for children over 5.	For immune response and tissue repair.

HERBS

❑ If necessary, catnip tea or garlic enemas can be used to lower fever. *See* ENEMAS in Part Three.

❑ Clove and peppermint tea aid in relieving symptoms.

❑ Alcohol-free goldenseal extract, placed directly under the tongue, aids in destroying bacteria and viruses and also relieves coughing. Use 3 drops for a child from three to ten years of age; for an adult or a child over ten, use one dropperful. Hold the extract under the tongue for a few minutes, then swallow. Repeat this three times daily for three days. As an alternative, use an echinacea and goldenseal combination extract, available in health food stores. Echinacea is good for the immune response.

❑ Take ½ teaspoon of lobelia extract every four to five hours for pain.
Caution: Do not take lobelia internally on an ongoing basis.

RECOMMENDATIONS

❑ Drink plenty of fluids such as water, juices, and vegetable broths.

❑ Avoid processed foods.

❑ Rest until the rash and fever have disappeared.

❑ Avoid contact with healthy individuals, especially women of childbearing age and their children, until one week after the rash disappears.

❑ *Do not* give aspirin to a child with German measles. *See* REYE'S SYNDROME in Part Two.

CONSIDERATIONS

❑ Antibiotics are useless against viruses, so they are not called for in the treatment of German measles.

❑ Persons who have had German measles have immunity to the disease for life.

❑ A woman who has had German measles will pass immunity to any child she has for the first year of his or her life.

❑ Immunity to German measles can be determined by a blood test. Any woman who wishes to become pregnant and who is not sure whether she has achieved immunity to German measles should be tested and vaccinated, if necessary. Pregnancy must then be avoided for at least three months following immunization.

❑ It is a good idea for any woman who is (or who may be) pregnant to take precautions to avoid exposure to anyone who has, or has recently been exposed to, German measles. A pregnant woman who suspects she may have been exposed to German measles and who knows she has not achieved immunity (either through vaccination or from having the disease) should consult her doctor immediately concerning a gamma-globulin injection. If given soon after exposure, gamma-globulin may reduce the severity of the illness or even prevent it from developing.

❑ Many doctors believe that children should be immunized against German measles at about 15 months of age and again a few years later. Nonpregnant women of childbearing age are advised to be immunized also. People who should *not* be immunized include women who may be pregnant and individuals with impaired immune function, such as those with AIDS or cancer, or those currently taking cortisone or anticancer drugs or undergoing radiation therapy. Those with an illness that causes a fever should defer vaccination until healthy.

Gingivitis

See under PERIODONTAL DISEASE.

Glaucoma

Glaucoma is a serious eye disease characterized by abnormally high intraocular pressure, which is the pressure that the fluids within the eyeball exert on the other parts of the eye. If this pressure is unrelieved, it damages the retina and ultimately destroys the optic nerve, resulting in vision loss and even total blindness. Glaucoma is one of the leading causes of blindness. The condition usually affects people over forty, and is more common in women than in men. Those with the highest risk of developing glaucoma are people of African ancestry; people with diabetes, high blood pressure, severe myopia (nearsightedness), or a family history of glaucoma; and those taking corticosteroid preparations. Many cases of glaucoma go undetected until vision loss begins.

There are two basic categories of glaucoma. The more severe (and, fortunately, less common) form of this disorder is called *closed-angle glaucoma*. Attacks of this type of glaucoma occur when the channel through which the eye's fluids normally drain become constricted or obstructed. This is usually due to narrowing or hardening of the exit channels from the eyes, and it results in extreme pain, poor vision, and even blindness. It is considered a medical emergency. Early warning signs that a problem may be developing include eye pain or discomfort mainly in the morning, blurred vision, seeing halos around lights, and inability of the pupils to adjust to a dark room. Symptoms of the acute attack itself include throbbing eye pain and loss of sight, especially peripheral vision; pupils that are fixed in a mildly dilated condition and do not respond to light properly; and a sharp increase in the pressure in the inner eye, especially on one side. These symptoms come on very rapidly and may be accompanied by nausea and even vomiting. Permanent vision damage can occur in as little as three to five days, making treatment within the first twenty-four to forty-eight hours imperative.

The most common form of glaucoma, accounting for 90 percent of all cases of this disorder, is *chronic open-angle glaucoma*. In open-angle glaucoma, there is no physical blockage and the structures of the eye appear normal, but the drainage of fluid nevertheless is inadequate to keep the intraocular pressure at a normal level. While the acute form of glaucoma is a frightening prospect, especially to those in high-risk categories, chronic glaucoma is much more insidious because *it almost never manifests any symptoms until very late in the condition.* By that time, vision may be irreversibly damaged. The most pronounced symptoms of open-angle glaucoma are the loss or "darkening" of peripheral vision and a marked decrease in night vision or the ability of the eye to adjust to darkness. Peripheral vision is the ability to see "out of the corner of the eye." The loss of this ability leaves a person with "tunnel vision." Other possible symptoms include chronic low-grade headaches (often mistaken for tension headaches), the need for frequent changes in eyeglass prescription, and/or seeing halos around electric lights.

Glaucoma probably has many causes, but it is closely related to stress and nutritional problems, and is often related to other disorders such as diabetes and high blood

pressure. Problems with collagen, the most abundant protein in the human body, have been linked to glaucoma.
Collagen acts to increase the strength and elasticity of tissues in the body, especially those of the eye. Collagen and
tissue abnormalities at the back of the eye contribute to the
"clogging" of the tissues through which intraocular fluid
normally drains. The result is elevated inner eye pressure
that leads to glaucoma and related vision loss. Conditions
characterized by errors of collagen metabolism are frequently associated with eye disorders.

NUTRIENTS

SUPPLEMENT	SUGGESTED DOSAGE	COMMENTS
Very Important		
Choline and inositol	1,000–2,000 mg daily.	Important B vitamins for the eyes and brain.
or lecithin	As directed on label.	A good source of choline and inositol.
Glutathione	500 mg twice daily, on an empty stomach. Take with 50 mg vitamin B$_6$ and 100 mg vitamin C for better absorption.	A powerful antioxidant that protects the lens and maintains the molecular integrity of the lens fiber membranes.
Omega-3 essential fatty acids	As directed on label. Take with meals.	Protects and aids repair of new tissues and cells.
Pantothenic acid (vitamin B$_5$)	100 mg 3 times daily.	Anti-stress vitamin needed for the adrenal glands, and an essential constituent of coenzyme A, needed for many vital metabolic processes.
Rutin	50 mg 3 times daily.	An important bioflavonoid that works with vitamin C and aids in reducing pain and intraocular pressure.
Vitamin A plus	50,000 IU daily. If you are pregnant, do not exceed 10,000 IU daily.	Needed for good eyesight. Essential in formation of visual purple, the substance necessary for night vision.
natural beta-carotene or	25,000 IU daily, with meals.	
carotenoid complex (Betatene)	As directed on label.	
Vitamin B complex	50 mg 3 times daily, with meals.	Use a sublingual form. Injections (under a doctor's supervision) may be necessary. Whenever stress is a factor, B-complex injections are a good idea.
Vitamin C with bioflavonoids	10,000–15,000 mg daily, in divided doses. Under a doctor's supervision, you can increase the dose to 30,000 mg daily.	Reduces intraocular pressure.
Vitamin E	400 IU daily.	Helpful in removing particles from the lens of the eye. Antioxidant properties protect the lens and other eye tissues.
Helpful		
Taurine Plus from American Biologics	As directed on label.	An antioxidant that protects the lens of the eye.
Multivitamin and mineral complex with	As directed on label.	All nutrients are needed to aid in healing and to reduce intraocular pressure.
selenium	200 mcg daily.	A potent antioxidant that works with vitamin E.
Zinc	50 mg daily. Do not exceed a total of 100 mg daily from all supplements.	Essential in activating vitamin A from the liver. Very beneficial in glaucoma therapy. Use zinc sulfate form.

HERBS

❑ Bilberry contains flavonoids and nutrients needed to
protect the eyes from further damage. Fresh blueberries and
red raspberry leaf can be used also.

❑ Chickweed and eyebright are good for all eye disorders.

❑ Eye baths using warm fennel tea, alternating with
chamomile and eyebright, are helpful. Or use an eye dropper
and apply three drops to each eye three times a day. Always
dilute any herbal preparations used in the eyes.

Caution: Do not use chamomile on an ongoing basis, as
ragweed allergy may result. Avoid it completely if you are
allergic to ragweed.

❑ A combination of ginkgo biloba extract and zinc sulfate
may slow progressive vision loss.

❑ Rose hips supply valuable flavonoids and vitamin C.

❑ *Avoid* the herbs ephedra (ma huang) and licorice.

RECOMMENDATIONS

❑ Follow the supplementation program outlined above.

❑ If your ophthalmologist recommends medication to
control glaucoma and it is working to your satisfaction,
continue to use it faithfully. Also take vitamin C in high
doses, but only under supervision.

❑ Avoid prolonged eye stress such as watching television,
reading, and using a computer for long periods. If you must
engage in close work for any length of time, take periodic
"focus breaks." Every twenty minutes or so, raise your eyes
and focus on something in the distance for a minute or so.

❑ Avoid tobacco smoke, coffee, alcohol, nicotine, and all
caffeine.

❑ Drink only small amounts of liquid at any given time.

❑ Avoid taking high doses of niacin (over a total of 200
milligrams daily).

CONSIDERATIONS

❑ There is no cure for glaucoma, and any damage to vision
is irreversible. Chronic open-angle glaucoma can often be
controlled through the use of medication, usually in the form
of eyedrops. Several types of these medications are available. Often an ophthalmologist has to experiment a little to
find the specific one that works most effectively for a particular individual. However, many people with glaucoma

find that the eyedrops cause severe headaches and other side effects. This problem can often be alleviated by changing the prescription. If headaches persist, it may help to adjust the schedule for taking the medication so that it interferes with normal activities as little as possible.

❑   If eyedrops fail to control intraocular pressure, a doctor may use a procedure called laser trabeculoplasty. With this technique, a laser beam makes tiny holes in the meshwork through which the aqueous fluid normally drains, opening up blocked drainage channels.

❑   Surgery has certain advantages over medication, such as reduced out-of-pocket costs. However, it has disadvantages as well. An estimated 40 percent of people who undergo surgery for glaucoma experience no improvement, and the procedure may have to be repeated; approximately 15 percent report a decline in their quality of life after surgery.

❑   The conventional treatment for acute closed-angle glaucoma is to immediately reduce eye pressure by employing an osmotic diuretic agent, followed by surgery. These osmotic agents (applied as eyedrops) almost always act immediately to alleviate symptoms. However, surgery is still recommended because without it, the attacks are likely to recur, and each attack can cause additional irreversible vision damage. Using only osmotic agents can lull a person into thinking that his or her condition is improving while in fact it is worsening rapidly.

❑   Agents that act to dilate the pupils, such as ephedra and belladonna, should be avoided at all costs.

❑   Vitamin C supplementation has been demonstrated to lower intraocular pressure in several clinical studies. Nearly normal tension levels have been achieved in some people who were unresponsive to conventional therapies. Intravenous administration of vitamin C has yielded even greater initial pressure reduction, but close monitoring by a physician is necessary to determine the required dosage. The role vitamin C plays in collagen formation may be the key to its action.

❑   Bioflavonoid supplementation prevents the breakdown of vitamin C in the body before it is metabolized. It also improves capillary integrity and stabilizes the collagen matrix by preventing free radical damage. The bioflavonoid rutin is known to help in lowering ocular pressure when used in conjunction with conventional drugs. Bilberry extract is particularly rich in this beneficial flavonoid compound. Is also good for diabetic retinopathy.

❑   Corticosteroids can induce glaucoma by destroying collagen structures in the eye. If you must take corticosteroids, you should take the smallest amount possible and for the shortest possible time. If you have glaucoma, you should avoid these medications entirely.

❑   Beta-blocking eyedrops, which are often prescribed for people with glaucoma, have a number of undesirable side effects. They tend to cause unfavorable changes in blood fats, lowering the proportion of high-density lipoproteins—the so-called "good" cholesterol—to low-density lipoproteins, or "bad" cholesterol. In addition, the incidence of hip fracture among beta-blocker users is roughly three times greater than that seen in the general population. This is attributed to the dizziness and fainting experienced by some people who take these medications. Vision loss compounds the risk of falls and other accidents. Hip fracture is a major health threat among postmenopausal women.

❑   Forskolin, an extract from the coleus plant, has been reported by Yale University to be effective for glaucoma, without causing side effects.

Glomerulonephritis

See under KIDNEY DISEASE.

Gout

Gout is a common type of arthritis that occurs when there is too much uric acid in the blood, tissues, and urine. Uric acid is the end product of the metabolism of a class of chemicals known as purines. In people with gout, the body does not produce enough of the digestive enzyme uricase, which oxidizes relatively insoluble uric acid into a highly soluble compound. As a result, uric acid accumulates in the blood and tissues and, ultimately, crystallizes.

When it crystallizes, uric acid takes on a shape like that of a needle and, like a needle, it jabs its way into the joints. It seems to prefer the joint of the big toe, but other joints can be vulnerable as well, including the mid-foot, ankle, knee, wrist, and even the fingers. Acute pain is usually the first symptom. Then the affected joints become inflamed, almost infected-looking—red, swollen, hot, and extremely sensitive to the touch.

Uric acid is a byproduct of certain foods, so gout is closely related to diet. Obesity and an improper diet increase the risk of developing gout. Gout has been called the rich man's disease, since it is associated with too much rich food and alcohol. But in fact it affects people from all walks of life, most commonly men between the ages of forty and fifty. It may be inherited or brought on by crash dieting, drinking, certain medications, overeating, stress, surgery, or injury to a joint. Approximately 90 percent of the people who suffer from gout are male. Uric acid kidney stones may be a related problem.

The best way to get a definitive diagnosis of gout is for a physician to insert a needle into the affected joint, remove some fluid, and examine the fluid under a microscope for the characteristic uric acid crystals.

NUTRIENTS

SUPPLEMENT	SUGGESTED DOSAGE	COMMENTS
Very Important		
Essential fatty acids	As directed on label. Take with meals.	Needed to repair tissues, aid in healing, and restore proper fatty acid balance. An excess of saturated fats is often behind this disorder.
Vitamin B complex	100 mg twice daily.	Needed for proper digestion and all bodily enzyme systems.
plus extra pantothenic acid (vitamin B$_5$) and	500 mg daily, in divided doses.	The anti-stress vitamin.
folic acid	200 mcg daily.	An important aid in nucleoprotein metabolism.
Vitamin C with bioflavonoids	3,000–5,000 mg daily, in divided doses.	Lowers serum uric acid levels.
Important		
AE Mulsion Forte from American Biologics	As directed on label.	Aids in reducing uric acid in the blood and is a potent antioxidant.
Kelp or alfalfa	1,000–1,500 mg daily.	Contains complete protein and vital minerals to reduce serum uric acid. *See under* Herbs, below.
Potassium	99 mg daily.	Needed for proper mineral balance.
Superoxide dismutase (SOD)	As directed on label, on an empty stomach (first thing in the morning is best). Take with a full glass of water.	An antioxidant and potent free radical destroyer.
Zinc	50–80 mg daily. Do not exceed a total of 100 mg daily from all supplements.	Important in protein metabolism and tissue repair. Use zinc gluconate lozenges or OptiZinc for best absorption.
Helpful		
Calcium and	1,500 mg daily.	To reduce stress caused by this disorder. Works well during sleep. Use chelate forms.
magnesium	750 mg daily.	
Sea cucumber (bêche-de-mer)	As directed on label.	Marine animals that have been used as an arthritis treatment in China for thousands of years.
Joint Support from Now Foods	As directed on label.	A combination of vitamins, minerals, herbs, and other nutrients that is excellent for joint problems.

HERBS

❑ Alfalfa is a good source of minerals and other nutrients that help to reduce serum uric acid. Take 2,000 to 3,000 milligrams daily in tablet or capsule form.

❑ Apply cayenne (capsicum) powder, mixed with enough wintergreen oil to make a paste, to affected areas to relieve inflammation and pain. This may cause a stinging sensation at first, but with repeated use, pain should diminish markedly. Cayenne can also be taken in capsule form.

❑ Other beneficial herbs include birch, burdock, colchicum tincture, hyssop, and juniper.

RECOMMENDATIONS

❑ When an attack of gout strikes, eat only raw fruits and vegetables for two weeks. Juices are best. Frozen or fresh cherry juice is excellent. Also drink celery juice diluted with distilled water—use distilled water only, not tap water. Cherries and strawberries neutralize uric acid, so eat lots of them. Also include grains, seeds, and nuts in your diet.

❑ Maintain a diet low in purines at all times. Purines are organic compounds that contribute to uric acid formation. Purine-rich foods to avoid include anchovies, asparagus, consommé, herring, meat gravies and broths, mushrooms, mussels, sardines, and sweetbreads.

❑ Consume plenty of quality water. Fluid intake promotes the excretion of uric acid.

❑ Eat no meat of any kind, including organ meats. Meat contains extremely high amounts of uric acid.

❑ Consume no alcohol. Alcohol increases the production of uric acid and must be eliminated from the diet.

❑ Do not eat any fried foods, roasted nuts, or any other foods containing (or cooked with) oil that has been subjected to heat. When heated, oils become rancid. Rancid fats quickly destroy vitamin E, resulting in the release of increased amounts of uric acid.

❑ Avoid rich foods such as cakes and pies. Leave white flour and sugar products out of your diet.

❑ Avoid the amino acid glycine. Glycine can be converted into uric acid more rapidly in people who suffer from gout.

❑ Limit your intake of caffeine, cauliflower, dried beans, lentils, fish, eggs, oatmeal, peas, poultry, spinach, and yeast products.

❑ If you are overweight, lose the excess pounds. Losing weight lowers serum uric acid levels. Avoid very restricted weight loss diets (crash diets), however. Abruptly cutting back on foods or fasting for longer than three days may result in increased uric acid levels.

CONSIDERATIONS

❑ Dimethylsulfoxide (DMSO) is helpful for flare-ups of gout. This oily liquid is applied topically, and is reportedly very effective at relieving pain and reducing swelling.
   Note: Only DMSO from a health food store should be used. Commercial-grade DMSO found in hardware stores is not suitable for healing purposes. The use of DMSO may result in a garlicky body odor. This is temporary, and is not a cause for concern.

❑ Treatment with honeybee venom has provided relief for some gout sufferers. In this practice, called *apitherapy*, honeybee venom is administered by injection, either with a hypodermic needle or by the bees themselves. The venom appears to act as both an anti-inflammatory and immune system stimulant. Further information is available from the American Apitherapy Society, Box 54, Hartland Four Corners, VT 05049; telephone 802–436–2708.

❑   Deficiencies of certain nutrients can provoke an attack. A deficiency of pantothenic acid (vitamin B5) produces excesssive amounts of uric acid. A study in animals found that a diet deficient in vitamin A can produce gout. Vitamin E deficiency causes damage to the nuclei of cells that produce uric acid, causing more uric acid to form.

❑   People who have candida infections, or who have taken antibiotics on and off for long periods, often have increased levels of uric acid in their blood.

❑   Because of the cellular destruction associated with chemotherapy in cancer treatment, uric acid is often released in extreme amounts, resulting in gouty arthritis.

❑   In rare cases, a secondary type of gout called saturnine gout can result from a toxic overload in the body.

❑   Allopurinol (Zyloprim), which inhibits uric acid synthesis, is often prescribed for gout. This drug has been linked directly to skin eruptions, inflammation of the blood vessels, and liver toxicity. If you have kidney problems, treatment with this drug should be carefully monitored.

❑   Colchicine, a drug derived from the autumn crocus (*Colchicum autumnale*), is used to both alleviate acute attacks and prevent further attacks from occurring. While often dramatically effective, this drug can cause serious side effects and toxicity, especially when taken in high doses and/or for prolonged periods.

❑   Cortisone is commonly prescribed for relief of acute attacks. However, this may put added strain on the adrenal glands, which are already under stress as a result of this painful disorder.

❑   *See also* ARTHRITIS in Part Two and PAIN CONTROL in Part Three.

Graves' Disease

See under HYPERTHYROIDISM.

Growth Problems

Growth problems usually occur when the pituitary gland fails to function as it should. The pituitary gland distributes hormones, including the growth hormone *somatotropin*, to various parts of the body. Somatotropin stimulates the growth of muscle and bone in growing children.

Either overproduction or underproduction of this hormone can cause growth abnormalities. The secretion of too little growth hormone by the pituitary causes dwarfism; too much causes the body to grow in an exaggerated fashion, resulting in abnormally large hands, feet, and jaw. Some cases of malfunction of the pituitary are caused by the growth of a tumor on the gland.

In some cases, growth problems are caused by the failure of the thyroid gland to function properly. The thymus gland may also be involved. If the thymus gland of an infant is damaged, development is retarded and the child has a greater than normal susceptibility to infection. Nutrition can also play a significant role in the growth and development of a child.

Unless otherwise specified, the dosages recommended here are for teenagers over age seventeen. For a child between ages twelve and seventeen, use three-quarters of the recommended amount. For a child between six and twelve, use half the recommended dose. For a child under six, use a quarter of the recommended dose.

NUTRIENTS

SUPPLEMENT	SUGGESTED DOSAGE	COMMENTS
Very Important		
Alfalfa		*See under* Herbs, below.
Cod liver oil	As directed on label.	Contains vitamins A and D, needed for proper growth and for strong tissues and bones.
Essential fatty acids or primrose oil	As directed on label. As directed on label.	For normal growth.
Kelp	As directed on label.	Contains natural iodine. An iodine deficiency can cause growth problems.
L-Lysine	As directed on label, on an empty stomach. Take with water or juice. Do not take with milk. Take with 50 mg vitamin B6 and 100 mg vitamin C for better absorption.	Needed for normal growth and bone development. *See* AMINO ACIDS in Part One. *Caution:* Do not take this supplement for longer than 6 months at a time.
Zinc	As directed on label. Do not exceed a total of 100 mg daily from all supplements.	Deficiency has been linked to growth problems. Use zinc gluconate lozenges or OptiZinc for best absorption.
Important		
Calcium and magnesium	As directed on label. As directed on label.	Needed for normal bone growth.
Free-form amino acid complex	As directed on label.	Deficiency has been linked to growth disorders.
Raw pituitary glandular	As directed on label.	For children. Stimulates growth.
Helpful		
L-Ornithine	As directed by physician.	Helps promote release of growth hormone. Use only under a physician's supervision.

Multiglandular complex	As directed on label.	For the endocrine, hormonal, and enzyme systems.
Bio-Bifidus from American Biologics	As directed on label.	For bowel flora replacement to improve assimilation and elimination.
Vitamin B complex plus extra	50 mg daily.	B vitamins work best when taken together.
vitamin B6 (pyridoxine)	50 mg 3 times daily, with meals.	Needed for uptake of the amino acids and for proper growth.

HERBS

❑ Alfalfa is a valuable source of vitamins, minerals, and other nutrients that promote the proper functioning of the pituitary gland. It can be taken in tablet or capsule form, as well as eaten in a natural form such as alfalfa sprouts.

RECOMMENDATIONS

❑ Eat a well-balanced diet high in healthful sources of protein. Protein is necessary for growth.

❑ Include in the diet foods high in the amino acid arginine. Arginine is used by the body to synthesize another amino acid, ornithine, which promotes the release of growth hormone. Good food sources of arginine include carob, coconut, dairy products, gelatin, oats, peanuts, soybeans, walnuts, wheat, and wheat germ.

CONSIDERATIONS

❑ When evaluating a child's growth, it is the overall growth pattern, rather than size, that is important. If a child seems to "fall off" a previously steady growth curve, he or she should be evaluated for possible nutritional deficiencies and other underlying health problems.

❑ If growth is slowed because of insufficient growth hormone production, a doctor may prescribe growth hormone therapy.

❑ If growth problems are the result of a tumor of the pituitary gland, surgical removal or treatment of the tumor with drugs or by other means, may be recommended.

❑ *Kwashiorkor* is a protein/calorie deficiency disorder that causes children to grow slowly and have very little resistance to disease. It is most common among very poor people in developing countries. However, it can occur anywhere if a child's protein and/or calorie requirements are not met over a period of time. If detected early, it can be treated. Malabsorption syndromes, such as that associated with celiac disease, can cause similar problems even though nutritional intake appears to be adequate.

❑ High levels of lead, a toxic metal, may cause growth problems. A hair analysis can be done to rule out this metal toxicity. (*See* LEAD POISONING in Part Two and HAIR ANALYSIS in Part Three.)

❑ *See also* HYPERTHYROIDISM and HYPOTHYROIDISM in Part Two.

Gum Disease

See PERIODONTAL DISEASE. *See also* Bleeding Gums *under* PREGNANCY-RELATED PROBLEMS.

Hair Loss

Baldness or loss of hair is referred to as alopecia. *Alopecia totalis* means loss of all the scalp hair. *Alopecia universalis* means loss of all body hair, including eyebrows and eyelashes. When the hair falls out in patches, it is termed *alopecia areata*. Factors that are involved in hair loss include heredity, hormones, and aging. Researchers have yet to determine the exact cause of hair loss, but some scientists believe the body's immune system mistakes hair follicles for foreign tissue and attacks them. Many suspect a genetic component.

A less dramatic but more prevalent type of hair loss is *androgenetic alopecia* (AGA), or male pattern baldness. AGA is common in men. As the name implies, a genetic or hereditary predisposition to the disorder and the presence of androgens—male sex hormones—are involved in this condition. Research indicates that the hair follicles of individuals susceptible to AGA may have receptors programmed to slow down or shut off hair production under the influence of androgens.

Women sometimes have the same type of hair loss, but it is not usually as extensive and most often does not occur until after menopause. All women experience some hair thinning as they grow older, especially after menopause, but in some it begins as early as puberty. In addition, most women lose some hair two or three months after having a baby because hormonal changes prevent normal hair loss during pregnancy.

In addition to heredity, factors that promote hair loss include poor circulation, acute illness, surgery, radiation exposure, skin disease, sudden weight loss, high fever, iron deficiency, diabetes, thyroid disease, drugs such as those used in chemotherapy, stress, poor diet, and vitamin deficiencies.

NUTRIENTS

SUPPLEMENT	SUGGESTED DOSAGE	COMMENTS
Very Important		
Bio Rizin from American Biologics		*See under* Herbs, below.
Essential fatty acids (flaxseed oil, primrose oil, and salmon oil are good sources)	As directed on label.	Improves hair texture. Prevents dry, brittle hair.
Raw thymus glandular	500 mg daily.	Stimulates immune function and improves functioning capacity of glands. *Caution:* Do not give this supplement to a child.

Ultra Hair from Nature's Plus	As directed on label.	Contains nutrients necessary to stimulate hair growth. If the condition is not severe, you can use this complex alone.
Vitamin B complex with		B vitamins are important for the health and growth of the hair.
vitamin B_3 (niacin) and	50 mg 3 times daily.	
pantothenic acid (vitamin B_5) and	100 mg 3 times daily.	
vitamin B_6 (pyridoxine) plus	50 mg 3 times daily.	
biotin and	50 mg 3 times daily. Also use hair care products containing biotin.	Deficiencies have been linked to skin disorders and hair loss.
inositol	100 mg twice daily.	Vital for hair growth.
Vitamin C	3,000–10,000 mg daily.	Aids in improving scalp circulation.
Vitamin E	Start with 400 IU daily and slowly increase to 800–1,000 IU daily.	Increases oxygen uptake, which improves circulation to the scalp. Improves health and growth of hair.
Zinc	50–100 mg daily. Do not exceed this amount.	Stimulates hair growth by enhancing immune function. Use zinc gluconate lozenges or OptiZinc for best absorption.
Important		
Coenzyme Q_{10}	60 mg daily.	Improves scalp circulation. Increases tissue oxygenation.
Dimethylglycine (DMG) (Aangamik DMG from FoodScience Labs)	100 mg daily.	Good for circulation to the scalp.
Kelp	500 mg daily.	Supplies needed minerals for proper hair growth.
Helpful		
Copper	3 mg daily.	Works with zinc to aid in hair growth. Use a chelate form.
Dioxychlor from American Biologics	5 drops in water twice daily.	Destroys harmful bacteria and supplies oxygen to the tissues.
L-Cysteine and L-methionine	500 mg each twice daily, on an empty stomach. Take with water or juice. Do not take with milk. Take with 50 mg vitamin B_6 and 100 mg vitamin C for better absorption.	Improves quality, texture, and growth of hair. Helps prevent hair from falling out. *See* AMINO ACIDS in Part One.
Silica or horsetail	As directed on label.	Helps to keep hair looking shiny and sleek. *See under* Herbs, below.

HERBS

❑ Use apple cider vinegar and sage tea as a rinse to help hair grow.

❑ Bio Rizin from American Biologics contains licorice extract and may help prevent hair loss. It can be taken orally and/or used topically.

❑ Horsetail is a good source of silica, necessary for strong, shiny hair.

RECOMMENDATIONS

❑ Eat plenty of foods high in biotin and/or take supplemental biotin as recommended under Nutrients, on this page. Biotin is needed for healthy hair and skin, and may even prevent hair loss in some men. Good food sources of biotin include brewer's yeast, brown rice, bulgur, green peas, lentils, oats, soybeans, sunflower seeds, and walnuts.

❑ Do not eat foods containing raw eggs. Raw eggs not only pose a risk of *Salmonella* infection (*see* FOOD POISONING in Part Two), but are high in avidin, a protein that binds biotin and prevents it from being absorbed. Cooked eggs are acceptable.

❑ Lie head down on a slant board fifteen minutes a day to allow the blood to reach your scalp. Massage your scalp daily.

❑ Be careful of using products that are not natural on the hair. Allergic reactions to chemicals in these products occur frequently. Alternate among several different hair care products, using only all-natural and pH-balanced formulas.

❑ Avoid rough treatment. Do not use a brush or fine-toothed comb, or towel-dry your hair. Also, do not use a blow dryer or other heated appliances on your hair; let it dry naturally. Do not comb your hair until it is dry, as wet hair tends to break off. Use a pick to put wet hair in place.

❑ If you are losing large amounts of hair, see a physician.

CONSIDERATIONS

❑ It is normal to lose 50 to 100 hairs a day.

❑ Taking large doses of vitamin A (100,000 IU or more daily) for a long period can trigger hair loss, but stopping the vitamin A will reverse the problem. Often the hair grows back when the cause is corrected.

❑ Rogaine, a topical solution developed by the Upjohn Company and containing 2 percent minoxidil, has been approved by the FDA for the treatment of male pattern baldness. This product is now available over the counter in drugstores. However, this drug may cause heart changes if used for long periods of time, researchers at the University of Toronto report. Also, although using minoxidil does result in hair growth, the quality of the hair is usually poor and hair growth ceases when use is discontinued.

❑ Hypothyroidism can cause hair loss. (*See* HYPOTHYROIDISM in Part Two.)

❑ Kombucha tea has been reported by some to help halt hair loss. (*See* MAKING KOMBUCHA TEA in Part Three.)

Halitosis (Bad Breath)

Halitosis is typically caused by poor dental hygiene. However, other factors may be involved, including gum disease, tooth decay, heavy metal buildup, nose or throat infection, improper diet, constipation, smoking, diabetes, foreign bacteria in the mouth, indigestion, inadequate protein digestion, liver malfunction, postnasal drip, stress, and too much unfriendly bacteria in the colon.

NUTRIENTS

SUPPLEMENT	SUGGESTED DOSAGE	COMMENTS
Very Important		
Aerobic Bulk Cleanse (ABC) from Aerobic Life Industries or oat bran or psyllium husks or rice bran	1 tbsp in juice or water twice daily, on an empty stomach. Take separately from other supplements and medications.	For needed fiber. Fiber removes toxins from the colon that can result in bad breath.
Chlorophyll (alfalfa liquid, wheatgrass, and barley juice are good sources)	1 tbsp in juice twice daily. Chlorophyll can also be used as a mouth rinse—add 1 tbsp to ½ glass of water.	"Green drinks" are one of the best ways to combat bad breath.
Vitamin C	2,000–6,000 mg daily.	Important in healing mouth and gum disease and in preventing bleeding gums. Also rids the body of excess mucus and toxins that can cause bad breath.
Important		
Acidophilus	As directed on label. Take on an empty stomach.	Needed to replenish "friendly" bacteria in the colon. Insufficient "friendly" bacteria and an overabundance of harmful bacteria can cause bad breath.
Alfalfa		*See under* Herbs, below.
Garlic (Kyolic)	2 capsules 4 times daily, with meals and at bedtime.	Acts as a natural antibiotic, destroying foreign bacteria in both the mouth and colon. Use an odorless form.
Zinc	30 mg 3 times daily. Do not exceed 100 mg daily.	Has an antibacterial effect and neutralizes sulfur compounds, a common cause of mouth odor.
Helpful		
Bee propolis	As directed on label.	Aids in healing the gums, aids control of infection in the body, and has an antibacterial effect.
Vitamin A	15,000 IU daily. If you are pregnant, do not exceed 10,000 IU daily.	Needed for control of infection and in healing of the mouth.
plus natural beta-carotene	10,000 IU daily.	
or carotenoid complex (Betatene)	As directed on label.	
Vitamin B complex	100 mg daily.	Needed for proper digestion.
plus extra vitamin B3 (niacin)	50 mg 3 times daily. Do not exceed this amount.	Dilates tiny capillaries to help blood flow to infection sites. *Caution:* Do not take niacin if you have a liver disorder, gout, or high blood pressure.
and vitamin B6 (pyridoxine)	50 mg daily.	Needed for all enzyme systems in the body.

HERBS

❑ Alfalfa supplies chlorophyll, which cleanses the bloodstream and colon, where bad breath often begins. Take 500 to 1,000 mg in tablet form or 1 tablespoon of liquid in juice or water three times daily.

❑ Gum disease is a major factor in bad breath. If infection is present, place alcohol-free goldenseal extract on a small piece of cotton and place the cotton over infected gums or mouth sores. Do this for two hours per day for three days. It should quickly heal the infected parts.

❑ Use myrrh (to brush your teeth and rinse your mouth), peppermint, rosemary, and sage.
Caution: Do not use sage if you suffer from epilepsy or other seizure disorder.

❑ Chewing a sprig of parsley after meals is an excellent treatment for bad breath. Parsley is rich in chlorophyll, the active ingredient in many popular breath mints.

RECOMMENDATIONS

❑ Go on a five-day raw foods diet. Eat at least 50 percent of your food raw every day.

❑ Avoid spicy foods, whose odors can linger for hours. Foods like anchovies, blue cheese, Camembert, garlic, onions, pastrami, pepperoni, Roquefort cheese, salami, and tuna leave oils in the mouth that can release odor for up to twenty-four hours, no matter how much you brush or gargle. Beer, coffee, whiskey, and wine leave residues that stick to the soft, sticky plaque on teeth and get into the digestive system. Each exhalation releases their odor back into the air.

❑ Avoid foods that get stuck between the teeth easily or that cause tooth decay, such as meat, stringy vegetables, and sweets, especially sticky sweets.

❑ Go on a cleansing fast with fresh lemon juice and water to detoxify the system. *See* FASTING in Part Three.

❑ Brush your teeth *and tongue* after every meal.

❑ Replace your toothbrush every month, as well as after any infectious illness, to prevent bacteria buildup.

❑ Use dental floss and a chlorophyll mouthwash daily.

❑ Use Stim-U-Dent wooden toothpicks, available in most drugstores, after every meal to massage between the teeth. This is important for the prevention of gum disease.

❑ Keep your toothbrush clean. Between uses, store it in hydrogen peroxide or grapefruit seed extract to kill germs (if using hydrogen peroxide, rinse it well before brushing). There are bacteria-destroying toothbrush sanitizers available that turn on automatically at intervals throughout the day.

❑ Do not use commercial mouthwashes. Most contain nothing more than flavoring, dye, and alcohol. While they may kill the bacteria that cause bad breath, the bacteria soon return in greater force. Mouthwashes can also irritate the gums, tongue, and mucous membranes in the mouth.

❑ Bad breath may be a sign of an underlying health problem. Consult your health care provider for a thorough checkup if the suggestions in this section do not improve the condition.

CONSIDERATIONS

❑ *See also* PERIODONTAL DISEASE; SINUSITIS; and/or SORE THROAT in Part Two.

Hay Fever

Hay fever (allergic rhinitis) is an allergic response to pollen that affects the mucous membranes of the nose, eyes, and air passages. Symptoms include itchy eyes, watery discharge from the nose and eyes, sneezing, and nervous irritability. Many of the symptoms of hay fever are similar to those of the common cold. However, allergies cause a distinctive clear, thin nasal discharge, whereas secretions caused by colds usually become thick and yellow-green as the illness progresses. Also, colds are often associated with mild fever and are usually gone within a week, while allergy sufferers often have a feeling of being "wiped out" for weeks on end.

At least 22 million Americans suffer from the seasonal sneezes, runny nose, and itchy eyes that come with hay fever. There are actually three hay fever seasons, distinguished by the different types of pollen present at different times. Tree pollens appear first, usually between February and May, depending on the local climate. The biggest problems come later in spring and in summer, when both tree and grass pollens—and people—are out at the same time. The fall is ragweed pollen season. Depending on which pollen or pollens an individual is allergic to, hay fever may be present at any or all of these times.

People who suffer from hay fever often also suffer from other so-called atopic disorders, such as asthma and dermatitis. Those who suffer from hay fever symptoms throughout the year are said to have *perennial rhinitis*. The symptoms may be triggered by animal hair, dust, feathers, fungus spores, or some other environmental agent.

People prone to allergies are most often aware of the time of year and conditions under which they are most sensitive. For a definitive diagnosis, the radioallergosorbent (RAST) test is easily done and gives reliable results.

The nutrient program outlined below is beneficial for hay fever. Hay fever sufferers should always choose hypoallergenic supplements.

NUTRIENTS

SUPPLEMENT	SUGGESTED DOSAGE	COMMENTS
Very Important		
Coenzyme Q$_{10}$	30 mg twice daily.	Improves oxygenation and immunity.
Quercetin	400 mg twice daily, before meals.	A bioflavonoid that stabilizes the membranes of the cells that release histamine, which triggers allergic symptoms. Contains quercetin plus bromelain and vitamin C for better absorption.
or		
Activated Quercetin from Source Naturals	As directed on label.	
or		
AntiAllergy formula from Freeda Vitamins	As directed on label.	A combination of quercetin, calcium pantothenate, and calcium ascorbate.
Raw thymus glandular	500 mg twice daily.	Promotes immune function. *Caution:* Do not give this supplement to a child under 16 years of age.
Vitamin A	100,000 IU daily for 1 month, then reduce to 25,000 IU daily. If you are pregnant, do not exceed 10,000 IU daily.	A powerful immunostimulant. An emulsion form is recommended for easier assimilation and greater safety at high doses.
Vitamin B complex plus extra	As directed on label.	All B vitamins are necessary for proper functioning of the immune system.
pantothenic acid (vitamin B$_5$) and	100 mg 3 times daily.	
vitamin B$_6$ (pyridoxine)	50 mg twice daily.	
Vitamin C with bioflavonoids	3,000–10,000 mg 3 times daily.	A potent immunostimulant and anti-inflammatory. Use an esterified or buffered form.
Important		
Proteolytic enzymes	As directed on label. Take with meals and between meals.	Necessary for digestion of essential nutrients that boost immune function. *Caution:* Do not give this supplement to a child.
Zinc	50–80 mg daily. Do not exceed a total of 100 mg daily from all supplements.	Boosts immune function. Use zinc gluconate lozenges or OptiZinc for best absorption.
Helpful		
Alfalfa		*See under* Herbs, below.
Aller Bee-Gone from CC Pollen	As directed on label.	A combination of herbs, enzymes, and nutrients to fight acute symptoms.
Bio Rizin from American Biologics		*See under* Herbs, below.
Calcium and	1,500 mg daily.	Minerals that have a calming effect on the system.
magnesium	1,000 mg daily.	
Dioxychlor from American Biologics	5 drops in water twice daily. Also use topically: mix 30 drops in 2 oz water and instill 1 dropperful in each nostril.	To supply stabilized oxygen and fight bacteria, fungi, and viruses.
or		
Aerobic 07 from Aerobic Life Industries	As directed on label.	
Manganese	5–10 mg daily. Take separately from calcium.	Aids in metabolism of vitamins, minerals, enzymes, and carbohydrates.
Pycnogenol	As directed on label.	A powerful free radical scavenger that also acts as an anti-inflammatory and enhances the activity of vitamin C.
Kelp	As directed on label twice daily.	A rich source of minerals.

Superoxide dismutase (SOD) (Cell Guard from Biotec Foods)	As directed on label.	A powerful antioxidant.
Vitamin E	400–800 IU daily.	Boosts the immune system.

HERBS

❑ Alfalfa supplies chlorophyll and vitamin K. Use a liquid form. Take 1 tablespoon in juice or water twice daily.

❑ Bio Rizin from American Biologics contains licorice extract, which improves energy levels and helps relieve allergy symptoms. Take 10 to 20 drops twice daily or as needed.
  Caution: Do not use licorice for more than seven days at a time. Avoid it completely if you have high blood pressure.

❑ Ephedra helps to relieve bronchial spasms, congestion, and coughing.
  Caution: Do not use this herb if you suffer from anxiety, glaucoma, heart disease, high blood pressure, or insomnia, or if you are taking a monoamine oxidase (MAO) inhibitor drug for depression.

❑ If your throat is itchy or you want to cough, use alcohol-free goldenseal extract. Hold a dropperful in your mouth for a few minutes, then swallow. This will halt a sore throat.
  Caution: Do not take goldenseal internally on a daily basis for more than one week at a time, as it may disturb normal intestinal flora. Do not use it during pregnancy, and use it with caution if you are allergic to ragweed.

❑ Horehound, mullein leaf, stinging nettle, and/or wild cherry bark help to ward off severe allergic reactions.

RECOMMENDATIONS

❑ Eat more fruits (especially bananas), vegetables, grains, and raw nuts and seeds. Stay on a high-fiber diet.

❑ Eat yogurt or any soured products three times a week. Homemade yogurt is best. However, beware of the possibility that you may be allergic to casein, the principal protein found in milk.

❑ Consume no cakes, chocolate, coffee, dairy products (except yogurt), packaged or canned foods, pies, soft drinks, sugar, tobacco, white flour products, or any junk food.

❑ When allergy season arrives, spend as little time as possible outdoors. Keep windows closed during the day, and use your car air conditioner when you drive. Especially avoid going outside in the afternoon. If you exercise or play sports outside, do it in the morning rather than in the afternoon; grasses pollinate in midday and the wind keeps the pollen floating until it drops to the ground at night.

❑ Shower and change your clothes when you come indoors after spending time outside. Pollen can stick to your hair, especially on a windy day. Washing your hair helps to keep the pollen from getting into your eyes.

❑ Perform a cleansing fast. *See* FASTING in Part Three.

❑ Keep pets either inside or outside. Dogs and cats can pick up pollen on their fur and bring it indoors with them.

❑ Try using an air purifier. The Air Supply personal air purifier from Wein Products is a miniature unit that is worn around the neck. It sets up an invisible pure air shield against microorganisms (such as viruses, bacteria, and mold) and microparticles (including dust, pollen, and pollutants) in the air. It also eliminates vapors, smells, and harmful volatile compounds in the air. The Living Air XL-15 unit from Alpine Industries is an ionizing unit that is good for purifying the air in the home or workplace.

CONSIDERATIONS

❑ The best and safest way to control allergies is the natural way—avoiding allergens and taking steps to normalize immune function and prevent or lessen the symptoms. Allergies can usually be controlled if you are willing to make changes in your lifestyle, diet, and mental state.

❑ A study at the University of California–Davis found that eating yogurt every day significantly reduced the incidence of hay fever attacks, especially those triggered by grass pollens.

❑ Researchers at Giessen University in Germany found that three bananas contain enough magnesium—180 milligrams—to quell a hay fever attack. Other foods rich in magnesium are kidney beans, soybeans, almonds, lima beans, whole-wheat flour, brown rice, molasses, and peas. Magnesium can also be taken in supplement form.

❑ Antihistamines are the most commonly recommended conventional treatment for hay fever. They can reduce itching in the eyes, ears, and throat; dry up a runny nose; and reduce sneezing attacks. However, they can also cause drowsiness, depression, and other side effects. Newer antihistamines, such as terfenadine (Seldane), astemizole (Hismanal), and loratidine (Claritin) do not cause drowsiness and depression. But they are expensive and available only by prescription, and they might not work for everyone.

❑ Steroid drugs are even more powerful suppressors of allergic reactions than antihistamines. Doctors often prescribe the steroid beclomethasone in nasal inhalers sold under the brand names Beconase and Vancenase. These can be very effective in relieving symptoms, but some of the steroids are bound to get into the rest of the body. Steroids suppress immune function.

❑ Some physicians recommend desensitization shots for people with hay fever. These are expensive, painful, and not risk-free. A disappointingly low percentage of people experience satisfactory relief, even after years of injections. The typical person requires weekly shots for up to a year and monthly shots for up to five years, at a total cost that can run into the thousands of dollars.

❑ *See also* ALLERGIES in Part Two and ASCORBIC ACID FLUSH in Part Three.

Headache

Virtually everyone gets a headache at one time or another. Common causes of headache include stress; tension; anxiety; allergies; constipation; coffee consumption; eyestrain; hunger; sinus pressure; muscle tension; hormonal imbalances; temporomandibular joint (TMJ) syndrome; trauma to the head; nutritional deficiencies; the use of alcohol, drugs, or tobacco; fever; and exposure to irritants such as pollution, perfume, or after-shaves.

Headache experts estimate that about 90 percent of all headaches are tension headaches and 6 percent are migraines. Tension headaches, as the name implies, are caused by muscular tension. Migraines result from a disturbance in the blood circulation to the brain. Another type of headache is the cluster headache. These are severe, recurring headaches that strike about 1 million Americans.

Headaches that occur often may be a sign of an underlying health problem. People who suffer from frequent headaches may be reacting to certain foods and food additives, such as wheat, chocolate, monosodium glutamate (MSG), sulfites (used in restaurants on salad bars), sugar, hot dogs, luncheon meats, dairy products, nuts, citric acid, fermented foods (cheeses, sour cream, yogurt), alcohol, vinegar, and/or marinated foods. Other possibilities to consider are anemia, bowel problems, brain disorders, bruxism (tooth-grinding), hypertension (high blood pressure), hypoglycemia (low blood sugar), sinusitis, spinal misalignment, toxic overdoses of vitamin A, vitamin B deficiency, and diseases of the eye, nose, and throat.

NUTRIENTS

SUPPLEMENT	SUGGESTED DOSAGE	COMMENTS
Helpful		
Bromelain	500 mg as needed.	An enzyme that helps to regulate the inflammatory response.
Calcium and magnesium	1,500 mg daily. 1,000 mg daily.	Minerals that help to alleviate muscular tension. Use chelated forms.
Coenzyme Q10	30 mg twice daily.	Improves tissue oxygenation.
Dimethylglycine (DMG) (Aangamik DMG from FoodScience Labs)	125 mg twice daily.	Improves tissue oxygenation. Use a sublingual form.
DL-Phenylalanine (DLPA)	750 mg daily.	For pain relief. *Caution:* Do not take this supplement if you are pregnant or nursing a baby, or if you suffer from panic attacks, diabetes, high blood pressure, or PKU.
Glucosamine sulfate	As directed on label.	A natural alternative to aspirin and other nonsteroidal anti-inflammatory drugs (NSAIDs).
L-Tyrosine plus L-glutamine plus quercetin	As directed on label. 500 mg twice daily. 500 mg twice daily.	For relief of cluster headaches. *Caution:* Do not take tyrosine if you are taking an MAO inhibitor drug, commonly prescribed for depression.
Potassium	99 mg daily.	For the proper sodium and potassium balance, which is needed to avoid water retention. Water retention may put undue pressure on the brain.
Primrose oil	500 mg 3–4 times daily.	Supplies essential fatty acids, which promote healthy circulation, help regulate the inflammatory response, and relieve pain.
Vitamin B3 (niacin) and niacinamide	Up to 300 mg combined daily. Do not exceed this amount. Stop and maintain the dosage that provides relief.	Improves circulation and aids in the functioning of the nervous system. Professional supervision is advised. *Caution:* Do not take niacin if you have a liver disorder, gout, or high blood pressure.
Vitamin B complex plus extra vitamin B6 (pyridoxine)	50 mg 3 times daily. 50 mg 3 times daily.	B vitamins work best when taken together. Use a yeast-free formula. In severe cases, injections (under a doctor's supervision) may be advisable. Removes excess water from tissues.
Vitamin C with bioflavonoids	2,000–8,000 mg daily, in divided doses.	Protects against harmful effects of pollution and aids production of anti-stress hormones. Use an esterified or buffered form.
Vitamin E	Start with 400 IU daily and increase slowly to 1,200 IU daily.	Improves circulation.

HERBS

❑ The following herbs may relieve headache pain: brigham, burdock root, fenugreek, feverfew, goldenseal, lavender, lobelia, marshmallow, mint, rosemary, skullcap, and thyme.

Caution: Do not use feverfew during pregnancy. Do not take goldenseal internally on a daily basis for more than one week at a time, do not use it during pregnancy, and use it with caution if you are allergic to ragweed. Do not take lobelia internally on an ongoing basis.

❑ A salve made from ginger, peppermint oil, and wintergreen oil rubbed on the nape of the neck and temples can help relieve tension headaches. For sinus headaches, rub the salve across the sinus area.

❑ Ginkgo biloba extract improves circulation to the brain, and may be helpful for certain types of headache.

RECOMMENDATIONS

❑ Eat a well-balanced diet. Avoid chewing gum, ice cream, iced beverages, salt, and excessive sunlight.

❑ Practice deep-breathing exercises. A lack of oxygen can cause headaches.

Types of Headaches

Headaches come in a number of forms, differentiated by their causes and specific symptoms. The appropriate treatment depends on the type of headache. The table below lists some of the more common types of headaches and possible treatments for them.

Type of Headache	Symptoms	Causes	Treatment
Arthritis headache	Pain at the back of the head or neck, made worse by movement; inflammation of joints and shoulder and/or neck muscles.	Unknown.	Take feverfew supplements. *Caution:* Do not use feverfew during pregnancy.
Bilious headache	Dull pain in forehead and throbbing temples.	Indigestion; overeating; lack of exercise.	Colon cleansing may be helpful (*see* COLON CLEANSING in Part Three).
Caffeine headache	Throbbing pain caused by blood vessels that have dilated.	Caffeine withdrawal.	Ingest a small amount of caffeine, then taper off.
Classic migraine	Similar to common migraine, but preceded by auras such as visual disturbances, numbness in arms or legs, smelling of strange odors, hallucinations.	Excessive dilation or contraction of blood vessels of the brain.	*See* MIGRAINE in Part Two.
Cluster headache	Severe, throbbing pain on one side of the head, flushing of the face, tearing of eyes, nasal congestion, occurring 1–3 times a day over a period of weeks or months and lasting from a few minutes to several hours each time.	Stress, alcohol, smoking.	Take supplemental L-tyrosine, DL-phenylalanine, ginkgo biloba extract, L-glutamine, quercetin. *Caution:* Do not take L-tyrosine if you are taking an MAO inhibitor drug. Do not take phenylalanine if you are pregnant or suffer from panic attacks, diabetes, high blood pressure, or phenylketonuria (PKU).
Common migraine	Severe throbbing pain, often on one side of the head; nausea; vomiting; cold hands; dizziness; sensitivity to light and sounds.	Excessive dilation or contraction of blood vessels of the brain.	*See* MIGRAINE in Part Two.
Exertion headache	Generalized headache during or after physical exertion such as running or sexual intercourse, or passive exertion such as sneezing or coughing.	Usually related to migraine or cluster headaches. About 10 percent are related to organic diseases such as tumors or blood vessel malformation.	Take nutritional supplements; apply ice packs at the site of pain.
Eyestrain headache	Usually bilateral, frontal pain.	Eye muscle imbalance; uncorrected vision; astigmatism.	Correct vision.
Fever headache	Headache develops with fever due to inflammation of blood vessels of the head.	Infection.	Reduce fever, apply ice packs.

Type of Headache	Symptoms	Causes	Treatment
Hangover headache	Migraine-like, with throbbing pain and nausea.	Alcohol causes dehydration and dilation of blood vessels in the brain.	Drink plenty of quality water and fruit juices. Apply ice to neck.
Hunger headache	Strikes just before mealtime due to low blood sugar, muscle tension, and rebound dilation of blood vessels.	Skipping meals; too-stringent dieting.	Eat regular meals with adequate amounts of complex carbohydrates and protein.
Hypertension headache	Dull, generalized pain affecting a large area of the head and aggravated by movement or exertion.	Severe high blood pressure.	Get blood pressure under control.
Menstrual headache	Migraine-type pain shortly before, during, or after menstruation, or at midcycle, at time of ovulation.	Variation in estrogen levels.	Take supplements of vitamin B$_6$, potassium, and extra magnesium.
Sinus headache	Gnawing, nagging pain over nasal/sinus area, often increasing in severity as the day goes by. Fever and discolored mucus may be present.	Allergies, infection, nasal polyps, food allergies. Often caused by blocked sinus ducts or acute sinus infection.	Increase intake of vitamins A and C; use moist heat to help get sinuses to drain.
Temporo-mandibular joint (TMJ) headache	Temporal, above-ear, or facial pain; muscle contraction of one side of face; clicking or popping of jaw; neck or upper back pain; temple pain upon awakening.	Stress, malocclusion (poor bite), jaw clenching, gum chewing.	Reduce stress; use relaxation techniques, biofeedback, nutritional supplements, ice packs.
Temporal headache	Jabbing, burning, boring pain; pain in temple or around ear on chewing; weight loss; problems with eyesight. Usually seen in people over 55.	Inflammation of temporal arteries.	Consult physician for steroid therapy.
Tension headache	Constant pain, in one area or all over the head; sore muscles with trigger points in neck and upper back; lightheadedness, dizziness. The most common type of headache.	Emotional stress, anxiety, worry, depression, anger, food allergies, poor posture.	Apply ice packs on neck and upper back; take supplements of vitamin C with bioflavonoids, DLPA, bromelain, magnesium, and primrose oil.
Tic douloureux	Short, jabbing pains around the mouth, jaw, or forehead. More common in women over 55 years old.	Unknown.	Take nutritional supplements. In some cases, surgery may be necessary.

❑ Try eliminating foods containing tyramine and the amino acid phenylalanine. Then reintroduce one food at a time and see which ones produce headaches. Phenylalanine is found in aspartame (Equal, NutraSweet), monosodium glutamate (MSG), and nitrites (preservatives found in hot dogs and luncheon meats). Foods that contain tyramine include alcoholic beverages, bananas, cheese, chicken, chocolate, citrus fruits, cold cuts, herring, onions, peanut butter, pork, smoked fish, sour cream, vinegar, wine, and fresh-baked yeast products. Tyramine causes the blood pressure to rise, resulting in a dull headache.

❑ Always seek and treat the cause of the headache, not the symptom. Long-term overreliance on aspirin, acetaminophen, and other nonprescription painkillers can make chronic headaches worse by interfering with the brain's natural ability to fight headaches. If you are using nonprescription painkillers more than four times a week, talk to your health care provider about other ways to control the pain.

❑ Use fiber daily and a cleansing enema weekly. *See* COLON CLEANSING and ENEMAS in Part Three.

Note: Always take supplemental fiber separately from other supplements and medications.

❑ When a headache strikes, take a cleansing enema. This removes the toxins that cause many headaches. If not eliminated, toxins can be absorbed into the bloodstream and circulated throughout the body. For a headache brought on by fasting, use a coffee retention enema. *See* ENEMAS in Part Three.

❑ Apply cold compresses to the spot from which the pain is radiating. This helps relieve headaches by constricting blood vessels and easing muscle spasms. Leave a damp washcloth in the freezer for ten minutes or use a cold gel-pack.

❑ Use a heating pad, hot water bottle, or hot towel to relax neck and shoulder muscles, which can cause muscle contraction headaches when they are too tight.

❑ For headaches caused by sinus congesion, try self-massage. By applying pressure to specific areas of the head, you can open up the sinuses and ease tension. Rub the area surrounding the bones just above and below the eyes, and massage the cheeks directly in line with these points. Lean your head forward slightly to facilitate sinus drainage. Applying heat to the sinuses, either with compresses or with steam inhalation, can also be beneficial.

❑ To help prevent headaches, eat small meals and eat between meals to help stabilize wide swings in blood sugar. Include almonds, almond milk, watercress, parsley, fennel, garlic, cherries, and pineapple in your diet.

❑ Be sure to get sufficient sleep. Inositol, tryptophan, and/or calcium, if taken before bedtime, aid sleeping. A grapefruit half also helps. Do not eat sweet fruit or anything else sweet after 5:00 p.m.

❑ If you suffer from headaches while taking birth control pills, talk to your doctor about switching to a low-estrogen formulation or going off the pills for a while. Oral contraceptives can cause a vitamin B6 deficiency that results in headaches and migraines.

❑ If you must eat a food to which you suspect you may be sensitive, use charcoal tablets (from a health food store). Take five tablets within an hour before eating, and three tablets after eating. As soon as possible, take a cleansing enema and a coffee retention enema. If you have severe headaches after consuming a food, this will relieve it quickly by eliminating the allergenic substances. Do not take charcoal tablets daily, however, as they also absorb the good nutrients.

❑ If any of the following symptoms accompany the headache, consult your health care provider: blurred vision, confusion or loss of speech, fever and stiffness in the neck, sensitivity to light, pressure behind the eyes that is relieved by vomiting, pressure in the facial sinus area, throbbing of the head and temples, a pounding heartbeat, visual color changes, and feeling as though your head will explode. Seek immediate medical attention if you experience a sudden, severe headache like a "thunderclap," or if you experience a headache after a head injury, even a minor fall or bump. Chronic headache pain that worsens after coughing, exertion, straining, or sudden movement is also reason to seek professional attention.

❑ If you suffer from more than the occasional tension headache, keep a headache log to help your health care provider diagnose your condition. Keep the log for at least two months, noting the time of each headache and describing the pain (throbbing or dull), its severity, location, and duration.

CONSIDERATIONS

❑ Headaches are often caused by allergies. A food allergy diary can help identify offending foods. (*See* ALLERGIES in Part Two.)

❑ Poor vertebral alignment may cause reduced blood flow to the brain. This is often caused by flat feet or by wearing high heels. Chiropractic adjustment can help.

❑ Regular exercise can help prevent headaches caused by tension and may also reduce the frequency and severity of migraines. But headaches with organic causes can be made worse by exercise. Talk to your health care provider about your headaches before using exercise to control the pain.

❑ Researchers are studying the possibility that the trigeminal nerve pathway (the site of the nerve responsible for sensation in the face, mouth, and nasal cavity) and the brain chemical serotonin are factors in severe headaches. Disturbances in serotonin levels are associated with most headaches. In migraines, serotonin levels increase before onset and then decrease during the headache phase. In chronic tension headaches, serotonin levels remain low all the time. As a result of lower serotonin levels, an impulse moves along the trigeminal nerve to blood vessels in the meninges, the brain's outer covering. This causes blood vessels in the meninges to dilate and become inflamed and swollen. The result is a headache.

❑ The drug sumatriptan (Imitrex) is sometimes prescribed for relief of migraines. This drug works by increasing the amount of serotonin in the brain. It is relatively expensive, however, and must be administered by injection (it is sold in the form of a home injection kit). Possible side effects include increased heart rate, elevated blood pressure, and a feeling of tightness in the chest, jaw, or neck.

❑ Some doctors prescribe the drug lidocaine (Anestacon, Xylocaine) for cluster headaches. Used in nose drop form, it gives relief in minutes.

❑ In one study, twenty adults suffering from long-term cluster headaches squirted a capsaicin solution in their noses daily for five days. Within ten days of the last dose, there was a 67 percent drop in the number of attacks.

There are a number of common misdiagnoses of headache, including sinus pain, allergies, and temporomandibular joint syndrome (TMJ). What many people think are sinus headaches are really migraines. Sinus infections can cause brief, intense bouts of head pain, but recurring headaches are more likely to be tension headaches, migraines, or cluster headaches. Facial pain, pain in the temples, or pain above the ear is sometimes diagnosed as temporomandibular joint (TMJ) headache, caused by the joint of the jawbone being out of alignment. But this too may actually be one of the common types of headache, which may be triggered or aggravated by the joint.

❑ Women who suffer from migraines may benefit from using progesterone cream topically.

❑ *See also* HYPOGLYCEMIA; MIGRAINE; and TMJ SYNDROME, all in Part Two.

❑ *See also* PAIN CONTROL in Part Three.

Hearing Loss

Loss of hearing occurs when the passage of sound waves to the brain is impaired. Hearing loss may be partial or complete, temporary or permanent, depending on the cause. Hearing loss affects more than 23.2 million Americans. Nearly 30 percent of adults over the age of sixty-five have sustained some degree of hearing impairment. Diagnosis and assessment of the degree of hearing loss is a complicated process involving a variety of different tests.

Doctors divide hearing loss into two basic categories: conductive hearing loss, which occurs when the passage of sound waves is impeded in the external or middle ear, and sensorineural hearing loss, which results from damage to the structures or pathways of the inner ear. Conductive hearing loss may result from factors such as earwax buildup, middle ear infection and inflammation, or excessive rigidity of the tiny bones in the middle ear that convey the vibrations of the eardrum to the inner ear structures. Sensorineural hearing loss may result from damage to the acoustic nerve (the eighth cranial nerve, also known as the auditory nerve), which carries information from the inner ear to the brain, or from damage to tiny cells called hair cells in the inner ear. The hair cells are responsible for translating sound waves into nerve impulses for transmission to the brain. If the hair cells die, they are unable to repair themselves and the resulting hearing loss is permanent. Sensorineural hearing loss can be present from birth, or it can be caused by certain drugs, illness (especially high fever), exposure to loud noises, smoking, or trauma. It can also be incurred in the aging process. This type of hearing loss affects both the acuity and clarity of hearing. Initially, it is noticed at higher pitches, and then, as it progresses, it is noticed at lower pitches, where speech is heard. It is also possible to have mixed hearing loss, in which both conductive and sensorineural loss are present.

Hearing loss can be sudden or gradual, occurring over a period of days, weeks, or years. Infection, trauma, changes in atmospheric pressure, and earwax buildup or impaction can cause a sudden loss of hearing. Infection and inflammation often follow an upper respiratory infection or trauma to the ear, such as from the overuse or improper use of cotton swabs. Bathing or swimming in water that is overly chlorinated or contains high levels of bacteria and/or fungi can also lead to ear infections. Persistent and recurrent ear infections are often linked to fungal infection (candidiasis) and are frequently seen in people with allergies, cancer, diabetes, or other chronic diseases.

If hearing loss develops gradually, the individual experiencing it may be unaware of it until it reaches a fairly advanced stage. In fact, it is not uncommon for friends and family members to notice signs of hearing loss before the person experiencing it does. Some signs that may point to a hearing problem include seeming inattentiveness, unusually loud speech, irrelevant comments, inappropriate responses to questions or environmental sounds, requests for statements to be repeated, a tendency to turn one ear toward sound, and unusual voice quality.

Hearing loss associated with ear pain may result from eardrum damage, strain, or perforation; an infected cyst in the eardrum or middle ear; mastoiditis (inflammation of the mastoid, the bone behind the ear); metabolic disorders such as hypothyroidism; vascular disorders such as hypertension; neurologic disorders such as multiple sclerosis; blood disorders such as leukemia; and even tooth and/or mouth disorders. Hearing loss without ear pain can be the result of an acoustic neuroma (a benign tumor in the cells covering the acoustic nerve); infection of the inner ear; osteosclerosis (overgrowth of bone in the middle ear); kidney dysfunction; Paget's disease of bone; or Ménière's disease. Hearing loss can also occur if the bones of the skull are out of alignment with one another.

Two of the most common hearing disorders in adults are *presbycusis* and *tinnitus*. Presbycusis is the gradual loss of hearing due to aging. It is prevalent in adults over the age of fifty. Tinnitus is a continuous buzzing or ringing in the ears with no obvious cause. It may occur by itself or as a symptom of another disorder, such as infection, obstruction of the ear canal, head trauma, noise-induced hearing loss, or Ménière's disease.

Suspected hearing deficits in infants deserve close and immediate attention, as an undiagnosed hearing impairment can lead to delayed and/or diminished acquisition of language skills and, possibly, learning disabilities. Risk factors for hearing loss in infancy include a family history of hearing loss; known hereditary disorders; congenital abnormalities of the ears, nose, or throat; maternal exposure to rubella or syphilis, or to ototoxic drugs such as tobramycin (Nebcin), streptomycin, gentamicin (Garamycin), quinine (Quinamm), furosemide (Lasix), or ethacrynic acid (Edecrin); and birth-related problems such as prematurity, trauma and/or lack of oxygen during delivery, low birth weight, or jaundice.

Otitis media (middle ear infection) is the most common cause of hearing loss in children. For the most part, this is temporary, but chronic or recurrent ear infection can cause permanent hearing loss due to inflammation and infection of the middle ear. Sensorineural hearing loss in children can also be caused by childhood diseases such as meningitis, mumps, and rubella.

Signs of hearing problems in infancy include failure to blink or startle at loud noises; failure to turn the head toward familiar sounds; a consistent ability to sleep through loud nosies; greater responsiveness to loud noises than to voices; a failure to babble, coo, or squeal; and monotonal babbling. In toddlers, warning signs include failure to speak clearly by age two, showing no interest in being read to or in playing word games, habitual yelling or shrieking when communicating or playing, greater responsiveness to facial expressions than to speech, shyness or withdrawal (often misinterpreted as inattentiveness, dreaminess, and/or stubbornness), and frequent confusion and puzzlement. In older children, signs of hearing loss are similar to those in adulthood—a failure to respond to verbal requests, inappropriate responses to questions or other sound stimuli, and a seeming inattentiveness.

Hearing loss caused by exposure to loud noises is an increasing problem in our society today. When the delicate mechanisms of the inner ear are assaulted by loud noises, a phenomenon called *temporary threshold shift* occurs. If you have ever walked away from a concert or a construction site with a buzzing or hissing in your ears, or with everything sounding as if you are underwater, you have experienced temporary threshold shift. While overnight rest usually restores normal hearing, this is a sign that damage has occurred to the hair cells in your inner ear, and if this type of damage is lengthy and/or repeated, permanent damage and hearing loss will be the eventual result. Most people who develop noise-related hearing loss say they were unaware that anything was wrong until they developed tinnitus or speech became inaudible, but in fact, the damage begins long before that and temporary threshold shift is a clear sign of it.

Noise-related hearing loss is common in train engineers, military personnel, and workers subjected to constant industrial noise, as well as in hunters and musicians, especially rock musicians. Recent National Institutes of Health (NIH) statistics indicate that as much as one-third of all hearing loss is associated with loud noises, and while conclusive data are as yet lacking, many researchers believe that more young people are losing their hearing today than in previous years. The National Center for Health Statistics reports that young people account for one-third of today's hearing loss statistics. They also report that in most cases, this type of hearing loss could have been prevented.

NUTRIENTS

SUPPLEMENT	SUGGESTED DOSAGE	COMMENTS
Important		
Coenzyme Q10	30 mg daily.	Powerful antioxidant. Crucial in the effectiveness of the immune system and circulation to the ears.
Manganese	10 mg daily.	Deficiency has been linked to ear disorders.
Multivitamin and mineral complex	As directed on label.	To provide a balance of all nutrients.
Potassium	99 mg daily.	Important for a healthy nervous system and transmission of nerve impulses.
Ultimate Oil from Nature's Secret	As directed on label.	Blend of essential fatty acids. Helps reduce tendency to produce excessive amounts of earwax.
Vitamin A plus natural beta-carotene	15,000 IU daily. If you are pregnant, do not exceed 10,000 IU daily. 15,000 IU daily.	To boost immunity, increase resistance to infection, and strengthen mucous membranes.
Vitamin B complex injections	As prescribed by physician.	Essential for healing; reduces ear pressure. Injections (under a doctor's supervision) are best. If injections are not available, use a sublingual form.
Vitamin C with bioflavonoids plus N-acetylcysteine	3,000–6,000 mg daily. As directed on label.	Needed for proper immune function and to aid in preventing ear infections. To remove excess fluids from the ear canal.
Vitamin D	400 IU daily.	Enhances immunity.
Vitamin E	600 IU daily.	Powerful antioxidant that increases circulation.
Zinc lozenges (Ultimate Zinc-C Lozenges from Now Foods)	50 mg daily. Do not exceed a total of 100 mg daily from all supplements.	Quickens immune response; aids in reducing infection.

HERBS

❑ Bayberry bark, burdock root, goldenseal, hawthorn leaf and flower, and myrrh gum purify the blood and counteract infection.

Caution: Do not take goldenseal internally on a daily basis for more than one week at a time, as it may disturb normal intestinal flora. Do not use it during pregnancy, and use it with caution if you are allergic to ragweed.

❑ Echinacea aids poor equilibrium and reduces dizziness. It also fights infection and helps reduce congestion. It can be taken in tea or capsule form.

❑ Ephedra, eucalyptus, hyssop, mullein, and thyme have decongestant properties, which may alleviate ringing in ears.

❑ Ginkgo biloba helps to reduce dizziness and improve hearing loss related to reduced blood flow. Other herbs that may help to improve circulation and blood flow to the ear area include butcher's broom, cayenne, chamomile, ginger root, turmeric, and yarrow.

❑ To soothe inflammation and fight infection, mullein oil can be used as ear drops. If mullein is not available, garlic oil or liquid extract may be substituted.

RECOMMENDATIONS

❑ Eat fresh pineapple frequently to reduce inflammation. Also include plenty of garlic, kelp, and sea vegetables.

❑ Limit your consumption of alcohol and sugars, which encourage the growth of yeast. This is particularly important if you have recurrent ear infections and have been treated with antibiotics. Also eliminate or keep to a minimum your intake of caffeine, chocolate, and sodium.

❑ Avoid saturated fats, which contribute to excess production of earwax.

❑ Eliminate from the diet any foods to which you may have an intolerance. Wheat and dairy products are common offenders. (See ALLERGIES in Part Two.)

❑ For earwax buidup, clean or irrigate your ears using either a solution of 1 part vinegar to 1 part warm water or a few drops of hydrogen peroxide. Using an eyedropper, place a few drops in your ear, allow them to settle for a minute, then drain. Repeat the process with the other ear. Do this two or three times a day. Do not use cotton swabs to clean inside the ear canal, as this can push wax further into the ear canal and exacerbate the problem. If the wax is hard and dry, apply garlic oil for a day or two to soften it. Then wash out the ear with a steady stream of warm water. Be patient, continue to irrigate the ear canal, and flush with warm water. Most cases of ear wax buildup can be treated by this method. Another method of removing excess ear wax, called ear candling, uses special candles available at health food stores. Instructions for the procedure are included with the candles. The candling procedure requires assistance, so do not attempt this by yourself.

❑ For an ear infection, put 2 to 4 drops of warm (not hot) liquid garlic extract in the affected ear. (If both ears are infected, do not use the same dropper for both ears, as it may spread infection.) This treatment is very helpful for children.

❑ If you are experiencing ear pain, tug on your earlobe. If this tug makes the ear hurt, you probably have an ear infection and should seek medical treatment. If the tug on the lobe does not hurt, the pain may be due to a dental problem.

❑ When flying, chew gum during the plane's descent to prevent the discomfort and hearing loss associated with changes in atmospheric pressure. Or pop your ears by holding your nose and *gently* blowing air through your closed mouth. This clears the eustachian tubes. A decongestant such as pseudoephedrine (found in Sudafed and other products) may also be helpful, but remember, these medications are dehydrating (and so is the lack of humidity in an airplane cabin). If you use them, be sure to drink plenty of water and juice during the flight, and skip the cocktail and coffee, as alcohol and caffeine also are dehydrating.

❑ Always wear ear protection (disposable plugs or earphone-style) when using loud appliances such as power tools or lawn mowers; and when you know you will be exposed to sudden loud noises, such as when shooting a gun. The U.S. Occupational Safety and Health Administration (OSHA) recommends using ear plugs rated for at least twice as many decibels as you need to ensure protection.

❑ Protect your hearing when listening to music. A general guideline is to keep the volume low enough that you can easily hear the telephone and other sounds over the music. If you are using a personal stereo unit with headphones, you should be the only one able to hear your music. If someone standing next to you can hear it, it's too loud.

❑ Take measures to reduce your cholesterol level. Studies suggest that people with high cholesterol levels have greater hearing loss as they age than people with normal cholesterol levels. See HIGH CHOLESTEROL in Part Two.

❑ If you are prone to ear infections, wear ear plugs while swimming.

❑ If you are planning to become pregnant, make sure you have achieved immunity to German measles, either through having had the disease or through vaccination. A doctor can perform a blood test to determine immunity. If vaccination is necessary, you must guard against becoming pregnant for at least three months to avoid the risk of serious birth defects, such as hearing loss.

❑ If you become ill during pregnancy and medication is required, question your doctor or pharmacist thoroughly about possible effects on the developing fetus and do some research on your own. This will reduce the risk of giving birth to a child with impaired hearing.

❑ If you have an infant, pay very close attention to his or her reactions to noises. If you have any doubt about your child's hearing, consult your physician. Be aware, however, that many physicians are not expert at picking up on hearing loss. If your doctor seems too quick to dismiss your concerns, talk to another doctor. Keep in mind that early detection is vitally important; detection of hearing loss before a child's first birthday greatly reduces the chances that he or she will be disadvantaged by hearing problems in the years to come.

❑ If you have experienced permanent hearing loss, advise family members, friends, and coworkers to speak slowly and distinctly, and avoid shouting. Depending on the nature of the hearing loss, a hearing aid may be helpful. Consult with your health care provider or a professional audiologist.

CONSIDERATIONS

❑ Appropriate treatment for hearing loss depends on the underlying cause.

❑ Food allergies, especially allergies to wheat and dairy products, can be the culprit in recurrent middle ear infections. (*See* ALLERGIES in Part Two.)

❑ You can minimize the level of hearing loss you will experience as you grow older if you reduce your exposure to loud noises in the earlier years of your life. Hearing can also be improved with proper diet and supplements.

❑ If you have to raise your voice to be heard over your surroundings, your environment is too noisy. You should try to limit your exposure to such places. If such exposure cannot be avoided, you should wear ear protection.

❑ Most cases of early childhood hearing deficit are first detected by the parents, not health care providers.

❑ The average rock concert or stereo headset set at full blast (about 100 decibels) can damage your hearing in as little as half an hour. Similar damage can occur after about two hours spent in a video game arcade.

❑ Any hearing loss that does not resolve on its own within two weeks should be evaluated by a professional. Some of the symptoms associated with hearing loss can be a sign of a serious health problem that requires treatment.

❑ *See also* EAR INFECTION and MÉNIÈRE'S DISEASE in Part Two.

Heart Attack

When the supply of blood to the heart is sharply reduced or cut off, the heart is deprived of needed oxygen. If blood flow is not restored within minutes, portions of the heart muscle begin to die, permanently damaging the heart muscle. This process is referred to as a *myocardial infarction*, more commonly known as a heart attack. Because this happens when the coronary arteries cannot provide the heart with sufficient oxygen, physicians also commonly refer to a heart attack as a "coronary."

With the onset of a heart attack, the primary symptom is a consistent deep, often severe, pain in the chest that can spread to the left arm, neck, jaw, or the area between the shoulder blades. The pain may be present for up to twelve hours. Many people who have had heart attacks describe it as a heavy, substernal pressure that makes it feel as if the chest is being squeezed. Other possible symptoms include shortness of breath, sweating, nausea, and vomiting. In addition, a heart attack can cause abnormal heartbeat rhythms called arrhythmias. Arrhythmias result in over 500,000 sudden deaths in the United States each year and the incidence is rising, despite much-improved cardiac resuscitative techniques.

There are three basic scenarios that can produce a heart attack. The first, and by far the most common, is partial or complete blockage of one of the arteries that supply the heart with oxygen, most often by a blood clot. Usually the arteries have been narrowed by years of coronary artery disease in which plaque, which is composed of cholesterol-rich fatty deposits, proteins, calcium, and excess smooth muscle cells, builds up on the arterial walls. The arterial walls thicken, inhibiting the flow of blood to the heart muscle. The roughening of arterial walls by deposits of plaque not only narrows the arteries, but also makes it easier for blood clots to form along their inner surfaces. When a clot grows, or detaches from its place of origin and travels through the blood vessels, it may block a coronary artery completely, resulting in a heart attack.

In the second heart attack scenario, an arrhythmia may set in, so that the heart is no longer pumping enough blood to ensure its own supply. In the third, a weak spot in a blood vessel, called an aneurysm, may rupture, causing internal bleeding and disrupting normal blood flow.

Anything that puts extra strain on the heart and/or blood vessels—an emotional crisis, a heavy meal, overexertion from exercise or heavy lifting—may act as a trigger for a heart attack, but such factors are not the underlying cause. Persons considered to be at greater than normal risk of heart attack are those with a family history of heart disease; those who smoke and/or abuse drugs; people with diabetes, high blood pressure, high blood cholesterol and/or triglyceride levels; sedentary people; and those who are under stress and/or who have "type A" personalities.

One third of all heart attacks occur without warning. The remainder are preceded by months or even years of symptoms, most commonly angina pectoris—chest pain that is typically aggravated by stress or physical exertion and relieved by rest. Like a heart attack, angina is caused by a lack of oxygen in the heart muscle, but the extent of oxygen deprivation is not sufficient to actually damage heart tissue. Many people complain of intermittent angina, shortness of breath, and/or unusual fatigue in the days or weeks leading up to a heart attack. A constant sensation of heartburn that persists for days and from which antacids provide no relief can be a sign of an impending heart attack.

NUTRIENTS

SUPPLEMENT	SUGGESTED DOSAGE	COMMENTS
Essential		
Choline and inositol	As directed on label, to supply up to 1,000 mg choline daily.	These substances aid in the removal of fat from the liver and bloodstream.
Coenzyme Q₁₀	100 mg daily.	Improves heart muscle oxygenation and may help prevent second heart attacks.
Vitamin E	Start with 200 IU daily, and increase slowly to 800 IU daily. If you are taking an anticoagulant drug, do not exceed 400 IU daily except under a doctor's supervision.	A powerful antioxidant that improves circulation and thins the blood, reducing the risk of clots.
Selenium	300 mcg daily.	Deficiency has been implicated in heart disease.

Grape seed extract	150–300 mg daily.	A powerful antioxidant. Best used in combination with phosphatidyl choline, a natural component of lecithin.

Very Important		
Acetyl-L-carnitine or L-carnitine plus L-cysteine and L-methionine	500 mg each daily, on an empty stomach. Take with water or juice. Do not take with milk. Take with 50 mg vitamin B_6 and 100 mg vitamin C for better absorption.	To reduce blood lipid levels, increase cellular glutathione and coenzyme Q_{10}, protect against lipid peroxidation, and assist in the breakdown of fats, preventing fatty buildup in the arteries, which helps restore blood flow to the heart.
Calcium and magnesium	1,500 mg daily. 1,000 mg daily, in divided doses, between meals and at bedtime.	Important for maintaining proper heart rhythm and blood pressure. Use chelate forms.
Chromium	100 mcg daily.	Helps raise levels of HDL ("good" cholesterol).
Essential fatty acids (primrose oil and salmon oil are good sources)	As directed on label.	Protects heart muscle cells.
Garlic (Kyolic)	2 capsules 3 times daily.	Beneficial for the heart, promotes circulation, and aids in reducing high blood pressure.
Glucosamine Plus from FoodScience Labs	As directed on label.	Plays an important role in the formation of heart valves.
Heart Science from Source Naturals	As directed on label.	Contains antioxidants, cholesterol-fighters, herbs, and vitamins that work together to promote cardiovascular function.
Multienzyme complex	As directed on label. Take with meals.	For proper digestion and to prevent heartburn.
Proteolytic enzymes	As directed on label 3 times daily. Take between meals.	Anti-inflammatory agents that prevent free radical damage to the arteries.
Sea mussel	As directed on label.	Aids in the functioning of the cardiovascular system, the lymphatic system, and the endocrine system.
Vitamin A plus natural beta-carotene	As directed on label. If you are pregnant, do not exceed 10,000 IU daily. 10,000 IU daily.	Helps prevent free radical damage to the arteries. Use emulsion form for easier assimilation. A precursor of vitamin A.
Zinc plus copper	50 mg daily. Do not exceed a total of 100 mg daily from all supplements. 3 mg daily.	Necessary for proper balance with copper and for thiamine utilization. Use a chelate form. Deficiency has been linked to heart disease.

Important		
Dimethylglycine (DMG) (Aangamik DMG from FoodScience Labs)	As directed on label.	Improves oxygenation of heart tissue.
Vitamin B complex plus extra vitamin B_1 (thiamine) and vitamin B_{12} and folic acid	50 mg 3 times daily. 500 mg 3 times daily, with meals. 2,000 mcg daily. 400 mcg daily.	B vitamins work best when taken together. Deficiency in the heart muscle leads to heart disease. Deficiencies have been linked to heart disease.

Pycnogenol	As directed on label.	Neutralizes free radicals, enhances the action of vitamin C, and strengthens connective tissue, including that of the cardiovascular system.
Vitamin C with bioflavonoids	3,000–6,000 mg daily.	Aids in thinning the blood. Prevents blood clots and free radical damage.

HERBS

❑ Alfalfa, borage seed, horsetail, nettle, and pau d'arco are rich in minerals necessary for proper regulation of heart rhythm.

❑ Black cohosh, oat straw, passionflower, valerian root, skullcap, and wood betony are calming herbs that may help to regulate arrhythmias.

❑ Butcher's broom, hawthorn berries and leaf, motherwort, and red sage strengthen the heart muscle.

❑ Cayenne (capsicum), ginger root, and ginkgo biloba strengthen the heart and are helpful for chest pain.

❑ Gotu kola, primrose, and rosemary are helpful in managing angina.

❑ Green tea has superb antioxidant properties. Drinking 10 to 20 cups a day can provide protection against heart disease and many other illnesses.

RECOMMENDATIONS

❑ Make sure your diet is high in fiber.

❑ Include in your diet almonds, brewer's yeast, grains, and sesame seeds.

❑ Add kelp and sea vegetables to your diet for necessary minerals. Drink fresh vegetable juices.

❑ Minimize your intake of vitamin D, and do not obtain it from whole milk or any dairy product that is high in fat. Consumption of these contributes to clogged arteries. Moderate consumption of skim milk and low-fat yogurt is acceptable.

❑ Do not eat red meat, highly spiced foods, salt, sugars, or white flour. Refined sugars produce adverse reactions in all cells by causing wide variations in blood sugar. The high surges are followed by hypoglycemic drops, causing dangerous instability in vital intracellular sugar levels.

❑ Eliminate fried foods, coffee, black tea, colas, and other stimulants from the diet.

❑ Do not smoke. Avoid secondhand smoke.

❑ Refrain from alcohol use, as it has a direct toxic effect on the heart. If you do occasionally drink, avoid cod liver oil.

❑ Drink steam-distilled water only.

❑ To relieve stress and promote relaxation, add a few drops of lavender, sandalwood, or ylang ylang essential oil to a bath, or simply place a few drops on a tissue and inhale the aroma from time to time throughout the day.

❑ Sip barley water throughout the day for its healing and fortifying properties. *See* THERAPEUTIC LIQUIDS in Part Three.

❑ Fast three days a month to cleanse and detoxify the body. *See* FASTING in Part Three, and follow the program.

CONSIDERATIONS

❑ Most people who have heart attacks experience the characteristic chest pain (see page 306). However, not all do. Some people have a sensation that feels like indigestion; others have no noticeable symptoms at all. This phenomenon is often referred to as a "silent" heart attack. Elderly people and people with diabetes are probably more likely than others to have this type of heart attack.

❑ In some cases, heart attacks are caused by spasms of the arteries that suddenly shut off the flow of blood to the heart.

❑ Sensible, moderate exercise and a proper diet with nutritional supplements can prevent arteriosclerosis of the coronary arteries and myocardial infarction.
Caution: If you are over thirty-five and/or have been sedentary for some time, consult with your health care provider before beginning an exercise program.

❑ Studies have shown that people who take supplemental coenzyme Q10 following a heart attack are less likely than those who did not to have a second attack within five years.

❑ Researchers have found that eating just an ounce of walnuts a day (about seven nuts) may reduce the risk of a heart attack by 8 to 10 percent.

❑ A heart attack is not the same thing as heart failure. In heart failure, the heart does not supply enough blood to the body; in a heart attack, the heart does not receive enough blood to meet its needs. However, the damage produced by a heart attack can lead to heart failure.

❑ *See also* ARTERIOSCLEROSIS; CARDIOVASCULAR DISEASE; and CIRCULATORY PROBLEMS in Part Two.

❑ *See also* CHELATION THERAPY in Part Three.

Heart Disease

See CARDIOVASCULAR DISEASE; HEART ATTACK.

Heartburn

Heartburn is a burning sensation in the stomach and/or chest. It often occurs when hydrochloric acid, which is used by the stomach to digest food, backs up into the esophagus, causing sensitive tissues to become irritated. Normally, the esophageal sphincter muscle pinches itself shut and prevents stomach acid from surging upward. However, if the

sphincter is not functioning properly, the acid can slip past it and into the esophagus. This phenomenon is referred to as *gastroesophageal reflux.*

People with hiatal hernia often experience heartburn. It can also be caused by excessive consumption of spicy foods, fatty or fried foods, alcohol, coffee, citrus fruits, chocolate, or tomato-based foods. Ulcers, gallbladder problems, stress, allergies, and enzyme deficiencies are other possible contributing factors.

NUTRIENTS

SUPPLEMENT	SUGGESTED DOSAGE	COMMENTS
Very Important		
Aloe vera		*See under* Herbs, below.
Pancreatin plus bromelain	As directed on label. Take with meals.	Enzymes necessary for proper digestion.
Papaya tablets	As directed on label.	To relieve symptoms. Use chewable tablets from a health food store.
Vitamin B complex plus extra vitamin B12	50 mg 3 times daily, with meals. 200 mcg 3 times daily.	Needed for proper digestion. Use a lozenge or sublingual form.
Helpful		
Acid-Ease from Prevail	As directed on label.	A soothing plant-enzyme and herb formula that aids in the breakdown and assimilation of foods.

HERBS

❑ Aloe vera juice aids healing of the intestinal tract.

❑ Catnip, fennel, ginger, marshmallow root, and papaya tea all aid in proper digestion and act as a buffer to stop heartburn.

RECOMMENDATIONS

❑ At the first sign of heartburn, drink a large glass of water. This often helps.

❑ Try raw potato juice. Do not peel the potato—just wash it and put it in the juicer. (*See* JUICING in Part Three.) Mix the juice with an equal amount of water. Drink it immediately after preparation, three times a day.

❑ Change your eating habits. Eat more raw vegetables. Chew your food well. Eat slowly and enjoy your food.

❑ Sip 1 tablespoon of raw apple cider vinegar, mixed with a glass of water, while eating a meal. Do not drink any other liquids with meals.

❑ Eat fresh papaya and/or pineapple to aid digestion. Chew a few of the papaya seeds as well.

❑ Do not eat for three hours before bedtime. Wait at least three hours after eating before lying down.

❑ Do not consume carbonated beverages, fats, fried foods, processed foods, sugar, or spicy or highly seasoned foods. These seem to be the main cause of heartburn.

❑ *See* FASTING in Part Three and follow the instructions. *Also see* the self-tests under ACIDOSIS and CARDIOVASCULAR DISEASE in Part Two.

❑ Do not take a multienzyme complex containing hydrochloric acid (HCl).

❑ As much as possible, avoid stress.

CONSIDERATIONS

❑ Estrogens can weaken the esophageal hiatus muscle, which keeps stomach acids in the stomach. Women who are pregnant and women who take birth control pills that contain estrogen and progesterone are therefore more likely to suffer from heartburn.

❑ People with certain illnesses, such as cancer, often have excessive amounts of acid in their systems. The consumption of too much processed and cooked food can also create an acidic environment in the body.

❑ Aspirin and ibuprofen can cause heartburn.

❑ Lying on your left side can help relieve heartburn. Lying on the left side keeps the stomach below the esophagus, helping to keep it acid-free.

❑ Antacids often provide relief of symptoms. However, in so doing, they may mask an underlying problem. In addition, many over-the-counter antacids contain excessive amounts of sodium, aluminum, calcium, and magnesium. With prolonged use of these products, dangerous mineral imbalances can occur. Excess sodium can aggravate hypertension, and excess aluminum has been implicated in Alzheimer's disease. Some of the most popular types of antacids and the products they are found in are:

• Aluminum salts or gels: AlternaGEL, Amphojel.

• Aluminum-magnesium mixtures: Aludrox, Di-Gel, Gaviscon, Gelusil, Maalox, Mylanta, Riopan.

• Calcium carbonate: Alka-Mints, Chooz, Titralac, Tums.

• Calcium-magnesium mixtures: Rolaids.

• Magnesium salts or gels: Phillips' Milk of Magnesia.

• Sodium bicarbonate: Alka-Seltzer, Bromo Seltzer, Citrocarbonate.

❑ Calcium carbonate works as an antacid and contains no aluminum.

❑ A product called Acid-Ease, from Prevail Corporation, has shown promising results. It can be purchased at health food stores. Acid-Ease is aluminum-free.

❑ Drugs that suppress the production of stomach acid are sometimes recommended for people who suffer from frequent heartburn. These include cimetidine (Tagamet), famotidine (Pepcid), and ranitidine (Zantac).

❑ The early symptoms of angina and heart attack sometimes mimic those of "acid stomach." If symptoms persist, if the pain begins to travel down into the left arm, or if the sensation is accompanied by a feeling of weakness, dizziness, or shortness of breath, emergency medical help should be sought at once. (*See* HEART ATTACK in Part Two.)

❑ *See also* HERNIA, HIATAL and ULCERS in Part Two.

❑ *See also under* PREGNANCY-RELATED PROBLEMS in Part Two.

Heel or Bone Spur

A bone spur is a pointed growth on a bone, most commonly in the heel. A bone spur may be caused by calcium deposits in unwanted areas of the body. Most people who have heel disorders are middle-aged or overweight. Heel spurs are also common in people who have arthritis, neuritis, alkalosis, and tendinitis. Uncomfortable shoes may contribute to the pain.

X-rays may reveal a bony spur within the heel. The presence of this may lead to the formation of tiny tumors at the end of several nerves, and these may be very painful.

NUTRIENTS

SUPPLEMENT	SUGGESTED DOSAGE	COMMENTS
Very Important		
Betaine hydrochloride (HCl)	As directed on label.	Needed for proper calcium uptake. A deficiency of HCl is more common in elderly people. *Caution:* Do not use HCl if you have a history of ulcers.
Calcium and magnesium	1,500 mg daily. 750 mg daily.	A proper balance of calcium and magnesium helps prevent abnormal calcium deposition. Use chelate or aspartate forms.
Important		
Proteolytic enzymes or Infla-Zyme Forte from American Biologics or Intenzyme Forte from Biotics Research	As directed on label. As directed on label. As directed on label.	To aid in absorption of nutrients and in control of inflammation and irritation. *Caution:* Do not give these supplements to a child.
Vitamin C	2,000–4,000 mg daily.	Acts as an anti-inflammatory; important for collagen and connective tissue.
Helpful		
Bioflavonoids	100 mg daily.	Vitamin C activators that also help relieve pain.
Vitamin B complex plus extra vitamin B6 (pyridoxine)	50–100 mg daily. 50 mg daily.	B vitamins work best when taken together. Necessary for production of hydrochloric acid, which helps prevent bone spurs by aiding proper calcium absorption.

HERBS

❑ Use arnica and chamomile to bathe the foot. You can also wrap the herbs in a cloth and apply it to the affected area as a poultice. *See* USING A POULTICE in Part Three.

RECOMMENDATIONS

❑ Do not eat any citrus fruits, expecially oranges. Eliminate alcohol, coffee, and sugar from your diet. These inhibit the healing process and upset the body's mineral balance.

❑ Drink steam-distilled water only.

❑ Select well-made, rubber-heeled shoes; these are better for the feet than leather. Choose footwear for comfort—not for looks. Some jogging shoes can be very comfortable. Adding heel cushions to footwear helps to relieve pain.

❑ Avoid walking on hard surfaces such as concrete, wood, or hard floors without carpeting.

❑ To relieve pain, use hot linseed oil packs. Place linseed oil in a pan and heat but do not boil it. Dip a piece of cheesecloth or other white cotton material into the oil until the cloth is saturated. Apply the cloth to the affected area and cover it with a piece of plastic that is larger in size than the cotton cloth. Place a heating pad over the plastic and use it to keep the pack warm. Keep the pack in place for one-half to two hours, as needed.

❑ Ice massages on the bottoms of the feet can be helpful. Alternate between hot and cold foot baths.

❑ If you normally walk or jog for exercise, try bicycling or swimming instead.

CONSIDERATIONS

❑ A two-week raw food fast or a cleansing fast can be beneficial. (*See* FASTING in Part Three.)

❑ Dimethylsulfoxide (DMSO), applied topically to the affected area, is good for relief of acute symptoms.

Note: Only DMSO from a health food store should be used. Commercial-grade DMSO found in hardware stores is not suitable for healing purposes. Using DMSO may result in a temporary garlicky body odor. This is not a cause for concern.

❑ It is best not to have a heel spur surgically removed unless it is extremely irritating or painful.

❑ *See also* ARTHRITIS in Part Two.

Hemophilia

In a healthy individual, a minor bump can damage a blood vessel, causing blood to leak into the surrounding tissue, producing a bruise. A process called hemostasis (coagulation) plugs the hole in the damaged vessel and forms a clot that stops the blood loss and limits the size of the bruise.

In people with hemophilia and related problems, bleeding can take a very different course. The blood does not clot normally because one or another of the blood proteins that collaborate to repair damaged vessels and form clots is defective, deficient, or totally absent.

The idea that people with hemophilia can bleed to death from a minor cut or injury is a misconception. In fact, external bleeding is seldom a serious problem for hemophiliacs. They may bleed somewhat longer than other people, but minor bleeding episodes can generally be controlled by ordinary first aid measures.

But injuries also commonly cause bleeding inside the body—bleeding we may neither see nor feel. Unchecked internal bleeding can be serious—even life threatening—for a person with hemophilia. Blood that leaks into the knee joint, a common site of internal bleeding, can cause painful swelling. Repeated bleeding eventually destroys the cartilage that enables the knee to work smoothly and easily. The joint becomes permanently stiff and painful, the result of hemophilic arthritis. Other joints—the ankle, wrist, or elbow—can be similarly affected by internal bleeding. People with hemophilia can also bleed into muscle and other soft tissue. Internal bleeding can ultimately obstruct air passages or damage the brain or other vital organs.

Hemophilia can be mild, moderate, or severe, depending on how impaired an individual's production of clotting factors is. In severe hemophilia, clotting factor activity is less than 1 percent of normal. Injury, surgery, or dental care can present significant problems for such people. Spontaneous bleeding can require infusion of clotting factor concentrate as often as several times a week. People with moderate hemophilia (factor levels between 1 and 5 percent of normal) do not usually experience spontaneous bleeding, but even a minor injury, if untreated, can cause prolonged bleeding. In mild hemophilia, factor activity ranges between 5 and 50 percent of normal. Bleeding can be expected from surgery, major dental care, or trauma. These individuals rarely bleed into joints, and their disease usually does not interfere with normal living.

The National Hemophilia Foundation estimates that nearly 450 babies with hemophilia are born each year in the U.S.— 1 in every 4,400 live male births. The number of female hemophiliacs is not known. Hemophilia is hereditary. It primarily affects males and is passed down through females. This is because it is linked to a defect in one of two genes that are involved in the production of clotting factors. These genes are located on the X chromosome, and while females have two X chromosomes, males have only one. For a female to develop the disease, both of her X chromosomes would have to carry the defective gene (which is unlikely), whereas a male has only a single X chromosome, so if one of its clotting factor genes is defective, he will be affected.

A woman who has one defective gene will not develop hemophilia herself, but is considered a *carrier* of the condition. All children of (female) carriers have a 50-percent chance of inheriting the defective gene. For sons, this means a 50-percent chance of developing the disease; for daughters, it means a 50-percent chance of being carriers, like their mothers. For the children of (male) hemophiliacs, the story is somewhat different. Sons are not affected (unless the mother is a carrier), but daughters always become carriers. For hemophilia to occur in a female, she would have to have both a father with the condition and a mother who is either a hemophiliac or a carrier.

People with hemophilia are commonly treated with plasma concentrates prepared from pooled blood plasma. As a result, as many as two thirds of all Americans with hemophilia became infected with HIV before the virus was identified and a screening test developed. Blood donors are now screened for HIV and clotting factor products are routinely subjected to heat to minimize, if not eliminate, the risk of transmission of the virus, but the chance of contracting HIV understandably remains a source of concern for people with hemophilia.

NUTRIENTS

SUPPLEMENT	SUGGESTED DOSAGE	COMMENTS
Helpful		
Calcium and	1,500 mg daily.	Essential for blood clotting.
magnesium	1,000 mg daily.	Needed to balance with calcium.
Liver extract injections or	1 cc once weekly or as prescribed by physician.	Contains vital nutrients for blood clotting.
raw liver extract	As directed on label.	
Multivitamin and mineral complex	As directed on label.	Provides necessary vitamins and minerals.
Vitamin B complex plus extra	As directed on label.	All B vitamins are essential in blood formation and clotting.
vitamin B₃ (niacin) and	As directed on label.	*Caution:* Do not take niacin if you have a liver disorder,
niacinamide	As directed on label.	gout, or high blood pressure.
Vitamin C with bioflavonoids	3,000 mg daily.	Important in normal blood coagulation.
Vitamin K or	300 mcg daily.	Essential in blood clotting mechanism.
alfalfa		*See under* Herbs, below.

HERBS

❑ Alfalfa is a good source of vitamin K. It can be taken in tablet form or eaten in a natural form, such as alfalfa sprouts.

RECOMMENDATIONS

❑ Eat a diet high in vitamin K. Foods that contain a measurable amount of this vitamin are alfalfa, broccoli, cauliflower, egg yolks, kale, liver, spinach, and all green leafy vegetables.

❑ "Green drinks" made from the vegetables listed above are very healthful. Drink one of these a day for vitamin K and other essential clotting factors.

❑ Be alert for early warning signs of internal bleeding, including a bubbling or tingling sensation or a feeling of warmth, tightness, or stiffness in the affected area. A blow to the head, headache, confusion, drowsiness, or other evidence of neurological impairment may signal intracranial bleeding.

❑ If you care for an infant or toddler with hemophilia, be alert for signs of joint or muscle pain caused by internal bleeding. The child may cry for no apparent reason, refuse to use an arm or leg, refuse to walk, or have swelling or excessive bruising. If you suspect internal bleeding, seek treatment immediately.

CONSIDERATIONS

❑ Treatment of hemophilia consists of intravenous infusion of the missing clotting factor. This is now usually done at home. How much antihemophilic factor an individual needs and when depends on the severity of his disease.

❑ Gene therapy may hold the key to curing hemophilia, but it has yet to be tried in humans. Studies in the laboratory and in experimental animals seem to show that the technique can work. Ongoing studies using a retrovirus as a "genetic bullet" to replace the hemophiliacs' defective clotting gene show promise for eventually curing this disease.

❑ More information about care for this disorder and the location of comprehensive treatment centers for hemophilia can be obtained from the National Hemophilia Foundation, 110 Greene Street, Suite 303, New York, NY 10012; telephone 212–219 8180. Information on dealing with AIDS is available from the Hemophilia and AIDS/HIV Network for Dissemination of Information (HANDI), which is operated by the Hemophilia Foundation. The number is 800–42–HANDI or 212–431–8541.

Hemorrhoids

Hemorrhoids are swollen veins around the anus and in the rectum (the very lowest portion of the colon) that may protrude from the anus. They are very much like varicose veins; they enlarge and lose their elasticity, resulting in saclike protrusions into the anal canal. They can be caused, and aggravated, by sitting or standing for prolonged periods, lifting heavy objects (or lifting even relatively light objects improperly), and straining at bowel movements (especially when constipated, although bouts of diarrhea accompanied by involuntary spasms can exacerbate the problem), as well as by pregnancy, obesity, lack of exercise, liver damage, food allergies, and insufficient consumption of dietary fiber.

The most common symptoms of hemorrhoids include itching, burning, pain, inflammation, swelling, irritation, seepage, and bleeding. The bleeding can be startling, even frightening, but although it does signal that something is amiss in the digestive system, rectal bleeding is not necessarily an indication of serious disease.

There are different types of hemorrhoids, depending on their location, severity, and the amount of pain, discomfort, or aggravation they cause. These are:

• *Internal.* Internal hemorrhoids are located inside the rectum and are usually painless, especially if located above the anorectal line. They do, however, tend to bleed. When they do, the blood appears bright red.

• *External.* "Piles" was the old-fashioned term to describe external hemorrhoids. These develop under the skin at the opening of the anal cavity. When an external hemorrhoid swells, the tissue in the area becomes firm but sensitive and turns blue or purple in color. This type of hemorrhoid can be extremely painful.

• *Prolapsed.* A prolapsed hemorrhoid is an internal hemorrhoid that collapses and protrudes outside the anus, often accompanied by a mucous discharge and heavy bleeding. Prolapsed hemorrhoids can become *thrombosed*—that is, they can form clots within that prevent their receding. Thrombosed hemorrhoids can also be excruciatingly painful.

Hemorrhoids are unique to human beings. No other creature develops this problem. This can be taken as an indication that our dietary and nutritional habits probably play a greater role in this disorder than anything else. Between 50 and 75 percent of this country's population develop hemorrhoids at one time or another, although many may be unaware of them. Hemorrhoids can occur at any age, but they tend to become more common as people age. Among younger people, pregnant women and women who have had children seem to be the most susceptible. The tendency to develop hemorrhoids also appears to be hereditary. Although hemorrhoids can be quite painful, they do not usually pose a serious threat to health.

NUTRIENTS

SUPPLEMENT	SUGGESTED DOSAGE	COMMENTS
Very Important		
Aerobic Bulk Cleanse (ABC) from Aerobic Life Industries	As directed on label. Mix with ½ fruit juice and ½ aloe vera juice, and drink it down quickly before the fiber thickens. Take separately from other supplements and medications.	Keeps the colon clean, relieving pressure on the rectum.
Calcium	1,500 mg daily.	Essential for blood clotting. Helps prevent cancer of the colon. Use calcium chelate or asporotate form.
and magnesium	750 mg daily.	Needed to balance with calcium.
Vitamin C plus bioflavonoids	3,000–5,000 mg daily. 100 mg daily.	Aids in healing and normal blood clotting.
Vitamin E	600 IU daily.	Promotes normal blood clotting and healing.

Important		
Vitamin B complex plus extra vitamin B6 (pyridoxine) and vitamin B12 plus choline and inositol	50–100 mg 3 times daily, with meals. 50 mg 3 times daily, with meals. 1,000 mcg twice daily. 50 mg each twice daily.	All B vitamins are vital for digestion. Improved digestion results in reduced stress on the rectum. Use a lozenge or sublingual form.

Helpful		
Coenzyme Q10	100 mg daily.	Increases cellular oxygenation and assists in healing.
Dimethylglycine (DMG) (Aangamik DMG from FoodScience Labs)	125 mg twice daily.	Improves cellular oxygenation.
Key-E suppositories from Carlson Labs	As directed on label.	Shrinks inflamed hemorrhoidal tissue.
Potassium	99 mg daily.	Constipation, which can cause hemorrhoids, is common in those with potassium deficiencies.
Shark cartilage (BeneFin)	1 gram per 15 lbs of body weight daily, divided into 3 doses. Can be taken either orally or rectally, in a retention enema.	Treats pain and inflammation.
Vitamin A plus natural beta-carotene or carotenoid complex (Betatene)	15,000 IU daily. If you are pregnant, do not exceed 10,000 IU daily. 15,000 IU daily. As directed on label.	Aids in healing of mucous membranes and tissues. Antioxidant and precursor of vitamin A.
Vitamin D	600 IU daily.	Aids in healing of mucous membranes and tissues. Also needed for calcium.

HERBS

❑ A paste made from powdered comfrey root can be used in a poultice to heal bleeding hemorrhoids.
Note: Comfrey is recommended for external use only.

❑ An elderberry poultice can relieve the pain associated with hemorrhoids. A mullein poultice can be used as well. *See* USING A POULTICE in Part Three.

❑ Other beneficial herbs include buckthorn bark, collinsonia root, parsley, red grape vine leaves, and stone root. These can be taken in capsule or tea form.

RECOMMENDATIONS

❑ If you decide to use a fiber supplement, start with a moderate amount and increase your intake gradually. If you take too much at first, this will cause painful bloating, gas, and possibly diarrhea.
Note: Always take supplemental fiber separately from other supplements and medications.

❑ Eat foods that are high in dietary fiber, such as wheat bran, fresh fruits, and nearly all vegetables. Apples, beets, Brazil nuts, broccoli, foods in the cabbage family, carrots, green beans, guar gum, oat bran, lima beans, pears, peas, psyllium seed, and whole grains are recommended. A high-fiber diet is probably the most important consideration in the treatment and prevention of hemorrhoids.

❑ Drink plenty of liquids, especially water (preferably steam-distilled). Water is the best, most natural stool softener in existence. It also helps prevent constipation.

❑ Avoid fats and animal products. Red meat and high-protein diets are especially hard on the lower digestive tract.

❑ Take 1 or 2 tablespoons of flaxseed oil daily. Flaxseed oil helps to soften stools.

❑ Learn not to strain when moving the bowels. Keep the bowels clean and avoid constipation.

❑ Cleanse the problem area frequently with warm water. A hot bath for fifteen minutes a day is quite helpful. Do not add bath beads, oils, or bubbles to the water, as this can irritate sensitive tissues. Many people add Epsom salts, but this has no proven clinical value. It is the warm water that reduces swelling and eases the pain.

❑ Warm sitz baths are especially beneficial. Take a mineral sitz bath daily. (*See* SITZ BATH in Part Three.) We recommend Batherapy from Para Laboratories/Queen Helene, a powder that contains many valuable minerals and is added to bath water. This can be found in many health food stores.

❑ Use cayenne (capsicum) and garlic enemas to keep the bowels clean. A plain warm water enema is fast acting and relieves discomfort in most cases. *See* ENEMAS in Part Three.

❑ Get regular moderate exercise.

❑ Use a peeled clove of garlic as a suppository three times a week. You can also use raw potato suppositories to help heal hemorrhoids and relieve pain. Peel a potato and cut it into small cone-shaped pieces.

❑ To help bleeding hemorrhoids, eat foods such as alfalfa, blackstrap molasses, and dark green leafy vegetables, which are high in vitamin K.

❑ If you are bothered by persistent bleeding, take vitamin and mineral supplements to prevent anemia. An iron supplement together with a powerful vitamin B complex and vitamin C will keep the blood healthy. A sublingual B complex, such as Perfect B from Pharmaceutical Purveyors of Oklahoma or Coenzymate B Complex from Source Naturals, is among the most efficiently absorbed forms of the B vitamins.

❑ Avoid use of strong or harsh laxatives. Most of these products induce unnecessary straining at bowel movements and often "overdo" their jobs by creating a condition similar to diarrhea. Also, using chemical laxatives does not provide the healthful benefits that natural substances provide. Laxative products can also cause the bowels to become dependent upon them for normal functioning, much like an addiction.

Instead of chemical preparations, use a stool softener if constipation or straining at defecation are a problem.

❑ Learn proper lifting techniques. Bend your knees, not your back. Do not hold your breath as you lift; this puts enormous strain and pressure upon the hemorrhoidal vessels. Instead, take a deep breath and exhale at the moment of lifting. Make your thighs do the work, not your back. Avoid heavy lifting as much as possible.

❑ Avoid sitting or standing for prolonged periods of time. If sitting for extended periods of time cannot be avoided, take frequent breaks to stretch and move around (this is also good for circulation, the back, and the legs). Above all, do not use the old-fashioned inflated doughnut cushion. This actually increases pressure upon the hemorrhoidal blood vessels, aggravating the swelling and bleeding.

❑ If home treatments bring no relief, consult your health care provider, especially if the problem is recurrent and bleeding persists. Although the amount of blood loss might seem insignificant, even a slow loss of blood will eventually result in anemia and its associated problems (*see* ANEMIA in Part Two). In addition, persistent rectal bleeding can lead to infections and even a compromised immune system.

CONSIDERATIONS

❑ Depending upon the location and severity of the problem, physicians today use the following treatment approaches in dealing with hemorrhoids:

• *Conservative measures.* A dietary regimen with fiber supplements and self-help treatments is helpful in most cases, except in instances where a hemorrhoid has thrombosed.

• *Infrared photocoagulation.* This involves the employment of infrared heat to treat minor internal hemorrhoids. It is less painful than ligation but is not always as effective.

• *Injection sclerotherapy.* In this procedure, used to shrink internal hemorrhoids and stop bleeding, a solution containing either quinine and urea or phenol is injected directly into the hemorrhoids.

• *Laser treatment.* This approach has gained popularity over the last several years as the easiest and least painful method of dealing with internal hemorrhoids. There is controversy about its efficacy, however. Repeated treatments are frequently required. Most researchers believe that more study should be done to improve effectiveness before laser treatment is routinely recommended.

• *Ligation.* This is now the most common treatment approach for internal hemorrhoids. A small rubber band is used to tie off the base of the blood vessel. Once blood circulation is eliminated from the offending vessel, it soon detaches and the rubber band is eliminated with body waste. This approach often requires repeat treatments and is painful.

• *Surgery.* Some hemorrhoids are not helped very much by any of the above approaches and respond to nothing short of aggressive surgery. If you have very painful hemorrhoids or are losing significant amounts of blood, you should receive a thorough examination from a physician, preferably a proctologist, as soon as possible. Improved surgical techniques have resulted in less painful operations and quicker recovery periods than in the past. Surgery is completely effective in about 95 percent of cases. However, additional surgery may be required if the hemorrhoids recur.

❑ Anurex is a drug- and chemical-free product that helps give prompt, soothing, and lasting relief from the burning, itching, and bleeding caused by hemorrhoids. It is a small plastic device that contains a permanently sealed cold-retaining gel. When placed at the site of pain, it imparts a controlled degree of cooling to the inflamed tissue. Each Anurex device is reusable for up to six months. This product can be found in many pharmacies and health food stores, or can be ordered directly from Anurex Labs, P.O. Box 414760, Miami, FL 33141; telephone 305–757–7733.

❑ Key-E suppositories from Carlson Labs are good for relief of itching and pain.

❑ Kombucha tea, which has antibacterial and immune-boosting properties, has been reported to be helpful. (*See* MAKING KOMBUCHA TEA in Part Three.)

❑ Eating certain foods, especially beets, can cause the stool to become reddish and can be mistaken for blood.

❑ The most common cause of anal itching is tissue trauma resulting from the use of harsh toilet paper. *Candida albicans*, allergies, and parasitic infections can also cause anal itching.

❑ *See also under* PREGNANCY-RELATED PROBLEMS in Part Two.

Hepatitis

Hepatitis is an inflammation of the liver, usually caused by a viral infection. The liver becomes tender and enlarged and is unable to function normally. As a result, toxins that would normally be filtered out by the liver build up in the body, and certain nutrients are not processed and stored as they should be. The symptoms of hepatitis include fever, weakness, nausea, vomiting, headache, appetite loss, muscle aches, joint pains, drowsiness, dark urine, light-colored stools, abdominal discomfort, and, often, jaundice (yellowing of the skin) and elevated liver enzymes in the blood. Flulike symptoms may be mild or severe.

There are different types of hepatitis, classified according to the virus that causes the condition. In the last fifteen years, scientists have identified the viruses responsible for three leading types of the disease, called hepatitis A, hepatitis B, and hepatitis C. There are also other, less common types known as hepatitis E, and non-A, non-B hepatitis. All are contagious.

Hepatitis A, also known as infectious hepatitis, is easily spread through person-to-person contact, and through contact with food, clothing, bed linen, and other items. It is contagious between two to three weeks before and one week after jaundice appears. After a bout with hepatitis A, the individual develops an immunity to it.

Hepatitis B, also referred to as serum hepatitis, is spread through contact with infected blood (for example, through the use of contaminated syringes, needles, and transfused blood) and some forms of sexual activity. It is estimated that up to 5 percent of all Americans, and as many as 85 percent of gay men, are infected with hepatitis B. However, most hepatitis B infections come and go unrecognized. In some 10 percent of cases, the disease becomes chronic, scarring the liver and making it more vulnerable to cancer. Hepatitis B is the ninth leading cause of death in the United States.

Hepatitis C accounts for 20 to 40 percent of all hepatitis and 90 to 95 percent of hepatitis contracted through blood transfusions. Tests can now detect antibodies against hepatitis C in donated blood, a major advance in ensuring a safe blood supply, but an infected individual may take up to six months to develop the antibodies, so it is still impossible to identify all infected blood. Hepatitis C can also be contracted through intravenous drug use, sexual contact, and broken skin or mucous membranes.

In addition to the various types of viral hepatitis, there is a form of the disease called toxic hepatitis, which can be caused by exposure to chemicals, principally the injection, ingestion, or absorption of toxins through the skin. Chlorinated hydrocarbons and arsenic are examples of severe hepatotoxic agents. In toxic hepatitis, the amount of exposure to the toxin determines the extent of liver damage.

NUTRIENTS

SUPPLEMENT	SUGGESTED DOSAGE	COMMENTS
Essential		
Free-form amino acid complex	As directed on label.	To supply necessary protein. The liver breaks down protein; taking free-form amino acids takes strain off the liver.
Glutathione plus	500 mg twice daily, on an empty stomach.	Protects the liver.
L-cysteine and L-methionine	500 mg each twice daily, on an empty stomach. Take with water or juice. Do not take with milk. Take with 50 mg vitamin B6 and 100 mg vitamin C for better absorption.	Detoxifies harmful hepatotoxins and protects glutathione. *See* AMINO ACIDS in Part One.
Milk thistle		*See under* Herbs, below.
Raw liver extract or desiccated liver	As directed on label. As directed on label.	Promotes liver function. *See* GLANDULAR THERAPY in Part Three. Consider injections (under a doctor's supervision).
Very Important		
Coenzyme Q10	60 mg daily.	Counteracts immunosuppression and enhances tissue oxygenation.

Dimethylglycine (DMG) (Aangamik DMG from FoodScience Labs)	As directed on label.	Improves cellular oxygen concentration.
Lecithin granules or capsules	1 tbsp 3 times daily, before meals. 1,200 mg 3 times daily, before meals.	Protects cells of the liver and is a fat mobilizer. Aids in preventing fatty liver.
Bifido Factor from Natren or LifeStart from Natren	As directed on label. As directed on label.	For adults. Needed for normal liver function and proper digestion. For infants and children.
Superoxide dismutase (SOD) or Cell Guard from Biotec Foods or Oxy-5000 Forte from American Biologics	As directed on label. As directed on label. As directed on label.	Powerful antioxidants that neutralize damaging superoxide free radicals, improving liver function.
Multivitamin complex with vitamin B complex plus extra vitamin B12 plus chloline and inositol	50–100 mg 3 times daily, with meals. Do not exceed a total of 100 mg vitamin B3 (niacin) in any one day until healing is complete. 1,000 mg twice daily. As directed on label.	All nutrients are necessary in balance. All B vitamins are absolutely essential for normal liver function. Sublingual forms are recommended. Injections (under a doctor's supervision) may be necessary, especially of vitamin B12 and folic acid.
Vitamin C with bioflavonoids	5,000–10,000 mg daily and up.	A powerful antiviral agent. Studies show improvement quickly with high doses.
Vitamin E	Start with 400 IU daily and increase to 1,200 IU daily over the course of 1 month.	A potent antioxidant.
Important		
Calcium and magnesium	1,500 mg daily. 1,000 mg daily.	Essential for blood clotting, which is a problem for people with liver disease. Use asporotate forms. Do not use bone meal.
Essential fatty acids (primrose oil and salmon oil are good sources) or shark liver oil	As directed on label. As directed on label.	Combats inflammation of the liver and lowers serum fats. Important source of essential lipids.
Multienzyme complex with betaine hydrochloride (HCl)	As directed on label.	Important for proper digestion.
Helpful		
Raw pancreas glandular	As directed on label.	Aids in digestion and pancreatic function.
Vitamin A	25,000 IU daily. If you are pregnant, do not exceed 10,000 IU daily.	Needed for healing. Use emulsion form for easier assimilation and greater safety. Avoid using beta-carotene or capsule forms of vitamin A until healing is complete.

Maitake or shiitake or reishi	As directed on label. As directed on label. As directed on label.	To boost the immune system and fight viral infection.

HERBS

❑ Burdock and dandelion are important in cleansing the liver and the bloodstream.

❑ Studies have shown licorice to be effecting in treating viral hepatitis, particularly chronic active hepatitis, due to its well-documented antiviral activity.

Caution: Do not use this herb on a daily basis for more than seven days in a row. Avoid if you have high blood pressure.

❑ Milk thistle extract contains silymarin, a flavonoid that has been shown to aid in healing and rebuilding the liver. It can be taken in capsule or alcohol-free extract form. Take 200 to 400 milligrams three times daily.

❑ Other herbs beneficial for hepatitis include black radish, goldenseal, green tea, red clover, and yellow dock.

Caution: Do not take goldenseal internally on a daily basis for more than one week at a time, do not use it during pregnancy, and use with caution if you are allergic to ragweed.

RECOMMENDATIONS

❑ Eat a raw vegetable and fruit diet for two to four weeks. Start this diet with a cleansing fast. *See* FASTING in Part Three.

❑ Include artichokes in the diet. Artichokes protect the liver. Globe artichoke extract also is available.

❑ Drink "green drinks," carrot juice, and beet juice. *See* JUICING in Part Three.

❑ Drink only steam-distilled water.

❑ Consume no alcohol.

❑ Avoid all fats, sugar, and highly processed foods.

❑ Avoid all raw fish and shellfish, and eat no animal protein. Also avoid chemicals and food additives.

❑ Get plenty of bed rest.

❑ Use a chlorophyll enema three times a week. Use one pint and retain it for fifteen minutes. *See* ENEMAS in Part Three.

❑ Apply warm castor oil packs over the liver area. Place castor oil in a pan and heat but do not boil it. Dip a piece of cheesecloth or other white cotton material in the oil until the cloth is saturated. Apply the cloth to the upper right abdomen and cover it with a piece of plastic that is larger in size than the cotton cloth. Place a heating pad over the plastic and use it to keep the pack warm. Keep the pack in place for one-half to two hours, as needed.

❑ Keep a person with hepatitis A in isolation to avoid spreading the infection. Wash hands and all clothing often. The clothing and bed linens of a person with hepatitis A require special handling. Wash them separately from other laundry in hot water with chlorine bleach or a disinfectant added. Because the feces are infectious, bathrooms should be decontaminated frequently. Clean toilets and floors with a disinfectant.

❑ Especially when traveling, beware of contaminated water or foods from polluted waters.

❑ Do not take any drugs that have not been prescribed by your doctor. Read package inserts carefully for information regarding liver toxicity.

CONSIDERATIONS

❑ One of the most important forms of hepatitis worldwide—hepatitis E—is rarely seen in the United States, but it has been linked to numerous large epidemics in Africa and Asia. Two outbreaks in Mexico in 1986 were the first to be identified in the Western Hemisphere. Sporadic cases have occurred among travelers, including some Americans. Hepatitis E is usually contracted from sewage-contaminated water, and it can be spread from person to person. It is more likely to cause symptoms in adults than in small children. No blood test is available, but the virus can be identified through a stool sample. The best known safeguard is to boil water before drinking it or washing with it.

❑ Taking excessive amounts of vitamin A over long periods may cause liver enzyme levels to become elevated. Anyone who has been taking over 50,000 international units of vitamin A daily for over a year should reduce his or her intake or switch to natural beta-carotene, which should not have any side effects.

❑ Catechin, a flavonoid found in green and black Indian teas, has been shown to decrease serum bilirubin levels in people with all types of acute viral hepatitis.

❑ According to researchers at the University of California, as many as 25 percent of Americans who receive blood transfusions develop hepatitis.

❑ A study reported in *The New England Journal of Medicine* indicated that high doses of the antiviral agent interferon alfa, given daily for four months, produced remission in a third of subjects with hepatitis B. People who had low levels of virus particles present in their bloodstreams benefited most. A version of interferon alfa (interferon alfa-2b) has been approved by the Food and Drug Administration for the treatment of hepatitis C.

❑ Studies have shown that the herb milk thistle can cure liver cancer in rats.

❑ Liver supplements contain a nutritional substance that aids liver regeneration. Only liver from organically raised beef should be used.

❑ In laboratory experiments, injections of whole liver cells have rapidly repaired liver tissue in experimental animals with lethal, acute liver failure.

❑ Vaccination against hepatitis B is recommended by the American Medical Association for all newborn babies, sexually active gay men, drug users, pregnant immigrants from Asia, babies whose mothers have hepatitis B, and medical and dental workers who may come in contact with blood.

Hernia, Hiatal

Hiatal hernia is a condition in which the stomach pushes, or herniates, upward through an opening in the diaphragm into the thorax. Usually a result of a congenital abnormality or trauma, this condition is associated with gastroesophageal reflux, in which the muscle that encircles the juncture of the stomach and the esophagus fails to keep food and acid from coming back up from the stomach into the esophagus as it should. If that happens, the tissues in the esophagus become irritated, causing heartburn and, sometimes, a coughing up of bloody mucus.

Common symptoms of hiatal hernia include heartburn and belching. If stomach acid comes up into the throat, it can cause a burning sensation and great discomfort behind the breastbone.

An estimated 50 percent of people over forty years of age have hiatal hernias. However, many people are unaware of the condition. Small hernias rarely cause any real trouble. It is the larger hernias that are most often linked to reflux problems. Ulcers often accompany a hiatal hernia. The acid reflux may lead to ulceration of the esophagus. Ulcers can also occur in the duodenum (the top of the small intestine) or the stomach.

NUTRIENTS

SUPPLEMENT	SUGGESTED DOSAGE	COMMENTS
Important		
Proteolytic enzymes plus pancreatin	As directed on label. Take between meals. As directed on label. Take with meals.	For improved digestion. *Caution:* Do not give these supplements to a child. *Do not* use a formula containing HCl.
Helpful		
Aloe vera		*See under* Herbs, below.
Multivitamin and mineral complex	As directed on label.	All nutrients are needed in balance. Use a hypoallergenic formula.
Papaya enzyme	2 tablets 3 or more times daily, before meals and/or as needed.	Good for digestion and healing. Use a chewable tablet form.
Zinc	50 mg daily. Do not exceed a total of 100 mg daily from all supplements.	Necessary for healing and repair of tissue. Use zinc gluconate lozenges or OptiZinc for best absorption.
Vitamin A	50,000 IU daily for 1 month, then 30,000 IU daily for 2 weeks, then reduce to 20,000 IU daily. If you are pregnant, do not exceed 10,000 IU daily.	Aids in combating excess acid and enhances immune function. Use emulsion form for easier assimilation and greater safety at higher doses.

Vitamin B complex	100 mg twice daily, with meals.	Needed for all enzyme systems in the body and for proper absorption of nutrients. Use a hypoallergenic formula.
plus extra vitamin B$_{12}$	200 mcg daily, between meals.	Use a lozenge or sublingual form.
Vitamin C	Up to 1,500 mg daily.	Needed for proper immune function and healing of tissues. Use a buffered form.

HERBS

❑ Aloe vera promotes healing of the intestinal lining. Drink ¼ cup of aloe vera juice in the morning and again at night. It can be added to juice or herbal tea if you wish.

❑ Other beneficial herbs include fenugreek, goldenseal, marshmallow root, red clover, and slippery elm.

Caution: Do not take goldenseal internally on a daily basis for more than one week at a time, do not use during pregnancy, and use it with caution if you are allergic to ragweed.

RECOMMENDATIONS

❑ At the first sign of heartburn, drink one or two large glasses of water. This often relieves heartburn by washing the acid out of the esophagus.

❑ Even if you are not thirsty, drink a large glass of water every three hours during the daytime.

❑ Eat several small meals daily.

❑ Include extra fiber in the diet.

❑ Do not consume spicy foods, and do not take enzyme supplements that contain hydrochloric acid (HCl).

❑ Avoid fats and fried foods. They delay digestion and prolong the stomach's emptying time. Also avoid coffee, tea, alcohol, colas, and smoking.

❑ Avoid heavy lifting and bending. Give the stomach at least two hours to empty before lifting or other exertion. Bend from the knees, not the waist, to avoid abdominal pressure.

❑ Do not wear clothing that is tight around the waist.

❑ Avoid becoming constipated and straining during bowel movements.

❑ Do not eat within three hours of bedtime. If you are regularly bothered by indigestion during the night, try raising the head of your bed six to ten inches.

❑ Do not lie down during the day if you are bothered by heartburn. Sitting or standing helps to keep the stomach acids in the stomach.

❑ Because heartburn causes symptoms similar to those of heart disease, see a physician if you have more than occasional bouts to rule out the possibility of heart problems.

CONSIDERATIONS

❑ Allergenic foods often magnify the symptoms and prolong healing. Symptoms of hiatal hernia often clear up when allergenic foods are avoided. (*See* ALLERGIES in Part Two.)

❑ Gastroesophageal reflux can also be caused by other factors as well as hiatal hernia, such as smoking or eating too close to bedtime. Obesity also can contribute to the problem.

❑ *See also* ULCERS and HEARTBURN in Part Two.

Herpesvirus Infection

There are more than ninety viruses that belong to a family of animal viruses called *herpes virdae*. Of this family of viruses, four are known to be important to humans. Varicella-zoster causes chickenpox and shingles; Epstein-Barr causes infectious mononucleosis; cytomegalovirus (CMV) often is carried without producing any symptoms, but can have devastating consequences for newborns and for people with compromised immune systems. This section addresses herpes simplex, which causes cold sores (fever blisters) and genital herpes.

There are two types of herpes simplex. Herpes simplex type I (HSV-1) typically causes cold sores and skin eruptions. In later life, it may erupt into a form of shingles. It can also cause *herpes keratitis*, an inflammation of the cornea of the eye. If herpes repeatedly flares up in the eye, it can lead to scarring and loss of vision.

Between 20 and 40 percent of the population in the United States has cold sores caused by HSV-1. As many as twice that number have been infected with the virus but may never have the sores. That means that 40 to 80 percent of the population is infected with this virus.

Herpes simplex type II (HSV-2) is the most prevalent sexually transmitted disease in the United States. More than 30 million Americans—one out of every six persons over the age of fifteen—have the type II infection, though more than half never develop.serious symptoms. This viral infection can range in severity from a silent infection to a serious inflammation of the liver with fever. It is especially dangerous to infants. A baby whose mother is infected can pick up the virus in the birth canal, creating a risk of brain damage, blindness, and death.

Both oral and genital herpes cause painful fluid-filled blisters that are highly infectious until they are completely healed, which can take up to three weeks. In oral herpes, sores usually appear within two to seven days after initial exposure to the virus. Recurrent eruptions are common. Some people are bothered by outbreaks once a year or less; others may get them every few weeks.

A mild tingling and burning in the vaginal area may be the first sign of genital herpes in women. Within a matter of a few hours, blisters develop around the rectum, clitoris, and cervix, and in the vagina. There is often a watery discharge from the urethra and pain when urinating. In men, blisters break out on the penis, groin, and scrotum, often with a urethral discharge and painful urination. Sometimes the penis and foreskin swell. A man may also have tender, swollen lymph nodes in the groin.

The first attack of genital herpes usually comes four to eight days after exposure to the virus. It may be so mild that it isn't noticed, or it may cause itching and burning at the site of viral entry as well as painful sores that can last a week or more, plus fever, headache, and other flulike symptoms. After a few days, pus erupts from the blisters and painful ulcers form. These sores crust over and dry while healing. Usually, they leave no scars.

Once they enter the body, herpesviruses never leave. They live in nerve cells, where the immune system cannot find them, and they become active from time to time as the immune system is depressed. The virus may lie dormant for long periods of time, until illness, sun exposure, fatigue, stress, or some other factor causes the virus to break out in open sores again. Fortunately, after a period of time, the virus seems to burn itself out. Outbreaks rarely appear after the age of fifty.

Until recently, it was assumed that genital herpes could be transmitted only during a visible outbreak of the disease, but recent research appears to refute this theory. The only sure way to avoid genital herpes is to avoid sex, or to remain in a monogamous relationship with an uninfected partner. Also, although HSV-1 principally causes cold sores and eye infections and HSV-2 principally causes genital herpes, both type I and II can infect either the mouth or the genitals—or both. Oral sex can spread the virus from one place to another.

NUTRIENTS

SUPPLEMENT	SUGGESTED DOSAGE	COMMENTS
Very Important		
L-Lysine	500–1,000 mg daily, on an empty stomach. Take with water or juice. Do not take with milk. Take with 50 mg vitamin B₆ and 100 mg vitamin C for better absorption.	When the amount of lysine present exceeds the amount of arginine, the growth of the herpes virus is inhibited. *See* AMINO ACIDS in Part One. *Caution:* Do not take this supplement for longer than 6 months at a time.
Oxy C-2 Gel from American Biologics	Apply to affected areas as directed on label.	A useful antiviral, antifungal, and bactericide.
Vitamin A	50,000 IU daily. If you are pregnant, do not exceed 10,000 IU daily.	Important for healing. Prevents spreading of infection. Use emulsion form for easier assimilation and greater safety at higher doses.
Vitamin B complex	50 mg and up, 3 times daily.	Combats the virus and helps to keep it from spreading. Also works with lysine to prevent outbreaks. Use hypoallergenic form.
Vitamin C	5,000–10,000 mg daily.	Needed to prevent sores and inhibit the growth of the virus. Use an esterified or buffered form.
plus bioflavonoids	30–60 mg daily, in divided doses.	Works with vitamin C.
Zinc	50–100 mg daily, in divided doses. Do not exceed 100 mg daily.	Boosts immune function. For genital herpes, use a chelate form. For oral herpes, use zinc gluconate lozenges.
Important		
Acidophilus	As directed on label, 3 times daily, on an empty stomach.	Needed for the production of the B vitamins. Prevents overgrowth of harmful microorganisms in the intestines.
Dioxychlor from American Biologics	As directed on label.	An important antiviral, antibacterial, and antifungal agent.
Egg lecithin	As directed on label.	Helps control the virus.
Essential fatty acids (primrose oil and salmon oil are good sources)	As directed on label.	Needed for cell protection.
Garlic (Kyolic)	3 tablets 3 times daily, with meals.	An immune system stimulant and a natural antibiotic.
Superoxide dismutase (SOD) or	As directed on label.	Reduces infection and speeds healing. A powerful free radical destroyer.
Cell Guard from Biotec Foods	As directed on label.	An antioxidant complex that contains SOD.
Vitamin E	600 IU daily.	Important in healing. Prevents spread of the infection. Use emulsion form for easier assimilation.
Helpful		
Calcium and	1,500 mg daily.	To relieve stress and anxiety. Use chelated forms.
magnesium	750 mg daily.	
Dimethylglycine (DMG) (Aangamik DMG from FoodScience Labs)	2 tablets dissolved in the mouth twice daily.	Enhances utilization of oxygen by tissue.
Maitake or	As directed on label.	Mushrooms that have immune-boosting and antiviral properties.
shiitake or	As directed on label.	
reishi	As directed on label.	
Multivitamin and mineral supplement	As directed on label.	Needed to enhance healing. Take a hypoallergenic form.
Proteolytic enzymes	As directed on label 2–3 times daily. Take between meals.	Helps protect against infection; works on undigested food remaining in the colon. *Caution:* Do not give this supplement to a child.
Raw thymus glandular	500 mg twice daily.	Enhances immune function. *Caution:* Do not give this supplement to a child.

HERBS

❑ Applying black walnut or goldenseal extract to the affected area may help.

❑ Herpes treatment should include cayenne (capsicum), echinacea, myrrh, red clover, and St. Johnswort.

❑ Tea tree oil is a powerful natural antiseptic. During a herpes outbreak, dab it lightly on the affected area several times a day, either full strength or, if that is too strong, diluted with distilled water or cold-pressed vegetable oil. Do not get tea tree oil close to the eye area.

❑ Goldenseal is a natural antibiotic. It can be taken in capsule or tea form.

Caution: Do not take goldenseal internally on a daily basis for more than one week at a time, do not use it during pregnancy, and use with caution if you are allergic to ragweed.

❑ Licorice root inhibits both the growth and cell-damaging effects of herpes simplex. If you are using licorice, increase your potassium intake.

Caution: Do not use this herb on a daily basis for more than seven days in a row. Avoid it completely if you have high blood pressure.

RECOMMENDATIONS

❑ Avoid alcohol, processed foods, colas, white flour products, sugar, refined carbohydrates, coffee, and drugs to lessen the chance of an outbreak. Herbal teas are beneficial (*see* Herbs, above), but all other teas should be avoided.

❑ Drink steam-distilled water.

❑ Eat the following in moderation during outbreaks: almonds, barley, cashews, cereals (grains), chicken, chocolate, corn, dairy products, meat, nuts and seeds, oats, and peanuts. These contain L-arginine, an amino acid that suppresses L-lysine, the amino acid that retards virus growth.

❑ Do not consume citrus fruits and juices while the virus is active.

❑ Get plenty of rest. Stress reduction is important.

❑ To ease swelling and pain in the genital area, use ice packs. Warm Epsom salts or baking soda baths help itching and pain. After the bath, pat dry gently and keep the lesions dry.

❑ Apply vitamin E and vitamin A, alternately, directly on the sores. Or try using L-lysine cream from a health food store.

❑ Wear cotton underwear. Practice good genital hygiene—keep clean and dry.

❑ If you have active lesions, refrain from sex until the sores have completely healed. Do not have intercourse with a person with visible genital lesions of any kind.

❑ If you are pregnant and know you have genital herpes, tell your health care provider. If an attack occurs late in the pregnancy, your baby may have to be delivered by cesarean section to protect against exposure during birth. If there are no lesions present, the risk to the baby is probably low.

❑ If an eye becomes infected, see your physician at once. This virus can cause encephalitis, a brain inflammation.

CONSIDERATIONS

❑ Genital herpes infections in women increase the risk of cervical cancer. Women with herpes should be conscientious about having a Pap smear done periodically.

❑ Excess serum cholesterol sets the stage for atherosclerosis, but it may get a hand from certain herpesviruses, including HSV-1. According to researchers at Cornell University Medical Center in New York City, the virus induces arterial changes that promote blood clotting and cholesterol buildup.

❑ In a study on rabbits, a vaccine to protect the eyes against HSV-1 cut active infections in half.

❑ A virus identified by the National Cancer Institute as the human B cell lymphotropic virus (HBLV) is believed to be a member of the herpesvirus family and may also be a factor in fatigue.

❑ Research suggests that capsaicin may be able to prevent outbreaks of herpes fever blisters or genital lesions.

❑ Dimethylsulfoxide (DMSO), a byproduct of wood processing, is a liquid that can be applied topically to relieve pain and promote the healing of herpes outbreaks.

Note: Only DMSO from a health food store should be used. Commercial-grade DMSO found in hardware stores is not suitable for healing purposes. The use of DMSO may result in a garlicky body odor. This is temporary, and is not a cause for concern.

❑ The antiviral drug acyclovir (Zovirax) has been shown to relieve symptoms and reduce the severity and frequency of outbreaks. This drug is available by prescription only and comes in capsule and lotion forms. It can be used for both oral and genital herpes. The capsules are usually taken every four hours for ten days. Applying the lotion when an imminent outbreak is first sensed usually weakens the attack. In studies conducted by the National Institutes of Health, taking 400 milligrams of acyclovir twice daily for four months reduced cold sore episodes by 52 percent, and when outbreaks did occur, the blisters healed approximately twice as fast as normal. Caution should be practiced if the drug is taken on a regular basis, however. When the drug is stopped, a "rebound" effect may result in a more serious outbreak than usual.

❑ Isotretinoin, a derivative of vitamin A, has given dramatic results with herpes simplex infections.

❑ Some physicians have used butylated hydroxytoluene (BHT) to treat herpes. This can have dangerous consequences, however, especially if taken on an empty stomach. Irritation and even perforation of the stomach can result. We do not recommend this treatment for herpes.

❑ *See also* COLD SORES; SEXUALLY TRANSMITTED DISEASE; and SHINGLES in Part Two.

Herpes Zoster

See SHINGLES. *See also under* EYE PROBLEMS.

Hiatal Hernia

See HERNIA, HIATAL.

High Blood Pressure (Hypertension)

When the heart pumps the blood through the arteries, the blood presses against the walls of the blood vessels. In people who suffer from hypertension, this pressure is abnormally high.

Whether blood pressure is high, low, or normal depends on several factors: the output from the heart, the resistance to blood flow of the blood vessels, the volume of blood, and blood distribution to the various organs. All of these factors in turn can be affected by the activities of the nervous system and certain hormones.

If blood pressure is elevated, the heart must work harder to pump an adequate amount of blood to all the tissues of the body. Ultimately, the condition often leads to kidney failure, heart failure, and stroke. In addition, high blood pressure is often associated with coronary heart disease, arteriosclerosis, kidney disorders, obesity, diabetes, hyperthyroidism, and adrenal tumors.

An estimated 50 million Americans have high blood pressure. According to the U.S. Public Health Service, hypertension affects more than half of all Americans over the age of sixty-five. The percentage of the African-American population with high blood pressure is approximately one-third higher than that for whites. African-Americans between the ages of twenty-four and forty-four are *eighteen times* more likely than whites to develop kidney failure due to hypertension. Men tend to develop hypertension more often than women, but the risk for women rises after menopause and soon approaches that of men. A woman's risk of high blood pressure also increases if she takes oral contraceptives or is pregnant.

Because high blood pressure usually causes no symptoms until complications develop, it is known as the "silent killer." Warning signs associated with advanced hypertension may include headaches, sweating, rapid pulse, shortness of breath, dizziness, and visual disturbances. In 1990, nearly 33,000 Americans died of hypertension-related diseases other than heart attack and stroke.

Blood pressure is usually divided into two categories, designated *primary* and *secondary*. Primary hypertension is high blood pressure that is not due to another underlying disease. The precise cause is unknown, but a number of definite risk factors have been identified. These include cigarette smoking, stress, obesity, excessive use of stimulants such as coffee or tea, drug abuse, high sodium intake, and the use of oral contraceptives. Because too much water retention can exert pressure on the blood vessels, those who consume foods high in sodium may be at a greater risk for high blood pressure. Elevated blood pressure is also common in people who are overweight. Blood pressure can rise due to stress as well, because stress causes the walls of the arteries to constrict. Also, those with a family history of hypertension are more likely to suffer from high blood pressure.

When persistently elevated blood pressure arises as a result of another underlying health problem, such as a hormonal abnormality or an inherited narrowing of the aorta, it is called secondary hypertension. A person may also have secondary hypertension because the blood vessels are chronically constricted or have lost elasticity from a buildup of fatty plaque on the inside walls of the vessel, a condition known as atherosclerosis. Arteriosclerosis and atherosclerosis are common precursors of hypertension. The narrowing and/or hardening of the arteries makes circulation of blood through the vessels difficult. As a result, blood pressure becomes elevated. Secondary hypertension can also be caused by poor kidney function, which results in the retention of excess sodium and fluid in the body. This increase in blood volume within the vessels causes elevated blood pressure levels. Kidneys may also elevate blood pressure by secreting substances that cause blood vessels to constrict.

To diagnose high blood pressure, a physician uses a device called a *sphygmomanometer*. Blood pressure is represented as a pair of numbers. The first is the *systolic* pressure, which is the pressure exerted by the blood when the heart beats, forcing blood into the blood vessels. This reading indicates blood pressure at its highest. The second reading is the *diastolic* pressure, which is recorded when the heart is at rest in between beats, when the blood pressure is at its lowest. Both figures represent the height (in millimeters, or mm) that a column of mercury (Hg) reaches under the pressure exerted by the blood. The combined blood pressure reading is then expressed as a ratio of systolic blood pressure to diastolic blood pressure. Thus, in a person with normal blood pressure, the systolic pressure measures 120 mm Hg and the diastolic pressure measures 80 mm Hg; together, this is expressed as 120 over 80, or 120/80. Both the systolic and diastolic readings are important; neither should be high. Normal blood pressure readings for adults vary from 110/70 to 140/90, while readings of 140/90 to 160/90 or 160/95 indicate borderline hypertension. Any pressure over 180/115 is severely elevated.

It is impossible for your health care provider to make a correct diagnosis of high blood pressure with a single reading. The test must be repeated throughout the day to be accurate. Home testing is best because it enables you to monitor your condition periodically. Measuring blood pressure at home on a regular schedule may:

• Help determine whether your blood pressure is high only when taken during a medical visit.

How to Measure Your Blood Pressure

Your blood pressure measurement actually tells you how much pressure it takes to stop the flow of blood through your arteries. This is assumed to be equivalent to the pressure at the pump end, the heart.

Blood pressure is measured at two points in the heart's pumping rhythm: *systolic pressure* is taken at the moment the heart beats; *diastolic pressure* is taken when the heart is at rest between beats. To measure blood pressure, the soft, inflatable cuff of the sphygmomanometer is wrapped around the upper arm and inflated. Systolic pressure is measured when there is no longer a pulse in the arm beyond the cuff. Then the cuff is deflated and the diastolic pressure is taken when the blood flows freely once more. The combined pressure is usually expressed as a fraction—120/80, for example.

Ideally, blood pressure should be taken with the arm bare. A tight sleeve may constrict the arm or make it impossible to apply the blood pressure cuff properly. The cuff should be placed around the arm about one inch above the bend in the elbow. Before beginning to work with the sphygmomanometer, check the following four items:

1. Be sure that the sphygmomanometer reads 0 when there is no pressure in the system.

2. Check to be sure that the needle stays in place when the valve is closed.

3. Check the valve screw to make sure that it operates smoothly.

4. Inspect your stethoscope for cracks or leaks in the tubing, earpieces, bell, or diaphragm.

You should first feel for the blood pressure. Find the radial pulse, on the thumb side of the wrist. Then inflate the cuff 30 mm Hg beyond the point where the pulse is obliterated. Open the valve and release 2–3 mm Hg per second. When the pulsations of the radial pulse again become palpable, this is the systolic pressure. The diastolic blood pressure occurs when vibrations in the artery cease. Diastolic pressure is much more difficult to obtain.

Next, use the stethoscope to take the blood pressure. Follow this procedure:

1. Position the disc of the stethoscope snugly against the skin where the elbow bends—a little to the left of center on the right arm, and a little to the right of center on the left arm. There should be no gaps between the stethoscope and the skin, but you should not apply any undue pressure. Make sure

that the stethoscope is not touching the cuff at any point.

2. Position the earpieces of the stethoscope in your ears (with the earpieces directed forward).

3. Hold the stethoscope disc snugly in position with one hand while you pump the cuff with the other hand.

4. Pump the cuff until the gauge registers about 30 mm Hg above the point where you felt the pulse disappear earlier, or about 200 mm Hg.

5. Loosen the valve slightly and permit the pressure to drop slowly. Listen carefully for the first sound of a beat—the number on the scale when you hear the first beat is the systolic pressure. (If you think that you missed the first beat or are unsure, tighten the valve again and pump the cuff up; repeat the process, listening carefully.)

6. Continue to deflate the cuff slowly until the last sound of blood pumping through the blood vessels is heard. When you hear no more blood flowing, the number on the scale is the diastolic pressure.

When taking your blood pressure, follow these general guidelines for best results:

• Avoid eating, smoking, or exercising for at least one-half hour before measuring your blood pressure.

• Test yourself at about the same times each day. Plan ahead to give yourself time to get over any feelings of anger or anxiety.

• Sit quietly and eliminate extraneous noise.

• Follow the manufacturer's instructions carefully.

• Position your arm at heart level, palm up. If you are using a cuff device, wrap the cuff just above the elbow—with your sleeve rolled up above the cuff—and be sure it is not too tight.

• Make sure the hoses from the cuff are not tangled or pinched.

• Take care not to move the hoses during the reading.

• Wait at least five minutes in between readings, with the cuff fully deflated.

• Take the device along on medical visits once a year or more to check its accuracy against your physician's measurements.

• Enable you to collaborate with your health care provider in controlling your high blood pressure.

• Reduce the frequency with which you need to visit your health care provider for blood pressure evaluation.

Blood pressure monitoring devices fall into two basic

categories: mechanical gauges and automated electronic gauges. The mechanical gauge is the type most often used in physicians' offices. It consists of an instrument to measure the pressure, an air bladder (inflatable cuff), and a pressure bulb with a release valve to pump up the cuff. The standard-size arm cuff on blood pressure monitors fits arms up to thirteen inches around (if your arm is larger than this, you will need to obtain a larger cuff). With most of these devices, the pressure is read on a gauge dial.

Mechanical gauges are much less expensive than electronic ones and many physicians feel they give more accurate readings, at least in the hands of an experienced user. However, if you use this type of device to take your own blood pressure, you must pump up the cuff with one hand, read a dial, and listen with a stethoscope more or less simultaneously (see How to Measure Your Blood Pressure on page 321). In other words, using these devices correctly requires dexterity, good eyesight, acute hearing, and some training and practice.

An alternative to the mechanical gauge is the digital sphygomanometer. With this device, the machine automatically gauges your blood pressure when the cuff is inflated and presents the result in a digital format. These are more expensive than the mechanical types, but because they are much easier to use accurately, they are generally preferred for home use.

There are also other electronic devices available, including wrist and finger cuff monitors. Although they are easy to operate, most doctors do not recommend them because they tend to be less accurate and also more sensitive to the effects of temperature and poor blood circulation.

NUTRIENTS

SUPPLEMENT	SUGGESTED DOSAGE	COMMENTS
Essential		
Calcium and	1,500–3,000 mg daily.	Deficiencies have been linked to high blood pressure.
magnesium	750–1,000 mg daily.	
Garlic (Kyolic)	2 capsules 3 times daily.	Effective in lowering blood pressure.
L-Carnitine	500 mg twice daily, on an empty stomach.	Transports long fatty acid chains. Together with L-glutamic acid and L-glutamine, aids in preventing heart disease.
plus L-glutamic acid and L-glutamine	500 mg each daily, on an empty stomach. Take with water or juice. Do not take with milk. Take with 50 mg vitamin B_6 and 100 mg vitamin C for better absorption.	To detoxify ammonia and aid in preventing heart disease. *See* AMINO ACIDS in Part One.
Selenium	200 mcg daily.	Deficiency has been linked to heart disease.
Very Important		
Coenzyme Q_{10}	100 mg daily.	Improves heart function and lowers blood pressure.
Essential fatty acids (black currant seed oil, flaxseed oil, olive oil, and primrose oil are good sources)	As directed on label. Take before meals.	Important for circulation and for lowering blood pressure.
Vitamin C	3,000–6,000 mg daily, in divided doses.	Improves adrenal function; reduces blood-clotting tendencies.

Important		
Lecithin granules or capsules or lipotropic factors	1 tbsp 3 times daily, before meals. 1,200 mg 3 times daily, before meals. As directed on label.	To emulsify fat, improving liver function and lowering blood pressure.
Vitamin E and/or octacosonol	Start with 100 IU daily and add 100 IU daily each month, until you reach 400 IU daily. As directed on label.	Improves heart function. Use emulsion form for easier assimilation and greater safety at high doses.
Helpful		
Bromelain	As directed on label.	An enzyme that aids in the digestion of fats.
Kelp	1,000–1,500 mg daily.	A good source of minerals and natural iodine.
Kyo-Green from Wakunaga	As directed on label twice daily.	This concentrated barley and wheatgrass juice contains important nutrients.
Maitake or shiitake or reishi	As directed on label. As directed on label. As directed on label.	To help reduce high blood pressure and prevent heart disease.
Multivitamin and mineral complex with vitamin A and zinc plus extra	15,000 IU daily. If you are pregnant, do not exceed 10,000 IU daily. 50 mg daily.	All nutrients are needed in balance.
potassium	99 mg daily.	If taking cortisone or high blood pressure medication, take extra potassium to counteract depletion of this mineral.
Proteolytic enzymes	As directed on label. Take with meals and between meals.	Aids in cleansing the circulatory system. Completes protein digestion.
Raw heart glandular plus	As directed on label.	Strengthens the heart.
Bio-Cardiozyme Forte from Biotics Research or	As directed on label.	A complex that strengthens the heart muscle.
Heart Science from Source Naturals	As directed on label.	Contains antioxidants, cholesterol-fighters, herbs, and vitamins that work together to promote cardiovascular function.
Vitamin B complex plus extra vitamin B_3 (niacin) and choline and inositol	100 mg twice daily, with meals. 50 mg twice daily. 50 mg twice daily. 50 mg twice daily.	Important for circulatory function and for lowering blood pressure. Take niacin only under the supervision of a physician.
Vitamin B_6	50 mg 3 times daily.	Reduces water content in tissues to relieve pressure on the cardiovascular system.

HERBS

❑ Use cayenne (capsicum), chamomile, fennel, hawthorn berries, parsley, and rosemary for high blood pressure.

Caution: Do not use chamomile on an ongoing basis, as ragweed allergy may result. Avoid it completely if you are allergic to ragweed.

❑ Hops and valerian root are good for calming the nerves.

❑ Drink 3 cups of suma tea daily.

❑ *Avoid* the herbs ephedra (ma huang) and licorice, as these herbs can elevate blood pressure.

RECOMMENDATIONS

❑ Follow a strict salt-free diet. This is essential for lowering blood pressure. Lowering your salt intake is not enough; eliminate all salt from your diet. Read labels carefully and avoid those food products that have "salt," "soda," "sodium," or the symbol "Na" on the label. Some foods and food additives that should be avoided on this diet include monosodium glutamate (Accent, MSG); baking soda; canned vegetables (unless marked sodium- or salt-free); commercially prepared foods; toothpastes containing saccharin or baking soda; over-the-counter medications that contain ibuprofen (such as Advil or Nuprin); diet soft drinks; foods with mold inhibitors, preservatives, and sugar substitutes; meat tenderizers; softened water; and soy sauce.

❑ Eat a high-fiber diet and take supplemental fiber. Oat bran is a good source of fiber.

Note: Always take supplemental fiber separately from other supplements and medications.

❑ Eat plenty of fruits and vegetables, such as apples, asparagus, bananas, broccoli, cabbage, cantaloupe, eggplant, garlic, grapefruit, green leafy vegetables, melons, peas, prunes, raisins, squash, and sweet potatoes.

❑ Include fresh "live" juices in the diet. The following juices are healthful: beet, carrot and celery, currant, cranberry, citrus fruit, parsley, spinach, and watermelon.

❑ Eat grains like brown rice, buckwheat, millet, and oats.

❑ Drink steam-distilled water only.

❑ Take 2 tablespoons of flaxseed oil daily.

❑ Avoid all animal fats. Bacon, beef, bouillons, chicken liver, corned beef, dairy products, gravies, pork, sausage, and smoked or processed meats are prohibited. The only acceptable animal foods are broiled white fish and skinless turkey or chicken, and these should be consumed in moderation only. Get protein from vegetable sources, grains, and legumes instead.

❑ Avoid foods such as aged cheeses, aged meats, anchovies, avocados, chocolate, fava beans, pickled herring, sour cream, sherry, wine, and yogurt.

❑ Avoid all alcohol, caffeine, and tobacco.

❑ If you are taking an MAO inhibitor (one of a class of drugs prescribed to counter depression, lower blood pressure, and treat infections and cancer), avoid the chemical tyramine and its precursor, tyrosine. Combining MAO inhibitors with tyramine causes the blood pressure to soar and could cause a stroke. Tyramine-containing foods include almonds, avocados, bananas, beef or chicken liver, beer, cheese (including cottage cheese), chocolate, coffee, fava beans, herring, meat tenderizer, peanuts, pickles, pineapples, pumpkin seeds, raisins, sausage, sesame seeds, sour cream, soy sauce, wine, yeast extracts (including brewer's yeast), yogurt, and other foods. In general, any high-protein food that has undergone aging, pickling, fermentation, or similar processes should be avoided. Over-the-counter cold and allergy remedies should also be avoided.

❑ Keep your weight down. If you are overweight, take steps to lose the excess pounds. *See* OBESITY in Part Two.

❑ Fast for three to five days each month. Periodic cleansing fasts help to detoxify the body. *See* FASTING in Part Three.

❑ Get regular light to moderate exercise. Take care not to overexert yourself, especially in hot or humid weather.

Caution: Consult with your health care provider before beginning a new exercise regimen, particularly if you have been sedentary for some time.

❑ Be sure to get sufficient sleep.

❑ Have your blood pressure checked at least every four to six months. Because hypertension often shows no signs, regular blood pressure checks by a professional are important, especially if you are in a high-risk category.

❑ If you are pregnant, have your blood pressure monitored frequently by your health care provider. Untreated hypertension in pregnancy can progress suddenly and pose a serious threat to both mother and child.

❑ Do not take antihistamines except under a physician's direction.

❑ Do not take supplements containing the amino acids phenylalanine or or tyrosine. Also avoid the artificial sweetener aspartame (Equal, NutraSweet), which contains phenylalanine.

❑ As much as possible, avoid stress.

CONSIDERATIONS

❑ Because the use of diuretic drugs causes increased urinary excretion of magnesium, it can cause hypomagnesemia in elderly people. Magnesium is needed in conjunction with calcium to prevent bone deterioration, as well as to maintain a normal heart rhythm and muscular contraction. Losses of potassium due to diuretics may be dangerous, causing heart malfunction. Herbal diuretics are far safer. Consult your physician before using diuretics.

❑ People with hypertension often suffer from sleep apnea, in which they stop breathing for ten seconds or more throughout the night. Apnea is associated with loud snoring and restless sleep, and can cause the individual to feel excessively sleepy during the day. Evaluation and treatment of apnea may help reduce high blood pressure.

Some risks for hypertension cannot be changed—a family history of the disease, for instance. However, many risk factors can be avoided by making changes in diet and lifestyle.

According to the National Stroke Association, hypertension is the most important controllable risk factor for stroke, increasing the risk of stroke by seven times.

Approximately 80 million Americans have increased sensitivity to dietary sodium. African-Americans in particular are prone to salt-sensitive hypertension.

Research has revealed that people with variations in two specific genes are twice as likely to develop high blood pressure from salt consumption. This discovery may make it possible to identify children prone to high blood pressure; if such people can be identified in early childhood, it may be possible to modify their diets so that they can avoid developing high blood pressure later in life.

Heavy snorers are more likely to have high blood pressure or angina than silent sleepers. Research suggests that snorers may suffer from a malfunctioning of the part of the brain responsible for fluent breathing; this can put an unnatural strain on the heart and lungs due to oxygen shortage.

Researchers at the State University of New York found that the lower the level of magnesium in the body, the higher the blood pressure. This double-blind, placebo-controlled trial showed that taking supplemental magnesium can result in a significant, dose-dependent reduction in both systolic and diastolic blood pressure.

Apple pectin aids in reducing blood pressure.

A synthetic heart hormone that appears to be very effective in lowering blood pressure is currently undergoing testing at some twenty-five medical centers.

Certain colors have a beneficial effect on blood pressure (see COLOR THERAPY in Part Three). Music also can be used to reduce stress and thereby lower blood pressure. (See MUSIC AND SOUND THERAPY in Part Three.)

See also ARTERIOSCLEROSIS and CARDIOVASCULAR DISEASE in Part Two.

High Cholesterol

Elevated blood cholesterol and triglyceride levels lead to plaque-filled arteries, with impeded blood flow to the brain, kidneys, genitals, extremities, and heart. High cholesterol levels are among the primary causes of heart disease, because cholesterol produces fatty deposits in arteries. High cholesterol levels are also implicated in gallstones, impotence, mental impairment, and high blood pressure. Colon polyps and cancer (especially prostate and breast cancer) have also been linked to high serum cholesterol levels.

Cholesterol levels are greatly influenced by diet. The consumption of foods high in cholesterol and/or saturated fat increases cholesterol levels, while a vegetarian diet, regular exercise, and the nutrients niacin and vitamin C can lower cholesterol (see Understanding Cholesterol on page 326).

CHOLESTEROL LEVEL SELF-TEST

A test called the Advanced Care Cholesterol Kit, produced by Johnson & Johnson, can be used to check your cholesterol level at home. It is available in drugstores without a prescription, and it gives a cholesterol reading in fifteen minutes.

The test contains pads that are the size of a credit card and have a chemical reagent zone. When a drop of blood is placed on the surface of the pad, the reagents react with enzymes in the blood and the treated zone changes color. The color of the zone is then matched against a color-coded chart to find the serum cholesterol level.

If you have high cholesterol, follow the nutritional guidelines and recommendations in this section, and consult your health care provider.

NUTRIENTS

SUPPLEMENT	SUGGESTED DOSAGE	COMMENTS
Very Important		
Apple pectin	As directed on label.	Lowers cholesterol levels by binding fats and heavy metals.
Calcium	As directed on label.	To prevent hypocalcemia, or low calcium levels. Use calcium aspartate form.
Chromium picolinate	400-600 mcg daily.	Lowers total cholesterol levels and improves HDL-to-LDL ratio.
Coenzyme Q_{10}	60 mg daily.	Improves circulation.
Fiber (oat bran and guar gum are good sources)	As directed on label, ½ hour before the first meal of the day. Take separately from other supplements and medications.	Helps to lower cholesterol.
Garlic (Kyolic)	2 capsules 3 times daily.	Lowers cholesterol levels and blood pressure.
Lecithin granules or capsules	1 tbsp 3 times daily, before meals. 1,200 mg 3 times daily, before meals.	Lowers cholesterol. A fat emulsifier.
Lipotropic factors	As directed on label.	Substances that prevent fat deposits (as in atherosclerosis).
Vitamin B complex plus extra vitamin B_1 (thiamine) plus choline and inositol	As directed on label. As directed on label. 100–300 mg 5 times daily.	B vitamins work best when taken together. Important in controlling cholesterol levels. Important in fat metabolism. Protects the liver from fat deposits.
Vitamin B_3 (niacin)	300 mg daily. Do not exceed this amount.	Lowers cholesterol. Do not use a sustained-release formula, and do not substitute niacinamide for niacin. *Caution:* Do not take niacin if you have a liver disorder, gout, or high blood pressure.

Vitamin C with bioflavonoids	3,000–8,000 mg daily, in divided doses.	Lowers cholesterol.
Vitamin E emulsion	Begin with 200 IU daily and slowly increase dosage to 1,000 IU daily.	Improves circulation. The emulsion form offers rapid assimilation.

Helpful		
Essential fatty acids (black currant seed oil, borage oil, and primrose oil are good sources)	As directed on label. Take with vitamin E as recommended above.	Reduces LDL level and thins the blood.
Heart Science from Source Naturals	As directed on label.	Contains antioxidants to lower cholesterol, plus herbs, vitamins, and other nutrients that protect the heart and promote healthy cardiovascular function.
Proteolytic enzymes	As directed on label. Take with meals and between meals.	Aids digestion. *Caution:* Do not give this supplement to a child.
Selenium	200 mcg daily.	Deficiency has been linked to heart disease.
Shiitake or reishi	As directed on label. As directed on label.	Helps to control and lower cholesterol levels.

HERBS

❑ Cayenne (capsicum), goldenseal, and hawthorn berries help to lower cholesterol.

Caution: Do not take goldenseal internally on a daily basis for more than one week at a time, do not use it during pregnancy, and use with caution if you are allergic to ragweed.

RECOMMENDATIONS

❑ Include in the diet the following foods, which aid in lowering cholesterol: apples, bananas, carrots, cold-water fish, dried beans, garlic, grapefruit, and olive oil.

❑ Make sure to take in plenty of fiber in the form of fruits, vegetables, and whole grains. Water-soluble dietary fiber is very important in reducing serum cholesterol. It is found in barley, beans, brown rice, fruits, glucomannan, guar gum, and oats. Oat bran and brown rice bran are the best foods for lowering cholesterol. Whole-grain cereals (in moderation) and brown rice are good as well. Since fiber absorbs the minerals from the food it is in, take extra minerals separately from the fiber.

❑ Drink fresh juices, especially carrot, celery, and beet juices. Carrot juice helps to flush out fat from the bile in the liver and this helps lower cholesterol.

❑ Go on a monthly spirulina fast, with carrot and celery juice or lemon and steam-distilled water. *See* FASTING in Part Three.

❑ Use only unrefined cold- or expeller-pressed oils. Cold-pressed oils are those that have never been heated above 110°F during processing—at this temperature, enzyme destruction begins. Use vegetable oils that are liquid at room temperature, such as olive, soybean, flaxseed, primrose, and black currant seed oil. Olive oil is recommended.

❑ Do not eat any nuts except for walnuts, which can be eaten in moderation. Eat walnuts only if they are raw and have been kept tightly sealed or refrigerated; do not eat them if they have been roasted (or otherwise subjected to heat) or exposed to air (such as those found in open bins in shopping mall kiosks and candy stores).

❑ Reduce the amount of saturated fat and cholesterol in your diet. Saturated fats include all fats of animal origin as well as coconut and palm kernel oils. Eliminate from the diet all hydrogenated fats and hardened fats and oils such as margarine, lard, and butter. Consume no heated fats or processed oils, and avoid animal products (especially pork and pork products) and fried or fatty foods. Always read food product labels carefully. You may consume nonfat milk, low-fat cottage cheese, and skinless white poultry meat (preferably turkey), but only in moderation.

❑ Do not consume alcohol, cakes, candy, carbonated drinks, coffee, gravies, nondairy creamers, pies, processed or refined foods, refined carbohydrates, tea, tobacco, or white bread.

❑ Avoid gas-forming foods such as Brussels sprouts, cabbage, cauliflower, and sweet pickles.

❑ Get regular moderate exercise. Always consult with your health care provider before beginning any new exercise program.

❑ Try to avoid stress and sustained tension. Learn stress-management techniques. *See* STRESS in Part Two.

CONSIDERATIONS

❑ It is considered healthier to have a total cholesterol reading of less than 200, and the higher the HDL fraction, the better (*see* Understanding Cholesterol on page 326).

❑ Meat and dairy products are primary sources of dietary cholesterol. Vegetables and fruits are free of cholesterol.

❑ Many people use margarine or vegetable shortening as substitutes for butter because they contain no cholesterol. However, these products contain compounds called cis- and trans-fatty acids that become oxidized when exposed to heat and can clog the arteries. They have been linked to the formation of damaging free radicals.

❑ In large amounts, coffee can elevate blood cholesterol levels, more than doubling the risk of heart disease. According to a report published in *The New England Journal of Medicine*, observation of 15,000 coffee drinkers revealed that as the intake of coffee rises, the amount of cholesterol in the blood goes up.

❑ Cream substitutes (nondairy coffee creamers) are actually poor alternatives to cholesterol-heavy dairy products. Many contain coconut oil, which is a highly saturated fat. Soymilk or almond milk is preferable.

Understanding Cholesterol

Pick up just about any newspaper or magazine these days and you will probably find mention of cholesterol. Everyone seems to be concerned with lowering his or her cholesterol level, and most people would like to know how they can do this. It is first helpful to know how cholesterol is produced and used by the body.

Cholesterol is a crystalline substance that is technically classified as a steroid. However, because it is soluble in fats rather than in water, it is also classified as a lipid, as fats are. It is found naturally in the brain, nerves, liver, blood, and bile of both humans and vertebrate animals. This is why persons who wish to decrease their cholesterol levels are told to stay away from meat and other foods containing animal products or derived from animals.

Despite its current unsavory reputation, cholesterol is actually necessary for the proper functioning of the body. About 80 percent of total body cholesterol is manufactured in the liver, while 20 percent comes from dietary sources. It is used by cells to build membranes, and it is also used in sex hormones and in the digestive process. Cholesterol travels from the liver through the bloodstream to the various tissues of the body by means of a special class of protein molecules called *lipoproteins*. The cells take what they need, and any excess remains in the bloodstream until other lipoproteins pick it up for transport back to the liver.

There are two main types of lipoproteins: low-density lipoproteins (LDLs) and high-density lipoproteins (HDLs). LDLs are often referred to as "bad cholesterol"; HDLs as "good cholesterol." An analysis of the function of each will explain why. Low-density lipoproteins are heavily laden with cholesterol, because they are the molecules that transport cholesterol from the liver to all the cells of the body. High-density lipoproteins, on the other hand, carry relatively little cholesterol, and circulate in the bloodstream removing excess cholesterol from the blood and tissues. After HDLs travel through the bloodstream and collect the excess cholesterol, they return it to the liver, where it may once again be incorporated into LDLs for delivery to the cells. If everything is functioning as it should, this system remains in balance. However, if there is too much cholesterol for the HDLs to pick up promptly, or if there are not enough HDLs to do the job, cholesterol can form plaque that sticks to artery walls and may eventually cause heart disease.

The precise ways in which lipoproteins perform their functions are not known, nor is it known whether or how they work with other elements in the body. It *is* known that persons with high HDL levels and relatively low LDL levels have a lower risk of heart disease. In those who already have clogged arteries or have had a heart attack, an increase in HDL levels and a decrease in LDL levels can result in improvement of arterial obstruction.

The National Cholesterol Education Program has set the "safe" level of total serum cholesterol (including both LDL and HDL) at 200 milligrams per deciliter of blood (mg/dl). A reading above 200 indicates an increased potential for developing heart disease. A level of 200 to 239 is borderline, and those with levels over 240 are considered to be at high risk.

The normal HDL level for adult men in the United States is 45 to 50 mm/dl, and that for women is 50 to 60 mg/dl. It is suggested that higher levels, such as 70 or 80 mg/dl, may protect against heart disease. An HDL level under 35 mg/dl is considered risky. So if you have a cholesterol reading of 200, with HDL at 80 and LDL at 120, you are considered at low risk for heart disease. On the other hand, even if you have a total cholesterol level well under 200, if your HDL level is under 35, you would still be considered at increased risk of developing cardiovascular disease. In other words, as your HDL decreases, your potential for heart problems intensifies, even if your total is on the low side.

Because LDLs are so undesirable, it is imperative to realize the effect of diet on cholesterol levels. It is only logical that we should decrease our intake of animal products and therefore decrease our overall cholesterol levels. However, dietary cholesterol is only a part of the story. There are other substances that affect cholesterol levels. Saturated fats, for example, have been shown to increase cholesterol levels even more than dietary cholesterol does—so even if a food product label proclaims "No Cholesterol!" the product may still have a negative effect on your cholesterol level. There are other substances that raise cholesterol, too. Sugar and alcohol both raise the level of *natural* cholesterol (that which the body produces). Although we do need this substance, we do not need to overproduce it, which is what happens when we consume sugar and alcohol. Stress also results in an overproduction of natural cholesterol. Therefore, preventing (or fighting) heart disease requires a comprehensive approach that includes avoiding the consumption of animal products, saturated fats, sugar, and alcohol, and eliminating stress.

❑ The body does need some fats, but they must be the right kind. Good fats supply essential fatty acids, which are a very important link in our health chain. Fats supply energy, and they stay in the digestive tract for longer periods than proteins or carbohydrates, giving a feeling of fullness. They act as an intestinal lubricant, generate body heat, and carry the fat-soluble vitamins A, D, E, and K in the body. The protective myelin sheaths that protect nerve fibers are composed of fats. All cell membranes are composed of fats as well. Unfortunately, most Americans consume much too much of the wrong fats—that is, saturated, hydrogenated, and heated fats—which are linked to obesity, cardiovascular disease, and certain types of cancer.

❑ Human growth hormone therapy has been found to decrease cholesterol levels. (*See* GROWTH HORMONE THERAPY in Part Three.)

❑ Kombucha tea, which has energizing, detoxifying, and immune-boosting properties, may help to lower cholesterol levels. (*See* MAKING KOMBUCHA TEA in Part Three.)

❑ Many fast-food restaurants use beef tallow (fat) to make their hamburgers, fish, chicken, and French-fried potatoes. Not only do these fried foods contain high amounts of cholesterol, but this fat is subjected to high temperatures in the deep-frying process, resulting in oxidation and the formation of free radicals. Heating fat, especially frying food in fat, also produces toxic trans-fatty acids, which seem to behave much like saturated fats in clogging the arteries and raising blood cholesterol levels.

❑ Certain drugs can elevate cholesterol levels. These include steroids, oral contraceptives, furosemide (Lasix) and other diuretics, and levodopa (L-dopa, sold under the brand names Dopar, Larodopa, and Sinemet), which is used to treat Parkinson's disease. Beta-blockers, often prescribed to control high blood pressure, can cause unfavorable changes in the ratio of LDL to HDL in the blood.

❑ Some people claim that taking charcoal tablets lowers blood cholesterol. However, charcoal also absorbs good nutrients along with the cholesterol. Activated charcoal should not be consumed daily, and it should not be taken at the same time as other supplements or medications. Other "experts" recommend taking fish oil capsules to lower cholesterol, but fish oil is 100-percent fat, and the evidence is lacking that the ingestion of fish oil reduces serum fats.

❑ Pure virgin olive oil appears to help reduce serum cholesterol. A monounsaturated-fatty-acid-rich diet that includes olive oil may be the reason for the low serum cholesterol levels found in people living in Italy and Greece.

❑ Studies have shown that so-called Third World diets, which consist of grains, fruits, and vegetables, result in lower blood cholesterol levels. In the United States and northern Europe, where people consume large amounts of meat and dairy products, extremely high rates of heart and circulatory disease are present. Even children in these nations show signs of progressive vascular disease due to hypercholesterolemia (an excess of cholesterol in the blood).

❑ There are a number of cholesterol-lowering drugs on the market. Available by prescription only, these tend to be costly and they can have serious side effects. We believe that these drugs should be used only as a last resort. The sensible way to keep the serum fats within a safe range is to follow a diet that excludes animal fats (including meat, milk, and all dairy products) and includes ample amounts of fiber and bulk (whole grains, fruits, and vegetables).

❑ Some people have hereditary disorders that prevent even the healthiest diet from lowering LDL levels. For these people, researchers are working on a device that uses an enzyme to break down LDL and accelerate its removal before it can fasten onto artery walls to form plaque. The device would be implanted under the skin to control the LDL levels in the blood.

❑ *See also* ARTERIOSCLEROSIS in Part Two.

❑ *See also* CHELATION THERAPY in Part Three.

HIV (Human Immunodeficiency Virus)

See AIDS.

Hives

Hives, called *urticaria* by the medical profession, is a skin condition that is characterized by sudden outbreaks of red, itchy welts on the skin. Any area of the body may be affected. The welts may vary in appearance, from tiny, goosebump-like spots to rashes that cover significant areas of the body.

Many cases of hives are brought on as allergic reactions and coincide with the release of histamine in the body. The release of histamine into the skin produces an inflammatory reaction, with itching, swelling, and redness. Hives can cause significant discomfort, but it does not cause injury or damage to any vital organs.

The skin is the largest organ of the body. It is an important part of the excretory system. The skin acts in conjunction with other systems in our body to remove toxins and waste. Hives can be a natural reaction to the presence of a foreign substance in the body. However, an offending substance need not enter the body to trigger an outbreak of hives. Merely coming into contact with various substances, such as pesticides, soaps, shampoos, hair sprays, residues from laundry products or dry cleaning chemicals on clothing, or any other of a vast array of other seemingly innocuous household items can unleash a maddening attack of hives.

The severity of a hives outbreak can vary from case to case as well as from person to person. Some people can break out in hives if they merely touch a certain type of plant or bush; others may develop hives only with considerable exposure, such as overconsumption of a certain food. Chemicals are a major cause of hives for many people; anything from perfumes to household cleaners can trigger a reaction, as can nervous conditions, stress, certain foods, and alcohol.

Viruses also can cause hives. Hepatitis B and Epstein-Barr virus, the virus that causes infectious mononucleosis, are the two most common culprits. Some bacterial infections likewise can cause outbreaks of hives, both chronic and acute. An association between *Candida albicans* and chronic hives has been established in several clinical studies over the past twenty years.

Antibiotics such as penicillin and related compounds are the most common cause of drug-induced hives. At least 10 percent of the American population is thought to be allergic to penicillin. Nearly one quarter of those people will develop hives, angioedema (a condition that is similar to hives but affects deeper layers of the skin and causes larger wheals), or anaphylaxis (a systemic allergic reaction causing generalized itching and difficulty breathing) if they ingest penicillin.

The following are some of the drugs and other substances that most commonly cause outbreaks of hives in susceptible people. This list is not exhaustive, and we do not mean to imply that these items *will* cause a hives outbreak, only that they at least contribute to the condition in some people:

- *Aspirin.*
- *Allopurinol* (Zyloprim), a gout medication.
- *Antimony,* a metallic element that is present in various metal alloys.
- *Antipyrine,* an agent used to relieve pain and inflammation.
- *Barbiturates.*
- *BHA and BHT,* preservatives used in many food products.
- *Bismuth,* another metallic element present in certain metal alloys.
- *Chloral hydrate,* a sedative used in the treatment of tetany.
- *Chlorpromazine* (Thorazine), a tranquilizer and antiemetic.
- *Corticotropin* (also known as adrenocorticotropic hormone, or ACTH, and sold for medicinal purposes under the brand names Acthar and Cortrosyn).
- *Eucalyptus,* a tree whose leaves yield an aromatic oil that is used in cough remedies and other medicines.
- *Fluorides,* which are found in certain dental care products and in fluoridated drinking water.
- *Food colorings.*
- *Gold.*

- *Griseofulvin* (Fulvicin, Grisactin, and others), an antifungal medication.
- *Insulin.*
- *Iodines,* used in certain antiseptics and dyes.
- *Liver extract.*
- *Menthol,* an extract of peppermint oil used in perfumes, as a mild anesthetic, and as a mint flavoring in candy and cigarettes.
- *Meprobamate* (Miltown, Equanil, Meprospan), a tranquilizer.
- *Mercury,* a toxic metallic element found in dental fillings, certain antacids, and some first-aid preparations, among other things.
- *Morphine.*
- *Opium.*
- *Para-aminosalicylic acid,* an anti-inflammatory drug.
- *Penicillin.*
- *Phenacetin,* an ingredient in some pain medications.
- *Phenobarbital,* a sedative and anticonvulsant.
- *Pilocarpine,* a glaucoma medication.
- *Poliomyelitis vaccine.*
- *Potassium sulfocyanate,* a preservative.

- *Preservatives.*
- *Procaine* (Novocain), an anesthetic.
- *Promethazine* (Phenergan), an antihistamine, sedative, and antiemetic.
- *Quinine,* used in quinine water and antimalaria medications.
- *Reserpine,* a heart medication.
- *Saccharin,* an artificial sweetener found in Sweet'n Low, many

toothpastes, and many dietetic and "sugarless" products.
- *Salicylates,* chemicals used as food flavorings and preservatives.
- *Sulfites,* chemicals used as food preservatives and in the production of dried fruits such as raisins.
- *Tartrazine,* a food dye and an ingredient in Alka-Seltzer.
- *Thiamine hydrochloride,* an ingredient in some cough medicines.

Other hives-provoking substances are being identified with increasing frequency. Meat, dairy, and poultry products, especially in frozen or fast foods, are increasingly being associated with hives, probably because many farmers and ranchers routinely give their livestock antibiotics in an effort to prevent disease or infection. These antibiotics are not affected by any subsequent amount of freezing, processing, or cooking. Allergic reactions have been traced to antibiotics in milk, soft drinks, and even frozen dinners.

NUTRIENTS

SUPPLEMENT	SUGGESTED DOSAGE	COMMENTS
Helpful		
Acidophilus	As directed on label. Take on an empty stomach.	Reduces allergic reactions and helps replenish "friendly" bacteria. Use nondairy formula.
Garlic (Kyolic)	10 drops of oil in water 3 times daily.	Aids in destroying bacteria.
Herpanacine from Diamond-Herpanacine Associates	As directed on label.	A nutrient and herb combination that supports overall skin health.
Multivitamin and mineral complex	As directed on label.	To correct any nutrient or mineral deficiencies that may be contributing to outbreaks.
Quercetin	As directed on label.	Reduces inflammation and reactions to substances that may cause hives.
or AntiAllergy formula from Freeda Vitamins	As directed on label.	A combination of quercetin, calcium pantothenate, and calcium ascorbate.
Vitamin B complex	As directed on label, with meals.	Needed for the functioning of the nervous system and for healthy skin.
plus extra vitamin B12	2,000 mcg daily.	Prevents nerve damage and promotes normal growth of the skin. Use a lozenge or sublingual form.
Vitamin C	1,000 mg 3 times daily.	Enhances immune response; acts as an anti-inflammatory.

Vitamin D	400 IU daily.	To reduce outbreaks.
Vitamin E	600 IU daily.	A powerful antioxidant that improves circulation to the skin tissues.
and		
zinc	50 mg daily. Do not exceed a total of 100 mg daily from all supplements.	Promotes a healthy immune system and healing of skin tissues. Needed for proper concentrations of vitamin E in the blood. Use zinc gluconate lozenges or OptiZinc for best absorption.

HERBS

❑ Alfalfa, cat's claw, chamomile, echinacea, ginseng, licorice, nettle, sarsaparilla, and yellow dock are all beneficial to the hives sufferer. Alfalfa can also be used as a preventive blood tonic. It cleanses the blood and helps keep the body free of toxins.

Caution: Do not use chamomile on an ongoing basis, and avoid it completely if you are allergic to ragweed. Do not use ginseng or licorice if you have high blood pressure.

❑ Applying aloe vera gel to the affected area can be helpful.

❑ Black nightshade leaves may help. Wash and boil the leaves in water, put them on a cloth, and apply as a poultice to the affected area. *See* USING A POULTICE in Part Three.

Caution: Do not take this herb internally, and avoid getting it in your eyes.

❑ The leaves and the bark of the red alder tree, when brewed into a strong tea, can help hives. Apply it locally to the affected area, and take a couple of tablespoons internally as well. Reapply several times daily until the hives abate. Red alder contains the astringent tannin.

RECOMMENDATIONS

❑ Avoid alcohol and all processed foods, which put added stress on the body by depleting nutrients. Also avoid dairy products, eggs, chicken, and nuts. Especially avoid foods high in saturated fats, cholesterol, and sugar.

❑ Try to identify the item or substance that caused the condition. Avoid anything you suspect may be causing outbreaks of hives.

❑ For the typical case of hives, avoid using prednisone or other steroids. Instead, use the nutrients and herbs listed above. Try nettle first.

❑ For topical treatment, use cornstarch or colloidal oatmeal added to bath water. A good oatmeal product for this purpose is Aveeno Bath Treatment, available at drugstores. Bathing in cool water with baking soda added also may relieve symptoms.

❑ If you have had hives for longer than six weeks, or if you are developing an acute case of hives, consult your health care provider.

❑ If hives develop in your mouth or throat, and especially if it causes swelling around the throat or interferes with swallowing or breathing *to any extent at all,* seek medical help immediately. Go to the emergency room of the nearest hospital or call for emergency assistance. Hives can signal or accompany the onset of anaphylaxis, a dangerous allergic reaction that can block the breathing passages. The possibility of anaphylaxis is what makes allergies to insect stings, such as those from bees, a potentially serious concern. If you have ever had this type of reaction, you should be under a physician's care and have an epinephrine injection kit on hand. Make sure you know how to use it, and keep the kit with you at all times.

CONSIDERATIONS

❑ Many people who suffer acute attacks find at least temporary relief from the symptoms of hives by taking antihistamines. Chronic sufferers have less success with this approach, as antihistamines are suppressive agents and may actually contribute to the persistence of hives.

❑ If a hives outbreak is the result of a food or drug that you have ingested, you obviously do not want that substance in your body again. If you cannot isolate whatever food or drug it might be that causes hives, having a physician do some blood work to find the allergen may be your only solution, even though this approach can be relatively expensive.

❑ Occasionally, hives can persist for weeks or even months, resisting all attempts at treatment. For this reason alone, it is best to learn what the cause of the outbreak is in order to avoid it. If you suffer from chronic hives and cannot isolate the cause, eliminating all the possible allergens from your home may be your only resort. This can be a long, drawn-out, and painstaking process. (*See* ALLERGIES in Part Two.)

❑ Chronic hives may be linked to *Candida albicans.* If you suspect this may be the cause of hives, adopting a yeast-free diet can be of some benefit. (*See* CANDIDIASIS in Part Two.)

❑ An elimination diet is important. (*See* ALLERGIES in Part Two.)

Hot Flashes

See under MENOPAUSE-RELATED PROBLEMS.

Human Immunodeficiency Virus (HIV)

See AIDS.

Hyperactivity

Hyperactivity, medically termed *attention deficit hyperactivity disorder (ADHD)*, is a disorder of certain mechanisms in the central nervous system. It primarily affects children and causes a variety of learning and behavior problems. Factors linked to hyperactivity include heredity, smoking during pregnancy, oxygen deprivation at birth, environmental pollutants, artificial food additives, lead poisoning, allergies, and prenatal trauma. Preservatives and foods containing salicylates also contribute to this disorder. A low-protein diet may be a contributing factor. Though the topic has been hotly debated for decades, studies have definitively shown that food additives do play a major role in hyperactivity.

Hyperactivity may be characterized by one or a combination of some the following:

- Head-knocking.
- Lack of concentration.
- A tendency to disturb other children.
- Self-destructive behavior.
- Emotional instability; daily or hourly mood swings.
- Disorders of speech and hearing.
- Temper tantrums.
- Impatience; difficulty waiting.
- Extreme distractibility.
- Forgetfulness.
- Absentmindedness.

- Inability to finish tasks.
- Difficulty solving problems or managing time.
- Low tolerance for stress and otherwise ordinary problems.
- Learning disabilities.
- A tendency to become frustrated quickly.
- An inability to sit still for any length of time, even at mealtimes.
- Clumsiness.
- Sleep disturbances.
- Failure in school despite average or above-average intelligence.

Not all symptoms are present in any one individual. Although hyperactivity is primarily a problem of childhood, adults can be affected, too.

Unless otherwise specified, the dosages recommended here are for adults. For a child between the ages of twelve and seventeen, reduce the dose to three-quarters the recommended amount. For a child between six and twelve, use one-half the recommended dose, and for a child under the age of six, use one-quarter the recommended amount.

NUTRIENTS

SUPPLEMENT	SUGGESTED DOSAGE	COMMENTS
Very Important		
Quercetin	As directed on label.	Prevents allergies from aggravating symptoms.
Calcium and magnesium	As directed on label, at bedtime.	Has a calming effect.
Gamma-aminobutyric acid (GABA)	750 mg daily.	Calms the body much in the same way as some tranquilizers, without side effects or danger of addiction. *See* AMINO ACIDS in Part One.
Vitamin B complex	50 mg 3 times daily.	B vitamins are needed for correct brain function and digestion. Also enhance adrenal gland function.
plus extra vitamin B₃ (niacin)	100 mg daily. Do not exceed a total of 300 mg daily from all supplements.	*Caution:* Do not take niacin if you have a liver disorder, gout, or high blood pressure.
and pantothenic acid (vitamin B₅)	100 mg daily.	The anti-stress vitamin.
and vitamin B₆ (pyridoxine)	50 mg daily.	Important for proper brain function.
Helpful		
Bio-Strath from Bioforce	As directed on label.	Contains yeast, herbs, and all B vitamins that have a calming effect.
Brewer's yeast	Start with ¼ tsp daily and slowly increase to the dose recommended on the label.	A natural source of the B vitamins.
L-Cysteine	As directed on label, on an empty stomach. Take with water or juice. Do not take with milk. Take with 50 mg vitamin B₆ and 100 mg vitamin C for better absorption.	Take this amino acid if a hair analysis reveals high levels of metals. *See* AMINO ACIDS in Part One.
Multivitamin and mineral complex	As directed on label.	High amounts of all nutrients are needed.
Taurine Plus from American Biologics	As directed on label.	The most important antioxidant and immune regulator, necessary for white blood cell activation and neurological function.
Vitamin C	1,000 mg 3 times daily.	An anti-stress vitamin.

HERBS

❑ Valerian root extract has been used for this disorder with dramatic results and no side effects. Mix the extract in juice (as directed on the product label according to age) and drink the mixture two to three times a day.

❑ Other herbs that may be beneficial for hyperactivity include catnip, chamomile, hops, lobelia, passionflower, skullcap, thyme, and wood betony.

Caution: Do not use chamomile or lobelia on an ongoing basis. Avoid chamomile completely if you are allergic to ragweed.

RECOMMENDATIONS

❑ Include in the diet all fruits and vegetables (except for those containing salicylates, listed below), plus breads, cereals, and crackers that contain only rice and oats.

❑ Remove from the diet all forms of refined sugar and any products that contain it. Also eliminate all foods that contain artificial colors, flavorings, or preservatives; processed and manufactured foods; and foods that contain salicylates. Certain foods naturally contain salicylates. These include almonds, apples, apricots, cherries, currants, all berries, peaches, plums, prunes, tomatoes, cucumbers, and oranges.

❑ Do not consume any of the following: apple cider vinegar, bacon, butter, candy, catsup, chocolate, colored cheeses, chili sauce, corn, ham, hot dogs, luncheon meat, margarine, meat loaf, milk, mustard, pork, salami, salt, soft drinks, soy sauce, sausage, tea, and wheat. Do not use antacid tablets, cough drops, perfume, throat lozenges, or commercial toothpaste. Use a natural toothpaste from a health food store instead.

❑ Avoid carbonated beverages, which contain large amounts of phosphates. Phosphate additives may be responsible for hyperkinesis (exaggerated muscle activity). High levels of phosphorus and very low calcium and magnesium levels (which can be revealed through a hair analysis) can indicate a potential for hyperactivity and seizures. Meat and fat also are high in phosphorus.

❑ Use an elimination diet to identify foods that may be causing or aggravating symptoms. *See* ALLERGIES in Part Two.

CONSIDERATIONS

❑ A hair analysis to rule out heavy metal intoxication is important. Lead and copper have both been linked to behavioral problems. (*See* HAIR ANALYSIS in Part Three.)

❑ A strong link has been established between learning disabilities and juvenile crime.

❑ Researchers who performed five-hour oral glucose tolerance tests on 261 hyperactive children found that 74 percent displayed abnormal glucose tolerance curves, suggesting a connection between hyperactive behavior and the consumption of sugar.

❑ Studies indicate that administration of gamma-aminobutyric acid (GABA) decreases hyperactivity, as well as tendencies toward violence, epilepsy, mental retardation, and learning disabilities.

❑ You can ask your health care provider to help you find a professional who specializes in treating people with attention deficit disorders, or seek a referral through one of the following groups:

Attention Deficit Disorder Association (ADDA)
PO Box 972
Mentor, OH 44061
800–487–2282

Children With Attention-Deficit Disorders (CHADD)
499 Northwest 70th Avenue
Suite 101
Plantation, FL 33317
305–587–3700

Learning Disabilities Association of America (LDA)
4156 Library Road
Pittsburgh, PA 15234
412–341–1515

For a list of attention disorder support groups in your area, you can write to the following address:

Public Relations Pharmaceuticals Division
CIBA-Geigy Corporation
556 Morris Avenue
Summit, NJ 07901
908–277–7082

Hypertension

See HIGH BLOOD PRESSURE.

Hyperthyroidism

This disorder occurs when the thyroid gland produces too much thyroid hormone, resulting in an overactive metabolic state. All of the body's processes speed up with this disorder. Symptoms of hyperthyroidism include nervousness, irritability, a constant feeling of being hot, increased perspiration, insomnia and fatigue, increased frequency of bowel movements, less frequent menstruation and decreased menstrual flow, weakness, hair and weight loss, change in skin thickness, separation of the nails from the nail bed, hand tremors, intolerance of heat, rapid heartbeat, goiter, and, sometimes, protruding eyeballs. Hyperthyroidism is sometimes also called *thyrotoxicosis*. The most common type of this disorder is *Graves' disease*, which affects about 2.5 million Americans.

The thyroid gland is the body's internal thermostat. It regulates the temperature by secreting two hormones that control how quickly the body burns calories and uses energy. If the thyroid secretes too much hormone, hyperthyroidism results; too little hormone results in hypothyroidism. Many cases of hypothyroidism and hyperthyroidism are believed to result from an abnormal immune response. The exact cause is not understood, but the immune system can produce antibodies that invade and attack the thyroid, disrupting hormone production. Hyperthyroidism can also be caused by lumps or tumors that form on the thyroid and disrupt hormone production. Infection or inflammation of the thyroid can cause temporary hyperthyroidism, as can certain prescription drugs.

Hyperthyroidism is not as common as hypothyroidism. Both of these thyroid disorders affect women more often than men. A malfunctioning thyroid can be the underlying cause of many recurring illnesses.

NUTRIENTS

SUPPLEMENT	SUGGESTED DOSAGE	COMMENTS
Very Important		
Multivitamin and mineral complex	As directed on label.	Increased amounts of vitamins and minerals are needed for this "hyper" metabolic condition. Use a super-high-potency formula.
Vitamin B complex	50 mg 3 times daily, with meals.	Needed for thyroid function. Injections (under a doctor's supervision) may be necessary.
plus extra vitamin B$_1$ (thiamine) and	50 mg twice daily.	Needed for blood formation and energy levels.
vitamin B$_2$ (riboflavin) and	50 mg twice daily.	Required for normal functioning of all cells, glands, and organs in the body.
vitamin B$_6$ (pyridoxine)	50 mg twice daily.	Activates many enzymes and is needed for immune function and antibody production.
Helpful		
Brewer's yeast	1–3 tbsp daily and up.	Rich in many basic nutrients, especially the B vitamins.
Essential fatty acids	As directed on label.	Needed for correct glandular function.
Lecithin granules or capsules	1 tbsp 3 times daily, before meals. 1,200 mg 3 times daily, before meals.	Aids in digestion of fats and protects the lining of all cells and organs.
Vitamin C	3,000–5,000 mg daily and up.	Especially important in this stressful condition.
Vitamin E	400 IU daily. Do not exceed this amount.	An antioxidant and necessary nutrient. However, excessive amounts may stimulate the thyroid gland.

RECOMMENDATIONS

❑ Eat plenty of the following foods: broccoli, Brussels sprouts, cabbage, cauliflower, kale, mustard greens, peaches, pears, rutabagas, soybeans, spinach, and turnips. These help to suppress thyroid hormone production.

❑ Avoid dairy products for at least three months. Also avoid stimulants, coffee, tea, nicotine, and soft drinks.

❑ Be wary of treatment with radioactive sodium iodine (iodine 131, or I-131), which is often recommended for this condition. Severe side effects have been known to accompany the use of I-131. Also, do not rush into surgery. Try improving your diet first.

CONSIDERATIONS

❑ Along with other bodily processes, digestion speeds up with this disorder. Malabsorption occurs, so a proper diet is important.

❑ Researchers in England studied ten people who were being treated for Parkinson's disease and found that all of them also had hyperthyroidism. Once the thyroid condition was treated, the Parkinson's disease improved dramatically.

❑ If a goiter affects breathing or swallowing, surgery may be needed to remove part or all of the thyroid. It may be necessary to take thyroid hormone pills after surgery.

❑ The pituitary gland, parathyroid glands, and sex glands all work together and are influenced by thyroid function. If there is a problem in one place, they all may be affected.

Hypoglycemia (Low Blood Sugar)

Hypoglycemia is a condition in which there is an abnormally low level of glucose (sugar) in the blood. Most often, this results from the oversecretion of insulin by the pancreas. Insulin facilitates the transport of glucose from the bloodstream into the cells, especially those of muscle and fatty tissue, and causes glucose to be synthesized in the liver. If the pancreas is not functioning properly, normal carbohydrate metabolism is impossible.

A person suffering from hypoglycemia may display any or all of the following symptoms: fatigue, dizziness, lightheadedness, headache, irritability, fainting spells, depression, anxiety, cravings for sweets, confusion, night sweats, weakness in the legs, swollen feet, a feeling of tightness in chest, constant hunger, pain in various parts of the body (especially the eyes), nervous habits, mental disturbances, and insomnia. People with hypoglycemia can become very aggressive and lose their tempers easily. Any or all of these symptoms may occur a few hours after eating sweets or fats. The onset and severity of symptoms are directly related to the length of time since the last meal was eaten and the type of foods that meal contained.

More and more Americans today may have this condition, due to poor dietary habits that include eating large quantities of simple carbohydrates, sugars, alcohol, caffeine, and soft drinks, and insufficient amounts of complex carbohydrates. High stress levels are believed to be a contributing factor in the increasing incidence of hypoglycemia.

Hypoglycemia can be inherited, but most often it is precipitated by an inadequate diet. This is referred to as *functional hypoglycemia (FH)*. Many other bodily disorders can cause hypoglycemic problems as well, among them adrenal insufficiency, thyroid disorders, pituitary disorders, kidney disease, and pancreatitis. Immune deficiency and candidiasis are strongly linked to hypoglycemia. Glucose intolerance and hyperinsulinemia (high blood insulin levels), producing hypoglycemia, frequently occur in people with chronic liver failure. Other common causes are smoking and the consumption of large amounts of caffeine, found in colas, chocolate, and coffee. Though it may seem paradoxical, low blood sugar can also be an early sign of diabetes (high blood sugar).

Diagnosis of hypoglycemia can be difficult because the

symptoms often mimic those of other disorders, including allergies, asthma, chronic fatigue syndrome, digestive or intestinal disorders, eating disorders, malabsorption syndrome, mental disorders, neurological problems, nutritional deficiencies, and weight problems. To diagnose hypoglycemia, a health care provider may perform a glucose tolerance test (GTT). However, many people have symptoms of hypoglycemia even though the results of a five-hour GTT are within normal limits. A useful diagnostic test may be to follow the dietary and nutritional supplement regimen outlined in this section and see if symptoms improve.

NUTRIENTS

SUPPLEMENT	SUGGESTED DOSAGE	COMMENTS
Very Important		
Brewer's yeast	As directed on label.	Aids in stabilizing blood sugar levels.
Chromium picolinate	300–600 mcg daily.	Vital in glucose metabolism. Essential for optimal insulin activity.
Pancreatin	As directed on label. Take with meals.	For proper protein digestion. Use a high-potency formula.
Proteolytic enzymes	As directed on label. Take between meals.	People with this disorder often fail to digest protein properly, resulting in "leaky gut syndrome" and allergies. *Caution:* Do not give this supplement to a child.
Vitamin B complex	50–100 mg daily and up.	Important in carbohydrate and protein metabolism, and proper digestion and absorption of foods; helps the body tolerate foods that produce low blood sugar reactions. Also helps counteract the effects of malabsorption disorders, common in people with hypoglycemia.
plus extra vitamin B$_1$ (thiamine)	100 mg daily.	Aids in the production of hydrochloric acid, needed for proper digestion.
and vitamin B$_3$ (niacin)	100 mg daily. Do not exceed this amount.	Aids in the functioning of the nervous system and in proper digestion. *Caution:* Do not take niacin if you have a liver disorder, gout, or high blood pressure.
and pantothenic acid (vitamin B$_5$)	1,000 mg daily, in divided doses.	Important in adrenal gland function and conversion of glucose to energy.
and vitamin B$_{12}$	300 mcg twice daily, on an empty stomach.	Crucial for prevention of anemia, common because malabsorption disorders result in deficiency.
Zinc	50 mg daily. Do not exceed a total of 100 mg daily from all supplements.	Needed for proper release of insulin. People with hypoglycemia are often zinc deficient. Use zinc gluconate lozenges or OptiZinc for best absorption.
Important		
Vitamin E	400 IU and up.	Improves energy and circulation.
Magnesium plus	750 mg daily, in divided doses, after meals and at bedtime.	Important in carbohydrate (sugar) metabolism.
calcium	1,500 mg daily, in divided doses, after meals and at bedtime.	Works with magnesium and aids in preventing colon cancer.
L-Carnitine plus	As directed on label.	Converts stored body fat into energy.
L-cysteine and	As directed on label.	Blocks the action of insulin, which lowers blood sugar.
L-glutamine	1,000 mg daily, on an empty stomach. Take with water or juice. Do not take with milk. Take with 50 mg vitamin B$_6$ and 100 mg vitamin C for better absorption.	Reduces cravings for sugar.
Manganese	As directed on label. Take separately from calcium.	Important for the maintenance of blood glucose levels. Most people with hypoglycemia have low levels of this trace mineral in their blood.
Vitamin C with bioflavonoids	3,000–8,000 mg daily, in divided doses.	For adrenal insufficiency, common in people with hypoglycemia.
Helpful		
Aerobic Bulk Cleanse (ABC) from Aerobic Life Industries or psyllium husks	As directed on label. Take with aloe vera juice on an empty stomach in the morning. Take separately from other supplements and medications.	Aids in slowing down blood sugar reactions and keeping the colon clean.
Liver extract injections or desiccated liver	1 cc twice weekly for 3 months, then once weekly for 2 months or more, or as prescribed by physician. As directed on label.	Liver glandulars supply B vitamins and other valuable nutrients.
Multivitamin and mineral complex	As directed on label.	All nutrients are required for healing.

HERBS

❑ Bilberry and wild yam aid in controlling insulin levels.

❑ Dandelion root is an excellent source of calcium and supports the pancreas and liver.

❑ Licorice nourishes the adrenal glands.
   Caution: Do not use this herb on a daily basis for more than seven days in a row. Avoid if you have high blood pressure.

❑ Milk thistle rejuvenates the liver.

RECOMMENDATIONS

❑ Remove from the diet all alcohol, canned and packaged foods, refined and processed foods, salt, sugar, saturated fats, soft drinks, and white flour. Also avoid foods that contain artificial colors or preservatives.

❑ Avoid sweet fruits and juices such as grape and prune. If you drink these, mix the juice with equal amount of water.

❑ Eat a diet high in fiber and include large amounts of vegetables, especially broccoli, carrots, Jerusalem artichokes, raw spinach, squash, and string beans. Vegetables should be eaten raw or steamed. Also eat beans, brown rice, lentils, potatoes, soy products (tofu), and fruits, especially apples, apricots, avocados, bananas, cantaloupes, grapefruits, lemons, and persimmons.

❑ For protein, eat low-fat cottage cheese, fish, grains, kefir, raw cheese, raw nuts, seeds, skinless white turkey or white chicken breast, and low-fat yogurt.

❑ Eat starchy foods such as corn, hominy, noodles, pasta, white rice, and yams in moderation only.

❑ Do not eat fatty foods such as bacon, cold cuts, fried foods, gravies, ham, sausage, or dairy products (except for low-fat soured products).

❑ Do not go without food. Eat six to eight small meals throughout the day. Some people find that eating a small snack before bedtime helps.

❑ Use a rotation diet; food allergies are often linked to hypoglycemia and can make the symptoms more pronounced. See ALLERGIES in Part Two.

❑ Try taking 200 micrograms of chromium picolinate daily. This can alleviate many symptoms and raise blood glucose levels if symptoms occur after sugar or a heavy meal is consumed. Chromium, also known as glucose tolerance factor or GTF, has been known to alleviate sudden shock.

❑ During a low blood sugar reaction, eat something that combines fiber with a protein food, such as bran or rice crackers with raw cheese or almond butter.

❑ Instead of eating applesauce, have a whole apple, which has more fiber. The fiber in the apple will inhibit fluctuations in blood sugar. Fiber alone (found in popcorn, oat bran, rice bran, crackers, ground flaxseed, and psyllium husks) will slow down a hypoglycemic reaction. Take fiber half an hour before meals. Spirulina tablets taken between meals further help to stabilize blood sugar.

❑ Fast once a month with live vegetable juices and a series of lemon juice enemas. See FASTING and ENEMAS in Part Three. To prevent a low blood sugar reaction while fasting, use spirulina or a protein powder supplement. Many people find this makes them start to feel better very quickly.

CONSIDERATIONS

❑ Avocados contain a seven-carbon sugar that depresses insulin production, which make them an excellent choice for people with hypoglycemia.

❑ The production of insulin is affected by the functioning of the adrenal glands. The adrenal glands produce epinephrine, which acts to "turn off" insulin production, among other things. If the adrenal glands are overstressed and exhausted, they cannot function properly and an overabundance of insulin may result. This causes the blood sugar level to sink below normal, creating a low energy syndrome in the body.

❑ Injections of vitamin B complex plus extra vitamin B$_6$ (pyridoxine) and liver extract have produced good results for those with hypoglycemia. Liver extract supplements contain a nutritional substance that aids liver regeneration. Only liver from organically raised beef should be used.

❑ It is estimated that half the people with hypoglycemia who are over fifty have reduced thyroid function and hypothyroidism. (See HYPOTHYROIDISM in Part Two.)

❑ Caffeine, alcohol, and tobacco cause profound swings in blood sugar levels. Insomnia can result if any type of sugar is consumed after dinner. Consuming sugar at any time tends to cause drowsiness and fatigue.

❑ Some studies have shown that reducing the amount of meat protein in the diet and adding some starches, such as potatoes, may be beneficial.

❑ Kombucha tea may help to normalize blood sugar. (See MAKING KOMBUCHA TEA in Part Three.)

❑ Milk allergy is common as this disorder progresses. Allergy testing is recommended. (See ALLERGIES in Part Two.)

Hypothyroidism

Hypothyroidism is caused by an underproduction of thyroid hormone. Symptoms include fatigue, loss of appetite, inability to tolerate cold, a slow heart rate, weight gain, painful premenstrual periods, a milky discharge from the breasts, fertility problems, muscle weakness, muscle cramps, dry and scaly skin, a yellow-orange coloration in the skin (particularly on the palms of the hands), yellow bumps on the eyelids, hair loss (including the eyebrows), recurrent infections, constipation, depression, difficulty concentrating, slow speech, goiter, and drooping, swollen eyes. The most common symptoms are fatigue and intolerance to cold. If you consistently feel cold while others around you are hot, you may be suffering from reduced thyroid function.

The thyroid gland is the body's internal thermostat, regulating the temperature by secreting two hormones that control how quickly the body burns calories and uses energy. If the thyroid secretes too much hormone, hyperthyroidism results; too little hormone results in hypothyroidism. Hypothyroidism affects about 5 million people in the U.S., about 90 percent of which are women. Thyroid problems can cause many recurring illnesses and fatigue.

A condition called *Hashimoto's disease* is believed to be the most common cause of underactive thyroid. In this disorder, the body in effect becomes allergic to thyroid hormone. Hashimoto's disease is a common cause of goiter, a swelling of the thyroid gland, among adults.

Measuring levels of different hormones in the blood can determine if the thyroid gland is working properly. A physician may order a blood test to measure levels of thyroid hormone or thyroid-stimulating hormone (TSH). This hormone is secreted by the pituitary gland and in turn helps regulate thyroid hormone production. Even a minuscule drop in thyroid function registers as a distinctly elevated TSH level. Most endocrinologists believe that TSH levels rise when a person is in the earliest stages of thyroid failure.

An iodine absorption test may also be performed. This test involves ingesting a small amount of radioactive iodine. An x-ray then shows how much of the iodine was absorbed by the thyroid. A low uptake of the iodine may indicate hypothyroidism.

THYROID SELF-TEST

To test yourself for an underactive thyroid, keep a thermometer by your bed at night. When you awaken in the morning, place the thermometer under your arm and hold it there for fifteen minutes. Keep still and quiet. Any motion can upset your temperature reading. A temperature of 97.6°F or lower may indicate an underactive thyroid. Keep a temperature log for five days. If your readings are consistently low, consult your health care provider.

NUTRIENTS

SUPPLEMENT	SUGGESTED DOSAGE	COMMENTS
Essential		
Kelp	2,000–3,000 mg daily.	Contains iodine, the basic substance of thyroid hormone.
L-Tyrosine	500 mg twice daily, on an empty stomach. Take with water or juice. Do not take with milk. Take with 50 mg vitamin B$_6$ and 100 mg vitamin C for better absorption.	Low plasma levels have been associated with hypothyroidism. *See* AMINO ACIDS in Part One.
Very Important		
Raw thyroid glandular	As prescribed by physician.	To replace deficient thyroid hormone (*see* GLANDULAR THERAPY in Part Three). Natural thyroid extract such as Armour Thyroid Tablets is best. Available by prescription only.
Important		
Vitamin B complex plus extra vitamin B$_2$ (riboflavin) and vitamin B$_{12}$	100 mg 3 times daily, with meals. 50 mg twice daily. 15 mg 3 times daily, on an empty stomach.	B vitamins improve cellular oxygenation and energy and are needed for proper digestion, immune function, red blood cell formation, and thyroid function. Use a lozenge or sublingual form for best absorption.
Helpful		
Brewer's yeast	As directed on label.	Rich in basic nutrients, especially B vitamins.
Essential fatty acids	As directed on label.	Necessary for proper functioning of the thyroid gland.
Iron	As directed by physician. Take with 100 mg vitamin C for better absorption.	Essential for enzyme and hemoglobin production. Use ferrous chelate form. *Caution:* Do not take iron unless anemia has been diagnosed.
or Floradix Iron + Herbs from Salus Haus	As directed on label.	A natural, nontoxic form of iron from food sources.
Vitamin A plus	15,000 IU daily. If you are pregnant, do not exceed 10,000 IU daily.	Needed for proper immune function and for healthy eyes, skin, and hair. May be taken in a multivitamin complex.
natural beta-carotene or	15,000 IU daily.	Antioxidant and precursor of vitamin A.
carotenoid complex (Betatene)	As directed on label.	*Note:* If you have diabetes, omit the beta-carotene; people with diabetes cannot convert beta-carotene into vitamin A.
Vitamin C	500 mg 4 times daily. Do not exceed this amount.	Needed for immune function and stress hormone production. *Caution:* Do not take extremely high doses of vitamin C—this may affect the production of thyroid hormone.
Vitamin E	400 IU daily. Do not exceed this amount.	An important antioxidant that improves circulation and immune response.
Zinc	50 mg daily. Do not exceed a total of 100 mg daily from all supplements.	An immune system stimulant. Use zinc gluconate lozenges or OptiZinc for best absorption.

HERBS

❑ Bayberry, black cohosh, and goldenseal can help this thyroid condition.

Caution: Do not take goldenseal internally on a daily basis for more than one week at a time, do not use it during pregnancy, and use it with caution if you are allergic to ragweed.

RECOMMENDATIONS

❑ Include in the diet molasses, egg yolks, parsley, apricots, dates, and prunes. Eat fish or chicken and raw milk and cheeses.

❑ Eat these foods in moderation: Brussels sprouts, peaches, pears, spinach, turnips, and cruciferous vegetables such as cabbage, broccoli, kale, and mustard greens. If you have severe symptoms, omit these foods entirely. They may further suppress thyroid function.

❑ Avoid processed and refined foods, including white flour and sugar.

❑ Drink steam-distilled water only.

❑ Do not take sulfa drugs or antihistamines unless specifically directed to do so by a physician.

❑ Avoid fluoride (including that found in toothpaste and tap water) and chlorine (also found in tap water). Chlorine, fluoride, and iodine are chemically related. Chlorine and fluoride block iodine receptors in the thyroid gland, resulting in reduced iodine-containing hormone production and finally in hypothyroidism.

CONSIDERATIONS

❑ Treatment for a regular morning temperature of 96°F is 3 to 4 grains of Armour Thyroid Tablets daily (available by prescription). A person with a regular morning temperature of 97°F should take 1 to 2 grains. If you have side effects, speak to your physician about reducing the dosage.

❑ A study done at the University of Massachusetts revealed that levothyroxine (Synthroid and others), a drug commonly used to treat thyroid conditions, can cause a loss of as much as 13 percent of bone mass. An estimated 19 million people in the United States take this drug for enlarged thyroid or thyroid cancer.

❑ Wilson's syndrome is a condition that results from a problem in the conversion of one thyroid hormone, thyroxine (T_4), to another thyroid hormone, triiodothyronine (T_3). This causes symptoms of decreased thyroid function, especially triggered by significant physicial or emotional stress. These symptoms can be debilitating, and may persist even after the stress has passed. People with Wilson's syndrome have many of the symptoms of hypothyroidism, including low body temperature, fatigue, headaches, menstrual dysfunction, memory loss, loss of concentration, loss of sex drive, anxiety and panic attacks, depression, unhealthy nails, dry skin, frequent infections, allergies, insomnia, intolerance to cold, and lack of energy and motivation. Their blood test results are often normal, however. For more information on Wilson's syndrome or to obtain the highly recommended *Wilson's Syndrome Doctor's Manual*, call the Wilson's Syndrome Foundation at 800–621–7006.

Hysterectomy-Related Problems

Hysterectomy is the surgical removal of the uterus. This is done for many different reasons. A common reason is fibroid tumors, benign growths in the uterus that can cause problems. Over 30 percent of the hysterectomies performed in the U.S. are done to remove fibroids. Other conditions for which hysterectomy is performed include endometriosis (20 percent) and prolapse of the uterus (16 to 18 percent).

The symptoms that lead women to consider hysterectomy are varied but include the following: a constant heavy, bloated feeling; urinary tract problems or incontinence; unusually long and heavy menstrual periods; unusual swelling in the abdominal region (due to fibroid tumors); infertility (due to fibroid tumors or endometriosis); and intolerance to the drug therapy usually prescribed for endometriosis.

There are three different ways in which hysterectomy may be performed:

• *Total hysterectomy.* In this procedure, the cervix is removed along with the uterus.

• *Partial hysterectomy.* In partial hysterectomy, the uterus is removed but the cervix and other female reproductive organs remain intact.

• *Pan hysterectomy.* In this, the most extensive form of hysterectomy, the ovaries, fallopian tubes, and uterus are removed.

Many women who have hysterectomies experience significant problems as a result. The most obvious of these occurs when the ovaries are removed together with the uterus; menopause begins abruptly, with its attendant difficulties and discomforts, because the body is suddenly deprived of estrogen. This hormonal loss in turn can lead to a greatly increased risk of bone mass loss, which often precedes osteoporosis, and to an increased likelihood of heart disease, as well as depression, urinary tract problems, joint pain, headaches, dizziness, insomnia, and fatigue.

Even women who retain their ovaries often experience a drastic reduction in estrogen production, and menopause comes earlier—sometimes years earlier—than it would have naturally. This is believed to be because the supply of blood to the ovaries is disrupted and decreased by removal of the uterus. Over half of women who have ovary-sparing "partial" hysterectomies experience early menopause.

Another problem common among women who have undergone hysterectomy is diminished sexual interest and desire after surgery. Research indicates that one third of all women who have hysterectomies find their sexual desire and enjoyment greatly diminished. Removal of the ovaries may result in loss of sexuality because they secrete about half of a woman's supply of androgens, hormones that are responsible for sex drive in both men and women. However, diminished sexuality may occur whether or not the ovaries are removed. In Finland, studies have shown that the removal of the cervix in hysterectomy also resulted in diminished capacity for orgasm.

Not all of the problems that can follow hysterectomy are directly hormone related. Some women experience depression because of the knowledge that once the uterus is gone, it is too late to change one's mind about having children. Also, no surgical procedure is entirely 100-percent safe, foolproof, or guaranteed. There is a 50-percent chance of at least one minor postoperative complication (usually fever, bleeding, or wound trouble). It is estimated that 1 woman in 1,000 who has a hysterectomy will die as a result of complications, and 10 percent of the women who have this surgery will require a blood transfusion, an unsettling prospect in this age of AIDS.

Many people question why over 600,000 hysterectomies are performed in the United States each year. Very few of these operations are performed because of a life-threatening situation, and it is likely that many of them are actually unnecessary. Per capita, half as many hysterectomies are performed in Great Britain as in the United States, and American women show no health benefits for their higher incidence of surgery. Outside the United States, very few hysterectomies are performed for what doctors often term "quality of life" reasons. Hysterectomy effectively and permanently causes sterility, and this may be a motive (conscious or subconscious) for some women and/or their doctors. Financial motives cannot be overlooked entirely, either. U.S. Department of Health and Human Services statistics show that far fewer hysterectomies are performed under managed care plans, in which doctors receive a set fee for their services each year, than when surgeons are compensated directly for each operation performed.

The following supplements can help to counteract the unpleasant side effects of hysterectomy.

NUTRIENTS

SUPPLEMENT	SUGGESTED DOSAGE	COMMENTS
Very Important		
Boron	3 mg daily. Do not exceed this amount.	Aids in calcium absorption and prevention of bone loss that can occur after hysterectomy.
Calcium	2,000 mg daily, at bedtime.	Lack of estrogen hinders calcium uptake. Needed for the central nervous system.
and		
magnesium	1,000 mg daily, at bedtime.	Enhances calcium absorption.
Essential fatty acids (primrose oil is a good source)	1,000 mg 3 times daily.	Helps the body manufacture estrogen.
Potassium	99 mg daily.	Needed if hot flashes occur to replace electrolytes lost through perspiration.
Raw thymus glandular	As directed on label.	Potentiates immune function.
Vitamin B complex	100 mg twice daily, with meals.	Needed for the nervous system and to redue stress. Use a high-stress formula. Injections (under a doctor's supervision) may be necessary.
Vitamin C	3,000–6,000 mg and up daily, in divided doses.	An anti-stress vitamin also needed for tissue repair.
Vitamin E	Start with 400 IU daily and increase slowly to 1,200 IU daily. For hot flashes, find the dosage that eases symptoms and stay at that level.	Important in estrogen production. *Caution:* Do not take this supplement for 2 weeks *prior* to surgery.
Important		
Vitamin A	50,000 IU daily.	Important in immune function and to promote tissue repair. Use emulsion form for easier assimilation and greater safety at higher doses.
plus		
zinc	50 mg daily. Do not exceed a total of 100 mg daily from all supplements.	Boosts the immune system. Use zinc gluconate lozenges or zinc methionate (OptiZinc) for best absorption.
L-Arginine and L-lysine	500 mg each daily, on an empty stomach. Take with water or juice. Do not take with milk. Take with 50 mg vitamin B$_6$ and 100 mg vitamin C for better absorption.	Essential amino acids important in recovery after surgery. Both are needed to avoid an imbalance in amino acids. *See* AMINO ACIDS in Part One.
Helpful		
Multiglandular complex (Cytozyme-F from Biotics Research)	As directed on label.	Aids in glandular function.
Multivitamin and mineral complex	As directed on label.	Restores the essential vitamins and minerals to balance.

HERBS

❑ Herbs that act as natural estrogen promoters include anise, dong quai, fennel, fenugreek, ginseng, licorice, red clover, sage, suma, and wild yam.

Caution: Do not use sage if you have any kind of seizure disorder.

RECOMMENDATIONS

❑ Adopt a hypoglycemic diet; eat plenty of foods that are high in fiber, such as vegetables, whole grains, and high-fiber fruits, plus fish, skinless white turkey or chicken breast, soy products, and low-fat yogurt, kefir, and cottage cheese for protein. Eat starchy foods in moderation only. Do not consume any refined sugar, white flour, alcohol, processed foods, saturated fats, or foods containing artificial colors, preservatives, or other additives. Eat six to eight small meals spaced regularly throughout the day, rather than two or three larger meals. *See* HYPOGLYCEMIA in Part Two for additional suggestions.

❑ Avoid caffeine, colas, dairy products (except for low-fat soured products), processed foods, red meat, and sugar.

❑ Use vitamin E to help prevent incisional scarring and relieve itching and discomfort in the area surrounding the stitches. Open a vitamin E capsule and apply the oil along the incision (but not on the stitches themselves).

❑ If you are pondering a hysterectomy, give the matter close and careful consideration. Seek wise counsel and second opinions. Check into alternative treatments. Remember, once the operation has been performed, it is impossible to restore the uterus if you find the symptoms unacceptable or unbearable. The results of a hysterectomy are irreversible.

CONSIDERATIONS

❑ Women over forty who have hysterectomies performed often have their ovaries removed as well, supposedly as a precaution against the later development of ovarian cancer. However, many health care professionals question the logic of doing this; ovarian cancer is relatively rare.

❑ Estrogen replacement therapy is often recommended following a hysterectomy. For some women, it is, unfortunately, unavoidable, because of severe posthysterectomy symptoms. Not all women can tolerate estrogen replacement. In our opinion, synthetic estrogens are potentially dangerous because they are strongly linked to breast cancer and cardiovascular disease (see Hormone Replacement Therapy on page 385). Natural estrogens, on the other hand, are safe and effective. Natural estrogen promoters include anise, dong quai, fennel, fenugreek, ginseng, licorice, primrose oil, red clover, sage, suma, and wild yam.

❑ A hysterectomy usually requires four or five days in the hospital followed by approximately six weeks of at-home recuperation. Recovery can be more painful if the surgeon makes a vertical incision as opposed to a horizontal one. In addition, the scar that results from a vertical incision acts as a lifelong reminder of the surgery (a horizontal incision can be hidden below the pubic hairline).

❑ Evidence is mounting that there is a higher incidence of cardiovascular disorders among women who have undergone hysterectomies.

❑ Some doctors advocate performing hysterectomies on women with fibroid tumors because they say that the fibroids block access to the ovaries during pelvic exams, which might delay a possible diagnosis of ovarian cancer. This position is no longer valid, however, because technology allows the use of ultrasound technology to examine the ovaries for any abnormality. If fibroid tumors need to be removed, a myomectomy should be considered and opted for if at all possible (see FIBROIDS in Part Two).

❑ There are instances in which hysterectomy proves advantageous. Some women manage to avoid the major hormonal changes that are so common after surgery, and in addition to no longer being bothered with monthly menses, they may feel liberated because they no longer need to fear becoming pregnant and have more fulfilling sex lives as a result. However, these women are probably in the minority.

❑ While over half of the women who have their ovaries left in place still experience drastic estrogen loss, this is not always permanent. A vitamin and mineral supplement regimen can reduce the risk of severe estrogen deprivation. Remember the natural estrogen promoters.

❑ If you do require hormone replacement to control symptoms after a hysterectomy, take the lowest dose possible. Ask your doctor for a combined hormone containing estrogen and progesterone to help reduce the risk of cancer.

❑ Dr. Betty Kamen, an expert in women's health problems, says that progesterone, not estrogen, should be the hormone of choice for replacement therapy.

❑ See also MENOPAUSE-RELATED PROBLEMS in Part Two.

❑ See also PREPARING FOR AND RECOVERING FROM SURGERY in Part Three.

Immune System, Weakened

See WEAKENED IMMUNE SYSTEM.

Impotence

If a man does not have the ability to achieve or maintain an erection adequate for normal sexual intercourse, he is said to be impotent. Erections result from a complex combination of brain stimuli, blood vessel and nerve function, and hormonal actions. Anything that interferes with any of these factors can cause impotence. Some of the factors that can lead to impotence include peripheral vascular disease; the use of certain medications, alcohol, or cigarettes; a history of sexually transmitted disease; and chronic illness such as diabetes or high blood pressure. Hormonal disturbances such as diminished levels of testosterone or elevated prolactin production, or over- or underproduction of thyroid hormone, may also cause impotence. Diabetes, which often leads to atherosclerosis and impaired circulation, is probably the most common physical cause of impotence.

Impotence may be chronic or recurring, or it may occur as a single isolated incident. It is estimated that as many as 30 million men in the United States suffer from at least occasional impotence. Most of these men are age forty or over (one in three men over sixty is affected), but those under forty may also have the problem.

In the past, it was assumed that impotence was primarily a psychological problem, but many therapists and physicians today believe that as many as 85 percent of all cases of impotence have some physical basis. The Association for Male Sexual Dysfunction recognizes over 200 drugs that may cause impotence. Some of the most common are alcohol, antidepressants, antihistamines, antihypertensives, diuretics, narcotics, nicotine, sedatives, stomach acid inhibitors, and ulcer medications. Atherosclerosis, or hardening of the arteries, poses a risk to the condition of both the heart and the penis. Most people today know smoking and eating fatty foods lead to the production of plaques that clog arteries and block the flow of blood to the heart. These plaques also can block the arteries leading to the genitals, interfering with the ability to attain an erection.

IMPOTENCE SELF-TEST

The appropriate treatment for impotence depends upon whether the cause is physical or psychological. A man whose impotence is psychologically based generally still has erections during sleep, whereas an individual whose impotence is physical in origin usually does not. One easy, inexpensive way to test for nocturnal erections is with postage stamps. Glue a strip of stamps around the shaft of the penis before going to bed. If the ring of stamps is broken in the morning, the cause of the impotence is likely psychological. If the strip is unbroken, the impotence is likely physiological.

You can also purchase a kit called Snap Gauge from UroHealth Corporation. This test is designed to detect and measure the rigidity of erections experienced during sleep. Call 800–328–1103 for more information.

NUTRIENTS

SUPPLEMENT	SUGGESTED DOSAGE	COMMENTS
Essential		
Prostata from Gero Vita	As directed on label.	Enhances libido and erectile function.
Vitamin E	Start with 200 IU daily and slowly increase to 400–1,000 IU daily.	Increases circulation.
Zinc	80 mg daily. Do not exceed this amount.	Important in prostate gland function and reproductive organ growth. Use zinc gluconate lozenges or OptiZinc for best absorption.
Important		
Dimethylglycine (DMG) (Aangamik DMG from FoodScience Labs)	As directed on label.	Increases oxygen supply in the blood to all tissues. Blood vessels must be dilated for an erection to occur. Use a sublingual form.
GH3 from Gero Vita	As directed on label.	Stimulates the activity of sex hormones. *Caution:* Do not use GH3 if you are allergic to sulfites.
Octacosanol	1,000–2,000 mcg 3 times weekly.	Natural source of vitamin E. Good for hormone production.
Helpful		
L-Tyrosine	500 mg twice daily, on an empty stomach. Take with water or juice. Do not take with milk. Take with 50 mg vitamin B_6 and 100 mg vitamin C for better absorption.	Helps stabilize moods and alleviate stress. *See* AMINO ACIDS in Part One. *Caution:* Do not take tyrosine if you are taking an MAO inhibitor drug.
Raw orchic glandular	As directed on label.	Glandular extracts from the male reproductive organs that promote their function. *See* GLANDULAR THERAPY in Part Three.
Vitamin A plus	15,000 IU daily.	Antioxidants that enhance immunity.
natural beta-carotene or	15,000 IU daily.	
carotenoid complex (Betatene)	As directed on label.	
Vitamin B complex	50 mg 3 times daily.	Needed for a healthy nervous system, and are important in all cell activity.
plus extra vitamin B_6 (pyridoxine)	50 mg 3 times daily.	Required for the synthesis of RNA and DNA, which govern cellular reproduction.

HERBS

❑ Damiana is good for improving blood flow to the genital area.

❑ Sarsaparilla contains a testosteronelike substance for men. Muscular men have higher testosterone levels.

❑ Wild yam contains natural steroids that rejuvenate and give vigor to lovemaking. Steroids are what help exercise to melt off more weight. This hormone is found in the human body as dehydroepiandrosterone (DHEA). Take twice the amount recommended on the label for two weeks, then stop for two weeks. Continue this on-and-off cycle, taking the recommended amount.

❑ Other herbs that may be beneficial include dong quai, gotu kola, hydrangea root, pygeum, saw palmetto, and/or Siberian ginseng.

❑ There are a number of herbal products on the market that claim to help sexual potency:

• Prostata from Gero Vita International normalizes prostate function, increasing libido and erectile ability.

• Saw Palmetto Supreme from Gaia Herbs is an herbal tincture that helps to normalize prostate function.

• SensualiTea from UniTea Herbs contains damiana, sarsaparilla, and licorice root. It can be found in many health food stores that sell bulk herbs.

• Virility Two from KAL contains damiana, gotu kola, Jamaican ginger, oak grass powder, sarsaparilla, and yohimbe.

RECOMMENDATIONS

❑ Eat a healthy, well-balanced diet. Include in the diet pumpkin seeds, bee pollen, or royal jelly.
Caution: Bee pollen may cause an allergic reaction in some individuals. Start with a small amount, and discontinue use if a rash, wheezing, discomfort, or other symptom occurs.

❑ Avoid alcohol, particularly before sexual encounters.

❑ Do not consume animal fats, sugar, fried or junk foods.

❑ Do not smoke. Avoid being around cigarette smoke.

❑ Avoid stress.

❑ Consult a urologist for testing to determine whether impotence is caused by an underlying illness that requires treatment.

❑ Consider possible psychological factors that may be contributing to impotence, especially repressed anger or a fear of intimacy. Exploring psychological issues with a qualified therapist can help.

❑ If you suspect impotence may be related to a drug you are taking, discuss this with your physician. There may be satisfactory alternatives that will not cause this problem. Certain blood pressure medications and tranquilizers often cause erectile difficulties. The drugs cimetidine (Tagamet) and ranitidine (Zantac), which are used to treat ulcers and heartburn, also have significant side effects in some men.

Caution: Do not stop taking a prescription drug or change the dosage without consulting your physician.

❑ Investigate the possibility of heavy metal intoxication. A hair analysis can reveal possible heavy metal poisoning. *See* HAIR ANALYSIS in Part Three.

❑ Keep in mind that sexual function changes with age. As you age, you may require more stimulation and a longer period of time to achieve an erection.

CONSIDERATIONS

❑ A study done at the Boston University School of Medicine linked overall health to impotence. Researchers studied the medical histories of 1,300 men aged forty to seventy years. They found some impotence in a total of 52 percent of those under study. Men who were being treated for heart disease, high blood pressure, or diabetes were one and a half to four times more likely than the overall group to be completely impotent later in life. The situation was even worse for men who had heart disease or hypertension and who smoked.

❑ Alcohol intake decreases the body's ability to produce testosterone. Research at Chicago Medical School revealed that drinking alcohol may cause the hormonal equivalent of menopause in men. Alcohol not only affects sexual function, but also helps set the stage for a heart attack and other dangerous conditions.

❑ Arteriosclerosis, which restricts blood supply to the penis and to the nerves that govern sexual arousal, may result in a "failure to perform." If impotence is related to clogged blood vessels, a diet low in fats can actually help reverse the problem. *See* ARTERIOSCLEROSIS/ATHEROSCLEROSIS, CARDIOVASCULAR DISEASE, and/or CIRCULATORY PROBLEMS in Part Two.

❑ A study done at Boston University showed that men who smoked one pack of cigarettes a day for five years were 15 percent more likely to develop clogging in the arteries that serve the penis, a situation that can cause impotence. In addition, heavy smoking decreases sexual capability by damaging the tiny blood vessels in the penis. The use of marijuana and cocaine also can result in impotence.

❑ Duplex ultrasonography, a noninvasive method of measuring penile blood flow, is a reliable method of determining whether arterial occlusion plays a role in impotence. If your doctor believes atherosclerosis to be the underlying problem, he or she may advise vascular surgery to improve blood flow to the penis.

❑ According to figures from impotence organizations, only about 5 percent of the estimated 30 million men affected are aware of therapy options.

❑ Urologists differ in the types of treatment they recommend for impotence, but many opt first for nonsurgical treatment.

❑ Injections of the drugs papaverine (Pavabid) and phentolamine (Regitine) or prostaglandin E1 (PGE1) into the base of the penis before intercourse have been shown to be roughly 80 percent effective in producing "satisfactory erection" in impotent men who have tried it. The drug alprostadil also is available in an injection kit (Caverject). These drugs work by relaxing smooth muscle, causing the blood vessels in the penis to dilate, promoting an erection that can last an hour or more. An estimated 300,000 men in the United States use this technique each year. Possible side effects include priaprism (prolonged, painful erections). Also, although the injections are done with a tiny needle, and are supposed to be painless when done properly (proper technique is crucial), this prospect is unappealing to many men. A less invasive technique, which involves instilling alprostadil into the urethra with a tiny plunger, is under development and is expected to become available in the near future.

❑ Yohimbine (sold under the brand names Dayto, Yocon, and Yohimex) is a prescription drug that has been approved by the FDA for treatment of impotence. Its effectiveness is questionable, however. Many experts consider it to be, in essence, a placebo. Yohimbine has an effect on the body similar to that of adrenaline; it speeds up the heartbeat and elevates blood pressure. Beware of yohimbine if you have high blood pressure.

❑ If impotence is linked to high levels of the hormone prolactin, bromocriptine (Parlodel) may be prescribed to correct the problem.

❑ A number of vacuum devices are used to promote erection. With these devices, a cylinder is placed over the penis and a hand pump is used to create a vacuum in the cylinder. This in turn causes blood to flow into the penis, creating an erection. The user then puts a constriction band around the base of the penis, causing the erection to last up to thirty minutes. These devices are available by prescription only. Some 100,000 men in the United States choose this treatment each year. Problems abound with this technique, however.

❑ Since the early 1970s, more than 250,000 American men have turned to inflatable penile implants to mechanically create erections. Penile implants are surgically installed devices that are made of silicone or polyurethane. One type is made of two semirigid but bendable rods; another type consists of a pump, a fluid-filled reservoir, and two cylinders into which the fluid is pumped to create an erection. Penile implants are now coming under FDA scrutiny. Since 1984, the FDA's Center for Devices and Radiological Health has logged more than 6,500 reports of problems with inflatable devices—a large number for a medical device, according to the FDA. With the development of more effective agents, implants are now considered to be a last resort, to be tried only when all other methods have failed.

❑ Dr. Robert Frankt of Budapest University in Hungary found a great increase in sexual vitality and energy in men using a combination of two herbs, green oats (*Avena sativa*) and stinging nettle. "Feeling one's oats" is an expression that originated centuries ago, and probably with good reason; a study by the Institute for Advanced Study of Human Sexuality found that men who sufferred from reduced sexual desire and diminished performance were helped by green oats. Nettle is full of vital minerals and is good also for hypoglycemia, allergies, depression, prostate and urinary tract disorders, and a host of other problems.

❑   *See also* HYPERTHYROIDISM and HYPOTHYROIDISM in Part Two.

Indigestion (Dyspepsia)

Indigestion may be a symptom of a disorder in the stomach or the intestines, or it may be a disorder in itself. Symptoms can include gas, abdominal pain, rumbling noises, a bloated feeling, belching, nausea, vomiting, and a burning sensation after eating.

Swallowing air—by chewing with the mouth open, talking while chewing, or gulping down food—can cause indigestion. Drinking liquids with meals contributes to indigestion because it dilutes the enzymes needed for digestion. Certain foods and beverages can cause indigestion because they are irritating to the digestive tract. These include alcohol, vinegar, caffeine, and greasy, spicy, or refined foods. Other factors that can cause or contribute to indigestion include intestinal obstruction, malabsorption, peptic ulcers, and disorders of the pancreas, liver, or gallbladder. Food allergies and intolerances (such as lactose intolerance) also can cause indigestion.

If food is not digested properly, it can ferment in the intestines, producing hydrogen and carbon dioxide. Foods high in complex carbohydrates, such as grains and legumes, are the primary foods responsible for gas because they are difficult to digest, and therefore more likely to yield undigested particles on which the intestinal bacteria act. Psychological factors such as stress, anxiety, worry, or disappointment can disturb the nervous mechanism that controls the contractions of stomach and intestinal muscles. A lack of digestive enzymes can also cause intestinal problems. Heartburn often accompanies indigestion.

STOMACH ACID SELF-TEST

Hydrochloric acid (HCl), which is produced by glands in the stomach, is necessary for the breakdown and digestion of many foods. Insufficient amounts of HCl can lead to indigestion. HCl levels often decline with age.

You can determine if you need more hydrochloric acid with this simple test. Take a tablespoon of apple cider vinegar or lemon juice. If this makes your indigestion go away, then you need more stomach acid. If it makes your symptoms worse, then you have too much acid, and you should take care not to take any supplements that contain HCl.

NUTRIENTS

SUPPLEMENT	SUGGESTED DOSAGE	COMMENTS
Very Important		
Aerobic 07 from Aerobic Life Industries	9 drops in water once daily.	Controls putrefying action of bacteria in the bowel.
Aloe vera		*See under* Herbs, below.
Glucomannan or Aerobic Bulk Cleanse (ABC) from Aerobic Life Industries	1 tbsp in liquid upon arising. Take separately from other supplements and medications.	Colon cleansers that aid in normal stool formation.
Proteolytic enzymes or Infla-Zyme Forte from American Biologics or pancreatin	As directed on label, with each meal. Take ½ the recommended dose with snacks.	To aid in the breakdown of protein for proper absorption. Important for combating gas and bloating. *Caution:* Do not give these supplements to a child.
Important		
Acidophilus or Kyo-Dophilus from Wakunaga	As directed on label, ½ hour before each meal. As directed on label.	Necessary for normal digestion. Use a nondairy formula such as Neo-Flora from New Chapter. Contains both garlic and acidophilus. Milk-free and heat-resistant.
Garlic (Kyolic)	2 capsules 3 times daily, with meals.	Aids in digestion and destroys unwanted bacteria in the bowel.
Vitamin B complex plus extra vitamin B$_1$ (thiamine) and vitamin B$_{12}$	100 mg 3 times daily, with meals. 50 mg 3 times daily. 1,000 mcg twice daily.	Essential for normal digestion. Enhances production of hydrochloric acid. Important for proper digestion. Use a lozenge or sublingual form.
Helpful		
Alfalfa		*See under* Herbs, below.
L-Carnitine	As directed on label.	Carries fat into the cells for breakdown into energy.
Lecithin granules or capsules or lipotropic factors	1 tbsp 3 times daily, before meals. 1,200 mg 3 times daily, before meals. As directed on label.	Fat emulsifiers that aid in the breakdown of fats.
L-Methionine	As directed on label, on an empty stomach. Take with water or juice. Do not take with milk. Take with 50 mg vitamin B$_6$ and 100 mg vitamin C for better absorption.	A potent liver detoxifier. *See* AMINO ACIDS in Part One.
Multienzyme complex	As directed on label. Take with meals.	To improve digestion. *Do not* use a formula containing HCl.

HERBS

❑   Acid-Ease from Prevail Corporation is an herbal formula that aids in the breakdown and assimilation of foods, and also contains natural plant enzymes to ease heartburn.

❑ Alfalfa supplies needed vitamin K and trace minerals. It can be taken in liquid or tablet form.

❑ Aloe vera is good for heartburn and other gastrointestinal symptoms. Take ¼ cup of aloe vera juice on an empty stomach in the morning and again at bedtime. George's Aloe Vera Juice from Warren Laboratories tastes like spring water.

❑ Anise seeds can help relieve a sour stomach. Chew the whole seeds or grind them and sprinkle on food.

❑ Catnip, chamomile, fennel, fenugreek, goldenseal, papaya, and peppermint are all good for indigestion.

Caution: Do not use chamomile on an ongoing basis, and avoid it completely if you are allergic to ragweed. Do not take goldenseal internally on a daily basis for more than one week, do not use it during pregnancy, and use it with caution if you are allergic to ragweed.

❑ Ginger is a time-honored remedy for nausea.

❑ A few sprigs of fresh parsley, or ¼ teaspoon of dried, taken with a glass of warm water, can help relieve indigestion.

❑ Slippery elm is good for inflammation of the colon; use it as an enema for fast relief. *See* ENEMAS in Part Three.

RECOMMENDATIONS

❑ If you are prone to indigestion, consume well-balanced meals with plenty of fiber-rich foods such as fresh fruits, vegetables, and whole grains.

❑ Include in the diet fresh papaya (which contains papain) and fresh pineapple (which contains bromelain). These are good sources of beneficial digestive enzymes.

❑ Add acidophilus to the diet. Acidophilus can be useful for indigestion, because a shortage of the "friendly" bacteria is often the cause. Open 10 capsules or use 1 tablespoon of powdered formula. Neo-Flora from New Chapter and Kyo-Dophilus from Wakunaga are nondairy products that can be used if you have a reaction to dairy products. Acidophilus used as an enema hardly ever results in a problem. You may experience some rumbling and slight disturbance for an hour or so, but it will subside. (*See* ENEMAS in Part Three.)

❑ For disorders such as gas, bloating, and heartburn, try brown rice and/or barley broth. Use 5 parts water to 1 part grain, and boil the mixture, uncovered, for ten minutes. Then put the lid on and simmer for fifty-five minutes more. Strain and cool the liquid. Sip this throughout the day.

❑ Limit your intake of lentils, peanuts, and soybeans. They contain an enzyme inhibitor.

❑ For upper gastrointestinal gas, take pancreatin; for lower gastrointestinal gas, take supplemental trace minerals. If you have gas, use the juice of one fresh lemon in a quart lukewarm water as an enema to balance the body's pH. If gas is constant for days, use a bifidus enema. This should relieve the problem within hours. *See* ENEMAS in Part Three.

❑ Avoid bakery products, beans, caffeine, carbonated beverages, citrus juices, fried and fatty foods, pasta, peppers, potato chips and other snack foods, red meat, refined carbohydrates (sugar), tomatoes, and salty or spicy foods.

❑ Do not eat dairy products, junk foods, or processed foods. These cause excess mucus formation, which results in inadequate digestion of protein.

❑ For relief of occasional digestive difficulties, use charcoal tablets, available in health food stores. These are good for absorbing gas and toxins. Because they can interfere with the absorption of other medications and nutrients, they should be taken separately, and they should not be taken for long periods of time. Occasional use is not harmful and has no side effects.

❑ If stools are foul-smelling and are accompanied by a burning sensation in the anus, follow a fasting program. This is often a sign that the colon contains toxic material. *See* FASTING in Part Three.

❑ If you have had abdominal surgery (such as a bowel shortened), take pancreatin to help digest foods. If you have hypoglycemia (low blood sugar), you also need pancreatin. After meals, if you have a stuffed feeling and a rumbling or gurgling with bloating and gas, use pancreatin.

❑ If the results of the stomach acid self-test showed that you need more hydrochloric acid, sip 1 tablespoon of pure apple cider vinegar in a glass of water with each meal to aid digestion.

❑ Always chew food thoroughly; do not gulp it down in a hurry.

❑ Do not eat when you are upset or overtired.

❑ Do not drink liquids while eating. This dilutes the stomach juices and prevents proper digestion.

❑ Find out which foods your body has trouble digesting, and stay away from foods that cause a reaction. *See* ALLERGIES in Part Two.

❑ If you develop heartburn and the symptoms persist, consult your health care provider. If the pain begins to travel down your left arm, or if the sensation is accompanied by a feeling of weakness, dizziness, or shortness of breath, seek emergency medical help. The early symptoms of a heart attack can be very much like those of indigestion, particularly heartburn, and as a result, many people mistakenly dismiss them. *See* HEART ATTACK in Part Two.

CONSIDERATIONS

❑ Drinking the juice of a lemon in a cup of water first thing in the morning is good for healing and for purifying the blood.

❑ Exercise, such as brisk walking or stretching, aids the digestive process. The herbal formula Tum-Ease from New Chapter also enhances digestion.

❑ Food combinations are important. Proteins and starches are a poor combination, as are vegetables and fruits. Milk should not be consumed with meals. Foods containing sugar, such as fruit, should not be consumed with proteins or starches.

❑ Older people often lack sufficient hydrochloric acid and pancreatin to digest foods properly.

❑ Many people take antacids to relieve the discomfort of indigestion and heartburn, but these medications may actually make matters worse. Antacids neutralize the acid in the stomach, preventing proper digestion and interfering with the absorption of nutrients. This only leads to continued indigestion. Antacids are useless for gas and bloating.

❑ Most antacids sold in the United States contain aluminum compounds, calcium carbonate, magnesium compounds, or sodium bicarbonate. Aluminum-based antacids can cause constipation. Calcium carbonate can cause a rebound effect in which the stomach produces more acid than before once the antacid's effects wear off. Magnesium compounds can cause diarrhea. Sodium bicarbonate can cause gas and bloating.

❑ Beano from AkPharma, Inc. and Be Sure from Wakunaga of America Company are good for preventing gas. These products must be taken with the first bite of food to be effective.

❑ *See also* ALLERGIES in Part Two and take the self-test.

❑ *See also* DIVERTICULITIS; FOOD POISONING; GALLBLADDER DISORDERS; HEARTBURN; HERNIA, HIATAL; IRRITABLE BOWEL SYNDROME; LACTOSE INTOLERANCE; MOTION SICKNESS; PANCREATITIS; PEPTIC ULCER; and/or ULCERATIVE COLITIS, all in Part Two.

Infertility

Infertility is usually defined as the failure to conceive after a year or more of regular sexual activity during the time of ovulation. It may also refer to the inability to carry a pregnancy to term. An estimated one in every five couples in the United States experiences infertility, and pinpointing the exact cause of the problem can be difficult. Ovulation, fertilization, and the journey of the fertilized ovum through the fallopian tube and finally into the uterus are highly intricate processes. Many events must work together perfectly for pregnancy to occur.

For men, infertility is most often the result of a low sperm count or an anatomical abnormality. A variety of factors can result in a low sperm count, including exposure to toxins, radiation, or excessive heat; testicular injury; endocrine disorders; alcohol consumption; recent acute illness or prolonged fever; and testicular mumps. The most common anatomical abnormality that leads to infertility in men is a varicocele, a dilated vein of the spermatic cord.

For women, the most common causes of infertility include ovulatory failure or defect, blocked fallopian tubes, endometriosis, and uterine fibroids. Some women develop antibodies to their partners' sperm, in effect becoming allergic to them. Chlamydia, a sexually transmitted disease that strikes 4 million Americans a year, causes many cases of infertility. Psychological issues, such as stress or fear of parenthood, may contribute to infertility as well.

OVULATION TIMING SELF-TEST

If you wish to become pregnant, there are a number of tests available over the counter that can help you determine the best time to attempt to conceive. These tests predict the time of ovulation by detecting the release of luteinizing hormone (LH), which in turn triggers the release of the egg.

A chemically treated dipstick detects the LH in urine samples. If the hormone has been released, the stick changes color. After a positive result, ovulation takes place within twelve to thirty-six hours. First Response from Hygeia Sciences and ClearPlan Easy from Whitehall Laboratories are test kits that can be purchased at your drugstore. Remember, however, that no test is 100-percent accurate.

Unless otherwise specified, the following nutrients are recommended for either or both partners.

NUTRIENTS

SUPPLEMENT	SUGGESTED DOSAGE	COMMENTS
Essential		
Selenium	200–400 mcg daily.	Deficiency leads to reduced sperm count and has been linked to sterility in men and infertility in women.
Vitamin C	2,000–6,000 daily, in divided doses.	Important in sperm production. Keeps the sperm from clumping and makes them more motile.
Vitamin E	Start with 200 IU daily and increase gradually to 400–1,000 IU daily.	Needed for balanced hormone production. Has been known as the "sex vitamin" that carries oxygen to the sex organs.
Zinc	80 mg daily. Do not exceed a total of 100 mg daily from all supplements.	Important for the functioning of the reproductive organs. Use zinc gluconate lozenges or OptiZinc for best absorption.
Important		
Dimethylglycine (DMG) (Aangamik DMG from FoodScience Labs)	As directed on label.	Increases oxygen supply in the blood to all tissues. Use a sublingual form.
Liver extract injections	As prescribed by physician, twice weekly.	Found to be beneficial in promoting function of the sex organs.
Octacosanol	As directed on label.	The heart of wheat germ. Aids in hormone production.
Helpful		
Essential fatty acids	As directed on label.	Essential for normal glandular function and activity, especially for the reproductive system.

L-Arginine plus	As directed on label.	Increases sperm count and plays a role in sperm motility.
L-cysteine and	As directed on label.	Sulfur-containing amino acids that are effective free radical
L-methionine plus	As directed on label.	destroyers and chelating agents that protect glandular and hormonal function.
L-tyrosine	500 mg daily, on an empty stomach. Take with water or juice. Do not take with milk. Take with 50 mg vitamin B$_6$ and 100 mg vitamin C for better absorption.	Alleviates stress and aids in stabilizing moods. See AMINO ACIDS in Part One. Caution: Do not take this supplement if you are taking an MAO inhibitor drug.
Manganese	As directed on label. Take separately from calcium.	Maintains sex hormone production.
Proteolytic enzymes	As directed on label. Take between meals.	Aids in the breakdown of foods. Facilitates absorption of nutrients.
Raw orchic glandular	As directed on label.	For men. Supports testicular function. See GLANDULAR THERAPY in Part Three.
Raw ovarian glandular	As directed on label.	For women. Supports ovarian function. See GLANDULAR THERAPY in Part Three.
Vitamin A plus	15,000 IU daily.	Important in reproductive gland function.
natural beta-carotene or	15,000 IU daily.	
carotenoid complex (Betatene)	As directed on label.	
Vitamin B complex plus extra	50 mg daily.	Important in reproductive gland function.
pantothenic acid (vitamin B$_5$) and	As directed on label.	Maintains sex hormone production. Helpful for stress.
vitamin B$_6$ (pyridoxine) and	50 mg 3 times daily.	Needed for the synthesis of RNA and DNA.
para-aminobenzoic acid (PABA)	50 mg daily.	Plays a role in restoring fertility in some women.

HERBS

❑ Astragalus extract has been reported to stimulate sperm motility.

Caution: Do not use this herb in the presence of a fever.

❑ Damiana, ginseng, sarsaparilla, saw palmetto, and yohimbe enhance sexual function in men. Damiana, dong quai, false unicorn root, ginseng, gotu kola, licorice root, and wild yam root are good for women.

Caution: Do not use ginseng or licorice if you have high blood pressure.

RECOMMENDATIONS

❑ Avoid vigorous exercise, hot tubs, and saunas, as they may lead to changes in ovulation and reduced sperm count.

❑ Avoid all alcohol; it reduces sperm count in men and can prevent implantation of the fertilized egg in women.

❑ Do not take any drugs except those prescribed by your physician.

❑ Do not smoke, and avoid being around cigarette smoke.

❑ A balanced diet is important. Do not consume animal fats, fried foods, sugar, or junk foods. Do eat pumpkin seeds, bee pollen, or royal jelly.

Caution: Bee pollen may cause an allergic reaction in some people. Start with a small amount, and discontinue use if a rash, wheezing, discomfort, or other symptom occurs.

❑ Investigate the possibility of heavy metal intoxication, which may affect ovulation. A hair analysis can reveal heavy metal poisoning. See HAIR ANALYSIS in Part Three.

❑ Infertility is stressful, but do all you can to reduce the stresses in your life. Learn stress management techniques to help you deal with stresses that cannot be avoided. See STRESS in Part Two.

CONSIDERATIONS

❑ Because there are so many causes of infertility, in most cases the opinion of a qualified health care professional is needed.

❑ Sperm factors account for approximately 40 percent of all cases of infertility. Some causes of sperm inadequacy (exposure to heat, recent illness, endocrine disorders) may be temporary or reversible, but others are not. Except for artificial insemination, orthodox drug therapy is ineffective in such cases.

❑ Varicoceles are treatable with surgery.

❑ The ulcer medications cimetidine (Tagamet) and ranitidine (Zantac) may decrease sperm count and even produce impotence.

❑ Strict adherence to a gluten-free diet has enabled some previously sterile men to become fathers. A gluten-free diet has also enabled women who were previously unable to conceive to become pregnant. See CELIAC DISEASE in Part Two for more information about a gluten-free diet.

❑ The transdermal use of natural progesterone cream may benefit infertile women.

❑ Researchers at Britain's Medical Research Council and Edinburgh University scientists have found a new clue to male infertility: gene defects that interfere with proper sperm production. Located on the Y chromosome, these genes are involved in producing a protein that contributes to fertility. Infertility results when a mutation disrupts its normal functioning. More research may lead to new infertility treatments, including gene therapy.

❑ A deficiency of selenium can lead to sterility in men and infertility in women.

❑ If a woman has developed antibodies to her partner's sperm, it may help to have him use a condom for at least thirty days. The sperm antibodies should then decrease, and intercourse without the use of a condom during the time of ovulation may lead to conception.

❑ A woman who suffers from premenstrual symptoms such as bloating and breast tenderness is probably ovulating, so if she is having difficulty becoming pregnant, the cause probably lies elsewhere.

❑ More women are waiting to bear children in later reproductive years. However, a woman's fertility begins to decrease when she reaches her thirties.

❑ Para-aminobenzoic acid (PABA) stimulates the pituitary gland and sometimes restores fertility to some women who cannot conceive.

❑ Caffeine consumption may prevent some women from becoming pregnant.

❑ Procedures known as transcervical balloon tuboplasty (TBT) and selective fallopian tube canalization have roughly 90-percent success rates in removing obstructions of the fallopian tubes. TBT is similar to the artery-clearing technique called angioplasty. A tiny balloon is inserted into the tube by means of a catheter; when the catheter reaches the blockage, the balloon is inflated to stretch and clear the blocked section of the tube. The procedure may be performed in about fifteen minutes under either local or general anesthesia. Because this procedure is relatively noninvasive (no incision is required), the risks involved are few. However, there is a chance that a tube may become blocked again. This happens in approximately 20 percent of the women who undergo the procedure. Fallopian tube canalization produces similar results to those of TBT.

❑ A University of Michigan study indicated that intense exercise may result in a drop in the production of hormones involved in potency, fertility, and sex drive.

❑ A study conducted at the University of Washington in Seattle found that stress may contribute to infertility. Researchers found that women with hormonal problems also reported less emotional support (close friends or family). The results suggest that stress resulting from a lack of emotional support may affect the hormones involved in fertility.

❑ Recent advances in the treatment of infertility have focused on making existing techniques more comfortable, as well as expanding treatments to include people who would not have been candidates in the past. One new development is the use of donor eggs to impregnate women who cannot conceive on their own, whether because of damage to the ovaries, age, or some other factor. This is a controversial procedure, and it is being done in only a few clinics in the United States. It is also extremely expensive.

❑ Your health care provider must get your consent before performing diagnostic tests to determine the cause of infertility. There may be risks involved any time you penetrate the body using a tube, needle, or viewing instrument, or expose the body to the radiation, drugs, anesthetics, and dye materials used in certain imaging techniques. The risks of any given procedure vary depending on your age and health status, and the skill of the practitioner.

Inflammation

Inflammation is a natural reaction to injury or infection. The affected tissues swell, redden, become warm and tender, and may be painful. Any organ or tissue of the body, internal or external, can become inflamed. Internal inflammation is often caused by bacterial infection, but can also be caused by disorders such as arthritis or allergies. External inflammation is most often the result of injury, but can also result from (or be aggravated by) infection, allergies, and other factors.

NUTRIENTS

SUPPLEMENT	SUGGESTED DOSAGE	COMMENTS
Essential		
Vitamin C with bioflavonoids	3,000–6,000 mg daily, in divided doses.	Essential to the healing process and in reducing inflammation.
Very Important		
Proteolytic enzymes or Infla-Zyme Forte from American Biologics	As directed on label, between meals and at bedtime, for 1 month. 2 tablets twice daily, between meals.	Aids in controlling inflammation.
Superoxide dismutase (SOD)	As directed on label.	A high-potency free radical scavenger that reduces infection and inflammation.
Zinc	50 mg daily. Do not exceed a total of 100 mg daily from all supplements.	Helps to control inflammation and promotes healing. Use zinc gluconate lozenges or OptiZinc for best absorption.
Important		
AE Mulsion Forte from American Biologics	As directed on label.	Supplies vitamins A and E in easily assimilable emulsion form to destroy free radicals, boost the immune system, and help the body to use oxygen efficiently.
Bromelain	As directed on label. Take on an empty stomach with 100–500 mg magnesium and 500 mg L-cysteine to enhance results. Take separately from copper and iron.	Has anti-inflammatory activity and increases the breakdown of fibrin, which forms around the inflamed area, blocking the blood and lymphatic vessels and leading to swelling.
Garlic (Kyolic)	2 capsules 3 times daily, with meals.	Has natural anti-inflammatory properties.
Multimineral complex	As directed on label.	Supplies important minerals. Needed to reduce stress. Use a formula high in calcium.
Silica or horsetail	As directed on label, twice daily.	Supplies silicon, which aids in absorption of calcium and repair of connective tissues. *See under* Herbs, on next page.

Helpful		
Kelp or alfalfa	1,000–1,500 mg daily.	Contains a balance of essential minerals plus chlorophyll, which cleanses the blood. *See under* Herbs, below.
Raw thymus glandular	As directed on label.	Improves thymus function—important for immune function.
VitaCarte from Phoenix BioLabs	As directed on label.	Contains bovine cartilage, which has been shown to be effective in reducing inflammation.

HERBS

❑ Alfalfa is a good source of minerals and chlorophyll.

❑ Bilberry contains flavonoids that reduce inflammation.

❑ Echinacea, goldenseal, pau d'arco, red clover, and yucca are all good for inflammation.

Caution: Do not take goldenseal internally on a daily basis for more than one week at a time, do not use during pregnancy, and use with caution if you are allergic to ragweed.

❑ A poultice that combines fenugreek, flaxseed, and slippery elm can be applied directly to the affected area to subdue inflammation. As an alternative, a goldenseal or mustard poultice can be used. *See* USING A POULTICE in Part Three.

❑ Horsetail extract is a good source of silica, beneficial for healing and repair of bones and connective tissue.

RECOMMENDATIONS

❑ Eat a diet composed of 75 percent raw foods, and drink plenty of herbal teas and juices.

❑ Consume half of a fresh pineapple daily. This is one of the best remedies for swelling and inflammation. It should reduce the pain and swelling in two to six days. Only fresh pineapple (not canned) is effective.

❑ Avoid cola, sugar, white flour products, and junk foods.

❑ For quick results, *see* FASTING in Part Three and follow the program.

CONSIDERATIONS

❑ Bacterial arthritis, which causes painful inflammation of the joints, is usually associated with an infection elsewhere in the body, such as in the lungs, kidney, or gallbladder.

❑ The traditional methods for relieving inflammation are positioning the affected part properly (including splinting, if necessary), applying heat and/or ice (heat and cold therapies), taking painkillers along with nutritional supplements, and getting plenty of rest.

❑ *See also* ABSCESS; ARTHRITIS; and SPRAINS, STRAINS, AND OTHER INJURIES OF THE MUSCLES AND JOINTS, all in Part Two.

❑ *See also* PAIN CONTROL in Part Three.

Influenza

Influenza, better known as "the flu," is a highly contagious viral infection of the upper respiratory tract. Because this illness can be spread easily by coughing and sneezing, influenza epidemics are very common, especially in winter. More than 200 different viruses can cause colds and flu, and strains of these viruses are constantly changing, so vaccinations against influenza have been only partly successful in preventing outbreaks of the disease.

The symptoms of influenza begin much like those of the common cold—headache, fatigue, and body aches. In many cases, a fever develops, and you may feel unbearably hot one moment and chilled and shaking the next. Most influenza sufferers have a dry throat and cough. Nausea and vomiting may occur as well. Often, a person with the flu is so weak and so uncomfortable that he or she does not feel like eating or doing anything else.

Influenza is rarely dangerous in healthy adults sixty years of age or younger, but it does make a person more susceptible to pneumonia, ear infections, and sinus trouble. Among people sixty-five or older, serious respiratory infections such as pneumonia and influenza are the fifth leading cause of death, so the flu is clearly a serious infection for older people.

NUTRIENTS

SUPPLEMENT	SUGGESTED DOSAGE	COMMENTS
Essential		
ACES + Zinc from Carlson Labs	As directed on label.	Contains vitamins A, C, and E, plus selenium and zinc. Take this supplement in addition to zinc lozenges as directed below.
Vitamin A plus natural beta-carotene or carotenoid complex (Betatene)	15,000 IU daily. If you are pregnant, do not exceed 10,000 IU daily. 15,000 IU daily. As directed on label.	A powerful antioxidant and immunity booster. A precursor of vitamin A.
Vitamin C with bioflavonoids	5,000–20,000 mg daily, in divided doses. *See* ASCORBIC ACID FLUSH in Part Three.	Strengthens the immune system by increasing the number and quality of white blood cells. For a child, use buffered vitamin C or calcium ascorbate.
Zinc lozenges (Ultimate Zinc-C Lozenges from Now Foods)	For adults and children over 6 years of age, one 15-mg lozenge every two hours for 2 days, starting at the first signs of the flu. Then reduce dosage to a total of 80 mg or less daily.	A potent immunostimulant that nourishes the cells. Keep these on hand and use them as soon as symptoms develop.
Important		
Free-form amino acid complex	As directed on label.	Helps to repair tissue and control fever. Free-form amino acids are rapidly absorbed into the body.

Garlic (Kyolic)	2 capsules 3 times daily.	Has antiviral and antibacterial properties.
L-Lysine	500 mg daily, on an empty stomach. Take with water or juice. Do not take with milk. Take with 50 mg vitamin B$_6$ and 100 mg vitamin C for better absorption.	Aids in combating viral infection and preventing outbreaks of cold sores in and around the mouth, common when the body is under stress from illness. See AMINO ACIDS in Part One. Caution: Do not take lysine longer than 6 months at a time.

Helpful		
Bifido Factor from Natren or	As directed on label.	For adults. Replaces "friendly" bacteria and acts as an antibiotic.
LifeStart from Natren	As directed on label.	For infants and children.
ClearLungs from Natural Alternatives		*See under* Herbs, below.
Dioxychlor from American Biologics	10–20 drops sublingually, 1–2 times daily. Also, add 20 drops to 1 oz water and instill a dropperful in each nostril daily.	An important antibacterial, antifungal, and antiviral agent. Especially good for elderly people.
Fenu-Thyme from Nature's Way		*See under* Herbs, below.
Maitake or	As directed on label.	Helps to boost immunity and fight viral infection.
shiitake or	As directed on label.	
reishi	As directed on label.	
Multivitamin and mineral complex with		All vitamins are needed for healing.
vitamin B complex	100 mg daily.	Necessary in all cellular and enzyme functions. Reduces stress caused by viral infection.
and selenium	100–200 mcg daily.	Boosts the immune response, enhancing the body's ability to fight infection.

HERBS

❑ If it is necessary to lower fever, take catnip tea enemas and ¼–½ teaspoon lobelia tincture every three to four hours until fever drops. This is good for children also.

Caution: Do not use this mixture if you are pregnant or breastfeeding, and do not give it to a child under one year old. Do not take lobelia internally on an ongoing basis.

❑ Echinacea, ginger, goldenseal, pau d'arco, slippery elm, and yarrow tea are good for influenza. Combining peppermint tea with any of these herbal teas is effective for helping to open up the nasal passages.

Caution: Do not take goldenseal internally on a daily basis for more than one week at a time, do not use it during pregnancy, and use it with caution if you are allergic to ragweed.

❑ Alcohol-free echinacea and goldenseal combination extract is recommended for children. Give a child 4 to 6 drops of combination extract in water or juice every four hours for three days. Echinacea is very effective at enhancing the body's own natural defenses. Goldenseal is a natural antibiotic and helps to relieve congestion.

❑ Cayenne (capsicum) helps to keep mucus flowing, aiding in preventing congestion and headaches. Simply add a bit of cayenne powder to soups and other foods.

❑ ClearLungs from Natural Alternatives is an herbal combination that reduces inflammation and protects the lungs. Take 2 capsules three times daily.

❑ At the first sign of a cough, place one dropperful of alcohol-free echinacea and goldenseal extract in your mouth and hold it there for five to ten minutes. Repeat this every hour for three to four hours. This stops the virus from multiplying.

❑ Ephedra (ma huang) is beneficial for relief of congestion and coughing.

Caution: Do not use this herb if you suffer from anxiety, glaucoma, heart disease, high blood pressure, or insomnia, or if you are taking a monoamine oxidase (MAO) inhibitor drug.

❑ Eucalyptus oil is beneficial for relieving congestion. Put 5 drops in a hot bath or 6 drops in a cup of boiling water, put a towel over your head, and inhale the vapors.

❑ Fenugreek breaks up phlegm and mucus, and slippery elm helps remove them from the body.

❑ Fenu-Thyme from Nature's Way helps to rid the nose and sinuses of mucus by loosening it so it can flow easily. It does not dry up the mucus, so healing is faster.

❑ For cough and sore throat, mix 1 tablespoon of slippery elm bark powder with 1 cup of boiling water and ½ cup honey. Take 1 teaspoon of this mixture every three to four hours. It can be taken either hot or cold, as you prefer.

RECOMMENDATIONS

❑ Consume plenty of fluids, especially fresh juices, herbal teas, soups, and quality water, to prevent dehydration and help flush out the body.

❑ Take hot chicken or turkey soup. This is grandmother's old remedy and it is still good today. Add a bit of cayenne pepper to help prevent and break up congestion.

❑ Sleep and rest as much as possible.

❑ Drink kombucha tea. This beverage has antiviral and immune-boosting properties. *See* MAKING KOMBUCHA TEA in Part Three.

❑ In treating a sore throat, avoid using aspirin chewing gum and aspirin gargles. Aspirin applied directly to mucous membranes does not reduce pain and can act as an irritant.

❑ Do not take zinc at the same time you eat or drink citrus fruits or juices. It will diminish the effectiveness of the zinc. Do consume a lot of other types of fruit.

❑ Do not give aspirin to a child who has the flu. The combination of aspirin and a viral illness has been linked to the development of Reye's syndrome, a potentially dangerous complication. (*See* REYE'S SYNDROME in Part Two.)

❑ If you consume alcoholic beverages even occasionally, or if you have liver or kidney disease, be cautious about using the painkiller acetaminophen (Tylenol, Datril, and others). The combination of alcohol and acetaminophen has been associated with serious liver problems.

❑ If you are over sixty-five, see your health care provider. Influenza can cause serious complications for people in this age group.

CONSIDERATIONS

❑ Antibiotics are useless against viral illnesses like influenza. The best way to get rid of the flu or any other infectious illness is to attack it head-on by strengthening the immune system. The thymus and the adrenal glands are the power seat of the immune system. When the body is getting sick, or already is sick, it is under stress, and stress taxes the immune system. Researchers have linked vulnerability to colds and flu to psychological stress.

❑ We do not recommend flu shots. Their usefulness is questionable, and the side effects may be worse than the flu would be. Enhancement of immune function is preferable—and safer.

❑ Dyslexia, a learning disability, appears to occur most often in summer babies than in babies born at other times of the year. Some researchers theorize this may be connected to flu contracted by women who are pregnant during the winter. Pregnant women should try to minimize their exposure to the virus.

❑ Children who have the flu frequently should be checked for thyroid malfunctions. (*See* HYPOTHYROIDISM in Part Two.)

❑ The term "stomach flu" is commonly used to refer to another condition, gastroenteritis. This is not influenza, but an acute inflammation of the lining of the stomach. Gastroenteritis is characterized by diarrhea, vomiting, and abdominal cramps that vary in severity, and may be accompanied by fever, chills, head and body aches, chest pain and cough, and extreme fatigue. It may be caused by a number of different factors, including food poisoning, viral infection, alcohol intoxication, sensitivity to drugs, and certain allergies. This type of illness usually runs its course in one or two days.

❑ *See also* COMMON COLD and PNEUMONIA, both in Part Two.

Insect Allergy

There are only a few stinging insects in the United States that can cause an allergic reaction: honeybees, hornets, yellow jackets, bumblebees, wasps, spiders, and ants. Insects of the group known as *hymenoptera*, which includes bees, wasps, hornets, and ants, cause an allergic reaction in 5 out of 1,000 people. This reaction is known as an insect venom allergy, and it can be dangerous, even life threatening. The yellow jacket and honeybee are the cause of most allergic reactions to insects.

Allergic reactions to stings can cause wheezing, tightness in the throat, nausea, diarrhea, hives, itching, pain and swelling in the joints, vascular swelling, and respiratory distress. A person who is highly allergic to insect venom can go into shock (circulatory collapse) and die within minutes. Signs that a dangerous reaction is developing include confusion, difficulty swallowing, hoarseness, labored breathing, severe swelling, weakness, and a feeling of impending disaster. A more severe reaction results in closing of the airway and/or shock, producing unconsciousness.

Some biting insects, such as mosquitos, can cause allergic skin reactions that appear as scaly and itchy eczema.

NUTRIENTS

SUPPLEMENT	SUGGESTED DOSAGE	COMMENTS
Essential		
Quercetin (Activated Quercetin from Source Naturals)	As directed on label.	A unique bioflavonoid that reduces allergic reactions.
Vitamin C	5,000–20,000 mg daily, in divided doses. *See* ASCORBIC ACID FLUSH in Part Three.	Acts as an anti-inflammatory and helps fight the toxicity of insect venom. For a child, use buffered vitamin C or calcium ascorbate.
Helpful		
Aller Bee-Gone from CC Pollen	As directed on label.	A combination of herbs, enzymes, and nutrients designed to fight acute allergic symptoms.

HERBS

❑ Herbal flea-repellent pet collars contain oils of cedar, citronella, eucalyptus, pennyroyal, rosemary, and rue. These herbs may be effective insect repellents for humans as well.

Caution: Do not use pennyroyal or rue during pregnancy. Avoid excessive and/or prolonged use.

❑ Tea tree oil can be rubbed on exposed areas of skin to deter insects. It can also be applied to bites. If pure tea tree oil is too strong, dilute it with canola oil or another low-fragrance vegetable oil until a tolerable strength is achieved.

RECOMMENDATIONS

❑ To avoid insect stings, wear plain, light-colored clothing when spending time outdoors—avoid wearing anything that is flowered or dark. Do not wear perfume, suntan lotion, hair spray, or shiny jewelry. Avoid wearing sandals or loose-fitting clothes.

❑ If you have ever had an allergic reaction to an insect sting, you should have access to an epinephrine (adrenaline) kit at all times. Have your physician prescribe an emergency treatment kit and instruct you in its proper use. Epinephrine raises the blood pressure and speeds the heart rate, counteracting the allergic response. It is best administered via a preloaded syringe found in injection kits.

❑ If you are bothered by a yellow jacket, do not squash it; doing so releases a chemical that attracts other yellow jackets and wasps. It is best to leave these insects alone, or to find and destroy the nest after dark, when they are less active.

❑ If you do get stung, *immediately and carefully* remove any stinger left in the skin. It is best not to pull the stinger out. Instead, gently and carefully scrape or tease it out with a sterilized knife. If no knife is readily available, you can use a fingernail or even the edge of a credit card instead. After a sting, be alert for signs that a reaction is developing. Reactions can occur in minutes or hours, and they can progress very quickly. If you have any doubts about your condition, seek treatment at once.

❑ As soon as possible after a bite or sting, soften charcoal tablets or capsules (these can be obtained from health food stores) in warm water and make a paste. Apply this paste to the site and cover it with a clean wet piece of gauze or cotton. It is a good idea to take a few charcoal tablets with you whenever you will spending time outdoors.

CONSIDERATIONS

❑ Sometimes brewer's yeast or garlic rubbed on the skin deters insects. Eating garlic may help also.

❑ A venom extractor called the Lil Sucker is available from International Reforestation Suppliers. It is small enough to fit inside a pocket or purse. If you get stung, it produces a vacuum that sucks the venom out within two minutes. The end of the extractor can also be used to remove a honeybee stinger. For more information about this product, call 800–321–1037.

❑ Antihistamines given by injection or by mouth following a sting can reduce later-appearing symptoms.

❑ *See also* BEE STING; INSECT BITE; and/or SPIDER BITE in Part Two.

Insect Bite

Many different insects bite, including mosquitoes, ants, fleas, gnats, and ticks. Spiders, while not technically insects, can cause similar bites. Most insect bites are a nuisance, causing localized itching and redness, but are relatively harmless. Others can be serious. Tick bites can spread diseases such as babesiosis, Lyme disease, or Rocky Mountain spotted fever. In some places (principally in developing countries), mosquito bites may transmit malaria and yellow fever, as well as viruses that cause encephalitis (inflammation of the brain).

NUTRIENTS

SUPPLEMENT	SUGGESTED DOSAGE	COMMENTS
Essential		
Quercetin (Activated Quercetin from Source Naturals)	As directed on label.	A unique bioflavonoid that reduces allergic reactions.
Vitamin C with bioflavonoids	5,000–20,000 mg daily, in divided doses. *See* ASCORBIC ACID FLUSH in Part Three.	An anti-inflammatory that is helpful for relieving the toxicity of bites. For a child, use buffered vitamin C or calcium ascorbate.

HERBS

❑ Calendula ointment is an excellent insect repellent and counterirritant.

❑ Citronella candles are good for repelling mosquitoes.

❑ Goldenseal and tea tree oil are natural insecticides and help to keep insects at bay.

❑ Poultices made with lobelia and charcoal are helpful for insect bites. *See* USING A POULTICE in Part Three.

❑ Pennyroyal oil helps to repel insects.
Caution: Do not use this herb during pregnancy. Avoid excessive and/or prolonged use.

RECOMMENDATIONS

❑ For ant, mosquito, or chigger bites, wash the area thoroughly with soap and water. For chigger bites, use a brush and scrub. Then apply a paste made of baking soda and water. Use ice packs if swelling occurs.

❑ For tick bites, remove the tick as quickly as you can. The sooner the tick is removed, the less chance there is of contracting any disease the tick may be carrying. Using tweezers, grasp the head of the tick firmly, as close to the skin as possible, and pull straight back with the tweezers. Try not to leave the head or any other part of the tick embedded in the skin. Do not touch the tick with your hands. Once it has been removed, scrub the bite with soap and water. *Do not* try to burn the tick out, or use home remedies like kerosene, turpentine, or petroleum jelly.

❑ Make a paste using a charcoal capsule and a few drops of goldenseal extract and place it on a piece of gauze. Apply the gauze to the bite and cover it with a bandage. This will draw out the poisons and aid in fast relief. Do this immediately after being bitten, if possible.

❑ To avoid mosquito bites, eat brown rice, brewer's yeast, wheat germ, blackstrap molasses, or fish before spending time outside. These foods are rich in vitamin B$_1$ (thiamine). Mosquitoes are attracted by carbon dioxide, estrogens, moisture, sweat, and warmth. They appear to be repelled by B vitamins, especially thiamine, which are excreted through the skin. As an alternative, take thiamine supplements.

❑ Apply calamine lotion to help relieve itching.

❑ To avoid many insect bites, try taking a chlorine bleach bath before going out. Add 1 cup of bleach per tub of water. Insects dislike the smell. Swimming in a pool treated with chlorine also works. Rubbing brewer's yeast or garlic on the skin may deter insects as well.

❑ Avoid all refined sugar, which causes the skin to give off a sweet smell that attracts mosquitoes.

❑ Avoid alcoholic drinks. Alcohol causes the skin to flush and the blood vessels to dilate, which attracts mosquitos and horseflies.

❑ Avoid using perfume, hair spray, and other cosmetics. These attract insects.

CONSIDERATIONS

❑ Diethyl toluamide (deet) works to repel chiggers, ticks, and mosquitos. It is probably the most effective insect repellent known, but it is also potentially quite toxic, and it can destroy substances such as plastics and synthetic fabrics, so it must be used with care and only in accordance with package directions.

❑ If you spend much time outdoors, you may want to purchase a vacuum pump called the Lil Sucker to extract the poison from insect bites. This pump is painless to use, and in one study, 94 percent of participants who used it had either no reaction or a minor one to an insect bite. Lil Sucker is sold by International Reforestation Suppliers. They can be contacted at 800–321–1037.

❑ *See also* BEE STING; INSECT ALLERGY; LYME DISEASE; and/or SPIDER BITE, all in Part Two.

Insomnia

Habitual sleeplessness, repeated night after night, is classified as insomnia. Insomnia can take the form of being unable to fall asleep when you first go to bed, or waking during the night and being unable to go back to sleep. An estimated 15 to 17 percent of the population suffers from insomnia at any given time. While insomnia can be very frustrating, it is hardly dangerous and is usually only a temporary annoyance, although in some cases sleep-related problems can last for months or even years.

Insomnia can result from a wide variety of causes, including hypoglycemia, muscle aches, indigestion, breathing problems, physical pain, anxiety, stress, grief, depression, jet lag, caffeine consumption, and the use of certain drugs, including the decongestant pseudoephedrine (found in many cold and allergy remedies), most appetite suppressants, many antidepressants, beta-blockers (medications used for high blood pressure and heart ailments), the antiseizure medication phenytoin (Dilantin), and thyroid hormone replacement drugs.

A lack of the nutrients calcium and magnesium can cause you to wake up after a few hours and not be able to return to sleep. Systemic disorders involving the lungs, liver, heart, kidneys, pancreas, digestive system, endocrine system, and brain all may affect sleep, as can poor nutritional habits and eating too close to bedtime. A sedentary lifestyle can be a major contributor to sleep disorders.

While one or two sleepless nights can cause irritability and daytime sleepiness, with decreased ability to perform creative or repetitive tasks, most people can adapt to short-term periods of sleep deprivation. After more than three days, however, sleep deprivation begins to cause a more serious deterioration in overall performance and can even result in mild personality changes. If chronic, inadequate sleep compromises productivity, creates problems in relationships, and can contribute to other health problems.

There are no hard and fast rules about how much sleep is enough, because every individual's requirements are different. Some people can function on as little as five hours of sleep a night, while others seem to perform better with nine, ten, or even more hours of sleep. Most adults need about eight hours of sleep nightly in order to feel refreshed and operate at peak efficiency during the day. Children, especially very young children and adolescents, generally require more sleep than adults to be at their best. It is not uncommon for people to sleep less as they get older, especially after the age of sixty.

Millions of people have trouble getting to sleep due to a condition commonly known as *restless leg syndrome*. For reasons unknown, when these people are in bed, their legs jerk, twitch, and kick involuntarily. Restless leg syndrome has also been linked to the painful nighttime leg muscle cramps that afflict so many people.

Sleep apnea is a potentially serious disorder that can cause repeated waking during the night. This problem is commonly associated with snoring and extremely irregular breathing throughout the night. In sleep apnea, breathing actually stops, for as long as two minutes at a time, while the individual is asleep. When breathing stops, the level of oxygen in the blood drops, resulting in oxygen deprivation. The individual then awakens, startled and gasping. A person with sleep apnea may awaken as many as 200 times throughout the night. The affected individual may not remember these awakenings, but anyone else who is awake at the time can naturally become alarmed when a person with sleep apnea stops breathing.

Aside from disrupting normal sleep and causing extreme sleepiness during the day, sleep apnea is associated with other, more serious, health problems. People who suffer from sleep apnea tend to have higher than normal blood pressure and are more likely to have strokes than the general population, and face an increased risk of heart disease, although the reason or reasons for these links are not known. People with sleep apnea also seem to have a higher than normal incidence of emotional and psychotic disorders. Experts attribute this to what they call a "dream deficit"—a lack of adequate rapid-eye-movement (REM) sleep, the stage of sleep in which dreaming occurs. A person with sleep apnea often cannot settle into REM sleep for even the eight to twelve seconds it takes to have a normal, healthy dream. While there is much about the phenomenon of dreaming that is not understood, it is known that prolonged periods of REM sleep deprivation can induce various psychoses and other serious emotional disorders.

NUTRIENTS

SUPPLEMENT	SUGGESTED DOSAGE	COMMENTS
Important		
Calcium	1,500–2,000 mg daily, in divided doses, after meals and at bedtime.	Has a calming effect. Use calcium lactate or calcium chelate form (do not use lactate form if you are allergic to dairy products.)
and magnesium	1,000 mg daily.	Needed to balance with calcium and relax the muscles.
Melatonin	Start with 1.5 mg daily, taken 2 hours or less before bedtime. If this is not effective, gradually increase the dosage until an effective level is reached (up to 5 mg daily).	A natural hormone that promotes sound sleep.
Helpful		
Vitamin B complex plus extra	As directed on label.	Helps to promote a restful state.
pantothenic acid (vitamin B5) and	50 mg daily.	Good for relieving stress.
inositol	100 mg daily, at bedtime.	Enhances REM sleep.

HERBS

❑ California poppy, hops, kava kava, passionflower, skullcap, and valerian root, taken in capsule or extract form, are all good for helping to overcome insomnia. It is best not to rely on one herb on a regular basis, but to rotate among several. Take these herbs before bedtime.

❑ Catnip and chamomile have mild sedative properties. These herbs are safe even for children if taken in tea form. For adults, drinking chamomile tea several times throughout the day helps to calm and tone the nervous system, promoting restful sleep.

❑ A combination herbal extract such as Slumber from Nature's Answer or Silent Night from Nature's Way can be helpful.

RECOMMENDATIONS

❑ Avoid alcohol. A small amount can help induce sleep initially, but it invariably disrupts deeper sleep cycles later.

❑ Avoid tobacco. While smoking may seem to have a calming effect, nicotine is actually a neurostimulant and can cause sleep problems.

❑ Avoid caffeine-containing beverages after lunch.

❑ In the evening, eat turkey, bananas, figs, dates, yogurt, milk, tuna, and whole grain crackers or nut butter. These foods are high in tryptophan, which promotes sleep. Eating a grapefruit half at bedtime also helps.

❑ Avoid bacon, cheese, chocolate, eggplant, ham, potatoes, sauerkraut, sugar, sausage, spinach, tomatoes, and wine close to bedtime. These foods contain tyramine, which increases the release of norepinephrine, a brain stimulant.

❑ Avoid taking nasal decongestants and other cold medications late in the day. While many ingredients in these preparations are known to cause drowsiness, they can have the opposite effect on some people and act as a stimulant.

❑ Establish a set of habits and follow them consistently to establish a healthy sleep cycle. Among them:

• Go to bed only when you are sleepy.

• Do not stay in bed if you are not sleepy. Get up and move to another room and read, watch television, or do something quietly until you are really sleepy.

• Use the bedroom only for sleep and sex—not for reading, working, eating, or watching television.

• Set an alarm clock and get out of bed at the same time every morning, no matter how you slept the night before. Once normal sleep patterns are reestablished, most people find that they have no need for an alarm clock.

• Do not nap during the day if this isn't a normal thing for you to do.

• Exercise regularly in the late afternoon or early evening—but not right before bedtime. Physical exertion is an excellent way to make your body tired so that sleep comes about more easily.

• Take a hot bath (not a shower) an hour or two before bedtime.

• Keep the bedroom comfortable and quiet. If *too much* quiet is the problem, try running a fan or playing a radio softly in the background. There are also devices available that generate "white noise" sounds like the ocean surf or a steady rain that help people who are "quiet-sensitive" to sleep.

• Learn to put worries out of your mind. If you have occasional trouble getting to sleep, concentrate on pleasant memories and thoughts. Recreate a pleasurable time or event in your life and relive it in your mind. Learning a relaxation technique such as meditation or the use of guided imagery is extremely helpful in getting sleep patterns back to normal for many people.

❑ For occasional sleeplessness, try using melatonin, Calcium Night from Source Naturals, or one of the herbs recommended above. These are effective and safe sleep-promoters.

CONSIDERATIONS

❑ A program of regular exercise improves sleep quality. provided the exercise is not undertaken too close to bedtime.

❑ Regardless of how many hours of sleep you get each night, if you wake up easily in the morning, and especially if you rarely (if ever) need the services of your alarm clock, and if you can make it through the entire day without seeming to run out of steam or feeling drowsy after sitting quietly or reading for a while, you are probably getting enough sleep.

❑ Research psychologist Dr. James Penland believes that a large number of women are suffering from copper and iron deficiencies, and that these deficiencies can cause insomnia. A hair analysis can reveal whether you have a deficiency. (*See* HAIR ANALYSIS in Part Three.)

❑ Various treatments have been attempted for restless leg syndrome, but nothing seems to work consistently for everyone. Some research strongly suggests that anemia may play a major role in this annoying disorder. We believe that taking the proper vitamin and mineral supplements is the best approach to this problem. The supplements that help this condition more than anything are calcium, potassium, magnesium, and zinc.

❑ Anyone who snores excessively should be evaluated for sleep apnea and be evaluated for treatment. Many cases of sleep apnea respond to measures such as allergy treatment, weight reduction, or a simple laser surgery procedure to remove obstructions in the nasal passages.

❑ Many people who suffer from insomnia resort to sleeping pills, whether over-the-counter or prescription medications. Sleeping pills do not cure insomnia, however, and they can interfere with REM sleep. The continued use of pharmacological sleeping aids can eventually lead to disruption of all the deeper stages of sleep. Researchers have found that up to 50 percent of people who take sleeping pills on a regular basis actually find that their insomnia becomes worse. The persistent use of sleeping pills also leads to dependency, either psychological or physical. The use of sleep medication should therefore be reserved for those whose insomnia has a physical basis, and then only as a temporary solution.

❑ Triazolam (Halcion), one of the most popular prescription sleep medications in the United States, can cause mental confusion and even amnesia. There have also been reports that the use of drugs such as temazepam (Restoril), secobarbital (Seconal), flurazepam (Dalmane), and diazepam (Valium) may lead to confusion, sluggishness, restlessness, and heightened anxiety, as well as prolonged sedation and drug dependency.

❑ People who take sleeping pills on a regular basis are 50 percent more likely than other people to die in accidents. Drowsiness accounts for 200,000 to 400,000 automobile accidents every year, and is responsible for two thirds of all industrial mishaps, most common among shift workers in the early morning hours. Sleeping pills are also the third most commonly used means in suicide and are implicated in one third of all drug-related suicide attempts and deaths.

❑ Dehydroepisterone (DHEA) is a naturally occurring hormone that improves the quality of sleep. (*See* DHEA THERAPY in Part Three.)

❑ A new sleeping pill is being investigated by researchers that may help to overcome insomnia without having the undesirable side effects associated with other sleep-inducing medications. Called zolpidem (Ambien), the drug is supposed to work differently than any other sleep aid on the market. In addition, its manufacturer claims that it does not inhibit or disrupt the deep sleep cycles, like REM.

❑ Millions of Americans consciously choose to skimp on their sleep in the mistaken belief that sleeping fewer hours allows them to be more productive. Many people even look on the fact that they can "get by" on so few hours of sleep as a badge of honor. In fact, however, they are likely doing themselves a great deal of harm in the long run. Moreover, the night owls who sleep less to accomplish more are actually less creative and less productive than those who get adequate amounts of sleep. Dr. Richard Bootzin, professor of psychology and director of the insomnia clinic at the University of Arizona Sleep Disorders Center, conducted long-term research into normal sleep habits and patterns. He discovered that people who get seven to eight hours of sleep each night live longer, happier, healthier lives than those who skimp on their sleep.

❑ Sleep therapists and other experts are greatly divided about the virtues of napping. While some maintain that napping is not necessary for people who are well rested, others say it is a natural human tendency and should not be discouraged. There have been studies that seem to demonstrate that productivity is higher and the incidence of accidents lower in countries where napping is common. Consistency is probably the most important factor. While it is usually most advisable to consolidate all sleeping into one time period, if you regularly take an afternoon nap and you do not suffer from any sleeping disorders, then giving up naps might actually cause a disruption in your sleeping habits. If you nap, keep your naps short—less than an hour—and make sure that they are a *regular* part of the daily routine, not a now-and-then proposition.

❑ Sleep experts advise that people with insomnia avoid caffeine, but many people who are accustomed to drinking coffee late in the day and in the evening hours have been known to have their sleep cycles disrupted if they give up their coffee. This seems to bear out the idea that maintaining a steady routine is the most important factor in establishing a healthy sleep pattern. Of course, this applies only to those who are not experiencing any difficulties with their sleeping habits. Anyone who develops a bout of insomnia should consider eliminating all caffeine from his or her diet.

❑ Over-the-counter sleep aids can cause a wide range of side effects, including agitation, confusion, depression, dry mouth, and worsening of symptoms of enlarged prostate.

❑ *See also under* PREGNANCY-RELATED PROBLEMS.

Intertrigo

Intertrigo is a type of dermatitis or skin inflammation caused by the repeated friction of skin rubbing against skin. It can appear anywhere two skin surfaces lie next to each other and rub together, but most often occurs in the skin folds of the groin and underarms, and between the ribs and the breasts. This condition is most common in warm climates and during the summer.

Intertrigo appears as a reddish rash that may be sore or itchy. It usually progresses gradually, beginning as a mild chafing, then slowly, with continued exposure to moisture and friction, develops into a persistent itchy rash. Occasionally, a secondary infection (bacterial or fungal) may develop, causing the formation of pustules and weeping and oozing of the skin, as well as severe itching and pain. Severe intertrigo on the groin or thighs can impede mobility.

Intertrigo primarily affects overweight women who perspire heavily. People with diabetes also are more disposed than others to developing intertrigo and accompanying secondary infections. Persons who suffer from urinary incontinence are at increased risk of developing intertrigo in the groin area.

NUTRIENTS

SUPPLEMENT	SUGGESTED DOSAGE	COMMENTS
Important		
AE Mulsion Forte from American Biologics and	As directed on label.	To aid in tissue repair and healing. Supplies vitamins A and E in emulsion form, which enters the system more rapidly.
natural carotenoid complex (Betatene)	As directed on label.	Contains free radical scavengers and immune enhancers.
Essential fatty acids (primrose oil and Ultimate Oil from Nature's Secret are good sources)	As directed on label.	Needed for tissue healing.
Free-form amino acid complex	As directed on label.	To supply protein, needed for tissue repair. Use a formula containing all the essential amino acids.
Garlic (Kyolic)	2 capsules 3 times daily, with meals.	Fights bacterial and fungal infection. Enhances immune function.
Silica gel	As directed on label.	To supply silicon, needed for repair of skin tissue.
Vitamin B complex	As directed on label.	Needed for protein metabolism, essential for healing and repair of skin tissue.
Vitamin C with bioflavonoids	10,000 mg daily and up.	Needed for tissue repair and healing. Also reduces scarring. Use an ascorbate form.
Zinc	50 mg daily. Do not exceed a total of 100 mg daily from all supplements.	Boosts the immune system and aids in tissue healing.

Helpful		
Aerobic 07 from Aerobic Life Industries or	9 drops in water 3 times daily.	For tissue oxygenation and to kill harmful bacteria and viruses.
Dioxychlor from American Biologics	As directed on label.	
All-Purpose Bactericide Spray from Aerobic Life Industries	Apply topically as directed on label.	Destroys bacteria on the skin, reducing the possibility of infection.
Aloe vera		*See under* Herbs, below.
Colloidal silver	Apply topically as directed on label.	An antiseptic to prevent infection, subdue inflammation, and promote healing.
Coenzyme Q10	60 mg daily.	An important free radical scavenger that supplies oxygen to the cells.
Dimethylglycine (DMG) (Aangamik DMG from FoodScience Labs)	As directed on label.	Increases oxygenation of tissue.
Herpanacine from Diamond-Herpanacine Associates	As directed on label.	A combination of vitamins, minerals, and herbs that is good for overall skin health.
Kelp	As directed on label.	Supplies balanced minerals needed for healthy skin.
Multivitamin and mineral complex	As directed on label.	All nutrients are necessary in balance.

HERBS

❑ Alfalfa, barley grass, dandelion root, horsetail, and parsley root nourish the skin and aid in healing.

❑ Aloe vera gel has excellent healing properties. Apply aloe vera gel to affected areas as directed on the product label or as needed.

❑ Calendula has anti-inflammatory properties, promotes cell formation, and stimulates tissue growth.

❑ Chamomile is an anti-inflammatory and antibacterial herb that soothes dry, blemished, and irritated skin.

❑ Tea tree oil has skin-healing properties. There are many personal hygiene products available that contain this ingredient.

RECOMMENDATIONS

❑ Add garlic, soured products, and acidophilus to the diet.

❑ Keep the skin surface clean, dry, and free of friction. Shower or bathe immediately following periods of heavy perspiration, and use a hair dryer on a cool setting instead of rubbing with a towel to dry the area. Then apply baby powder. Do this several times daily, or as often as needed.

❑ Use only natural, chemical-free soaps, deodorants, and other personal care preparations. Most health food stores carry such products. Avoid commercial products, which may contain substances that can further irritate the inflamed areas.

❑ Avoid sugar and other refined carbohydrates. Both bacteria and fungi thrive on sugar.

❑ Wear loose-fitting 100-percent-cotton clothing that does not rub against the skin.

❑ Avoid sitting in one position for prolonged periods.

CONSIDERATIONS

❑ Many intertrigo sufferers find relief by remaining unclothed whenever possible.

❑ Calamine lotion can be used to soothe irritated areas.

❑ Intertrigo usually responds quickly to treatment. However, if it is left untreated, it can become infected and painful.

❑ If intertrigo is complicated by a bacterial or fungal infection, an antibiotic may be prescribed. If you must take antibiotics, you should be sure to take some form of acidophilus to replace the necessary "friendly" bacteria.

❑ If itching is severe, an antihistamine may be prescribed.

❑ *See also* CANDIDIASIS in Part Two.

Irritable Bowel Syndrome

Irritable bowel syndrome (IBS) is the most common digestive disorder seen by physicians. It is estimated that about one in five adult Americans has symptoms of IBS, although fewer than half of them seek help for it. Twice as many women suffer from the condition as men. This disorder is also sometimes called intestinal neurosis, mucous colitis, spastic colitis, or spastic colon.

In IBS, the normally rhythmic muscular contractions of the digestive tract become irregular and uncoordinated. This interferes with the normal movement of food and waste material, and leads to the accumulation of mucus and toxins in the intestine. This accumulated material sets up a partial obstruction of the digestive tract, trapping gas and stools, which in turn causes bloating, distention, and constipation. IBS may affect the entire gastrointestinal tract, from the mouth through the colon.

Symptoms of IBS may include constipation and/or diarrhea (often alternating), abdominal pain, mucus in the stools, nausea, flatulence, bloating, anorexia, and intolerances to certain foods. Pain is often triggered by eating, and may be relieved by a bowel movement. Because of the pain, diarrhea, nausea, and sometimes severe headaches and even vomiting, a person with IBS may dread eating. Whether or not an individual with IBS eats normally, malnutrition may result, as nutrients often are not absorbed properly. As a result, people with IBS require as much as 30 percent more protein than normal, as well as an increased intake of minerals and trace elements, which can quickly be depleted by diarrhea.

There are no physical signs of disease in bowel tissue with this disorder, and its cause or causes are not well understood. Some scientists believe a virus or bacterium may play a role. Lifestyle factors such as stress and diet are probably common causes. The overuse of antibiotics, antacids, or laxatives, which disturb the bacterial microflora of the bowel, may also be a factor.

Many other diseases can be related to IBS, including candidiasis, colon cancer, diabetes mellitus, gallbladder disease, malabsorption disorders, pancreatic insufficiency, ulcers, and the parasitic infections amebiasis and giardiasis. Over 100 different disorders may be linked to the systemic effects of IBS. One disorder that is linked in about 25 percent of adults with IBS is arthritis, usually peripheral arthritis, which affects the ankles, knees, and wrists. Less frequently, the spine is affected. IBS can also be related to skin disorders, but this is unusual. Some people with IBS have abnormalities in the levels of liver enzymes in their blood.

Diagnosis of irritable bowel syndrome requires ruling out disorders that can cause similar symptoms, such as Crohn's disease, diverticulitis, lactose intolerance, and ulcerative colitis. A physician may recommend one or more of a variety of procedures to do this, including barium enema, colonoscopy, rectal biopsy, sigmoidoscopy, and stool examination to check for the presence of bacteria, blood, and/or parasites.

Irritable bowel syndrome is painful, but not serious, and most people who have it can lead active, productive lives if they change their diets, get regular exercise, and replace needed nutrients.

NUTRIENTS

SUPPLEMENT	SUGGESTED DOSAGE	COMMENTS
Very Important		
Alfalfa		*See under* Herbs, below.
Vitamin B complex plus extra vitamin B12	50–100 mg 3 times daily, with meals. 200 mcg twice daily.	Needed for proper muscle tone in the gastrointestinal tract. Needed for proper absorption of foods, protein synthesis, and metabolism of carbohydrates and fats, and to prevent anemia. Use a lozenge or sublingual form.
Important		
Acidophilus	As directed on label.	To replenish the "friendly" bacteria. Needed for digestion and for the manufacture of the B vitamins. Use a nondairy formula.
or Bio-Bifidus from American Biologics	As directed on label.	
or Kyo-Dophilus from Wakunaga	As directed on label.	
Aloe vera		*See under* Herbs, below.
Garlic (Kyolic)	As directed on label.	Aids in digestion and destruction of toxins in the colon. Liquid form is best.

Fiber (oat bran, flaxseeds, psyllium seeds, and Aerobic Bulk Cleanse (ABC) from Aerobic Life Industries are good sources)	As directed on label. Take separately from other supplements and medications.	Has both a healing and cleansing effect. Avoid wheat bran, as it may be too irritating.
Free-form amino acid complex	As directed on label.	Necessary for repair of mucous membranes of the intestines.
L-Glutamine	500 mg twice daily, on an empty stomach. Take with water or juice. Do not take with milk. Take with 50 mg vitamin B$_6$ and 100 mg vitamin C for better absorption.	A major metabolic fuel for the intestinal cells; maintains the villi, the absorption surfaces of the gut. See AMINO ACIDS in Part One.
Multivitamin and mineral complex	As directed on label.	Supplies those nutrients lost or not absorbed. Use a hypoallergenic formula.
N-Acetylglucosamine (N-A-G from Source Naturals)	As directed on label.	A major constituent of the intestinal lining and of the barrier layer that protects the intestinal lining from digestive enzymes and other potentially damaging intestinal contents.
Primrose oil or flaxseed oil	As directed on label. As directed on label.	To supply essential fatty acids needed to protect the intestinal lining.
Proteolytic enzymes with pancreatin	As directed on label.	To aid in protein digestion and prevention of "leaky gut syndrome." Also aids in reducing inflammation. Use a formula that is low in HCl and high in pancreatin.
Ultra Clear Sustain from Metagenics	As directed on label.	A complex that provides nutritional support for gastrointestinal mucosa. Available only through health care professionals.
Helpful		
Calcium and magnesium	2,000 mg daily. 1,000 mg daily.	Helps the "nervous stomach" and the central nervous system. Aids in preventing colon cancer. Use chelate forms.
Dioxychlor from American Biologics	As directed on label.	Destroys foreign bacteria in the digestive tract and carries oxygen to the tissues.
Shark cartilage (BeneFin)	As directed on label. If you cannot tolerate taking it orally, it can be administered rectally in a retention enema.	Fights growth and metastasis of cancerous tumors. IBS is associated with an increased risk of colon cancer.

HERBS

❑ If you have IBS, it is wise to treat your liver as well as your digestive tract, preferably with silymarin (milk thistle extract). Licorice can also be used. Other beneficial herbs are burdock root and red clover, which are good for cleansing the bloodstream, and thereby the liver.

Caution: If overused, licorice can elevate blood pressure. Do not use this herb on a daily basis for more than seven days in a row. Avoid it completely if you have high blood pressure.

❑ Alfalfa contains vitamin K, needed to build intestinal flora for proper digestion, and chlorophyll for healing and cleansing of the bloodstream. It can be taken in liquid or tablet form.

❑ Aloe vera is healing to the digestive tract. Used in combination with Aerobic Bulk Cleanse (ABC) from Aerobic Life Industries, it helps to keep the colon walls clean of excess mucus and slow down food reactions. Take ½ cup of aloe vera juice three times daily, on an empty stomach.

❑ Peppermint aids in healing and digestion, and also relieves upset stomach and gas or that "too-full" feeling. It must be taken in enteric-coated capsule form to prevent the oil from being released before it reaches the colon. Do not take any other form, or heartburn may result.

❑ Skullcap and valerian root are helpful for the nerves that regulate intestinal muscle function. These are good taken at bedtime or when an upset occurs.

❑ Other herbs that can be beneficial for irritable bowel syndrome include balm, chamomile, fenugreek, ginger, goldenseal, lobelia, marshmallow, pau d'arco, rose hips, and slippery elm.

Caution: Do not use chamomile or lobelia on an ongoing basis. Avoid chamomile completely if you are allergic to ragweed. Do not take goldenseal internally on a daily basis for more than one week at a time, do not use it in large quantities during pregnancy, and use it with caution if you are allergic to ragweed.

RECOMMENDATIONS

❑ Eat a high-fiber diet including plenty of fruits and vegetables, plus whole grains (especially brown rice) and legumes.

❑ Use supplemental fiber. Psyllium powder regulates bowel movements and should be used daily. Also use oat bran and ground flaxseeds daily, on an alternating basis.

❑ Avoid animal fats, butter, all carbonated beverages, coffee and all other substances containing caffeine, candy, chocolate, all dairy products, fried foods, ice cream, all junk foods, the additives mannitol and sorbitol, margarine, nuts, orange and grapefruit juices, pastries, all processed foods, seeds, spicy foods, sugar, sugar-free chewing gum, and wheat bran and wheat products. These foods encourage the secretion of mucus by the membranes and prevent the uptake of nutrients.

❑ Avoid alcohol and tobacco; these irritate the linings of the stomach and colon.

❑ When an intestinal upset occurs, switch to a bland diet. Put vegetables and nonacidic fruits through a food processor or blender. Organic baby food is good. If you are on a soft diet, take some type of fiber and a protein supplement.

❑ To relieve occasional gas and bloating, use charcoal tablets (available in health food stores). Take 5 tablets as soon as this problem arises. Do not use charcoal daily, however, because it also absorbs needed nutrients, and do not take it at the same time as other supplements or medications.

❑ For excessive gas and bloating that lingers, read the section on ENEMAS in Part Three and follow the instructions for the *L. bifidus* retention enema. This will replace the "friendly" bacteria very quickly and resolve the problem. Exercise, such as stretching exercises, swimming, or walking, is also important.

❑ Check to see if you have food allergies; they are important factors in this disorder. Eliminating allergenic foods from the diet relieves symptoms in many cases. *See* ALLERGIES in Part Two.

❑ Chew your food well. Do not overeat or eat in a hurry.

❑ Practice deep breathing exercises. Shallow breathing reduces the oxygen available for proper bowel function.

❑ Wear loose-fitting clothing. Do not wear anything that is tight around the waist.

❑ Do not eat right before going to bed. Wait one or two hours after eating before lying down.

❑ *See* ACIDOSIS in Part Two and take the self-test. Significant acidosis may occur with IBS.

CONSIDERATIONS

❑ Eating the correct diet, using supplemental fiber, and drinking plenty of quality water are very important in controlling IBS. Early recognition of the disease, good nutrition, and a positive outlook help minimize complications.

❑ Enteric-coated peppermint capsules are used successfully in Europe for IBS.

❑ Certain foods irritate the wall of the intestinal tract. Lactose (milk sugar) is a common culprit, as are all dairy products.

❑ IBS should not be confused with the more serious bowel disorders, such as Crohn's disease and ulcerative colitis. These are also inflammatory bowel diseases but, unlike IBS, they result in demonstrable lesions in the digestive tract. Crohn's disease affects the entire length and thickness of the wall of the large and/or small intestine; ulcerative colitis affects the lining of the large intestine, the last five to seven feet of the digestive tract. (*See* CROHN'S DISEASE and/or ULCERATIVE COLITIS, both in Part Two.)

❑ People with IBS should receive regular physical examinations. This disorder has been linked to a higher than normal incidence of colon cancer and diverticulitis.

❑ If IBS causes chronic diarrhea, electrolyte and trace mineral deficiencies are likely. *See* DIARRHEA in Part Two for suggested mineral supplementation. *Also see* MALABSORPTION SYNDROME in Part Two.

❑ Certain drugs can aggravate the malabsorption problems often present with IBS. These include antibiotics, corticosteroids, cholestyramine (Questran), and sulfasalazine (Azulfidine), among others. These drugs increase the need for nutritional supplements.

❑ Research and testing have found not only that breathing exercises can control IBS, but that people who practice stress management have fewer and less severe attacks. Stress management also relieves symptoms. (*See* STRESS in Part Two.)

❑ The symptoms of IBS are similar to those of many other disorders, including cancer. If dietary modification and natural remedies yield no relief, it is wise to consult a physician to rule out some other underlying problem. We recommend this only after natural remedies have been tried, however.

❑ *See also* HEARTBURN; INDIGESTION; and/or DIVERTICULITIS in Part Two.

Jaundice

Jaundice is a yellowing of the skin and eyes that is caused by a buildup of bilirubin in the blood. Bilirubin is a yellow-brown substance that results from the breakdown of old red blood cells. If this waste product is not removed from the bloodstream by the liver, as it should be, a backup of bilirubin in the blood occurs, producing a yellowing of the skin and the whites of the eyes. The urine may be darker than normal, while the stools may appear lighter.

Jaundice is not a disease in itself, but a sign of any one of several blood or liver disorders. Among the conditions that can cause jaundice are cirrhosis of the liver, pernicious anemia, hepatitis, and hemolysis (abnormal destruction of red blood cells). Jaundice can also be a sign of an obstruction in the path of the bile flow, from the liver through the bile ducts to the gallbladder and then to the intestinal tract. If the biliary tract is obstructed, the bile (which contains bilirubin) passes back into the bloodstream instead of into the digestive system, producing jaundice. Occasionally, jaundice is caused by some form of parasitic infestation such as tapeworm or hookworm, or a bite from a flea or mosquito that carries a viral, bacterial, or parasitic infection. It can also be caused by a tumor, a gallstone, or inflammation.

Some degree of jaundice is common in newborn babies, especially premature babies, and is not considered serious. It occurs because a new baby's liver is limited in its ability to process bilirubin, and in most cases soon resolves itself.

NUTRIENTS

SUPPLEMENT	SUGGESTED DOSAGE	COMMENTS
Very Important		
Burdock root or red clover		*See under* Herbs, on next page.

Dandelion extract	*See under* Herbs, below.	
Milk thistle extract or Liv-R-Actin from Nature's Plus	*See under* Herbs, below.	
L-Glutathione and L-methionine	500 mg each daily, on an empty stomach. Take with water or juice. Do not take with milk. Take with 50 mg vitamin B_6 and 100 mg vitamin C for better absorption.	Substances that work together to protect the liver. *See* AMINO ACIDS in Part One.

HERBS

❑ Burdock root and red clover aid in cleansing the blood.

❑ Dandelion extract aids in proper liver function.

❑ Silymarin, an active flavonoid extracted from the herb milk thistle, is known to repair damaged tissues in the liver. Liv-R-Actin from Nature's Plus is a good source of silymarin.

RECOMMENDATIONS

❑ Eat only raw vegetables and fruits for one week. Then eat a diet consisting of 75 percent raw food for a month. Take fresh lemon enemas daily during this period. *See* ENEMAS in Part Three.

❑ Drink the following juices: lemon juice and water, beet and beet greens, and dandelion or black radish extract. All are good for rebuilding and cleansing the liver.

❑ Never consume raw or undercooked fish, meat, or poultry. All raw fish pose a risk of infection from bacteria, parasites, and viruses.

❑ Do not consume *any* alcohol. Alcohol places a great strain on the liver, which can aggravate the condition further.

CONSIDERATIONS

❑ If jaundice is a result of a tumor or gallstone, surgery may be necessary to correct the problem.

❑ *See* CIRRHOSIS OF THE LIVER and HEPATITIS, both in Part Two, for additional nutritional and dietary suggestions.

Jock Itch

See under FUNGAL INFECTION.

Kaposi's Sarcoma

See under SKIN CANCER.

Kidney Disease

There are a number of different kidney problems that may occur. The kidneys may be damaged by exposure to certain drugs or toxins, including heavy metals, solvents, chemotherapy agents, snake or insect venom, poisonous mushrooms, and pesticides. Impaired kidney function can also accompany or result from many other disorders, such as diabetes, lupus, hypertension, and liver disease.

Bright's disease is a kidney disease marked by the presence of blood protein in the urine, along with hypertension and edema (retention of water in the tissues). *Glomerulonephritis* is an inflammation of the filtering units within the kidney. This may occur as a result of an immunological response to infection, such as a *Streptococcus* throat infection. *Pyelonephritis* is a kidney infection. Both glomerulonephritis and pyelonephritis can be chronic or acute, and can be serious. *Hydronephrosis* is a condition in which the kidney and the renal pelvis (the structure into which urine is discharged from the kidney) become filled with urine due to an obstruction of urinary flow. *Kidney stones* are mineral accumulations (primarily calcium) in the kidneys. In *renal tubular acidosis,* the kidneys fail to reabsorb bicarbonate normally, causing impaired ammonia production and acid excretion. Severe dehydration, acidosis, potassium depletion, and bone disorders may result. *Nephrotic syndrome* is not a disease in itself, but can be a sign of kidney disease. It is marked by edema and excess protein in the urine. It can be caused by lesions of glomeruli (small structures in the kidney made of capillaries) that become inflamed, or by chronic diseases such as diabetes or lupus.

If the kidneys cannot function properly to excrete salt and other wastes, edema results. Toxic wastes may accumulate in the bloodstream due to kidney malfunction, a condition known as *uremia.* Symptoms of kidney problems include chills, fever, urinary urgency, fluid retention (bloating), abdominal pain, appetite loss, back pain, nausea, and vomiting. The urine may be cloudy or bloody. Back pain may be sudden and intense, occurring just above the waist and running down the groin.

The following supplements aid in controlling urinary tract infection and help maintain proper kidney function.

NUTRIENTS

SUPPLEMENT	SUGGESTED DOSAGE	COMMENTS
Essential		
Cranberry		*See under* Herbs, below.
Very Important		
Acidophilus	As directed on label, 3 times daily. Take on an empty stomach.	Especially important if taking antibiotics.

Vitamin B₆ (pyridoxine)	50 mg 3 times daily.	To reduce fluid retention.
plus choline	50 mg daily.	
and inositol	100 mg daily.	
Vitamin C with bioflavonoids	2,000–4,000 mg daily.	Acidifies the urine, boosts immune function, and aids healing.

Important	
Dandelion root	See under Herbs, below.

Helpful		
Calcium	1,500 mg daily.	For proper mineral balance; calcium and magnesium should be in a 2-to-1 ratio in the body. Do not use bone meal, oyster shells, or dolomite as a source.
and magnesium	750 mg daily.	Important in water absorption.
L-Arginine	500 mg 4 times daily.	For kidney disease.
and L-methionine	As directed on label, on an empty stomach. Take with water or juice. Do not take with milk. Take with 50 mg vitamin B₆ and 100 mg vitamin C for better absorption.	For improved kidney circulation. See AMINO ACIDS in Part One.
Lecithin granules or capsules	1 tbsp 3 times daily, before meals. 1,200 mg 3 times daily, before meals.	Needed for nephritis.
Multienzyme complex	As directed on label.	Necessary for digestion. Caution: Do not give this supplement to a child under 16 years except as directed by physician. Particularly important for elderly people, who tend to be deficient. Caution: Do not take HCl if you have a history of ulcers.
plus hydrochloric acid (HCl)	As directed on label.	
Multimineral complex	As directed on label.	Corrects mineral depletion, common with kidney disease. Use high-potency formula.
Potassium	99 mg daily.	Acts as a kidney stimulant. Needed for nephritis. Note: Omit this supplement if serum potassium is elevated.
Vitamin A	100,000 IU daily for 3 days, then 50,000 IU daily for 5 days, then reduce to 25,000 IU daily. If you are pregnant, do not exceed 10,000 IU daily.	Important in healing of urinary tract lining and in immune function. Use emulsion form for easier assimilation and greater safety at high doses. Do not take this amount in pill form.
Vitamin B complex	100 mg daily.	B vitamins work best when taken together. Use a high-potency formula. Needed for nephritis.
plus extra vitamin B₂ (riboflavin)	25 mg 3 times daily.	
Vitamin E emulsion or capsules	800 IU daily. Start with 200 IU daily and gradually increase to 1,000 IU daily.	Promotes immune function. An important free radical destroyer.
Zinc	50–80 mg daily. Do not exceed 100 mg daily.	An immunostimulant necessary for healing and an important inhibitor of crystallization and crystal growth. Use zinc gluconate lozenges or OptiZinc for best absorption.

HERBS

❑ Buchu tea is good. Do not boil it, however.

❑ Celery and parsley seeds are natural diuretics. Taken in combination, they are especially helpful if high uric acid levels are present in the blood. Eating large amounts of animal proteins makes one susceptible to high levels of uric acid. These two herbs help keep them in check.

❑ Cranberries contain substances that acidify the urine, destroy bacteria buildup, and promote healing of the bladder. Drink at least 8 ounces of cranberry juice three times daily. Use only pure, unsweetened juice (available at health food stores). Do not substitute a commercial cranberry juice cocktail product; these contain large amounts of sugar. If natural cranberry juice is not available, cranberry capsules can be used as a substitute.

❑ Dandelion root extract aids in excretion of the kidney's waste products and is very beneficial for nephritis.

❑ The herbs hydrangea and uva ursi are excellent natural diuretics. One of the best first steps in cleaning out the urinary tract and keeping it healthy is to help it flush itself. Voiding the urinary tract keeps harmful deposits of calcium or other mineral salts from forming obstructions. Uva ursi is also slightly germicidal, so if there are any bacteria present, they will likely be destroyed by it.

❑ Marshmallow tea helps to cleanse the kidneys. Drink 1 quart daily.

❑ SP-6 Cornsilk Blend from Solaray helps reduce water retention. KB formula from Nature's Way is also a good herbal diuretic.

❑ Other herbs that are beneficial for kidney problems include goldenrod tea, juniper berries, marshmallow root, nettle, parsley, red clover, and watermelon seed tea.

RECOMMENDATIONS

❑ Consume a diet composed of 75 percent raw foods. Eat garlic, potatoes, asparagus, parsley, watercress, celery, cucumbers, papaya, and bananas. Watermelon and pumpkin seeds are also beneficial. Watermelon should be eaten by itself so that it passes through the system quickly; if it stays in the body too long, toxins begin to form. Also eat sprouts and most green vegetables.

❑ Include in the diet legumes, seeds, and soybeans. These foods contain the amino acid arginine, which is beneficial for the kidneys.

❑ Reduce your intake of potassium and phosphates. Do not use any salt or potassium chloride, a salt substitute. Also avoid beet greens, chocolate, cocoa, eggs, fish, meat, spinach, rhubarb, Swiss chard, and tea.

❑ If you have symptoms of kidney problems, especially blood in the urine or severe back pain, consult your health care provider promptly. You may need medical treatment.

❑ Drink 6 to 8 ounces of steam-distilled water every waking hour. Quality water is essential for urinary tract function.

❑ Reduce your intake of animal protein, or eliminate it altogether. A diet high in animal protein puts stress on the kidneys. Excess accumulation of protein can result in uremia. Protein is easiest to utilize if it has been broken down into free-form amino acids. Other good protein sources include peas, beans, lentils, millet, soybeans, and whole grains.

❑ Avoid all dairy products except for those that are soured, such as low-fat yogurt, buttermilk, and cottage cheese.

❑ Try a raw goat's milk diet for two weeks, consuming nothing but 4 quarts of raw goat's milk, warmed to body temperature, each day. Add 1 tablespoon of crude blackstrap molasses to each quart. During this period, take 1,000 international units of vitamin E and 75,000 international units of vitamin A emulsion.

❑ Try a three-day cleansing and juice fast, and coffee or catnip tea enemas. *See* FASTING AND ENEMAS in Part Three.

❑ If you are taking antibiotics for a kidney problem, do not take iron supplements as long as the problem exists.

CONSIDERATIONS

❑ Lead and other metallic poisons are very harmful to the kidneys. Anyone who works with lead, or who is exposed to lead regularly, should take precautions to protect his or her kidneys from damage. (*See* LEAD POISONING in Part Two.)

❑ Infectious diseases, such as measles, scarlet fever, and tonsillitis, can damage the kidneys if not treated properly and completely.

❑ A study at the pharmaceutical department of Chiba University in Japan found that spirulina reduced kidney poisoning caused by mercury and drugs. Researchers discovered that adverse effects of certain drugs on the kidneys also may be decreased by the use of spirulina.

❑ Human growth hormone treatment can improve kidney function. (*See* GROWTH HORMONE THERAPY in Part Three.)

❑ Recurrent urinary tract infections indicate the possibility of a serious underlying problem. See your health care provider.

❑ High doses of the painkiller ibuprofen (Advil, Nuprin, and others) can lead to kidney dysfunction.

❑ *See also* BLADDER INFECTION and KIDNEY STONES in Part Two.

Kidney Stones

Kidney stones, medically termed *renal calculi,* are accumulations of mineral salts that can lodge anywhere along the course of the urinary tract. Human urine is often saturated to the limit with uric acid, phosphates, and calcium oxalate.

Normally, due to the secretion of various protective compounds and natural mechanisms that control the pH of urine, these substances remain suspended in solution. However, if the protective compounds are overwhelmed or immunity becomes depressed, the substances may crystallize and the crystals may begin to clump together, eventually forming stones large enough to restrict urinary flow. Symptoms of kidney stones include pain radiating from the upper back to the lower abdomen and groin, frequent urination, pus and blood in the urine, absence of urine formation, and sometimes chills and fever. In milder cases, the symptoms may mimic a bad case of stomach flu or other gastrointestinal ailment.

Stones can range in size from microscopic specks to the size of a fingertip. There are four kinds of kidney stones: *calcium stones* (composed of calcium oxalate); *uric acid stones*; *struvite stones* (composed of magnesium ammonium phosphate); and *cystine stones*.

About 80 percent of all stones are calcium stones. High blood calcium levels lead to *hypercalciuria*—excessive absorption of calcium from the intestine—which increases the level of calcium in the urine. This excess calcium eventually forms a stone. High blood calcium levels can also result from malfunctioning parathyroid glands (tiny glands in the neck that regulate blood calcium levels), vitamin D intoxication, and multiple myeloma. The consumption of refined carbohydrates, especially sugar, can help precipitate kidney stones as well, because the sugar stimulates the pancreas to release insulin, which in turn causes extra calcium to be excreted in the urine. Mild chronic or recurrent dehydration can also be a factor in kidney stones; it concentrates the urine, increasing the likelihood of stone formation.

Uric acid stones form when the volume of urine excreted is too low and/or blood levels of uric acid are abnormally high. The latter condition is commonly associated with symptoms of gout. Unlike other types of kidney stones, struvite stones are unrelated to metabolism; these stones are caused by infection. Women often get them with recurrent urinary tract infections. Cystine stones are caused by a condition called cystinuria, a rare congenital defect that can cause stones composed of the amino acid cystine to form in the kidney or bladder.

Calcium stones often run in families because the tendency to absorb too much calcium is hereditary. Also, in people with a family history of kidney stones, there seems to be a stronger than normal correlation between the intake of either vitamin C or oxalic acid and the urinary excretion of oxalate. Apparently, such individuals either absorb more oxalate from their diets or metabolize greater amounts of oxalate precursors. People who have Crohn's disease or irritable bowel syndrome, or who eat diets high in oxalic acid, may have an increased risk of kidney stones as well, as these factors can cause the excretion of oxalate in the urine to increase. Other risk factors for kidney stones include low urine volume, low bodily pH, and reduced production of natural urinary inhibitors of crystal formation.

Kidney stones are ten times as common now as they were at the start of the twentieth century. While the consumption of foods high in oxalic acid (mostly eggs, fish, and certain vegetables) has declined markedly in this country in that time, the amount of animal fats and protein in the average American's diet has increased significantly. The ratio of plant to animal protein in the typical diet at the beginning of this century was roughly 1 to 1. This ratio has since declined to 1 to 2. The consumption of animal protein is strongly associated with oxalate absorption.

Kidney stones affect approximately 1 in 1,000 Americans. They are most common in white men between the ages of thirty and fifty, and rare in children and in African-Americans. Kidney stones are more prevalent in the southeastern United States (known to doctors as the "Stone Belt") than in other parts of the country. The reason for this is not known, but it is theorized that the hot climate, which promotes dehydration, and/or regional dietary habits may be to blame. An estimated 10 percent of American men and 3 percent of American women develop kidney stones at some point in their lives.

NUTRIENTS

SUPPLEMENT	SUGGESTED DOSAGE	COMMENTS
Very Important		
L-Methionine	500 mg daily, on an empty stomach. Take with water or juice. Do not take with milk. Take with 50 mg vitamin B6 and 100 mg vitamin C for better absorption.	Reduces the incidence of kidney stones by destroying free radicals associated with stone formation. See AMINO ACIDS in Part One.
Magnesium	500 mg daily.	Reduces calcium absorption and can lower urinary oxalate, a mineral salt common in kidney stones. Use magnesium oxide, magnesium hydroxide, or magnesium chloride form.
Vitamin B complex plus extra vitamin B6 (pyridoxine)	50 mg 3 times daily, with meals. 50 mg twice daily.	B vitamins work best when all are taken together. Taken with magnesium, reduces oxalate.
Zinc	50–80 mg daily. Do not exceed 100 mg daily.	An important inhibitor of crystallization, which can lead to stone formation. Use zinc gluconate lozenges or OptiZinc for best absorption.
Helpful		
Multivitamin complex	As directed on label.	To maintain a balance of all nutrients.
L-Arginine	500 mg daily.	Aids kidney disorders.
Potassium	99 mg daily.	Inhibits crystallization, which can lead to stone formation. Use potassium citrate form.
Proteolytic enzymes	As directed on label. Take between meals.	Aids normal digestion.
Raw kidney glandular	500 mg daily.	Strengthens the kidneys. See GLANDULAR THERAPY in Part Three.
Vitamin A	25,000 IU daily.	Promotes healing of the urinary tract lining, which is often damaged by stones. If you are pregnant, use a natural carotenoid complex such as Betatene in place of vitamin A.
Vitamin C	3,000–6,000 mg daily, in divided doses.	Acidifies urine. Most stones will not form in acidic urine.
Vitamin E	600 IU daily.	A powerful antioxidant.

HERBS

❑ Aloe vera juice, taken at levels that do not produce a laxative effect, can be useful in preventing stone formation and in reducing the size of a stone during an acute attack.

❑ Ginkgo biloba and goldenseal, taken in extract form, aid circulation to the kidneys and have anti-inflammatory properties. They are both also powerful antioxidants.

❑ A combination of lobelia tincture (3 to 4 drops) and wild yam tincture (15 drops) in a glass of warm water helps to relax the ureters, relieve pain, and hasten the passing of stones. Sip this mixture throughout the day.

❑ Marshmallow root tea daily helps to to cleanse the kidneys and to expel kidney stones. Drink 1 quart daily.

❑ Uva ursi helps to relieve pain and bloating.

RECOMMENDATIONS

❑ For pain relief, drink the juice of half a fresh lemon in 8 ounces of water every half hour until the pain subsides. You can alternate between lemon juice and fresh apple juice.

❑ To maintain good kidney function, drink plenty of quality water—at least 3 quarts daily. By far the single most important measure one can take to prevent kidney stones from forming is to increase water consumption. Water dilutes urine and helps prevent concentrations of the minerals and salts that can form stones. Also drink unsweetened cranberry juice to help acidify the urine (unless you are prone to uric acid stones). Drinking the juice of a fresh lemon in a glass of warm water first thing each morning can help prevent stones from forming.

❑ Increase your consumption of foods rich in vitamin A. Vitamin A is beneficial to the urinary tract and helps to discourage the formation of stones. Good sources of vitamin A include alfalfa, apricots, cantaloupes, carrots, pumpkin, sweet potatoes, and squash.

❑ Use distilled water only for drinking and cooking. Add trace mineral drops to your drinking water.

❑ Minimize your consumption of animal protein, or eliminate it from your diet altogether. A high-animal-protein diet causes the body to excrete calcium, producing excessive amounts of calcium, phosphorus, and uric acid in the kidneys and often resulting in painful kidney stones.

❑ Limit your calcium intake and avoid dairy products.

Also avoid aluminum compounds and alkalis, such as those in antacids. The consumption of milk and antacids may cause kidney stones in susceptible individuals.

❑ Reduce your intake of potassium and phosphates. Do not use any salt or potassium chloride, a salt substitute, and avoid carbonated soft drinks.

❑ Avoid foods that contain or lead to the production of oxalic acid, including asparagus, beets, beet greens, eggs, fish, parsley, rhubarb, sorrel, spinach, Swiss chard, and vegetables of the cabbage family. Also avoid alcohol, caffeine, chocolate, cocoa, dried figs, nuts, pepper, poppy seeds, and black tea.

❑ Avoid all refined sugar and products that contain it. Sugar stimulates the pancreas to release insulin, which in turn causes extra calcium to be excreted in the urine.

❑ Stay active. People who are sedentary tend to accumulate high levels of calcium in the bloodstream. Exercise helps pull calcium from the blood into the bones, where it belongs.

❑ If you have a history of cystine stones, avoid the amino acid L-cystine. If you must take a supplement containing L-cystine, take at least three times as much vitamin C at the same time. Otherwise, cystine can crystallize in the kidneys and form large stones that fill the interior of the kidney.

CONSIDERATIONS

❑ Long-term overconsumption of dairy products and antacids often results in the development of kidney stones. Experts refer to this as the "milk-alkali syndrome."

❑ In Japan, the incidence of kidney stones has been rising steadily since the middle of this century, when dietary changes typical of an industrialized nation began to occur. People in Japan who form kidney stones consume far more proteins, refined carbohydrates, fats, oils, and calcium than did their forebears.

❑ Most kidney stones eventually pass by themselves. Depending on the type and size of stone, your physician may recommend the use of electroshock wave lithotripsy (ESWL) to break up the stones, or the use of a laser or other tiny device that is threaded up the urinary tract to break up stones.

❑ Once kidney stones have formed and have been treated, the risk of recurrence increases; once a person has formed a stone, there is a 20- to 50-percent chance that he or she will form another in the next ten years. Once a second incidence has occurred, the risk increases markedly.

❑ Prescription medications containing sodium cellulose phosphate are effective on calcium-based stones. Potassium citrate is effective on stones not of calcium origin.

❑ Taking up to 100 milligrams of zinc daily can help inhibit the formation of crystals that later accumulate into stones. While the recommended amount of zinc helps to enhance immune function, anything over 100 milligrams per day tends to depress immunity.

❑ Excessive intake of vitamin D can lead to an excess of calcium in the body.

❑ To control calcium stones, the pH of the body should be raised, while to control uric acid stones, bodily pH should be lowered. (*See* ACIDOSIS and/or ALKALOSIS, both in Part Two.)

❑ Diet alone cannot remove kidney stones, but it can be very effective at preventing them. Kidney stones are primarily an affliction of well-fed societies in which people consume large quantities of animal protein. A vegetarian diet can be of great benefit to anyone prone to kidney stones. A strict vegan diet that contains no animal proteins whatsoever, is almost entirely devoid of processed foods, and is low in sodium and high in fiber and water, is generally considered conducive to kidney stone prevention.

❑ Measures used to treat kidney stones and to prevent recurrences depend on the nature of the stone, so it is important to take any stone you pass to your health care provider for analysis.

❑ Kombucha tea may be helpful for kidney stones. (*See* MAKING KOMBUCHA TEA in Part Three.)

Lactose Intolerance (Lactase Deficiency)

Lactose intolerance is the inability to digest milk sugar. It is caused by a lack or deficiency of lactase, an enzyme manufactured in the small intestine that splits lactose into glucose and galactose. When a person with lactose intolerance consumes milk or other dairy products, some or all of the lactose they contain remains undigested, retains fluid, and ferments in the colon, resulting in diarrhea, gas, and abdominal cramps. Symptoms usually begin between thirty minutes and two hours after consumption of dairy foods.

The degree of lactose intolerance varies in individuals. For most of the world's adults, lactose intolerance is actually a normal condition. Only Caucasians of northern European origin generally retain the ability to digest lactose after childhood. Lactose deficiency can also occur as a result of a gastrointestinal disorder that damages the digestive tract, such as celiac disease, irritable bowel syndrome, regional enteritis, or ulcerative colitis. It can also develop on its own. There is no known way to prevent it.

Although far less common, lactose intolerance can occur in children as well as adults. In infants, lactose intolerance can occur after a severe bout of gastroenteritis, which damages the intestinal lining. Symptoms of lactose intolerance in an infant can include foamy diarrhea with diaper rash, slow weight gain and development, and vomiting.

Lactose intolerance can cause discomfort and digestive disruption, but it is not a serious threat to health and it can easily be managed through dietary modification.

NUTRIENTS

SUPPLEMENT	SUGGESTED DOSAGE	COMMENTS
Very Important		
Charcoal tablets	For an acute attack, take 4 tablets every hour with water until symptoms subside. Take separately from other medications and supplements.	Absorbs toxins and relieves diarrhea.
Acidophilus	1 tsp in distilled water twice daily, on an empty stomach.	Replaces lost "friendly" bacteria and promotes healthy digestion. Use a nondairy formula only.
Helpful		
Bone Defense from KAL or	As directed on label.	To supply necessary calcium and nutrients needed for calcium absorption.
Bone Support from Synergy Plus	As directed on label.	
LactAid from Lactaid, Inc.	As directed on label.	To supply the enzyme lactase, needed for digesting milk sugar.
Magnesium	1,000 mg daily.	Needed for calcium uptake. Promotes pH balance.
Multivitamin and mineral complex	As directed on label.	All nutrients are needed for optimal health.
Ultra Clear Sustain from Metagenics	As directed on label.	Promotes favorable bacteria in the digestive tract and provides additional nutritional support for the digestive system. Available only through health care professionals.
Vitamin D	400 IU daily.	Needed for calcium uptake.
Vitamin E	400–1,000 IU daily.	Protects the cell membranes that line the colon wall.
Zinc	30 mg 3 times daily. Do not exceed a total of 100 mg daily from all supplements.	To maintain immune system and proper mineral balance. Use zinc gluconate lozenges or OptiZinc for best absorption.

RECOMMENDATIONS

❑ Avoid milk and all dairy products except yogurt. This is the most important dietary measure for anyone who is intolerant to lactose. Use soymilk or Rice Dream in place of milk and soy cheese instead of dairy cheese. Especially avoid consuming lactose-containing foods on an empty stomach.

❑ Include yogurt in your diet. Yogurt is the one dairy product that can be good for a person with lactose intolerance. The cultures present in yogurt digest the lactose it contains, so it is no longer a problem. They also aid in overall digestion. Be sure to eat only yogurt that contains active live yogurt cultures. Homemade yogurt is best.

❑ Be sure to eat plenty of foods that are high in calcium. Good choices include apricots, blackstrap molasses, broccoli, calcium-fortified orange juice, dried figs, rhubarb, spinach, tofu, and yogurt. Calcium supplements may be beneficial.

❑ Check with your pharmacist before taking any medications. Many pills are formulated using lactose as a filler.

❑ During an acute attack, do not eat any solid food, but do drink plenty of quality water and replace lost minerals. *See* DIARRHEA in Part Two for dietary suggestions.

❑ Read food product labels carefully, and avoid any that contain lactose or "milk solids." Lactose is added to many different types of processed food, including breads, canned and powdered soups, cookies, pancake mixes, powdered drink mixes such as flavored coffees, and processed meats.

❑ If you are pregnant and have a family history of lactose intolerance, give serious consideration to breastfeeding your baby. If that is not possible, choose a nondairy baby formula, such as a soy-based product.

CONSIDERATIONS

❑ Lactose intolerance is not the same as milk allergy. Lactose intolerance specifically refers to a syndrome caused by the failure to digest milk sugar; a person with a milk allergy may be able to digest milk normally, but his or her immune system then has an allergic response to one or more of the milk's components. (*See* ALLERGIES in Part Two.)

❑ Hard, aged cheeses, such as Parmesan cheese, are relatively low in lactose, and may be easier to tolerate than other dairy products.

❑ Ice cream is particularly difficult for a person with lactose intolerance to digest. Not only is ice cream made from milk, but many brands add extra lactose to achieve the desired texture, and the cold temperature can be shocking to the digestive system as well.

❑ The symptoms of lactose intolerance are similar to those of celiac disease, and the two disorders may occur together. (*See* CELIAC DISEASE in Part Two.)

❑ LactAid, available in most pharmacies, is a commercial formula that provides the enzyme lactase. It can be taken before consuming dairy products to avoid discomfort.

Lead Poisoning

Lead is one of the most toxic metal contaminants known. It is a cumulative poison that is retained in the body. Even at low levels, lead that is not excreted through the digestive system accumulates in the body and is absorbed directly from the blood into other tissues. When lead leaves the bloodstream, it is stored, along with other minerals, in the bones, where it continues to build up over a lifetime. Lead from the bones may then reenter the bloodstream at any time as a result of severe biologic stress, such as renal failure, pregnancy, menopause, or prolonged immobilization or illness.

Unlike some metallic elements, lead has no known functions or health benefits for humans. It is considered a metabolic poison, which means that it inhibits some basic enzyme functions. Lead reacts with selenium and sulfur-containing antioxidant enzymes in the cells, seriously diminishing the ability of these substances to protect against free radical damage. When present in toxic amounts, it can damage the kidneys, liver, heart, and nervous system.

The body cannot distinguish between calcium and lead. Once lead enters the body, it is assimilated in the same manner as calcium. Because young children and pregnant women absorb calcium more readily to meet their extra needs, they also absorb more lead than other people. Children absorb 25 to 40 percent more lead per pound of body weight than adults do. People with deficiencies of calcium are more susceptible to lead toxicity as well.

Symptoms of lead poisoning typically come on over the course of several weeks in adults and several days in children. Children's symptoms also tend to be more severe. People with lead poisoning commonly have days of severe gastrointestinal colic. Their gums often turn blue and they may experience muscle weakness. Other possible symptoms include diarrhea, anxiety, loss of appetite, chronic fatigue, tremors, seizures, gout, vertigo, insomnia, learning disabilities, confusion, a metallic taste in the mouth, and arthritis. Lead poisoning can eventually lead to paralysis of the extremities, blindness, mental disturbances, loss of memory, mental retardation, and even coma and death. Chronic lead poisoning can also cause impotence, reproductive disorders, infertility, and liver failure.

Lead is one of the most widely used metals in the U.S. today, and it is estimated that a large number of people have high levels of lead in their bodies. Sources of lead exposure include lead-based paints, ceramic glazes, lead crystal dishes and glassware, leaded gasoline, lead-acid batteries used in automobiles, tobacco, liver, water, some domestic and imported wines, canned fruit (the lead from lead-soldered cans leaches out and is absorbed by fruits), garden vegetables (if grown in lead-contaminated soil), bone meal, and insecticides. Recently, such innocuous-seeming items as vinyl mini-blinds and porcelain-glazed sinks and bathtubs have been implicated in lead exposure.

Another potential source of lead poisoning is water supplied through lead piping. Lead piping was used in most homes built before 1930. Newer homes use copper pipes; however, even if you have copper pipes in your home, the chances are very good that they were assembled with lead solder, which is 50 percent lead. Solder can leach a significant amount of lead into the water supply, especially in the first few years after installation. Due to mounting concern over the amount of lead leaching into the water, the use of lead solder was banned in 1986.

Lead poisoning first gained widespread public attention when large numbers of children, especially children in inner cities, were found to have been poisoned by chips of lead-based paint that had peeled off the walls. Some children acquired high lead levels from playing in lead-contaminated dirt, which would get on their hands and then into their mouths. Since then, it has been learned that pregnant women who have high levels of lead in their bodies can give birth to babies with high lead levels. An estimated 90 percent of the lead stored in the mother's body is free to cross the placenta to the fetus. Children born to women who have toxic amounts of lead in their bodies generally suffer from growth retardation and nervous system disorders. Even low-level lead exposure in young children may be associated with impaired intellectual development and behavioral problems. According to the U.S. Centers for Disease Control and Prevention (CDC), 16 percent of all American children have blood lead levels that exceed the acceptable norm. Around 200 children in the United States die each year from lead-induced encephalopathy, 800 suffer permanent brain damage, and over 3,000 experience temporary mental impairment as a result of lead exposure.

NUTRIENTS

SUPPLEMENT	SUGGESTED DOSAGE	COMMENTS
Essential		
Apple pectin	As directed on label.	Binds toxins and metals, removing them from the body.
Calcium	2,000 mg daily.	Prevents lead from being deposited in the body tissues. Use calcium chelate form. Do not obtain calcium from dolomite, bone meal, or cow's milk, which can contain lead.
and magnesium	1,000 mg daily.	Needed to balance with calcium. Use magnesium chelate form.
Garlic (Kyolic)	2 tablets 3 times daily, with meals.	Protects the body's immune system. Helps to bind and excrete lead.
Kelp and/or alfalfa	As directed on label.	Contains essential minerals, especially calcium and magnesium. Also removes unwanted metal deposits. *See under* Herbs, below.
L-Lysine plus	500 mg daily, on an empty stomach.	Assists calcium absorption.
L-cysteine and L-cystine	500 mg each daily, on an empty stomach. Take with water or juice. Do not take with milk. Take with 50 mg vitamin B$_6$ and 100 mg vitamin C for better absorption.	Sulfur-containing amino acids that act as detoxifiers and remove heavy metals. *See* AMINO ACIDS in Part One.
Vitamin C with bioflavonoids	5,000–20,000 mg daily, in divided doses. *See* ASCORBIC ACID FLUSH in Part Three.	Helps to neutralize the effects of lead.
Zinc	80 mg daily. Do not exceed a total of 100 mg daily from all supplements.	Can displace lead and lower the body burden. Low levels of zinc have been found in people with high lead levels.
Very Important		
Lecithin granules or capsules	1 tbsp 3 times daily, before meals. 1,200 mg 3 times daily, before meals.	Protects cell membranes.
Selenium	200 mcg daily.	A potent antioxidant.

Glutathione plus L-methionine	As directed on label, on an empty stomach. Take with water or juice. Do not take with milk. Take with 50 mg vitamin B_6 and 100 mg vitamin C for better absorption.	Powerful antioxidants that protect the liver, kidneys, heart, and central nervous system. *See* AMINO ACIDS in Part One.
Important		
Vitamin B complex plus extra vitamin B_1 (thiamine) and vitamin B_6 (pyridoxine)	100 mg 3 times daily, with meals. 100 mg daily. 50 mg daily.	B vitamins work best when taken together. These B vitamins are vital in cellular enzyme function and important in brain metabolism; they help to remove lead from the brain.
Helpful		
Vitamin A plus vitamin E	Start with 25,000 IU daily and increase slowly to 50,000 IU daily for 2 months. If you are pregnant, do not exceed 10,000 IU daily. Start with 400 IU daily and increase slowly to 800 IU for 2 months.	Potent antioxidants that destroy free radicals and protect the cells from damage due to lead poisoning.
or AE Mulsion Forte from American Biologics	As directed on label.	An emulsified form of vitamins A and E that enters the system rapidly.

HERBS

☐ Alfalfa is rich in vitamins, minerals, and other valuable nutrients, and has a detoxifying effect on the body.

☐ Try using aloe vera juice. Take ½ cup in the morning and ½ cup before bedtime. This softens bowel movements and aids in removing metals from the digestive tract.

RECOMMENDATIONS

☐ Make sure that your diet is high in fiber and that you supplement it with pectin (found in apples).

Note: Always take supplemental fiber separately from other supplements and medications.

☐ Eat legumes, beans, eggs, onions, and garlic. These help to rid the body of lead.

☐ Drink steam-distilled water only.

☐ Do not smoke, and avoid secondhand smoke.

☐ If you suspect lead poisoning, have a hair analysis done to determine long-term accumulation of lead. Blood tests reveal only the most recent exposure. *See* HAIR ANALYSIS in Part Three.

CONSIDERATIONS

☐ A new drug, succimer (Chemet), has been approved by the FDA to chelate lead from children. This drug may reduce illness and death from lead poisoning. Succimer has been approved for use only in children who have significantly high blood lead levels (above 45 mg/dl).

☐ The CDC recommends routine blood testing for lead in all children at one and two years of age. When small children have blood lead levels above 10 micrograms per deciliter (mg/dl)—the highest level the CDC considers acceptable—their intelligence suffers. Numerous studies show an average decrease of one-quarter point in intelligence quotient (IQ) for each 1-mg/dl increase in blood lead level.

☐ One way to get an indication if your child may be at risk of developing lead poisoning is to have a veterinarian check the lead level in your family dog. Long before children show symptoms of lead poisoning, dogs can get colic, then diarrhea or vomiting, and even seizures. Dogs ingest lead the way small children do—licking toys covered with lead-filled dust, chewing old paint on walls or furniture, or putting things covered with old lead paint flakes in their mouths.

☐ Chelation with EDTA can help prevent accumulation of lead. Chelating agents work by binding to lead in the bloodstream and expediting its elimination from the body in urine. (*See* CHELATION THERAPY in Part Three.)

☐ Children with above-average levels of lead in their blood are half an inch shorter, on average, than other children. According to one researcher, lead levels are significantly higher in infants who die of sudden infant death syndrome (SIDS) than in infants who die of other causes.

☐ A study reported in *The New England Journal of Medicine* suggested that even low levels of lead in children may lead to lifelong problems, such as severe reading difficulties, learning disabilities, poor eye-hand coordination, retarded growth, and slowed reflexes. High levels of lead in the body have also been implicated in hyperactivity, behavioral problems, and juvenile delinquency.

☐ Even though leaded gasoline has been almost completely replaced with unleaded fuel, there is still an estimated 4 to 5 million metric tons of lead in American soil that accumulated as a result of leaded gasoline use in the past. Anyone who grows crops or garden produce near busy roads or highways should check the lead level in the soil.

☐ Any building fifty years old or older should be inspected by a professional, and if there is lead-based paint on the walls, it should be removed by someone with the proper expertise and equipment. Simply painting over old lead-based paint can release tiny particles containing lead into the air, posing a possible lead hazard.

☐ A previously underreported source of lead poisoning may be lead-based hair colorings used by men. According to the Cosmetic, Toiletry, and Fragrance Association, 80 percent of the hair coloring products designed for men use so-called progressive coloring agents, which are made of lead acetate. It is known that some lead is absorbed through the scalp, raising questions about the risk of lead poisoning.

☐ The U.S. Food and Drug Administration (FDA) considers children and pregnant women at highest risk for lead poisoning.

Tips for a Lead-Free Environment

Once lead accumulates in the body, it remains there for life. Prevention is therefore much better than treatment when it comes to lead poisoning. The following are simple measures you can take to avoid exposure to lead:

• Do not buy foods in cans sealed with lead solder, which leaches into foods. Lead-soldered cans often have remnants of solder and indentations along the seam. If you buy canned foods, look for lead-free cans that have no side seams. Be wary of imported canned foods. Other countries may have no regulations governing the use of lead solder.

• Make sure children's hands are clean before they eat.

• Keep painted surfaces in good repair, so that older layers of paint are not exposed, chipping, or peeling. Although lead-based paints have been banned for use in residences, numerous older homes and public housing units still contain these paints. Do not allow children to eat paint chips. Hire a professional to remove lead-based paint from any surface; people can poison themselves by burning or scraping off layers of paint.

• Have your water tested to ensure a safe level of lead and other minerals. National Testing Labs sells a kit for testing impurities in your water. To order one of these kits, call 800–H20–TEST. Your state health department may also conduct tests for water contaminants at a reasonable price. Culligan International provides a WaterWatch Hot Line at 800–285–5442 (Monday through Friday, 8:15 a.m. to 5:00 p.m. Central Standard Time). They will put you in contact with a local Culligan dealer, who will provide a free water-testing service. You may also send away for a free booklet entitled *Water Quality Answers* by writing to the Water Quality Association, 4151 Naperville Road, Lisle, IL 60532. Enclose a stamped, self-addressed envelope.

• Never use the first water drawn from your tap in the morning. Let it run for at least three minutes before you use it. Better yet, use only steam-distilled, filtered, deionized water for drinking and cooking. If safe drinking water is not available, treat water with grapefruit seed extract (available in health food stores) before using it. Add 10 drops of extract per gallon of water and shake or stir vigorously.

• Never boil water longer than necessary. Five minutes is enough. Boiling concentrates contaminants in water, including lead.

• Be careful about buying imported ceramic products. The amount of lead allowable in ceramic ware manufactured in the United States is strictly regulated, but there are often no rules governing the glazing techniques of foreign producers. Standards for acceptable lead levels are relatively strict in countries where many of our dishes are manufactured—Great Britain and Japan, for example—but they are often more lax in other countries, such as Mexico and China. The FDA is unable to check a significant number to insure safety.

• Antiques and other collectibles may look attractive, but this type of dinnerware is more likely to leach lead than dishes made more recently. If you buy such items, use them for decorative purposes only.

• Do not store alcoholic beverages, or acidic foods or beverages such as vinegar, fruit juices, or foods made with tomatoes, in lead crystal glassware for any length of time. The lead that gives fine crystal its sparkle and brilliance leaches into foods and beverages served or stored in it. Babies and children should not be fed from crystal dishes or glassware at all.

• If you are pregnant, avoid drinking hot coffee or other hot acidic beverages, such as tomato soup, from lead-glazed ceramic cups or mugs.

• Do not turn bread bags inside out and use them to store other foods. The ink used to print labels on many bread bags contains considerable amounts of lead. While the lead on the labels doesn't get through the plastic to the bread inside, it can contaminate food if you turn the bags inside out and use them to store other foods.

• If you drink wine, always wipe the mouth of the bottle well (inside and out) with a damp cloth before pouring the wine. The foil wrappers around the corks of wine bottles can deposit lead around the mouth of a bottle and contaminate the beverage. The Bureau of Alcohol, Tobacco, and Firearms analyzed more than 500 samples of wine and found that samples poured directly from bottles often contained more lead than samples drawn from bottles with strawlike instruments.

❑ An easy way to test dishes for lead is to use LeadCheck Swabs from Hybrivet Systems. The same company also makes a kit for testing for lead in water. For further information, contact Hybrivet Systems, P.O. Box 1210, Framingham, MA 01701; telephone 800–262–LEAD.

Leg Cramps

See MUSCLE CRAMPS. *See also under* PREGNANCY-RELATED PROBLEMS.

Leg Ulcers

Ulcers are open sores that develop on deteriorated patches of skin. When poor circulation in the legs restricts blood flow, the skin tissue begins to erode; it is thus more susceptible to the development of an open sore. The broken skin can be very slow to heal. Leg ulcers are more likely to develop in persons with poor circulation, thrombophlebitis, and/or varicose veins.

NUTRIENTS

SUPPLEMENT	SUGGESTED DOSAGE	COMMENTS
Important		
Coenzyme Q10	60 mg daily.	Increases resistance to leg ulcers by increasing tissue oxygenation.
Dimethylglycine (DMG) (Aangamik DMG from FoodScience Labs)	As directed on label.	Enhances utilization of oxygen to improve blood flow to the legs.
Garlic (Kyolic)	2 capsules 3 times daily.	Improves circulation and aids the healing process.
Grape seed extract	As directed on label.	A powerful antioxidant that prohibits free radical damage.
Vitamin C with bioflavonoids	5,000–10,000 mg daily, in divided doses.	Improves circulation and aids in healing process. Also keeps infection in check.
Vitamin E emulsion or capsules	800 IU daily.	Helps the body use oxygen efficiently and speeds healing.
	Start with 400 IU daily and increase slowly to 1,600 IU daily.	Emulsion form is preferable; it provides easier assimilation and greater safety at higher doses.
Helpful		
Colloidal silver	Take orally and apply topically to the affected area as directed on label.	A broad-spectrum antiseptic that promotes rapid healing and subdues inflammation.
Flaxseed oil or Ultimate Oil from Nature's Secret	2 tsp daily.	To minimize clot formation and help keep veins soft and pliable.
	As directed on label.	
Free-form amino acid complex	As directed on label. Take on an empty stomach.	Promotes healing and tissue repair.
Iron	As directed by physician. Take with 100 mg vitamin C for better absorption.	Important for cell growth and healing. *Caution:* Do not take iron unless anemia is diagnosed.
or Floradix Iron + Herbs from Salus Haus	As directed on label.	A natural and nontoxic source of iron.
Multivitamin and mineral complex	As directed on label, with meals.	Necessary for proper healing and to remedy and/or prevent nutritional deficiencies.
Vitamin A emulsion	25,000 IU daily for 1 month. If you are pregnant, do not exceed 10,000 IU daily.	Necessary for healing and protection of tissues. Use emulsion form for more rapid and complete assimilation.
Vitamin B complex	As directed on label.	B vitamins work best when taken together. Use a high-potency formula.
plus extra vitamin B12	1,000 mcg twice daily.	Allows proper tissue enzyme function for healing. Helps prevent anemia. Use a lozenge or sublingual form.
and folic acid	1 10-mg tablet 3 times daily, plus injections (under a doctor's supervision) twice weekly or as prescribed by physician.	Vital for proper utilization of protein during the healing process.
Vitamin K	As directed on label.	Needed for blood clotting and healing.
Zinc	50 mg daily. Do not exceed a total of 100 mg daily from all supplements.	Aids in the healing of ulcers and boosts immune function. Use zinc gluconate lozenges or OptiZinc for best absorption.

HERBS

❑ Alfalfa, in capsule or tablet form, is a good source of vitamin K. Red clover tea or capsules are also beneficial.

❑ Echinacea improves immune function and aids healing.

❑ Goldenseal is a natural antibiotic and promotes healing. It can be taken in tea or capsule form. It can also be used as a poultice. Moisten a piece of sterile gauze with alcohol-free goldenseal extract and use this to cover the ulcer.

❑ Make comfrey tea and use it as a compress; soak a clean cloth in it and apply the cloth to aching, inflamed leg ulcers. *Note:* Comfrey is recommended for external use only.

RECOMMENDATIONS

❑ Go on a diet of raw foods with lightly steamed vegetables for one month to help the healing process.

❑ Eat dark green leafy vegetables to obtain vitamin K.

❑ Include plenty of fresh garlic and onions in your diet. These promote circulation and healing, and also contain the trace element germanium, which boosts the immune system and improves tissue oxygenation.

❑ *See* FASTING in Part Three and follow the program.

❑ To speed healing, apply vitamin E oil to the sore and bandage it lightly with a sterile gauze pad. Change the bandage daily until the sore is healed.

❑ Keep the ulcer clean and germ-free to prevent infection.

❑ See your physician if you have this medical problem. Sometimes antibiotics are necessary for the sores to heal.

❑ If you must take antibiotics, be sure to take acidophilus liquid or tablets. You can also obtain acidophilus from yogurt and soured milk products.

CONSIDERATIONS

❑ Dimethylsulfoxide (DMSO) can be applied topically to the sores. It helps to relieve pain and promote healing. *Note:* Only DMSO from a health food store should be used. Commercial-grade DMSO found in hardware stores is not suitable for healing. The use of DMSO may result in a temporary garlicky body odor, which is not a cause for concern.

❑ *See also* CIRCULATORY PROBLEMS and VARICOSE VEINS in Part Two and CHELATION THERAPY in Part Three.

Legionnaires' Disease

This is a serious lung and bronchial tube infection caused by bacteria of the genus *Legionella*, especially *Legionella pneumophila*. It was first identified following an outbreak that affected 182 people attending an American Legion convention in 1976. The bacteria live primarily in water and are transmitted through airborne vapor droplets, although they are sometimes found in excavation sites and newly plowed soil. The incubation period is from two to ten days after exposure to the bacteria. The disease does not spread from one person to another.

The first signs of illness may resemble those of the flu—achiness, fatigue, headache, and moderate fever. The disease then progresses to include high fever (up to 105°F), chills, coughing, diarrhea, disorientation, nausea and vomiting, severe chest pain, shortness of breath, and, as a result of inadequate oxygen, a bluish tinge to the lips, nails, or skin. The coughing begins without sputum but eventually produces sputum that is gray or blood-streaked. Laboratory blood studies and cultures of sputum aid in diagnosis.

The risk of contracting Legionnaire's disease increases with chronic illness such as diabetes, emphysema, or kidney failure, and with immune-suppressing lifestyle habits such as smoking and alcohol consumption. Young adults usually recover fully from the disease, whereas elderly people, especially those in poor health, are at greater risk of developing respiratory failure.

NUTRIENTS

SUPPLEMENT	SUGGESTED DOSAGE	COMMENTS
Essential		
Garlic (Kyolic)	2 capsules 3 times daily, with meals.	Aids in destroying bacteria.
Natural beta-carotene or	25,000 IU daily.	A precursor of vitamin A that protects the lungs.
carotenoid complex (Betatene)	As directed on label.	
Vitamin C plus	3,000 mg 3 times daily.	Powerful antioxidants that help to kill bacteria. Intravenous treatment (under a doctor's supervision) may be beneficial.
bioflavonoids	100 mg twice daily.	
Very Important		
Coenzyme Q10	60 mg daily.	Increases and regulates immunity. Carries oxygen to the cells.
Lactobacillus bulgaricus (Digesta-Lac from Natren)	As directed on label.	Aids digestion and destroys bacteria.
L-Carnitine plus L-cysteine	500 mg each daily, on an empty stomach. Take with water or juice. Do not take with milk. Take with 50 mg vitamin B6 and 100 mg vitamin C for better absorption.	Important in immune function. Protect lung tissues. See AMINO ACIDS in Part One.
Vitamin B complex	100 mg daily.	A complex of vital coenzymes needed for cellular function and protection.
Important		
Intenzyme from Biotics Research	2 tablets 3 times daily, on an empty stomach.	Stimulates the immune system and reduces inflammation in the body.

ClearLungs from Natural Alternatives		See under Herbs, below.
Raw thymus and raw lung glandulars	As directed on label. As directed on label.	Glandulars that potentiate thymus and lung function and enhance immune function.
Vitamin A	Up to 100,000 IU daily for 1 week, then reduce to 25,000 IU daily. If you are pregnant, do not exceed 10,000 IU daily.	Boosts the immune system and protects and repairs lung tissue. Use emulsion form for easier assimilation and greater safety at high doses.
Vitamin E emulsion or capsules	Up to 400 IU twice daily. 400 IU daily.	An important antioxidant that protects lung tissue. Emulsion form is easier to assimilate.
Zinc	80 mg daily. Do not exceed a total of 100 mg daily from all supplements.	Important for immune response. Zinc gluconate in lozenge form is best.
Helpful		
Aerobic 07 from Aerobic Life Industries or	As directed on label.	To destroy infectious bacteria but not "good" bacteria.
Dioxychlor from American Biologics	As directed on label.	

HERBS

❑ Catnip tea is good for reducing fever.

❑ ClearLungs from Natural Alternatives is a Chinese herbal formula that protects the lungs. Take 2 capsules three times daily.

❑ Echinacea is a powerful immune stimulant.

❑ Eucalyptus helps to open up air passages.

❑ Goldenseal is a natural antibiotic.

Caution: Do not take goldenseal internally on a daily basis for more than a week at a time, do not use it during pregnancy, and use it with caution if you are allergic to ragweed.

RECOMMENDATIONS

❑ Eat a diet consisting of 75 percent raw foods and very lightly steamed vegetables.

❑ Consume no alcohol, dairy products, fried foods, sugar, or tobacco.

❑ Use a cool mist humidifier to increase the amount of moisture in the air and to thin lung secretions.

❑ Keep warm—do not get chilled, as this will worsen the disease.

❑ Practice deep breathing exercises.

❑ Use a heating pad or a hot water bottle on the chest to relieve pain.

❑ Be aware that recovery from Legionnaire's disease takes time. Allow yourself two to four weeks for recovery, and be sure to get adequate rest. Do not push yourself to resume normal activities prematurely.

CONSIDERATIONS

❑ Legionnaire's disease progresses rapidly and can be very dangerous. Hospitalization and aggressive treatment with intravenous antibiotics and oxygen may be necessary.

❑ *Legionella* bacteria may inhabit heating and cooling systems. It is wise to have the heating and cooling systems in your home cleaned and inspected regularly, and to change the filters often.

Leukorrhea

Leukorrhea is a thick, whitish vaginal discharge. It is often a symptom of vaginal infection, such as that caused by the one-celled microorganism *Trichomonas vaginalis*, chlamydia, or monilia (yeast, or *Candida albicans*). It can also be caused by excessive douching, a vitamin B deficiency, the use of antibiotics or oral contraceptives, or intestinal worms. Leukorrhea is common in women who have diabetes or are pregnant. The amount of discharge increases when estrogen levels are elevated.

Leukorrhea may be associated with other symptoms, principally burning and itching of the vulva. Blood present in the discharge may indicate a more serious disorder.

NUTRIENTS

SUPPLEMENT	SUGGESTED DOSAGE	COMMENTS
Essential		
Essential fatty acids or	As directed on label.	Effective as an antifungal substance.
Caprystatin from Ecological Formulas	As directed on label.	
Garlic (Kyolic)	2 capsules 3 times daily.	Acts as a natural antibiotic and kills fungi.
Very Important		
Acidophilus	2 capsules 3 times daily, on an empty stomach.	Reestablishes normal bacterial flora. Especially needed if you are taking antibiotics. Also has antifungal properties.
Vitamin B complex	100 mg 3 times daily.	Deficiencies are common in those with this condition. Use a high-potency, yeast-free formula.
plus extra vitamin B₆ (pyridoxine)	50 mg 3 times daily.	Necessary for optimal immunity.
Important		
Vitamin C with bioflavonoids	3,000–8,000 mg daily.	Vital in immune system function.
Helpful		
Multivitamin and mineral complex with		For balanced nutrients.
vitamin D	400 IU daily.	Necessary for calcium uptake.
Vitamin E	400 IU capsules daily.	Necessary for optimal immunity.
Calcium and	1,500 mg daily.	Relieves nervousness and irritability.
magnesium	750 mg daily.	Needed to balance with calcium. Use magnesium asporotate or chelate form.
Vitamin A	20,000 IU daily for 1 month. If you are pregnant, do not exceed 10,000 IU daily.	Aids healing of mucous membranes and enhances immunity.
plus natural beta-carotene or	15,000 IU daily.	Antioxidant and precursor of vitamin A.
carotenoid complex (Betatene)	As directed on label.	

HERBS

❑ Pau d'arco is a natural antibiotic agent. Drink 3 cups of pau d'arco tea daily.

❑ Tea tree oil (10 drops in a quart of warm water) makes a good douche and works well to destroy yeast and bacteria.

RECOMMENDATIONS

❑ *See* CANDIDIASIS in Part Two and follow the dietary instructions there.

❑ Include yogurt and soured products in your diet.

❑ Douche with 6 capsules of acidophilus or with plain yogurt to restore healthy vaginal flora. Also douche with Kyolic or the juice of fresh garlic and water.

❑ For itching, open a vitamin E capsule and apply the oil to the affected area. A vitamin E cream can also be used. Natureworks Marigold Ointment from Abkit is good for severe itching.

❑ Wear white cotton underwear so that air can circulate freely. Keep clean and dry.

❑ Do not use bubble baths, scented toilet tissue or sanitary products, "feminine hygiene sprays," or other potentially irritating substances.

❑ Use a mild laundry detergent.

❑ If you have frequent yeast infections, consult your health care provider to check for a possible underlying illness, such as diabetes or an immune system defect.

CONSIDERATIONS

❑ Any abnormal vaginal discharge should be evaluated by a physician.

❑ *See also* VAGINITIS and YEAST INFECTION in Part Two.

Liver Disease

See CIRRHOSIS OF THE LIVER; HEPATITIS.

Lumbago

See BACKACHE.

Lupus

Lupus is a chronic inflammatory disease that can affect many of the body's organs. It is an autoimmune disease—that is, it occurs when the immune mechanism forms antibodies that attack the body's own tissues. Many experts believe that it is due to an as-yet-unidentified virus. According to this theory, the immune system develops antibodies in response to the virus that then turn on the body's own organs and tissues. This produces inflammation of the skin, blood vessels, joints, and other tissues. Heredity and sex hormones are two other possible factors.

This disease was named *lupus*, which means "wolf," because many people who get it develop a butterfly-shaped rash over the cheeks and nose that gives them something of a wolflike appearance. At least 90 percent of those who contract lupus are women, and women of Asian background appear to be at greater risk of developing lupus than other women. It usually develops between the ages of fifteen and thirty-five, although it may occur at any age.

There are two types of lupus: *systemic lupus erythematosus* (SLE) and *discoid lupus erythematosus* (DLE). As the name implies, SLE is a systemic disease that affects many different parts of the body. The severity can range from mild to life threatening. The first symptoms of many cases of SLE resemble those of arthritis, with swelling and pain in the fingers and other joints. The disease may also appear suddenly, with acute fever. The characteristic red rash may appear across the cheeks; there may also be red, scaling lesions elsewhere on the body. Sores may form in the mouth. The lungs and kidneys are often involved. Approximately 50 percent of those with SLE develop nephritis, inflammation of the kidneys. In serious cases, the brain, lungs, spleen, and/or heart may be affected. SLE can cause anemia and inflammation of the surface membranes of the heart and lungs. It can also cause excessive bleeding and increased susceptibility to infection. If the central nervous system is involved, seizures, amnesia, psychosis, and deep depression may be present.

The discoid type of lupus is a less serious disease that primarily affects the skin. The characteristic butterfly rash forms over the nose and cheeks. There may also be lesions elsewhere, commonly on the scalp and ears, and these lesions may recur or persist for years. The lesions are small, soft yellowish lumps. When they disappear, they often leave scars. If these scars form on the scalp, permanent bald patches may result. While DLE is not necessarily dangerous to overall health, it is a chronic and disfiguring skin disease. Some experts have related it to a reaction to infection with the tubercle bacillus.

Both types of lupus follow a pattern of periodic flare-ups alternating with periods of remission. Exposure to the sun's ultraviolet rays can result in a flare-up of DLE and may even induce the first attack. Fatigue, pregnancy, childbirth, infection, some drugs, stress, unidentified viral infections, and chemicals may also trigger a flare-up. Drug-induced cases usually clear up when the drug is discontinued.

According to the American Rheumatism Association, four of the following eight symptoms must occur, either serially or at the same time, before a diagnosis can be made:

1. Abnormal cells in the urine.

2. Arthritis.

3. Butterfly rash on the cheeks.

4. Sun sensitivity.

5. Mouth sores.

6. Seizures or psychosis.

7. Low white blood cell count, low platelet count, or hemolytic anemia.

8. The presence in the blood of a specific antibody that is found in 50 percent of people with lupus.

A kidney biopsy may be needed to diagnose lupus-related nephritis.

NUTRIENTS

SUPPLEMENT	SUGGESTED DOSAGE	COMMENTS
Very Important		
Calcium and magnesium	1,500–3,000 mg daily. 750 mg twice daily.	Necessary for pH balance and for protection against bone loss due to arthritis.
L-Cysteine and L-methionine	500–1,000 mg each daily, on an empty stomach. Take with water or juice. Do not take with milk. Take with 50 mg vitamin B$_6$ and 100 mg vitamin C for better absorption.	Assist in cellular protection and preservation; important in skin formation and in white blood cell activity.
plus L-lysine	500–1,000 mg daily, on an empty stomach.	Aids in preventing mouth sores and offers protection against viruses. *See* AMINO ACIDS in Part One.
Proteolytic enzymes	As directed on label. Take with meals.	Powerful anti-inflammatory and antiviral agents.
Important		
Essential fatty acids (black currant seed oil, flaxseed oil, and primrose oil are good sources)	As directed on label.	Aids in arthritis prevention, protects skin cells, and needed for reproduction of all body cells.
Glucosamine sulfate or N-Acetylglucosamine (N-A-G from Source Naturals)	As directed on label. As directed on label.	Important for healthy skin, bones, and connective tissue. May help to prevent lupus erythematosus.

Garlic (Kyolic)	2 capsules 3 times daily, with meals.	An immune system enhancer that protects enzyme systems.
Raw thymus and raw spleen glandulars	As directed on label. As directed on label.	Glandulars that enhance thymus and spleen immune function. See GLANDULAR THERAPY in Part Three.
Vitamin C	3,000–8,000 mg daily.	Aids in normalizing immune function.
Zinc	50–100 mg daily. Do not exceed this amount.	Aids in normalizing immune function; protects the skin and organs and promotes healing. Use zinc gluconate lozenges or OptiZinc for best absorption.

Helpful		
Acidophilus	As directed on label. Take on an empty stomach.	Protects against intestinal bacterial imbalances. Use a nondairy formula.
Herpanacine from Diamond-Herpanacine Associates	As directed on label.	Contains a balance of antioxidants, amino acids, and herbs that promote skin health.
Kelp or alfalfa	1,000–1,500 mg daily.	Supplies commonly deficient minerals. See under Herbs, below.
Multivitamin and mineral complex with vitamin B complex	50 mg 3 times daily, with meals.	To supply commonly deficient nutrients. Use a high-quality, hypoallergenic formula. Heals mouth sores, protects against anemia, and protects the skin tissues. Important for brain function and digestion.
Pycnogenol or grape seed extract	As directed on label. As directed on label.	Powerful antioxidants and free radical scavengers that protect the cells.
Vitamin A plus natural beta-carotene or carotenoid complex (Betatene)	25,000 IU daily. If you are pregnant, do not exceed 10,000 IU daily. 15,000 IU daily. As directed on label.	Potent antioxidant and free radical scavenger needed for tissue healing. Use emulsion form for easier assimilation. An antioxidant and vitamin A precursor.
Vitamin E	400–800 IU daily.	Powerful antioxidant that helps the body use oxygen more efficiently and promotes healing.

HERBS

❑ Alfalfa is a good source of minerals needed for healing.

❑ Alcohol-free goldenseal extract is good for mouth sores or inflammation. Place a few drops on a small piece of gauze or cotton before bedtime and leave it on overnight for fast healing.

Caution: Do not take goldenseal internally on a daily basis for more than one week at a time, do not use it during pregnancy, and use it with caution if you are allergic to ragweed.

❑ Other herbs beneficial in treating lupus include echinacea, feverfew, pau d'arco, and red clover.

Caution: Do not use feverfew during pregnancy.

❑ Milk thistle cleanses and protects the liver.

❑ Yucca is good for arthritis-type symptoms.

RECOMMENDATIONS

❑ Eat a diet low in fat, salt, and animal protein—this kind of diet is easy on the kidneys. Use only canola or olive oil. Consume sardines often; they are a good source of essential fatty acids.

❑ Eat asparagus, eggs, garlic, and onions. These foods contain sulfur, which is needed for the repair and rebuilding of bone, cartilage, and connective tissue, and aids in the absorption of calcium.

❑ Include in the diet brown rice, fish, green leafy vegetables, nonacidic fresh fruits, oatmeal, and whole grains.

❑ Eat fresh (not canned) pineapple frequently. Bromelain, an enzyme present in fresh pineapple, is excellent for reducing inflammation.

❑ Use some form of fiber daily.

❑ Do not consume milk, dairy products, or red meat. Also avoid caffeine, citrus fruits, paprika, salt, tobacco, and everything that contains sugar.

❑ Avoid the nightshade vegetables (peppers, eggplant, tomatoes, white potatoes). These foods contain a substance called solanine, which can contribute to inflammation and pain.

❑ Get your iron from food sources, not supplements. Taking iron in supplement form may contribute to pain, swelling, and joint destruction.

❑ Avoid eating alfalfa sprouts. They contain canavain, a toxic substance that is incorporated into protein in place of arginine.

❑ Get plenty of rest and regular moderate exercise.

❑ Avoid strong sunlight and use protection from the sun. Go out in the sun only when absolutely necessary.

❑ Avoid large groups of people and those with colds or other viral infections. Autoimmune diseases such as lupus render an individual more susceptible to viral infections.

❑ Avoid using birth control pills. They may cause lupus to flare up.

CONSIDERATIONS

❑ A test for food allergies is helpful and often very revealing in cases of lupus. (See ALLERGIES in Part Two.)

❑ Some researchers believe that faulty genes are the ultimate culprit behind this disorder, but that outside factors can trigger it. Substances that are common contributing factors include chemicals, environmental pollutants, food additives, and some foods.

❑ Up to 10 percent of lupus cases are probably caused by drug reactions, according to an article that was published in The New England Journal of Medicine. Certain drugs, such as hydralazine (Apresoline), a blood pressure medication, and procainamide (Procan), used for irregular heartbeat, seem to be able to cause lupus in susceptible individuals. Drug-related lupus usually does not affect the kidneys or nervous system. It is likely to be milder, and the condition usually subsides when the drug is stopped.

❑ Many people with lupus also have Raynaud's disease. (*See* RAYNAUD'S PHENOMENON in Part Two.) Some have been treated for syphilis because the condition can lead to false positive blood test results.

❑ Many different treatments are used for lupus. Anti-in-flammatory drugs are usually used first. Antimalarial drugs such as hydroxychloroquine (Plaquenil) may alleviate the skin problems and sun sensitivity that afflict those who have lupus. In severe cases, physicians may have to use cortisone and immunosuppressive agents to induce remission. Corticosteroids, such as prednisone (Deltasone and others) are adrenal hormones that are considered important in the treatment of lupus. Anticonvulsants, drugs used to control seizures, and warfarin (Coumadin), an anticoagulant used to prevent blood clotting and reduce the possibilty of stroke or heart attack, may also be prescribed. All of these drugs, especially the corticosteroids, have potentially serious side effects.

❑ Dehydroepiandrosterone (DHEA) therapy has been found to help in treating lupus. (*See* DHEA THERAPY in Part Three.)

❑ Radiation treatment for lupus is in the experimental stages. It involves using low doses of radiation to the lymph nodes to suppress the immune system. Anticancer drugs are sometimes used to decrease both the immune system's responsiveness and the need for steroids. Anticancer drugs may be toxic to the bone marrow and must be used with caution. Another experimental treatment for lupus involves plasmapheresis, a process in which harmful anti-antigen complexes are filtered out of the blood plasma.

❑ Mild cases of lupus respond well to supplements that build up the immune system. (*See* WEAKENED IMMUNE SYSTEM in Part Two.)

❑ Further information on lupus can be obtained from the Lupus Foundation of America. They can be reached at 800–558–0121.

❑ *See also* ARTHRITIS in Part Two.

Lyme Disease

This disease takes its name from the town of Lyme, Connecticut, where it was first identified in the mid-1970s. Since that time, the locations and the number of cases of Lyme disease have continued to increase. In 1983, the year after national surveillance began, 48 cases were reported to the national Centers for Disease Control and Prevention (CDC) in Atlanta. By 1991, this number had risen to 9,344—a nearly 200-fold increase in eight years—with only Alaska, Arizona, Hawaii, Montana, and Nebraska remaining free of the disease. Approximately 90 percent of all known cases in the United States have occurred in California, Connecticut, Massachusetts, Minnesota, New Jersey, New York, Rhode Island, and Wisconsin. It also occurs in Europe, Russia, China, Japan, and Australia.

Lyme disease is the most common tick-borne illness in the United States. The bacteria that cause it, spirochetes called *Borrelia burgdorferi*, are transmitted by the deer tick (carried by deer and mice) in most places. In California, however, they are transmitted by the closely related black-legged tick, which is also carried by wood rats. Both deer ticks and black-legged ticks are very tiny; an adult tick is less than one-tenth of an inch long, and the nymph is the size of a pinhead. They are hard to spot because they are so much smaller than the common dog tick. Because they are so tiny, they often go undetected. The nymphs and larvae feed primarily on white-footed mice, and the adults on white-tailed deer, although they may feed on many other animals as well, including birds, chipmunks, cows, horses, cats, dogs, lizards, and jackrabbits. The ticks fall off one host animal into grasses in marshes or fields, or into brush in wooded areas, from which they can be picked up by an unsuspecting passerby, whether human or animal, who becomes the next host. Not surprisingly, those most likely to be affected are people who spend time outdoors in or near wooded areas, where the ticks are prevalent, and the majority of cases occur in the summer and fall. Household pets like dogs and cats can pick up ticks and carry them into the home, where they can be transmitted to humans.

After a tick bites, it waits several hours before it begins to feed on the host's blood, and once it does, it feasts for three or four days. As it feeds, it may deposit its infectious cargo in the host's bloodstream. The longer the tick remains attached, the greater the risk of disease.

The symptoms of Lyme disease are extremely variable, as is the incubation period, which may take anywhere from two to thirty-two days. The first sign may be the appearance of a red, circular lesion or rash on the skin. This is caused by the migration of the infecting organism outward through the skin, and it may appear anywhere from a few days to a few weeks after the bite. The lesion gradually expands in a circular pattern, while the center appears to clear up. For this reason, it is often referred to as a bull's-eye rash. In addition to the rash (or, in some cases, instead of the rash), fatigue, flulike symptoms, difficulty sleeping, muscle weakness, achiness, headache, stiff neck, backache, and, occasionally, nausea and vomiting may occur. The disease then usually progresses through three stages, although not everyone experiences all three:

1. Three days to three weeks after a tick bite, small raised bumps on the skin and/or a rash appears and may cover the entire torso, for as little as a day or two or as much as several weeks, and then fade. (If a rash appears

immediately at the site of the tick bite, it may be a reaction to the bite itself and not to the bacteria that causes Lyme disease.) Fever, chills, nausea, sore throat, and vomiting may also occur.

2. Facial paralysis may occur weeks to months later. Enlargement of the spleen and lymph glands, severe headaches, enlargement of the heart muscle, and abnormal heart rhythm may also occur about this time.

3. Over the long term, persistent backache, stiff neck, joint pains that attack the knees, swelling and pain in other joints, and even degenerative muscle disease may be caused by Lyme disease.

Because tick bites are usually painless, the incubation period is so long, and the symptoms of Lyme disease are so varied, the disorder may go unrecognized for weeks or even months. A physician may fail to diagnose the disease before it is in its advanced stages. Lyme disease produces symptoms that resemble those of multiple sclerosis, gout, lupus, and chronic fatigue syndrome, and misdiagnosis is not uncommon. Once arthritis appears, the joint pain and stiffness can come and go, recurring even years later. An estimated 10 percent of those with Lyme disease arthritis are left with permanent stiffness in their joints.

Lyme disease is treatable and almost always curable if found in its early stages. If the disease is not treated in the early stages, however, enlargement of the spleen and lymph nodes, irregular heart rhythm, arthritis, and damage to the cardiovascular and central nervous systems can occur. Some people find that their symptoms slowly subside over two to three years; others develop chronic problems. Often, symptoms leave and recur without another tick bite.

A test has been developed to identify Lyme disease. A blood sample is used to measure the levels of certain antibodies that usually increase in number from three days to three weeks after infection.

NUTRIENTS

SUPPLEMENT	SUGGESTED DOSAGE	COMMENTS
Very Important		
Essential fatty acids	As directed on label.	Reduces inflammation and joint stiffness.
Pancreatin and bromelain or Infla-Zyme Forte from American Biologics	As directed on label 2–3 times daily, between meals and at bedtime.	To aid protein digestion and reduce inflammation.
Primrose oil	1,000 mg 2–3 times daily.	Helps to combat pain and inflammation by promoting the production of anti-inflammatory prostaglandins.
Helpful		
Garlic (Kyolic)	2 capsules 3 times daily.	A powerful immune system stimulator; acts as an antibiotic.

Goldenseal		See under Herbs, below.
Kelp	1,000–1,500 mg daily.	Contains essential vitamins and minerals and aids in detoxifying the body.
Multivitamin and mineral complex	As directed on label.	For necessary vitamins. Use a high-potency formula.
Selenium	200 mcg daily.	A free radical scavenger.
Taurine Plus from American Biologics	As directed on label.	An important antioxidant and immune system regulator necessary for white blood cell activation and neurological function. Use the sublingual form.
Vitamin A	50,000 IU daily. If you are pregnant, do not exceed 10,000 IU daily.	An important antioxidant.
Vitamin C	6,000–10,000 mg daily, in divided doses.	Needed for adequate immune function.
Vitamin E	600 IU daily.	An important antioxidant.
Zinc lozenges (Ultimate Zinc-C Lozenges from Now Foods) plus	1 15-mg lozenge every 3 waking hours for 4 days. Do not repeat this regimen for at least 30 days.	Necessary for immune function.
copper	3 mg daily.	Needed to balance with zinc.

HERBS

❑ Alfalfa supplies needed minerals.

❑ Dandelion root, ginseng, hawthorn, horsetail, and marshmallow root are all good for helping to rebuild the blood and damaged tissues.

❑ Echinacea is an immune enhancer.

❑ Goldenseal is a natural antibiotic. Take ½ dropperful of alcohol-free goldenseal extract three times a day for one week. It can be taken under the tongue for fast results, or added to tea.

Caution: Do not take goldenseal internally on a daily basis for more than one week at a time, do not use it during pregnancy, and use it with caution if you are allergic to ragweed.

❑ Milk thistle extract protects the liver.

❑ Red clover cleanses the bloodstream.

RECOMMENDATIONS

❑ Include plenty of garlic in your diet or take garlic supplements. It is a natural antibiotic and immune-booster.

❑ Use barley grass, bee pollen, and/or royal jelly to supply nutrients needed to repair tissue and rebuild the blood.

❑ Use "green drinks" to provide chlorophyll, which aids in detoxification, and other valuable nutrients and enzymes. Kyo-Green from Wakunaga is an excellent choice.

❑ If you develop a bull's-eye-type rash anywhere on your body, see your health care provider as soon as possible, even if you have no memory of being bitten by a tick. Early treatment is essential.

❑ If antibiotics are prescribed, be sure to take some form of acidophilus supplement daily.

❑ Take hot baths or whirlpool treatments. Heat relieves joint pain.

❑ Take precautionary measures to help prevent tick bites:

• When spending time in or near wooded areas, wear long pants and tuck them into your socks. Wear a long-sleeved shirt with a high neck or a scarf, plus a hat and gloves. Wear light-colored clothing so that any ticks will be more visible.

• Use an insect repellent containing diethyl toluamide (deet) on your clothing, your neck, and any other exposed area except your face. Deet lasts longer and is safer when used on clothing than on exposed skin, so cover as much of the body with clothing as you can. Do not use excessive amounts of deet. Follow product label directions carefully, and wash the repellent off as soon as you go indoors.

Caution: Deet is extremely toxic and can be deadly if ingested. Be extremely careful when using it, especially if you are around small children. Do not use it on clothing or other items containing plastic or synthetics such as nylon or polyester, as it can permanently damage such materials (it can even dissolve certain types of paint and nail polish).

• After spending time outdoors, check yourself carefully for any small raised bumps and for pinpoint-sized specks on clothing. Do this right away; the longer a tick is attached, the greater the risk of Lyme disease.

• Check children before they go to bed during the summer if they spend a lot of time outdoors. Look closely at their hair, ears, underarms, trunks, groins, and the backs of their knees. Have them shower when they come in from outdoors, and wash their clothes immediately.

• Dry your laundry in an electric clothes dryer for a half hour to kill any ticks that may be present. Washing clothes, even in hot water and bleach, will not necessarily kill ticks.

• Inspect pets before letting them indoors. They may carry ticks into the house that can fall off and bite family members.

• In a wooded or overgrown area, try to stay near the centers of trails and out of wooded areas.

• Keep your lawn mowed and remove leaf litter and brush. Move woodpiles away from the house during the summer.

❑ If you find a tick on your body, do the following:

1. Remove the tick with a pair of tweezers. Grasp the tick with the tweezers as close to the skin as possible and pull the tick straight out. Do not twist the tweezers as you pull, and do not squeeze the tick's body, or bacteria may be injected into the skin. If possible, save the tick in a small bottle or jar. *Do not* use a match to try to burn the tick out, or resort to other home remedies like kerosene or petroleum jelly.

2. Once the tick is removed, thoroughly wash your hands and the bite area, and apply rubbing alcohol or another topical antiseptic to the bite. If you suspect the tick may be a deer tick, see your health care provider promptly. Take the tick with you for identification.

3. For the three weeks following a tick bite, be alert for any of the symptoms described in this section. If you have any doubts about your condition, consult your health care provider.

❑ If you are being treated for Lyme disease but are not getting better, consider having yourself tested again. False-positive results are possible, and you may actually have a different problem.

CONSIDERATIONS

❑ Prompt treatment with antibiotics can halt the course of Lyme disease. Many physicians do not like to prescribe antibiotics unless a person develops the characteristic symptoms of Lyme disease—a small red bump at the site of the tick bite, and a bull's-eye rash surrounding it, and flulike symptoms such as fatigue, chills, and joint pain. If treatment is deferred until the onset of more advanced symptoms, such as involvement of the heart, brain, or joints, antibiotic therapy is not as effective.

❑ One study showed that of 788 people diagnosed with Lyme disease, over half actually had other problems. Physicians blame current laboratory tests for the false-positive results. A urine test that may be more accurate should soon become available. It will detect the presence of the *Borrelia burgdorferi* bacteria that cause Lyme disease.

❑ Pets can get Lyme disease, too. Call your veterinarian if your pet exhibits any of the following:

• Fever of 103°F to 106°F.

• One or more swollen, hot joints.

• A tendency to sit or lie in one place for longer periods of time than usual.

• Lameness that seems to come and go.

• Reluctance to move.

• Poor appetite.

• A hot, dry nose.

❑ Recorded information on Lyme disease is available by calling the U.S. Centers for Disease Control and Prevention (CDC) at 404–332–4555. The CDC provides information on Lyme disease to health professionals and the public. CDC also works with state health departments to track cases of Lyme disease. Your state or local health department can tell you if Lyme disease has been reported in your area.

Macular Degeneration

See under EYE PROBLEMS.

Malabsorption Syndrome

Malabsorption is the failure of the body to properly absorb vitamins, minerals, and other nutrients from food. Even though his or her diet is adequate, an individual with malabsorption develops various nutritional deficiencies. This problem can result from impaired digestion, impaired absorption of nutrients into the bloodstream from the digestive tract (especially the small intestine), or both.

Common symptoms of malabsorption syndrome include constipation or diarrhea, dry skin, fatigue, gas, mental difficulties such as depression or an inability to concentrate, muscle cramps and/or weakness, premenstrual syndrome (PMS), steatorrhea (pale, bulky, fatty stools), a tendency to bruise easily, thinning hair, unexplained weight loss, and visual difficulties, especially problems with night vision. Abdominal discomfort may be present as well. A combination of anemia, diarrhea, and weight loss is typical. However, in some individuals, paradoxically, obesity may result, if fats are deposited in the tissues rather than being utilized properly by the body. In addition, in an attempt to get the nutrients it needs but is not absorbing, the body may begin to crave more and more food, often leading to the consumption of many empty and/or fat calories.

Digestive disorders are among the most common health problems in America today. Impaired digestion leads to malabsorption because if food is not broken down properly, the nutrients it contains cannot be absorbed through the lining of the intestines. The intestinal tract, pancreas, liver, and gallbladder all have parts to play in the uptake of nutrients. Consequently, anything that interferes with the proper functioning of any of these can lead to impaired digestion. Some factors that can contribute to impaired digestion are a lack of adequate levels of digestive enzymes; food allergies; a diet deficient in nutrients, such as the B vitamins, that are needed to produce digestive enzymes; and diseases of the pancreas, gallbladder, liver, and bile ducts that result in a lack of bile and essential enzymes. Although any type of nutrient may be affected by poor digestion, lipids (fats) are affected most often. In addition to causing nutritional deficiencies, the failure to digest food properly causes gastrointestinal problems. Undigested food ferments in the intestinal tract, causing gas, bloating, and abdominal pain and discomfort.

Even if food is properly digested, there may be a problem that prevents nutrients from being taken up by the bloodstream and used to nourish the body tissues. Damage to the intestinal walls, through which nutrients are absorbed, is one such problem. Disorders such as celiac disease, colitis, Crohn's disease, diverticulitis, irritable bowel syndrome, lactose intolerance, parasitic infestation, and excessive consumption of alcohol, antacids, or laxatives can all cause intestinal damage. Chronic constipation and/or diarrhea can have the same result. Another problem is too-rapid intestinal transit time, which results in nutrients being passed out of the body as waste before they can be absorbed. Radiation therapy, digitalis treatment, and surgery that shortens the intestinal tract all reduce the absorptive area, and therefore the absorptive capacity, of the small bowel.

Other factors that can contribute to a malfunction of the absorption mechanism include a poor diet; excess mucus covering the intestinal lining (most commonly a result of the overconsumption of mucus-forming and processed foods); an imbalance in intestinal bacterial flora, such as in candidiasis; the use of certain medications, such as neomycin (an antibiotic), colchicine (an anti-gout drug), and cholestyramine (a cholesterol-lowering drug); food allergies; and illnesses such as cancer and AIDS. People with AIDS are particularly prone to malabsorption problems because of chronic diarrhea, loss of appetite, and an overgrowth of *Candida albicans* in the digestive tract. Obstructions in the lymphatic system may also interfere with nutrient absorption.

Regardless of how good your diet is or how many supplements you take, if you suffer from malabsorption syndrome, you will have nutritional deficiencies. These in turn lead to other problems. The impaired absorption of protein can induce edema (swelling of the tissues due to fluid retention). A lack of potassium can result in muscle weakness and cardiovascular problems. Anemia results from a lack of needed iron and folic acid. Calcium and vitamin D deficiency result in bone loss and tetany, a condition characterized by painful muscular spasms and tremors. Bruising easily results from a lack of vitamin K, night blindness from a deficiency of vitamin A. Malabsorption is also self-perpetuating; the failure to absorb B vitamins and to transfer amino acids across the intestinal lining interferes with the production of needed digestive enzymes and causes further malabsorption, since these nutrients are essential in the absorption process itself. A vicious circle results.

Besides being a serious condition in itself, malabsorption is a factor in other medical and physical problems. The body needs all nutrients in balance because they work in concert. If there is a deficiency in even a single nutrient, the body can no longer function as it should, and all kinds of things can go awry. The result is disease. Malabsorption is a common contributing factor to a wide range of disorders, including cancer, heart disease, osteoporosis, and—because immune function is damaged by a lack of necessary nutrients—all types of infection.

Malabsorption is also a significant factor in the overall aging process, and it may account for the fact that some people seem to age more rapidly than others. As we age, the intestinal tract gets "out of shape" and the lining becomes covered with hard fecal matter and mucus, which makes absorption of nutrients more difficult. This is one reason why older people need to consume greater amounts of nutrients. It is also why it is so important to keep the colon clean. Fecal deposits can irritate the nerve endings in the colon, leading to spastic colon or inflamed colon. Both of these conditions interfere with bowel function and with the proper absorption of nutrients. In addition, the impacted deposits decay after a time, releasing toxins that can seep into the boodstream, poisoning the organs and tissues.

Those suffering from malabsorption must take in more nutrients than the average person to compensate, and to treat and correct the problem. In supplying these nutrients, it is best to bypass the intestinal tract as much as possible. When choosing supplements, sustained-release and large, hard tablets should be avoided. Many people with malabsorption problems are unable to break down supplements taken in hard pill form; some even discharge pills whole in the stool. Injections, powders, liquids, and lozenges provide nutrients in forms that are more easily assimilated and therefore are preferred.

NUTRIENTS

SUPPLEMENT	SUGGESTED DOSAGE	COMMENTS
Very Important		
Acidophilus	1 tsp 3 times daily, on an empty stomach.	Needed for uptake and manufacture of many nutrients. Use a nondairy formula.
Dioxychlor from American Biologics	As directed on label.	Destroys harmful bacteria in the intestinal tract and cleanses the bloodstream.
Vitamin B complex injections	2 cc twice weekly, or as prescribed by physician.	To correct deficiencies. B vitamins must be replenished daily. Injections (under a doctor's supervision) are best. If injections are not available, use a sublingual form.
plus extra vitamin B12 and liver extract	1 cc twice weekly, or as prescribed by physician. 1 cc twice weekly, or as prescribed by physician.	Needed for normal digestion and to prevent anemia. A good source of B vitamins and other valuable nutrients.
plus vitamin B12	1,000 mcg 3 times daily, on an empty stomach.	Use a lozenge, sublingual, or spray form.
Important		
Free-form amino acid complex	As directed on label 3 times daily, on an empty stomach.	Needed because protein is not broken down properly into amino acids, which are needed for virtually all life functions.
Garlic (Kyolic)	As directed on label. Take with meals.	Aids digestion and promotes healing of the digestive tract. Use the liquid form.
Infla-Zyme Forte from American Biologics	2 tablets with each meal.	Needed to heal the colon and to aid protein uptake.
Vitamin C	2,000–8,000 mg daily, in divided doses. Take with juice.	Needed to stimulate immune function and to aid uptake of nutrients. Use a buffered powder form.
Helpful		
Essential Fatty Acid Complex from Ecological Formulas	As directed on label.	To repair the cells along the intestinal walls and to assist in proper utilization of fats.
Liquid Liver Extract #521 from Enzymatic Therapy	As directed on label.	Prevents anemia and supplies necessary B vitamins in natural form.
Multivitamin and mineral complex	As directed on label.	To replace lost nutrients. Minerals are the key to protein and vitamin utilization. Use a powdered form that is yeast- and allergen-free.
Proteolytic enzymes or multienzyme complex with pancreatic enzymes	As directed on label 3–6 times daily. Take with meals and between meals. As directed on label, 3 times daily, with meals.	Needed for protein digestion and breakdown of carbohydrates and fats.
Zinc lozenges (Ultimate Zinc-C Lozenges from Now Foods)	1 15-mg lozenge 3 times daily for 1 month. Do not exceed a total of 100 mg daily from all supplements.	Aids in the manufacture of digestive enzymes and in protein uptake.

HERBS

❑ Alfalfa, dandelion root, fennel seed, ginger, and nettle are rich in minerals and can aid the body in absorbing nutrients.

❑ Aloe vera and peppermint aid digestion.

❑ Buchu decreases inflammation of the colon and mucous membranes.

❑ Goldenseal promotes the functioning capacity of the colon, liver, and pancreas.

❑ Irish moss and rhubarb are good for colon disorders.

❑ Yellow dock improves colon and liver function.

RECOMMENDATIONS

❑ Follow the dietary recommendations in this section for at least thirty days to give the colon a chance to heal and to cleanse its walls of hard matter and mucus. After thirty days, you may gradually reintroduce the foods that you have eliminated back into your diet; however, do not add them back too quickly or all at once. Instead, add small amounts of these foods, one at a time, back into your diet.

❑ Eat a diet that is high in complex carbohydrates and low in fats. Include in the diet well-cooked brown rice, millet, oatmeal, and steamed vegetables.

❑ Eat plenty of fruits (except for citrus fruits).

❑ Consume fresh papaya and pineapple often. Chew four to six papaya seeds after meals.

❑ Eat broiled, steamed, or baked white fish three times a week.

❑ Drink six to eight glasses of liquids daily, including juices, quality water, and herbal teas (*see* Herbs, above, for suggestions). Use barley malt, a small amount of honey, or nut or soy milk for sweeteners, if necessary.

❑ Do not consume wheat products until healing is complete.

❑ Avoid products containing caffeine, which interferes with iron absorption. These include teas, coffee, colas, chocolate, many processed foods, and some over-the-counter medications (read labels).

❑ Keep fats and oils to an absolute minimum. Do not consume any animal products (including butter), fried or fatty foods, or margarine. The fats these foods contain exacerbate malabsorption problems by coating the stomach and small intestines, blocking the passage of nutrients. For the same reason, avoid all dairy products and processed food products, which encourage the secretion of mucus.

❑ Eliminate citrus fruits, shellfish, and white rice from the diet.

❑ Do not eat meat or meat products. Meats are difficult to digest and are acid-forming.

❑ Strictly avoid all junk foods, such as potato chips and candy, as well as other products containing sugar, salt, monosodium glutamate (MSG), and preservatives.

❑ See COLON CLEANSING in Part Three and follow the program.

❑ Follow the fasting program once monthly. See FASTING in Part Three.

❑ Avoid using mineral oil or other laxatives. Especially avoid using them for extended periods, as dependence and damage to the colon may result.

❑ If diarrhea or other symptoms of digestive disturbance occur for longer than three days, call your health care provider. Also consult a professional if you notice black and tarry or bright-red stools, or if digestive problems are accompanied by severe abdominal pain or a fever of over 101°F.

❑ If a change of diet and the correct supplements do not improve your health status in a few months, consult your physician. You may have a malabsorption problem that requires medical attention.

CONSIDERATIONS

❑ Chronic pancreatic insufficiency is a condition in which the pancreas does not secrete enough enzymes for proper digestion. Serious pancreatic disease can lead to malabsorption severe enough to damage the nervous system. Gallbladder and/or liver problems can lead to trouble in the digestion and absorption of essential fatty acids, which are necessary for good health. Impaired absorption of fats in turn can lead to deficiencies of fat-soluble nutrients, such as beta-carotene and vitamins A, D, E, and K.

❑ Treatment of malabsorption requires recognition and, if possible, correction of the underlying cause of the problem, plus a healthful dietary regimen and supplementation. Appropriate medical consultation is needed in cases related to the use of cancer drugs, pancreatic insufficiency, and special problems associated with gastric or intestinal surgery.

❑ Certain drugs interfere with the absorption of nutrients. Examples include corticosteroids, cholestyramine (Questran), sulfasalazine (Azulfidine), and especially antibiotics. Corticosteroids depress protein synthesis, inhibit normal calcium absorption, and increase the amount of vitamin C lost through excretion. Cholestyramine interferes with the absorption of the fat-soluble vitamins A, D, E, and K. Sulfasalazine inhibits the transport of folate and iron, causing anemia. Antibiotics disrupt the essential bacterial flora of the intestine. All of these drugs increase the need for nutritional supplements.

Malnutrition

See MALABSORPTION SYNDROME; UNDERWEIGHT.

Manic-Depressive Disorder

Manic-depressive disorder—medically termed *bipolar mood disorder*—is a variant of classic depression. It typically begins as depression and then develops into alternating periods of depression and mania. A person with severe manic-depressive disorder may go from feeling unrealistically (and dangerously) invincible and elated to being overwhelmed with misery and despair, even suicidal. Some of the symptoms of manic-depressive disorder are changes in sleep pattern, withdrawal from society, extreme pessimism, a sudden loss of interest in and failure to finish projects that were started with enthusiasm, chronic irritability, sudden attacks of rage when crossed, loss of inhibition, and changes in sexual behavior that may range from a complete loss of sex drive to sexual excess. It is estimated that 3 percent of the population of the United States suffers from some form of this disorder.

The course of manic-depressive disorder is highly variable. Both mania and depression can vary in severity, and the length of the cycles, from depression to mania and back again, can occur over the course of a few days or over many months—even, in some cases, years. The depressive phase is characterized by low self-esteem and feelings of hopelessness. A person experiencing depression may lack motivation to do anything, even to get out of bed. Some people simply sleep for weeks, withdraw from social activities, avoid relationships with others, and become unable to work. Others may seem to be living normal lives—going to work, interacting with others—but inwardly feel a deadening sadness and are unable to experience genuine pleasure.

The periods of mania often start suddenly and without warning. Some people experience what is called *hypomania*, excitement that does not necessarily appear to be a sign of mental illness—just great enthusiasm and energy. Others experience *full-blown manic psychosis*, in which they have seemingly boundless energy and are ceaselessly active and easily distracted. They may not want to rest or sleep for twenty-four hours or more. Mental activity is sharply accelerated, and delusions of grandeur, persecution, or invincibility are not uncommon. Most people in this condition seem to be utterly elated for no apparent reason, but some become unreasonably irritable and hostile. They may even have hallucinations. Despite all this, a person experiencing full-blown mania generally believes that he or she is functioning at peak efficiency.

The cause of this disorder is not well understood, but there are several theories as to its origin. It may be triggered by extreme stress. Heredity may be a factor in some cases. Some researchers believe that early experiences, such as the loss of a parent or other early childhood trauma, play an important role. Others believe that the manic phase is used (unconsciously) as a kind of psychological compensation for the depression that otherwise engulfs the individual. Biological factors are also possible. There is evidence that concentrations of intracellular sodium increase during the mood swings of manic-depressive disorder, then return to normal after recovery. It is also known that in depressed individuals, brain chemicals called monoamines are depleted.

NUTRIENTS

SUPPLEMENT	SUGGESTED DOSAGE	COMMENTS
Very Important		
Free-form amino acid complex	As directed on label twice daily, on an empty stomach.	To supply protein, needed for normal brain function and to combat depression.
L-Tyrosine	500 mg twice during the day and again at bedtime. Take with water or juice on an empty stomach. Do not take with milk. Take with 50 mg vitamin B$_6$ and 100 mg vitamin C for better absorption.	Important in treating depression. Stabilizes mood swings. *See* AMINO ACIDS in Part One. *Caution:* Do not take this supplement if you are taking an MAO inhibitor drug.
Taurine	500 mg 3 times daily, on an empty stomach.	Deficiency can result in hyperactivity, anxiety, and poor brain function.
Vitamin B complex or liver extract injections plus extra vitamin B$_6$ (pyridoxine) and vitamin B$_{12}$	2 cc twice a week or as prescribed by physician. ½ cc twice a week or as prescribed by physician. 1 cc twice a week or as prescribed by physician.	To supply B vitamins essential for normal brain function and a healthy nervous system. All injectables can be combined in a single injection.
or vitamin B complex plus vitamin B$_{12}$	100 mg 3 times daily. 15 mg twice daily, on an empty stomach.	Use a hypoallergenic formula. A sublingual form is best. Important in making myelin, the substance of which the sheaths covering the nerves are made. Use a lozenge or sublingual form.
Zinc	50 mg daily. Do not exceed a total of 100 mg daily from all supplements.	Protects the brain cells. Use zinc gluconate lozenges or OptiZinc for best absorption.
Important		
Lithium	As prescribed by physician.	A trace mineral that alters the manic-depressive cycles, producing greater mood stability. Available by prescription only.
Helpful		
Essential fatty acids	As directed on label.	Important for improved cerebral circulation and blood pressure stability.
Multivitamin and mineral complex with calcium and magnesium	1,500 mg daily. 750 mg daily.	Mineral imbalances may cause depression. Use a high-potency formula. Has a calming effect; enhances sleep if taken at bedtime.
Vitamin C	3,000–6,000 mg daily.	To aid in brain function and to protect the immune and nervous systems.

RECOMMENDATIONS

❑ Eat a diet consisting of vegetables, fruits, nuts, seeds, beans, and legumes. Whole grains and whole grain products are recommended, except for those that contain gluten, which should be consumed in moderation only. (*See* CELIAC DISEASE for more information on a gluten-restricted diet.) Eat white fish and turkey twice a week.

❑ Consume no sugar or sugar byproducts (read food product labels carefully). Also avoid alcohol, dairy products, caffeine, carbonated beverages, and all foods with colorings, flavorings, preservatives, and other additives.

❑ Be aware that food allergies may aggravate mood swings. Use an elimination diet to find which foods may be causing problems, and eliminate them from the diet. *See* ALLERGIES in Part Two.

❑ Take high doses of B-complex vitamins, approximately 100 mg of each B vitamin three times daily. The B complex is very important for all mood disorders. Use injections (under a doctor's supervision) or a sublingual form for best absorption. Persons with manic-depressive disorder do not absorb the B-complex vitamins easily, and often have deficiencies of these vitamins.

❑ Avoid choline and the amino acids ornithine and arginine. These substances may make symptoms worse.

CONSIDERATIONS

❑ Injections of vitamin B$_{12}$ and megadoses of the B vitamins often bring about an improvement. The B vitamins have a lithium-like effect on the brain.

❑ Amino acids, especially taurine and tyrosine, are important in the treatment of this disorder.

The trace mineral lithium is known to alter the period of the rhythmic cycling of the brain, and helps to even out the moods in persons with manic-depressive disorder. The high doses of lithium used in the treatment of manic-depressive disorder may cause side effects, however, including nausea, vomiting, tremors, kidney dysfunction, and thyroid enlargement.

According to an article in *The New England Journal of Medicine*, individuals with depression and manic-depressive disorder appear to be hypersensitive to the neurotransmitter acetylcholine. Therefore, choline should not be taken in a dose that exceeds the amount in a multiple vitamin.

Manic-depressive disorder may be aggravated by an overgrowth of yeast in the intestinal tract and by nutritional deficiencies. Food allergies, such as an allergy to wheat products, and the consumption of large amounts of caffeine and/or refined sugar, can make symptoms worse.

According to Richard S. Wilkinson, M.D., of Yakima, Washington, an expert in environmental medicine, manic-depressive disorder may be caused by environmental sensitivities or allergies.

Certain systemic disorders can cause depression, including Alzheimer's disease, diabetes mellitus, encephalitis, hyper- and hypothyroidism, multiple sclerosis, and Parkinson's disease. Any depression diagnosis should be made only after a thorough physical examination to rule out an underlying illness.

See also DEPRESSION in Part Two.

Mastitis

See under BREASTFEEDING-RELATED PROBLEMS.

Measles

Measles, known to doctors as *rubeola*, is a viral infection that attacks the respiratory tract, eyes, and skin. Although it is typically a childhood disease, adults are also susceptible. Measles is very contagious and is easily spread by coughing and sneezing.

Illness usually sets in between seven and fourteen days after exposure to the virus. The first symptoms include fever, cough, sneezing, runny nose, and red eyes that may be sensitive to light. Several days later, Koplik's spots (tiny red spots with white centers) appear in the mouth and throat, the throat becomes sore, and a raised red rash erupts on the forehead and ears. Over a period of five to seven days, the rash spreads to all parts of the body.

In previously healthy children, measles usually runs its course in about ten days. However, it can be followed by a number of complications, some of them potentially serious. These include middle ear infection (especially in children with a history of repeated ear infections), bronchitis, croup, pneumonia, strep throat, and even, in rare cases, encephalitis or meningitis. Adults who develop measles tend to suffer more serious cases of the disease than children do.

Unless otherwise specified, the dosages recommended here are for adults. For a child between the ages of twelve and seventeen, reduce the dose to three-quarters the recommended amount. For a child between six and twelve, use one-half the recommended dose, and for a child under the age of six, use one-quarter the recommended amount.

NUTRIENTS

SUPPLEMENT	SUGGESTED DOSAGE	COMMENTS
Helpful		
AE Mulsion Forte from American Biologics or	As directed on label.	For adults. Needed to reduce infection and to repair tissues.
vitamin A	10,000 IU twice daily for 1 week, then reduce to 10,000 IU once daily. Do not exceed this dosage. If you are pregnant, do not exceed 10,000 IU daily.	For children.
or cod liver oil	As directed on label.	For children unable to swallow capsules.
Bio-Strath from Bioforce	As directed on label.	Acts as a tonic. Contains the vitamin B complex. Use the liquid form.
Calcium and magnesium	As directed on label. As directed on label.	Needed for tissue repair.
Proteolytic enzymes	As directed on label 2–3 times daily, between meals.	Reduces infection and aids digestion.
Raw thymus glandular	500 mg twice daily.	Stimulates the immune system.
Vitamin C	For children. 3,000–10,000 mg daily, in divided doses. For adults, 1,000–3,000 mg daily, in divided doses,	Very important for immune function. Controls fever and infection. Has antiviral properties. Use an ascorbate or esterified form.
Vitamin B complex	100 mg 3 times daily or as directed on label.	Important in all bodily functions, including immune response and proper healing. For a child under 8, use a formula designed specifically for children.
Vitamin E	200–800 IU daily for children over 6.	Neutralizes harmful free radicals, which can destroy cell membranes.
Zinc lozenges (Ultimate Zinc-C Lozenges from Now Foods)	1 15-mg lozenge 3 times daily for 4 days. Then reduce to 1 lozenge daily.	For immune response and tissue repair. Reduces symptoms and speeds healing. Also relieves itchy throat and coughing.

HERBS

❑ Catnip tea or garlic enemas can be used to help to lower fever if necessary. *See* ENEMAS in Part Three.

❑ Lobelia extract helps to relieve pain. Take ½ teaspoon of lobelia extract every four to five hours.

Caution: Do not take lobelia internally on an ongoing basis.

RECOMMENDATIONS

❑ If you suspect that you or a member of your family has measles, see your health care provider. This is important for a correct diagnosis and to prevent serious complications.

❑ Drink plenty of fluids such as water, juices, and vegetable broths.

❑ Avoid processed foods.

❑ Rest until the rash and fever have disappeared.

❑ Keep the lights dim. Do not read or watch television while your eyes are sensitive to light.

❑ Do not send a child who has had measles to school until seven to nine days after the fever and rash have disappeared.

CONSIDERATIONS

❑ Doctors generally recommend that children receive two measles vaccinations, the first at the age of about fifteen months and the second either before entering school or at approximately twelve years of age. A second vaccination is now considered necessary because there have been outbreaks of measles among college students who received a single immunization in childhood. However, certain individuals should *not* be immunized against measles, including anyone who has cancer or a weakened immune system, is on cortisone or anticancer drugs, is undergoing radiation therapy, or has any type of illness with fever. A person who has had and recovered from measles does not require immunization; a single attack of measles gives lifelong immunity to the disease.

❑ Antibiotics are useless against viruses, so they are not called for unless complications occur.

Melanoma

See under SKIN CANCER.

Memory Problems

Memory is as natural to us as breathing. It is an ability we all have, yet rarely ever think of—unless we perceive that we are losing that ability. Memory lapses are an annoyance in themselves, but worse is the anxiety that often comes along with them. We begin asking ourselves if they are a symptom of some other problem, such as midlife depression or arteriosclerosis. Probably the greatest fear provoked by lapses in memory is that of Alzheimer's disease, a progressive and debilitating disease that usually starts in midlife with minor defects in memory and behavior. Although this is a fairly common disorder among older people, it is important to realize that most memory lapses have nothing to do with Alzheimer's disease.

People have come to expect that, as they age, their ability to remember will begin to deteriorate; that their powers of recall will diminish. This is not necessarily true. The aging process itself has little, if any, bearing on the ability to recall information. Occasional memory lapses are a natural, normal part of life at virtually any age, but with proper diet and nutrition, the memory should remain sharp and active well into one's nineties or beyond.

One reason many people suffer from memory loss is an insufficient supply of necessary nutrients to the brain. The life of the body is in the blood. It literally feeds and nourishes every cell within our bodies. The brain is surrounded by a protective envelope known as the blood-brain barrier, which allows only certain substances to pass from the bloodstream into the brain. If the blood is "thick" with cholesterol and triglycerides, the amount of nutrient-rich blood that can pass through the blood-brain barrier decreases. Over time, this can result in the brain becoming malnourished.

In addition, the functioning of the brain depends upon substances called neurotransmitters. Neurotransmitters are brain chemicals that act as electrical switches in the brain and, through the functioning of the nervous system, are ultimately responsible for all the functions of the body. If the brain does not have an adequate supply of neurotransmitters, or the nutrients from which to make them, it begins to develop the biochemical equivalent of a power failure or a short circuit. If your mind goes blank when you are trying to recall a specific fact or piece of information, or it begins to plug into some other, irrelevant memory instead, it is likely that such a "short circuit" has occurred.

There are numerous other factors involved in the deterioration of memory. One of the most important is probably exposure to free radicals, which can wreak enormous damage to the memory if unchecked. Nutritional deficiencies, especially deficiencies of the B vitamins and amino acids, account for memory loss in some individuals. Alcoholics and drug addicts often suffer a great deal from memory loss. Alcoholics are notorious for "blackouts"—huge memory gaps that occur even though they are conscious. Allergies, candidiasis, stress, thyroid disorders, and poor circulation to the brain may be contributing factors. Hypoglycemia (low blood sugar) can play a role in memory loss as well, because to function properly, the brain requires that the level of glucose in the blood fall within a very specific narrow range. Wide swings in blood sugar levels affect brain function and memory.

NUTRIENTS

SUPPLEMENT	SUGGESTED DOSAGE	COMMENTS
Very Important		
Acetylcholine	As directed on label.	Most important of the neurotransmitters. Maximizes mental ability and prevents memory loss in adults.
Choline	100 mg 3 times daily.	Increases levels of acetylcholine.
Manganese	As directed on label. Take separately from calcium.	Helps nourish the brain and nerves. Aids in the utilization of choline.
Superoxide dismutase (SOD)	As directed on label.	Known for its ability to eliminate free radicals.
Vitamin B complex	100 mg daily.	Needed for improved memory. Injections (under a doctor's supervision) may be necessary.
plus extra pantothenic acid (vitamin B_5) and	50 mg 3 times daily.	Helps in transformation of the amino acid choline to the neurotransmitter acetylcholine.
vitamin B_6 (pyridoxine)	50 mg 3 times daily.	Needed for proper brain function.
Vitamin B_3 (niacin) and	As directed on label.	To promote proper circulation to the brain and aid in brain function.
niacinamide	As directed on label.	*Caution:* Do not take niacin if you have a liver disorder, gout, or high blood pressure.
Vitamin C	3,000–10,000 mg daily.	A powerful antioxidant that also improves circulation.
Vitamin E	Start with 400 IU daily and slowly increase to 1,200 IU daily.	Causes dilation of blood vessels, improving blood flow to the brain.
Zinc	50–80 mg daily. Do not exceed 100 mg daily.	Important in binding toxic substances and removing them from the brain. Use zinc gluconate lozenges or OptiZinc for best absorption.
Important		
Lecithin granules or capsules	1 tbsp 3 times daily, before meals. 1,200 mg 3 times daily, before meals.	Improves brain function. Lecithin is high in choline and inositol, important B vitamins.
L-Glutamine and L-phenylalanine plus L-aspartic acid	As directed on label, on an empty stomach. Take with water or juice. Do not take with milk. Take with 50 mg vitamin B_6 and 100 mg vitamin C for better absorption.	Amino acids necessary for normal brain function; serve as fuel for the brain and prevent excess ammonia from damaging the brain. *Caution:* Do not take phenylalanine if you are pregnant or nursing, or if you suffer from panic attacks, diabetes, high blood pressure, or PKU.
L-Tyrosine	Up to 100 mg per kg of body weight daily. Take on an empty stomach with 1,000 mg vitamin C and 50 mg vitamin B_6.	Helps sharpen learning, memory, and awareness; elevates mood and motivation; aids in preventing depression. *Caution:* Do not take this supplement if you are also taking an MAO inhibitor drug.
Helpful		
Coenzyme Q_{10}	100 mg daily.	Improves brain oxygenation.
Dimethylglycine (DMG) (Aangamik DMG from FoodScience Labs)	As directed on label.	Improves brain oxygenation.
Melatonin	2–3 mg daily, taken 2 hours or less before bedtime.	A powerful antioxidant that may prevent memory loss.
RNA and DNA	As directed on label.	Increases energy production for memory transfer in the brain. *Caution:* Do not take this supplement if you have gout.

HERBS

❑ Ginkgo biloba has been attracting attention from researchers because of its ability to increase blood flow to the brain. Ginkgo is available in capsule or extract form at most health food stores. Products vary, depending on the brand. For memory enhancement, take capsules as directed on the product label, or place 6 drops of an alcohol-free extract under your tongue and hold it there for a few minutes, then swallow. Do this twice daily.

❑ Other herbs that are helpful for memory include anise, blue cohosh, ginseng, and rosemary.

Caution: Do not use ginseng if you have high blood pressure.

RECOMMENDATIONS

❑ Eat a diet high in raw foods. Consume the following often: brewer's yeast, brown rice, farm eggs, fish, legumes, millet, nuts, soybeans, tofu, wheat germ, and whole grains.

❑ Combine complex carbohydrates with foods containing 10 percent protein and 10 percent essential fats. All-carbohydrate meals have an adverse effect on the memory.

❑ Avoid dairy and wheat products (except for wheat germ) for one month. If there is no memory improvement, slowly add these foods back to your diet.

❑ Avoid refined sugars—these "turn off" the brain.

❑ Practice holding your breath for thirty seconds every hour for thirty days. This improves mental alertness.

❑ Consider having a hair analysis done to rule out intoxication by heavy metals such as aluminum and lead. Either of these conditions can lead to impaired mental functioning. *See* HAIR ANALYSIS in Part Three.

❑ If already taking a multivitamin and mineral supplement, you may wish to try Cognitex from Prolongevity or Fuel for Thought from Nature's Plus. Bee pollen may also be helpful.

Caution: Bee pollen may cause an allergic reaction in some people. Start with a small amount, and discontinue use if a rash, wheezing, discomfort, or other symptom occurs.

❑ Make sure to focus on things that you may wish to remember. Often, we blame our inability to recall something on a failing memory when the problem is that we did not really pay attention in the first place.

CONSIDERATIONS

❑ Supplementation with the hormone dehydroepian-drosterone (DHEA) may help to improve memory. (See DHEA THERAPY in Part Three.) Human growth hormone (HGH) has also been shown to improve brain function. (See GROWTH HORMONE THERAPY in Part Three.)

❑ The keys to having a good memory are in attitude and approach. As we age, our attitudes change. Our ability to remember isn't affected as much as we think. It is the change in our motivation to remember things that is probably the larger factor.

❑ See also AGING; ALZHEIMER'S DISEASE; ARTERIOSCLEROSIS; HYPOGLYCEMIA; and/or SENILITY, all in Part Two.

Ménière's Disease

Ringing in the ears, variable loss of hearing, loss of balance, dizziness, and nausea and vomiting are symptoms of the inner ear disturbance known as Ménière's disease. The condition may affect one or both ears. The exact cause or causes are unknown, but many experts believe it results from a metabolic problem caused by a disturbed carbohydrate metabolism like that associated with hypoglycemia. Impaired blood flow to the brain from clogged arteries and poor circulation may also be involved. Allergies, stress, exposure to loud noises, and excessive salt intake may contribute to this disorder.

In the semicircular canals of the inner ear, increased fluid retention produces pressure, which may disturb balance and hearing, resulting in bouts of dizziness, nausea, and even vomiting. Fluid retention during the premenstrual period in women, allergies, and spasms of the blood vessels that supply the inner ear may be related to Ménière's disease. Drug use, smoking, trauma, and temporomandibular joint syndrome (TMJ) may also be involved.

NUTRIENTS

SUPPLEMENT	SUGGESTED DOSAGE	COMMENTS
Essential		
Manganese	5 mg daily. Take separately from calcium.	Deficiency may be the cause of Ménière's syndrome.
Very Important		
Bio-Strath from Bioforce	As directed on label.	A natural source of the B vitamins. Acts as a tonic and enhances brain function.
Chromium picolinate	200 mcg daily.	Aids in controlling blood sugar levels, which are often high in those with this disorder.
Coenzyme Q$_{10}$	100 mg daily.	Improves circulation.
Vitamin B$_3$ (niacin)	100 mg twice daily. Do not exceed this amount.	Improves circulation. If you are uncomfortable with the flush caused by niacin, use part niacinamide. *Caution:* Do not take niacin if you have a liver disorder, gout, or high blood pressure.
Important		
Vitamin B complex	As directed on label.	Important for the nervous system. Use a high-stress formula.
plus extra vitamin B$_6$ (pyridoxine)	100 mg twice daily.	Reduces fluid retention.
Vitamin C with bioflavonoids	3,000–6,000 mg daily, in divided doses.	Boosts immune function. Use an esterified or buffered form.
Helpful		
Calcium and magnesium	1,500 mg daily. 1,000 mg daily.	Needed for stability of the nervous system and for muscle contraction. Chelated forms are the most effective.
Essential fatty acids (primrose oil and salmon oil are good sources)	As directed on label 3 times daily, with meals.	To correct metabolic disturbances.
Lecithin granules or capsules	1 tbsp 3 times daily, before meals. 1,200 mg 3 times daily, before meals.	For cellular protection and brain function.
Vitamin E	400–800 IU daily. If you have high blood pressure, start with 100 IU daily and increase slowly to 400 IU daily.	Promotes efficient oxygen use.

HERBS

❑ Butcher's broom combats fluid retention and improves circulation.

❑ Ginkgo biloba, taken in extract or tablet form, increases circulation to the brain.

RECOMMENDATIONS

❑ Try a hypoglycemic diet for two weeks. If you experience an improvement, remain on the diet. See HYPOGLYCEMIA in Part Two.

❑ Do not consume any fats, fried foods, salt, sugar (in any form), or anything containing caffeine.

❑ Check for food allergies. See ALLERGIES in Part Two.

CONSIDERATIONS

❑ Some doctors recommend a high-protein, low-refined-carbohydrate diet because they have found that people with this disorder have high blood insulin levels. High insulin levels impair circulation. (See ARTERIOSCLEROSIS and CIRCULATORY PROBLEMS, both in Part Two.) Other factors, such as obesity, alcohol use, smoking, and high blood cholesterol may contribute to this syndrome as well.

Meningitis

Meningitis is an infection of the three membranes, called the meninges, that lie between the brain and the skull. The thin membranes that cover the spinal cord may also be involved. Meningitis can be caused by many different infectious agents, including any of a number of different viruses, such as the polio or rubella viruses; fungi, such as yeast; and bacteria, such as *Neisseria meningitidis* (meningococcus), *Streptococcus pneumoniae* (pneumococcus), *Hemophilus influenzae* type B, and group B *Streptococcus*. The infection may spread to the meninges from the nose and throat, or it may spread through the bloodstream from elsewhere in the body. This disease is contagious.

The most common type of meningitis is a viral infection that causes comparatively mild symptoms, such as headache and malaise, and usually improves on its own in a week or two. Bacterial meningitis is a more serious infection and requires prompt, aggressive medical treatment. Meningitis caused by a fungal infection progresses more slowly, but still requires medical treatment.

The early symptoms of meningitis include sore throat, red or purple skin rash, and signs of a recent respiratory disorder. Other classic symptoms include stiff neck, headache, irritability, high fever, chills, nausea, vomiting, delirium, and sensitivity to light. A blotchy red skin rash may appear. In infants, the signs include fever, vomiting, poor muscle tone, difficulty feeding, irritability, a high-pitched cry, and a bulging fontanel (soft spot). Changes in temperament and extreme sleepiness signal dangerous changes in the cerebrospinal fluid, the fluid that surrounds and cushions the brain.

Meningitis is more common in children than in adults. A higher risk of meningitis is also associated with alcoholism, brain cancer, brain surgery, chronic exposure to chemical toxins, head injury, Lyme disease, pneumonia, syphilis, tuberculosis, as well as with anything that damages the immune system, such as chemotherapy or radiation treatment, HIV disease, long-term steroid therapy, and certain types of cancer. Diagnosis of meningitis requires microscopic analysis and culture of the cerebrospinal fluid.

The recommendations in this section are designed to support medical treatment, not replace it. Meningitis can progress very quickly and become life threatening in a matter of twenty-four hours for adults, much less for children. If untreated, this disease can cause permanent brain damage and paralysis, even coma and death.

Unless otherwise specified, the dosages recommended here are for adults. For a child between the ages of twelve and seventeen, reduce the dose to three-quarters the recommended amount. For a child between six and twelve, use one-half the recommended dose, and for a child under the age of six, use one-quarter the recommended amount.

NUTRIENTS

SUPPLEMENT	SUGGESTED DOSAGE	COMMENTS
Helpful		
Acidophilus	As directed on label. Take on an empty stomach.	Needed to replenish the friendly bacteria antibiotics destroy.
Dimethylglycine (DMG) (Aangamik DMG from FoodScience Labs)	125 mg twice daily.	Carries oxygen to the cells, relieving many symptoms. Use a sublingual form.
Free-form amino acid complex	As directed on label.	Needed for tissue repair and protection of membranes.
Garlic (Kyolic)	2 capsules 3 times daily, with meals.	An immune system stimulant that also acts as a natural antibiotic.
Maitake or	As directed on label.	To help to build immunity and fight viral infection.
shiitake or	As directed on label.	
reishi	As directed on label.	
Multivitamin and mineral complex	As directed on label.	Needed for tissue protection and healing. Use a high-potency formula.
Raw thymus glandular	500 mg twice daily.	Enhances immune response.
Vitamin A emulsion or	50,000 IU daily.	A powerful antioxidant and immune booster. Needed for protection and healing of all membranes. Emulsion form is recommended for easier absorption and greater safety at higher doses.
capsules	50,000 IU daily for 5 days, then 25,000 IU daily for 7 days, then reduce to 15,000 IU daily. If you are pregnant, do not exceed 10,000 IU daily.	
Vitamin C with bioflavonoids	3,000–10,000 mg daily.	Reduces infection and aids in cleansing the bloodstream.
Zinc lozenges (Ultimate Zinc-C Lozenges from Now Foods)	1 15-mg lozenge 3 times daily. Do not exceed a total of 100 mg daily from all supplements.	An immune system booster.

HERBS

❑ For fever, use catnip tea enemas. *See* ENEMAS in Part Three. Catnip tea is also good for sipping.

❑ Echinacea boosts the immune system.

❑ Goldenseal is a natural antibiotic.

Caution: Do not take goldenseal internally on a daily basis for more than one week, as it may disturb normal intestinal flora. Do not use it in large quantities during pregnancy, and use it with caution if you are allergic to ragweed.

❑ St. Johnswort is good for viral infections.

RECOMMENDATIONS

❑ If you develop symptoms characteristic of meningitis, see a physician or go to the emergency room of the nearest hospital immediately.

❑ Avoid aspirin, which increases bleeding tendencies.

❏ Once the acute phase of the illness has passed and recovery has begun, eat a well-balanced diet including fresh fruits and vegetables (50 percent of them raw), grains, nuts, seeds, and yogurt and other soured products.

❏ Consume fresh pineapple and papaya frequently. Pineapple reduces inflammation; papaya is good for digestion. Only the fresh forms are effective.

❏ Avoid the following foods, which encourage the formation of mucus: animal protein and its byproducts, caffeine, dairy products (except for yogurt), processed foods, salt, sugar, and white flour products.

❏ Rest in bed in a dimly lit room. Drink plenty of high-quality liquids.

❏ Take cool sponge baths.

CONSIDERATIONS

❏ Without complications, recovery from meningitis generally takes three weeks under a physician's care.

❏ For bacterial meningitis, aggressive treatment with antibiotics is necessary. For viral meningitis, antibiotics are ineffective and therefore inappropriate. If meningitis is caused by a fungal infection, treatment with an antifungal drug is used.

❏ Corticosteroids may be prescribed to reduce inflammation. Antinausea and strong pain medication may also be needed.

❏ It is wise to seek prompt treatment for a bacterial infection anywhere in the body, such as strep throat or an ear infection.

❏ Antibiotics may be prescribed as a preventive for those who have been in close contact with a person who has bacterial meningitis.

Menopause-Related Problems

Menopause, also referred to as the "change of life," is the point at which a woman stops ovulating and menstruation ceases, indicating the end of fertility. When a woman stops ovulating, her ovaries largely stop producing the hormones estrogen and progesterone. Estrogen is commonly thought of as a sex hormone strictly tied to reproduction, but it also acts on many different organs in the body. Cells in the vagina, bladder, breasts, skin, bones, arteries, heart, liver, and brain all contain estrogen receptors, and require this hormone to stimulate these receptors for normal cell function. Estrogen is needed to keep the skin smooth and moist, the body's internal thermostat operating properly, and the arteries unclogged, for example. It is also necessary for proper bone formation.

Although estrogen levels drop sharply after menopause, the hormone does not disappear entirely. Other organs take over from the ovaries and continue to produce some estrogen and other hormones. The organs known as endocrine glands secrete hormones to maintain proper bodily functions.

The menopausal period is different for each individual woman. Some start earlier and some later, but the average age at menopause is about fifty. The transition usually lasts up to five years. A woman who undergoes a hysterectomy but who keeps at least one of her ovaries stops menstruating after surgery, but she will still go through menopause. If the ovaries are removed during hysterectomy, menopause occurs suddenly, and symptoms may be more severe.

Some women go through menopause with few or no noticeable symptoms. However, many women experience short-term or acute symptoms such as hot flashes, night sweats, mood swings, fatigue, dizziness, headaches, anxiety, depression, poor libido, bladder problems, vaginal dryness and itching, burning and discomfort during sexual intercourse, breast tenderness, dryness and aging of the skin, shortness of breath, heart palpitations, and insomnia. All of these symptoms are due to estrogen and progesterone deficiency. Over the long term, the diminished supply of estrogen increases the likelihood of cardiovascular disease, osteoporosis, and vaginal atrophy. Osteoporosis in particular is a major problem for women after menopause. An estimated 80 percent of the 250,000 hip fractures that occur in the United States every year are due to osteoporosis.

It is important to remember that menopause is *not* a disease. It is a natural process in a woman's life. How a woman views this time of her life can have a lot to do with how frequent and severe her symptoms are. If menopause is viewed as the end of youth and sexuality, this time will be much more difficult than if it is viewed as the next, natural phase of life. With a proper diet, nutritional supplements, and exercise, most of the unpleasant side effects of menopause can be minimized, if not eliminated.

NUTRIENTS

SUPPLEMENT	SUGGESTED DOSAGE	COMMENTS
Very Important		
Lecithin granules or capsules	1 tbsp 3 times daily, before meals. 1,200 mg 3 times daily, before meals.	Important as an emulsifier for vitamin E, which reduces hot flashes and related symptoms.
Multienzyme complex with hydrochloric acid (HCl)	As directed on label. Take with meals.	To aid digestion. HCl production declines with age. *Caution:* Do not give use HCl if you have a history of ulcers.
Primrose oil or black currant seed oil	As directed on label. As directed on label.	Act as sedatives and diuretics. Good for hot flashes. Important for production of estrogen.

Vitamin B complex	As directed on label.	For improved circulation and cellular function. Use a sublingual form for best absorption. Or consider injections (under a doctor's supervision).
plus extra pantothenic acid (vitamin B₅) and	100 mg 3 times daily.	A powerful anti-stress vitamin needed for adrenal function.
vitamin B₆ (pyridoxine)	50 mg 3 times daily.	Minimizes water retention and eases symptoms.
Vitamin E	Start with 400 IU daily and slowly increase the dosage until hot flashes are relieved, up to 1,600 IU daily.	Reduces hot flashes and many other symptoms. Use emulsion form for easier assimilation and greater safety at high doses.

Important		
Boron	3 mg daily. Do not exceed this amount.	Enhances calcium absorption.
Calcium and	2,000 mg daily.	To relieve nervousness and irritability, and to protect against bone loss. Use chelate forms.
magnesium	1,000 mg daily.	
Silica	As directed on label.	Supplies silicon, needed for connective tissue and for calcium uptake.
Zinc	50 mg daily. Do not exceed a total of 100 mg daily from all supplements.	Aids in protecting against bone loss and reducing symptoms. Use zinc gluconate lozenges or OptiZinc for best absorption.

Helpful		
L-Arginine and	500 mg twice daily.	Detoxifies the liver and ammonia.
L-lysine	500 mg daily, on an empty stomach. Take with water or juice. Do not take with milk. Take with 50 mg vitamin B₆ and 100 mg vitamin C for better absorption.	Aids liver function. See AMINO ACIDS in Part One.
Meno-Fem from Prevail	As directed on label.	Contains gamma-oryzanol, a component of rice brain oil effective in controlling uncomfortable symptoms of menopause.
Multiglandular complex	As directed on label.	For hormonal stability. See GLANDULAR THERAPY in Part Three.
Multivitamin and mineral complex with	As directed on label. Take with meals.	All nutrients are needed for normal hormone production and function.
potassium	99 mg daily.	To replace potassium lost through perspiration during hot flashes.
and selenium	200 mcg daily.	An important trace mineral linked to normal hormonal balance.
Vitamin C	3,000–10,000 mg daily.	For hot flashes.

HERBS

❑ A paste made from aloe vera gel and slippery elm powder, mixed to the consistency of toothpaste and inserted into the vagina at night, can relieve vaginal dryness.

❑ Damiana enhances sexual desire and pleasure.

❑ Amaranth, chickweed, dandelion greens, nettle, seaweed, and watercress are rich in calcium and can help prevent osteoporosis.

❑ Anise, black cohosh, fennel, licorice, raspberry, sage, sarsaparilla, squawvine, unicorn root, and wild yam root are natural estrogen promoters.

Caution: Do not use licorice on a daily basis for more than seven days in a row, and avoid it completely if you have high blood pressure. Do not use sage if you suffer from any type of seizure disorder.

❑ Chamomile and valerian root help to calm the body and promote restful sleep.

Caution: Do not use chamomile on an ongoing basis, and avoid it completely if you are allergic to ragweed.

❑ Gotu kola and dong quai relieve hot flashes, vaginal dryness, and depression.

❑ Siberian ginseng aids in relieving depression and in the production of estrogen.

Caution: Do not use this herb if you have hypoglycemia, high blood pressure, or a heart disorder.

RECOMMENDATIONS

❑ Eat a diet consisting of 50 percent raw foods and take a protein supplement to help stabilize blood sugar. Add black-strap molasses, broccoli, dandelion greens, kelp, salmon with bones, sardines, and white fish to your diet.

❑ Do not consume any animal products except for those recommended in this section. Avoid dairy products—limit your consumption to small amounts of low-fat yogurt or buttermilk. Dairy products and meat promote hot flashes. They also contribute to a loss of calcium from the bones.

❑ Avoid alcohol, caffeine, sugar, spicy foods, and hot soups and drinks; they can trigger hot flashes, aggravate urinary incontinence, and make mood swings worse. They also make the blood more acidic, which prompts the bones to release calcium to act as a buffering agent. This is an important factor in bone loss.

❑ Get regular moderate exercise.

❑ Avoid stress as much as possible.

❑ Substitute garlic or onion powder for salt when cooking. Consuming salt increases urinary excretion of calcium.

❑ Drink 2 quarts of quality water each day to help prevent drying of the skin and mucous membranes.

❑ For itching in the vaginal area, use vitamin E cream (with no fragrance added) or open a vitamin E capsule and apply the oil. Natureworks Marigold Ointment from Abkit stops itching almost immediately.

❑ If sexual intercourse is painful, try using vitamin E oil or aloe vera gel to lubricate the vagina.

Hormone Replacement Therapy

Although highly controversial, hormone replacement therapy (HRT) is one option many women consider to help ease themselves through the symptoms of menopause. However, it is up to each woman to give careful consideration to the risks as well as the potential benefits of HRT.

The goal of HRT is to restore a woman's hormonal balance, primarily her estrogen level, to something closer to her normal premenopausal state. In addition to relieving temporary premenopausal and menopausal symptoms, estrogen replacement appears to be an effective preventive against some of the longer term effects of estrogen deficiency, including osteoporosis and heart disease. However, HRT also has a serious dark side, which includes a possible connection to several forms of cancer. A 1995 report by *The New England Journal of Medicine* reaffirmed the suspected link between estrogen-replacement therapy and breast cancer, while another alarming report suggested that long-term use of estrogen may increase the risk of ovarian cancer. And results of a recent study, analyzed by doctors at the Robert Breck Brigham Multipurpose Arthritis and Muskuloskeletal Disease Center in Boston, Massachusetts, indicate a possible connection between the long-term use of estrogen and lupus, a serious autoimmune disorder.

Ultimately, the decision to use hormone replacement therapy is up to each individual. If you are considering estrogen treatment, it is critical to analyze your medical history while weighing the benefits against the possible risks. It is inadvisable to take estrogen if you have a personal or family history of breast cancer, uterine cancer, or fibroid tumors; if you have cystic breasts diagnosed as "atypical hyperplasia"; or if you suffer from liver or gallbladder disease.

It is also important to understand the difference between natural and synthetic forms of estrogen. *Synthetic estrogens* are manufactured in laboratories and they are not easily broken down by the body's natural enzymes. Because of this, they tend to accumulate in the body. Synthetic estrogens can also cause metabolic changes in the liver, resulting in an increased incidence of such side effects as high blood pressure, fluid retention, and blood clots. Most *natural estrogens,* on the other hand, although also produced in laboratories, are chemically identical to the ones produced by the ovaries. One popular type of natural estrogen, equine estrogen (sold under the brand names Estratab and Premarin), is extracted from the urine of pregnant mares. Generally, it is an effective form of replacement estrogen for menopausal women; however, it is extremely potent and may cause metabolic changes in the liver. Equine estrogen probably should not be used by women who are obese, who smoke cigarettes, or who suffer from high blood pressure, high cholesterol, or varicose veins. The most common truly natural estrogens are estropipate (Ogen) and estradiol (Emcyt, Estrace, Estraderm). These natural estrogens are easily metabolized. Any woman who makes the choice to use HRT should use the safer natural estrogens. We recommend that if you do decide to take estrogen, you should use the smallest possible dose of oral estrogen and take it every other day, rather than every day.

Recent research suggests that replacing progesterone may be more important than replacing estrogen. A safe way to replace progesterone is to use a natural progesterone cream. This can often provide effective relief of menopausal symptoms, and also stimulate the body's production and regulation of estrogen and other hormones.

CONSIDERATIONS

❑ If a woman has hypoglycemia, her symptoms often become more pronounced during menopause. Stress puts a burden on the adrenal glands, causing them to work harder than they should. The adrenals therefore produce smaller amounts of the hormones that are needed to help reduce the effects of declining estrogen in the body.

❑ Japanese women generally experience far fewer symptoms of menopause than do Western women. An article in the British medical journal *The Lancet* reported that the reason may be that Japanese women consume more phytoestrogens (plant estrogens). These estrogenlike compounds are found in foods such as soybeans, tofu, miso, flaxseeds, pomegranites, and dates. When these substances are eaten, they act like the estrogens produced in the body.

❑ Gamma-oryzanol, a nutrient derived from rice bran, has been shown to be effective in treating symptoms of menopause. A daily dose of 20 milligrams reduced symptoms by 50 percent in 67 percent of the women studied.

❑ Kombucha tea has detoxifying, energizing, and immune-boosting properties. Many women have found that using it regularly helps to increase vitality and diminish unpleasant menopausal symptoms. (*See* MAKING KOMBUCHA TEA in Part Three.)

❑ Smoking is associated with early menopause.

❑ Frequent sexual intercourse can help relieve vaginal dryness.

❑ Many physicians recommend hormone replacement therapy (HRT) to control severe symptoms caused by estrogen deficiency in menopausal and postmenopausal women. Although hormone therapy appears to be effective, it does have possible serious risks, which should be carefully considered. *See* Hormone Replacement Therapy above.

❑ After menopause, a reduction in the amount of the sex hormone estrogen can cause shrinkage of urethral and vaginal membranes, promoting incontinence. There may be a continuous dribbling of urine. Urethral dilation helps stretch a contracted urethra.

❑ It may be more important to replace progesterone than estrogen. Natural progesterone cream is a good way to do this.

❑ A good source of information on available strategies for coping with menopause is *Smart Medicine for Menopause* by Dr. Sandra Cabot (Avery Publishing Group, 1995).

❑ Hypothyroidism is common in menopausal women. Many symptoms ascribed to menopause may be due to improper thyroid function. (*See* HYPOTHYROIDISM in Part Two.)

❑ *See also* HYPOGLYCEMIA and HYSTERECTOMY-RELATED PROBLEMS in Part Two.

Menstrual Cramps

See under PREMENSTRUAL SYNDROME.

Mercury Toxicity

Mercury is one of the most toxic metals—even more so than lead. This poison is found in our soil, water, and food supply, as well as in sewage sludge, fungicides, and pesticides. Some grains and seeds are treated with methyl mercury chlorine bleaches, which seep into the food supply. Because methyl mercury contaminates our waters, large amounts are found in fish, particularly larger ones that are further up in the food chain. Mercury is also present in a wide variety of everyday products, including cosmetics, dental fillings, fabric softeners, inks used by printers and tattooists, latex, some medications, some paints, plastics, polishes, solvents, and wood preservatives.

Mercury is a cumulative poison. There is no barrier that prohibits mercury from reaching the brain cells, and it is retained in the pain center of the brain and in the central nervous system. Its presence there can prevent both the normal entry of nutrients into the cells and the removal of wastes from the cells. It can bind to immune cells, distorting them and interfering with normal immune responses. This may be one factor behind autoimmune disorders. Significant amounts of mercury in the body can produce arthritis, depression, dermatitis, dizziness, fatigue, gum disease, hair loss, insomnia, memory loss, muscle weakness, and excessive salivation. High levels can also interfere with enzyme activity, resulting in blindness and paralysis. The symptoms of mercury poisoning can mimic those of multiple sclerosis and amyotrophic lateral sclerosis (ALS, also known as Lou Gehrig's disease). Many food and environmental allergies may be directly attributable to mercury poisoning. The U.S. Environmental Protection Agency has linked exposure to mercury vapor to menstrual disorders and spontaneous abortion (miscarriage) as well.

Signs that indicate the presence of toxic mercury levels include behavioral changes, depression, irritability, and hyperactivity. People with this toxicity may also experience allergic reactions or asthma. They may complain about a metallic taste in the mouth, and their teeth may loosen.

According to the World Health Organization, amalgam dental fillings are a prime source of mercury exposure. More than 180 million Americans have mercury amalgam dental fillings. When dentists refer to "silver" fillings, they are usually referring to amalgams, which are silver in color but actually contain approximately 50 percent mercury, 25 percent silver, and 25 percent other materials, such as copper, tin, and nickel. While all the metals used in fillings can be toxic, none is as harmful as the mercury. One amalgam filling can release 3 to 17 micrograms of mercury each day. The mercury vapor released from dental amalgams combines with chemicals in the mouth to create minute amounts of toxic methyl mercury, which is absorbed through the tissues of the mouth and air passages and transported in the blood to the brain and other body tissues. Many people have suffered for years from various health problems—including candidiasis, muscle spasms, chronic fatigue, and recurring infections—that cleared up after they had their amalgam dental fillings removed.

NUTRIENTS

SUPPLEMENT	SUGGESTED DOSAGE	COMMENTS
Essential		
Glutathione plus L-methionine and L-cysteine	As directed on label, on an empty stomach. Take with water or juice. Do not take with milk. Take with 50 mg vitamin B_6 and 100 mg vitamin C for better absorption.	Needed for sulfur. Also helps to detoxify harmful metals and toxins. *See* AMINO ACIDS in Part One.
Selenium	200 mcg daily, in divided doses.	Neutralizes the effects of mercury.
Vitamin E	400–800 IU daily.	Works with selenium to neutralize mercury.
Very Important		
Apple pectin	As directed on label.	Aids in removing toxic metals from the body.
Garlic (Kyolic)	2 capsules 3 times daily.	Acts as a detoxifier.
Kelp or alfalfa	1,000–1,500 mg daily.	Aids the body in removing toxins. *See under* Herbs, below.
Vitamin A plus	50,000 IU daily for 1 month, then reduce to 25,000 IU daily. If you are pregnant, do not exceed 10,000 IU daily.	A powerful antioxidant; destroys free radicals.
natural beta-carotene or	15,000 IU daily.	A powerful free radical scavenger.
carotenoid complex (Betatene)	As directed on label.	
Vitamin C with rutin	4,000–10,000 mg daily.	Helps remove metals and strengthens the immune system.

Important		
Vitamin B complex	100 mg twice daily.	Important for the functioning and protection of the brain.
Helpful		
Brewer's yeast	As directed on label.	A good source of B vitamins.
Hydrochloric acid (HCl)	As directed on label.	To aid digestion. Take this supplement if you are over 40 and deficient in HCl (see INDIGESTION in Part Two).
Lecithin granules or capsules	1 tbsp 3 times daily, before meals. 1,200 mg 3 times daily, before meals.	Protects brain cells from mercury poisoning.

HERBS

❑ Alfalfa contains valuable nutrients and helps the body to eliminate toxins.

RECOMMENDATIONS

❑ Eat organically grown foods, especially beans, onions, and garlic, for added sulfur, which helps protect the body against toxic substances.

❑ Drink water only if it is steam-distilled. Drink plenty of pure fresh fruit and vegetable juices.

❑ Supplement your diet with plenty of fiber (oat bran is a good source) and pectin (found in apples).

Note: Always take supplemental fiber separately from other supplements and medications.

❑ Eat fish in moderation, and always broil it; do not baste it in its juices. While some fish may contain mercury, fish also contains compounds called alkylglycerols, which help to remove mercury from the body. If there is mercury in the fish, it is primarily stored in the fat. By broiling the fish and draining the juices, you will get rid of much of the fat and retain the beneficial alkylglycerols.

❑ If you suspect mercury toxicity, have a hair analysis performed. This can detect toxic levels of mercury. Mercury does not show up in urine or blood samples. See HAIR ANALYSIS in Part Three.

❑ Do not rush to have amalgam dental fillings removed until you have tests done that show elevated levels of mercury. Removal of the fillings should be tried only after other measures, such as the program outlined in this section, have been tried.

CONSIDERATIONS

❑ Chelation therapy removes toxic metals from the body. (See CHELATION THERAPY in Part Three.)

❑ Hal A. Huggins, D.D.S., has done extensive research on the toxic effects of mercury from dental amalgams. He has found links between mercury toxicity and many debilitating and degenerative diseases, including multiple sclerosis,

Alzheimer's disease, Parkinson's disease, arthritis, and lupus. Dr. Huggins has written an informative book describing the dangers of dental amalgams called It's All in Your Head (Avery Publishing Group, 1993).

❑ In response to concern about the health hazards of mercury amalgam fillings, the Swedish government has taken steps to ban their use.

❑ High mercury levels have been linked to candidiasis. (See CANDIDIASIS in Part Two.)

❑ See also CHEMICAL ALLERGIES and ENVIRONMENTAL TOXICITY in Part Two.

Migraine

A migraine is a vascular headache that involves the excessive dilation or contraction of the brain's blood vessels. There are two types of migraine, common and classic. The common migraine occurs slowly, producing a throbbing pain that may last for two to seventy-two hours. The pain is severe and is often centered at the temple or behind one ear. Alternatively, it can begin at the back of the head and spread to one entire side of the head (the word "migraine" comes from the Greek hemikrania, which means "half a skull"). It is usually accompanied by nausea, vomiting, blurred vision, and tingling and numbness in the limbs that can last up to eighteen hours.

A classic migraine is similar to a common migraine, but it is preceded by a set of symptoms referred to as an aura, which can consist of speech disorders, weakness, and disturbances in the senses of vision and/or smell. An aura can also consist of brilliant stars, sparks, flashes, or simple geometric forms passing across the visual field. The most common symptom is an inability to see clearly. Visual disturbances may last only a few seconds or may persist for hours, then disappear.

Migraines are a relatively common disorder, affecting about 10 percent of the population. An estimated 8.7 percent of females and 2.6 percent of males in the United States suffer from migraines. They may occur anywhere from once a week to once or twice a year, and they often run in families. One factor behind the higher incidence of migraine in women may be fluctuations in the level of the hormone estrogen; women typically get migraines around the time of menstruation, when estrogen levels are low. Migraines occur most often in people between the ages of twenty and thirty-five, and tend to decline with age. However, children too can suffer from migraines. In children, migraine pain tends to be more diffuse, rather than localized. Migraine can first show up in childhood not as headaches, but as colic, periodic abdominal pains, vomiting, dizziness, and severe motion sickness. According to the U.S. Centers for Disease Control and Prevention (CDC), the incidence of migraine headaches has increased by nearly 60 percent in all age groups in recent years.

Any number of things can trigger a migraine in a susceptible individual, including allergies, constipation, stress, liver malfunction, too much or too little sleep, emotional changes, hormonal changes, sun glare, flashing lights, lack of exercise, and changes in barometric pressure. Dental problems may also be a factor. Low blood sugar is frequently associated with migraine; studies have shown that blood sugar levels are low during a migraine attack, and the lower the blood sugar level, the more severe the headache. Smoking can cause an attack because the nicotine and carbon monoxide cigarette smoke contains affects the blood vessels—the nicotine constricts them while the carbon monoxide tends to expand them. Many different foods may precipitate an attack. Some of the most common offenders are chocolate, citrus fruits, alcohol (especially red wine), and any food that is aged, cured, pickled, soured, yeasty, or fermented.

NUTRIENTS

SUPPLEMENT	SUGGESTED DOSAGE	COMMENTS
Very Important		
Calcium and magnesium	2,000 mg daily. 1,000 mg daily.	Minerals that help to regulate muscular tone and to transmit nerve impulses throughout the body and to the brain. Use chelate forms.
Coenzyme Q10	60 mg daily.	Increases blood flow to the brain and improves circulation.
Dimethylglycine (DMG) (Aangamik DMG from FoodScience Labs)	125 mg twice daily.	Improves brain oxygenation.
Essential fatty acids or primrose oil	As directed on label. As directed on label.	Needed for brain cells and for fat metabolism. An anti-inflammatory agent to keep the blood vessels from constricting.
Multivitamin and mineral formula	As directed on label.	All nutrients are necessary in balance.
Vitamin B3 (niacin) plus niacinamide	200 mg 3 times daily. Do not exceed this amount. 800 mg daily.	Increases blood flow to the brain. Caution: Do not take niacin if you have a liver disorder, gout, or high blood pressure.
Rutin	200 mg daily.	Removes toxic metals, which may cause migraines.
Helpful		
Bio Rizin from American Biologics		See under Herbs, below.
Garlic (Kyolic)	2 capsules 3 times daily, with meals.	A potent detoxifier.
Pantothenic acid (vitamin B5) or royal jelly	100 mg twice daily. 1 tsp twice daily.	Needed by the adrenal glands when the body is under stress. Royal jelly is high in pantothenic acid. Use royal jelly from a natural source.
Quercetin and bromelain or Activated Quercetin from Source Naturals	500 mg daily, before meals. As directed on label.	Helps control food allergies. Needed for a variety of enzyme functions. Contains quercetin plus bromelain and vitamin C to aid absorption.
Taurine Plus from American Biologics	10–20 drops daily.	An important antioxidant and immune regulator, needed for white blood cell activation and neurological function. Use the sublingual form.
Vitamin B complex	As directed on label.	Needed for a healthy nervous system. Use a hypoallergenic form. Injections (under a doctor's supervision) may be necessary.
Vitamin B6 (pyridoxine)	50 mg 3 times daily.	Required for normal brain function. Use a hypoallergenic form.
Vitamin C	3,000–6,000 mg daily.	Aids in producing anti-stress adrenal hormones and enhances immunity. A buffered or esterified form is best.

HERBS

❑ Bio Rizin from American Biologics contains licorice extract, which improves energy levels and helps to relieve allergy symptoms that can trigger migraines.

Caution: Do not use this herb on a daily basis for more than seven days in a row. Avoid it completely if you have high blood pressure.

❑ Feverfew helps to alleviate pain.

Caution: Do not use feverfew during pregnancy.

❑ Ginkgo biloba extract enhances cerebral circulation.

❑ Other herbs effective for the treatment of migraines include cayenne (capsicum), chamomile, ginger, peppermint, rosemary, valerian, willow bark, and wormwood.

Caution: Do not use wormwood during pregnancy. It is not recommended for long-term use.

RECOMMENDATIONS

❑ Adopt a diet that is low in simple carbohydrates and high in protein. *See* HYPOGLYCEMIA in Part Two and follow the dietary guidelines.

❑ Include almonds, almond milk, watercress, parsley, fennel, garlic, cherries, and fresh pineapple in the diet.

❑ Omit from the diet foods that contain the amino acid tyramine, including aged meats, avocados, bananas, beer, cabbage, canned fish, dairy products, eggplant, hard cheeses, potatoes, raspberries, red plums, tomatoes, wine, and yeast. Also avoid alcoholic beverages, aspirin, chocolate, monosodium glutamate (MSG), nitrites (preservatives found in hot dogs and luncheon meats), and spicy foods.

❑ Get regular moderate exercise.

❑ Massage the neck and back of the head daily.

❑ Avoid salt and acid-forming foods such as meat, cereal, bread, and grains. Also avoid fried foods and fatty and greasy foods.

❑ Eat small meals, and eat small, nutritious snacks between meals if needed, to help stabilize wide swings in blood sugar that may precipitate a migraine. Especially avoid missing meals.

❑ Take only hypoallergenic supplements.

❑ See your dentist for treatment of any tooth problems, such as gum disease, tooth decay, bacterial infection, temporomandibular joint syndrome (TMJ), or tooth-grinding, that may be contributing to the problem.

❑ Try coffee as a migraine treatment. At the first sign of a migraine attack, drink 1 or 2 cups of strong coffee, then lie down in a dark, quiet room. For this treatment to be effective, you must not otherwise consume caffeine. Eliminate the following from your daily diet: coffee (even decaffeinated; it still contains some caffeine) and all other sources of caffeine, including chocolate, soft drinks, and over-the-counter and prescription medications that contain caffeine (but do not discontinue a prescription medication or change the dosage without consulting with your physician).

❑ Do not smoke, and avoid secondhand smoke.

CONSIDERATIONS

❑ Researchers believe many migraine attacks are caused by chemical imbalances in the brain. Levels of the brain chemical serotonin drop during a headache. This triggers an impulse along the trigeminal nerve to blood vessels in the meninges, the brain's outer covering. In the meninges, the blood vessels become inflamed and swollen. The result is a headache.

❑ The frequent use of over-the-counter painkillers may actually increase the likelihood of migraine attacks.

❑ A study reported in the British medical journal *The Lancet* found that when allergenic foods were eliminated from the diets of migraine sufferers, as many as 93 percent of them found relief.

❑ Migraine headaches in women may result from hormonal changes during the menstrual cycle. After menopause, the headaches usually decrease.

❑ Researchers in France have identified a gene linked to a rare, severe type of migraine called *familial hemiplegic migraine.*

❑ Studies have shown biofeedback training to be useful in lessening the frequency and severity of attacks. Typically, a person's hands cool to as low as 65°F before an attack, signaling a constriction of the blood vessels. Raising the temperature of the hands can prevent this and avert the attack. Those trained in biofeedback learn to relax, thus raising their temperature in seconds and preventing vessel constriction. Taking a hot bath also can be helpful.

❑ Music has a calming effect and can help to relieve migraines (*see* MUSIC AND SOUND THERAPY in Part Three).

❑ Some find migraine relief by taking lecithin (a soybean derivative). In one study, those who took between three and six 1,200-milligram capsules when they felt a headache coming on had fewer, milder migraine attacks.

❑ Many people who suffer from migraines end up perpetuating their pain by trying to relieve it with daily use of over-the-counter painkillers. Once the medication wears off, the headache often returns, and may be more severe, prompting the person to take yet more medication—setting in motion a cycle of pain, pills, more pain, and more pills. Anyone who thinks his or her headaches may be related to medication should see a physician.

❑ A study on the herb feverfew conducted at the University of Nottingham in England found that participants who took the herb got an average of 24 percent fewer migraines than those who did not, and also that vomiting was reduced, with no side effects.

❑ Women who suffer from migraines may benefit from the use of natural progesterone cream.

❑ The drug most commonly prescribed for relief of migraine, ergotamine (sold under the brand names Cafergot, Ergostat, and Wigraine), can be addicting, and should not be taken for more than two days in any one week. Cafergot and Wigraine also contain caffeine.

❑ A relatively new drug, sumatriptan (Imitrex), relieves acute migraine attacks by increasing the amount of serotonin in the brain. In clinical studies, 82 percent of people with migraines who took sumatriptan improved within two hours of treatment; 65 percent were pain-free. This drug currently must be administered by injection (it is sold in the form of a home injection kit), and it can cause side effects, including dizziness, drowsiness, anxiety, and malaise. It is not appropriate for all migraine sufferers, and because it has the potential to cause coronary artery constriction, it should not be taken by people with ischemic heart disease (angina or a history of heart attack). Also, treatment with sumatriptan may result in a rise in blood pressure, so people with uncontrolled hypertension should not use it.

❑ Other drugs that are sometimes prescribed for people who get migraines include amitriptyline (Elavil, Endep), diazepam (Valium), methysergide (Sansert), and propranolol (Inderal). These are used as a preventive rather than as therapy for an acute attack.

❑ The following agencies offer information about how to deal with headaches:

National Headache Foundation
5252 North Western Avenue
Chicago, IL 60625
800–843–2256
Send a self-adressed, stamped business-size envelope with two first-class stamps and a brief note explaining your questions.

American Council for Headache Education (ACHE)
875 Kings Highway Suite 200
Woodbury, NJ 08096
800–255–ACHE

☐ *See also* HEADACHE in Part Two and PAIN CONTROL in Part Three.

Miscarriage

See under PREGNANCY-RELATED PROBLEMS.

Mononucleosis

Mononucleosis ("mono") is an infectious viral disease. The vast majority of cases of mono are caused by the Epstein-Barr virus (EBV), a member of the herpes virus family. More rarely, it may be caused by cytomegalovirus (CMV). Once the virus enters the body, it multiplies in lymphocytes (white blood cells). Mono affects the respiratory system, the lymphatic tissues and glands in the neck, groin, armpits, bronchial tubes, spleen, and liver. Symptoms include depression, fatigue, fever, generalized aching, headache, jaundice, sore throat, swollen glands, and, sometimes, a bumpy red rash. The spleen may become enlarged, and liver function may be affected.

The virus that causes mono is contagious, and can be transmitted from person to person by close contact such as kissing or sharing food or utensils, although it can also spread during sexual contact or through the air like the common cold. The incubation period is about ten days in children and thirty to fifty days in adults. This disorder is most common among children and adolescents.

Because the symptoms are often so similar, mononucleosis is often mistaken for influenza. However, with mono, the symptoms tend to be more persistent. The acute symptoms usually last from two to four weeks, and fatigue can persist for three to eight weeks after the other symptoms disappear. A few individuals may experience a more chronic form in which symptoms persist for months or even years.

A diagnosis of mono is made through a blood test called a heterophil antibody test. This reveals the presence of specific antibodies against EBV and confirms the presence of mono. A liver function test may aid in diagnosis.

NUTRIENTS

SUPPLEMENT	SUGGESTED DOSAGE	COMMENTS
Very Important		
Acidophilus	As directed on label.	"Friendly" bacteria are important. Use a nondairy formula.
Proteolytic enzymes	As directed on label 3–4 times daily, between meals and at bedtime, on an empty stomach.	Reduces inflammation and aids in absorption of nutrients.
Vitamin A and vitamin E	50,000 IU daily for 2 weeks, then slowly reduce to 15,000 IU daily. If you are pregnant, do not exceed 10,000 IU daily. 400–800 IU daily for 4 weeks, then slowly reduce to 400 IU daily.	Essential for the immune system. Use emulsion forms for easier assimilation and greater safety at high doses.
Vitamin C with bioflavonoids	5,000–10,000 mg daily, in divided doses.	Destroys the virus and boosts the immune system. A buffered or esterified form is best.
Important		
Dimethylglycine (DMG) (Aangamik DMG from FoodScience Labs)	125 mg twice daily.	An immune stimulant that enhances oxygenation.
Free-form amino acid complex	¼ tsp 2–3 times daily, on an empty stomach.	To provide protein, necessary for healing and to rebuild tissues. Use a powdered form.
Garlic (Kyolic)	2 capsules 3 times daily, with meals.	A powerful immune booster. Acts as a natural antibiotic.
Vitamin B complex	100 mg 3 times daily, with meals.	B vitamins increase energy and are needed for every bodily function, including proper digestion and brain function. Use a high-stress, hypoallergenic formula. A sublingual form is recommended. Injections (under a doctor's supervision) may be necessary.
plus extra vitamin B$_{12}$	15 mg twice daily.	Required for proper digestion and to prevent anemia. Use a lozenge or sublingual form.
Helpful		
Maitake or	As directed on label.	Has immune-boosting and antiviral properties.
shiitake or	As directed on label.	
reishi	As directed on label.	
Multivitamin and mineral complex with		Necessary for normal cellular function and repair. Use a high-potency formula.
calcium and	1,000 mg daily.	
magnesium and	75–1,000 mg daily.	
potassium	99 mg daily.	
Raw thymus glandular plus	500 mg 3 times daily.	To enhance immune response. *See* GLANDULAR THERAPY in Part Three.
multiglandular complex	As directed on label.	

HERBS

☐ Astragalus and echinacea boost the immune system.

☐ Dandelion and milk thistle protect the liver.

☐ Goldenseal fights infection. If a sore throat is present, place a dropperful of alcohol-free goldenseal extract in the mouth and hold it there for a few seconds, then swallow. Do this every four hours for three to five days.

Caution: Do not take goldenseal internally on a daily basis for more than one week at a time, do not use it during pregnancy, and use it with caution if you are allergic to ragweed.

❑ Pau d'arco balances the bacteria in the colon.

RECOMMENDATIONS

❑ Eat a diet composed of at least 50 percent raw foods. Consume as much of your food as possible raw. Also emphasize wholesome soups, root vegetables, and whole grains, including brown rice.

❑ Each day, drink eight 8-ounce glasses of distilled water, plus fresh juice.

❑ Do not consume any coffee, fried foods, processed foods, soft drinks, stimulants, sugar, tea, and white flour products. These depress immune function.

❑ Eat four to six small meals daily. Avoid overeating at any one meal.

❑ Get plenty of rest. Round-the-clock bed rest is a good idea during the acute phase of the disorder.

❑ Use a protein supplement from a vegetable source. Spiru-tein from Nature's Plus is a good protein drink for between meals.

❑ Use chlorophyll in tablet form, or in a liquid form such as "green drinks" made from leafy green vegetables or wheatgrass. Kyo-Green from Wakunaga is a highly concentrated natural barley and wheatgrass source of amino acids, vitamins, minerals, carotene, chlorophyll, and enzymes. It is also available in powder form containing chlorella, kelp, and brown rice.

❑ Do not strain when having a bowel movement, as this may injure an enlarged spleen.

❑ Do not give aspirin to a child or adolescent with mononucleosis, as it may lead to complications such as Reye's syndrome. *See* REYE'S SYNDROME in Part Two.

❑ Avoid close physical contact with others as much as possible. Flush all tissues after use, and do not share food, eating utensils, or towels. Wash your hands frequently.

❑ If you have a fever over 102°F, or if you develop severe pain in the upper left abdomen that lasts for five minutes or more, or if breathing and/or swallowing becomes difficult as a result of throat inflammation, consult your health care provider promptly. These can be signs that a more serious condition is developing.

CONSIDERATIONS

❑ Once contracted, both EBV and CMV remain in the body for life, but the acute illness eventually runs its course in nearly all cases. Because there is no cure for mononucleosis,

a proper diet and supplements, plus adequate rest, are especially important for this disorder.

❑ Antibiotics are of no use unless there is a secondary infection such as ear infection or strep throat. However, in approximately 20 percent of cases, strep throat is also present, and antibiotic therapy may be prescribed.

❑ Adequate rest, exercise, and nutrition are essential for the maintenance of general health and the prevention of mononucleosis. Protein is needed to stimulate the formation of antibodies that protect against complications such as hepatitis and jaundice.

❑ *See also* CHRONIC FATIGUE SYNDROME in Part Two.

Morning Sickness

See under PREGNANCY-RELATED PROBLEMS.

Motion Sickness

Motion sickness occurs when motion causes the eyes, the sensory nerves, and the vestibular apparatus of the ear to send conflicting signals to the brain. Anxiety, genetics, overeating, poor ventilation, and traveling immediately after eating are common contributing factors.

People suffering from motion sickness experience symptoms that range from severe headache to queasiness to nausea and vomiting while flying, sailing, or traveling in automobiles or trains. Other symptoms of motion sickness include cold sweats, dizziness, excessive salivation and/or yawning, fatigue, loss of desire for food, pallor, severe distress, sleepiness, and weakness. If severe, an attack can make the sufferer completely uncoordinated. Women are affected by this condition more frequently than men are. Elderly people and children under the age of two usually are not affected.

Natural remedies have been used with great success for motion sickness. Prevention is the key; motion sickness is far easier to prevent than it is to cure. Once excessive salivation and nausea set in, it is often too late to do anything but wait for the trip to be over so recovery can begin.

NUTRIENTS

SUPPLEMENT	SUGGESTED DOSAGE	COMMENTS
Important		
Charcoal tablets	5 tablets 1 hour before travel. Take separately from other medications and supplements.	A detoxifier.
Ginger		*See under* Herbs, on next page.

Magnesium	500 mg 1 hour before trip.	Acts as a nerve tonic.
Peppermint		*See under* Herbs, below.
Vitamin B$_6$ (pyridoxine)	100 mg 1 hour before trip, then 100 mg 2 hours later.	Relieves nausea.

HERBS

❑ Ginger is an excellent treatment and preventive for nausea and upset stomach. Take 2 ginger capsules (approximately 1,000 milligrams) every three hours, starting one hour before the beginning of the trip.

❑ Peppermint tea soothes and calms the stomach. A drop of peppermint oil on the tongue provides excellent relief from nausea and motion sickness. Peppermint can also be taken in lozenge form.

RECOMMENDATIONS

❑ When traveling, take whole-grain crackers with you on trips. Olives can help ward off nausea because they have the effect of decreasing salivation.

❑ Pay special attention to your diet. If a certain dish disagrees with you at home, it will most certainly disagree with you on the road.

❑ Do not eat spicy, heavy, fatty, processed, or junk foods, especially fried foods, before or during travel. They can contribute to nausea.

❑ Avoid alcohol. Alcohol disrupts the delicate operations that occur in the inner ear. If you are prone to motion sickness, alcohol consumption will only aggravate the problem by further disrupting communication between the eyes, the inner ears, and the brain.

❑ Avoid odors and aromas that can bring about nausea. Aside from obvious things such as smoke and engine exhaust, certain food odors can make you ill, as can paint fumes, nail polish, or animal waste. Even otherwise pleasant smells, such as those from perfume or after-shave, can cause a problem if you are prone to motion sickness.

❑ Sit still and breathe deeply. Your brain is already thoroughly confused without extra motion on your part. Especially try to keep your head still.

❑ Stay cool, if possible. Fresh air can assist in battling motion sickness. If in a car, roll down a window. If on a ship, standing on deck and taking in the sea breezes can help. In an airplane, open the overhead vent.

❑ Limit or eliminate visual input. This will cut down on the conflicting information assaulting the brain. Traveling at night helps many people, simply because visual acuity is diminished, so that they do not perceive motion to the same degree as during the day. At sea, lying down and closing your eyes at the first sign of motion sickness can be helpful. In an automobile, set your eyes on a distant, stationary object, such as the horizon.

CONSIDERATIONS

❑ Symptoms of nausea may indicate that the liver needs attention.

❑ A homeopathic liver remedy may help reduce nausea.

❑ Chewable papaya tablets can be helpful.

❑ There are numerous over-the-counter products available that may help to prevent motion sickness, including cyclizine (Marezine), dimenhydrinate (Dramamine), and Meclizine (Bonine). These drugs are not always effective, however, and can cause side effects, especially drowsiness.

❑ If motion sickness is debilitating, and herbal, homeopathic, and over-the-counter medications do not bring relief, a physician can prescribe scopolamine, available in a dime-sized patch (Transderm-V or Transderm-Scop), which delivers the drug through the skin for up to three days. It should be applied at least four hours before embarking. The patch can be worn on any part of the body that is free of hair. Possible side effects of scopolamine include dry mouth, drowsiness, blurred vision, and a dilated pupil on the side the patch is worn. This drug should not be used by anyone with glaucoma, as it raises pressure within the eye.

❑ To a certain extent, motion sickness is psychological. In many cases, it can be prevented if you consciously tell yourself that you *will not* get sick.

Mouth and Gum Disease

See HALITOSIS; PERIODONTAL DISEASE. *See also* Bleeding Gums *under* PREGNANCY-RELATED PROBLEMS.

Multiple Sclerosis

Multiple sclerosis (MS) is a progressive, degenerative disorder of the central nervous system, including the brain, the optic nerve, and the spinal cord. The disease affects various parts of the nervous system by destroying the myelin sheaths that cover the nerves and leaving scar tissue called plaques, ultimately resulting in destruction of the nerves. This process is known as sclerosis.

Symptoms vary in individuals, depending on which portion or portions of the nervous system are most affected. In the earlier stages, a person may experience episodes of dizziness; emotional changes such as mood swings and/or depression; eye problems such as blurred or double vision; a feeling of tingling and/or numbness, especially in the hands and feet; loss of balance and/or coordination; muscular stiffness; nausea and vomiting; slurred speech; tremors; a vague feeling of weakness and/or fatigue; difficulty breathing; and, for men, impotence. As the disease progresses, a person with MS may have trouble walking and develop a staggering gait. In the advanced stages, movements may become more spastic, and paralysis and breathing difficulty may occur. Bowel and bladder problems, especially chronic urinary incontinence or urgency, are not uncommon, and extreme fatigue—one of the most disabling symptoms of MS—may set in.

The disease follows a pattern of periodic flare-ups, called exacerbations, followed by periods in which symptoms diminish or even disappear. MS is variable in its rate of progression. It can be relatively benign, with only a few minor attacks spread over decades, or it can be rapidly and completely disabling. Most commonly, it progresses slowly, disappearing for periods of time but returning intermittently, often in progressively more severe attacks.

The cause of MS is not known, but it is widely believed to be an autoimmune disease in which white blood cells attack the myelin sheaths as if they were a foreign substance. Stress and malnutrition, whether from poor absorption or poor diet, often precede the onset of the disease. Some experts suspect that an as-yet-unidentified virus may be involved. Heredity may also be a factor. Another theory is that this disease is caused by food intolerances or allergies, especially allergies to dairy products and gluten.

Chemical poisoning of the nervous system by pesticides, industrial chemicals, and heavy metals may also play a part in the development of MS. Environmental toxins can cause disturbances in the body's normal metabolic pathways that result in damage to the nerves' protective myelin sheaths. Even substances that are not necessarily toxic to everyone can be a problem for susceptible individuals. Toxins such as those produced by bacteria and fungi in the body have been known to produce symptoms like those of MS.

Many experts suspect that mercury poisoning is behind many cases of MS. Mercury has been shown to bind to the DNA of cells and cell membranes, causing cellular distortion and inhibited cell function. The installation of mercury amalgam dental fillings (the chief source of mercury exposure for most people in the United States) has been known to produce symptoms indistinguishable from those of multiple sclerosis in some people. Further, the levels of mercury in people with MS have been found to be an average of seven times higher than those in healthy people.

Finally, diet may play a key role in the development of MS. This is suggested by the fact that MS is fairly common in the United States and almost unheard of in some other countries, such as Japan, Korea, and China. The consumption of saturated fats, cholesterol, and alcohol, so common in Western countries, leads to the production of a hormonelike substance called prostaglandin 2 (PG2), which promotes the inflammatory response and worsens symptoms of multiple sclerosis. People in Asian countries typically consume much less fat than people in North America and northern Europe do. Their diets are also rich in marine foods, seeds, and fruit oils, which are high in essential fatty acids, including the omega-3 essential fatty acids, which have an inhibitory effect on the inflammatory response.

MS is usually diagnosed between the ages of twenty-five and forty. Women are affected nearly twice as often as men are. MS is rarely diagnosed in children and in people over sixty years of age. Magnetic resonance imaging (MRI) may be used to diagnose MS. However, there is no single diagnostic test for the disease, and diagnosis must be done indirectly, by ruling out other possible causes of symptoms.

There is no known cure for this disease, but the supplement and dietary programs outlined in this section have been shown to be helpful. Long-term sufferers of MS may not benefit as much, but younger people who are just starting to exhibit symptoms may find that the correct supplements slow or even stop the progression of the disease.

NUTRIENTS

SUPPLEMENT	SUGGESTED DOSAGE	COMMENTS
Very Important		
Coenzyme Q10	90 mg daily.	Needed for improved circulation and tissue oxygenation. Strengthens the immune system.
Gamma-linolenic acid (GLA) or flaxseed oil or primrose oil or omega-3 essential fatty acids	As directed on label 3 times daily, with meals. As directed on label 3 times daily, with meals.	An essential fatty acid needed to control symptoms. Deficiency is common in people with MS. If GLA is not available, use one of these supplements for essential fatty acids.
Sulfur or garlic (Kyolic)	500 mg 2–3 times daily. 2 capsules 3 times daily.	Protects against toxic substances. An excellent source of sulfur.
Vitamin B complex	100 mg 3 times daily.	Aids immune system function and maintains healthy nerves. Use hypoallergenic formulas for all the B vitamins.
plus extra vitamin B6 (pyridoxine)	50 mg 3 times daily.	Promotes red blood cell production; aids the nervous system and immune function. Deficiency may cause MS in susceptible persons.
and vitamin B12	1,000 mcg twice daily.	Aids in cellular longevity and helps prevent nerve damage by maintaining the protective myelin sheaths. Use a lozenge or sublingual form.
and choline and inositol	As directed on label.	To stimulate the central nervous system and aid in protecting the myelin sheaths from damage.
Important		
Amino-LIV from Carlson Labs	¼ tsp twice daily, on an empty stomach.	A combination of the branched-chain amino acids, which aid in use of nutrients by the muscles. *See* AMINO ACIDS in Part One.
plus L-glycine	500 mg twice daily, on an empty stomach.	Aids in supporting the myelin sheaths.

Acidophilus	1 tsp twice daily, on an empty stomach.	Helps to detoxify harmful substances, enhances absorption of nutrients, and aids digestion. Use a powdered form.
Calcium	2,000–3,000 mg daily.	Deficiency may create a predisposition to developing MS. Use chelate form for best assimilation.
and magnesium	1,000–1,500 mg daily.	Needed for calcium absorption and for proper muscular coordination.
Free-form amino acid complex	As directed on label 3 times daily, between meals.	Helps maintain good absorption of nutrients needed for proper brain function.
Grape seed extract	As directed on label.	A powerful antioxidant and anti-inflammatory.
Multienzyme complex or	As directed on label. Take with meals.	For proper breakdown of foods.
Infla-Zyme Forte from American Biologics	3–4 tablets before each meal and 2 tablets between meals 2–3 times daily.	To reduce inflammation.
Multiglandular complex	As directed on label.	Needed for the endocrine, hormonal, and enzyme systems. See GLANDULAR THERAPY in Part Three.
Potassium	300–1,000 mg daily.	Needed for normal muscle function.
Raw thymus glandular	500 mg twice daily.	Enhances immune function.
Selenium	150–300 mcg daily.	An antioxidant and immune system stimulant.
Vitamin A plus	25,000 IU daily. If you are pregnant, do not exceed 10,000 IU daily.	Important antioxidants. Use emulsion forms for easier assimilation.
natural beta-carotene or	15,000 IU daily.	
carotenoid complex (Betatene)	As directed on label.	
Vitamin C	3,000–5,000 mg daily.	Promotes production of the antiviral protein interferon in the body. Also an antioxidant and immune stimulant. Use buffered ascorbic acid or an esterified form such as Ester C Plus Bioflavonoids from Natrol.
Vitamin D	800 IU daily.	Aids in calcium absorption.
Vitamin E	Begin with 400 IU daily and increase slowly to 1,800 IU daily.	Important for circulation, destroys free radicals, and protects the nervous system. Emulsion form is recommended for easier assimilation and greater safety at high doses.
Vitamin K or alfalfa	200 mcg 3 times daily, with meals.	Helps prevent nausea and vomiting. See under Herbs, below.
Helpful		
Brewer's yeast	Start with ¼ tsp daily and slowly increase to 2 tsp daily.	Improves blood sugar metabolism when taken with chromium. Aids in lowering cholesterol and improving HDL/LDL ratio.

Kyo-Green from Wakunaga	1 tsp in liquid 3 times daily.	A good source of organic chlorophyll, live enzymes, vitamins, and minerals plus amino acids.
Lecithin granules or capsules	1 tbsp 3 times daily, before meals. 1,200 mg 3–4 times daily, before meals.	Protects the cells. Needed for normal brain function.
Manganese	5–10 mg daily. Take separately from calcium.	An important mineral often deficient in people with MS.
Multimineral complex	As directed on label.	Needed for all enzyme systems in the body and to supply needed nutrients. Use a high-potency formula.
Phosphorus	900 mg daily.	Needed for transfer of energy within cells.

HERBS

❑ Alfalfa is a good source of vitamin K. It can be taken in liquid or tablet form.

❑ Burdock, dandelion, echinacea, goldenseal, pau d'arco, red clover, St. Johnswort, sarsaparilla, and yarrow are effective detoxifiers.

Caution: Do not take goldenseal internally on a daily basis for more than one week at a time, do not use it during pregnancy, and use it with caution if you are allergic to ragweed.

❑ Lobelia, skullcap, and valerian root relax the nervous system. Taken at bedtime, they aid in preventing insomnia. Lobelia is good also for daytime use.

Caution: Do not take lobelia internally on an ongoing basis.

RECOMMENDATIONS

❑ Eat only organically grown foods with no chemical treatments or additives, including eggs, fruits, gluten-free grains, raw nuts and seeds, vegetables, and cold-pressed vegetable oils. The best diet for people with this disorder is totally vegetarian.

❑ Eat plenty of raw sprouts and alfalfa, plus foods that contain lactic acid, such as sauerkraut and dill pickles. Also good are "green drinks" that contain plenty of chlorophyll.

❑ Eat plenty of dark leafy greens. These are good sources of vitamin K.

❑ Drink at least eight 8-ounce glasses of quality water each day to prevent toxic buildup in the muscles.

❑ Do not consume any alcohol, barley, chocolate, coffee, dairy products, fried foods, highly seasoned foods, meat, oats, refined foods, rye, salt, spices, sugar, tobacco, wheat, or processed, canned, or frozen foods.

❑ Take a fiber supplement. Fiber is important for avoiding constipation. Periodically take warm cleansing enemas with the juice of a fresh lemon. A clean colon is important for keeping toxic waste from interfering with muscle function. *See* COLON CLEANSING and ENEMAS in Part Three.

❑ Never consume saturated fats, processed oils, oils that have been subjected to heat (either in processing or in cooking), or oils that have been stored without refrigeration.

❑ Have yourself tested for possible food allergies. *See* ALLERGIES in Part Two. We believe that food allergies are a major factor in the development and progression of multiple sclerosis. Unfortunately, all too often the allergies are not discovered until irreversible nerve damage has occurred. Early detection is therefore vital. Eliminating offending foods from your diet may slow down the progression of the disease and help you avoid further damage.

❑ Avoid stress and anxiety. Attacks of MS are often precipitated by a trauma or a period of emotional distress.

❑ Avoid exposure to heat, such as hot baths, showers, sunbathing, and overly warm surroundings, and avoid becoming overheated when working or exercising. Avoid exhaustion and viral infections. All of these may trigger an attack or worsen symptoms.

❑ Utilize massage, get regular exercise, and keep mentally active. These are extremely valuable in maintaining muscle function and bringing about remission of symptoms. However, exercises that may increase body temperature can decrease the function of the nerves involved and make symptoms worse. Swimming is the best activity. Doing other exercises in cool water is good as well because body temperature is kept lower and the body's weight is supported by the water. Stretching exercises help to prevent muscle contractures. Physical therapy is often needed.

❑ When an exacerbation begins, take at least two days of complete bed rest. This can often stop a mild attack.

❑ Educate yourself and your family about the disease, and seek out sources of emotional support. Contact the National Multiple Sclerosis Society at 733 Third Avenue, New York, NY 10017; telephone 212–986–3240 or 800–344–4867.

❑ If your physician makes you feel that you cannot get better, find another physician. Such negative input can have a disastrous effect on your health.

CONSIDERATIONS

❑ A strong immune system may help to prevent multiple sclerosis by helping the body avoid infection, which often precedes the onset of this disease.

❑ While the effects of MS on pregnancy seem to be minimal, slightly more flare-ups occur during the six months following childbirth.

❑ Gluten intolerance may make a person more susceptible to MS.

❑ Oral corticosteroids, such as prednisone (Deltasone and others), are often used to hasten remission and to reduce the severity of attacks. Giving cortisone intravenously for a short period (five days) eliminates the side effects that come with the use of oral medication. The same drugs now used by transplant patients to keep their bodies from rejecting donated organs can be used to control symptoms. These immunosuppressant drugs are not without side effects, however; people who take them commonly experience nausea, vomiting, and hair loss, and they run a greater risk of cancer as well.

❑ A doctor may prescribe an antispasmodic or a tranquilizer such as diazepam (Valium) to relax spastic muscles and provide pain relief; amantadine (Symmetrel) to help counteract fatigue; and/or an antidepressant to help alleviate depression associated with MS.

❑ Injections of interferon beta may be prescribed. This is a synthetic form of the naturally occurring immune system protein beta interferon that can reduce the severity and frequency of attacks. A two-year multicenter study reported in the *Archives of Neurology* found that spinal injections of natural human beta interferon can relieve exacerbations of MS. Vitamin C promotes the production of natural interferon in the body.

❑ A tiny pump implanted in the abdomen is bringing new hope to some people with multiple sclerosis. The tiny machine delivers controlled doses of a drug called baclofen (Lioresal) directly into the spinal cord to control MS spasms. The drug supply lasts one to three months, and then the pump is refilled with a syringe. This new delivery system eliminates side effects such as weakness, drowsiness, and dizziness that often occur when the drug is taken in pill form.

❑ A new drug called 4-aminopyridine, which increases the conduction of nerve impulses, has been shown to improve motor skills in some people with MS. This drug is relatively inexpensive and has minimal side effects. Another relatively new drug, copolymer 1 (Copaxone) may prevent MS flare-ups and slow or halt the progression of the disease. It appears to present no serious health risks.

❑ According to the New Jersey College of Medicine, x-ray irradiation to the lymph glands and the spleen may halt the progress of MS in some cases. However, radiation exposure depresses the immune system.

❑ Short fasts are helpful. (*See* FASTING in Part Three.)

❑ Researchers in Scandinavia have long used essential fatty acid supplementation to treat MS and to reduce the frequency of new events.

❑ Although its use is controversial in the United States, hyperbaric oxygen therapy has been used with success for people with multiple sclerosis in some other countries. (*See* HYPERBARIC OXYGEN THERAPY in Part Three.)

❑ Some people with MS have had success with treatment involving honeybee venom. In this practice, called *apitherapy*, honeybee venom is administered by injection, either with a hypodermic needle or by the bees themselves. The venom apparently acts as an anti-inflammatory and immune system stimulant, and can relieve the fatigue, cramping, and weakness that mark MS. Further information is available from the American Apitherapy Society, Box 54, Hartland Four Corners, VT 05049; telephone 800–823–3460.

❑ Recent studies point to a possible link between MS and candida infection. A significant proportion of people with MS show evidence of imbalanced bowel flora, which is characteristic of candidiasis. Further, chronic fatigue is a symptom of candidiasis, and it is also one of the most common complaints of people with multiple sclerosis. Treatments to reduce candida activity have been found to reduce the fatigue experienced by many people with MS. (See CANDIDIASIS in Part Two.)

❑ The symptoms of Lyme disease may mimic those of multiple sclerosis. (See LYME DISEASE in Part Two.)

Mumps

Mumps is a common viral illness of childhood. It is an acute, contagious viral infection of the parotid glands, the salivary glands located at the jaw angles below the ears. Symptoms include swelling of one or both glands, plus headache, fever, sore throat, and pain when swallowing or chewing. Often, one of the parotid glands swells before the other, and as swelling in one gland subsides, the other begins to swell.

Mumps is transmitted from person to person by means of infected droplets of saliva or direct contact with contaminated materials. The incubation period of the virus can vary from fourteen to twenty-four days (the average is eighteen days). A person with mumps is contagious any time from forty-eight hours before the onset of symptoms to six days after the symptoms have started. This illness is not as contagious as measles or chickenpox, and one attack usually affords lifetime immunity. Mumps is most common in children between the ages of three and sixteen. It can occur after puberty, however, and when it does, the ovaries or testes may become involved and sterility may result. If the testicles are affected, they become swollen and painful; if the ovaries or pancreas is affected, abdominal pain results.

Unless otherwise specified, the dosages recommended here are for adults. For a child between the ages of twelve and seventeen, reduce the dose to three-quarters the recommended amount. For a child between six and twelve, use one-half the recommended dose, and for a child under the age of six, use one-quarter the recommended amount.

NUTRIENTS

SUPPLEMENT	SUGGESTED DOSAGE	COMMENTS
Very Important		
Vitamin C	500 mg every 2 hours until improvement is noted, up to 3,000–10,000 mg daily.	Destroys the virus and eliminates toxins. For children, use sodium ascorbate form to lessen diarrhea.
Lactobacillus bifidus	As directed on label.	"Friendly" bacteria contain antibiotic substances that inhibit pathogenic organisms.
Zinc lozenges (Ultimate Zinc-C Lozenges from Now Foods)	1 15-mg lozenge every 4–6 hours. Do not exceed a total of 100 mg daily.	Aids healing. Lozenges are fast acting. Do not chew them, but allow them to dissolve slowly in the mouth.
Important		
Acidophilus	As directed on label.	For adults and children. Contains antibiotic substances that inhibit pathogenic organisms.
Free-form amino acid complex plus	As directed on label.	Important for tissue repair and healing.
vitamin B complex plus	100 mg 3 times daily.	Needed for healing.
potassium	99 mg daily.	To restore electrolytes depleted by fever. Potassium levels are depressed by fever over 101°F.
Vitamin A and vitamin E	For children under 12, 15,000 IU daily. For adults, 50,000 IU daily. If you are pregnant, do not exceed 10,000 IU daily. For children, 200 IU daily for 1 week. For adults, 400–800 IU daily for 1 week.	Vitamins A and E potentiate immune function. Use emulsion forms for easier assimilation.
Helpful		
Kelp	1,000–1,500 daily.	Contains essential minerals, iodine, and vitamins.

HERBS

❑ Catnip and chamomile teas are good calming agents and help to induce sleep. Catnip tea enemas help reduce fever. See ENEMAS in Part Three.

❑ Taken as a tea, dandelion cleanses and supports the liver. Ground into a powder and combined with a little aloe vera gel in a poultice, it helps to reduce swelling.

❑ Echinacea helps to reduce swelling and cleanses the blood and lymphatic system. Take it in tea form, mixed with a little juice, four times a day or more.

❑ Elder flower tea helps to reduce fever.

❑ Lobelia extract is good for pain. Take ½ teaspoon every three to four hours.
    Caution: Do not take lobelia internally on an ongoing basis.

❑ Mullein poultices are good for relieving pain and swelling of the salivary glands. See USING A POULTICE in Part Three.

❑ Peppermint tea soothes an upset stomach and helps to flush infection from the body.

❑ Adding powdered slippery elm bark to barley water makes a drink that is nourishing and soothing to the throat and digestive tract. See THERAPEUTIC LIQUIDS in Part Three.

❑ Yarrow reduces fever and inflammation and is a good lymphatic cleanser.

RECOMMENDATIONS

❑ As long as the glands are swollen, eat mostly raw fruits and vegetables that are juiced or softened. Sticking to a diet of soft foods helps to minimize the pain of chewing.

❑ Drink plenty of pure water and fresh juices to keep the body well hydrated and to flush the system clean.

❑ Do not consume coffee, dairy products, tobacco, or white flour or sugar. Avoid acidic foods, such as pickles and citrus fruits or juices, as they are likely to cause discomfort.

❑ Follow a fasting program to detoxify the body. *See* FASTING in Part Three.

❑ Stay warm and dry, and get plenty of rest.

❑ Intermittently apply warmth or cold, whichever feels best, to the swollen glands. Use hot towels, hot water bottles, and ice packs with caution.

❑ If testicular swelling and pain occurs, support the scrotum by means of an adhesive tape "bridge" between the thighs and use cool compresses to help relieve pain.

CONSIDERATIONS

❑ Complete recovery from mumps usually can be expected in about ten days if no complications occur.

❑ Because complications are more common when this disease is contracted in adulthood, immunization should be considered for any adult who has not had mumps or who has not already been vaccinated against it.

❑ The mumps virus may be contagious even during incubation. Anyone who has come in contact with a person who had or who developed mumps should be on the lookout for symp-toms for a fourteen- to twenty-eight-day period following exposure, and should minimize his or her contact with persons who may be susceptible during this period.

❑ A doctor may advise the use of corticosteroids to diminish testicular pain and swelling. These are powerful drugs, and should be used with caution.

❑ If nausea and/or pain on swallowing is so severe that a person with mumps becomes unable to eat, intravenous administration of dextrose and fluids may be required.

❑ Swelling of the parotid and/or other salivary glands can also be caused by a number of other factors, including cirrhosis of the liver; a bacterial infection such as strep throat; poor oral hygiene; a salivary gland tumor or a calcium-based stone in one of the salivary ducts; and Mikulicz's syndrome, which is characterized by swelling (usually painless) of the parotid glands and, sometimes, the tear glands, and which can occur in people with a number of different diseases, including leukemia, lupus, non-Hodgkin's lymphoma, and tuberculosis. Swollen salivary glands can also be related to the use of certain drugs. Consequently, an isolated case of mumps (a case not associated with a local outbreak of the disease) warrants extra care in diagnosis.

Muscle Cramps

Most common muscle cramps occur at night and affect the legs, especially the calf muscles, and the feet. These kinds of cramps occur more frequently in elderly people. Children may experience a type of muscle and leg pain often called "growing pains."

Muscle cramping is most commonly caused by an imbalance in the levels of calcium and magnesium in the body and/or a deficiency of vitamin E. Anemia, the use of tobacco, inactivity, fibromyalgia, arthritis, and even arteriosclerosis can also result in cramping, as can dehydration, heat stroke, hypothyroidism, or varicose veins, or, more rarely, the early stages of amyotrophic lateral sclerosis (ALS, or Lou Gehrig's disease).

The use of diuretic drugs for high blood pressure or heart disorders may lead to electrolyte imbalances, causing muscle cramps. Poor circulation also contributes to leg cramps.

NUTRIENTS

SUPPLEMENT	SUGGESTED DOSAGE	COMMENTS
Essential		
Calcium and magnesium	1,500 mg daily. 750 mg daily and up.	Deficiencies are most often the cause of cramping in the legs and feet at night. Use chelate or citrate forms.
Vitamin E	Start with 400 IU daily and increase slowly to 1,000 IU daily.	Improves circulation. Deficiency may cause leg cramps while standing or walking. Especially good if cramping is related to varicose veins.
Very Important		
Bone Support from Synergy Plus	As directed on label.	Contains minerals that aid in absorption of calcium.
Malic acid and magnesium	As directed on label.	Malic acid is involved in the production of energy in muscle cells; magnesium is a cofactor in cellular energy production.
Potassium	99 mg daily.	Needed for proper calcium and magnesium metabolism; aids in relieving muscle cramps.
Silica	As directed on label.	Supplies silicon, which aids in calcium absorption.
Vitamin B complex plus extra vitamin B$_1$ (thiamine) and vitamin B$_3$ (niacin)	50 mg 3 times daily, with meals. 50 mg 3 times daily, with meals. 50 mg 3 times daily, with meals. Do not exceed this amount.	For improved circulation and cellular function. Enhances circulation and may aid in maintaining proper muscle tone. Increases circulation. *Caution:* Do not take niacin if you have a liver disorder, gout, or high blood pressure.
Vitamin C with bioflavonoids	3,000–6,000 mg daily.	Improves circulation.
Vitamin D	400 IU daily.	Needed for calcium uptake.

Important		
Dimethylglycine (DMG) (Aangamik DMG from FoodScience Labs)	As directed on label.	Improves tissue oxygenation.

Helpful		
Coenzyme Q10	100 mg daily.	Improves heart function and circulation. Lowers blood pressure.
Lecithin granules or capsules	1–2 tbsp 3 times daily, before meals. 1,200–2,400 mg 3 times daily, before meals.	Reduces cholesterol levels.
Multivitamin and mineral complex	As directed on label.	All nutrients are necessary for healthy muscles.
Zinc	50 mg daily. Do not exceed a total of 100 mg daily from all supplements.	Needed for absorption of calcium and action of B vitamins. Use zinc gluconate lozenges or OptiZinc for best absorption.

HERBS

❑ Alfalfa, dong quai, elderberry extract, ginkgo biloba extract, horsetail grass, and saffron are good for circulation.

❑ Rubbing lobelia extract on the affected area helps to relieve muscle spasms.

❑ Taking valerian root at bedtime helps to relax the muscles.

RECOMMENDATIONS

❑ Eat alfalfa, brewer's yeast, plenty of dark-green and leafy vegetables, cornmeal, and kelp.

❑ Drink a large glass of quality water (preferably steam-distilled) to flush out toxins stored in the muscles. Do this every three hours throughout the day.

❑ Massage the muscles and use heat to relieve pain.

❑ If you are on diuretic medication for high blood pressure or a heart disorder, be sure to take supplemental potassium daily.

❑ Rub pure, unprocessed olive or flaxseed oil into your muscles before and after strenuous exercise. Add 25 drops of oil to a hot bath and soak. Canola oil is also good for this purpose.

❑ Take a hot bath using mineral salts before bedtime to increase blood flow to the muscles.

❑ If you have cramps during the day, while you are active, consult your health care provider. This can be a sign of impaired circulation or arteriosclerosis. (*See* CIRCULATORY PROBLEMS in Part Two.)

❑ If cramping occurs after walking and is relieved when you stop, suspect impaired circulation. *See* ARTERIOSCLEROSIS/ATHEROSCLEROSIS in Part Two and take the artery function self-test.

Muscle Injuries

See SPRAINS, STRAINS, AND OTHER INJURIES OF THE MUSCLES AND JOINTS.

Myocardial Infarction

See HEART ATTACK.

Nail Problems

The nails protect the nerve-rich fingertips and tips of the toes from injury. Nails are a substructure of the epidermis (the outer layer of the skin) and are composed mainly of keratin, a type of protein. The nail bed is the skin on top of which the nails grow. Nails grow from 0.05 to 1.2 millimeters (approximately $\frac{1}{500}$ to $\frac{1}{20}$ inch) a week. If a nail is lost, it takes about seven months to grow out fully.

Healthy nail beds are pink, indicating a rich blood supply. Changes or abnormalities in the nails are often the result of nutritional deficiencies or other underlying conditions. The nails can reveal a great deal about the body's internal health.

The following are some of the changes that nutritional deficiencies can produce in the nails:

• A lack of protein, folic acid, and vitamin C causes hangnails. White bands across the nails are also an indication of protein deficiency.

• A lack of vitamin A and calcium causes dryness and brittleness.

• A deficiency of the B vitamins causes fragility, with horizontal and vertical ridges.

• Insufficient intake of vitamin B12 leads to excessive dryness, very rounded and curved nail ends, and darkened nails.

• Iron deficiency may result in "spoon" nails (nails that develop a concave shape) and/or vertical ridges.

• Zinc deficiency may cause the development of white spots on the nails.

• A lack of sufficient "friendly" bacteria (lactobacilli) in the body can result in the growth of fungus under and around nails.

• A lack of sufficient hydrochloric acid (HCl) contributes to splitting nails.

The following table lists supplements that promote healthy nail growth.

NUTRIENTS

SUPPLEMENT	SUGGESTED DOSAGE	COMMENTS
Very Important		
Free-form amino acid complex plus extra L-cysteine and L-methionine	As directed on label, on an empty stomach. Take with water or juice. Do not take with milk. Take with 50 mg vitamin B₆ and 100 mg vitamin C for better absorption.	The building materials for new nails. Also supplies sulfur, which is necessary for skin and nail growth. *See* AMINO ACIDS in Part One.
Silica or horsetail or oat straw	As directed on label.	Supplies silicon, needed for hair, bones, and strong nails. *See under* Herbs, below. *See under* Herbs, below.
Vitamin A emulsion or capsules	50,000 IU daily. If you are pregnant, do not exceed 10,000 IU daily. 25,000 IU daily. If you are pregnant, do not exceed 10,000 IU daily.	The body cannot utilize protein without vitamin A. Emulsion form is recommended for easier assimilation and greater safety at higher doses.
Helpful		
Black currant seed oil	500 mg twice daily.	Helpful for weak, brittle nails.
Calcium and magnesium and vitamin D	As directed on label. As directed on label. As directed on label.	Necessary for nail growth. Needed to balance with calcium. Enhances calcium absorption.
Iron (ferrous fumarate from Freeda Vitamins) or Floradix Iron + Herbs from Salus Haus	As directed by physician. Take with 100 mg vitamin C for better absorption. *Do not* take with vitamin E. As directed on label.	Deficiency produces "spoon" nails and/or vertical ridges. *Caution:* Do not take iron unless anemia is diagnosed. A natural source of iron.
Ultimate Oil from Nature's Secret	As directed on label.	A combination of essential fatty acids necessary for the health of skin, hair, and nails.
Ultra Nails from Nature's Plus	As directed on label.	Contains calcium, gelatin, amino acids, magnesium, iron, and other nutrients important for healthy nails.
Vitamin B complex plus extra vitamin B₂ (riboflavin) and vitamin B₁₂ and biotin and folic acid	As directed on label. 50 mg 3 times daily. 100 mcg 3 times daily. 2.5 mg daily for 9 months. 50 mg 3 times daily.	Deficiencies result in fragile nails. Useful for treating brittle nails. Reduces splitting and other nail irregularities.
Vitamin C	3,000–6,000 mg daily.	Hangnails and inflammation of the paronychia (the tissue surrounding the nail) may be linked to vitamin C deficiency.
Zinc	50 mg daily. Do not exceed a total of 100 mg daily from all supplements.	Affects absorption and action of vitamins and enzymes. Use zinc gluconate lozenges or OptiZinc for best absorption.

HERBS

❑ Alfalfa, black cohosh, burdock root, dandelion, gotu kola, and yellow dock are rich in minerals, including silica and zinc, as well as B vitamins, all of which strengthen the nails. Horsetail and oat straw also are good sources of silica.

❑ Borage seed, flaxseed, lemongrass, parsley, primrose, pumpkin seed, and sage are all good sources of essential fatty acids, which nourish the nails.

Caution: Do not use sage if you suffer from any kind of seizure disorder.

❑ Butcher's broom, chamomile, ginkgo biloba, rosemary, sassafras, and turmeric are good for circulation, which nourishes the nails.

RECOMMENDATIONS

❑ For healthy nails, be sure to get plenty of quality protein, and take a protein supplement. Eat grains, legumes, oatmeal, nuts, and seeds. Eggs also are a good source of protein, as long as your blood cholesterol levels are not too high.

❑ Eat a diet composed of 50 percent fresh fruits and raw vegetables to supply necessary vitamins, minerals, and enzymes. Eat foods that are rich in sulfur and silicon, such as broccoli, fish, onions, and sea vegetables. Also include in the diet plenty of foods that are high in biotin, such as brewer's yeast, soy flour, and whole grains.

❑ Drink plenty of quality water and other liquids. Cuts and cracks in the nails may indicate a need for more liquids.

❑ Drink fresh carrot juice daily. This is high in calcium and phosphorus and is very good for strengthening the nails.

❑ Consume citrus fruits, salt, and vinegar in moderation, if at all. Excessive intake of these foods can result in a protein/calcium imbalance that may adversely affect the health of the nails.

❑ Supplement your diet with royal jelly, a good source of essential fatty acids, and spirulina or kelp, which are rich in silica, zinc, and B vitamins, and help to strengthen nails.

❑ For splitting nails and/or hangnails, take 2 tablespoons of brewer's yeast or wheat germ oil daily.

❑ To restore color and texture to brittle, yellowed nails, make a mixture of equal parts of honey, avocado oil, and egg yolk, and add a pinch of salt. Rub the mixture into your nails and cuticles. Leave it on for half an hour, then rinse it off. Repeat this treatment daily. You should begin to see results after about two weeks.

❑ To strengthen the nails, try soaking them in warm olive oil or cider vinegar for ten to twenty minutes daily.

❑ Treat your nails gently. Using them to pry, pick, scrape, or perform tasks such as removing staples can damage them.

❑ Keep your nails relatively short. Nails longer than one-quarter inch beyond the fingertip break and bend easily.

❑ Do *not* cut the cuticles. Uncovering the nails this way is harsh and irritating, and may cause infection. Use baby oil or cream and gently push the cuticles back.

Disorders That Show Up in the Nails

Nail changes may signify a number of disorders elsewhere in the body. These changes may indicate illness before any other symptoms do. Seek medical attention if any of the following symptoms are suspected.

- **Black, splinterlike bits under the nails** can be a sign of infectious endocarditis, a serious heart infection; other heart disease; or a bleeding disorder.

- **Brittle nails** signify possible iron deficiency, thyroid problems, impaired kidney function, and circulation problems.

- **Brittle, soft, shiny nails without a moon** may indicate an overactive thyroid.

- **Dark nails and/or thin, flat, spoon-shaped nails** are a sign of vitamin B_{12} deficiency or anemia. Nails can also turn gray or dark if the hands are placed in chemicals such as cleaning supplies (most often bleach) or a substance to which one is allergic.

- **Deep blue nail beds** show a pulmonary obstructive disorder such as asthma or emphysema.

- **Downward-curved nail ends** may denote heart, liver, or respiratory problems.

- **Flat nails** can denote Raynaud's disease.

- **Greenish nails,** if not a result of a localized fungal infection, may indicate an internal bacterial infection.

- **A half-white nail with dark spots at the tip** points to possible kidney disease.

- **An isolated dark-blue band in the nail bed,** especially in light-skinned people, can be a sign of skin cancer.

- **Nail beading** (the development of bumps on the surface of the nail) is a sign of rheumatoid arthritis.

- **Nails that broaden toward the tip and curve downward** are a sign of lung damage, such as from emphysema or exposure to asbestos.

- **Nails that chip, peel, crack, or break easily** show a general nutritional deficiency and insufficient hydrochloric acid and protein. Minerals are also needed.

- **Nails raised at the base, with small, white ends,** show a respiratory disorder such as emphysema or chronic bronchitis. This type of nail may also simply be inherited.

- **Nails separated from the nail bed** may signify a thyroid disorder or a local infection.

- **Nails that have pitting resembling hammered brass** indicate a tendency toward partial or total hair loss.

- **Pitted red-brown spots and frayed and split ends** indicate psoriasis; vitamin C, folic acid, and protein are needed.

- **Red skin around the cuticles** can be indicative of poor metabolism of essential fatty acids or of a connective tissue disorder such as lupus.

- **Ridges** can appear in the nails either vertically or horizontally. Vertical ridges indicate poor general health, poor nutrient absorption, and/or iron deficiency; they may also indicate a kidney disorder. Horizontal ridges can occur as a result of severe stress, either psychological or physical, such as from infection and/or disease. Ridges running up and down the nails also indicate a tendency to develop arthritis.

- **Thick nails** may indicate that the vascular system is weakening and the blood is not circulating properly. They may also be a sign of thyroid disease.

- **Thinning nails** may signal lichen planus, an itchy skin disorder.

- **Two white horizontal bands that do not move as the nail grows** are a sign of hypoalbuminemia, a protein deficiency in the blood.

- **Unusually wide, square nails** can suggest a hormonal disorder.

- **White lines** show possible heart disease, high fever, or arsenic poisoning.

- **White lines across the nail** may indicate a liver disease.

- **If the white moon area of the nail turns red,** it may indicate heart problems; **if it turns slate blue,** then it can indicate either heavy metal poisoning (such as silver poisoning) or lung trouble.

- **White nails** indicate possible liver or kidney disorders and/or anemia.

- **White nails with pink near the tips** are a sign of cirrhosis.

- **Yellow nails or an elevation of the nail tips** can indicate internal disorders long before other symptoms appear. Some of these are problems with the lymphatic system, respiratory disorders, diabetes, and liver disorders.

❑ Soak your nails before trimming them. Nails are most likely to split and peel when they are dry. Apply hand cream each morning and evening to prevent nails from drying out.

❑ Do not repeatedly immerse your hands in water that contains detergents or chemicals such as bleach or dish soap; this results in split nails. Wear cotton-lined gloves when doing housework such as dishes and laundry or when using furniture polish. This protects your hands and nails against harsh chemicals. Wearing gloves is especially important for people who work in jobs where their hands are exposed to chemicals. Not only does this damage the nails, but it causes the skin surrounding the nail bed to dry out and crack. This can lead to bleeding and can be quite painful.

❑ Do not pull at hangnails. Cut them with sharp clippers or scissors. Keep your hands moisturized to help prevent hangnails.

❑ If you are diabetic, see your health care provider if your cuticles become inflamed, because the infection can spread.

❑ If you wear nail polish, use a base coat underneath it to prevent yellowing.

❑ Use nail polish removers as little as possible. They contain solvents that leach lipids from the nails and make them brittle. These solvents are also potentially highly toxic, and can be absorbed through the skin.

❑ Never apply artificial nails over your own. They may look nice for a while, but they destroy the underlying nail. The chemicals and glue used are dangerous to the body, and are readily absorbed through the damaged nail and nail bed. The use of artificial nails has also been known to contribute to the development of fungal infection of the fingernails.

CONSIDERATIONS

❑ If you expose your hands to too much water and soap, the nail may become loose from the nail bed. Water causes the nails to swell. They then shrink as they dry, resulting in loose and brittle nails.

❑ Discolored nails can be caused by prolonged illness, stress, nicotine, allergies, or diabetes. If your nails are green, you may have a bacterial infection or a fungal infection between the nail and the nail bed. If you have a fungal or bacterial infection, and especially if you are taking antibiotics, acidophilus is needed.

❑ Physicians often prescribe a regimen of 250 milligrams of griseofulvin (Fulvicin), four times daily, for a fungal infection of the nails. The white blood cell count must be monitored during this treatment. Another prescription antifungal agent is ketoconazole (Nizoral), which is available as a cream or shampoo, as well as in tablet form.

❑ Anticancer medications can cause bands and streaks of color to appear in the nails. These conditions disappear when the medication is stopped.

❑ Poor thyroid function may be reflected in the nails. (*See* HYPOTHYROIDISM in Part Two.)

Narcolepsy

Narcolepsy is a rare neurological disorder that may affect as many as 250,000 Americans. There are four classic symptoms that define this syndrome: sleep attacks, cataplexy, sleep paralysis, and sleep-related hallucinations. A person with narcolepsy may experience any or all of these classic phenomena.

The best known symptom of narcolepsy is the sleep attack. A person with narcolepsy can suddenly fall into a sleep state with almost no warning whatsoever. Sleep attacks can occur at any time, even in mid-conversation, as many as ten times a day (even more, in some cases). These periods of sleep usually last only a matter of minutes, but in some cases sleep can continue for an hour or more. Afterwards, the person may feel refreshed, yet he or she may fall asleep again in a few minutes.

While the sleep that results from narcolepsy looks like ordinary sleep, researchers have found at least one key difference. Normal sleep is a cyclical process that alternates between periods of rapid-eye-movement (REM) and non-rapid-eye-movement (NREM) sleep. During the NREM part of the cycle, the entire body slows down—pulse, breathing, blood pressure, and brain wave activity are all lowered. When the REM cycle begins, the body remains asleep, but the brain becomes significantly active; brain waves as recorded by an electroencephalograph (EEG) more closely resemble those of the waking brain. It is during REM sleep that most dreaming occurs.

In healthy individuals, sleep begins with the NREM phase. After sixty minutes or so of NREM sleep, REM sleep begins. A short time later, the entire cycle begins again. In a narcoleptic sleep attack, in contrast, researchers have found that REM sleep begins almost instantly, with no introductory NREM sleep. The precise significance of this is not yet understood, but it does provide a useful diagnostic tool as well as a clue for researchers to pursue in trying to understand this mysterious disorder.

The second classic symptom of narcolepsy is cataplexy. This is a type of paralysis that usually occurs in response to some type of heightened emotion, such as anger, fear, or excitement. The individual does not lose consciousness, but experiences a sudden and temporary loss of muscle tone. Often, only the legs and/or arms are affected. These episodes normally last less than a minute, and they seem to be most likely to occur if the person is surprised in some way.

Sleep paralysis is the third classic symptom of narcolepsy. Just as you are falling asleep, or as you are beginning to awaken, you try to move or say something but find that you cannot, even though you are fully conscious. This lasts for only a second or two, but it can be frightening, especially the first time it happens. These episodes usually end either on their own or when someone touches or speaks to you. Many doctors feel that sleep paralysis is similar to cataplexy and to the state that accompanies REM sleep, in which motor activity is inhibited even though the brain is active. This phenomenon is not strictly limited to people with narcolepsy; many otherwise healthy people may experience it occasionally.

Like sleep paralysis, sleep-related hallucinations—medically termed *hypnagogic phenomena*—usually occur just prior to sleep, or sometimes upon awakening. The affected individual may hear sounds that aren't there and/or see illusions. These visual and auditory illusions are very vivid. This phenomenon also can occur in individuals who do not suffer from narcolepsy, particularly in children.

Because the symptoms of narcolepsy vary from individual to individual (it is estimated that only 10 percent of people with narcolepsy experience all four of the classic symptoms), this disorder is frequently misdiagnosed. Further compounding the problem is the fact that other sleep disorders, such as sleep apnea, also can produce spells of marked daytime drowsiness. Narcolepsy is not a particularly dangerous problem, unless one experiences a sleep attack while operating a motor vehicle or other machinery. It can, however, be embarrassing and extremely inconvenient. The cause or causes of this disorder are unknown, but brain infection, head trauma, or brain tumors may be behind some cases. It is known that narcolepsy is almost never the result of insomnia or sleep deprivation. There is currently no cure for this disorder, so the focus must be on treating the symptoms.

NUTRIENTS

SUPPLEMENT	SUGGESTED DOSAGE	COMMENTS
Essential		
Calcium and magnesium	2,000 mg daily, at bedtime. 400 mg twice during the day and at bedtime.	Needed for energy production and the nervous system.
Choline or lecithin granules or capsules	300 mg daily. 1 tbsp 3 times daily, before meals. 1,200 mg 3 times daily, before meals.	Acts as a neurotransmitter and is important for brain function. A good source of choline.
Chromium picolinate	100 mcg daily.	Boosts energy and regulates sugar metabolism.
Coenzyme Q10	As directed on label.	Promotes circulation to the brain.
Free-form amino acid complex	As directed on label.	Increases energy levels; needed for proper brain function. Use a formula that contains all the essential amino acids.
L-Glutamine	As directed on label, on an empty stomach. Take with water or juice. Do not take with milk. Take with 50 mg vitamin B$_6$ and 100 mg vitamin C for better absorption.	Promotes mental ability. Known as brain fuel because it can pass the blood-brain barrier freely. *See* AMINO ACIDS in Part One.
L-Tyrosine	As directed on label. Take at bedtime.	Important in thyroid function. Low levels have been associated with narcolepsy. *Caution:* Do not take tyrosine if you are taking an MAO inhibitor drug.
Multivitamin and mineral complex	As directed on label.	All nutrients are needed to balance body functioning.
Octocosanol	100 mg daily.	Increases oxygen utilization and boosts endurance.
Omega-3 essential fatty acids (fish oil and flaxseed oil are good sources)	As directed on label.	To protect cell membranes.
Vitamin C	2,000–6,000 mg daily, in divided doses.	Increases energy and promotes production of interferon in the body to protect against free radical damage.
Vitamin D	400 IU daily.	Essential for calcium absorption.
Vitamin B complex (Coenzymate B Complex from Source Naturals) plus extra vitamin B$_6$ (pyridoxine)	150 mg daily. 200 mg daily.	B vitamins boost metabolism and are essential for increased energy levels and normal brain function.
Vitamin E	400–600 IU daily.	Increases circulation and protects heart functioning and brain cells.

HERBS

❑ Ephedra, gotu kola, and St. Johnswort boost energy levels and possess antioxidant properties as well.

❑ Ginkgo biloba improves circulation to the brain and is a powerful antioxidant protecting cells.

RECOMMENDATIONS

❑ Eat a low-fat diet high in cleansing foods such as leafy green vegetables and sea vegetables. Also eat foods high in the B vitamins, such as brewer's yeast and brown rice.

❑ Eat foods high in protein (meats, poultry, cheese, nuts, seeds, and soy products) in the middle of the day, and save the complex carbohydrates (fresh fruits and vegetables, legumes, natural whole grains, and pasta) for the evening meal. High-protein foods increase alertness, whereas carbohydrates have a calming effect and can promote sleepiness.

❑ Include in the diet foods rich in the amino acid tyrosine. Good choices include eggs, oats, poultry, and wheat germ.
Caution: If you are taking an MAO inhibitor drug, *avoid* foods containing tyrosine, as drug and dietary interactions can cause a sudden, dangerous rise in blood pressure. Discuss food and medicine limitations thoroughly with your health care provider or a qualified dietitian.

❑ Avoid alcohol and sugar. They may seem stimulating initially, but will only make you tired later.

❑ Exercise daily to improve circulation and oxygenate tissues.

❑ Napping can rejuvenate you when you have lost sleep. Take up to a forty-five-minute nap in the early afternoon.

❑ Make sure your home and workplace are well lit, either by natural sunlight or overhead lighting. Light suppresses the production of melatonin, which is the hormone that produces drowsiness. Full-spectrum light bulbs are best.

CONSIDERATIONS

❑ Irregular sleep patterns are just as likely to cause drowsiness as lack of sleep. Jet lag, shift work, inconsistent bedtimes, and weekend partying can all disturb our natural sleep/wake cycles. America is a nation of sleep-starved yawners fighting a daily battle against the sandman. We live in a world where people drive themselves on relentless schedules that leave insufficient time for quality sleep.

☐ There have been some documented cases in which persons who suffered from narcolepsy were cured by eliminating allergenic foods from the diet. One person, for instance, was found to have an allergy to potatoes. When he removed potatoes from his diet, he no longer experienced the symptoms. (*See* ALLERGIES in Part Two.)

☐ There is some evidence that the immune systems of people who suffer from narcolepsy may react abnormally to the chemical processes in the brain that cause sleep.

☐ Certain dogs, mainly Doberman pinschers, have been observed to sleep excessively and to collapse when overstimulated. Research has revealed a withering away of axons (the "communication cables" that convey signals between nerve cells) in the brains of these animals, especially in three regions of the brain that have been linked to sleep inhibition, motor control, and the processing of emotions. If similar degeneration can be demonstrated in human brains, this may offer further clues as to the causes of narcolepsy.

☐ *See also* the discussion of sleep apnea under INSOMNIA in Part Two.

Nausea and Vomiting

See FOOD POISONING; INDIGESTION. *See also under* INFLUENZA.

Nephritis

See under KIDNEY DISEASE.

Nervousness

See ANXIETY DISORDER; STRESS.

Neuritis

Neuritis is the inflammation and/or deterioration of a nerve or group of nerves. It is often part of a degenerative illness such as leukemia. Neuritis can result in muscle weakness and atrophy, loss of sensation, and loss of reflexes. Muscles served by the affected nerve are usually quite tender to pressure. The skin over the affected muscle group may become glossy-looking, and the affected area of the body may cease to perspire normally. A condition known as footdrop may occur, in which the toes drag on the ground

as the individual walks, caused by weakness or paralysis of muscles in the foot and ankle.

The causes of neuritis are varied and can include nutritional deficiencies, especially a lack of the B vitamins; metabolic imbalances; a direct blow or nearby bone fracture; infection involving a nerve; diseases such as diabetes, gout, and leukemia; ingestion of methyl alcohol; and toxic levels of metals such as lead and mercury. Neuritis can occur in persons of any age and either sex, but the incidence is highest in men between the ages of thirty and fifty. It can begin rapidly, especially in cases caused by severe and/or chronic infection or by alcohol intoxication, but that is not the norm. Symptoms usually develop slowly and can include pain, tingling, and loss of sensation in the affected nerve area; swelling and redness; and, in severe cases, convulsions. The onset is not always readily apparent. Often, a person may compensate for the muscle weakness by overusing unaffected muscles.

Optic neuritis occurs when inflammation affects the optic nerve in the eye, causing gradual or sudden blurring and loss of vision. In severe cases, blindness may occur, although this is usually temporary, especially with prompt treatment. The eye may also be painful.

NUTRIENTS

SUPPLEMENT	SUGGESTED DOSAGE	COMMENTS
Essential		
Essential fatty acids (flaxseed oil and Ultimate Oil from Nature's Secret are good sources)	As directed on label.	To rebuild and repair nerve damage.
Glutathione	500–1,000 mg daily.	Deficiency affects the brain and nervous system.
L-Asparagine	As directed on label, on an empty stomach. Take with water or juice. Do not take with milk. Take with 50 mg vitamin B$_6$ and 100 mg vitamin C for better absorption.	To help maintain balance in the central nervous system. *See* AMINO ACIDS in Part One.
Lecithin granules or capsules	2 tbsp twice daily, with meals. 2,400 mg twice daily, with meals.	Important in nerve protection and repair.
Vitamin B complex	100 mg daily and up.	Deficiencies are common. Use a high-stress formula. Injections (under a doctor's supervision) are best. If injections are not available, use a sublingual form.
plus extra vitamin B$_1$ (thiamine) and	100 mg twice daily.	Deficiency is common in people with neuritis.
vitamin B$_3$ (niacin)	50 mg twice daily. Do not exceed this amount.	Helps maintain healthy nerves. *Caution:* Do not take niacin if you have a liver disorder, gout, or high blood pressure.
and vitamin B$_{12}$	2,000 mcg twice daily.	Use a lozenge or sublingual form.
Taurine	As directed on label.	Suppresses neuronal activity in the brain and reduces stress.

Multivitamin and mineral complex with	As directed on label.	Nutritional deficiencies are common. Neuritis is often the first sign. Use a high-potency formula. If you have diabetes, use a formula without beta-carotene.
vitamin A and natural beta-carotene	If you are pregnant, do not exceed 10,000 IU vitamin A daily.	
Vitamin C with bioflavonoids	3,000–6,000 mg daily, in divided doses.	Has anti-inflammatory and antiviral properties. Also necessary for nerve impulse transmission.
Zinc	50–80 mg daily. Do not exceed a total of 100 mg daily from all supplements.	Important for proper immune function. Use zinc gluconate lozenges or OptiZinc for best absorption.

Very Important		
Calcium and	2,000 mg daily.	Important in nerve impulse conduction. Use a chelate form.
magnesium	400–1,000 mg daily.	Important in nerve impulse conduction. Use magnesium chloride form.
Free-form amino acid complex	As directed on label.	Necessary in nerve repair and function.

Important		
Grape seed extract	As directed on label.	A powerful antioxidant and anti-inflammatory.
Proteolytic enzymes or Infla-Zyme Forte from American Biologics	As directed on label 3 times daily. Take on an empty stomach.	Potent anti-inflammatory agents.
Quercetin plus	500 mg twice daily.	To improve digestion and reduce swelling.
bromelain	100 mg twice daily.	Enhances absorption of quercetin.

HERBS

❑ Bilberry, calendula, chamomile, marshmallow root, St. Johnswort, yarrow, and yucca have anti-inflammatory properties, and can be helpful in the management of neuritis.

❑ Blue vervain, hops, rosemary, wild lettuce, and wood betony can be used to relax muscles.

❑ Feverfew, kava kava, lobelia, passionflower, skullcap, valerian, and white willow bark are what herbalists call "nervines"—they have analgesic properties; they calm and tone the nerves. They come in capsule, tea, or extract form.

RECOMMENDATIONS

❑ Eat a diet consisting of fruits, vegetables, nuts, seeds, and whole grains.

❑ Get some type of mild exercise daily to relieve nerve trauma and oxygenate tissues.

❑ Avoid stimulants such as coffee, carbonated beverages, caffeine, and cigarettes.

❑ If you are having a problem with your vision that suggests optic neuritis, see your physician right away. Prompt treatment is essential.

❑ Increase your fluid intake.

CONSIDERATIONS

❑ Neuritis treatment consists of pain relief measures, rest, and physical therapy, if indicated. In severe cases, electrotherapy may be recommended to stimulate nerves and muscles. For treatment to be successful, however, the underlying cause must first be identified and corrected. Removal of toxic agents and appropriate nutritional supplementation can improve the condition and are part of the treatment.

❑ After the pain subsides, massage may be beneficial.

❑ Some people with neuritis have benefitted from osteopathy, a form of medicine that combines physical therapy, joint manipulation, and postural education.

❑ Fasting and chelation therapy may be helpful to remove toxins. (*See* CHELATION THERAPY and FASTING in Part Three.)

Nickel Toxicity

Small amounts of nickel are useful in certain bodily functions. For example, minute amounts of nickel are important in DNA and RNA stabilization. Nickel also helps to activate certain important enzymes, such as trypsin and arginase. A nickel deficiency may affect iron and zinc metabolism.

Too much nickel can be toxic, however. Although toxic levels of nickel have not been established, it is known that the presence of excess amounts of nickel can cause dermatitis (skin rash and inflammation) and respiratory illness, and can interfere with the Kreb's cycle, a series of enzymatic reactions necessary for cellular energy production. Significant levels of nickel may also contribute to heart attack, or myocardial infarction.

Many foods naturally contain some amount of nickel. These include buckwheat, legumes, oats, and cabbage. Nickel can also be present in hydrogenated fats and oils, refined and processed foods, stainless steel cookware, superphosphate fertilizers, and tobacco smoke. Using cooking utensils containing nickel may add unnecessarily to your dietary intake of nickel.

NUTRIENTS

SUPPLEMENT	SUGGESTED DOSAGE	COMMENTS
Important		
Apple pectin	As directed on label.	Binds toxic metals and removes them from the body.
Garlic (Kyolic)	As directed on label.	Acts as a detoxifier and aids in removing harmful metals.
Kelp	1,000–1,500 mg daily.	Supplies minerals and iodine to aid in removing toxic metals.
Vitamin A	25,000 IU daily. If you are pregnant, do not exceed 10,000 IU daily.	A powerful antioxidant that destroys free radicals.
plus natural beta-carotene	15,000 IU daily.	A free radical scavenger.

Vitamin C with rutin	4,000–10,000 mg daily.	Helps to remove metals from the body and strengthens immunity.
Vitamin E	400 IU daily.	A powerful free radical scavenger that also improves circulation.
L-Cysteine and L-methionine	As directed on label, on an empty stomach. Take with water or juice. Do not take with milk. Take with 50 mg vitamin B$_6$ and 100 mg vitamin C for better absorption.	Helps to detoxify the body, including the liver, of harmful metals. See AMINO ACIDS in Part One.
Selenium	200 mcg daily.	A powerful free radical destroyer.

RECOMMENDATIONS

❑ If you suspect you may have symptoms of metal toxicity, have a hair analysis to detect toxic levels of nickel and other minerals. See HAIR ANALYSIS in Part Three.

❑ Avoid processed food products, as well as any products containing hydrogenated fats and oils.

❑ Do not smoke, and avoid those who do.

❑ Beware of metal cookware, especially when preparing acidic foods, such as tomato sauce. Use glass cookware instead. Also avoid using metal cooking utensils. Use utensils made from plastic or wood instead (wood is best).

❑ Ask your dentist about the metal content of the materials he or she uses. Nickel toxicity can result from nickel alloys used in dental surgery and appliances.

❑ If your job or hobby involves using nickel to plate metals, use a face mask while working. Inhalation of nickel can cause pulmonary edema (accumulation of fluid in the lungs).

CONSIDERATIONS

❑ Chelation can remove toxic metals from the body. (See CHELATION THERAPY in Part Three.)

❑ Aside from being potentially toxic, nickel is often allergenic. The nickel in watchbands, zippers, bra closures, pierced earrings, and other everyday items has been associated with many allergic reactions. A high incidence of allergic reactions to nickel in pierced earrings has been reported among children. Many earrings and posts contain nickel. Gold (14-karat or higher) is probably the safest metal for pierced earrings. (See CHEMICAL ALLERGIES in Part Two.)

Nosebleed

Any injury to the tissues inside the nose can cause a nosebleed. Injury can result from a blow to the nose; the intrusion of foreign objects (including fingers); a sudden change in atmospheric pressure; or simply blowing the nose too forcefully. Winter often brings about nosebleeds because heated air tends to be dry. Excessive dryness can cause the nasal membranes to crack, form crusts, and bleed.

In some cases, nosebleeds—medically termed *epistaxis*—can be associated with an underlying illness. Arteriosclerosis, high blood pressure, malaria, scarlet fever, sinusitis, and typhoid fever are all known to cause nosebleeds, some of which can be serious and result in significant blood loss. Conditions that cause increased bleeding tendencies, such as hemophilia, leukemia, thrombocytopenia (a below-normal concentration of platelets in the blood), aplastic anemia, or liver disease, also may be implicated in nosebleeds.

Nosebleeds are much more common in children than in adults. This is no doubt largely due to the fact that children are prone to inserting their fingers and other objects into their nostrils. In addition, children's tissues, including the mucous membranes lining the nose, are thinner than those of adults and therefore more susceptible to damage.

There are two classifications of nosebleeds, depending on where in the nose the blood is coming from. *Posterior nosebleeds* primarily afflict elderly people and those with high blood pressure. In this type of nosebleed, blood comes from the rear of the nose and runs down the back of the mouth into the throat, no matter what position the person is in. The blood is usually dark red in color, although it can be bright red. If the bleeding is severe, blood can flow from the nostrils as well.

The overwhelming majority of nosebleeds are *anterior nosebleeds*, in which bright-red blood flows from the front part of the nose. Most often they are the result of some type of trauma to the nasal tissues. If the person stands or sits, the flow of blood comes out of one or both nostrils. If the person lies on his or her back, the blood may flow backward, into the throat. This type of nosebleed can be frightening, and it may look as if there is a lot of blood, but in reality it is not usually serious and very little blood is actually lost.

NUTRIENTS

SUPPLEMENT	SUGGESTED DOSAGE	COMMENTS
Helpful		
Bioflavonoid complex with rutin	As directed on label.	Deficiencies have been linked to nosebleeds.
Vitamin C	3,000 mg when bleeding starts and 1,000 mg every hour thereafter until bleeding has completely stopped.	Promotes healing.

HERBS

❑ If your nasal membranes become sore from dryness, use comfrey ointment or aloe vera gel as needed.

❑ A snuff made from finely ground oak bark is soothing and healing.

❑ To promote healing, rub a small amount of Natureworks Marigold Ointment from Abkit into each nostril once the bleeding subsides. Repeat as needed.

RECOMMENDATIONS

❑ To stop an anterior nosebleed, do the following:

1. Gently blow all the clots out of both sides of the nose.

2. Sit up in a chair and lean forward (*do not* tilt the head back).

3. Pinch all the soft parts of the nose together between your thumb and index finger. The pressure should be firm but not painful. Hold this position for ten minutes.

4. Apply crushed ice or cold washcloths to the nose, neck, and cheeks. This can be done both as you apply pressure (*see* No. 3, above) and afterwards.

5. Then lie back until the bleeding subsides. Refrain from any physical activity for a few hours and any vigorous exercise for at least two days.

❑ If you suspect a posterior nosebleed, consult your doctor. This type of nosebleed requires the care of a physician.

❑ Do not blow your nose for at least twelve hours after a nosebleed stops. Doing so may dislodge the blood clots that stanch bleeding.

❑ Once bleeding is controlled and healing has begun, apply a small amount of vitamin E to the affected tissues— open a capsule and *gently* apply the oil inside the nose. If vitamin E is unavailable, use a little petroleum jelly. If you wish, pack the nose with gauze to prevent leakage.

❑ While healing, eat plenty of foods high in vitamin K, which is essential for normal blood clotting. Good sources include alfalfa, kale, and all dark green leafy vegetables.

❑ Avoid foods high in salicylates, aspirinlike substances found in tea, coffee, most fruits, and some vegetables. Foods to avoid include apples, apricots, almonds, all berries, cloves, cherries, cucumbers, currants, grapes, mint, oil of wintergreen, bell peppers, peaches, pickles, plums, raisins, tangelos, and tomatoes.

❑ To counteract dryness in the nasal passages, especially during the winter, use nasal irrigation. Spray inside the nostrils with plain warm water from time to time.

❑ To prevent nosebleeds, increase the environmental humidity, especially in winter. Use a cool mist humidifer, a vaporizer, or even a pan of water placed near a radiator.

❑ When you sneeze, keep your mouth open.

❑ If you have frequent nosebleeds, see your doctor. The cause of frequent nosebleeds is often an underlying problem such as hypertension, which should be treated.

❑ If you are prone to nosebleeds, an iron supplement may help to rebuild the blood. Iron is an important component in hemoglobin, which is a vital element in red blood cells.

Caution: Do not take iron supplements unless anemia has been diagnosed.

CONSIDERATIONS

❑ If packing the nose with gauze or cotton is necessary to stem the flow of blood, some medical authorities recommend moistening the packing material with white vinegar. They contend that the acid in white vinegar gently cauterizes broken blood vessels and aids in stopping the bleeding.

❑ Sometimes the use of drugs that thin the blood, such as the anticoagulants warfarin (Coumadin) or heparin, may cause nosebleeds. Even aspirin can act as an anticoagulant and interfere with blood clotting, which is necessary in stopping nosebleeds.

❑ High estrogen levels increase the flow of blood from the mucous membranes in the nose. This is why nosebleeds are more common during pregnancy. Oral contraceptives also can contribute to nosebleeds.

❑ The risk of serious nosebleeds increases with hemophilia, Hodgkin's disease, rheumatic fever, vitamin C deficiency, or the prolonged use of nose drops or nasal sprays.

❑ Nosebleeds are common among alcoholics. As alcohol dilates blood vessels, including those in the nasal cavities, the vessels bleed more easily. Heavy alcohol use can also create problems with blood clotting because of the toxic effects of alcohol on the liver and bone marrow.

❑ People with hypertension are especially prone to nosebleeds. A low-fat, low-cholesterol diet is recommended for keeping blood pressure under control. (*See* HIGH BLOOD PRESSURE in Part Two.)

❑ *See also under* PREGNANCY-RELATED PROBLEMS in Part Two.

Obesity

Obesity is, quite simply, an excess of body fat. Usually, anyone who is 20 percent over the normal weight for his or her age, sex, build, and height is considered obese. According to the Mayo Clinic in Rochester, Minnesota, a person's weight is healthy if it falls within the acceptable range for his or her height and age; if the pattern of fat distribution does not place the person at increased risk for certain diseases; and if the person has no medical problem for which a physician recommends that he or she lose weight.

How much a person weighs is only part of the story, however. Perhaps more important than weight is the percentage of fat in the body. For healthy women, fat can account for as much as 25 percent of body weight; 17 percent is a healthy percentage for men. Women's bodies are designed to carry a higher proportion of fat tissue to ensure that there is plenty of fuel for pregnancy and nursing, even if food is scarce.

The average human body has 30 to 40 billion fat cells. Most of the extra calories we eat that we do not need for immediate energy are stored as fat. If we were still "hunter/gatherers" like our early ancestors, the fat would provide a needed food store for times when no food is readily available. In fact, some researchers believe that our seemingly innate love of high-calorie (especially fatty) foods may be a remnant of a survival tactic from ancient times, when we needed to store food for energy. But in modern society, storing energy as fat is no longer necessary for most people. Most Americans wait no more than four hours between meals and snacks. So instead of being a valuable survival mechanism, the body's ability to store fat now is more likely to have a profoundly negative effect on health. As fat accumulates, it crowds the space occupied by the internal organs. Obesity—even moderate overweight— puts an undue stress on the back, legs, and internal organs, and this can eventually exacerbate many physical problems and compromise health. Obesity increases the body's resistance to insulin and susceptibility to infection, and puts one at a higher risk for developing coronary artery disease, diabetes, gallbladder disease, high blood pressure, kidney disease, stroke, and other serious health problems that can result in premature death. Complications of pregnancy and liver damage also are more common in overweight individuals. Obese persons suffer psychologically as well as physically, because our society tends to equate beauty, intelligence, and even success with thinness.

The most common causes of obesity are poor diet and/or eating habits and a lack of exercise. Other factors that can lead to obesity include glandular malfunctions, diabetes, hypoglycemia, emotional tension, boredom, and a simple love of food. Obesity has also been linked to food sensitivities and/or allergies. Food your body cannot use or that is a poison to your system is stored in the tissues and causes water retention. Ironically, poor nutrition may be an important factor in obesity. When there is inadequate intake of certain essential nutrients, fat is not easily or adequately burned and can accumulate in the body.

Obesity is a serious health problem and, according to the U.S. Centers for Disease Control and Prevention, it is on the rise in the United States. At least one third of Americans are 20 percent or more overweight. Even though this country has gone through several fitness crazes in recent years, Americans today are fatter, more stressed out, and no likelier to get regular exercise than we were ten years ago. And if we are getting fatter, it isn't because we have stopped trying to lose weight. National surveys estimate that at any given time, 25 to 50 percent of adult Americans are on some sort of diet, and we spend more than $30 billion each year on diet aids and remedies. Unfortunately, even those who lose weight often put it back on. It is estimated that two thirds of those who lose weight regain the lost pounds within three to five years.

Traditionally, there are three basic approaches to weight management through nutritional supplementation. The first is the use of diuretic herbs and nutrients to reduce water retention. The second is the use of lipotropic vitamins, which have the ability to reduce cholesterol and fat. Third is the use of natural appetite suppressants. Permanent weight loss, however, requires a lifetime commitment to a healthier lifestyle in general.

NUTRIENTS

SUPPLEMENT	SUGGESTED DOSAGE	COMMENTS
Very Important		
Aerobic Bulk Cleanse (ABC) from Aerobic Life Industries or psyllium husks	As directed on label. Always take supplemental fiber separately from other supplements and medications. 1 tbsp ½ hour before meals with a large glass of liquid. Drink it quickly.	Especially good for high or low blood sugar problems and also provides fiber. Gives a full feeling, cutting down hunger pangs.
Chromium picolinate	200–600 mcg daily.	Reduces sugar cravings by stabilizing the metabolism of simple carbohydrates (sugars).
Essential fatty acids (flaxseed oil, primrose oil, and salmon oil are good sources)	As directed on label.	Use these with a low-fat diet to provide essential fatty acids, needed by every cell in the body and for appetite control.
Kelp	1,000–1,500 mg daily.	Contains balanced minerals and iodine. Aids in weight loss.
Lecithin granules or capsules	1 tbsp 3 times daily, before meals. 1,200 mg 3 times daily, before meals.	A fat emulsifier; breaks down fat so it can be removed from the body.
Spirulina or Spiru-tein from Nature's Plus	As directed on label 3 times daily. Take between meals.	Excellent sources of usable protein. Contains needed nutrients and stabilizes blood sugar. Can replace a meal.
Vitamin C with bioflavonoids	3,000–6,000 mg daily.	Necessary for normal glandular function. Speeds up a slow metabolism, prompting it to burn more calories.
Helpful		
Calcium	1,500 mg daily.	Involved in activation of lipase, an enzyme that breaks down fats for utilization by the body.
Choline and inositol	As directed on label.	Helps the body burn fat.
Coenzyme Q$_{10}$	As directed on label.	Necessary for energy.
Dehydroepiandrosterone (DHEA)	As directed on label.	Inhibits an enzyme that is involved in fat production.
Gamma-aminobutyric acid (GABA)	As directed on label.	Suppresses cravings and has antidepressant qualities. *See* AMINO ACIDS in Part One.
L-Arginine and L-ornithine plus L-lysine	500 mg each or as directed on label, before bedtime. Take on an empty stomach with water or juice. Do not take with milk. Take with 50 mg vitamin B$_6$ and 100 mg vitamin C for better absorption.	These amino acids decrease body fat. *See* AMINO ACIDS in Part One. *Caution:* Do not take these if you have diabetes. Do not take arginine or ornithine without lysine.

L-Carnitine	500 mg daily.	Has the ability to break up fat deposits and aids in weight loss.
L-Glutamine	As directed on label.	Lessens carbohydrate cravings.
L-Methionine	As directed on label.	Assists in the breakdown of fat.
L-Phenylalanine	As directed on label, on an empty stomach.	An appetite suppressant that tells the brain you are not hungry. See AMINO ACIDS in Part One. Caution: Do not take this supplement if you are pregnant or nursing, or suffer from panic attacks, diabetes, high blood pressure, or PKU.
L-Tyrosine	As directed on label. Take at bedtime.	Suppresses cravings and has antidepressant qualities. See AMINO ACIDS in Part One. Caution: Do not take tyrosine if you are taking an MAO inhibitor drug.
Maitake	As directed on label.	Aids in weight loss.
Multivitamin and mineral complex with	As directed on label.	Obesity and nutritional deficiency are parts of the same syndrome.
potassium	99 mg daily.	Important in the production of energy. Sodium and potassium levels must be balanced.
Vitamin B complex plus extra	50 mg 3 times daily.	Needed for proper digestion.
vitamin B_2 (riboflavin) and	50 mg 3 times daily.	Required for efficiency in burning calories.
vitamin B_3 (niacin)	50 mg 3 times daily. Do not exceed this amount.	Lessens sugar cravings. Caution: Do not take niacin if you have a liver disorder, gout, or high blood pressure.
and vitamin B_6 (pyridoxine) and	50 mg 3 times daily.	Boosts metabolism.
vitamin B_{12}	50 mg 3 times daily.	Needed for proper digestion and absorption.
Zinc	80 mg daily. Do not exceed a total of 100 mg daily from all supplements.	Enhances the effectiveness of insulin and boosts immune function. Use zinc gluconate lozenges or OptiZinc for best absorption.

HERBS

❑ Alfalfa, corn silk, dandelion, gravel root, horsetail, hydrangea, hyssop, juniper berries, oat straw, parsley, seawrack, thyme, uva ursi, white ash, and yarrow can be used in tea form for their diuretic properties.

❑ Aloe vera juice improves digestion and cleanses the digestive tract.

❑ Astragalus increases energy and improves nutrient absorption.
Caution: Do not use this herb in the presence of a fever.

❑ Butcher's broom, cardamom, cayenne, cinnamon, Garcinia cambogia, ginger, green tea, and mustard seed are thermogenic herbs that improve digestion and aid in the metabolism of fat.
Caution: Do not use cinnamon in large quantities during pregnancy.

❑ Bladderwrack, borage seed, hawthorn berry, licorice root, and sarsaparilla stimulate the adrenal glands and improve thyroid function.
Caution: If overused, licorice can elevate blood pressure. Do not use this herb on a daily basis for more than seven days in a row. Avoid it completely if you have high blood pressure.

❑ Ephedra, guarana, and kola nut are appetite suppressants.
Caution: Do not use ephedra if you suffer from anxiety, glaucoma, heart disease, high blood pressure, or insomnia, or if you are taking a monoamine oxidase (MAO) inhibitor drug for depression.

❑ Fennel removes mucus and fat from the intestinal tract, and is a natural appetite suppressant.

❑ Fenugreek is useful for dissolving fat within the liver.

❑ Siberian ginseng aids in moving fluids and nutrients throughout the body, and reduces the stress of adjusting to new eating habits.
Caution: Do not use this herb if you have hypoglycemia, high blood pressure, or a heart disorder.

RECOMMENDATIONS

❑ Do not worry so much about the number of calories you consume as about eating the proper foods. Rotate your foods, and be sure to eat a variety of foods. Eat meals that consist of a balance of proteins, complex carbohydrates, and some fat. Proteins can increase your metabolic rate by as much as 30 percent, and help to balance the release of insulin by prompting secretion of the pancreatic hormone glucagon. Protein-induced glucagon mobilizes fats from the tissues in which it is stored, thus aiding in weight loss. By eating balanced meals you get more steady blood sugar levels and the ability to burn stored body fat for long-term weight loss.

❑ Eat more complex carbohydrates that also offer protein, such as tofu, lentils, plain baked potatoes (no toppings, except for vegetables), sesame seeds, beans, brown rice, whole grains, skinless turkey or chicken breast, and whitefish (no shellfish). Poultry and fish should be broiled or baked, never fried.

❑ Eat fresh fruits and an abundance of raw vegetables. Have one meal each day that consists entirely of vegetables and fruits. Use low-calorie vegetables such as broccoli, cabbage, carrots, cauliflower, celery, cucumbers, green beans, kale, lettuce, onions, radishes, spinach, and turnips. Low-calorie, low-carbohydrate fruits include apples, cantaloupe, grapefruit, strawberries, and watermelon. The following are higher in calories and should be consumed in moderation: bananas, cherries, corn, figs, grapes, green peas, hominy, pears, pineapple, sweet potatoes, white rice, and yams.

❑ Eat foods raw, if possible. If foods are heated, they should be baked, broiled, steamed, or boiled. Never consume fried or greasy foods.

❑ Drink six to eight glasses of liquids daily. Herbal teas and steam-distilled water with trace minerals (such as Concentrace from Trace Minerals Research) added are good. They are nonfattening fillers that also help to dilute toxins and flush them out of the body. Herbal teas mixed with unsweetened fruit juice are very satisfying low-calorie drinks and are also very filling. Use these between meals and when a desire for sweets hits you. Drink sparkling water mixed with fruit juice in place of sodas.

❑ Pay particular attention to the fat in your diet. Some fat is necessary, but it must be the right kind. Avocados, olives, olive oil, raw nuts and seeds, and wheat and corn germ are sources of "good" fats that contain essential fatty acids. Use these foods in moderation—no more than twice a week. Eliminate saturated fats from the diet completely. Never consume animal fat, found in butter, cream, gravies, ice cream, mayonnaise, meat, rich dressings, and whole milk. Do not eat any fried foods.

❑ Consume the following foods in moderation: apples, brown rice, buckwheat, chestnuts, corn, grapes, oatmeal, white potatoes, and yellow vegetables. These foods contain small amounts of essential fatty acids, but they should not be overused.

❑ If you must eat snacks occasionally to ward off hunger, make sure they are healthy. Good choices include:

• Celery and carrot sticks.

• Low-fat cottage cheese topped with fresh applesauce and walnuts.

• Unsweetened gelatin made with fruit juice in place of sugar and water.

• Natural sugar-free whole-grain muffins.

• Freshly made unsalted popcorn.

• Rice cakes topped with nut butter (but not peanut butter).

• Watermelon, fresh fruit, or frozen fruit popsicles.

• Unsweetened low-fat yogurt topped with granola or nuts and fresh fruit.

❑ Do not eat any white flour products, salt, white rice, or processed foods. Also, avoid fast food restaurants and all junk foods.

❑ Do not consume sweets such as soda, pastries, pies, cakes, doughnuts, or candy. Omit all forms of refined sugar (including white sugar, brown sugar, and corn sweetener) from the diet. Sugar triggers the release of insulin, which then activates enzymes that promote the passage of fat from the bloodstream into the fat cells.

❑ Follow a fasting program once monthly. See FASTING in Part Three.

❑ For a quick energy boost, try taking a spirulina tablet.

❑ Use wheatgrass to calm the appetite. This is a very nutritious fuel from whole food that assists metabolic functions. Kelp is also beneficial.

❑ Do not consume alcohol in any form, including beer and wine. Alcohol not only adds calories, but it inhibits the burning of fat from fat deposits. It can also interfere with your judgment, so you may find yourself eating things you ordinarily would not.

❑ Use powdered barley malt sweetener (found in health food stores) instead of sugar. This is highly concentrated but not dangerous. It contains only 3 calories per gram (approximately 2 teaspoons). This sweetener is also beneficial for people with diabetes or hypoglycemia.

❑ Use extra fiber daily. Guar gum and psyllium husks are good sources. Take fiber with a large glass of liquid one-half hour before meals.
Note: Always take supplemental fiber separately from other supplements and medications.

❑ Move your bowels daily. A clean colon is important in stabilizing your weight. See COLON CLEANSING in Part Three.

❑ Be active. Take a brisk walk every day before breakfast or dinner to burn off fat. Make a habit of using the stairs instead of the elevator. Walk or ride a bicycle instead of driving whenever possible. Exercise increases the metabolic rate as well as burning off calories.

❑ Be sure to get regular aerobic exercise, such as walking, running, bicycling, or swimming, *and* do exercises for strength and flexibility, such as yoga or stretching exercises. Exercise is better than an overly strict diet for maintaining your health and controlling your weight. It is the best way to rid the body of fat and to maintain good muscle tone. Be sure to drink water during exercise to prevent dehydration and muscle cramps.
Caution: If you are over thirty-five and/or have been sedentary for some time, consult your health care provider before beginning an exercise program.

❑ If you have been sedentary for some time, try exercising in water. Water aerobics are excellent for those who are overweight or who find running or walking difficult. They are also good for arthritis sufferers. Water aerobics tone the body and strengthen the heart without straining the joints. Start by taking a class at a local fitness center or YMCA. Sedentary individuals should consult their health care providers before starting an exercise program.

❑ Change your eating habits. This is extremely important not only for losing weight, but for maintaining weight loss. Begin with the following:

• Always eat breakfast. It jump-starts the metabolism at the beginning of the day. Eat small but nutrient-dense meals every three to four hours throughout the day to keep your metabolism stable, to maintain a full feeling, and to avoid wide swings in blood sugar. Good choices might include a 2-ounce portion of protein food (beans, an egg, poultry) with ½ cup fresh salad dressed with apple cider vinegar; or ½ cup of a steamed vegetable with some type of grain (½ cup brown rice or a piece of whole- or multi-grain bread).

• Don't skip meals. This only intensifies hunger and food cravings.

• Make your main meal lunch, not dinner. Some people have had excellent results consuming no food after 3:00 p.m.

• At meals, put less food on your plate. Chew slowly. Stop eating as soon as you are no longer hungry—don't wait until you feel full.

• Try eating a small amount (200 calories or so) of complex carbohydrate prior to having a high-protein meal. This will help supply tryptophan to the brain, which in turn helps to reduce food cravings.

❑ If you get the urge to eat, put on a tight belt. This will make you uncomfortable and remind you that you want to lose that excess fat.

❑ Learn to ride out your food cravings. They peak and subside like ocean waves. When you get an urge to eat, tell yourself that you can satisfy the craving if you *really* want to. Then wait ten minutes. This ensures that your eating is conscious, not compulsive. Keep in mind that most cravings last only a few minutes. Try doing something to distract yourself. Also remember that food addiction is the same as any other addiction: That first bite only makes you want more. If you ultimately decide that you really do want that food, then decide how much is reasonable and enjoy it. *Really* enjoy it. Take one bite and savor the taste. Eat slowly.

❑ Find out what causes your cravings. If you get a strong urge to snack while you're watching television, try reading a book, drinking a large glass of liquid, or taking a walk instead. If your cravings are triggered by where you are, move. If you're in the kitchen, go outside to relax, take a walk, or do yard work. If you're in the mall, avoid the food court.

❑ Consider having yourself tested for food allergies. Many people who have eliminated allergenic foods from their diets have stabilized their weight quickly.

❑ Do not chew gum. Chewing gum starts the digestive juices flowing and makes you feel hungry.

❑ Do not grocery shop on an empty stomach. You will be tempted to buy forbidden foods and will often buy more food than you need or can use before it loses its freshness.

❑ Avoid crash dieting. A very low calorie diet causes the metabolism to slow down, resulting in fewer calories being burned. Instead, increase your activity level. This will raise your metabolic rate, burn fat, and help prevent the loss of lean tissue.

❑ To maintain weight loss, calculate how many calories you need daily by multiplying your weight by 10. Then add 30 percent (about one third) of that amount to the result. Assuming a moderate activity level, consuming anything less than that number of calories should allow you to lose weight. This is the number of calories you can consume daily without gaining the weight back.

CONSIDERATIONS

❑ The basic arithmetic of weight loss is that each pound of body fat is worth 3,500 calories. Thus, to lose 1 pound a week (a safe, reasonable goal), you must tip the calorie consumption/expenditure balance in your favor by 500 calories each day. To do this, you can, for example, lose 250 calories by drinking a glass of water flavored with lemon or lime juice instead of a can of regular soda and leaving the cheese off your sandwich at lunch, and then make up the other 250 calories by walking two and a half miles.

❑ The best way to lose weight—and virtually the only way to maintain weight loss—is to adopt a healthier, more active lifestyle. A lifestyle that includes a natural, healthy diet and regular exercise will keep you healthy; give you more energy; lower your risk of heart disease, stroke, and cancer; and still allow you to lose weight. Those who choose fad diets over such a lifestyle can count on gaining back their lost weight and more. Almost 95 percent of all dieters regain their lost weight within a year and have to diet all over again.

❑ Repeated crash dieting is not healthy and can increase the risk of heart disease. Quick weight loss tends to come back rapidly. This rapid weight gain often results in elevated cholesterol levels and can also damage vital organs. In one study, a third of people who had gone on crash diets of 500 calories or less per day were found to have developed gallstones. The fourteen-year Framingham Heart Study showed that those whose weight changed a lot or changed often had higher death rates than other people. They also ran a greater risk of coronary heart disease. The study showed that weight fluctuation seemed to pose as great a risk of heart disease and premature death as being overweight.

❑ A study by the U.S. Department of Agriculture showed that one of every four teenagers carries enough excess weight to put him or her at high risk of heart attack, stroke, colon cancer, gout, and other health problems later in life—regardless of whether the individual slims down as an adult.

❑ The American Cancer Society has found that people who regularly use artificial sweeteners tend to gain, not lose, weight. These substances seem to increase the appetite and slow down the digestive process.

❑ Researchers at Rockefeller University in New York discovered a gene in mice that, if defective, leads to obesity. When activated, the gene apparently produces a hormonelike protein that is secreted by the fat cells into the bloodstream. The mouse gene is said to be 85 percent identical to its human counterpart. Its discovery may eventually lead to the development of effective drugs to battle obesity. It also lends credence to the theory that some people truly are predisposed to put on more weight than others.

❑ A person whose body has a high ratio of muscle to fat will have a higher metabolic rate than a person of the same weight with a lower muscle-to-fat ratio, and therefore will require more calories. This is because it takes more calories to maintain muscle tissue than fat tissue. Conversely, obese persons tend to have lower than normal metabolic rates. Unfortunately, this can make the battle to lose weight that much more difficult and frustrating.

❑ Calories derived from fat are more easily converted into flab than calories from other sources. Only 3 percent of fat calories are burned in the digestive process. By contrast, 25 percent of calories from complex carbohydrates (fruits, vegetables, whole grains) are burned in the course of digestion.

❑ Many people feel the need to eat something sweet after meals, but this is an acquired habit and it *can* be broken. In many cultures, sweetened foods are reserved only for rare special occasions (and even then are less sweet-tasting than many of the foods Americans eat every day). It may take some time to break the cycle, but if you stick with it you will eventually realize that you no longer even want sweets very often. You will also probably find that virtually all other foods taste much better. In fact, once your taste buds recover from years of overexposure to sugar, you will be surprised to discover just how heavily sweetened many food products are.

❑ Eating a low-fat diet that is high in complex carbohydrates does *not* mean eating tasteless, bland foods. There are many delicious and healthy foods available that can be eaten. The goal is to reduce the total fat, saturated fat, and cholesterol in the diet and to increase the amount of complex carbohydrates. Potatoes, pasta, breads, corn, rice, and other complex-carbohydrate-rich foods are not the cause of obesity, as some people think. They are the cure. The exception to this rule involves people who are addicted to carbohydrates. Carbohydrate addicts respond to carbohydrates the way alcoholics respond to alcohol. When they consume carbohydrates, it results in a release of insulin that is even greater than is needed, which in turn leads to even less of a feeling of satisfaction, so the urge to eat sets in again. Because of this, carbohydrate addicts end up trying to satisfy their hunger by eating more and more carbohydrates. People who are addicted to carbohydrates should limit their intake of foods high in complex carbohydrates and avoid *all* simple carbohydrates. They should consume two low-carbohydrate meals each day and save all of their carbohydrate-rich foods for a third "reward" meal. Keeping a daily record of what you eat and when, and how you feel afterward, is a simple way to reveal possible carbohydrate addiction.

❑ Hydroxycitric acid (HCA), a substance extracted from the rind of fruit of the *Garcinia cambogia* tree, is proving very effective for weight management. Not only does it suppress hunger, but it helps to prevent the body from turning carbohydrate calories into fat by inhibiting the action of an enzyme called ATP-citrate lyase. HCA is available in supplement form and is an ingredient in various diet products.

❑ Gamma-linolenic acid (GLA), the active ingredient in borage oil, black currant seed oil, flaxseed oil, and primrose oil, helps to control the metabolism of fats. Taking at least 250 IU of GLA a day helps to control the appetite.

❑ Diet Esteem Plus from Esteem is a diet product that contains many of the nutrients recommended in this section plus the herbal extract HCA. Along with good nutrition and regular exercise, this product has helped many people to lose weight and maintain weight loss.

❑ A 1994 study sponsored by the U.S. Department of Agriculture revealed that the trace mineral boron may speed the burning of calories. Raisins and onions are good food sources of boron.

❑ Some people have had good results taking 1 tablespoon of natural apple cider vinegar in 1 cup of pure, unsweetened cranberry juice every morning upon arising. Kombucha tea has also shown good results, and helps to boost energy. (*See* MAKING KOMBUCHA TEA in Part Three.)

❑ In human studies, the hormone dehydroepiandrosterone (DHEA) has led to a loss of body fat by blocking an enzyme that is known to produce fat tissue. (*See* DHEA THERAPY in Part Three).

❑ A weight-loss diet research center in England reported on using one part vegetable oil to two parts apple cider vinegar in massage to rid the body of fat. We recommend using pure virgin olive oil because it needs no refrigeration. Knead lightly but firmly over the fat areas at least three times weekly. This treatment is also good for sore and stiff joints.

❑ Researchers have found that weight reduction can be improved with the use of a combination of the amino acids L-ornithine and L-arginine, enhanced by L-lysine (see the Nutrients table in this entry for recommended dosages). L-Ornithine helps to release growth hormone, normally lacking in adults, which burns fat and builds muscle. This combination works best while the body is at rest.

Note: Never take an amino acid that contains L-arginine but not L-lysine. Too much L-arginine without L-lysine can cause an imbalance of amino acids, possibly causing an outbreak of cold sores or previously dormant herpes.

❑ Numerous ongoing studies using genetically engineered human growth hormone (HGH), have been effective in causing weight reduction in animals. An injection or capsule for humans is years away, however. The long-term consequences of using HGH are yet unknown.

❑ An ancient Ayurvedic herbal remedy that uses the extract of the guggulu tree has proven effective in normalizing blood cholesterol and triglyceride levels. It also has a mildly stimulating effect on the thyroid.

❑ Phenylpropanolamine, a common ingredient in over-the-counter appetite suppressants (and many commercial cold remedies), acts on the central nervous system and increases blood pressure. Persons with diabetes, high blood pressure, or hyperthyroidism, or who have difficulty urinating, should consult a doctor before using a product containing this drug.

❑ As a last resort, morbid (life-threatening) obesity may be treated surgically.

❑ The U.S. Food and Drug Administration has approved the use of a synthetic fat called olestra in snack foods. A synthetic compound of fatty acids and sugar, olestra is neither absorbed nor digested by the body and therefore contributes no calories. For the same reason, however, it can cause indigestion, gas, and diarrhea. Scientists have also raised concerns over its safety because it may inhibit the absorption of necessary fat-soluble vitamins.

❑ More detailed information and dietary suggestions helpful for weight loss, including nutritional information and recipes, may be found in *Prescription for Dietary Wellness* by Phyllis A. Balch, C.N.C., and James F. Balch, M.D.

Oily Skin

Oily skin occurs when the sebaceous (oil-secreting) glands produce more oil than is needed for proper lubrication of the skin. This excess oil can clog pores and cause blemishes. Oily skin is probably largely a matter of heredity, but it is known to be affected by factors such as diet and hormone levels. Humidity and hot weather also stimulate the sebaceous glands to produce more oil. Because skin tends to become dryer with age, and because of the hormonal shifts of adolescence, oily skin is common in teenagers, but it can occur at any age. Many people have skin that is oily only in certain areas and dry or normal in others, a condition known as combination skin. In general, the forehead, nose, chin, and upper back tend to be oilier than other areas.

Oily skin has its positive aspects. It is slow to develop age spots and discoloration, fine lines, and wrinkles. It doesn't freckle or turn red in the sun—on the contrary, it tans evenly and beautifully. On the negative side, oily skin is prone to "breakouts" well past adolescence and has a chronically shiny appearance, an oily or greasy feeling, and enlarged pores.

NUTRIENTS

SUPPLEMENT	SUGGESTED DOSAGE	COMMENTS
Very Important		
Flaxseed oil capsules or	1,000 mg daily.	Supplies needed essential fatty acids.
liquid or	1 tsp daily.	
primrose oil	Up to 500 mg daily.	A good healer for most skin disorders. Contains linoleic acid, which is needed by the skin.
Vitamin A	25,000 IU daily for 3 months, then reduce to 15,000 IU daily. If you are pregnant, do not exceed 10,000 IU daily.	Necessary for healing and construction of new skin tissue.
Vitamin B complex plus extra	As directed on label.	B vitamins are important for healthy skin tone.
vitamin B12	100 mcg 3 times daily.	

Important		
Kelp	1,000–1,500 mg daily.	Supplies balanced minerals needed for good skin tone.
Vitamin E	Start with 400 IU daily and increase slowly to 800 IU daily.	Protects against free radicals.
Zinc	50 mg daily. Do not exceed a total of 100 mg daily from all supplements.	For tissue repair. Enhances immune response. Use zinc gluconate lozenges or OptiZinc for best absorption.
Helpful		
Aloe vera		*See under* Herbs, below.
GH3 cream from Gero Vita	Apply topically as directed on label.	Good for acne. Also good for any discoloration of the skin.
Grape seed extract	As directed on label.	A powerful antioxidant that protects skin cells.
Herpanacine from Diamond-Herpanacine Associates	As directed on label.	Contains antioxidants, amino acids, and herbs that promote overall skin health.
L-Cysteine	500 mg daily, on an empty stomach. Take with water or juice. Do not take with milk. Take with 50 mg vitamin B6 and 100 mg vitamin C for better absorption.	Contains sulfur, needed for healthy skin. *See* AMINO ACIDS in Part One.
Lecithin granules or capsules	1 tbsp 3 times daily, before meals. 1,200 mg 3 times daily, before meals.	Needed for better absorption of the essential fatty acids.
Superoxide dismutase (SOD)	As directed on label.	A free radical destroyer.
Tretinoin (Retin-A)	As prescribed by physician.	Acts as a gradual chemical peel; unclogs pores and speeds up sloughing off of top layers of skin, exposing new, fresh skin. Available by prescription only.

HERBS

❑ Aloe vera has excellent healing properties. Apply aloe vera gel topically, as directed on product label or as needed.

❑ Burdock root, chamomile, horsetail, oat straw, and thyme nourish the skin.

❑ Lavender is very good for oily skin. Mist your skin with lavender water several times daily.

❑ A facial sauna using lemongrass, licorice root, and rosebuds is good for oily skin. Two or three times a week, simmer a total of 2 to 4 tablespoons of dried or fresh herbs in 2 quarts of water. When the pot is steaming, place it on top of a trivet or thick potholder on a table, and sit with your face at a comfortable distance over the steam for fifteen minutes. You can use a towel to trap the steam if you wish. After fifteen minutes, splash your face with cold water and allow your skin to air dry or pat it dry with a towel. After the sauna, you can allow the herbal water to cool and save it for use as a toning lotion to be dabbed on your face with a cotton ball after cleansing.

RECOMMENDATIONS

❑ Drink plenty of quality water to keep the skin hydrated and flush out toxins.

❑ Reduce the amount of fat in your diet. Consume no fried foods, animal fats, or heat-processed vegetable oils such as those sold in supermarkets. Do not cook with oil, and do not eat any oils that have been subjected to heat, whether in processing or cooking. If a little oil is necessary, such as in salad dressing, use cold-pressed canola or olive oil only.

❑ Do not drink soft drinks or alcoholic beverages. Avoid sugar, chocolate, and junk food.

❑ Keep your skin very clean. Wash your face two or three times in the course of a day, but do not use harsh soaps or cleansers. Use a pure soap with no artificial additives, such as E•Gem Skin Care Soap from Carlson Laboratories. Do not use cleansers or lotions that contain alcohol. After cleansing, apply a natural *oil-free* moisturizer to keep the skin supple.

❑ Alpha-hydroxy acids are a group of naturally occurring acids (found mostly in fruits) that help to stimulate cell renewal, aid the skin in retaining water, and give it a smoother, less oily appearance. Oily skin can benefit from the use of products containing alpha-hydroxy acids because they aid in removal of the top layer of dead skin cells, which stimulates healthy skin growth and may diminish large pores. Glycolic acid is probably the best of the alpha-hydroxy acids for this purpose. If you decide to try an alpha-hydroxy acid product, begin with a product containing 5 percent alpha-hydroxy acid (not more), and apply it at night only. First wash your face, then wait five minutes before applying a small amount of the product. After two or three weeks of nighttime application, you can begin applying the product in the morning as well. As your skin becomes accustomed to the effects of alpha-hydroxy acids, you may wish to work your way up to higher-concentration products.

❑ Two or three times a week, use a loofah sponge for the face (available in health food stores) and warm water to boost circulation, remove dead skin cells, and remove many of the impurities found in oily skin. Avoid using the loofah around your eyes, and do not use it on areas with open sores.

❑ To clear away excess oil, use a clay mask. Blend together well 1 teaspoon green clay powder (available in health food stores) and 1 teaspoon raw honey. Apply the mixture to your face, avoiding the eye area. Leave it on for fifteen minutes, then rinse well with lukewarm water. Do this at least three times a week—or more often if necessary.

❑ Once or twice daily, mix equal parts of lemon juice and water together. Pat mixture on your face and allow it to dry, then rinse with warm water. Follow with a cool-water rinse.

❑ For combination skin, simply treat the oily areas as oily skin and the dry areas as dry skin. *See* DRY SKIN in Part Two.

❑ Do not smoke. Smoking promotes enlargement of the pores and impairs the overall health of the skin.

CONSIDERATIONS

❑ Caring for oily skin does *not* mean trying to dry the skin out. Despite having excess oil, skin may still lack moisture. Moisture is a term that is used to refer to the amount of water inside the skin cells, not the amount of oil on the surface of the skin. While oil and moisture levels are related (the oil helps prevent loss of moisture through evaporation), the two are not the same. There are products available that help to supply and protect moisture without adding oil. Vitamin A Moisturizing Gel from Derma-E Products is a good non-greasy moisturizer. Using such a moisturizer may help prevent the development of wrinkles in the long run.

❑ *See also* ACNE in Part Two.

Optic Neuritis

See under NEURITIS.

Osteoarthritis

See under ARTHRITIS.

Osteomalacia

See RICKETS/OSTEOMALACIA.

Osteoporosis

Osteoporosis is a progressive disease in which the bones gradually become weaker and weaker, causing changes in posture and making the individual extremely susceptible to bone fractures. The term *osteoporosis*, derived from Latin, literally means "porous bones." Because of the physiological, nutritional, and hormonal differences between males and females, osteoporosis primarily affects women. Indeed, this debilitating disease afflicts more women than heart disease, stroke, diabetes, breast cancer, or arthritis. Fully half of all women between the ages of forty-five and seventy-five show signs of some degree of osteoporosis. Over a third of that group suffer from serious bone deterioration. Treatment and care for people with osteoporosis in the United States costs approximately $3.8 billion annually.

Bone mass—the amount of mineral in the bone—generally reaches its peak when a woman is between the ages of thirty and thirty-five. After that, it then begins to decline. Between the ages of fifty-five and seventy, women typically

Calcium and Osteoporosis

People in the United States consume more dairy products and other foods high in calcium per capita than the citizens of any other two nations on earth put together. We even have orange juice and antacids that are fortified with calcium. Yet we eat far less total food, take in less calcium, and get less exercise that stimulates bone growth than our grandparents did. At the same time, we consume more animal protein and phosphate-containing foods such as soft drinks. Perhaps not surprisingly, therefore, we also have the world's highest rates of osteoporosis and bone fractures among elderly people. Obviously, we need to eat more of the right foods and take high-quality supplements in some form as well.

Drugstores and health food stores carry a bewildering array of vitamin and mineral supplements in a variety of brands and forms. While it is now easy to find a high-quality calcium supplement, this was not always the case. In 1987, more than half of the eighty brands of calcium tablets tested by the University of Maryland School of Pharmacy failed to meet the dissolution criteria set by the U.S. Pharmacopeial Convention (USP). Fortunately, formulations have changed since then. A 1995 study conducted by *Consumer Reports* tested twenty-one supplements using the USP dissolution test, and found that all brands and all types—calcium carbonate, calcium lactate, calcium citrate, and calcium gluconate—dissolve well. No form of calcium, in fact, was found to dissolve more reliably than another.

However, there are still significant nutritional differences between the various supplements available. Where calcium is concerned, the number on the label does not necessarily reflect the amount of calcium you can expect to absorb from the product. For example, if a label says "calcium lactate 600 milligrams," this may mean that each tablet weighs 600 milligrams—but out of 600 milligrams of calcium lactate, only 60 milligrams are actually calcium that is available for absorption. This is because minerals cannot be turned into tablets in their pure state; they must be combined with some other substance or substances to make a stable compound. In the case of calcium lactate, the compound consists of calcium plus lactic acid. The important information to look for is the amount of *elemental* calcium that is present in the supplement. Calcium carbonate contains a higher percentage of elemental calcium than do the other forms.

If you are in doubt about your calcium tablets, you can do a home test to determine whether the supplement will dissolve readily in your body. Place a tablet in a cup of vinegar and stir it every few minutes. The tablet should be completely dissolved within half an hour. If it isn't, it will not dissolve in your stomach, either, and you should choose another supplement.

---

experience a 30- to 40-percent bone loss. Unfortunately, bone loss causes no symptoms while it is occurring, so it goes unnoticed until significant loss has occurred. It is very common for a woman to be completely unaware of having osteoporosis until what should have been a minor accident causes her to break a bone, often a wrist or hip. If osteoporosis becomes quite advanced, even an enthusiastic hug can result in cracked or broken ribs. As bone loss advances, the vertebrae are subject to what are called compression fractures, crowding the nerves of the spine and various internal organs and causing a loss of height. This can be very painful. It is this compression that causes the "dowager's hump" that many women develop as they age. Osteoporosis can also be a contributing factor in tooth loss; when the structure of the jawbone weakens, it can no longer hold the teeth firmly in place.

Many people have the impression that osteoporosis is caused solely by a dietary calcium deficiency and that it therefore can be remedied by taking calcium supplements. This is not quite correct. While calcium supplementation is important in dealing with osteoporosis, there are other considerations as well. Vitamins C, D, E, and K all play vital roles in battling osteoporosis, as does protein. Regulating the amounts of certain minerals, such as magnesium, phosphorus, silicon, boron, zinc, manganese, and copper, in the body are also important in maintaining proper calcium levels. Exercise is another vital factor.

There are two basic types of osteoporosis. Type I is believed to be caused by hormonal changes, particularly a loss of estrogen, which causes the loss of minerals from the bones to accelerate. Type II is linked to dietary deficiency, especially a lack of sufficient calcium and of vitamin D, which is necessary for the absorption of calcium. Many women mistakenly believe that osteoporosis is something they need be concerned about only after menopause. However, recent evidence indicates that osteoporosis often begins early in life and is *not* strictly a postmenopausal problem. Although bone loss accelerates after menopause, as a result of the drop in estrogen levels, it begins in the premenopausal years.

A number of factors are known to influence an individual's risk of developing osteoporosis. The first, and probably the most important, is the peak bone mass achieved in adulthood; the larger and denser the bones are to begin with, the less debilitating bone loss is likely to be. Small, fine-boned women therefore have more reason for concern than women with larger frames and heavier bones. Race and ethnicity also appear to play a role. Women of northern European or Asian extraction are more likely to develop osteoporosis, while women of African descent are less likely to be affected.

Dietary and lifestyle habits are important as well. Insufficient calcium intake is one factor, but equally important are other dietary practices that affect calcium metabolism. A diet high in animal protein, salt, and sugar causes the body to excrete increased amounts of calcium. The body then is forced to "steal" calcium from the bones to meet its requirements. Caffeine, alcohol, and many other drugs have a similar effect. Too much magnesium and/or phosphorus (found in most sodas and many processed food products) can inhibit the body from absorbing calcium properly, because these minerals compete with calcium for absorption in the blood and bone marrow. Bone density also depends on exercise. When it gets regular weight-bearing exercise (such as walking), the body responds by depositing more mineral in the bones, especially the bones of the legs, hips, and spine. Conversely, a lack of regular exercise accelerates the loss of bone mass. Other factors that make one more likely to develop osteoporosis include smoking, late puberty, early menopause (natural or artificially induced), a family history of the disease, hyperthyroidism, chronic liver or kidney disease, and the long-term use of corticosteroids, antiseizure medications, or anticoagulants.

While osteoporosis causes no specific symptoms until it is advanced, there are some early warning signs that may signal bone loss is occurring. These include a gradual loss of height, a stooping or rounding of the shoulders, and generalized aches and pains. If you notice that your clothes seem to be getting longer, that may be a clue.

NUTRIENTS

SUPPLEMENT	SUGGESTED DOSAGE	COMMENTS
Essential		
Bone Builder from Ethical Nutrients or	As directed on label.	A highly absorbable nutritional supplement containing minerals and the organic matrix that makes up bone.
Bone Defense from KAL or	As directed on label.	Contains calcium, magnesium, phosphorus and other valuable bone-reinforcing nutrients.
Bone Support from Synergy Plus or	As directed on label.	A complex containing many of the nutrients listed in this section.
Bone Builder with Boron from Metagenics or	As directed on label.	A bone complex that is effective for reducing the risk of osteoporosis. Available through health care professionals only.
Joint Support from Now Foods or	As directed on label.	Contains vitamins, minerals, and herbs for bone and joint health.
Osteo-B-plus from Biotics Research	As directed on label.	Contains calcium, magnesium, zinc, and other vitamins and minerals.
Boron	3 mg daily. Do not exceed this amount.	Improves calcium absorption. *Note:* If you are taking a complex containing boron, omit this supplement.
Calcium	1,500–2,000 mg daily.	Necessary for maintaining strong bones. Use chelate form. Injections (under a doctor's supervision) may be needed.
Glucosamine Plus from FoodScience Labs	As directed on label.	Contains glucosamine and other nutrients necessary for the development of bone and connective tissue.
Silica	As directed on label.	Supplies silicon, for calcium utilization and bone strength.

Copper	3 mg daily.	Aids in the formation of bone.
Floradix Iron + Herbs from Salus Haus	As directed on label.	Provides organic iron and other nutrients needed for optimum health.
Magnesium	1,000 mg daily.	Important in calcium uptake.
Very Important		
L-Lysine and L-arginine	As directed on label, on an empty stomach. Take with water or juice. Do not take with milk. Take with 50 mg vitamin B$_6$ and 100 mg vitamin C for better absorption.	Aid calcium absorption and connective tissue strength. *See* AMINO ACIDS in Part One.
Multienzyme complex with betaine hydrochloride (HCl) plus proteolytic enzymes	As directed on label. Take with meals. Take between meals.	Needed for proper absorption of calcium and all nutrients.
Sulfur	As directed on label.	Necessary for calcium uptake. Increases bone and connective tissue strength.
Vitamin A and vitamin E plus vitamin D	50,000 IU daily for 1 month, then reduce to 25,000 IU daily. 400 IU daily. 400 IU daily.	Important in retarding the aging process. Use emulsion forms for easier assimilation. Plays a role in calcium uptake.
Zinc	50 mg daily. Do not exceed a total of 100 mg daily from all supplements.	Important for calcium uptake and immune function. Use zinc gluconate lozenges or OptiZinc for best absorption.
Helpful		
Chromium picolinate	400–600 mcg daily.	Improves insulin efficiency, which improves bone density.
Cod liver oil	3 tsp twice daily.	A natural source of vitamins A and D.
DL-Phenylalanine	As directed on label, on an empty stomach. Take with water or juice. Do not take with milk. Take with 50 mg vitamin B$_6$ and 3,000 mg vitamin C for better absorption.	Good for bone pain. *See* AMINO ACIDS in Part One. *Caution:* Do not take this supplement if you suffer from panic attacks, diabetes, high blood pressure, or PKU.
Kelp	2,000–3,000 mg daily.	A rich source of important minerals.
Manganese	As directed on label. Take separately from calcium.	Vital in mineral metabolism.
Multivitamin and mineral complex	As directed on label.	To supply essential minerals. Use a high-potency formula.
Vitamin B$_{12}$	1,000 mcg daily.	Promotes normal growth. Use a lozenge or sublingual form. Consider injections (under a doctor's supervision).
Vitamin C	3,000 mg and up daily.	Important for collagen and connective tissue formation.

HERBS

❑ Feverfew is good for pain relief and acts as an anti-inflammatory.

Caution: Do not use feverfew during pregnancy.

❑ Alfalfa, barley grass, black cohosh, boneset, dandelion root, nettle, parsley, poke root, rose hips, and yucca help to build strong bones.

Caution: Do not use boneset on a daily basis for more than one week, as long-term use can lead to toxicity.

❑ Horsetail and oat straw contain silica, which helps the body absorb calcium.

RECOMMENDATIONS

❑ Eat plenty of foods that are high in calcium and vitamin D. Good sources of easily assimilable calcium include broccoli, chestnuts, clams, dandelion greens, most dark green leafy vegetables, flounder, hazelnuts, kale, kelp, molasses, oats, oysters, salmon, sardines (with the bones), sea vegetables, sesame seeds, shrimp, soybeans, tahini (sesame butter), tofu, turnip greens, and wheat germ.

❑ Consume whole grains and calcium foods at different times. Whole grains contain a substance that binds with calcium and prevents its uptake. Take calcium at bedtime, when it is best absorbed and also aids in sleeping.

❑ Include garlic and onions in the diet, as well as eggs (if your cholesterol level is not too high). These foods contain sulfur, which is needed for healthy bones.

❑ Limit your intake of almonds, asparagus, beet greens, cashews, chard, rhubarb, and spinach. These foods are high in oxalic acid, which inhibits calcium absorption.

❑ Avoid phosphate-containing drinks and foods such as soft drinks, high-protein animal foods, and alcohol. Avoid smoking, sugar, and salt. Limit your consumption of citrus fruits and tomatoes; these foods may inhibit calcium intake.

❑ Avoid yeast products. Yeast is high in phosphorus, which competes with calcium for absorption by the body.

❑ If you are over fifty-five, include a calcium lactate (if you are not not allergic to milk) or calcium phosphate supplement in your daily regimen, and take hydrochloric acid (HCl) supplements. In order for calcium to be absorbed, there must be an adequate supply of vitamin D as well as sufficient HCl in the stomach. Older people often lack sufficient stomach acid.

❑ If you take thyroid hormone or an anticoagulant drug, increase the amount of calcium you take by 25 to 50 percent.

❑ If you take a diuretic, consult your physician before beginning calcium and vitamin D supplementation. Thiazide-type diuretics increase blood calcium levels, and complications may result if these drugs are taken in conjunction with calcium and vitamin D supplements. Other types of diuretics increase calcium requirements, however.

❑ Keep active, and exercise regularly. A lack of exercise can result in the loss of calcium, but this can be reversed with sensible exercise. Walking is probably the best exercise for maintaining bone mass.

CONSIDERATIONS

❑ Manganese may help prevent osteoporosis, according to a report presented at an American Chemical Society meeting in Anaheim, California. Biologist Paul Saltman of the University of California–San Diego found that rats on a low-manganese diet developed porous bones.

❑ Both men and women slowly lose bone as they age. A woman may lose 30 to 50 percent of her cortical bone thickness over a lifetime.

❑ A study conducted by *The Journal of Clinical Nutrition* reported that women who are vegetarians experience significantly less bone loss than women who consume meat.

❑ A study reported in the *Journal of the American Medical Association* revealed that senior citizens who took tranquilizers suffered 70 percent more hip fractures than did other people their age.

❑ Caffeine has been linked to calcium loss. In one study, adults given 300 milligrams of caffeine excreted more than the normal amount of calcium in their urine. Another study revealed that caffeine is associated with decreased bone minerals in women.

❑ Carbonated soft drinks contain high amounts of phosphates. These cause the body to eliminate calcium as the phosphates themselves are excreted, even if calcium must be taken from the bones to do this.

❑ Bone disintegration with pain in the hips, lower back, or legs and vertebral fractures (usually affecting people over fifty years old) is common. The best way to monitor bone loss is with a bone mineral density test. X-rays do not detect bone loss until 25 percent or more of bone mass has been lost.

❑ The use of sodium fluoride, which was once thought to be helpful in building bone, has been shown to be ineffective for the treatment of osteoporosis. While sodium fluoride does increase bone mass in the vertebral column, the bone itself is of inferior quality. Women participating in a study at the Mayo Clinic in Rochester, Minnesota, were three times as likely to suffer from a fracture of the arm, leg, or hip if they took sodium fluoride than if they took a placebo. Some of the participants also suffered from unusual lower leg pain, perhaps due to stress fractures.

❑ The prescription drug calcitonin (sold under the brand names Calcimar, Cibacalcin, and Miacalcin) is sometimes prescribed for people with osteoporosis. It is said to have no side effects even with long-term use. Studies show that calcitonin prevents further loss of bone mass in 70 percent of the people who take it. It should not be taken by anyone with a history of kidney stones.

❑ Dehydroepiandrosterone (DHEA) and human growth hormone (HGH) are two hormones whose production progressively declines with age. Research suggests that supplementation with either of these hormones may help increase bone strength and treat osteoporosis. (*See* DHEA THERAPY and GROWTH HORMONE THERAPY in Part Three.)

❑ Estrogen therapy is often recommended for women at high risk of osteoporosis, and it can be very effective. However, we recommend against it in most cases because of the increased risk of cancer it entails.

❑ *See also* RICKETS in Part Two.

Paget's Disease of the Nipple

See under BREAST CANCER.

Paget's Disease of Bone

Paget's disease of bone (named for Sir James Paget, who first described it) is a slowly progressive bone disease characterized by disorganized and alternating bone-destructive and bone-constructive processes. The consequence is that sound bone is gradually replaced by excessive amounts of abnormal bone that is deficient in calcium and lacks the proper architecture for maximum strength. Paget's disease most often affects the bones of the pelvis, the spine, the thighs, the skull, the hips, the shins, and the upper arms. It is most common in men over the age of forty, but women are affected, too, and in rare instances it has been reported in young adults.

In the early stages, the disease usually causes no symptoms, although there may be mild pain in the affected bones. As it progresses, bone pain tends to become more severe and persistent, especially at night, and to worsen with exertion. Paget's disease can also lead to neck and/or back pain; pain and/or stiffness in affected joints; warming of the skin over the area of the affected bones; unexplained bone fractures; hearing loss; headaches; dizziness; ringing in the ears; and impaired mobility. The disease follows a pattern of alternating remissions and flare-ups. Over time, the flare-ups gradually become worse. Sometimes joints adjacent to the affected bone become involved, and osteoarthritis may develop. Over time, deformities such as bowed legs, an increasingly barrel-shaped chest, a bent spine, and an enlarged forehead may develop as well. Other possible late complications include kidney stones (caused by immobilization), congestive heart failure, deafness or blindness (caused by the skull pressing on the brain), high blood pressure, and gout. In approximately 5 percent of

cases, the affected bone undergoes malignant changes, leading to osteosarcoma (bone cancer). The life expectancy of individuals with Paget's disease is somewhat reduced, but most live with the disease for at least ten to fifteen years.

Because this disease usually does not cause significant symptoms, especially in the early stages, most cases go undetected unless discovered accidentally when x-rays or blood tests are taken for another reason. The cause is unknown, although some researchers suspect a viral infection may be involved. Multiple cases of the disease have been recorded as occurring within families. However, it does not appear to be transmitted from one generation to another, a finding more consistent with an infectious disorder than with a hereditary condition.

Paget's disease is often confused with other disorders, including hyperthyroidism and other disorders that cause bone lesions, such as bone cancer, fibrous dysplasia, and multiple myeloma. Doctors use x-rays, bone scans, CT scans, MRI, blood and urine tests, and bone biopsy to verify a diagnosis of Paget's disease.

NUTRIENTS

SUPPLEMENT	SUGGESTED DOSAGE	COMMENTS
Essential		
Calcium plus	1,500 mg daily.	For the formation of strong bones. Use a chelate form.
boron and	3 mg daily. Do not exceed this amount.	Nutrients that are needed for calcium absorption.
magnesium and	750 mg daily.	
vitamin D	400 IU daily.	
Copper	3 mg daily.	Aids in the formation of bone.
Glucosamine Plus from FoodScience Labs	As directed on label.	Contains nutrients necessary for healthy development of bone and connective tissues.
Manganese	2 mg daily.	Required for normal bone growth.
Phosphorus	1,200 mg daily.	Required for bone formation.
Silica	As directed on label.	Necessary for bone formation.
Primrose oil or	As directed on label.	To supply essential fatty acids vital for proper growth and cell formation.
Ultimate Oil from Nature's Secret	As directed on label.	
Vitamin B complex plus extra	50 mg 3 times daily, with meals.	Involved in energy production.
vitamin B$_{12}$ and	300 mcg daily.	Assists in food absorption and aids in cell formation.
folic acid	400 mcg daily.	Needed for energy production.
Vitamin C	3,000–6,000 mg daily, in divided doses.	Enhances immunity and aids in proper bone growth.
Vitamin A plus	10,000 IU daily.	To improve immune function and promote proper bone growth.
natural beta-carotene	10,000 IU daily.	
Zinc	30 mg daily. Do not exceed a total of 100 mg daily from all supplements.	Promotes a healthy immune system. Use zinc gluconate lozenges or OptiZinc for best absorption.

Helpful		
Bone Builder from Ethical Nutrients	As directed on label.	Contains minerals and the organic matrix that makes up bone.
DL-Phenylalanine (DLPA)	As directed on label.	Alleviates chronic pain. *Caution:* Do not take this supplement if you are pregnant or nursing, or suffer from panic attacks, diabetes, high blood pressure, or PKU.
Floradix Iron + Herbs from Salus Haus	As directed on label.	Provides organic iron and other nutrients needed for optimum health and fitness.
Joint Support from Now Foods	As directed on label.	Contains vitamins and minerals necessary for bone and joint health.
Shiitake or reishi	As directed on label. As directed on label.	To help reduce inflammation.

HERBS

❑ Alfalfa and horsetail contain minerals needed for proper bone formation and that help to reduce inflammation.

❑ Angelica, cayenne (capsicum), feverfew, hops, passionflower, skullcap, valerian root, and white willow bark work well for pain.
Caution: Do not use feverfew during pregnancy.

❑ Black cohosh and St. Johnswort help both to reduce inflammation and to alleviate pain.
Caution: Do not use black cohosh during pregnancy.

❑ Boneset, dandelion root, nettle, parsley, poke root, rose hips, and yucca help to build strong bones.
Caution: Do not use boneset on a daily basis for more than one week, as long-term use can lead to toxicity.

❑ Echinacea, goldenseal, and licorice aid in reducing inflammation.
Caution: Do not take goldenseal internally on a daily basis for more than one week at a time, do not use it during pregnancy. Use with caution if you are allergic to ragweed. Do not use licorice on a daily basis for more than seven days in a row, and avoid it if you have high blood pressure.

RECOMMENDATIONS

❑ Eat plenty of calcium-rich foods. These include brewer's yeast, buttermilk, carob, goat's milk, all leafy greens, salmon (with the bones), sardines, seafood, tofu, whey, and yogurt.

❑ Include plenty of garlic in the diet. Garlic is beneficial for circulation and helps to keep inflammation down.

❑ Eat fresh papaya and pineapple frequently. These fruits contain enzymes that help to reduce inflammation.

❑ Avoid nightshade vegetables. These include tomatoes, potatoes, eggplant, cayenne peppers, chili peppers, sweet peppers, paprika, and pimiento. These vegetables are high in alkaloids, chemical substances with strong physiological

effects. They affect the metabolism of calcium and, through a mechanism not yet understood, cause calcium from the bones to be deposited in other areas of the body where it does not belong, such as the arteries, joints, and kidneys.

❑ Use barley grass and/or kelp to supply valuable minerals and other nutrients needed for bone formation.

❑ Use heat to alleviate pain. Hot soaks, hot compresses, and heat lamps are all effective.

❑ Follow an exercise program recommended by your health care provider to combat immobility.

❑ Sleep on a very firm mattress or use a bed board. This will lessen the chance of developing spinal deformities.

❑ During active phases of the disease, rest in bed and move or turn often to prevent pressure sores.

❑ Accident-proof your home to help prevent fractures. Remove throw rugs and avoid slippery flooring. Install hand rails next to the bathtub and toilet.

❑ Avoid placing extreme physical stress on the bones.

❑ Get regular medical checkups to screen for early bone cancer and to detect hearing loss. If hearing loss occurs, consider a hearing aid.

CONSIDERATIONS

❑ There is no known cure for Paget's disease. However, most patients never develop symptoms and so do not require treatment. For those who do, drug treatment can relieve and manage symptoms. Drug therapy for Paget's disease may include:

• *Calcitonin (Calcimar, Cibacalcin, Miacalcin)*, a natural hormone given by injection, and *etidronate (Didronel)*, a calcium regulator, which both slow the progression of the disease.

• *Fluoride*, which is sometimes used to correct deformities, relieve pinched nerves, and prevent or reduce fractures.

• *Pliamycin (Mithracin)*, an anti-tumor drug, which can produce a remission of symptoms within two weeks, and further improvement in two months. However, this drug can also cause kidney damage and destruction of red blood cells.

Pancreatitis

Pancreatitis is an inflammation of the pancreas resulting from an obstruction of the pancreatic duct. This obstruction can be caused by the presence of gallstones, scarring (often from alcohol-related damage), or a cancerous tumor. Alcoholism is by far the leading underlying cause of pancreatitis in men. In women, it is most commonly linked to bile tract disease. Pancreatitis can also come about as a result of viral infection, abdominal injury, obesity, poor nutrition, and the use of certain drugs.

The disease can be either acute or chronic. Acute pancreatitis usually causes severe pain that comes on suddenly, starting in the area of the navel and radiating to the back. The pain is typically exacerbated by movement and relieved by sitting, and may be accompanied by nausea and vomiting, sometimes severe. Other symptoms include upper abdominal swelling and distension, excessive gas, upper abdominal pain described as burning or stabbing, fever, sweating, hypertension, muscle aches, and abnormal, fatty stools.

Chronic pancreatitis is a condition in which the inflammation has caused irreversible changes in the microscopic structure of the gallbladder tissue. Repeated episodes of gallbladder infection and gallstones are often involved. The symptoms of chronic pancreatitis may be hard to distinguish from those of acute pancreatitis, except that the pain tends to be chronic rather than coming on suddenly. In addition, chronic pancreatitis may be punctuated with periodic episodes of acute disease.

Because the pancreas is the gland that produces the hormones insulin and glucagon, which regulate blood sugar levels and contribute to digestion, pancreatitis—especially if chronic—often leads to glucose intolerance (diabetes) and digestive difficulties.

NUTRIENTS

SUPPLEMENT	SUGGESTED DOSAGE	COMMENTS
Essential		
Chromium picolinate	300 mcg daily.	Important in maintaining stable blood sugar levels.
Very Important		
Calcium and	1,500 mg daily.	Works closely with magnesium.
magnesium	1,000 mg daily.	Counteracts glandular disorders. Use chelate forms.
Pancreatin	As directed on label. Take with food.	Pancreatic enzyme deficiency is common in people with pancreatitis.
Proteolytic enzymes	As directed on label. Take between meals and at bedtime, on an empty stomach.	Aids in reducing inflammation; reduces strain on the pancreas by aiding protein digestion. *Caution:* Do not give this supplement to a child.
Raw pancreas glandular	As directed on label.	Contains certain proteins needed to repair the pancreas. *See* GLANDULAR THERAPY in Part Three.
Vitamin B complex plus extra	50 mg 3 times daily.	Anti-stress vitamins.
vitamin B3 (niacin) and pantothenic acid (vitamin B5)	50 mg 3 times daily. Do not exceed this amount. 100 mg 3 times daily.	Niacin and pantothenic acid are important in fat and carbohydrate metabolism. *Caution:* Do not take niacin if you have a liver disorder, gout, or high blood pressure.
Important		
Vitamin C	1,000 mg 4 times daily and up.	A potent free radical scavenger. Use a buffered form.
Choline and inositol and/or	As directed on label.	Fat emulsifiers that aid in fat digestion.
lecithin and/or	As directed on label.	
lipotropic factors	As directed on label.	
Helpful		
Coenzyme Q10	75 mg daily.	A powerful antioxidant and oxygen carrier.
CTR Support from PhysioLogics	As directed on label.	Helps diminish damage caused by inflammation and protects against future damage.
Detoxygen from Nature's Plus	As directed on label.	Herbal formula that detoxifies the body and oxygenates cells.
Digesta-Lac from Natren	As directed on label.	Replenishes "friendly" bacteria in intestines.
DL-Phenylalanine	As directed on label.	To relieve pain in acute cases. *Caution:* Do not take this supplement if you are pregnant or nursing , or if you suffer from panic attacks, diabetes, high blood pressure, or PKU.
Grape seed extract	As directed on label.	A powerful anti-inflammatory.
L-Cysteine	As directed on label.	Protects the liver.
Vitamin E	Start with 200 IU daily and increase slowly to 400–800 IU daily.	A powerful antioxidant and oxygen carrier. Important in tissue repair.
Zinc	50 mg daily. Do not exceed a total of 100 mg daily from all supplements.	Facilitates proper enzyme activity for cell division, growth, and repair. Plays a role in the manufacture of insulin. Use zinc gluconate lozenges or OptiZinc for best absorption.

HERBS

❑ Cedar berries, echinacea, gentian root, and goldenseal stimulate and strengthen the pancreas.

Caution: Do not take goldenseal internally on a daily basis for more than one week at a time, do not use it during pregnancy, and use it with caution if you are allergic to ragweed.

❑ Dandelion root stimulates bile production and improves the health of the pancreas.

❑ Licorice root supports all glandular functions.

Caution: If overused, licorice can elevate blood pressure. Do not use this herb on a daily basis for more than seven days in a row. Avoid it if you have high blood pressure.

RECOMMENDATIONS

❑ If you develop symptoms of pancreatitis, call your physician. This is an extremely serious condition that requires medical attention.

❑ Eat a diet low in fat and sugar. This is very important for recovery. *See* DIABETES in Part Two and follow the dietary guidelines.

❑ Consume no alcohol in any form.

❑ If antibiotics are prescribed, be sure to consume butter-milk, kefir, and yogurt, and add some form of acidophilus to the program.

❑ If you smoke, stop, and try to avoid secondhand smoke. Recent studies point to a distinct link between chronic pancreatitis and cigarette smoking.

❑ *See* FASTING in Part Three and follow the program. Fasting can improve the health of all organs, including the pancreas.

CONSIDERATIONS

❑ Pancreatic cancer is the fourth leading cause of cancer deaths in the United States. Pancreatitis can lead to the development of this type of cancer. Conversely, improving the health of the pancreas may help to prevent it.

❑ A high level of triglycerides (fat) in the blood is a factor in pancreatitis.

Panic Attack

See under ANXIETY DISORDER.

Parkinson's Disease

Also called *shaking palsy* or *paralysis agitans,* Parkinson's disease is a degenerative disease affecting the nervous system. The underlying cause is unknown, but symptoms appear when there is a lack of dopamine in the brain. Dopamine is a neurotransmitter that carries messages from one nerve cell to another. In healthy persons, it exists in balance with another neurotransmitter, acetylcholine. In people with what is called primary Parkinson's disease, the cells that manufacture dopamine are lost, and the brain can no longer manufacture this chemical. There is also a secondary form of the disorder, in which dopamine receptors in the brain are blocked in some way, interfering with the action of the brain chemical.

The disease may start with a mild to moderate tremor of the hand or hands while at rest, a general slow and heavy feeling, muscular stiffness, and a tendency to tire more easily than usual. Later symptoms may include muscular rigidity; drooling; loss of appetite; a stooped, shuffling gait; tremors, including a characteristic "pill-rolling" movement in which the thumb and forefinger rub against each other; impaired speech; and a fixed facial expression. The body gradually becomes rigid and the limbs stiffen. Depression and/or dementia may accompany the physical symptoms.

Parkinson's disease is one of the most common debilitating diseases in the United States. It runs its course over a period averaging ten years, ultimately resulting in death,

usually from infection or aspiration pneumonia. It affects men more often than women. Recent statistics indicate that 1 in every 100 persons after the age of sixty is afflicted.

While the cause of the loss of brain cells that causes Parkinson's disease remains unknown, a number of different theories have been developed. One hypothesis is that the cells are destroyed by toxins within the body that the liver is unable to filter out, metabolize, or detoxify because as the body ages, the liver loses its ability to work as effectively and as efficiently as it once did. Another theory is that exposure to environmental toxins, such as herbicides and pesticides that leach into ground water, is responsible. The discovery that a chemical known as N-MPTP (n-methyl-1,2,3,4 tetrahydropyridine), a byproduct of the production of a type of heroin used by heroin addicts, can kill brain cells and cause Parkinsonism has also helped direct current research. Malnutrition also is believed to be an important underlying factor.

NUTRIENTS

SUPPLEMENT	SUGGESTED DOSAGE	COMMENTS
Essential		
Vitamin C and	3,000–6,000 mg daily, in divided doses.	Antioxidants that may slow progression of the disease and
vitamin E plus	3,200 IU daily.	postpone the need for drug therapy.
selenium	200 mcg daily.	A powerful antioxidant.
Very Important		
Aangamik DMG from FoodScience Labs	50 mg twice daily.	Enhances tissue oxygenation.
Calcium and	1,500 mg daily.	Needed for nerve impulse transmission. These important
magnesium or	750 mg daily.	minerals work together.
Bone Support from Synergy Plus	As directed on label.	Contains calcium, magnesium, zinc, phosphorus, and other nutrients.
Dimethylamino-ethanol (DMAE)	As directed on label.	Stimulates the production of choline for brain function. Improves memory and learning ability.
Floradix Iron + Herbs from Salus Haus	As directed on label.	Contains iron derived from natural food sources, beneficial in the treatment of Parkinson's disease.
Gamma-ami-nobutyric acid (GABA)	As directed on label.	Functions as a neurotransmitter that stabilizes neuron activity. *See* AMINO ACIDS in Part One.
Grape seed oil (Salute Santé Grapeseed Oil from Lifestar International)	As directed on label.	Contains a high level of vitamin E as well as the essential fatty acid linoleic acid.
Lecithin granules or capsules and/or phosphatidyl choline	1 tbsp 3 times daily, before meals. 1,200 mg 3 times daily, before meals. As directed on label.	To supply choline, important in transmission of nerve impulses.
L-Glutamic acid	As directed on label.	Improves nerve impulse transmission. *See* AMINO ACIDS in Part One.

Supplement	Suggested Dosage	Comments
L-Phenylalanine	100–500 mg daily.	Alleviates symptoms (see AMINO ACIDS in Part One). Caution: Do not take this supplement if you are pregnant or nursing; if you take an MAO inhibitor drug; or if you suffer from panic attacks, diabetes, high blood pressure, or PKU.
L-Tyrosine	As prescribed by physician.	Helps to regulate mood (see AMINO ACIDS in Part One). Caution: Do not take this supplement if you take an MAO inhibitor drug.
Pycnogenol or grape seed extract	As directed on label. As directed on label.	Potent bioflavonoids and free radical scavengers.
Superoxide dismutase (SOD)	As directed on label.	An enzyme that retards oxidation, protecting neurons and sparing neurotransmitters like dopamine.
Vitamin B complex	50 mg 3 times daily, with meals.	Extremely important in brain function and enzyme activity. Use a high-potency sublingual formula. Consider injections (under a doctor's supervision).
plus extra pantothenic acid (vitamin B5)	25 mg 3 times daily.	Aids in speeding messages from one nerve cell to another.
Vitamin B3 (niacin) or niacinamide	50 mg 3 times daily, with meals. Do not exceed this amount. As directed on label.	Improves brain circulation. Flushing may occur from niacin use—this is normal. Caution: Do not take niacin if you have a liver disorder, gout, or high blood pressure. Niacinamide does not cause flushing.
Vitamin B6 (pyridoxine)	50–75 mg 3 times daily, with meals.	Brain dopamine production depends on adequate supplies of this vitamin. Consider injections (under a doctor's supervision). Caution: Do not take this supplement if you are taking a levodopa preparation.
Helpful		
Multienzyme complex	As directed on label.	To aid digestion and assimilation of all nutrients, especially the B vitamins.
Multivitamin and mineral complex with potassium	As directed on label. 99 mg daily.	To correct nutritional deficiencies, common in people with Parkinson's disease.
Primrose oil	2,000–4,000 mg daily, in divided doses.	May reduce the severity and frequency of tremors.
Raw brain glandular	As directed on label.	A glandular extract that improves brain function. See GLANDULAR THERAPY in Part Three.

HERBS

❑ Degenerative disease is often facilitated by the accumulation of toxins in the body. The following herbs have detoxifying properties:

• Burdock root, dandelion root, ginger root, and milk thistle detoxify the liver.

• Cayenne (capsicum), goldenseal, mullein, Siberian ginseng, and yarrow stimulate the thymus and lymphatic system.
Caution: Do not take goldenseal internally on a daily basis for more than one week at a time, do not use it during pregnancy, and use it with caution if you are allergic to ragweed. Do not use Siberian ginseng if you have hypoglycemia, high blood pressure, or a heart disorder.

• Hawthorn, licorice, red clover, and sarsaparilla cleanse the blood.
Caution: Do not use licorice on a daily basis for more than seven days in a row. Avoid it completely if you have high blood pressure.

• Yellow dock cleanses the blood and detoxifies the liver.

❑ Black cohosh, catnip, lemon balm, passionflower, skullcap, and valerian root have anti-stress properties and can help nourish the nervous system.
Caution: Do not use black cohosh during pregnancy.

❑ Ginkgo biloba helps to improve memory and brain function. Source Naturals offers an excellent extract.

RECOMMENDATIONS

❑ Eat a diet consisting of 75 percent raw foods, with seeds, grains, nuts, and raw milk.

❑ Include in the diet foods containing the amino acid phenylalanine, such as almonds, Brazil nuts, fish, pecans, pumpkin, sesame seeds, lima beans, chickpeas, and lentils.

❑ Reduce your intake of protein, especially if you are taking levodopa. This can help with control of coordination and muscle movements. Try to limit your protein consumption to 7 grams per day, consumed mostly at dinner. Eat barley, tofu, yogurt, beans, lentils, and other sources of protein instead of meat and poultry.

❑ If you must take the drug levodopa (see under Considerations, below), consume the following foods in moderation only: bananas, beef, fish, liver, oatmeal, peanuts, potatoes, and whole grains. These foods contain vitamin B6, which interferes with the drug's potency. Do not take supplemental vitamin B6, as it counteracts the drug's therapeutic effects (be careful with multivitamin supplements). Also, because some of the amino acids contained in food proteins can prevent this drug from reaching the brain, where it is needed, eat protein foods only in the evening, and not at the same time as the drug is taken. Once on medication, discuss with your physician any dietary change you plan to make, as dosage adjustments may be needed.

❑ If your work or a hobby exposes you to chemicals or metals such as lead or aluminum, always wear protective clothing, including gloves and a face mask.

CONSIDERATIONS

❑ Hand tremors are common in middle age and later. There are different types of tremors. Parkinsonian tremors are most pronounced during rest, can be aggravated by tension or fatigue, and disappear during sleep. *Intention tremors* occur only when a muscle is being used, rather than at rest. *Essential tremors* are more or less continuous up-and-down tremors that seem to run in families. These usually affect both hands, and become milder with rest, more severe with activity and/or stress. Attempts to stop this type of tremor through willpower often seem to make the trembling worse. Any persistent or recurrent tremor deserves investigation, especially if it interferes with normal activity, but it should be kept in mind that most tremors are *not* an indication of Parkinson's disease.

❑ There is no known cure for Parkinson's disease. Treatment is focused on relieving the symptoms and maintaining independence as long as possible. Drug therapy, physical therapy, and surgery (in severe cases) are among the treatment methods used.

❑ The drug most often used to treat this disease is levodopa (sold under the brand names Dopar and Larodopa). This drug is not effective alone, however, and can have serious side effects, including paranoia and hallucinations. A combination of levodopa and a drug called carbidopa (Sinemet) is also used. This drug also reduces stiffness.

❑ Fasting and chelation are both beneficial and may help to halt the progression of Parkinson's disease. (*See* FASTING and CHELATION THERAPY in Part Three.)

❑ Physical therapy, including active and passive range-of-motion exercises, plus daily moderate exercise like walking can help to maintain normal muscle tone and function.

❑ "Green drinks" may significantly reduce symptoms. (*See* JUICING in Part Three.)

❑ Octocosanol, a substance found in wheat germ oil, has been shown to have beneficial effects on neuron membranes, and may make it possible to reduce the dosage of levodopa required.

❑ Some people with Parkinson's disease have been found to have high levels of lead in their brains. Chelation therapy is the only way to remove lead from the body. (*See* CHELATION THERAPY in Part Three.)

❑ Because there are no definitive tests for Parkinson's disease, people with hypoglycemia are sometimes misdiagnosed as having the condition. (*See* HYPOGLYCEMIA in Part Two.)

❑ Iron supplementation appears to be beneficial to some people with Parkinson's disease. The production of tyrosine hydroxylase, an enzyme involved in the production of dopa (the precursor of dopamine), apparently can be stimulated by iron supplementation.

❑ A study published in *The New England Journal of Medicine* concluded that when the drug selegiline (Eldepryl), also known as deprenyl, is taken in the early stages of the disease, the onset of the more disabling symptoms seems to be delayed. The drug's mechanism of action is unclear, however, and it has not been proved that it can actually delay or slow the disease process, as opposed to easing symptoms.

❑ Treatment with the hormone dehydroepiandrosterone (DHEA) may help to prevent Parkinson's disease. *See* DHEA THERAPY in Part Three.

❑ The use of antioxidant supplements may delay the need for the levodopa therapy in people with Parkinson's disease, in some cases by as much as two to three years. In one study, people with Parkinson's disease were given 3,000 milligrams of vitamin C and 3,200 international units of vitamin E daily. The results strongly suggested that the progression of the disease can be slowed significantly by the administration of high dosages of antioxidants. If Parkinson's disease is related to free radical damage of dopamine-producing brain cells, in theory, a person who takes antioxidants while still healthy might never develop Parkinson's disease. Other research is exploring the role of a naturally occurring substance, glial-cell-line-derived neutrotrophic factor (GDNF), which nourishes the neurons that produce dopamine.

❑ Additional information is available from the National Parkinson's Foundation (NPF), 1501 NW 9th Avenue, Miami, FL 33136; telephone 800–433–7022.

Pellagra

Pellagra is a vitamin deficiency disease. It is caused by a long-term shortage of B vitamins, particularly vitamin B3 (niacin). It is prevalent in populations for whom corn, which is devoid of niacin, is the basis of the diet. Pellagra is rare in the United States, thanks to our more varied diet. When it does occur, it is most often the result of diseases that deplete the body of niacin, riboflavin, and thiamine, such as chronic gastrointestinal disturbances or alcoholism. It also can follow a long course of treatment with the antibiotic isoniazid (INH, Laniazid, Nydrazid, Tubizid), which is used to treat tuberculosis. Poor and/or homeless people, recent immigrants, and individuals in special circumstances, such as repatriated prisoners of war, may be at some risk due to poor diet.

The symptoms of pellagra include anxiety, depression, dementia, diarrhea, dizziness, headaches, an inflamed and sore red tongue, loss of appetite, weakness, and weight loss. Itchy dermatitis on the hands and neck is a prominent characteristic of the disease. Symptoms of subclinical pellagra are sometimes misinterpreted as mental illness. Disturbed or hyperactive behavior in children might signal a deficiency of niacin and other B vitamins.

All that is needed to prevent pellagra is a diet that provides adequate amounts of niacin, thiamine, riboflavin, folic acid, and vitamin B12.

NUTRIENTS

SUPPLEMENT	SUGGESTED DOSAGE	COMMENTS
Essential		
Vitamin B complex plus extra	100 mg daily.	All B vitamins are needed to correct deficiencies. B vitamins work best when taken together. Sublingual forms are recommended. Injections (under a doctor's supervision) may be necessary. *Caution:* Do not take niacin if you have a liver disorder, gout, or high blood pressure.
vitamin B$_1$ (thiamine) and	50 mg 3 times daily, with meals.	
vitamin B$_2$ (riboflavin) and	50 mg 3 times daily, with meals.	
vitamin B$_3$ (niacin)	100 mg daily. Do not exceed this amount.	
and		
vitamin B$_{12}$ plus	1,000 mcg twice daily, on an empty stomach.	Use a lozenge or sublingual form.
folic acid or	400 mcg daily.	
brewer's yeast or	As directed on label.	A good source of B vitamins.
Bio-Strath from Bioforce	As directed on label.	Natural source of the B complex.

RECOMMENDATIONS

❑ Eat plenty of foods that are high in B vitamins, such as avocados, bananas, broccoli, collards, figs, legumes, nuts and seeds, peanut butter, potatoes, prunes, tomatoes, and whole grain or enriched bread and cereal.

❑ Include in the diet halibut, salmon, sunflower seeds, swordfish, tuna, and white skinless breast of chicken and turkey. These foods are good sources of the amino acid tryptophan, which is converted into niacin in the body.

CONSIDERATIONS

❑ Individuals with diabetes should take supplementary niacin with caution, as it can raise blood sugar levels. Long-term niacin therapy may also increase the risk of gout. At least one study has pointed out the danger of taking too much niacin, especially for elderly people. The short-term side effects of niacin overdosage include flushing, itching, and skin disorders. Over the long term, high doses of niacin can be dangerous. Taking as little as 500 milligrams per day over a period of several months may result in liver damage.

Peptic Ulcer

A peptic ulcer is a spot where the lining of the stomach and the tissues beneath—and sometimes part of the stomach muscle itself—have been eroded, leaving an open wound inside the stomach. The surrounding tissue is usually swollen and irritated. Ulcers can occur anywhere along the gastrointestinal tract, but are most common in the stomach (gastric ulcers) and duodenum (duodenal ulcers). They affect approximately 10 percent of the U.S. population.

The symptoms of a peptic ulcer include chronic burning or gnawing stomach pain that usually begins forty-five to sixty minutes after eating or at night, and that is relieved by eating, taking antacids, vomiting, or drinking a large glass of water. The pain may range from mild to severe. It may cause the individual to awaken in the middle of the night. Other possible symptoms include lower back pain, headaches, a choking sensation, itching, and possibly nausea and vomiting.

An ulcer results when the lining of the stomach fails to provide adequate protection against the effect of digestive acids, and the acids in effect start to digest the stomach itself. This may be caused by an excess of stomach acid, insufficient production of protective mucus, or both.

Many factors affect the secretion of stomach acid. Stress and anxiety cause an increase in acid production, which is why ulcers are so closely related to stress levels. Certain drugs and supplements may also increase acid production. Taking aspirin or nonsteroidal anti-inflammatory drugs, especially over a long period of time, can increase stomach acidity and lead to ulcers. Steroids, such as those taken for arthritis, and even vitamin C supplements can contribute to stomach ulcers. Heavy smokers are more prone to developing ulcers, and have greater trouble getting ulcers to heal.

Although ulcers have long been known to be closely related to stress, recent evidence has also implicated a common type of bacteria, *Helicobacter pylori*. This organism is almost always found in persons who have ulcers and is seldom found in persons who do not. Further, eradication of these bacteria often results in healing of the ulcers. *H. pylori* may also be a risk factor for stomach cancer. The presence of *H. pylori* can be documented by direct biopsy of the stomach lining, by a blood test, or by a breath test.

STOMACH ACID SELF-TEST

If you suffer from stomach pain, you can determine whether the problem is caused by excess stomach acid with this simple test. When you have the pain, take a tablespoon of apple cider vinegar or lemon juice. If this makes the pain go away, you most likely have too little stomach acid, not too much. If it makes your symptoms worse, then you may have an overly acidic stomach. The suggestions in this section should help to correct the problem.

NUTRIENTS

SUPPLEMENT	SUGGESTED DOSAGE	COMMENTS
Important		
Acid-Ease from Prevail	As directed on label.	Balances acidity in the body, reducing symptoms. For some people, may be able to replace ulcer medications such as ranitidine (Zantac).
Pectin	As directed on label.	Helps relieve duodenal ulcers by creating a soothing protective coating in the intestines.

L-Glutamine	500 mg daily, on an empty stomach. Take with water or juice. Do not take with milk. Take with 50 mg vitamin B$_6$ and 100 mg vitamin C for better absorption.	Important in the healing of peptic ulcers. See AMINO ACIDS in Part One.
Vitamin E	400–800 IU daily.	A potent antioxidant that aids in reducing stomach acid and in relieving pain. Helps promote healing.

Helpful

Aloe vera juice		See under Herbs, below.
Kyo-Dophilus from Wakunaga	2–3 capsules, 1–3 times daily.	Human-cultured flora for the small intestine that improves assimilation of nutrients.
Bromelain	250 mg 3 times daily.	An enzyme from papaya that improves digestion and relieves symptoms. Chewable papaya tablets are also good.
Curcumin	250–500 mg 2–3 times daily, between meals.	Promotes healing.
Essential fatty acids (MaxEPA, primrose oil, and salmon oil are good sources)	As directed on label.	Protects the stomach and intestinal tract from ulcers.
Iron	As directed by physician. Take with 100 mg buffered or esterified vitamin C for better absorption.	Helps prevent anemia, which may occur with bleeding ulcers. Use ferrous chelate or ferrous fumarate form. Caution: Do not take iron unless anemia is diagnosed.
or Floradix Iron + Herbs from Salus Haus	As directed on label.	A nontoxic form of iron from food sources.
Licorice		See under Herbs, below.
Multivitamin and mineral complex	As directed on label.	To provide a balance of essential nutrients.
Proteolytic enzymes or Infla-Zyme Forte from American Biologics or Wobenzym N from Marlyn Nutraceuticals	As directed on label. Take between meals. As directed on label. As directed on label.	Works on undigested food remaining in the colon, and helps reduce inflammation. Caution: Do not use a formula containing HCl.
Pycnogenol or grape seed extract	As directed on label. As directed on label.	Powerful free radical scavengers that also act as anti-inflammatories and strengthen tissues.
Vitamin A emulsion or capsules	100,000 IU daily for 1 month; then 50,000 IU daily for 1 month; then 25,000 IU daily; then reduce to 10,000 IU daily. 25,000 IU daily. If you are pregnant, do not exceed 10,000 IU daily.	Needed for healing. Protects the mucous membranes of the stomach and intestines.
Vitamin B complex plus extra vitamin B$_6$ (pyridoxine)	50 mg 3 times daily. Do not exceed a total of 25 mg vitamin B$_3$ (niacin) daily from all sources. 50 mg 3 times daily.	Needed for proper digestion. A sublingual type is best. Needed for enzyme production and wound healing.
Vitamin C	3,000 mg daily.	Promotes wound healing and protects against infection. Use a buffered or esterified form.
Vitamin K	100 mcg daily.	Needed for healing and to prevent bleeding; promotes nutrient absorption and has a neutralizing effect on the intestinal tract. Deficiency is common in those with digestive disorders.
Zinc	50–80 mg daily. Do not exceed a total of 100 mg daily from all supplements.	Promotes healing. Use zinc gluconate lozenges or OptiZinc for best absorption.

HERBS

❑ Alfalfa is a good source of vitamin K.

❑ Aloe vera aids in pain relief and speeds healing. Take 4 ounces of aloe vera juice or gel daily. Be sure to buy a food-grade product such as George's Aloe Vera Juice from Warren Laboratories.

❑ Cat's claw is cleansing and healing to the digestive tract. Cat's Claw Defense Complex from Source Naturals is a combination of cat's claw and other herbs, plus antioxidant nutrients such as beta-carotene, N-acetylcysteine, vitamin C, and zinc.

Caution: Do not use cat's claw during pregnancy.

❑ Licorice promotes healing of gastric and duodenal ulcers. Take 750 to 1,500 milligrams of deglycyrrhizinated licorice two to three times daily, between meals, for eight to sixteen weeks.

Caution: Do not substitute ordinary licorice root for the deglycyrrhizinated variety. Ordinary licorice can elevate blood pressure if used on a daily basis for more than seven days in a row, and should be avoided completely by persons with high blood pressure. Deglycyrrhizinated licorice has had a component known as glycyrrhizinic acid removed, which should eliminate this side effect.

❑ Marshmallow root and slippery elm soothe irritated mucous membranes.

❑ Other beneficial herbs include bayberry, catnip, chamomile, goldenseal, hops, myrrh, passionflower, sage, and valerian. All of these can be taken in tea form.

Caution: Do not use chamomile on an ongoing basis, as ragweed allergy may result. Avoid it completely if you are allergic to ragweed. Do not take goldenseal on a daily basis for more than one week at a time, as it may disturb normal intestinal flora. Do not use it during pregnancy, and use it with caution if you are allergic to ragweed. Do not use sage if you suffer from any type of seizure disorder.

RECOMMENDATIONS

❑ Eat plenty of dark green leafy vegetables. These contain vitamin K, which is needed for healing and is likely to be deficient in people with digestive problems.

❑ Do not consume coffee (even decaffeinated) or alcoholic beverages.

❑ Drink freshly made cabbage juice daily. Drink it immediately after juicing. *See* JUICING in Part Three.

❑ If symptoms are severe, eat soft foods such as avocados, bananas, potatoes, squash, and yams. Put vegetables through a blender or food mill. Eat vegetables like broccoli and carrots occasionally—well steamed.

❑ Eat frequent small meals; include well-cooked millet, cooked white rice, raw goat's milk, and soured milk products such as yogurt, cottage cheese, and kefir.

❑ Drink barley, wheat, and alfalfa juice. They contain chlorophyll, making them potent anti-ulcer treatments.

❑ If you have a bleeding ulcer, consume organic baby foods and add nonirritating fiber such as guar gum and/or psyllium seed. These foods are easy to digest and nutritious, and they contain no chemicals.

❑ For rapid relief of pain, drink a large glass of water. This dilutes the stomach acids and flushes them out through the stomach and duodenum.

❑ Avoid fried foods, tea, caffeine, salt, chocolate, strong spices, animal fats of any kind, and carbonated drinks. Instead of drinking soda, sip distilled water with a bit of lemon juice added.

❑ Do not drink cow's milk. Even though it neutralizes existing stomach acid, the calcium and protein it contains actually stimulate the production of more acid. Almond milk is a good substitute.

❑ Allow teas and other hot beverages to cool before drinking them. Otherwise, they may trigger gastric discomfort.

❑ Keep the colon clean. Make sure the bowels move daily, and take cleansing enemas periodically. *See* COLON CLEANSING and ENEMAS in Part Three.

❑ Do not smoke. Smoking can delay or even prevent healing, and makes relapse more likely.

❑ Avoid painkillers such as aspirin. Aspirin is present in many over-the-counter remedies; read labels carefully. Also avoid ibuprofen (in Advil, Nuprin, and other products).

❑ Try to avoid stressful situations. Learn stress management techniques (*see* STRESS in Part Two). Music therapy may be helpful (*see* MUSIC AND SOUND THERAPY in Part Three).

CONSIDERATIONS

❑ While prescribed and over-the-counter drugs may relieve the symptoms of ulcers, they do not get to the root of the problem, which is damaged tissue. They offer short-term relief by temporarily decreasing stomach acid. In the long run, they may make the problem worse because they create the illusion that the ulcer has been cured. They also disrupt the normal digestive processes and alter the structure and functioning of the tissues that line the digestive tract.

❑ With treatment, most peptic ulcers heal, but it may take eight weeks or longer for healing to be complete.

❑ Antacids are often recommended for people with ulcers. If you must take antacids, avoid products containing aluminum, which has been linked to Alzheimer's disease (*see* ALZHEIMER'S DISEASE in Part Two).

❑ Persons who take cimetidine (Tagamet) or ranitidine (Zantac) for ulcers should be cautious about ingesting alcohol. These drugs magnify the effects of alcohol on the brain.

❑ A simple procedure using Kool-Aid to test for the presence of stomach ulcers has been developed by the Cabrini Medical Center in New York City. The person being tested is given two glasses of Kool-Aid made with extra sugar. After a short period, he or she takes a urine test. In people with ulcers, the sugar leaks across the stomach wall and shows up in the urine as undigested sugar. If there is no ulcer, the sugar is broken down normally by the body.

❑ Researchers in Europe have found that a dual-drug treatment approach using the antibiotic clarithromycin (Biaxin) and the ulcer medication omeprazole (Prilosec) was successful in eliminating *H. pylori* in 83 percent of ulcer patients studied, and prevented the recurrence of ulcers in 96 percent of those individuals.

❑ Many experts believe that food allergies are a prime cause of ulcers. *See* ALLERGIES in Part Two and follow the self-test program to identify possible problem foods.

Periodontal Disease

Periodontal disease is second only to the common cold as the most prevalent infectious ailment in the United States. It is the major cause of adult tooth loss. The rate of periodontal disease increases with age, ranging from 15 percent at age ten to more than 50 percent at age fifty.

Periodontal means "located around a tooth." *Periodontal disease* therefore can refer to any disorder of the gums or other supporting structures of the teeth. *Gingivitis* (inflammation of the gums) is the early stage of periodontal disease. It is caused by plaque—sticky deposits of bacteria, mucus, and food particles—that adheres to the teeth. The accumulation of plaque causes the gums to become infected and swollen. As the gums swell, pockets form between the gums and the teeth that act as a trap for still more plaque. Other factors that contribute to the development of gingivitis include breathing through the mouth, badly fitting fillings and prostheses that irritate surrounding gum tissue, and a diet consisting of too many soft foods that rob the teeth and gums of much needed "exercise." The gums become red, soft, and shiny, and they bleed easily. In some cases, there is pain, but gingivitis can also be essentially painless.

If left untreated, gingivitis can lead to a condition called *pyorrhea* or *periodontitis*. This is an advanced stage of periodontal disease in which the bone supporting the teeth begins to erode as a result of the infection. Abscesses are common. Pyorrhea causes halitosis, with bleeding and often painful gums. Poor nutrition, improper brushing, wrong foods, sugar consumption, chronic illness, glandular disorders, blood disease, smoking, drugs, and excessive alcohol consumption make an individual more likely to develop pyorrhea. It is often related to a deficiency of vitamin C, bioflavonoids, calcium, folic acid, or niacin. Smokers are more susceptible than nonsmokers to periodontitis and tooth loss. Periodontal disease can be made worse by missing teeth, food impaction, malocclusion, tongue-thrusting, tooth-grinding, and toothbrush trauma.

Stomatitis is inflammation of the oral tissues, and may affect the lips, palate, and insides of the cheeks. It often occurs as part of another disease. Stomatitis produces swollen gums that bleed easily. Sores may develop in the mouth and eventually become blisterlike lesions that can affect the gums. Two common types of stomatitis are *acute herpetic stomatitis* (better known as oral herpes) and *aphthous stomatitis* (canker sores).

Problems in the mouth often are reflections of deficiencies or underlying disorders in the body. Bleeding gums may signal a vitamin C deficiency; dryness and cracking at the corners of the mouth may indicate a deficiency of vitamin B_2 (riboflavin). Both conditions may also signal a generalized nutritional deficiency. Dry or cracked lips can be the result of an allergic reaction. Raw, red mouth tissue may be a sign of stress; a smooth, reddish tongue can indicate anemia or poor diet. Sores under the tongue can be an early warning sign of mouth cancer. Regular dental checkups can help detect these conditions early.

NUTRIENTS

SUPPLEMENT	SUGGESTED DOSAGE	COMMENTS
Essential		
Coenzyme Q₁₀	100 mg daily.	Increases tissue oxygenation.
Goldenseal		*See under* Herbs, below.
Vitamin C with bioflavonoids	4,000–10,000 mg daily, in divided doses throughout the day.	Promotes healing, especially of bleeding gums. Bioflavonoids retard plaque growth.
Very Important		
Bone Support from Synergy Plus	As directed on label.	Contains calcium, magnesium, phosphorus, zinc, and other nutrients that are easily absorbed by the body to rebuild bone.
or calcium and	1,500 mg daily.	Helps prevent bone loss around the gums.
magnesium	750 mg daily.	Works with calcium. Use a chelate form.
Vitamin A	25,000 IU daily for 1 month, then reduce to 10,000 IU daily. If you are pregnant, do not exceed 10,000 IU daily.	Needed for healing of gum tissue. Emulsion form is recommended for easier assimilation and greater safety at high doses.
plus natural beta-carotene or carotenoid complex (Betatene)	As directed on label.	An antioxidant used by the body to manufacture vitamin A as needed.
Vitamin E	Start with 400 IU daily and increase slowly to 1,000 IU daily. Also open a capsule and rub the oil on the gums 2–3 times daily.	Needed for healing of gum tissue.
plus selenium (E•SEL from Carlson Labs)	200 mcg daily.	A powerful antioxidant that works with vitamin E to ward off cancer.
Important		
Grape seed extract	As directed on label.	A powerful antioxidant and anti-inflammatory.
Proteolytic enzymes with pancreatin	As directed on label. Take between meals and at bedtime.	Aids in keeping down inflammation and aids proper digestion.
Vitamin B complex	50 mg 3 times daily, with meals.	Needed for proper digestion and healthy mouth tissues.
Zinc	50–80 mg daily. Do not exceed a total of 100 mg daily from all supplements.	Enhances immune function. Needed to prevent infection and promote healing. Use zinc gluconate lozenges or OptiZinc for best absorption.

HERBS

❑ Applying aloe vera gel directly to inflamed gums eases discomfort and soothes the tissues.

❑ Clove oil is good for temporary relief of tooth and/or gum pain. Simply rub a drop or two of clove oil on the affected area. If the oil is too strong in its pure form, it can be diluted with a drop or two of olive oil.

❑ Echinacea, hawthorn berries, myrrh gum, and rose hips help to keep down inflammation and enhance immune function. You can apply these herbs directly to the inflamed areas as a poultice or drink them in tea form.

❑ Goldenseal destroys the bacteria that cause periodontal disease. Place a dropperful of alcohol-free goldenseal extract in your mouth, swish it around for three minutes, then swallow. For inflamed gums, place a dropperful of alcohol-free goldenseal extract on a piece of gauze or pure cotton and place this on the inflamed area. Do this immediately whenever mouth sores or inflammation starts, and you will be amazed at the results. In severe cases it may take three to five nights for sores to heal.

Caution: Do not take goldenseal internally on a daily basis for more than one week at a time, as it may disturb normal intestinal flora. Do not use it during pregnancy, and use it with caution if you are allergic to ragweed.

RECOMMENDATIONS

❑ Eat a varied diet of fresh fruits, green leafy vegetables, meat, and whole grains to provide the teeth and gums with needed exercise and supply the body with the vitamins and minerals that are essential for dental health. Although all vitamins and minerals are essential for the proper formation and continued health of the teeth, adequate vitamin C intake is particularly important for the prevention of gingivitis and pyorrhea. Vitamin A seems to control the development and general health of the gums; a lack of this vitamin often results in gum infection. Vitamin A is also necessary for healthy tooth development in children. Minerals important for healthy teeth include sodium, potassium, calcium, phosphorus, iron, and magnesium.

❑ Eat plenty of high-fiber foods, such as whole grains, vegetables, and legumes.

❑ Avoid sugar and all refined carbohydrates. Sugar causes plaque buildup and inhibits the ability of white blood cells to fight off bacteria.

❑ Brush your teeth with goldenseal powder every day for at least one month. After one month, change brands of toothpaste. Don't stay with the same brand; some brands may irritate the gums.

❑ Change toothbrushes every month to keep the disease in check, and keep your toothbrush clean between uses. Bacteria live on toothbrushes.

❑ Floss your teeth daily. Use a product called Stim-U-Dent (available in drugstores) between meals to clean and stimulate the gums with a massaging motion. Do this faithfully every day.

❑ Try using a dental rinse called Plax to help loosen plaque. Unlike mouthwashes, this is designed to be used before brushing. Listerine also helps to remove plaque.

❑ Use a *very* soft natural-bristle toothbrush. Be sure to brush your gums and tongue as well as your teeth. The most effective way to get under the gum line is to tilt the toothbrush so that the bristles are at a 45-degree angle to the gum, and brush in a forward and backward motion using short strokes across the gums to remove bacteria.

❑ If inflammation is present, run very hot water over the toothbrush to soften it before brushing, and be gentle until healing is complete.

❑ Open a capsule of vitamin E and rub the oil on inflamed gums. This is very healing and helps to alleviate soreness.

❑ For relief of toothache pain until you can get to your dentist, apply ice to the gums. Clove oil can also be helpful (*see under* Herbs, above).

❑ Avoid taking antibiotics. The mouth is the hardest place for them to work, and they destroy needed friendly bacteria in the colon. Try goldenseal first; it works faster and has no side effects (*see under* Herbs, above).

❑ In addition to the products described above, we recommend the following tooth and gum products. Most of these can be bought at health food stores.

• *Nature de France (Pierre Cattier).* Contains a clay base for healing.

• *Nature's Gate.* Contains baking soda and sea salt, which is effective against plaque and gum disease. Also contains vitamin C.

• *Peelu.* Contains a natural tooth whitener derived from the small peelu tree, native to the Middle East and Asia. People have chewed its branches for centuries to keep their teeth white. Also contains natural flavor, fruit pectin, sodium lauryl sulfate (from coconut oil), and vegetable glycerine.

• *Tom's Natural Toothpaste.* Contains a natural calcium base. Features myrrh (an astringent herb) and propolis.

• *Weleda Salt Toothpaste.* Contains baking soda and salt formulation with medicinal herbs and silica.

• *Vicco Pure Herbal Toothpaste.* Contains extracts from plants, bark, roots, and flowers used in Ayurvedic medicine.

❑ Be sure your dentist is taking the proper steps to avoid transmitting disease. The dentist's office and waiting room should be clean. Dentists, hygienists, and dental assistants should wash their hands and change gloves between patients. Every reusable instrument should be sterilized between patients, and large equipment and all surfaces in the treatment room should be cleaned and disinfected periodically. If you have questions about your dentist's procedures, do not hesitate to ask.

CONSIDERATIONS

❑ Severe cases of periodontal disease may necessitate surgery to remove the infected tissue from the gum and reshape the bone.

❑ Certain illnesses, such as diabetes and several kinds of blood disorders, create a higher risk for developing gum disease.

❑ A simple blood test can detect gum disease up to eight months before symptoms appear, according to Dr. Jeffrey Ebersole, associate professor of periodontics at the University of Texas Health Science Center. A dentist can draw a drop of blood from a finger and have it analyzed for the bacteria that cause gum disease.

❑ Regular intimate contact with an infected person can transmit the bacteria that cause periodontal disease.

❑ Some people appear to be more susceptible than others to the bacteria that cause gum disease because of a genetic predisposition.

❑ Dry mouth, a condition in which there is not enough saliva in the mouth, can promote tooth decay and periodontal disease. Saliva is essential for ridding the mouth of plaque, sugar, and debris. Dry mouth problems increase with age; more than half of people over the age of fifty-five are affected by it. It can also be caused by alcohol consumption or by prescription or over-the-counter drugs, especially those for high blood pressure, depression, colds, and allergies. Diabetes is also associated with dry mouth. The best treatment for dry mouth is to draw more moisture from the salivary glands by chewing carrots, celery, or gum; sipping liquids; chewing ice chips; or breathing through the nose.

❑ Dental implants look more natural than dentures, and many people are opting for them. Unfortunately, improperly inserted dental implants can cause or exacerbate periodontal disease. If you are interested in implants, consult an implant specialist.

❑ Air abrasion technology, a dental technique that painlessly removes tooth decay without drilling, allows dentists to make smaller fillings and save more of the natural tooth. The new technique, considered to be a major breakthrough, does not necessitate numbing drugs or anesthesia.

❑ Regular dental checkups are important in detecting oral cancer, a disease that strikes 30,000 Americans each year. If oral cancer is caught early, nine out of ten people survive.

❑ One advantage (perhaps the only one) to having allergies is that people who suffer from allergies are less likely to lose teeth to periodontal disease. The reason apparently is that the allergy sufferer's overactive imune system is better at fighting off the bacteria that cause periodontal disease.

❑ There is a tablet you can purchase at most drugstores that shows areas your toothbrush missed. Chew a tablet after brushing, then brush until the color is gone.

❑ Electric toothbrushes, such as the Braun or Oral B systems, help to remove plaque.

❑ An automatic toothbrush sanitizer has been proven effective in keeping toothbrushes free of bacteria. The device automatically turns on every half-hour for two minutes to sanitize the bristles twenty-four hours a day. As an alternative, you can store your toothbrush in hydrogen peroxide or grapefruit seed extract to kill germs (if using hydrogen peroxide, rinse it well before brushing).

❑ *See also* CANKER SORES and HERPESVIRUS INFECTION, both in Part Two.

❑ *See also Bleeding Gums under* PREGNANCY-RELATED PROBLEMS in Part Two.

Phlebitis

See THROMBOPHLEBITIS.

Photophobia

See under EYE PROBLEMS.

Pinkeye

See under EYE PROBLEMS.

PMS

See PREMENSTRUAL SYNDROME.

Pneumonia

Pneumonia is a serious infection of the lungs that can be caused by any of a number of different infectious agents, including viruses, bacteria, fungi, protozoa, and mycoplasma. The infection causes tiny air sacs in the lung area to become inflamed and filled with mucus and pus. Although symptoms can vary in intensity, they usually include fever, chills, cough, bloody sputum, muscle aches, fatigue, sore throat, enlarged lymph glands in the neck, cyanosis (a bluish cast to the skin and nails), pain in the chest, and rapid, difficult respiration.

Pneumonia is typically preceded by an upper respiratory infection such as a cold, influenza, or measles. Factors that increase the risk of pneumonia include being either under one year or over sixty years of age, a weakened immune system, cardiovascular disease, diabetes, HIV infection, seizure or stroke, aspiration under anesthesia, alcoholism, smoking, kidney failure, sickle cell disease, malnutrition, foreign bodies in the respiratory passages, exposure to chemical irritants, and even allergies. A positive diagnosis of the disease can be made only with a chest x-ray.

Bacterial pneumonia is very dangerous and comes on suddenly, usually as a complication of some other illness. Symptoms usually include shaking, chills, and a high temperature. The cough is dry at first. Then a rust-colored sputum is produced, and breathing becomes rapid and labored. Chest pain that worsens upon inhalation, abdominal pain, and fatigue are also common. This type of pneumonia is unlikely to spread from one person to another.

Viral pneumonia is more variable in course and severity. It can come on suddenly or gradually, and symptoms can be mild, severe, or anywhere in between. It is less serious than bacterial pneumonia, but if not cared for properly, a second, bacterial infection can set in.

Fungal pneumonia is much less common than either the bacterial or viral variety, and is often associated with a weakened or suppressed immune system. People with HIV, AIDS, or certain types of cancer, or who are taking immunosuppressive drugs following organ transplantation, are most likely to be affected.

About 2 million cases of pneumonia are diagnosed in the United States every year, and 40,000 to 70,000 people die of the disease, making it the sixth leading cause of death in this country. No matter what the cause, pneumonia usually leaves the sufferer with weakness that persists for four to eight weeks after the acute phase of the infection has resolved.

Unless otherwise specified, the dosages recommended here are for adults. For a child between the ages of twelve and seventeen, reduce the dose to three-quarters the recommended amount. For a child between six and twelve, use one-half the recommended dose, and for a child under the age of six, use one-quarter the recommended amount.

NUTRIENTS

SUPPLEMENT	SUGGESTED DOSAGE	COMMENTS
Essential		
Betatene	15,000 IU daily.	A mixture of beta-carotene and other carotenoids to protect the lungs from free radical damage.
Colloidal silver	As directed on label.	Reduces inflammation and promotes healing of lesions in lung tissue.
Vitamin A	Up to 100,000 IU daily.	Enhances immunity and promotes repair of lung tissue. Use emulsion form for easier assimilation and greater safety at high doses. Do not take such high doses in capsule form.
Vitamin C plus	5,000–20,000 mg daily, in divided doses. *See* ASCORBIC ACID FLUSH in Part Three.	Very important for immune response and for reducing inflammation.
bioflavonoids	100 mg twice daily.	Needed to activate vitamin C.
Very Important		
Digesta-Lac from Natren	As directed on label. Take on an empty stomach.	For replacement of "friendly" bacteria.
L-Carnitine plus L-cysteine plus glutathione	As directed on label, on an empty stomach. Take with water or juice. Do not take with milk. Take with 50 mg vitamin B$_6$ and 100 mg vitamin C for better absorption.	To protect the lungs from free radical damage and break down mucus in the respiratory tract.
Free-form amino acid complex	As directed on label.	To supply protein, important in tissue repair.
Pycnogenol and/or grape seed extract	As directed on label. As directed on label.	Boosts the immune system and protects lung tissue; reduces the frequency and severity of colds and flu.
Vitamin B complex	100 mg 3 times daily.	Needed for normal digestion, production of antibodies and formation of red blood cells, and for healthy mucous membranes. Use a sublingual form.
Important		
Raw thymus and raw lung glandulars	500 mg each twice daily.	Stimulates immune response and promotes healing of lung tissue. *See* GLANDULAR THERAPY in Part Three.
Vitamin E emulsion or capsules	1,500 IU daily. 400 IU twice daily, before meals.	A potent antioxidant that protects the lung tissues and enhances oxygen utilization. Emulsion form is recommended.
Zinc	80 mg daily. Do not exceed a total of 100 mg daily from all supplements.	Needed for tissue repair and immune function. Zinc gluconate lozenges are very effective.
Helpful		
Body Language Super Antioxidant from Oxyfresh	As directed on label.	To protect against free radical damage and environmental stresses and pollutants.
Coenzyme Q$_{10}$	100 mg daily.	Enhances cellular oxygen utilization.
Essential fatty acids (flaxseed oil, primrose oil, salmon oil, and Ultimate Oil from Nature's Secret are good sources)	As directed on label.	Needed to build new lung tissue and to reduce inflammation. Improves stamina, speeds recovery, and boosts immunity.
Garlic (Kyolic)	As directed on label.	Protects against respiratory infections. Destroys unwanted bacteria in the body.
Infla-Zyme Forte from American Biologics	As directed on label 4 times daily, between meals and at bedtime.	Helps keep the infection in check.
Maitake or shiitake or reishi	As directed on label. As directed on label. As directed on label.	Helps to build immunity and fight infection.
Melatonin	1.5–5 mg daily, taken 2 hours or less before bedtime.	To improve sleep. This is a natural hormone produced by the pineal gland that controls the body's sleep/wake cycle.
Multivitamin and mineral complex	As directed on label.	To maintain a balance of all necessary nutrients in the body.
Proteolytic enzymes	As directed on label 3 times daily, on an empty stomach.	Aids in absorption of nutrients and reduces inflammation.

HERBS

☐ ClearLungs from Natural Alternatives is an herbal combination that helps provide relief from shortness of breath, tightness in the chest, and wheezing due to bronchial congestion. It is available in two formulas: one with ephedra and the other without. They appear to be equally effective.

☐ Echinacea enhances immunity.

☐ Ginger is an effective antimicrobial agent and is helpful for fever.

☐ Goldenseal and licorice root are natural antibiotics.
Caution: Do not take goldenseal internally on a daily basis for more than one week at a time, do not use it during pregnancy, and use it with caution if you are allergic to ragweed. Do not use licorice on a daily basis for more than seven days in a row, and avoid it completely if you have high blood pressure.

RECOMMENDATIONS

☐ See your health care provider if you suspect pneumonia. This is a potentially dangerous disease.

☐ Eat a diet consisting of raw fruits and vegetables.

☐ Take a protein supplement from a vegetable source, such as a free-form amino acid complex.

❑ Drink plenty of fresh juices. Liquids help to thin the lung secretions. Fast on pure juices, fresh lemon juice, and distilled water. *See* FASTING and JUICING, both in Part Three.

❑ Include "green drinks" in the diet or take chlorophyll in tablet form. Earthsource Greens & More from Solgar is a good product that contains immune-building shiitake, reishi, and maitake mushrooms; chlorophyll-rich organic grasses and sea algae; and phytonutrients.

❑ If you are taking antibiotics, take acidophilus in capsule or liquid form three times each day. Do not take the acidophilus at the same time as the antibiotics, however.

❑ Exclude from the diet dairy products, sugar, white flour products, coffee, and all tea except herbal teas.

❑ Do not smoke.

❑ Use a cool mist from a humidifier or vaporizer to help ease breathing.

❑ Place a heating pad or a hot water bottle on your chest to relieve pain.

❑ Consider using a device called Air Supply from Wein Products. This is a personal air purifier that is worn around the neck. It kills and deactivates airborne viruses, bacteria, molds, and spores.

❑ To avoid passing the infection along to others, dispose of secretions properly. Sneeze and/or cough into disposable tissues. Flush used tissues to discard them.

CONSIDERATIONS

❑ Vitamin A is necessary for maintaining the health of the lining of the respiratory passages. A deficiency of this vitamin increases susceptibility to respiratory infections, which in turn can lead to pneumonia.

❑ Pneumococcal vaccine provides protection against more than twenty different strains of microorganisms that can cause pneumonia. It is recommended for anyone without a spleen, anyone with a chronic disease (especially diseases that affect the lungs), and everyone over the age of sixty-five.

❑ The use of antibiotics for minor infections such as colds may lead to the development of antibiotic-resistant bacteria in the upper airway, which can cause pneumonia.

❑ *See also* INFLUENZA and COMMON COLD, both in Part Two.

Poison Ivy/Poison Oak/ Poison Sumac

Poison ivy, poison oak, and poison sumac are probably the most common allergenic plants in the United States. These plants grow in every state except Alaska, and are common along roadsides, in forests and pastures, and along streams—even, in the case of poison ivy, in suburban back yards.

Poison ivy and poison oak are members of the same botanical family. Poison ivy is more prevalent east of the Rocky Mountains; poison oak is more common to the west and southwest. Poison sumac is common in southern swamps and northern wetlands. All three plants produce similar symptoms, and as a result all three are often referred to simply as poison ivy.

It is estimated that 65 percent of Americans are sensitive to these plants, and about 2 million people each year have a reaction from contact with them. Sensitivity to poison ivy is acquired and is at its peak during childhood. Most susceptible are people who are sensitive to sunlight. The irritating substance in poison ivy is urushiol, a substance present in the oily sap in the leaves, flowers, fruit, stem, bark, and roots. Urushiol is one of the most potent toxins on earth; less than 1 ounce would be enough to affect every living person. The blisters, swelling, and itching are caused by an immune system response to this poisonous sap. The plant is poisonous even long after it has dried out, but it is particularly irritating in the spring and early summer, when it is full of sap. Every part of these plants is toxic.

The first symptom of poison ivy is a burning and itching sensation. This is followed by the development of a red, intensely itchy rash, often accompanied by swelling, oozing, and crusting blisters. A mild case may involve only a few small blisters, while a severe case may cause many large blisters, acute inflammation, fever, and/or inflammation affecting the face or genitals. Symptoms can appear anywhere from a few hours to seven days after contact, and tend to be at their worst between the fourth and seventh days. The rash often forms a linear pattern. Exposed parts of the body, such as the hands, arms, and face, are the areas most likely to be affected. Scratching can then spread the inflammation to other parts of the body. Itching, redness, and swelling begin to heal by the second day after the appearance of the rash, and most people are completely healed within seven to fourteen days.

Direct contact with the plant is the most common means of contracting poison ivy, but the poisons can be conveyed to the skin in other ways. Some people have contracted poison ivy by petting an animal that has been in contact with it. It can also be transmitted by clothing or objects that have come in contact with the plant. People who are highly sensitive to poison ivy can develop a reaction if the plant is burned and they inhale the smoke. Severe cases of mouth poisoning have occurred in children who have eaten the plant's leaves or grayish berries.

Unless otherwise specified, the dosages recommended here are for adults. For a child between the ages of twelve and seventeen, reduce the dose to three-quarters the recommended amount. For a child between six and twelve, use one-half the recommended dose, and for a child under the age of six, use one-quarter the recommended amount.

NUTRIENTS

SUPPLEMENT	SUGGESTED DOSAGE	COMMENTS
Important		
Vitamin C	3,000–8,000 mg daily.	To prevent infection and spreading of the rash. A natural antihistamine that reduces swelling.
Helpful		
All-Purpose Bactericide Spray from Aerobic Life Industries	Apply topically as directed on label.	Destroys bacteria. Prevents spreading of the rash.
Calamine lotion	Apply topically as directed on label.	Contains calamine, phenol, and zinc oxide. Has drying properties for faster healing.
Natureworks Marigold Ointment from Abkit or aloe vera	Apply topically as directed on label.	To help relieve itching. *See under* Herbs, below.
Rhus toxicodendron or Poison Ivy/Oak Tablets from Hylands	As directed on label. As directed on label.	The classic homeopathic remedy for poison ivy. Relieves itching and promotes healing. A homeopathic combination remedy for poison ivy.
Shark cartilage (BeneFin)	1 gram per 15 lbs of body weight daily, divided into 3 doses.	Reduces inflammation.
Vitamin A	25,000 IU daily. If you are pregnant, do not exceed 10,000 IU daily.	Needed for healing of skin tissue. Also boosts the immune system.
Vitamin E oil or cream	Apply topically as directed on label. Apply topically as directed on label.	To aid in healing and prevent scarring.
Zinc	80 mg daily. Do not exceed a total of 100 mg daily from all supplements.	Needed for repair of skin tissues. Use zinc gluconate lozenges or OptiZinc for best absorption.

HERBS

❑ Aloe vera helps relieve burning and itching. Apply pure aloe vera gel as directed on the product label or as needed.

❑ A strong tea made of equal parts lime water and white oak bark is very good for poison ivy, poison oak, or poison sumac. Apply a compress wet with this solution. Replace the compress with a fresh one as often as it becomes dry.

❑ The following herbs can be used topically as remedies for poison ivy, poison oak, or poison sumac: black walnut extract, bloodroot, echinacea, goldenseal, and myrrh. Black walnut has antiseptic properties and helps to fight infection; bloodroot reduces swelling; echinacea promotes healing of skin wounds; goldenseal is good for skin inflammation; myrrh is a powerful antiseptic. Echinacea can also be taken internally to boost the immune system.

Caution: Do not use bloodroot during pregnancy. Use goldenseal with caution if you are allergic to ragweed.

RECOMMENDATIONS

❑ Treat a mild case of poison ivy with one or more of the following:

• Apply compresses made with very hot plain water for brief intervals.

• Apply compresses soaked in a diluted Burow's solution (use 1 pint to 15 pints of cool water). You can purchase Burow's solution at most drugstores.

• Soak the affected skin in cool water with colloidal oatmeal (Aveeno) added, available at most drugstores.

• For relief of itching, apply a paste made from water, cornstarch, baking soda, oatmeal, or Epsom salts. Use 1 teaspoon of water to 3 teaspoons of the dry ingredient.

• Apply aloe vera juice, tofu, or watermelon rind to the area for cooling relief. Using 1 pint of buttermilk with 1 tablespoon of sea salt added may be helpful.

• Use an herbal preparation suggested under Herbs, above.

❑ For a severe case of poison ivy, consult a physician. Symptoms that warrant medical attention include an extensive rash that covers more than half of the body; extreme swelling and redness; and fever. You should also consult your health care provider if poison ivy occurs near the eyes, mouth, or genitals.

❑ Stay cool. Sweating and heat can make itching worse.

CONSIDERATIONS

❑ Oral prednisone is sometimes prescribed to relieve itching and reduce swelling. However, this treatment should be reserved only for very severe cases involving fever, difficulty urinating, dangerous facial or genital swelling, or other symptoms of acute illness. Oral steroids are extremely powerful drugs and can cause serious side effects.

❑ Topical steroids are not helpful for poison ivy and should be avoided.

❑ The toxin urushiol does not affect dogs or cats, but they can bring the irritating substance home on their fur and pass it to you. If you suspect your pet may have walked through poison ivy or poison oak, wash the animal thoroughly (wear rubber gloves and protective clothing).

❑ Prevention is better than treatment when it comes to poison ivy, poison oak, and poison sumac:

• Lightweight fabrics do not provide adequate protection against poison ivy or oak, because the sap can easily penetrate them. Wear gloves and heavier clothing if you may be exposed to the plant.

• Everyone, even children, should learn to recognize, and avoid, these harmful plants. Poison ivy usually grows as a vine, but it can also take the form of a shrub, growing anywhere from two to seven feet high. Its leaves always grow in clusters of three, one at the end of the stalk, the other two opposite each other. Poison oak grows as a shrub exclusively, and its leaves are lobed, like oak leaves. Like those of poison ivy, they grow in threes. Poison sumac grows as a shrub or small tree that has multiple leaflets growing on both sides of a stem. The number of leaflets may range from seven to thirteen, but it is always an odd number.

• Appropriate protective clothing should be worn for activities that take you into forests or through thick underbrush—long pants, a long-sleeved shirt, shoes, socks, and gloves. These items should be washed after they are worn; if they come into contact with poison ivy, they are not safe to wear again until they have been laundered or dry-cleaned.

• If you know or suspect that you may have come in contact with poison ivy, remove all clothing and shoes, and *immediately* scrub your skin using brown or yellow laundry soap (such as Fels Naptha) and water or alcohol to remove the irritating oil. Lather several times and rinse in running water after each sudsing. This procedure is useless if not done within ten minutes; after that time, the oil will have penetrated the skin and cannot be washed off. Wash clothing, gear, or pack material in plenty of hot, soapy water, with chlorine bleach added, if possible. Stubborn cases of poison ivy that do not respond to proper treatment are often due to repeated contact with contaminated clothing.

Poisoning

There are literally thousands of substances, both natural and synthetic, that can cause poisoning. Many of these are present in everyday items and products, including drugs, cleaning products, pesticides, paints and varnishes, hobby and art supplies, batteries, cosmetics, and house plants. Some are poisonous only if ingested; others can cause problems if inhaled or absorbed through the skin or eyes.

Most cases of accidental poisoning involve young children, especially children under the age of five. Young children are very curious, and their preferred method of exploring often involves putting things in their mouths. However, there are also many cases of poisoning every year among elderly people and hospital patients (most commonly the result of overmedication or drug mix-ups), as well as adolescents, who may experiment with the ingestion of toxic substances, including recreational drugs. Other causes of poisoning include exposure to environmental pollutants and toxic substances used in the workplace. Toxins in food can also cause poisoning.

Poison Control Centers

The following are telephone numbers for local Poison Control Centers in the United States and Canada. It is a good idea to post the number of your local center near your telephone, especially if you have young children. If you can program your telephone for automatic dialing, you may wish to add the number to your phone's programming as well. Please note that all phone numbers are subject to change.

UNITED STATES

ALABAMA

205–939–9201
205–933–4050
800–292–6678 (AL only)

ALASKA

907–261–3193

ARIZONA

Statewide
800–362–0101 (AZ only)
Phoenix Area
602–253–3334
Tucson Area
602–626–6016

ARKANSAS

501–686–6161

CALIFORNIA

Davis Area
916–734–3692
800–342–9293 (No. CA only)
Fresno Area
209–445–1222
800–346–5922 (CA only)
Orange County Area
714–634–5988
800–544–4404 (So. CA only)
San Diego Area
619–543–6000
800–876–4766 (619 area code)
San Francisco/Bay Area
415–476–6600
San Jose/Santa Clara Valley
408–299–5112
800–662–9886 (CA only)

COLORADO

303–629–1123

CONNECTICUT

203–679–1000
800–343–2722 (CT only)

DELAWARE

302–655–3389

DISTRICT OF COLUMBIA

202–625–3333
202–784–4660 (TTY*)

FLORIDA

813–253–4444
800–282–3171 (FL only)

GEORGIA

404–589–4400
800–282–5846 (GA only)

HAWAII

808–941–4411

IDAHO

208–378–2707
800–632–8000

ILLINOIS

217–753–3330
800–543–2022 (IL only)
800–942–5969

INDIANA

317–929–2323
800–382–9097 (IN only)

IOWA

800–272–6477 (IA only)
800–362–2327 (IA only)

KANSAS

Topeka/Northern KS
913–354–6100
Wichita/Southern KS
316–263–9999

KENTUCKY

502–629–7275
800–722–5725 (KY only)

LOUISIANA

800–256–9822 (LA only)

MAINE

800–442–6305 (ME only)

MARYLAND

Statewide
410–528–7701
800–492–2414 (MD only)

D.C. Suburbs
202–625–3333
202–784–4660 (TTY*)

MASSACHUSETTS

617–232–2120
800–682–9211

MICHIGAN

Statewide
800–632–2727 (MI only)
800–356–3232 (TTY*)

Detroit Area
313–745–5711

MINNESOTA

Statewide
800–222–1222

Duluth/Northern MN
218–726–5466

Minneapolis/St. Paul Area
612–347–3141
612–337–7474 (TDD**)
612–221–2113

MISSISSIPPI

601–354–7660

MISSOURI

314–772–5200
800–366–8888

MONTANA

303–629–1123

NEBRASKA

Statewide
800–955–9119 (NE only)

Omaha Area
402–390–5555

NEVADA

702–732–4989

NEW HAMPSHIRE

603–650–5000
800–562–8236 (NH only)

NEW JERSEY

800–962–1253

NEW MEXICO

505–843–2551
800–432–6866 (NM only)

NEW YORK

Albany Area
800–336–6997

Binghamton/Southern Tier
800–252–5655

Buffalo/Western NY
716–878–7654
800–888–7655

Long Island
516–542–2323
516–542–2324
516–542–2325
516–542–3813

New York City
212–340–4494
212–POISONS
212–689–9014 (TDD**)

Nyack/Hudson Valley
914–353–1000

Syracuse/Central NY
315–476–4766

NORTH CAROLINA

Statewide
800–672–1697

Charlotte Area
704–355–4000

NORTH DAKOTA

800–732–2200 (ND only)

OHIO

Statewide
800–682–7625

Columbus/Central OH
614–228–1323
614–461–2012
614–228–2272 (TTY*)

Cincinnati Area
513–558–5111
800–872–5111 (OH only)

OKLAHOMA

800–522–4611 (OK only)

OREGON

503–494–8968
800–452–7165 (OR only)

PENNSYLVANIA

Hershey/Central PA
800–521–6110

Philadelphia/Eastern PA
215–386–2100

Pittsburgh/Western PA
412–681–6669

PUERTO RICO

809–754–8535

RHODE ISLAND

401–277–5727

SOUTH CAROLINA

803–777–1117

SOUTH DAKOTA

800–952–0123 (SD only)

TENNESSEE

Memphis/Western TN
901–528–6048

Nashville/Eastern TN
615–322–6435

TEXAS

214–590–5000
800–441–0040 (TX only)

UTAH

801–581–2151
800–456–7707 (UT only)

VERMONT

800–562–8236 (VT only)

VIRGINIA

Statewide
800–451–1428

Charlottesville/Blue Ridge
804–925–5543

D.C. Suburbs
202–625–3333
202–784–4660 (TTY*)

WASHINGTON

800–732–6985 (WA only)

WEST VIRGINIA

304–348–4211
800–642–3625 (WV only)

WISCONSIN

Madison/Southwestern and
Northern WI
608–262–3702

Milwaukee/Southeastern WI
414–255–2222

WYOMING

800–955–9119 (WY only)

CANADA

ALBERTA

403–670–1414

BRITISH COLUMBIA

604–682–5050

MANITOBA

204–787–2591

NEW BRUNSWICK

Fredericton
506–452–5400

St. John
506–648–6222

NEWFOUNDLAND

709–722–1110

NOVA SCOTIA

902–428–8161

ONTARIO

Provincewide
800–267–1373 (ON only)

Eastern Ontario
613–737–1100

PRINCE EDWARD ISLAND

902–428–8161

QUEBEC

800–463–5060 (QB only)

SASKATCHEWAN

306–359–4545

*TTY= teletype (for the hearing impaired)
**TDD= telecommunications device for the deaf

RECOMMENDATIONS

❑ If you suspect that you or another have been poisoned, call your local Poison Control Center and follow their directions. The appropriate measures to take depend on the toxin involved and the method of ingestion. The professionals who staff these centers will be able to tell you what to do.

❑ Keep the telephone number of your local Poison Control Center posted near your telephone (*see* Poison Control Centers on previous pages). This is particularly important if you have children. Also, keep a bottle of syrup of ipecac, available in drugstores, on hand at all times. However, *do not* use syrup of ipecac unless specifically directed to do so by a physician or your Poison Control Center.

❑ If you are directed to go to the nearest hospital emergency room, take the container of the suspected poison with you, if possible. This can help medical personnel to deal with the situation and save precious time.

CONSIDERATIONS

❑ When dealing with suspected poisoning, it is better to rely on the advice of Poison Control Center staff rather than the information on product packaging. Poison Control Centers keep up to date with the latest knowledge and practices; information provided by manufacturers may not be as current or reliable.

❑ *See also* ALUMINUM TOXICITY; ARSENIC POISONING; CADMIUM TOXICITY; CHEMICAL POISONING; COPPER TOXICITY; ENVIRONMENTAL TOXICITY; FOOD POISONING; LEAD POISONING; MERCURY TOXICITY; NICKEL TOXICITY.

Polyps

Polyps are benign (noncancerous) growths of various sizes that are found on stalklike structures growing from the epithelial lining of the large intestine, cervix, bladder, nose, and other structures. They are most common in the rectum and sigmoid colon, and usually occur in groups.

Most polyps of the colon and/or rectum cause no symptoms at all, and are discovered only during routine physical examinations that include examination of the colon, or during examination or treatment of other disorders. If they are very large, however, they may cause rectal bleeding, cramping, or abdominal pain. The relationship between polyps and cancer is not fully understood. Some physicians believe most colon cancers begin as polyps. However, most polyps probably do not turn into cancer. On the other hand, it is true that many people who have a cancerous growth in the colon also have multiple polyps surrounding that growth, and it does appear that the larger a polyp grows, the greater the chance that it will become malignant.

Familial polyposis is a hereditary disease in which large numbers of growths (100 or more), develop in the colon. If removed, they grow back. Rectal bleeding and a mucous drainage are common symptoms. This disorder is more closely linked to cancer than ordinary polyps are; unless it is treated, it virtually always leads to colon cancer.

Cervical polyps line the inside of the cervix, the passage from the vagina into the uterus. Symptoms indicative of cervical polyps include a heavy, watery, bloody discharge from the vagina. Bleeding may occur after sexual intercourse, between periods, and after menopause. The growth of cervical polyps may be caused by infection, injury to the cervix, or hormonal changes during pregnancy. Polyps are more common in women who have not had children. Women with diabetes also have a higher than normal chance of developing polyps. A pap smear may or may not detect cervical polyps. They rarely return once removed.

Bladder polyps produce blood in the urine. Unless they are removed, cancer of the bladder may follow.

Nasal polyps usually form in the back of the nose, near the openings into the sinuses. They too can bleed, and can interfere with normal breathing. People with hay fever and other nasal allergies are most prone to nasal polyps, as are people who overuse nose drops and nasal sprays.

Polyps on the vocal cords are caused by abuse (such as from repeated and prolonged episodes of screaming or, among singers especially, improper vocal technique), usually in the presence of an infection. People who smoke or have allergies are more susceptible. Vocal cord polyps usually cause painless hoarseness.

NUTRIENTS

SUPPLEMENT	SUGGESTED DOSAGE	COMMENTS
Essential		
Betatene	As directed on label.	A mixture of beta-carotene and other carotenoids to protect the epithelial linings (mucous membranes) of body cavities.
Multivitamin and mineral complex plus extra	As directed on label.	Provides a balance of necessary nutrients.
calcium and	1,000–1,500 mg daily.	Protects against colorectal polyps and colon cancer.
magnesium	750 mg daily.	Assists in the absorption of calcium.
Vitamin A	25,000 IU daily. If you are pregnant, do not exceed 10,000 IU daily.	Protects the membranous linings. Use emulsion form for easier assimilation.
Vitamin C	5,000–10,000 mg daily, in divided doses.	Can reduce the number of polyps, and may eliminate them altogether.
Very Important		
Digesta-Lac from Natren	As directed on label.	Replenishes "friendly" bacteria in the intestines.
Vitamin E	Start with 400 IU daily and increase slowly to 800 IU daily.	A potent antioxidant. Protects against the effects of lipid peroxidation; if deficiency occurs, cells are vulnerable to damage.

Important		
Aerobic Bulk Cleanse (ABC) from Aerobic Life Industries	As directed on label. Use with aloe vera juice.	Cleanses the colon, assisting in normal stool formation to aid in removing harmful toxins.

Helpful		
Coenzyme Q10	60 mg daily.	An important antioxidant. Increases cellular oxygen levels.
Concentrace trace mineral drops from Trace Minerals Research	As directed on label.	Normalizes electrolytes after bowel cleansing.
Garlic (Kyolic)	2 capsules 3 times daily, between meals.	Acts as a natural antibiotic and enhances immune function.
Homozon from Aerobic Life Industries	As directed on label.	Supplies oxygen to the intestines to cleanse the colon.
Superoxide dismutase (SOD) or	As directed on label.	An important antioxidant and free radical destroyer.
Cell Guard from Biotec Foods	As directed on label.	An antioxidant complex that contains SOD.

HERBS

❑ Aloe vera juice improves digestion and cleanses the digestive tract.

❑ Butcher's broom, cardamom, cayenne, cinnamon, *Garcinia cambogia*, ginger, green tea, and mustard seed are thermogenic herbs that improve digestion.

Caution: Do not use cinnamon in large quantities during pregnancy.

❑ Coloklysis-7 by PhysioLogics contains herbs and a blend of soluble and insoluble fiber to support healthy digestion.

RECOMMENDATIONS

❑ A high-fiber diet with no animal fats is important. Include in the diet apricots, broccoli, brown rice, cabbage, cantaloupe, carrots, cauliflower, garlic, oatmeal, onions, green peppers, sweet potatoes, sesame seeds, spinach, sunflower seeds, and whole grains. Fruits with edible seeds, such as figs, raspberries, strawberries, and even bananas, tend to contain lots of fiber. *See* CANCER in Part Two and follow the diet recommended there.

❑ Take some form of supplemental fiber daily. Barley, legumes, oat bran, psyllium husks (in Aerobic Bulk Cleanse), and rice bran are good sources of fiber.

Note: Always take supplemental fiber separately from other supplements and medications.

❑ Be sure to increase your water intake when increasing fiber consumption. If you do not, it may result in bloating, gas, pain, and constipation.

❑ Exclude from the diet fried foods, highly processed foods, caffeine, and alcohol. Do not use tobacco.

❑ Regular physical examinations are important, particularly after age forty. A digital rectal exam is easily performed in the physician's office and can quickly determine if there are any abnormalities along the colon wall.

❑ If you experience rectal bleeding, or if blood appears in the stool, consult your physician. A fecal occult blood test (FOBT) should be done to identify the source of the blood. Bleeding can be a symptom of polyps, but it also can be a sign of cancer.

CONSIDERATIONS

❑ The treatment of choice for most polyps, regardless of location, is surgical removal. In most cases this is a relatively minor procedure, often performed on an outpatient basis.

❑ Vocal cord polyps may be treated with humidification, speech therapy, and rest. Surgical removal of the polyps may be necessary.

❑ For familial polyposis, a surgical procedure called a colectomy may be necessary involving the removal of the entire colon. In some cases, the rectum is left in place and connected to the small intestine to allow for bowel evacuation. However, in most cases, polyps return in the rectum.

❑ Jerome J. DeCosse, M.D., Ph.D., and his colleagues at the University of Wisconsin's Department of Surgery and Pathology discovered that when vitamin C was added to the treatment, polyps were either reduced in number or completely eliminated in five out of eight people.

❑ Research has found that men with the highest consumption of saturated fat were twice as likely to develop potentially malignant polyps as men who limited their fat intake.

Pregnancy-Related Problems

Pregnancy is the time between conception and childbirth in which a fetus grows and matures for forty weeks (approximately nine months) inside the womb until it is ready to be born. There are many problems that can occur during a pregnancy. Many, like stretch marks and gas, are merely annoying. Others, such as miscarriage, are quite serious.

Most of the problems that occur during pregnancy are the result of hormonal changes within the body, nutritional deficiencies, or the shift in weight distribution caused by sudden weight gain. This entry addresses some of the most common pregnancy-related problems and offers natural remedies as well as helpful hints and suggestions for maintaining maximum health during pregnancy. For a healthy pregnancy and birth, it is necessary to consult and work with a qualified health care professional, be it a physician, nurse, nurse practitioner, or midwife.

Tests Performed During Pregnancy

There are many tests that can be performed during pregnancy to assess the health and development of the fetus. However, many of these tests involve an element of risk for both mother and child. Therefore, they should be done only when medically indicated, and not used routinely or for the mother's or the health care provider's convenience. If a test is suggested, be sure that you are fully aware of why it is needed and of any dangers that may be involved before deciding to have it done.

AMNIOCENTESIS

This medical procedure is performed during pregnancy to determine the health of the fetus. A local anesthetic is administered and then a long, hollow needle is inserted through the mother's abdomen into the uterus to remove amniotic fluid for cellular analysis. Although it has become fairly common, this procedure entails risks for both the pregnant woman and the fetus. Specifically, there is some chance of blood exchange between the mother and the fetus, infection of the amniotic fluid, peritonitis, the development of blood clots, placental hemorrhage, needle injury to the fetus, and premature labor. Therefore, great care must be taken in recommending, and then in performing, amniocentesis.

This test can determine the sex of the fetus. However, it definitely should *not* be performed only to find this out. This test should be performed only if you plan to terminate the pregnancy if an abnormality is found, or if knowledge of any problem is necessary for proper prenatal care.

CHORIONIC VILLUS SAMPLING (CVS)

The chorionic villi are fingerlike projections of the embryonic sac that contain cells with the same genetic composiiton as the embryo. In this test, a small sample of this chorionic tissue is taken and analyzed to determine genetic abnormalities in the fetus. It can be performed earlier than amniocentesis, usually between the eighth and tenth weeks of pregnancy, and takes about a half hour to complete.

Possible dangers from CVS include infection, maternal or fetal bleeding, spontaneous abortion, Rh immunization, birth defects, and perforation of the membrane surrounding the embryo. CVS is generally considered to be slightly riskier than amniocentesis. The chief advantage is that it can be performed earlier in pregnancy, when termination, if deemed necessary, is a simpler and less dangerous procedure. As with all tests, you should weigh all the pluses and minuses carefully before making a decision.

ULTRASOUND

Ultrasound is a procedure in which high-frequency sound waves are bounced off objects to create images of those objects. This technology was originally developed for the space program, but later found uses in medical diagnostics, including prenatal care.

One form of ultrasound, the sonogram or B-scan, directs intermittent sound waves toward the pregnant woman's abdomen. An outline of the fetus, placenta, and other structures involved in pregnancy is transmitted to a video screen. In this way, the physician can determine fetal size and position, estimate the maturity of the fetus, confirm a multiple pregnancy, find the location of the placenta, check the fetal heart rate, and estimate the baby's due date.

Ultrasound is effective and is far safer for the fetus than x-ray. Like all medical tests, it should be used only when medically indicated.

ESTRIOL EXCRETION STUDIES, NONSTRESS TEST, OXYTOCIN CHALLENGE TEST

These tests are also used to determine the health of the fetus. The estriol excretion study determines the best time for delivery of the baby in cases of diabetes or other difficulties in pregnancy. The nonstress test determines fetal well-being, and the oxytocin challenge test helps to predict how well the baby will fare during the stress of labor.

If it is determined that any of these tests is necessary, your health care provider should discuss it with you in depth. When considering any type of prenatal testing, always remember that it is your body and your baby. You should be fully informed of all the advantages and all the risks of any procedure before agreeing to it.

PREGNANCY SELF-TEST

Over-the-counter pregnancy test kits are sold in most drugstores. Studies show that home pregnancy testing is only 77.1-percent accurate. You should always see your health care provider to confirm a positive result.

BACKACHE

Backache is common with pregnancy, often rooted in poor posture. The increase in body weight, the muscle-relaxing effects of the hormone progesterone, and the shift in one's center of gravity contribute to the problem.

Recommendations

❑ To minimize back pain during pregnancy, do not stay in any one position for a long period of time.

❑ Pay attention to your posture. Keep your shoulders relaxed and your back as straight as possible at all times.

❑ Include two to three minutes of gentle stretching exercises in your daily routine. Do not do any forward-bending or strongly upward-stretching exercises, however.

❑ Do not wear high-heeled shoes. High heels throw your body off balance and put extra strain on your back. Instead, wear well-fitting, well-padded flat or low-heeled shoes that support your feet and provide ample room for your toes. Be aware that you may require a different size shoe than normal while you are pregnant.

❑   When your back hurts, try soaking a small towel in cider vinegar. Squeeze off any excess and lie down on your side in bed. Spread the towel directly across your back. Relax this way for fifteen to twenty minutes.

❑   *See also* BACKACHE in Part Two.

BLEEDING GUMS

During pregnancy, increasing estrogen levels cause the gums to swell and become somewhat softer than normal, and the circulation of blood to them increases. This makes the gums more prone to bleeding and infection, especially if good oral hygiene is not maintained.

Recommendations

❑   Be sure your diet contains enough calcium and high-quality, complete proteins.

❑   Increase your intake of foods rich in vitamin C, as a deficiency in this vitamin can contribute to bleeding gums.

❑   If you smoke, quit—preferably *before* you get pregnant. Cigarette smoking reduces the oxygen supply to the developing fetus, and also drains vitamin C from the body.

❑   Brush your teeth three to four times daily (remembering to rinse your mouth well), and massage your gums with clean fingers when necessary. Floss your teeth daily.

❑   See your dentist at least once during the pregnancy, but *do not* have any x-rays taken.

CONSTIPATION

Hormonal changes during pregnancy have a relaxing effect on the muscles, including those of the digestive tract. The increasing level of progesterone in your system makes the bowels less efficient. The normal rhythmic contractions of the intestines slow down, and the result can be constipation.

Recommendations

❑   Eat fresh and dried fruit such as prunes, raisins, and figs.

❑   Eat fresh vegetables and salads containing a variety of raw green and colored vegetables daily.

❑   Increase the amount of fiber in your diet. Whole-grain breads, cereals, and bran are helpful. Begin by taking 2 teaspoons of bran in a glass of apple juice twice daily. The bran may cause some gas until your system is used to it, but after that you should not have any difficulty.

❑   Drink six to eight 8-ounce glasses of liquid, including water, each day.

❑   Walk at least a mile a day, and set a regular time each day for bowel movement. This is very helpful for digestion and elimination. Elevate your feet and legs during elimination to relax the anal muscles.

❑   If all else fails, an enema, using body-temperature water, may be used occasionally.

❑   *Do not* take over-the-counter laxatives unless specifically recommended by your health care provider.

❑   *See also* CONSTIPATION in Part Two.

DIZZINESS

During pregnancy, especially during the second trimester, blood pressure often drops as the expanding uterus presses on major blood vessels. This can cause dizziness.

Recommendation

❑   Do not change positions quickly. Always go from lying down to sitting to standing slowly. Take your time and focus on what you are doing.

EDEMA (SWELLING) OF THE HANDS AND FEET

The rise in estrogen in the body during pregnancy increases the tendency to retain fluids. This can cause some swelling of the hands and feet and is considered normal.

Recommendations

❑   Remove any rings you wear on a regular basis. Do not wait, or the rings may have to be cut off.

❑   As soon as you notice your hands, legs, or feet getting puffy or larger than usual, tell your health care provider. While some swelling is acceptable, the condition should nevertheless be evaluated by a professional, as edema can also be the first sign of toxemia, a potentially serious complication of pregnancy.

❑   Avoid salt and all highly processed foods, while maintaining a well-balanced high protein diet. *Do not* take diuretics (water pills).

❑   Wear loose, comfortable clothing and properly fitting shoes. You may require a larger size shoe than normal. Once the baby arrives, your feet will return to normal.

❑   Do not sit with a weight, such as another child, on your lap, as this impedes circulation.

❑   Walk one mile each day. This helps to keep this condition under control.

❑   *See also* EDEMA in Part Two.

GAS (FLATULENCE)

Gas, like other digestive upsets, is a common complaint during pregnancy. Even foods that cause no difficulties at other times may begin to cause trouble.

Recommendations

❑ Keep a food diary to help you determine which foods, or combinations of foods, seem to be causing the gas. Avoid any suspect foods.

❑ Eat four to five small meals a day, instead of three big meals. Chew your food slowly and well.

❑ Eat four or more servings of fresh fruits and vegetables every day.

❑ Cook vegetables quickly using a perforated steamer instead of boiling them for long periods of time.

❑ To reduce gas-causing sulfur compounds in beans (garbanzo, pinto, navy, and so on), use the following cooking method: Place 1 cup of beans in 5 cups of water and bring them to a boil. Boil the beans for one minute. Then drain them and add 5 cups of fresh water. Bring the water to a boil and continue cooking the beans according to directions.

GROIN SPASM, STITCH, OR PRESSURE

When the round ligaments connecting the corners of the uterus to the pubic area kink and go into spasm, it feels like a "stitch" on the right side. In the later months of pregnancy, lower groin pressure may develop.

Recommendations

❑ Exercise daily, using exercises recommended by your health care provider. This can help alleviate this condition.

❑ During spasms, breathe deeply and bend toward the point of pain in order to allow the ligament to relax. Rest in bed on one side until the spasm is over.

HEARTBURN

Heartburn occurs more often than normal during pregnancy. This is because the expanded size of the uterus promotes the reentry of stomach fluids into the esophagus.

Recommendations

❑ To prevent heartburn, do not consume spicy or greasy foods, alcohol, coffee, baking soda, or antacids containing sodium bicarbonate (such as Alka-Seltzer).

❑ Remain active.

❑ Refrain from bending or lying flat for several hours after eating.

❑ To relieve discomfort, try using Acid-Ease from Prevail Corporation. This product, found in health food stores, contains natural plant enzymes, and can be taken with meals and/or between meals, as needed. It is safe and effective for reducing heartburn.

❑ *See also* HEARTBURN in Part Two.

HEMORRHOIDS

Hemorrhoids are common during pregnancy. A number of factors contribute to the development of hemorrhoids, including constipation and the pressure exerted by the uterus as the fetus gains in size and weight.

Recommendations

❑ Increase your intake of roughage. Eat plenty of raw vegetables, fruits, dried fruits, bran, and whole-grain breads. This helps to soften stools and make elimination easier. Hard stools can be very painful to pass and can cause bleeding. Also, drink six to eight 8-ounce glasses of liquid each day, including water, juices, and herbal teas.

❑ Keep your feet and legs elevated on a high footstool while eliminating. This helps to move the bowels by relaxing the anal muscles. Do not strain and do not sit on the toilet for too long.

❑ Use cold witch hazel compresses to help shrink hemorrhoids.

❑ Walk one mile a day to help digestion and elimination.

❑ *See also* HEMORRHOIDS in Part Two.

INSOMNIA

Insomnia is very common during the last weeks of pregnancy when finding a comfortable sleeping position is difficult. Deficiencies of the B vitamins also can cause insomnia. The emotional changes that accompany pregnancy often contribute to sleep difficulties as well.

Recommendations

❑ Increase your intake of foods rich in the B vitamins (*see* VITAMINS in Part One).

❑ Do not force yourself to sleep if you are not really tired. Read or do nonstrenuous chores until you feel sleepy.

❑ Try drinking a cup of hot herbal tea with honey or lemon before bed or in the middle of the night. Herbal teas such as chamomile, marjoram, lemon balm, and passionflower are known for their sleep-inducing qualities.

Caution: Do not use chamomile on an ongoing basis, as ragweed allergy may result. Avoid it completely if you are allergic to ragweed.

❑ Arrange pillows behind or under your abdomen to relieve breathlessness.

❑ *See also* INSOMNIA in Part Two.

LEG CRAMPS

Leg cramps are often a result of nutritional deficiencies and/or electrolyte imbalances, in addition to the strain placed on the legs by the extra weight.

438

Recommendations

❑ Increase your calcium and potassium intake by eating foods such as almonds, bananas, grapefruit, low-fat cottage cheese, oranges, salmon, sardines, sesame seeds, soy products (such as tofu), and low-fat yogurt to help avert leg cramps. Adequate calcium is also needed to help prevent high blood pressure, often seen in late pregnancy, as well as for fetal development.

❑ While sleeping or sitting, elevate your legs so that they are higher than your heart.

❑ Do not stand in one place for too long. Shift your weight from one leg to the other every few minutes.

❑ Do not point your toes.

❑ Walk at least a mile every day to stimulate the circulation of blood through the legs.

❑ To relieve cramps, flex your feet, with your toes pointing upward.

❑ When experiencing a cramp, apply a hot water bottle or heating pad to the cramping area and apply pressure with your hands.

❑ *See also* MUSCLE CRAMPS in Part Two.

MISCARRIAGE (SPONTANEOUS ABORTION)

Some pregnancies are not carried to full term, resulting in a miscarriage, or spontaneous abortion. There are many reasons for this, including abruptio placentae (separation of the placenta from the wall of the uterus), cervical incompetence, ectopic pregnancy (implantation of the fertilized egg outside the uterine cavity, most commonly in one of the fallopian tubes), emotional stress, general malaise, infection, glandular disorders, malnutrition, placenta previa (implantation of the placenta over the cervical opening), and pregnancy-induced hypertension. In many cases, the miscarriage may be the result of some abnormality in the fetus.

Recommendations

❑ If you experience bleeding or cramping during pregnancy, contact your health care provider immediately and follow his or her advice.

Considerations

❑ Some women who have had repeated miscarriages may be able to boost their chances of a full-term pregnancy with a new immunization procedure. Doctors at the University of Michigan have discovered that injecting two vaccines containing white blood cells from the father into the mother can prevent an abnormal reaction in the woman's immune system that results in rejection of the growing fetus as a "foreign transplant."

❑ Premature labor is the onset of rhythmic uterine contractions before fetal maturity. It usually occurs between the twentieth and thirty-seventh weeks of gestation. Around 5 to 10 percent of pregnancies end prematurely; 75 to 85 percent of infant deaths and many birth defects are associated with prematurity.

❑ Ectopic pregnancy is a potentially dangerous condition that may produce cramping and light bleeding, but in some cases may result in no symptoms other than mild abdominal pain, making diagnosis difficult. If a fallopian tube ruptures as a result of ectopic pregnancy, life-threatening hemorrhage and infection may result. This condition requires immediate surgical treatment.

MOOD CHANGES

Mood changes are quite common during pregnancy. They are thought to be caused by hormonal changes and deficiencies of the B vitamins, as well as the stress of physical discomforts and psychological issues that arise as a result of bodily changes and the awareness of impending motherhood.

Recommendations

❑ Increase your intake of foods rich in the B vitamins and iron, such as alfalfa, blackstrap molasses, brown rice, eggs, enriched whole-grain cereals, fish, green leafy vegetables, kidney beans, oats, poultry, soy products, and wheat germ. Inadequate iron intake causes anemia, which can make you feel tired, irritable, and unhappy.

❑ If mood changes are severe and/or are interfering with your life, consider counseling. Making an effort to explore and understand underlying emotions can help you to cope with your feelings as well.

❑ Keep in mind that mood changes during pregnancy are normal, and most likely temporary.

MORNING SICKNESS

Approximately 50 percent of all pregnant women experience some degree of nausea and vomiting between the sixth and twelfth weeks of pregnancy. This is normal. Although it is commonly called morning sickness, it can occur at any time of day.

Abnormal vomiting—severe, continual nausea and vomiting after the twelfth week—occurs in approximately 1 in 200 pregnancies. It can result in dehydration, acidosis, malnutrition, and substantial weight loss. Possible causes of abnormal vomiting include bile duct disease, drug toxicity, pancreatitis, inflammatory bowel disorders, vitamin deficiencies (mainly a lack of vitamin B_6), and the production of high levels of a hormone called human chorionic gonadotropin. This may occur due to the presence of cysts in the uterus or multiple pregnancy.

NUTRIENTS

SUPPLEMENT	SUGGESTED DOSAGE	COMMENTS
L-Methionine	1,000 mg daily.	Effective in preventing nausea. Used to prevent toxemia in pregnancy.
Vitamin B$_6$ (pyridoxine) plus	50 mg every 4 hours.	A combination of nutrients that helps to prevent and alleviate nausea.
magnesium	400 mg daily, upon arising.	Caution: Take this combination only as long as needed. Do not take it for longer than 6 weeks.

Herbs

❑ Ginger, taken in capsule or tea form, is helpful for relieving nausea. Other beneficial herbs include catnip, dandelion, peppermint, and red raspberry leaf.

Recommendations

❑ Keep crackers or whole wheat toast near your bed and eat some before arising.

❑ Eat small, frequent meals and snack on whole-grain crackers with nut butters (but not peanut butter) or cheese. It helps to keep some food in the stomach at all times.

❑ Do not go without food or drink because of the nausea.

❑ Keep in mind that morning sickness usually does not last beyond the first thirteen weeks of pregnancy. If you suffer from persistent nausea or vomiting later in pregnancy, consult your health care provider. With appropriate treatment, the prognosis is good.

NOSEBLEEDS AND NASAL CONGESTION

During pregnancy, increased blood volume often causes some of the tiny capillaries in the nasal passages to rupture, causing a nosebleed. Inner nasal passages normally swell as well. A lack of vitamin C and the bioflavonoids may be a contributing factor. These conditions disappear with the birth of the baby.

Recommendations

❑ Increase your intake of foods rich in vitamin C, including broccoli, cabbage, grapefruits, lemons, oranges, peppers, and strawberries.

❑ If congestion is a problem, eat fewer dairy products and supplement your diet with calcium and magnesium. Dairy products tend to stimulate the secretion of mucus.

❑ Use a humidifier to help keep nasal tissues moisturized.

❑ Do not use nasal sprays or nose drops. Instead, use an empty nasal spray container filled with warm water to spray into the nostrils. This helps to moisten the nose and shrink the membranes.

❑ See also NOSEBLEED in Part Two.

SCIATICA

The sciatic nerve is the longest nerve in the body. It arises from the sacral plexus, in the lower back, threads downward through the pelvis through an opening called the greater sciatic foramen, and runs through the hip joint and down the back of the thigh. Irritation of this nerve is common during pregnancy and usually disappears with the birth of the baby.

Recommendations

❑ Ask your health care provider to recommend a registered physical therapist or a chiropractor who has been specially trained to deal with pregnancy problems. A competent practitioner is best able to deal with this problem.

SKIN PROBLEMS

Common skin problems during pregnancy include pimples, acne, red marks, and mask of pregnancy (dark blotches on the skin of the face). These skin changes usually disappear with the birth of the baby.

NUTRIENTS

SUPPLEMENT	SUGGESTED DOSAGE	COMMENTS
Folic acid	5 mg before each meal.	May help to make pregnancy mask disappear.

Recommendations

❑ Keep your skin clean. Do not use makeup if your skin is broken out.

❑ See also ACNE and OILY SKIN, both in Part Two.

SORENESS IN THE RIB AREA

This soreness comes from the pressure of the expanding uterus.

Recommendations

❑ Change positions frequently.

❑ Keep in mind that this problem is temporary. It often disappears in the last six weeks of pregnancy, once the baby drops into position to be born.

STRETCH MARKS

Stretch marks are wavy stripes appearing on the abdomen, buttocks, breasts, and thighs. They start out reddish in color and gradually turn white. They are caused by rapid weight gain such as that typically associated with pregnancy, and appear when the skin becomes overstretched and the fibers in the deep layers tear. Once they appear, they are permanent, but they do become much less noticeable with time.

Recommendations

❑ Try the following recipe for preventing stretch marks:

1/2 cup virgin olive oil
1/4 cup aloe vera gel
6 capsules vitamin E, cut open
4 capsules vitamin A, cut open

1. Mix all the ingredients together in a blender.
2. Pour the mixture into a jar and store it in the refrigerator.

Once a day, apply the oil externally all over the abdomen, hips, and thighs—the places where stretch marks commonly appear. If you do this diligently, every day, you may be able to prevent stretch marks.

❑ Apply cocoa butter and/or elastin cream topically as directed on the product label. These substances are very good for stretch marks.

SWEATING

While you are pregnant, your body makes sure that its temperature is perfect for your baby's development. In addition, as your size increases, the amount of effort it takes to walk, climb stairs, and do many everyday things also increases. As a result, you may find yourself sweating more than you did before.

Recommendations

❑ Wear loose, light, comfortable clothing. Choose clothing made of "breathable" natural fibers.

❑ Do not use a hot tub during pregnancy. This increase in body temperature can cause fetal distress. For the same reason, be careful about strenuous exercise, especially in hot weather.

URINATION, FREQUENT

Frequent urination is a natural byproduct of the early and late months of pregnancy. It is primarily a result of changes in kidney function and pressure from the expanding uterus. Many women find it most common during the night.

Recommendation

❑ Although it may seem that drinking liquids aggravates this problem, *do not* cut down on fluid intake in an attempt to minimize it. Drink 6 to 8 full glasses of liquid each day.

VARICOSE VEINS

Varicose veins are enlarged veins close to the surface of the skin. In many cases they disappear after the baby's birth.

Recommendations

❑ As often as possible, sit with your feet elevated, higher than your heart.

❑ Change positions frequently. Do not stand for long periods of time or sit in cross-legged positions.

❑ Wear support hose if your health care provider recommends them. Keep them near your bed and put them on before you get out of bed.

❑ Walk one mile each day to promote circulation.

❑ Do not wear elastic-topped knee socks, garters, belts, or high-heeled shoes.

❑ *See also* VARICOSE VEINS in Part Two.

NUTRITIONAL HEALTH IN PREGNANCY

During pregnancy, it is more important than ever to have a balanced diet that is high in nutrients and fiber and low in bad fats and cholesterol. The following are recommendations for maintaining health in pregnancy.

NUTRIENTS

SUPPLEMENT	SUGGESTED DOSAGE	COMMENTS
Very Important		
Vitamin B complex plus extra	As directed on label.	To prevent deficiencies.
folic acid	800 mcg daily.	Adequate levels of folic acid reduce the chance of birth defects such as spina bifida.
Iron	30 mg daily, or as directed by physician. Take with 100 mg vitamin C for better absorption.	Extra iron is needed during pregnancy.
or Floradix Iron + Herbs from Salus Haus	As directed on label.	A natural, nontoxic source of iron.
Protein supplement	As directed on label.	A lack of protein has been linked to birth defects. Use protein from a vegetable source, such as soy.
Quercetin	500 mg daily.	A valuable bioflavonoid that promotes proper circulation.
Vitamin C	2,000–4,000 mg daily, in divided doses.	Larger doses taken before delivery may help reduce labor pain.
Zinc	15–25 mg daily. Do not exceed 75 mg daily.	Insufficient zinc intake may be a cause of low birth weight. Use zinc gluconate lozenges or OptiZinc for best absorption.
Helpful		
Acidophilus	As directed on label. Take on an empty stomach.	Provides necessary "friendly" bacteria to prevent candidiasis (yeast infection), protect the baby at birth, and ensure proper assimilation of nutrients.
Body Language Essential Green Foods from OxyFresh	As directed on label.	Promotes health and protects the intestinal tract and blood cells.
Calcium	1,500 mg daily.	Necessary for formation of healthy bones and teeth. May prevent hypertension and premature birth.
and magnesium	750 mg daily.	Needed to balance with calcium.

Coenzyme Q10	As directed on label.	Helps the body convert food to energy, enhances circulation, and protects the heart.
Kelp	As directed on label.	Rich in necessary minerals.
Multimineral and trace mineral complex with	As directed on label.	For optimal health and to provide a balance of nutrients needed for fetal development.
selenium	3 mcg per lb of body weight daily.	May play a role in protecting the lung tissue after birth.
Natural beta-carotene	25,000 IU daily.	Precursor of vitamin A. *Caution:* Do not substitute vitamin A for beta-carotene. Excessive intake of vitamin A during pregnancy has been linked to birth defects.
Vitamin D	1,000 IU daily.	Needed for calcium absorption and bone formation.
Vitamin E	400 IU daily.	Premature and low birth weight infants are often deficient in vitamin E.
Vitamin K or	As directed on label.	Take for excessive bleeding.
alfalfa		*See under* Herbs, below.

Herbs

❑ Alfalfa is a good source of vitamins and minerals, especially vitamin K, which is essential for normal blood clotting.

❑ Blessed thistle, blue cohosh, false unicorn root, and squawvine are beneficial taken in the last four weeks of pregnancy. They help to prepare the body for an easier birth and aid contractions. These herbs should *not* be taken in the first two trimesters of pregnancy, however.

❑ Burdock root, dandelion, ginger, and nettle help to enrich a mother's milk.

❑ Red raspberry leaf tea helps the uterus contract more effectively. It also helps to enrich mother's milk. Drink no more than 1 cup per day until the last four weeks of pregnancy. Then drink 1 quart daily.

❑ St. Johnswort and shepherd's purse help uterine contractions at birth.

❑ Avoid the following herbs during pregnancy: angelica, barberry, black cohosh, bloodroot, cat's claw, celandine, cottonwood bark, dong quai, feverfew, goldenseal, lobelia, Oregon grape, pennyroyal, rue, and tansy.

Recommendations

❑ Eat a well-balanced, nutritious diet and be sure to get moderate exercise, fresh air, and plenty of rest.

❑ Do not consume junk food, highly seasoned or fried foods, or coffee.

❑ Avoid eating rare or undercooked meat, poultry, or fish. Do not eat grilled meats. Grilling has been shown to produce carcinogens in meat.

❑ Do not smoke, consume alcohol in any form, or use drugs, except as prescribed by your health care provider.

❑ Do not take supplements containing the amino acid phenylalanine. Phenylalanine may alter brain growth in the fetus. Also avoid food products containing the sweetener asparatame (Equal, NutraSweet), which contains high levels of phenylalanine. (*See* Is Aspartame a Safe Sugar Substitute? on page 9.)

❑ Keep your intake of vitamin A below 10,000 international units daily.

❑ Avoid the following medications, which can stunt fetal growth: acetaminophen (Tylenol, Datril, and others), antacids (Alka-Seltzer, Di-Gel, Gelusil, Maalox, Pepto-Bismol, Rolaids, Tums), antihistamines, aspirin, cold pills, cough remedies, decongestants, and estrogens. Do not take mineral oil, which blocks the absorption of the fat-soluble vitamins. Consult your health care provider about the use of any supplements and over-the-counter medications.

❑ Avoid activities that may endanger the abdomen, or that involve jarring, bouncing, or twisting movements. Also avoid activities involving rapid starts and stops, because during pregnancy, the body's center of gravity changes, and it is easy to lose your balance. After the fourth month, do not exercise on your back, as this can interrupt the blood flow to the uterus and slow the fetal heart rate.

❑ Do *not* take any preparations containing shark cartilage during pregnancy. Shark cartilage inhibits the formation of new blood vessels, which is essential during pregnancy.

❑ Do not use an electric blanket. Several experts warn that the invisible electromagnetic field emanating from an electric blanket may increase the risk of miscarriage and developmental problems.

Considerations

❑ Researchers at the University of Washington found that pregnant women with previous health problems who used electric blankets, particularly in the first three months of pregnancy, were five times as likely as others to give birth to children with urinary tract defects.

❑ An estimated 3 to 5 percent of all pregnant women develop gestational diabetes. This occurs during the second half of pregnancy. A screening for gestational diabetes should therefore be performed between the twenty-fourth and twenty-eighth weeks of pregnancy.

❑ Lack of zinc, manganese, and folic acid, as well as amino acid imbalances, have been linked to fetal deformities and mental retardation.

❑ Aspirin has been linked with fetal deformities, bleeding, and complications during delivery.

❑ Isotretinoin (Accutane), a drug prescribed for acne, can cause birth defects, as can etretinate (Tegison), which is used for psoriasis.

❑ All women of childbearing age should take a daily supplement of 400 micrograms of folic acid. Folic acid deficiency is linked to such neurologic birth defects as spina bifida and anencephaly. In order to prevent these disorders, this B vitamin must be present in the body during the first six weeks following conception, a crucial early phase in fetal neurological development. Since most women do not know they have conceived until several weeks afterward, the best way to prevent these birth defects is for women who have any chance of becoming pregnant to have an adequate supply of this nutrient at all times. Supplementation is recommended because many women do not get enough folic acid from dietary sources. Folic acid also helps alleviate heavy menstrual bleeding and hemorrhaging in childbirth and improves lactation.

❑ Taking the drug phenytoin (Dilantin) or phenobarbital, used to control epileptic seizures, creates four times the usual risk of producing a baby with heart defects. In addition, the antibiotics ampicillin (Omnipen, Polycillin) or tetracycline may cause heart malformations.

❑ Large quantities of caffeine can cause birth defects.

❑ Excessive intake of vitamin A has been linked with cleft palate, heart defects, and other congenital defects. Foods rich in vitamin A may also cause problems. Foods containing natural beta-carotene, however, are not harmful because the body converts beta-carotene to vitamin A only as needed, and not in amounts that may be toxic to the body.

❑ One of the best things you can do for your child is to breastfeed your baby for at least the first three months of life—longer if possible. Mother's milk is not only the most nutritious food for a baby, but it also provides crucial disease-fighting agents. A new mother should consume 500 more calories per day when nursing than she ate during pregnancy. The diet should include a substantial amount of liquids and extra portions of calcium-rich foods. If nursing is not possible and you must bottlefeed, use a well-balanced soy-based product. Cow's milk does not supply a human infant with enough iron, linoleic acid, or vitamin E, and babies who are fed cow's milk have a greater chance of developing allergies to milk and dairy products later in life.

Premenstrual Syndrome

Premenstrual syndrome (PMS) is a disorder that affects many women during the one to two weeks before menstruation begins. Symptoms can include any or all of the following: abdominal bloating, acne, anxiety, backache, breast swelling and tenderness, cramps, depression, food cravings, fainting spells, fatigue, headaches, insomnia, joint pain, nervousness, skin eruptions, water retention, and personality changes such as drastic mood swings, outbursts of anger, violence, and thoughts of suicide.

While there are no hard statistics, it is estimated that as many as 70 to 75 percent of all women experience some premenstrual symptoms at one time or another. Approximately 5 percent of women have symptoms so severe as to be incapacitating, and 30 to 40 percent report symptoms severe enough to interfere with their day-to-day lives.

For many years, PMS was dismissed as a purely psychological problem, and some women were even diagnosed as mentally ill. We now know that this is indeed a physically based problem. One of the causes of PMS is hormonal imbalance—excessive levels of estrogen and inadequate levels of progesterone. Hormonal fluctuations lead to fluid retention, which affects circulation, reducing the amount of oxygen reaching the uterus, ovaries, and brain. Eating red meat and dairy products may cause or contribute to such a hormonal imbalance. Unstable blood sugar levels are an important factor as well. PMS has also been linked to food allergies, changes in carbohydrate metabolism, hypoglycemia, and malabsorption. Diet is an important contributing factor. Other suspected causes of PMS symptoms include erratic levels of beta-endorphin (a narcotic-like substance produced by the body), vitamin and/or mineral deficiencies, and clinical depression. When the workings of the brain's hormones are better understood, we may understand why this disorder can produce such a multitude of symptoms.

NUTRIENTS

SUPPLEMENT	SUGGESTED DOSAGE	COMMENTS
Very Important		
A.M./P.M. Ultimate Cleanse from Nature's Secret	As directed on label.	A cleansing program that enhances the liver's ability to metabolize estrogen.
Black currant seed oil or flaxseed oil or primrose oil	As directed on label 3 times daily. As directed on label 3 times daily. 1,000 mg 3 times daily.	To supply gamma-linolenic acid (GLA), an essential fatty acid that is important in relieving symptoms and aiding proper glandular function.
Calcium and magnesium	1,500 mg daily. 1,000 mg daily.	Relieves cramping, backache, and nervousness. Use calcium chelate form. Deficiency may be associated with PMS. Use magnesium chloride or chelate form.
Vitamin B complex plus extra pantothenic acid (vitamin B5) and vitamin B6 (pyridoxine) and vitamin B12	100 mg 3 times daily. 100–200 mg daily. 50 mg 3 times daily. 200 mcg twice daily.	B vitamins work best when taken together. Reduces stress and is needed by the adrenal gland. Reduces water retention and increases oxygen flow to the female organs. Also aids in restoring estrogen levels to normal. Reduces stress, prevents anemia, and is needed for all bodily functions. Use a lozenge or sublingual form.

Vitamin E	Start with 400 IU daily and increase slowly to 800 IU daily.	Good for sore breasts and other PMS symptoms; improves oxygen utilization and limits free radical damage. Also helps to relieve nervous tension, irritability, and depression.
Helpful		
Choline and inositol or lecithin	1,000 mg each daily. As directed on label.	To aid in nerve impulse transmission and help prevent estrogen-related cancers.
Chromium picolinate	200 mcg daily.	Stabilizes blood sugar levels.
DL-Phenylalanine (DLPA)	375 mg 3–4 times daily.	Helpful for alleviating headaches and pain. *Caution:* Do not take this supplement if you suffer from panic attacks, diabetes, high blood pressure, or PKU.
Floradix Iron + Herbs from Salus Haus	As directed on label. Do not take at the same time as vitamin E; iron depletes vitamin E in the body.	To supply iron in easily assimilable natural formula. Women with heavy menstrual flow are often anemic.
Gamma-aminobutyric acid (GABA)	750 mg daily.	Assists in controlling anxiety and restlessness.
Kelp	1,000–1,500 mg daily.	A good source of needed minerals. Helps protect thyroid function.
L-Tyrosine	500 mg twice daily, on an empty stomach. Take with water or juice. Do not take with milk. Take with 50 mg vitamin B6 and 100 mg vitamin C for better absorption.	Reduces anxiety, depression, and headache. *Caution:* Do not take this supplement if you are taking an MAO inhibitor drug.
Melatonin	2–3 mg daily, taken 2 hours or less before bedtime.	Helps to alleviate symptoms and also aids sleep.
Multivitamin and mineral complex	As directed on label.	All nutrients are needed for relief of symptoms.
Vitamin A plus natural beta-carotene	10,000 IU daily. 15,000 IU daily.	Deficiency has been linked to PMS. An antioxidant and precursor of vitamin A.
Vitamin C with bioflavonoids	3,000–6,000 mg daily, in divided doses.	Aids in relief of discomfort and breast swelling. Also boosts the immune system.
Vitamin D	As directed on label.	Needed for uptake of calcium and magnesium.
Zinc	50 mg daily. Do not exceed a total of 100 mg daily from all supplements.	Needed for proper immune function. Diuretics deplete zinc. Use zinc gluconate lozenges or OptiZinc for best absorption.

HERBS

❑ Angelica root, cramp bark, kava kava, and red raspberry, have antispasmodic properties and may alleviate cramps.

❑ Black haw and rosemary are good for cramps and help to calm the nervous system.

❑ Black cohosh, peppermint, strawberry leaf, and valerian root help to stabilize mood swings and tone the nervous system.
   Caution: Do not use black cohosh if you are pregnant or have any type of chronic disease.

❑ Blessed thistle, dong quai, false unicorn root, fennel seed, sarsaparilla root, and squawvine are hormone-balancing herbs effective in the treatment of PMS.

❑ Corn silk or an herbal combination such as SP-6 Cornsilk Blend from Solaray aids in releasing excess water from the tissues and relieves many premenstrual symptoms. Dandelion and hawthorn also act as natural diuretics.

❑ Feverfew is good for migraines.

❑ Milk thistle cleanses the liver and helps improve liver function, thus enhancing the liver's ability to metabolize estrogen. For best results, this herb should be taken on a daily basis for a period of three months.

❑ Pau d'arco tea is good for protecting against candidiasis (yeast infection).

❑ Wild yam extract contains natural progesterone and has proved effective in alleviating many symptoms of PMS, including cramps, headache, mood swings, depression, irritability, and insomnia.

RECOMMENDATIONS

❑ Eat plenty of fresh fruits and vegetables, whole-grain cereals and breads, beans, peas, lentils, nuts and seeds, and broiled chicken, turkey, and fish. Have high-protein snacks between meals.

❑ Drink 1 quart of distilled water daily, starting a week before the menstrual period and ending one week after.

❑ Do not consume salt, red meats, processed foods, or junk or fast foods. At the very least, omit these foods from the diet for at least one week before the expected onset of symptoms. Eliminating sodium (principally salt and foods that contain it) is especially important for preventing bloating and water retention.

❑ Eat fewer dairy products. Dairy products block the absorption of magnesium and increase its urinary excretion. Refined sugars also increase magnesium excretion.

❑ Avoid caffeine. Caffeine is linked to breast tenderness and is a central nervous system stimulant that can make you anxious and jittery. It also acts as a diuretic and can deplete many important nutrients.

❑ Do not consume alcohol or sugar in any form, especially during the week before symptoms are expected. These foods cause valuable electrolytes, particularly magnesium, to be lost through the urine.

❑ Fast on fresh juices and spirulina for several days before the anticipated onset of menstruation to help minimize symptoms. *See* FASTING in Part Three.

❑ Get regular exercise. Walking, even if only one-half to one mile per day, can be very helpful. Exercise increases the oxygen level in the blood, which helps in nutrient absorption and efficient elimination of toxins from the body. It also helps to keep hormone levels more stable.

❑ To relieve cramping, use warm sitz baths, a heating pad, or a hot water bottle. Warmth increases blood flow to the pelvic region and relaxes the muscles. *See* SITZ BATH in Part Three.

❑ See a physician to rule out an underlying medical condition that may be causing symptoms, such as abnormal thyroid function, endometriosis, or a genuine psychological problem such as clinical depression. A food allergy test and a hair analysis to rule out heavy metal intoxication are also recommended.

❑ Do not smoke.

CONSIDERATIONS

❑ Premenstrual depression may be due to a miscue of the biological clock that results in lower than normal levels of certain brain chemicals. Research at the University of California–San Diego suggests that some women who suffer from PMS may be deficient in melatonin, a hormone secreted at night by the pineal gland.

❑ Studies have shown that women who regularly consume caffeine are four times more likely than others to have severe PMS.

❑ Some physicians recommend oral contraceptives for women with PMS, especially if they also are interested in reliable birth control. If you take oral contraceptives, be aware that their effectiveness at preventing pregnancy can be sharply reduced if you also take antibiotics. Oral contraceptives and other preparations containing estrogen-type substances should *not* be used if you are pregnant or if you have breast cancer, abnormal vaginal bleeding, or phlebitis (inflammation of leg veins).

❑ Proper diet is extremely important in treating PMS. Meals high in complex carbohydrates have been found to help in dealing with stress. Researchers speculate that such a diet may increase the body's production of serotonin, a brain chemical with antidepressant properties. Conversely, eating red meat and dairy products promotes the type of hormonal imbalance that causes PMS—excessive estrogen levels and inadequate progesterone levels.

❑ Wild yam cream, which contains a natural form of the hormone progesterone, has been helpful for many women. You rub the cream into the skin on your chest, inner arms, thighs, and abdomen just after ovulation, and the active ingredient is absorbed through the skin.

❑ The amino acid L-glutamine, either alone or in combination with DL-phenylalanine (DLPA), may help to reduce food cravings.

❑ Research has discovered that many women with PMS also suffer from some form of immune system disorder or frequently suffer from some variety of yeast infection. (*See* CANDIDIASIS in Part Two.)

❑ A significant number of women who suffer from PMS have some sort of thyroid dysfunction. (*See* HYPOTHYROIDISM in Part Two.)

❑ Kombucha tea, an energizing and immune-boosting drink, has been reported to be helpful for some women who suffer from PMS. (*See* MAKING KOMBUCHA TEA in Part Three.)

❑ Clinics specializing in the treatment of PMS are springing up all over the country. Experience and expertise can vary greatly among these establishments, however. Ask your health care provider for a referral or recommendation, or look for a clinic that is affiliated with a major local hospital. Beware of clinics that promote only one type of treatment or a quick-fix approach to this complicated disorder.

❑ *See also* ALLERGIES in Part Two and HAIR ANALYSIS in Part Three.

Prolapse of the Uterus

Uterine prolapse is a condition that develops when muscular support for the uterus is lost. The uterus is normally held in place by the pelvic muscles and supporting ligaments. When these muscles become weakened or injured, uterine prolapse can occur. In mild cases, a portion of the uterus descends into the top of the vagina. In more serious cases, the uterus may even protrude through the vaginal opening, and can be accompanied by a cystocele (a bladder that bulges into the front wall of the vagina) or a urethrocele (a urethra that does the same). In some instances, the rectum may bulge into the back wall of the vagina, a condition known as rectocele.

Symptoms of prolapse of the uterus can include backache, abdominal discomfort, a feeling of heaviness, and urinary incontinence, especially stress incontinence (the involuntary passage of urine when straining, sneezing, or otherwise putting pressure on the abdomen). Other symptoms can include excessive menstrual bleeding, abnormal vaginal discharge or bleeding, painful intercourse, and constipation. However, a woman with a prolapsed uterus may not exhibit any symptoms at all.

Women who have borne several children and/or who have gone through difficult and prolonged labor are more prone to prolapse. Other factors that can increase the likelihood of uterine prolapse include obesity, uterine cancer, diabetes, chronic bronchitis, asthma, heavy lifting or straining (particularly if the pelvic muscles are already weakened), and a retroverted uterus (a uterus that is tilted toward the back of the body). Two thirds of all women who prolapse do so before the age of fifty-five.

NUTRIENTS

SUPPLEMENT	SUGGESTED DOSAGE	COMMENTS
Important		
Calcium and	1,500 mg daily.	Essential minerals needed for muscle tone and metabolism.
magnesium or	1,000 mg daily.	
Bone Defense from KAL	As directed on label.	A good source of necessary minerals and other nutrients.
L-Carnitine plus	500 mg twice daily, on an empty stomach.	Improves muscle strength in the uterus.
L-glycine	500 mg twice daily, on an empty stomach. Take with water or juice. Do not take with milk. Take with 50 mg vitamin B_6 and 100 mg vitamin C for better absorption.	Retards muscle degeneration.
plus branched-chain amino acid complex	As directed on label.	Promotes healing of muscle tissue.
Cranberry		*See under* Herbs, below.
Multivitamin and mineral complex with natural beta-carotene and vitamin B complex	As directed on label.	All nutrients work together for healing and tissue repair.
Vitamin C	3,000–5,000 mg daily, in divided doses.	Important for keeping bladder infections under control and to enhance immune function. Use an esterified form for best absorption.
Zinc	50 mg daily. Do not exceed a total of 100 mg daily from all supplements.	Needed for proper immune function, bone support, and all bodily enzyme systems. Use zinc gluconate lozenges or OptiZinc for best absorption.

HERBS

❑ Cranberry aids in bladder function and helps to prevent urgency incontinence. It can be taken in capsule form. Pure, unsweetened cranberry juice is good also.

RECOMMENDATIONS

❑ Eat a diet consisting of 75 percent raw fruits and vegetables plus whole grains such as brown rice and millet.

❑ Use a fiber supplement daily to prevent constipation.

❑ Do not wear tight pants, belts, or girdles.

❑ Do not strain during bowel movements or urination.

❑ Drink 8 to 10 full glasses of quality water daily.

CONSIDERATIONS

❑ Doing Kegel's exercises to tone the pelvic and vaginal muscles when prolapse is beginning may prevent the condition from getting worse. These exercises can be done in two ways:

1. Tighten and squeeze the vagina and rectum by drawing the muscles inward and upward. Hold this position for five to ten seconds, then relax. Repeat as many times as possible, preferably at least 100 times a day.

2. When urinating, start and stop the flow of urine as many times as possible. This form of the exercise is particularly useful for stress incontinence.

❑ If the prolapse causes no symptoms, no treatment is needed, other than perhaps adopting an exercise program designed for the individual problem and situation.

❑ Estrogen replacement therapy for postmenopausal women may help build genital muscle strength and slow the rate of prolapse. However, we do not recommend hormone therapy because it poses an increased risk of developing certain types of cancer.

❑ Natural progesterone replacement may be more beneficial than estrogen therapy.

❑ A vaginal device (a ring-shaped pessary) can be inserted to hold the uterus in place. This approach can have undesirable results, however. It can interfere with sexual intercourse and may also cause an irritating discharge with an unpleasant odor and even infection.

❑ It is possible to surgically resuspend the uterus into its normal position. This procedure is usually performed on women who wish to bear children in the future. For women who have completed childbearing, or who do not wish to have children, vaginal hysterectomy is a viable option for this condition. Women pondering a hysterectomy should give the matter close and careful consideration. *See* HYSTERECTOMY-RELATED PROBLEMS in Part Two.

Prostate Cancer

The prostate is a walnut-sized gland at the base of the bladder that encircles the urethra, the tube through which urine is voided. The prostate produces prostatic fluid, which makes up the bulk of the male ejaculate and nourishes and transports the sperm. Cancer of the prostate gland is the second leading cause of cancer death among men. It is primarily a disease of aging. Men in their thirties and forties rarely develop prostate cancer, but the incidence increases steadily after the age of fifty-five. Approximately 80 percent of all cases occur in men over the age of sixty-five, and by the age of eighty, 80 percent of all men have prostate cancer to some degree. The American Cancer Society estimates that more than 244,000 new cases of prostate cancer were diagnosed in 1995. In that same year, 40,400 men died from the disease. A male baby born today has a 13 percent chance of developing prostate cancer at some time in his life, and a 3 percent chance of dying from the disease. Many experts feel that every man will eventually develop prostate cancer if he lives long enough.

Although it is relatively common, in most cases prostate cancer is, fortunately, a slow-growing cancer. Most prostate cancers arise in the rear portion of the prostate gland; the rest originate near the urethra. Prostate cancers double in mass every six years, on average (by comparison, breast cancers commonly double every three and a half years). Possible symptoms of prostate cancer can include one or more of the following: pain or a burning sensation during urination, frequent urination, a decrease in the size and force of urine flow, an inability to urinate, blood in the urine, and continuing lower back, pelvic, or suprapubic discomfort. However, the disease often causes no symptoms at all until it reaches an advanced stage and/or spreads outside the gland. In addition, these symptoms most often are caused not by cancer, but by benign enlargement or inflammation of the prostate. Professional evaluation and diagnosis is therefore necessary.

The rate of prostate cancer in the United States is rising. In part, this is due to the aging of our population. Just a generation ago, the life expectancy for white men in the United States was sixty-five years; today, it is close to eighty years. However, the rate of prostate cancer is rapidly rising in all men, even those under age fifty. This is significant because, in general, the younger a man is when he is diagnosed with prostate cancer, the worse his prognosis. The increase in prostate cancer among younger men points to the role of diet and exposure to environmental toxins in the development of the disease.

African-American men have the highest incidence of prostate cancer, while Asian-Americans have the lowest. Men with a family history of prostate cancer also run a higher risk of developing the disease. The incidence is higher among married men than it is among unmarried men. Also at increased risk are men who have had recurring prostate infections, those with a history of venereal disease, and those who have taken testosterone. Researchers have also found a link between a high-fat diet and prostate cancer. This may be due to the fact that heavy fat consumption raises testosterone levels, which could then stimulate growth of the prostate, including any cancer cells it may be harboring. Exposure to cancer-causing chemicals increases risk as well. Some experts believe that vasectomy may increase a man's chances of developing prostate cancer.

There is no known way to prevent this disease, but early detection can make it possible to catch the cancer before it spreads to other sites in the body. A careful rectal exam of the prostate is the simplest and most cost-effective approach for detecting prostate cancer. The American Cancer Society recommends that every man have an annual exam beginning at age forty; the American Urologic Association suggests beginning at age fifty. A blood test to detect elevated levels of a substance called prostate-specific antigen (PSA) is an excellent screening test for prostate cancer. PSA is currently the most valuable "tumor marker" available to diagnose and evaluate the effectiveness of therapy for prostate cancer. A PSA test result between 0 and 4 is considered to be within the normal range; a PSA over 10 is assumed to indicate cancer until proven otherwise. High PSA levels can be caused by factors other than cancer, including benign enlargement or inflammation of the prostate, an activity as innocuous as bicycle riding, or even the rectal exam itself. If a man's PSA level is found to be high, the test should always be repeated, because it does yield false-positive or false-negative results an estimated 10 to 20 percent of the time. Having the test repeated every year may help a physician to better interpret the results; in healthy men, PSA levels tend to remain relatively stable, rising only gradually from year to year, while cancer causes the levels to rise more dramatically.

Ultrasound scanning of the prostate is often done to follow up on an abnormal rectal exam or PSA test. Other diagnostic tests, including computerized tomography (CT) scans, bone scans, and magnetic resonance imaging (MRI) may be necessary, but are costly. Ultimately, if test results point consistently to the presence of cancer, a tissue diagnosis must be done to confirm it. This can be done only by microscopic examination of a needle biopsy, preferably directed under ultrasound control. Repeated biopsies may be needed in some cases. This invasive procedure may itself cause complications. Bleeding, urinary retention, impotence, and sepsis ("blood poisoning") have been reported.

NUTRIENTS

SUPPLEMENT	SUGGESTED DOSAGE	COMMENTS
Essential		
Coenzyme Q$_{10}$	100 mg daily.	Improves cellular oxygenation.
Dimethylglycine (DMG) (Aangamik DMG from FoodScience Labs)	As directed on label.	Enhances oxygen utilization.
Proteolytic enzymes or Wobenzym N from Marlyn Nutraceuticals	As directed on label. Take with meals. As directed on label.	To keep down inflammation and destroy free radicals.
Selenium	200 mcg daily.	Powerful free radical scavenger. Aids in protein digestion.
Shark cartilage (BeneFin)	1 gm per 2 lbs of body weight daily, divided into 3 doses. If you cannot tolerate taking it orally, it can be administered rectally in a retention enema.	Inhibits tumor growth and stimulates the immune system.
Superoxide dismutase (SOD)	As directed on label.	Destroys free radicals. Consider injections (under a doctor's supervision).
Vitamin A plus natural beta-carotene or carotenoid complex (Betatene) plus vitamin E	50,000–100,000 IU daily for 10 days or as long as on the program. 10,000 IU daily. As directed on label. Up to 1,000 IU daily.	Powerful antioxidants that destroy free radicals. Use emulsion forms for easier assimilation, and greater safety at higher doses.

Vitamin B complex plus extra	100 mg daily.	B vitamins necessary for normal cell division and to improve
vitamin B3 (niacin) and	100 mg daily. Do not exceed this amount.	circulation, build red blood cells, and aid liver function.
choline and	500–1,000 mg daily.	*Caution:* Do not take niacin if you have a liver disorder, gout,
folic acid plus	180 mcg daily.	or high blood pressure.
vitamin B6 (pyridoxine) and	100 mg daily.	Enhances the efficacy of zinc.
vitamin B12	2,000 mcg daily.	Prevents anemia. Use a lozenge or sublingual form. Consider injections (under a doctor's supervision).
Vitamin C with bioflavonoids	5,000–20,000 mg daily, in divided doses. *See* ASCORBIC ACID FLUSH in Part Three.	Powerful anticancer agent.
Garlic (Kyolic)	2 capsules 3 times daily.	Enhances immune function.
Prostata from Gero Vita	As directed on label.	A natural supplement formulated for prostate health.

Important		
Maitake	4,000–8,000 mg (4–8 gm) daily.	Inhibits the growth and spread of cancerous tumors. Also boosts immune response.

Helpful		
Acidophilus or Kyo-Dophilus from Wakunaga	As directed on label. Take on an empty stomach.	Has an antibacterial effect on the body. Use a nondairy formula.
Aerobic 07 from Aerobic Life Industries or Dioxychlor (DC3) from American Biologics	As directed on label. As directed on label.	Antimicrobial agents.
Glutathione plus L-cysteine and L-methionine	As directed on label. As directed on label, on an empty stomach. Take with water or juice. Do not take with milk. Take with 50 mg vitamin B6 and 100 mg vitamin C for better absorption.	Protects against environmental toxins. Sulfur-containing amino acids that act as detoxifiers and protect the liver and other organs. *See* AMINO ACIDS in Part One.
Kelp or seaweed	1,000–1,500 mg daily.	For mineral balance.
L-Carnitine	As directed on label.	Protects against free radical damage and toxins. Use a form from fish liver (squalene).
Multimineral complex with calcium and magnesium and potassium	1,500 mg daily. 750–1,000 mg daily. 99 mg daily.	Essential for normal cell division and function.
Multiglandular complex plus raw thymus glandular	As directed on label. As directed on label.	To stimulate glandular function, especially that of the thymus, site of T lymphocyte production. *See* GLANDULAR THERAPY in Part Three.

Multienzyme complex	As directed on label. Take with meals.	To aid digestion.
Multivitamin complex	As directed on label.	Many nutrients in this table may be found in a combination multivitamin. Do not use a sustained-release formula. Choose a product that is iron-free.
Selenium	As directed on label.	Destroys free radicals and is needed for proper prostate function.
Taurine	As directed on label.	Functions as foundation for tissue and organ repair.
Zinc	50–100 mg daily. Do not exceed this amount.	Plays a role in the prevention of prostate cancer. Use zinc gluconate lozenges or OptiZinc for best absorption.

HERBS

❑ Black radish, dandelion, and red clover are good for cleansing the liver and the blood.

❑ Buchu, Carnivora, echinacea, goldenseal, pau d'arco, and suma have all shown anticancer properties. Take them in tea form, using two at a time and alternating among them.

❑ Damiana and licorice root have the ability to balance hormones and glandular function.

❑ Gravel root, hydrangea, oat straw, parsley root, uva ursi, and yarrow are diuretics that also dissolve sediment.

❑ Pygeum and saw palmetto are helpful. European studies suggest pygeum may prevent prostate cancer.

RECOMMENDATIONS

❑ Maintain a whole-foods diet. Eat plenty of whole grains, raw nuts and seeds, and unpolished brown rice. Millet cereal is a good source of protein. Eat wheat, oats, and bran. Also eat plenty of cruciferous vegetables, such as broccoli, Brussels sprouts, cabbage, and cauliflower, and yellow and deep orange vegetables, such as carrots, pumpkin, squash, and yams. This type of diet is important for the prevention of cancer as well as for healing.

❑ Include in the diet apples, fresh cantaloupe, all kinds of berries, Brazil nuts, cherries, grapes, legumes (including chickpeas, lentils, and red beans), and plums. All of these foods help to fight cancer.

❑ Consume freshly made vegetable and fruit juices daily. Carrot and cabbage juices are good choices.

❑ Include in the diet foods that are high in zinc, such as mushrooms, pumpkin seeds, seafood, spinach, sunflower seeds, and whole grains. Zinc nourishes the prostate gland and is vital for proper immune function.

❑ Restrict your intake of dairy products. Moderate consumption of soured products such as low-fat yogurt and kefir is acceptable.

❑ If you experience difficulty urinating or notice an increasing trend toward waking up to urinate during the night, consult your health care provider. This may indicate prostatic obstruction.

❑ Use cold-pressed organic oils such as sesame, safflower, or olive oil to obtain essential fatty acids.

❑ Do not eat red meat. There is a definite correlation between high red meat consumption (five servings a week or more) and the development of prostate cancer.

❑ Eliminate from the diet alcoholic beverages, coffee, and all teas except for caffeine-free herbal teas.

❑ Strictly avoid the following foods: junk foods, processed refined foods, salt, saturated fats, sugar, and white flour. Instead of salt, use a kelp or potassium substitute. If necessary, a small amount of blackstrap molasses or pure maple syrup can be used as a natural sweetener in place of sugar. Use whole wheat or rye instead of white flour.

❑ Unless otherwise recommended in the table above, take vitamins and other supplements daily with meals, with the exception of vitamin E, which should be taken before meals.

❑ Try to avoid *all* known carcinogens. Eat only organic foods, if possible. Avoid tobacco smoke, polluted air, polluted water, noxious chemicals, and food additives. Use only distilled water or reverse-osmosis-filtered water. Municipal and well water can contain chlorine, fluoride, and agricultural chemical residue.

❑ Do not take any drugs except those that are prescribed by your physician. Always seek counsel and alternative opinions before deciding which treatments, if any, you will pursue.

CONSIDERATIONS

❑ If the disease is caught early, treatment for prostate cancer is usually successful. If the cancer has spread beyond the prostate, however, it is difficult to treat and cure. Unfortunately, prostate cancer can be difficult to diagnose in its early stages. Many cases are diagnosed only after the cancer has spread outside the gland. Once the cancer has spread outside the gland's capsule, the survival rate over the next five years is about 40 percent. If the disease spreads to the lymph nodes, bones, or other organs, the chances of survival drop to 20 percent.

❑ Berries help protect DNA from damage and mutation that may result in cancer.

❑ Experimental therapies such as cryoablation (freezing of cancer cells) and laser surgery are sometimes used in prostate cancer treatment.

❑ If the cancer has spread into the capsule of the gland, the standard approach is some form of radiation therapy. Ten-year survival rates are 50 to 60 percent. Radiation therapy leaves men impotent 50 percent of the time. It may also adversely affect the bladder and rectum.

❑ If the disease is confined to the prostate and a man is healthy and under seventy years old, removal of the gland (radical prostatectomy) is often recommended. About 50 percent of men who have radical prostatectomy, even with the new "nerve sparing" techniques, become impotent. Significant incontinence occurs in up to 25 percent of cases. Watchful waiting, with nutritional support and lifestyle changes, is becoming the preferred approach if the cancer is in the early stages.

❑ If the cancer has spread outside the gland, treatment is aimed at trying to block production of testosterone, which fuels the cancer. This can be done by means of orchiectomy (surgical removal of the testes) or by suppressing the production and action of hormones. For the latter, either goserelin (Zoladex) or leuprolide (Lupron) is given by monthly injections (they are fundamentally the same drug); in addition, flutamide (Eulexin) is taken orally. Together, these agents effectively shut down testosterone production and use by the body. Both orchiectomy and hormone suppression cause impotence in nearly 100 percent of the cases.

❑ Estrogens have been used effectively for the treatment of prostate cancer for sixty years. However, they can cause breast growth and other feminizing effects, as well as cardiac complications.

❑ Many consider prostate cancer to be one of the most overtreated diseases in America. Physicians in Europe have long used a conservative approach with comparable results. In addition, a 1994 report in *The New England Journal of Medicine* reported on a large group of men who refused traditional treatment. Surprisingly, they fared just as well as—and possibly better than—men who did accept medical treatment. In our experience, a conservative approach to prostate cancer has great merit, but we recommend making critical lifestyle and dietary changes and using nutritional supplementation.

❑ Dr. Hans Nieper, a German cancer specialist, uses Carnivora, a substance derived from a South American plant, to treat prostate cancer. Fresh cabbage and carrot juice are used in clinics worldwide in cancer therapy.

❑ A high-fat, low-fiber diet is linked not just to heart disease, but also to prostate cancer. Chemical reactions occur when fat is cooked, leading to the production of free radicals, which play a major role in certain cancers. It is logical to assume that the accelerating increase in prostate cancer since the 1950s must be attributable at least in part to a parallel increase in fat consumption in the United States. According to the *Journal of the National Cancer Institute*, men who eat red meat five times a week may have a risk of prostate cancer that is nearly three times higher than that for men who eat red meat less than once a week. Butter consumption also appears to contribute to this disease. Researchers theorize that a diet high in fat raises the levels of testosterone and other hormones in the body, which stimulates the prostate—and any cancerous cells in it—to grow.

A high intake of milk and coffee may also increase the risk of developing prostate cancer.

❑ Research has shown that soybeans and soy products, such as tofu, soy flour, and soymilk, have cancer-fighting powers due to the presence of a protein called genistein. Genistein apparently retards tumor growth by preventing the growth of new blood vessels to feed the tumor. It appears to be particularly effective against prostate cancer, but also works against breast cancer in women and colon cancer in both sexes.

❑ A man who is impotent as a result of treatment for prostate cancer may be able to remain sexually active through penile prostheses and other devices (*see* IMPOTENCE in Part Two).

❑ Studies from Israel indicate shark cartilage may be effective in treating prostate cancer. Its antiangiogenic potential seems to inhibit new blood vessel formation, especially in highly malignant vascular cancers.

❑ It is unclear whether benign enlargement of the prostate, a common condition in men over fifty, can eventually lead to cancer.

❑ In 1993, the *Journal of the American Medical Association* revealed a connection between vasectomy and an increased risk of prostate cancer. Reported studies of 48,000 and 29,000 men who had vasectomies showed a 66-percent and 56-percent higher rate of prostate cancer, respectively. The risk increased with age and the number of years since the vasectomy was performed. Since then, a panel called by the National Institutes of Health found no biological cause-and-effect relationship between vasectomy and prostate cancer. Not all experts accept that finding, however.

❑ A man with prostate cancer needs support and understanding from family members, friends, and physicians. Besides coming to grips with cancer and its treatments, he also has to deal with the possible loss of sexual potency, which can be very difficult. A book entitled *Coping With Prostate Cancer* by Robert H. Phillips, Ph.D. (Avery Publishing Group, 1994) provides a great deal of detailed information and practical advice to help the man with prostate cancer and his family to deal with the many different aspects of this disease.

❑ Diet and nutrition are important not only for treatment, but for prevention. An anticancer diet is composed primarily of brown rice, fresh raw fruits and vegetables, fresh juices, legumes, raw nuts and seeds, and whole grains, and *excludes* alcohol, coffee, refined carbohydrates, and strong tea. Regular intake of zinc (50 milligrams daily) and essential fatty acids (in supplement form or from cold-pressed sesame, safflower, or olive oil) in later life also may help to prevent the development of problems.

❑ *See also* PROSTATITIS/ENLARGED PROSTATE in Part Two.

❑ *See also* PAIN CONTROL in Part Three.

Prostatitis/Enlarged Prostate

The prostate is a doughnut-shaped male sex gland, positioned beneath the urinary bladder. It encircles the urinary outlet, or urethra. Contraction of the muscles in the prostate squeeze fluid from the prostate into the urethral tract during ejaculation. Prostatic fluid makes up the bulk of semen.

The prostate is the most common site of disorders in the male genitourinary system. Two of the most common prostate problems are prostatitis and benign prostatic hypertrophy (BPH), or enlarged prostate.

Prostatitis, common in men of all ages, is the inflammation of the prostate gland. The usual cause is infectious bacteria that invade the prostate from another area of the body. Hormonal changes associated with aging may also be a cause. The inflammation can result in urine retention. This causes the bladder to become distended, weak, tender, and itself susceptible to infection. Infection in the bladder is in turn easily transmitted up the ureters to the kidneys.

Prostatitis can be either acute or chronic. Symptoms of acute prostatitis include pain between the scrotum and rectum, fever, frequent urination accompanied by a burning sensation, a feeling of fullness in the bladder, and blood or pus in the urine. Symptoms of chronic prostatitis are frequent and burning urination with blood in the urine, lower back pain, and impotence. As prostatitis becomes more advanced, urination becomes more difficult.

Benign prostatic hypertrophy is the gradual enlargement of the prostate. It occurs in approximately half of all men over the age of fifty and three quarters of men over seventy years of age—a total of about 10 million American men—and is largely attributable to hormonal changes associated with aging. After the age of fifty or so, a man's testosterone and free testosterone levels decrease, while the levels of other hormones, such as prolactin and estradiol, increase. This creates an increase in the amount of dihydrotestosterone—a very potent form of testosterone—within the prostate. This causes a hyperplasia (overproduction) of prostate cells, which ultimately results in prostate enlargement.

While not cancerous, an enlarged prostate can nevertheless cause problems. If it becomes too large, it obstructs the urethral canal, interfering with urination and the ability to empty the bladder completely. Because the bladder cannot empty completely, the kidneys also may not empty as they should. Dangerous pressure on the kidneys can result. In severe cases, the kidneys may be damaged both by pressure and by substances in the urine. Bladder infections are associated with both prostatitis and enlarged prostate.

The major symptom of enlargement of the prostate is the need to pass urine frequently, with frequency increasing as time goes on. A man may find himself rising several times during the night to urinate. There can also be pain, burning, and difficulty in starting and stopping urination. The presence of blood in the urine is not uncommon.

Testing for prostatitis and enlarged prostate usually involves a digital rectal exam plus a blood test that screens for levels of prostate-specific antigen (PSA), a protein secreted by the prostate.

NUTRIENTS

SUPPLEMENT	SUGGESTED DOSAGE	COMMENTS
Essential		
Prostata from Gero Vita	1 capsule 4 times daily.	Contains all the essential nutrients for normal prostate function, plus the herbs saw palmetto and pygeum.
Vitamin B complex plus extra vitamin B$_6$ (pyridoxine)	50 mg 3 times daily. 50 mg twice daily.	Necessary for all cellular functions. Anti-stress vitamins. Has anticancer properties.
Zinc	80 mg daily. Do not exceed a total of 100 mg daily from all supplements.	Deficiency has been linked to BPH, prostatitis, and even prostate cancer. Use zinc gluconate lozenges or OptiZinc for best absorption.
Very Important		
Essential fatty acids (fish oil)	As directed on label 3 times daily.	Important in prostate function.
Garlic (Kyolic)	2 capsules 3 times daily.	Acts as a natural antibiotic.
L-Alanine and L-glutamic acid and L-glycine	As directed on label, on an empty stomach. Take with water or juice. Do not take with milk. Take with 50 mg vitamin B$_6$ and 100 mg vitamin C for better absorption.	Amino acids needed for maintaining normal prostate function. *See* AMINO ACIDS in Part One.
Pumpkin seeds		*See under* Recommendations, below.
Raw prostate glandular	As directed on label.	To normalize prostate function.
Vitamin A plus natural carotenoid complex	5,000–10,000 IU daily. As directed on label.	Potent antioxidants and immune system enhancers.
Vitamin E	600 IU daily.	Potent antioxidant and immune system enhancer.
Helpful		
Kelp	1,000–1,500 mg daily.	Supplies necessary minerals for improved prostate function.
Lecithin granules or capsules	1 tbsp 3 times daily, before meals. 1,200 mg 3 times daily, before meals.	For cellular protection.
Magnesium plus calcium	As directed on label. As directed on label.	Necessary minerals for improved prostate function.
Vitamin C	1,000–5,000 mg daily.	Promotes immune function and aids healing.

HERBS

❑ Chinese ginseng is beneficial for prostate health and sexual vitality.

❑ Teas made from the diuretic herbs buchu and corn silk are helpful. Juniper berries, parsley, slippery elm bark, and uva ursi are also natural diuretics and urinary tract tonics.

❑ Goldenseal root is a diuretic and antiseptic.
Caution: Do not take goldenseal internally on a daily basis for more than one week at a time, and use it with caution if you are allergic to ragweed.

❑ A decoction of equal quantities of gravel root, hydrangea root, and sea holly helps to ease inflammation and reduce the discomfort of urination. Take 3 to 4 teaspoonfuls three times daily. Marshmallow leaves may be added to this mixture for their demulcent properties if burning persists.

❑ Horsetail is astringent and can be used if small amounts of blood are passed, as well as for frequent urination at night. Combine it with hydrangea for even greater effect.

❑ Pygeum (*Pygeum africanum*) has been proven effective in the treatment and prevention of BPH and prostatitis in many worldwide studies. It has become a primary therapy for these conditions in Europe.

❑ Saw palmetto has been used to treat prostate enlargement and inflammation, painful ejaculation, difficult urination, and enuresis (the inability to control urination). It reduces prostatic enlargement by reducing the amount of hormonal stimulation of the prostate gland.

❑ Siberian ginseng is a tonic for the male reproductive organs.
Caution: Do not use Siberian ginseng if you have hypoglycemia, high blood pressure, or a heart disorder.

❑ Other herbs beneficial for the prostate include cayenne (capsicum) and false unicorn root.

RECOMMENDATIONS

❑ *See* Herbs, above, and try one or more of the recommended combinations. Acute inflammation or enlargement of the prostate gland often responds to certain herbal teas. If no improvement takes place or if the symptoms recur, consult a urologist.

❑ Take steps to reduce your blood cholesterol level. *See* HIGH CHOLESTEROL in Part Two. Studies have shown a connection between high cholesterol and prostate disorders. Cholesterol has been shown to accumulate in enlarged or cancerous human prostates.

❑ Use hydrotherapy to increase circulation in the prostate region. One method involves sitting in a tub that contains the hottest water tolerable for fifteen to thirty minutes once or twice a day. Another form of hydrotherapy involves spraying the lower abdomen and pelvic area with warm and cold water, alternating between three minutes of hot water and one minute of cold. Still another technique involves sitting in hot water while immersing the feet in cold water for three minutes, and then sitting in cold water while immersing the feet in hot water for one minute.

❑ Eat 1 to 4 ounces of raw pumpkin seeds every day. Pumpkin seeds are helpful for almost all prostate troubles because they are rich in zinc. As an alternative, pumpkin seed oil can be taken in capsule form.

❑ Eliminate from your lifestyle such items as tobacco, alcoholic beverages (especially beer and wine), caffeine (especially coffee and tea), chlorinated and fluoridated water, spicy and junk foods, and tomato and tomato products. Limit your exposure to pesticides and other environmental contaminants.

❑ If you have prostatitis, increase your fluid intake. Drink two to three quarts of spring or distilled water daily to stimulate urine flow. This helps to prevents cystitis and kidney infection as well as dehydration.

❑ Get regular exercise. Do not ride a bicycle, however; this may put pressure on the prostate. Walking is good exercise.

❑ If your prostate is enlarged, be cautious about using over-the-counter cold or allergy remedies. Many of these products contain ingredients that can inflame the condition and cause urinary retention.

❑ Avoid exposure to very cold weather.

CONSIDERATIONS

❑ If the prostate is infected, treatment with antibiotics and analgesics may be necessary.

❑ Enlarged prostate may be treated surgically with a procedure called transurethral resection of the prostate (TURP). About 350,000 TURPs were done in the United States in 1990. The procedure is twice as likely than are drugs or other treatments to provide long-term relief. Side effects of the procedure include retrograde ejaculation (in which the semen is pumped back up into the bladder) and in some cases impotence or incontinence. About 15 percent of men who have the procedure need another operation within eight years. Newer surgical procedures using laser technology and other technologies are available, but TURP remains the standard treatment. TURP is not used for prostatitis.

❑ The drug finasteride (Proscar) may be used to treat moderate prostate enlargement. It blocks an enzyme that converts the male hormone testosterone into dihydrotestosterone, which promotes the growth of prostate tissue. The drug has been shown to increase urine flow in 30 percent of test cases and to reduce the size of the prostate by 20 percent in more than half the test cases. But it also causes impotence and reduced libido in many cases. In addition, because it reduces the amount of prostate tissue, it can skew the results of the blood test used to detect prostate cancer.

❑ Engaging in sexual intercourse while the prostate is infected and irritated may further irritate the prostate and delay recovery.

❑ Vasectomy for sterilization has been linked to prostate disorders and even cancer.

❑ Although antibiotics are often used to treat prostatitis, the long-term use of such drugs can lead to bacterial resistance, which in turn necessitates more potent drugs, more expense, and more medical complications.

❑ Zinc deficiency is linked to enlargement of the prostate. Soil used for farming is often deficient in zinc, and unless you eat husks of cereals or brewer's yeast, it is difficult to get enough zinc in the diet. Alcohol causes a deficiency of zinc and other serious nutritional deficiencies. However, too much zinc (over 100 milligrams a day) can depress immune function.

❑ The injectable drug leuprolide (Lupron) may shrink an enlarged prostate. Side effects that can occur with the use of leuprolide include impotence, decreased libido, and even hot flashes. You should take this drug only if you are not concerned with potency. It is available by a doctor's prescription only.

❑ All men aged forty or over should have a yearly rectal examination, during which the prostate gland is checked.

Psoriasis

Psoriasis appears as patches of silvery scales or red areas on the legs, knees, arms, elbows, scalp, ears, and back. Toes and fingernails can lose their luster and develop ridges and pits. Often hereditary, this condition is linked to a rapid growth of cells in the skin's outer layer. These growths on the epidermis never mature. Whereas a normal skin cell matures and passes from the bottom layer of the skin to the epidermis in about twenty-eight days, psoriatic cells form in about eight days, causing scaly patches that spread to cover larger and larger areas. The condition is not contagious.

Psoriasis generally follows a pattern of periodic flare-ups alternating with periods of remission, most commonly begining between the ages of fifteen and twenty-five. Among other things, attacks can be triggered by nervous tension, stress, illness, injury, surgery, cuts, poison ivy, viral or bacterial infection, sunburn, overuse of drugs or alcohol, or the use of nonsteroidal anti-inflammatory drugs, lithium (Eskalith and others), chloroquine (Aralen), and beta-blockers, a type of medication frequently prescribed for heart disease and high blood pressure. Some people experience an associated arthritis that is similar to rheumatoid arthritis and that is difficult to treat.

The underlying cause of the condition is not known, but it may result from a faulty utilization of fat; psoriasis is rare in countries where the diet is low in fat. Current research points also to an immune system role in psoriasis. People with HIV or AIDS often have severe psoriasis. The buildup of toxins in an unhealthy colon also has been linked to the development of psoriasis.

NUTRIENTS

SUPPLEMENT	SUGGESTED DOSAGE	COMMENTS
Essential		
Flaxseed oil or	As directed on label 3 times daily.	To supply essential fatty acids, important for all skin disorders. Aids in preventing dryness.
primrose oil or	As directed on label 3 times daily.	
Ultimate Oil from Nature's Secret	As directed on label.	
Milk thistle		*See under* Herbs, below.
Natural beta-carotene or	25,000 IU daily.	Protects the skin tissue. *Note:* If you have diabetes, omit this supplement; people with diabetes cannot utilize beta-carotene.
carotenoid complex	As directed on label.	
Zinc	50–100 mg daily. Do not exceed this amount.	Protein metabolism depends on zinc. Protein is needed for healing. Use zinc gluconate lozenges or OptiZinc for best absorption.
Very Important		
Proteolytic enzymes	As directed on label. Take between meals.	Stimulates protein synthesis and repair.
Selenium	200 mcg daily.	Has powerful antioxidant properties.
Shark cartilage (BeneFin)	1 gm per 15 lbs of body weight daily, divided into 3 doses. If you cannot tolerate taking it orally, it can be administered rectally, in a retention enema.	Inhibits the growth of blood vessels to stop the spread of psoriasis. Itching and scaling clear first, then redness gradually fades. Allow 2–3 months to see results.
Vitamin A	As directed on label. If you are pregnant, do not exceed 10,000 IU daily.	Essential for healthy skin and nails. Use an emulsion form for easier assimilation and greater safety at higher doses.
Vitamin B complex	50 mg 3 times daily.	Necessary for all cellular functions; anti-stress vitamins that help to maintain healthy skin.
plus extra vitamin B$_1$ (thiamine) and	50 mg 3 times daily.	Needed for repair and healing of skin tissue.
pantothenic acid (vitamin B$_5$) and	100 mg 3 times daily.	Aids in proper adrenal function, relieving stress on this organ.
vitamin B$_6$ (pyridoxine) and	50 mg 3 times daily.	Aids in reducing fluid retention, keeping down infection.
vitamin B$_{12}$ and	2,000 mcg daily.	Use a lozenge or sublingual form.
folic acid	400 mcg daily.	
Vitamin C	2,000–10,000 mg daily.	Important for formation of collagen and skin tissue, and for enhancing the immune system.
Vitamin D	As directed on label.	Needed for healing of skin and for calcium uptake.
Vitamin E	400–1,200 IU daily.	Neutralizes free radicals that damage the skin. Use an emulsion form for and easier assimilation.
Important		
Kelp	1,000–1,500 mg daily.	Supplies balanced minerals. A good source of iodine.

SUPPLEMENT	SUGGESTED DOSAGE	COMMENTS
Helpful		
Herpanacine from Diamond-Herpanacine Associates	As directed on label.	Contains antioxidants, amino acids, and herbs that promote overall skin health.
Glutathione	500 mg twice daily, on an empty stomach.	A powerful antioxidant that inhibits the growth of psoriatic cells.
Lecithin granules or	1 tbsp 3 times daily, with meals.	Fat emulsifiers. Lecithin also protects the cells.
capsules or	1,200 mg 3 times daily, with meals.	
lipotrophic factors	200–500 mg daily.	
Multivitamin and mineral complex with	As directed on label.	Needed for basic vitamins and minerals.
calcium and	1,500 mg daily.	Use a chelate form.
magnesium	750 mg daily.	
VitaCarte from Phoenix Biolabs	As directed on label.	Contains pure bovine cartilage, which has been shown to be effective in improving psoriasis.

HERBS

❑ Burdock root, sarsaparilla, and yellow dock are good detoxifiers.

❑ Poultices made from chaparral, dandelion, and yellow dock can help psoriasis. *See* USING A POULTICE in Part Three.

❑ Add 2 teaspoons of ginger to bath water.

❑ To reduce redness and swelling, lightly brush off scales with a loofah and apply alcohol-free goldenseal extract.

❑ Lavender is good to use in a sauna or steam bath. It fights inflammation, and soothes and heals irritated skin.

❑ Silymarin (milk thistle extract) increases bile flow and protects the liver, which is important in keeping the blood clean. Take 300 milligrams three times daily.

RECOMMENDATIONS

❑ Eat a diet that is composed of 50 percent raw foods and includes plenty of fruits, grains, and vegetables. Include fish in the diet as well.

❑ Get plenty of dietary fiber. Fiber is critical for maintaining a healthy colon. Many fiber components, such as apple pectin and psyllium husks, are able to bind to bowel toxins and promote their excretion in the feces. Also follow the program for colon cleansing. *See* COLON CLEANSING in Part Three. A clean colon is very important.

❑ Use fish oil, flaxseed oil, or primrose oil supplements. They contain ingredients that interfere with the production and storage of arachidonic acid (AA), a natural substance that promotes the inflammatory response and makes the lesions of psoriasis turn red and swell. Red meat and dairy products contain AA. Avoid these foods.

❑ Apply seawater to the affected area with cotton several times a day.

❑ Use cold-pressed flaxseed, sesame, or soybean oils.

❑ Do not consume citrus fruits, fried foods, processed foods, saturated fats (found in meat and dairy products), sugar, or white flour.

CONSIDERATIONS

❑ There is no known cure for psoriasis. Treatment is aimed at reducing the symptoms and includes the use of ointments and creams to soften the scales combined with gentle scrubbing to remove them. Sometimes ultraviolet light therapy is used to retard the production of new skin cells. UVL therapy is sometimes combined with tar therapy; tar is applied to the scaly patches, which are then exposed to the UV light. A similar treatment involves using a drug called anthralin (Drithocreme, Dritho-Scalp) instead of tar in tandem with the UV light. Only the scales and skin debris, which can be quite itchy, can be removed.

❑ Outbreaks of psoriasis seem to lessen during the summer months. It may even go away on its own, but once you have had psoriasis, it is always possible that it will return.

❑ Recent research has led some to believe that rapid growth of psoriatic cells can be attributed to problems with prostaglandin regulation, and a deficiency of sulfur and fatty acids. In a study at Marselisborg Hospital in Denmark, Dr. Knud Kragballe used a mixture of omega-3 and omega-6 essential fatty acids to treat people with psoriasis. At the end of the twelve-week test, there was a moderate improvement of the skin condition in most cases. Some researchers disagree, but we have found fatty acid supplementation to benefit skin disorders.

❑ The drug methotrexate (also sold as Rheumatrex) is effective for severe psoriasis. However, this drug can cause liver damage, especially with long-term use. Another drug, hydroxyurea (Hydrea), and drugs called retinoids, are under study. Cyclosporine (Sandimmune) therapy has been tested with good results. A study by Boston University of a drug called calcitriol (Rocaltrol) found it resulted in improvement when applied directly to the skin. All of these drugs have potentially serious side effects.

❑ The freezing of moderately sized psoriatic lesions using liquid nitrogen has been tested, with good results.

❑ Cortisone creams, which discourage skin cells from multiplying, are often prescribed for psoriasis, but long-term use makes the skin thin and delicate.

❑ A skin patch called Actiderm, manufactured by ConvaTec/Squibb, can be applied over most topical psoriasis medications, especially steroid (cortisone) ointments, to make them more effective. The patch allows one to achieve better results with milder steroids and fewer doses.

❑ Activated vitamin D_3 ointment (Dovonex), available by prescription only, has produced good results for many people with severe forms of psoriasis.

❑ The drug etretinate (Tegison), a retinoid used for stubborn cases of psoriasis, can cause bone spurs in the knees and ankles. One study found that 84 percent of those who used this drug for five years had bony buildups causing stiffness and restriction of movement.

❑ Long-wave ultraviolet light has been effectively used to treat psoriasis, but it may increase the likelihood of skin cancer. Exposure to the sun for fifteen minutes to half an hour (not longer) may reduce the scaling and redness. A liquid drug called methoxsalen (Oxsoralen-Ultra) is also widely used.

❑ Further study must be done on the subject, but researchers believe that shark cartilage may be very effective for the treatment of psoriasis, without the risk of toxicity that standard drugs entail.

❑ For more information about psoriasis, you can contact the National Psoriasis Foundation at 6600 SW 92nd Avenue, Suite 300, Portland, OR 97223; telephone 503–244–7404 or 800–723–9166.

Pyelonephritis

See under KIDNEY DISEASE.

Pyorrhea

See under PERIODONTAL DISEASE.

Radiation Sickness

Radiation sickness is caused by exposure to radioactive substances. These are elements made up of unstable atoms that give off energy as the result of spontaneous decay of their nuclei. If the energy released by a radioactive element is strong enough to dislodge electrons from other atoms or molecules in its path, it can damage or even kill living tissue. This type of radiation is called ionizing radiation. Even if only one cell is exposed to radiation, the radiation can destroy, damage, or alter the makeup of that cell. The alteration of cell structure by radioactive particles can lead to the development of cancer. If a cell's DNA is damaged, this can cause genetic mutations that can be passed down to offspring.

The type and extent of damage done by exposure to radiation depends on the total dose of radiation received; the length of time over which it was received; and the size and location of the body area involved. Damage obviously tends to be worse with greater degrees of exposure. This may be modified, however, by the length of time involved.

A relatively high total dose of radiation might be fatal if received in the space of a few minutes, but considerably less harmful if accumulated over weeks or months. Similarly, radiation may be better tolerated if it affects only a small percentage of the body's tissues, and/or if certain key organs are not affected. Some types of tissue are more susceptible than others to radiation damage. Generally, cells that are replaced relatively rapidly are more sensitive than those that reproduce over longer periods of time.

Radioactive elements are structurally similar to their nonradioactive counterparts, differing only in the number of neutrons the atoms contain. This is why nutrition is important in preventing or blocking damage from exposure to radioactive elements. If you do not obtain sufficient amounts of calcium, potassium, and other minerals in your diet, your body may absorb radioactive elements that are similar in structure to these nutrients. For example, if you do not obtain enough calcium, your body will absorb radioactive strontium 90 or other elements that are similar in structure to calcium, if they are available. Similarly, if you obtain sufficient potassium from your diet, your body will be less likely to retain any radioactive cesium 137 it encounters, as this element is similar to potassium. If the cells are able to obtain all nutrients they need from your diet, they will be less likely to absorb radioactive substitutes, which are then more likely to be discarded from the body.

The effects of radiation exposure can be acute, following a single, relatively high-intensity exposure, or they can be delayed or chronic. Acute reactions to radiation are extremely dangerous. They cause symptoms of listlessness, nausea, vomiting, weakness, and loss of coordination, leading to dehydration, convulsions, shock, and even death. Fortunately, the amount and type of exposure that causes such serious reactions is rare. Much more common is chronic and/or low-level exposure. Symptoms associated with this type of radiation exposure include cataracts, dizziness, fatigue, headache, and nausea. Among the most frequent sources of low-level radiation exposure are medical and dental x-rays (see X-Ray Radiation in this section), as well as other diagnostic and therapeutic procedures involving the use of radioactive materials. Many people are injected with radioactive elements designed to trace a problem area so that an accurate diagnosis can be made. Other sources of radiation exposure include radon or uranium in soil or building materials; tobacco smoke; and such devices as cellular phones, computers with video display terminals, electronic games, microwave ovens, radar devices, satellite dishes, and smoke detectors. Workers in certain industries, such as nuclear power generation and the production of radioactive materials for medical and industrial applications, are more likely than most people to be exposed to problematic levels of radiation.

Radiotherapy treatment for cancer involves the administration of fairly high doses of radiation specifically targeted at cancerous cells. The idea underlying this treatment is that the radiation kills the cancer, but healthy tissue, which is not targeted, is only minimally affected. Not sur-

prisingly, the major side effect of this type of treatment is radiation sickness, with the classic symptoms of nausea, vomiting, headache, weakness, loss of appetite, and hair loss.

The specific dietary and nutritional approach to minimizing the effects of radiation depends on the particular type of radiation involved.

RADIOACTIVE IODINE

Iodine is needed by the thyroid to produce hormones that help to regulate body processes. If the amount of iodine in the diet is insufficient, the body may instead supply the thyroid with radioactive iodine 131 (I-131), which is fairly widespread in the environment due to atmospheric contamination of food and water. For example, I-131 is prevalent in milk due to exposure of cows and goats to radioactive (and acid) rain in the fields. The presence of radioactive I-131 in the thyroid can damage the cells, decreasing the functioning ability of the thyroid and possibly leading to cancer.

Many people were exposed to radioactive iodine fallout as a result of the 1986 nuclear disaster in Chernobyl, Ukraine. In an effort to protect them from this dangerous radioactive element, Soviet health authorities gave people likely to have been exposed large amounts of (nonradioactive) iodine. This was done to prevent the absorption of at least some of the radioactive iodine salts; if the body is saturated with iodine, it is more likely to excrete and less likely to absorb the radioactive element.

The destructive power of radioactive iodine can be used in medical treatment, as in the treatment of thyroid cancer. I-131 may be employed to destroy any malignant thyroid tissue left behind after surgery to remove a cancerous tumor. If thyroid cancer is inoperable, I-131 may be used in conjunction with external radiation treatment.

NUTRIENTS

SUPPLEMENT	SUGGESTED DOSAGE	COMMENTS
Very Important		
Calcium and magnesium	1,500 mg daily. 750 mg daily.	Protects against radiation.
Coenzyme Q10	60 mg daily.	Protects against many chemicals and radiation.
Kelp	2,000–3,000 mg daily.	Contains essential minerals, especially iodine, that protect against radiation sickness.
Vitamin C with citrus bioflavonoids and rutin	5,000–20,000 mg daily, in divided doses. See ASCORBIC ACID FLUSH in Part Three.	A powerful free radical scavenger. A noncitrus bioflavonoid that neutralizes acidic wastes.
Vitamin E	Start with 400 IU daily and increase slowly to 800 IU daily.	Neutralizes harmful free radicals.

Important		
Garlic (Kyolic)	2 capsules 3 times daily.	A powerful immunostimulant and protector.
Grape seed extract	As directed on label.	A powerful antioxidant. Protects against free radicals.
L-Cysteine and L-methionine	500 mg each daily, on an empty stomach. Take with water or juice. Do not take with milk. Take with 50 mg vitamin B_6 and 100 mg vitamin C for better absorption.	Potent detoxifiers that help protect the liver. Important for protection against radiation and pollution. See AMINO ACIDS in Part One.
Lecithin granules or capsules	1 tbsp 3 times daily, before meals. 1,200 mg 3 times daily, before meals.	Necessary for cellular protection.
Raw thyroid glandular	As directed on label.	To protect and support the thyroid. See GLANDULAR THERAPY in Part Three.
Vitamin B complex	100 mg twice daily, with meals.	For cellular function and protection.
Helpful		
Multivitamin and mineral complex	As directed on label.	For cellular protection.

Recommendations

❑ Eat plenty of cruciferous vegetables, such as broccoli, Brussels sprouts, cabbage, and cauliflower.

❑ Include in the diet soured milk products such as yogurt, buttermilk, and kefir. These contain the *Lactobacillus* bacteria that protect the gastrointestinal tract. They have also been found to protect against radiation.

❑ Supplement your diet with pectin, found in apples and kelp. Kelp is an iodine-rich food. The element sodium alginate, which is also found in seaweed, acts as a chelating agent. It protects the body from the harmful effects of radiation by binding with the radioactive elements, and then excreting them from the body.

STRONTIUM 90

Strontium 90 (Sr-90) is a radioactive element that is similar in structure to calcium. Due to nuclear testing, Sr-90 has contaminated the earth and has been passed on to us in water and foods, especially milk and milk products. Cattle feed is often made from crops irrigated with water contaminated with Sr-90. This radioactive element accumulates in the bones and teeth.

Making sure that your diet contains adequate amounts of calcium can protect the body from Sr-90; studies indicate that the body retains Sr-90 only if sufficient amounts of calcium are not available. Contamination with Sr-90 is associated with anemia as well as with bone cancer (osteosarcoma), leukemia, and many other forms of cancer. To protect against Sr-90, include the following supplements in your program.

NUTRIENTS

SUPPLEMENT	SUGGESTED DOSAGE	COMMENTS
Helpful		
Apple pectin	As directed on label.	Binds with Sr-90 and removes it from the body.
Calcium and magnesium	2,000 mg daily. 1,000 mg daily.	Counteracts Sr-90. Take calcium and magnesium in a 2-to-1 ratio. Use chelate forms.
Coenzyme Q_{10}	60 mg daily.	Important free radical scavenger.
Garlic (Kyolic)	2 capsules 3 times daily.	A potent immunostimulant.
Grape seed extract	As directed on label.	A powerful antioxidant.
Kelp	1,000–1,500 mg daily.	Contains necessary minerals, especially iodine, to protect against accumulation of Sr-90.
L-Cysteine and L-methionine	As directed on label, on an empty stomach. Take with water or juice. Do not take with milk. Take with 50 mg vitamin B_6 and 100 mg vitamin C for better absorption.	To protect against the harmful effects of radioactivity and pollution. See AMINO ACIDS in Part One.
Lecithin granules or capsules	1 tbsp 3 times daily, with meals. 1,200 mg 3 times daily, with meals.	Protects cell membranes.
Multivitamin and mineral complex	As directed on label.	Essential to basic radiation protection. Use a high-potency formula.
Selenium	200 mcg daily.	An important antioxidant.
Superoxide dismutase (SOD)	As directed on label.	A powerful free radical scavenger.
Vitamin B complex	100 mg daily.	For cellular enzyme systems. Use high-stress formula.
Vitamin C	2,000–10,000 mg daily, in divided doses.	Neutralizes and destroys free radicals formed by radiation, especially in combination with vitamin E.
Vitamin E	Start with 200 IU daily and increase slowly to 800 IU daily.	Neutralizes and destroys free radicals formed by radiation, especially in combination with vitamin C.

Recommendations

❑ Eliminate from the diet all dairy products, except for yogurt and soured products. Milk and dairy products are major sources of dietary Sr-90 in the United States.

❑ Supplement your diet with pectin (found in apples), seaweed, and sunflower seeds. Pectin binds with Sr-90.

X-RAY RADIATION

Dental checkups today typically include x-rays to locate cavities. Physicians take x-rays to determine whether a bone is broken, to check cardiovascular and respiratory health, and to locate tumors and areas of dysfunction. Women are urged to have regular mammograms for early detection of breast cancer. Despite the widespread use of x-rays, dentists, physicians, chiropractors, and hospitals have often ignored the potential danger and long-term effects of even small amounts of radiation. Sterility, tissue damage, and cancer are among the risks for those exposed to low levels of radiation from x-rays. Women who are exposed to x-rays while pregnant are at a higher risk of having a miscarriage or delivering a baby with birth defects.

Cancer research indicates that a significant percentage of women in the United States have inherited a gene, dubbed *oncogene AC*, that is sensitive to x-ray exposure. For these women, even short periods of x-ray exposure can lead to the development of cancer.

The level of radiation from x-rays is measured in units called roentgens (pronounced RENT-gins). The National Academy of Science has reported that exposure (single or cumulative) to 10 milliroentgens of radiation from x-rays increases the risk of cancer. This is the same amount of radiation that the chest is exposed to during a tuberculosis chest x-ray. Mammography uses a much lower dose. However, there is mounting evidence to suggest that there may be *no* safe level of radiation. Prolonged exposure to radiation also destroys the body's immune system.

To protect against radiation from x-rays, follow the supplement program below.

NUTRIENTS

SUPPLEMENT	SUGGESTED DOSAGE	COMMENTS
Very Important		
Coenzyme Q10	100 mg daily.	Protects the body from harmful radiation.
Glutathione plus L-cysteine and L-methionine	500 mg each daily, on an empty stomach. Take with water or juice. Do not take with milk. Take with 50 mg vitamin B_6 and 100 mg vitamin C for better absorption.	To detoxify harmful substances and protect against the harmful effects of radiation.
Kelp	1,000–1,500 mg daily.	Protects against radiation. Take kelp in tablet form or eat sea vegetables.
Important		
Garlic (Kyolic)	2 capsules 3 times daily.	Stimulates and protects the immune system.
Grape seed extract	As directed on label.	A powerful antioxidant.
Oxy-5000 Forte from American Biologics	As directed on label.	This antioxidant is high in superoxide dismutase (SOD), a powerful antioxidant.
Pantothenic acid (vitamin B_5)	200 mg before and after x-ray exposure; 50 mg daily thereafter.	Protects against the harmful effects of radiation.
Selenium	200 mcg daily.	A free radical scavenger that protects against cancer.
Vitamin C with bioflavonoids	3,000–10,000 mg daily.	Protects immune system. A vitamin C complex that contains 200 mg of rutin per capsule is best.
Helpful		
Brewer's yeast	As directed on label.	A natural source of pantothenic acid, as well as the other B vitamins.
Lecithin granules or capsules	1 tbsp 3 times daily, with meals. 1,200 mg 3 times daily, with meals.	Protects cell membranes from radiation.
Vitamin A	25,000 IU daily. If you are pregnant, do not exceed 10,000 IU daily.	Protects and strengthens the immune system, especially in combination with vitamin E.
Vitamin B complex plus extra inositol	50 mg 3 times daily. 100 mg daily.	Helps to protect against the harmful effects of radiation.
Vitamin E	400–1,000 IU daily.	Protects and strengthens the immune system, especially in combination with vitamin A.
Zinc	50–80 mg daily. Do not exceed a total of 100 mg daily from all supplements.	Helps increase immunity. Use zinc gluconate lozenges or OptiZinc for best absorption.

Herbs

❑ The herb chaparral helps protect against harmful radiation.

Caution: Do not use this herb on a regular basis, and do not take it daily for longer than one week. Long-term use may be harmful to the liver.

Recommendations

❑ Include apples in the diet; they are a good source of pectin, which binds with radioactive particles.

❑ Eat buckwheat, which is high in rutin, a bioflavonoid that protects against radiation.

❑ Consume avocados, lemons, and cold-pressed safflower and olive oils. These supply essential fatty acids.

❑ Drink plenty of steam-distilled water.

❑ Avoid x-rays unless absolutely necessary.

Considerations

❑ A study at the University of Medicine and Dentistry of New Jersey in Newark showed that rats given orange juice before exposure to low-level radiation (1 to 50 rads) suffered two times less damage than rats given water before exposure.

❑ *See also* WEAKENED IMMUNE SYSTEM in Part Two.

Rash

See SKIN RASH.

Raynaud's Phenomenon

Raynaud's phenomenon is a circulatory disorder that results in the hands, and sometimes feet, being hypersensitive to the cold. When the hands are exposed to cold temperatures, the small arteries that supply the toes and fingers suddenly contract and go into spasm. As a result, the fingers and toes are deprived of adequate amounts of oxygenated blood, and become whitish or bluish in color. The symptoms come on quickly, and may also be triggered by emotional stress. Over time, the condition may result in a general shrinkage of the affected area. Ultimately, ulcers may form, damaging the tissues and resulting in chronic infection under and around the fingernails and toenails. In severe cases, gangrene may result from prolonged and persistent contraction of the arteries.

Raynaud's phenomenon is more common in women than in men. It may occur by itself or it may be a complication of another underlying illness. Some of the disorders that can lead to Raynaud's phenomenon include arteriosclerosis and Buerger's disease, a chronic inflammation of the blood vessels in the extremities that is most common in people who smoke. Certain drugs that affect the blood vessels—such as calcium channel blockers, ergot preparations, and alpha- and beta-adrenergic blockers—have been known to produce symptoms similar to those of Raynaud's as a side effect. Recent research has also linked Raynaud's with other conditions involving abnormal constriction of blood vessels, including migraine and Prinzmetal's angina (angina caused by spasms in the coronary arteries). If symptoms occur on their own, and are not related to any other condition, a person is said to have *Raynaud's disease*.

NUTRIENTS

SUPPLEMENT	SUGGESTED DOSAGE	COMMENTS
Essential		
Coenzyme Q10	100–200 mg daily.	Improves tissue oxygenation.
Vitamin E	Start with 200 IU daily and increase slowly to 1,000 IU daily.	Improves circulation; acts as an anticoagulant, dissolving clots in the legs, heart, and lungs. Use emulsion form for easier assimilation and greater safety at higher doses.
Very Important		
Calcium and	1,500 mg daily, at bedtime.	To protect the arteries from stress caused by sudden blood pressure changes.
magnesium and	750 mg daily.	
zinc	50 mg daily. Do not exceed a total of 100 mg daily from all supplements.	
Lecithin granules or	1 tbsp 3 times daily, with meals.	Lowers blood lipid levels.
capsules	1,200 mg 3 times daily, with meals.	
Chlorophyll or	As directed on label.	Helps to fight infection and enhance blood flow.
Kyo-Green from Wakunaga	As directed on label.	A fresh "green drink" made from leafy greens that supplies chlorophyll and other nutrients.
Choline and inositol	As directed on label.	Lowers cholesterol and helps circulation.
Dimethylglycine (DMG) (Aangamik DMG from FoodScience Labs)	1 tablet 3 times daily.	Improves tissue oxygenation.
Vitamin B complex plus extra	100 mg daily.	B vitamins are necessary for metabolism of fat and cholesterol. Use a high-potency formula.
vitamin B6 (pyridoxine) and	50 mg daily.	
folic acid plus	400 mcg daily.	
vitamin B3 (niacin)	100 mg daily. Do not exceed this amount.	Dilates small arteries, improving circulation. *Caution:* Do not take niacin if you have a liver disorder, gout, or high blood pressure.
Important		
Aerobic 07 from Aerobic Life Industries	As directed on label.	Improves tissue oxygenation.
Bee propolis or	As directed on label.	To strengthen the cardiovascular system and act as a natural antibiotic.
royal jelly	As directed on label.	
Flaxseed oil or	1,000 mg daily.	To supply essential fatty acids, which are necessary for circulation and help prevent hardening of the arteries.
primrose oil or	1,000 mg daily.	
salmon oil	As directed on label.	

HERBS

❑ Butcher's broom, cayenne (capsicum), ginkgo biloba, and pau d'arco can be used separately or in combination to improve circulation and strengthen blood vessels.

RECOMMENDATIONS

❑ Eat a diet composed of 50 percent raw foods. *See* NUTRITION, DIET, AND WELLNESS in Part One, and follow the dietary guidelines.

❑ Avoid fatty and fried foods.

❑ Avoid caffeine. This stimulant constricts the blood vessels.

❑ Keep your hands and feet warm. A warm climate is best. Wear comfortable shoes and do not go barefoot outdoors. Always wear gloves in cold weather.

❑ Avoid stress as much as possible.

❑ Avoid drugs that constrict the blood vessels, such as birth control pills and migraine headache medicine.

❑ Do not smoke. Nicotine constricts the blood vessels.

CONSIDERATIONS

❑ The calcium channel blocker nifedipine (Adalat, Procardia) is a generally accepted treatment for Raynaud's phenomenon. Like all drugs, this can have side effects.

❑ *See also* CIRCULATORY PROBLEMS in Part Two.

Repetitive Motion Injury

See CARPAL TUNNEL SYNDROME.

Retinitis Pigmentosa

See under EYE PROBLEMS.

Reye's Syndrome

Reye's syndrome is a serious disease that affects many internal organs, particularly the brain and liver. It primarily strikes children between the ages of four and fifteen. Most cases of Reye's syndrome occur after a viral infection such as the flu or chickenpox. It has also been associated with Epstein-Barr virus, influenza B, and enteroviruses (viruses that infect mainly the gastrointestinal tract).

Four to six days after the onset of the viral illness, the child suddenly develops a fever and severe vomiting. Other symptoms include mental and personality changes that may manifest themselves as confusion, drowsiness, lethargy, memory lapses, and/or unusual belligerence and irritability. In addition, the child may experience weakness and paralysis in the arms or legs, double vision, palpitations, speech impairment, impaired skin integrity, and/or hearing loss. Convulsions, coma, brain damage, and even death may follow, usually the result of cerebral edema or respiratory failure. Fortunately, due to increased awareness of the disease, and especially of the importance of early detection and prompt treatment, the mortality rate for this illness has been declining. It currently stands at approximately 5 percent.

The exact cause of Reye's syndrome is unknown, but as a result of research conducted in the early 1980s, it is known that the combination of aspirin and viral illness dramatically increases the risk of developing this dangerous disorder. This is why aspirin is no longer recommended for routine use as a pain reliever for children.

The following supplements are designed for use once appropriate medical measures, including hospitalization, have been taken and recovery has begun. Discuss any supplements with a health care professional before using them. Unless otherwise specified, the doses recommended here are for persons age eighteen and over. For a child between twelve and seventeen, use three-quarters the rec-

ommended dose; for a child between six and twelve, use one-half the recommended dose; and for a child under six, use one-quarter the recommended dose.

NUTRIENTS

SUPPLEMENT	SUGGESTED DOSAGE	COMMENTS
Important		
Branched-chain amino acid complex	As directed on label.	Prevents muscle depletion. *See* AMINO ACIDS in Part One.
Flaxseed oil	As directed on label.	To supply essential fatty acids, vital for maintaining and restoring skin suppleness and moisture.
Garlic (Kyolic)	As directed on label.	Increases energy and enhances immune function.
Lecithin granules	1 tbsp 3 times daily.	To supply choline, important in transmission of nerve impulses and in energy production.
or		
capsules	1,200 mg 3 times daily.	
or		
phosphatidyl choline	As directed on label.	
L-Methionine	As directed on label.	Powerful antioxidants that protect and detoxify the liver.
plus		
glutathione	As directed on label.	
Raw brain glandular	As directed on label.	To improve brain function.
Vitamin A	5,000 IU daily.	Helps in formation of healthy skin cells.
plus		
natural beta-carotene	15,000 IU daily.	Used by the body to make vitamin A as needed.
Vitamin B complex	50–100 mg daily.	Needed for all enzyme systems and to support healing.
Vitamin E	400 IU daily.	To protect against free radical damage.

HERBS

❑ The following are herbal remedies that can be useful once the acute phase of the illness has passed and recovery has begun:

• Alfalfa, hawthorn berry, hyssop, milk thistle, pau d'arco, Siberian ginseng, and wild yam help to rebuild and strengthen the liver.

Caution: Do not use Siberian ginseng if you have hypoglycemia, high blood pressure, or a heart disorder.

• A lotion containing aloe vera, calendula, and/or chamomile can be used to nourish and heal the skin.

• Catnip or chamomile tea helps to reduce anxiety.

Caution: Do not use chamomile on an ongoing basis, and avoid it completely if you are allergic to ragweed.

• Ginger and peppermint are good for relief of nausea.

• Gravel root, hydrangea, oat straw, parsley root, and uva ursi have diuretic properties.

• Korean (or Chinese) ginseng (*Panax ginseng*) helps to reduce fatigue.

Caution: Do not use this herb if you have high blood pressure.

Before administering them, discuss any herbal remedies you wish to use with your health care provider.

❑ *Do not* give white willow bark to a child. It contains a chemical very similar to aspirin.

RECOMMENDATIONS

❑ Be alert for the following warning signs any time your child is recovering from a viral infection such as a cold, the flu, an ear infection, or chickenpox:

• Prolonged and heavy vomiting, followed by drowsiness.

• Agitation, disorientation, and delirium.

• Fatigue, lethargy, and lapses in memory.

If you have *even a suspicion* that you (or your child) may be developing the disease, seek professional help at once. Reye's syndrome progresses rapidly and is extremely dangerous. Some health care providers, however, may dismiss your concerns, telling you to use aspirin (or acetaminophen) and to call back if there is no improvement. *Do not* be put off. Go to the nearest hospital emergency room immediately and explain the situation.

❑ If Reye's syndrome is diagnosed, follow your health care provider's recommendations regarding treatment and care, both during the period of hospitalization and afterwards, at home.

❑ *Never* give aspirin to a child with a fever or other sign of viral illness. To be safe, many experts recommend against giving children aspirin for any reason. Use acetaminophen (Tylenol, Datril, and others) or ibuprofen (Advil, Nuprin, and others) instead.

CONSIDERATIONS

❑ Treatment for Reye's syndrome depends upon the stage of the disease, but it involves hospitalization. Typical hospital care includes the administration of intravenous fluids to restore blood electrolytes and glucose levels, and sometimes a diuretic to reduce inflammation and help eliminate waste and excess fluid. In some cases, surgery may be performed to reduce swelling and pressure on the brain.

❑ If a person with Reye's syndrome receives an intravenous solution of glucose (sugar) and electrolytes (mineral salts) within twelve to twenty-four hours after the heavy vomiting starts, the chance of recovery is excellent. This treatment is safe.

❑ The British aspirin industry withdrew all children's aspirin products from the British market a number of years ago in response to the discovery of the link with Reye's syndrome.

❑ A study done by the U.S. Centers for Disease Control and Prevention found that 96 percent of the children who had Reye's syndrome had been given aspirin in the presence of a viral illness. The study also indicated a direct correlation between the amount of aspirin taken and the severity of the disease. The makers of aspirin are now required to alert users to the link between aspirin and this potentially life-threatening condition.

❑ Research is being conducted concerning a possible connection between Reye's syndrome and the drug trimethobenzamide (Tigan), which is used in suppository form to control nausea and vomiting.

❑ *See also* CHICKENPOX, COMMON COLD, and INFLUENZA, all in Part Two.

Rheumatic Fever

Rheumatic fever is a complication of a streptococcal infection. It typically develops following strep throat, tonsillitis, scarlet fever, or ear infection. It most often affects children aged three to eighteen. It may affect one or several parts of the body, among them the heart, brain, and joints. If the heart is affected, permanent damage to one or more heart valves may result.

The first signs of rheumatic fever are typically pain, inflammation, and stiffness in a large joint such as the knee, accompanied by fever. The pain and swelling can travel from one joint to another. There may be an accompanying skin rash. After one occurrence, the disease tends to recur.

Unless otherwise specified, the following recommended dosages are for persons over the age of eighteen. For a child between twelve and seventeen years old, reduce the dose to three-quarters the recommended amount. For a child between six and twelve, use one-half the recommended dose, and for a child under six years old, use one-quarter the recommended amount.

NUTRIENTS

SUPPLEMENT	SUGGESTED DOSAGE	COMMENTS
Important		
Acidophilus or	As directed on label. Take on an empty stomach.	Especially important if antibiotics are prescribed.
Bifido Factor from Natren or	As directed on label.	For adults.
LifeStart from Natren	As directed on label.	For children.
Garlic (Kyolic)	2 capsules 3 times daily.	A natural antibiotic.
L-Carnitine	500 mg twice daily, on an empty stomach.	Protects the heart.
L-Methionine	500 mg daily, on an empty stomach. Take with water or juice. Do not take with milk. Take with 50 mg vitamin B_6 and 100 mg vitamin C for better absorption.	An important free radical fighter. *See* AMINO ACIDS in Part One.
Vitamin C	5,000–20,000 mg daily, in divided doses. *See* ASCORBIC ACID FLUSH in Part Three.	Boosts immune function and aids in reducing pain and swelling.

Helpful		
Calcium plus	1,500 mg daily.	Important nutrients that work together. Use chelate forms.
magnesium	1,000 mg daily.	
Coenzyme Q10	100 mg daily.	Boosts immune function.
Concentrace from Trace Minerals Research	As directed on label.	To supply trace minerals needed for bone and joint health. Increases energy.
Dimethylsulfoxide (DMSO)	Apply topically as directed on label.	To relieve joint pain. Should be used by adults only. Use only DMSO from a health food store.
Flaxseed oil	As directed on label.	Reduces pain and inflammation.
Free-form amino acid complex	As directed on label.	To supply protein, needed to strengthen body and for tissue repair. Use a formula containing all essential amino acids.
Joint Support from Now Foods	As directed on label.	Contains vitamins, minerals, and herbs to nourish and protect the joints.
Kelp	1,000–1,500 mg daily.	Contains essential nutrients.
Multivitamin and mineral complex	As directed on label.	To maintain a balance of all necessary nutrients.
Proteolytic enzymes	As directed on label. Take between meals.	An important antioxidant.
Raw thymus glandular	500 mg twice daily.	Stimulates immune response.
Vitamin A plus	10,000 IU daily.	Important antioxidants. Use emulsion forms for easier assimilation.
natural beta-carotene or	15,000 IU daily.	
carotenoid complex (Betatene)	As directed on label.	
Vitamin B complex	50 mg 3 times daily.	For healing and improved immune function.
Vitamin D or	400 IU or more daily.	Needed for healing and absorption of minerals, especially calcium.
cod liver oil	As directed on label.	
Vitamin E emulsion or	800 IU daily.	Increases tissue oxygenation and reduces fever. Emulsion form is recommended for easier assimilation.
capsules	Start with 200 IU daily and increase slowly to 800 IU daily.	

HERBS

❑ Bayberry bark, burdock root, milk thistle, nettle, pau d'arco, sage, and yellow dock purify the blood, fight infection, and aid in recuperation after the trauma of illness.
Caution: Do not use sage if you suffer from any kind of seizure disorder.

❑ Birch leaves and lobelia both help to reduce pain.
Caution: Do not take lobelia internally on an ongoing basis.

❑ Catnip tea is a nerve tonic. It can also be used as an enema to reduce fever. *See* ENEMAS in Part Three.

❑ Echinacea, hawthorn leaf, myrrh gum, and red clover detoxify and de-acidify the blood.

❑ Dandelion has a long history in the treatment of fever.

❑ Goldenseal is a natural antibiotic.
Caution: Do not take goldenseal internally on a daily basis for more than one week at a time, do not use it during pregnancy, and use it with caution if you are allergic to ragweed.

❑ Wintergreen oil can be applied to the chest in compress form to relieve pain.

RECOMMENDATIONS

❑ Drink plenty of fresh juices and distilled water.

❑ Eat no solid food until the fever subsides and joint pain begins to ease. Then keep to a light diet, including fresh fruits and vegetables, yogurt, cottage cheese, and fruit juices.

❑ Do not consume any caffeine, carbonated soft drinks, fried foods, processed or refined foods, salt, or sugar in any form during the recovery period. These foods slow healing.

❑ Get plenty of bed rest. This is vital for recovery.

❑ If antibiotics are prescribed, take acidophilus to replace the needed "friendly" bacteria. Antibiotics may be necessary to combat the underlying *Streptococcus* infection and help prevent permanent heart damage. Do not take the acidophilus at the same time as the antibiotics, however.

CONSIDERATIONS

❑ Massage therapy and mild exercise such as yoga can be helpful for preventing muscle atrophy during bed rest.

❑ *See also* ARTHRITIS; FEVER; and/or SORE THROAT, all in Part Two.

Rheumatoid Arthritis

See under ARTHRITIS.

Rickets/Osteomalacia

Rickets and osteomalacia are two terms for the disorder caused by vitamin D deficiency. In children, this disease is called rickets, and results either from inadequate intake of vitamin D or from too little exposure to sunlight (sunlight causes vitamin D to be synthesized in the skin). The lack of vitamin D in turn affects the body's ability to absorb calcium and phosphorus. Early signs include nervousness, painful muscle spasms, leg cramps, and numbness in the extremities. Ultimately, bone malformations may develop due to softening of the bones—bowed legs, knock-knees, scoliosis (abnormal curvature of the spine), a narrow rib cage, a protruding breastbone, and/or beading at the ends of the ribs—as well as decaying teeth, delayed walking, irritability, restlessness, and profuse sweating.

In adults, vitamin D deficiency disease is referred to as osteomalacia, and is usually related to the body's inability to absorb vitamin D properly. It is most likely to occur in pregnant women and nursing mothers, whose nutritional requirements are higher than normal, or in people with malabsorption problems. It may also affect individuals who do not get enough exposure to sunshine or those whose diets are so low in fat that adequate bile cannot be manufactured and vitamin D cannot be absorbed. Osteomalacia is difficult to diagnose, and is often misdiagnosed as osteoporosis.

Unless otherwise specified, the dosages recommended in this section are for adults. For a child between the ages of twelve and seventeen, reduce the dose to three-quarters the recommended amount. For a child between six and twelve, use one-half the recommended dose, and for a child under the age of six, use one-quarter the recommended amount.

NUTRIENTS

SUPPLEMENT	SUGGESTED DOSAGE	COMMENTS
Essential		
Boron	3 mg daily. Do not exceed this amount.	Enhances calcium absorption.
Calcium	1,500 mg daily.	Necessary to remineralize bone. Do not use bone meal or dolomite as a source of calcium, as these may contain lead.
Phosphorus	As directed on label.	Needed for bone and tooth formation.
Silica	500 mg daily.	Supplies silicon, which strengthens bones and connective tissue. Aids calcium absorption.
Vitamin D	400–600 IU daily. Do not exceed this amount.	Necessary for utilization of calcium and phosphorus.
Important		
Betaine hydrochloride (HCl)	As directed on label.	May be needed for proper digestion.
Cod liver oil	As directed on label.	A good source of vitamins A and D.
Multivitamin and mineral complex plus extra vitamin B$_{12}$	As directed on label. 300 mcg daily.	If malabsorption is a problem, take higher amounts of all vitamins and minerals.
Proteolytic enzymes	As directed on label. Take between meals.	Important in digestion.
Vitamin A	10,000 IU daily.	Necessary for growth.
Zinc	30 mg daily.	Needed for calcium absorption. Use zinc gluconate lozenges or OptiZinc for best absorption.

HERBS

❑ Dandelion root, horsetail, nettle, and oat straw promote bone building and are all good sources of calcium and magnesium.

RECOMMENDATIONS

❑ Change your diet. Eat more raw fruits and vegetables, raw nuts and seeds, yogurt, and cottage cheese. A diet high in calcium is essential.

❑ Do not consume sugar, junk foods, or carbonated beverages.

❑ Have a hair analysis done to check for mineral deficiencies. *See* HAIR ANALYSIS in Part Three.

❑ Be watchful if a child has severe allergies, celiac disease, asthma, bronchitis, or colon disturbances. These conditions can result in absorption problems. This may be difficult to detect at first because growth and weight are normal with these conditions.

CONSIDERATIONS

❑ Food allergy testing may be beneficial.

❑ There are a number of combination supplement products available that contain many of the nutrients recommended in the table above. Bone Builder from Ethical Nurients, Bone Defense from KAL, Bone Support from Synergy Plus, Cal Apatite from Metagenics, and Joint Support from Now Foods are all good products for promoting proper bone growth.

❑ *See also* OSTEOPOROSIS in Part Two.

Ringworm

See under FUNGAL INFECTION.

Rosacea

Rosacea is a chronic skin disorder that most often affects the forehead, nose, cheekbones, and chin. Groups of capillaries close to the surface of the skin become dilated, resulting in blotchy red areas with small bumps and, sometimes, pimples. The redness can come and go, but eventually may become permanent. The skin tissue can swell and thicken, and may be tender and sensitive to the touch.

The inflammation of rosacea can look a great deal like acne, but it tends to be more chronic, blackheads and whiteheads are almost never present, and it usually begins in middle age or later. It is a fairly common disorder—about one in every twenty Americans is afflicted with it—but many never realize they have it. Rosacea usually begins with frequent flushing of the face, particularly the nose and cheeks. The flushing is caused by the swelling of the blood vessels under the skin. This "red mask" can serve as a flag for attention. Rosacea can also cause a persistent burning and feeling of grittiness in the eyes or inflamed and swollen eyelids. In severe cases, vision can be impaired.

The underlying cause or causes of rosacea are not understood, but certain factors are known to aggravate the condition, including the consumption of alcohol, hot liquids, and/or spicy foods; exposure to sunlight; extremes of temperature; and the use of makeup and skin care products containing alcohol. Stress, vitamin deficiencies, and infection can be contributing factors. The things that aggravate one person's rosacea may have no effect on another person.

Rosacea is most common in white women between the ages of thirty and fifty. When it does occur in men it tends to be more severe, and is usually accompanied by rhinophyma (a nose that becomes chronically red and enlarged). Fair-skinned individuals seem to be more susceptible to this condition than darker skinned people. People who flush easily seem to be more prone than others to develop rosacea.

In rare cases, rosacea may affect the skin in other parts of the body as well as the face. It is not a dangerous condition, but it is chronic and can be distressing for cosmetic reasons. Without proper care, it can develop into a disfiguring condition.

NUTRIENTS

SUPPLEMENT	SUGGESTED DOSAGE	COMMENTS
Very Important		
Primrose oil	500 mg 3 times daily.	A good healer for many skin disorders. Contains linoleic acid, which is needed by the skin.
Vitamin A	25,000 IU daily for 3 months, then reduce to 15,000 IU daily. If you are pregnant, do not exceed 10,000 IU daily.	Necessary for healing and construction of new skin tissue.
Vitamin B complex plus extra vitamin B$_{12}$	As directed on label. 100 mcg 3 times daily.	Anti-stress vitamins that are necessary in all cellular functions and help to maintain healthy skin.
Important		
Kelp	1,000–1,500 mg daily.	Supplies balanced minerals needed for good skin tone.
Multivitamin and mineral complex	As directed on label.	To ensure optimum nutrition and guard against deficiencies.
Vitamin E	Start with 400 IU daily and increase slowly to 800 IU daily.	Protects against free radicals.
Zinc	50 mg daily. Do not exceed a total of 100 mg daily from all supplements.	For tissue repair. Enhances immune response. Use zinc gluconate lozenges or OptiZinc for best absorption.
Helpful		
Ageless Beauty from Biotec Foods	As directed on label.	Protects the skin from free radical damage.
Aloe vera		*See under* Herbs, below.
Chlorophyll or alfalfa	As directed on label.	Aids in cleansing the blood, preventing infections. Also supplies needed balanced minerals. *See under* Herbs, below.
Flaxseed oil capsules or liquid	1,000 mg daily. 1 tsp daily.	To supply needed essential fatty acids.
GH3 cream from Gero Vita	Apply topically as directed on label.	Good for any discoloration of the skin. Also helps prevent wrinkles.
Herpanacine from Diamond-Herpanacine Associates	As directed on label.	Contains antioxidants, amino acids, and herbs that promote skin health.
L-Cysteine	500 mg daily, on an empty stomach. Take with water or juice. Do not take with milk. Take with 50 mg vitamin B$_6$ and 100 mg vitamin C for better absorption.	Contains sulfur, needed for healthy skin. *See* AMINO ACIDS in Part One.
Lecithin granules or capsules	1 tbsp 3 times daily, before meals. 1,200 mg 3 times daily, before meals.	Aids absorption of the essential fatty acids.
Proteolytic enzymes	As directed on label. Take between meals.	Helps to reduce inflammation.
Selenium	200 mcg daily.	Encourages tissue elasticity and is a powerful antioxidant.
Superoxide dismutase (SOD)	As directed on label.	A free radical destroyer.
Vitamin C with bioflavonoids	3,000–5,000 mg daily, in divided doses.	Promotes immune function, strengthens capillaries, and acts as a mild anti-inflammatory.

HERBS

❑ Alfalfa is a good source of chlorophyll, which has detoxifying properties. It also supplies many needed vitamins and minerals.

❑ Aloe vera has excellent healing properties. Apply pure aloe vera gel topically to dry skin as directed on the product label or as needed.

Note: Some people with rosacea may experience irritation as a result of using aloe. If this occurs, discontinue use.

❑ Borage seed, dandelion root, dong quai, parsley, sarsaparilla, and yellow dock root improve skin tone.

❑ Burdock root and red clover are powerful blood cleansers. Burdock also helps to improve skin tone.

❑ Calendula, cayenne (capsicum), fennel seed, ginger, marshmallow root, sage, and slippery elm nourish the skin and promote healing.

Caution: Do not use sage if you suffer from any kind of seizure disorder.

❑ Milk thistle aids the liver in cleansing the blood.

❑ Nettle and rosemary improve skin tone, nourish the skin, and promote healing.

RECOMMENDATIONS

❑ Eat a clean diet that emphasizes raw vegetables and grains.

❑ Avoid fats, especially saturated fats, and all animal products. Saturated fats promote inflammation. Also avoid alcohol, dairy products, caffeine, cheese, chocolate, cocoa, eggs, fat, fish, salt, sugar, and spicy foods.

❑ Do not drink hot beverages such as coffee or tea. Allow your food to cool to room temperature before eating it.

❑ Investigate the possibility of food allergies. Keep a food diary for one month to see which foods may be aggravating the condition. Then avoid those foods. *See* ALLERGIES in Part Two for further information.

❑ Once a month, follow a fasting program. *See* FASTING in Part Three.

❑ Keep the skin scrupulously clean, but treat it gently. Use a mild natural soap and lukewarm to cool (never cold or hot) water for cleansing. Pat the skin dry after washing—do not rub it. Avoid touching the skin except when cleansing it.

❑ Avoid extremes of temperature, especially heat. Keep baths and showers short, and use water that is as cool as you can tolerate comfortably. Avoid saunas (including the type used for facials and steam inhalations), steam baths, and hot tubs. If you need to increase the humidity in your home, use only a cool mist humidifier.

❑ As much as possible, avoid wearing makeup. If you do use cosmetics, choose all-natural, water-based products.

❑ *Do not* use topical steroid creams. These only make the condition worse.

❑ Friction is extremely irritating, so avoid wearing tight clothing such as turtlenecks that can rub against the skin. Be careful about anything that comes close to or into contact with your face. Even holding the telephone receiver against your face for a while can raise the local temperature and irritate sensitive skin.

❑ In severe cases, a laser or electrical device can be used to remove the excess tissue. Dermabrasion also has helped some people with rosacea.

CONSIDERATIONS

❑ There is no known cure for rosacea. Topical and/or oral antibiotics, usually tetracycline, are often prescribed to keep the inflammation under control. As with any drug, these can have side effects, especially with long-term use. Moreover, if you stop taking the antibiotics, the condition may rebound.

❑ An underlying vascular disorder may be involved in the development of rosacea. Several findings support this theory. First, there are structural abnormalities in the small blood vessels in the facial skin of people with rosacea. Second, the condition is exacerbated by the use of drugs that dilate blood vessels, such as theophylline and nitroglycerin. Finally, people with rosacea are more likely than most to suffer from migraines, a type of headache also linked to vascular malfunction.

❑ *Demodex folliculorum*, a type of microscopic mite that lives on cast-off skin cells and is normally present on human skin, has been found in significantly higher than normal numbers in skin samples taken from people with rosacea. Researchers speculate that this organism, or some type of reaction to it, may be involved in rosacea.

Rubella

See GERMAN MEASLES.

Scabies

Scabies is a parasitic infection that causes a persistent, itchy rash. It is caused by a tiny mite that burrows into the top layer of the skin to lay its eggs. This results in groups of small red lumps. When the rash first appears, you may see fine, wavy lines emanating from some of the lumps if you look closely. The skin may then become dry and scaly, and the itching can be intense, especially at night. Scratching can set the stage for a bacterial infection as well.

Scabies can be a particular problem in institutional settings such as nursing homes and day care centers. It is spread primarily by skin-to-skin contact, and it is highly contagious. The areas most commonly affected are the buttocks, genitals, wrists, and armpits, as well as the skin between the toes and fingers.

To diagnose the condition, a physician usually takes a scraping of skin from the affected area and examines it under a microscope. If one family member develops scabies, all the members of the household should be checked (and possibly treated). Children under the age of fifteen have the highest incidence of scabies and are usually the first in the family to contract it.

NUTRIENTS

SUPPLEMENT	SUGGESTED DOSAGE	COMMENTS
Very Important		
Garlic (Kyolic)	2 capsules 3 times daily, with meals.	Has antiparasitic and antibiotic properties.
Primrose oil	1,000 mg 3 times daily.	A good healer for most skin disorders.
Vitamin A	25,000 IU daily for 3 months, then reduce to 15,000 IU daily. If you are pregnant, do not exceed 10,000 IU daily.	Necessary for healing and for construction of new skin tissue.

Important		
Kelp	1,000–1,500 mg daily.	Supplies balanced minerals.
Zinc	50 mg daily. Do not exceed a total of 100 mg daily from all supplements.	For tissue repair. Enhances immune response. Use zinc gluconate lozenges or zinc methionate (OptiZinc) for best absorption.

Helpful		
Aloe vera		*See under* Herbs, below.
Colloidal silver	Apply topically as directed on label.	To prevent secondary infection.
Vitamin E	600 IU daily.	Promotes healing.

HERBS

❑ Aloe vera has excellent healing properties. Apply gel topically to the affected area as directed on the product label.

❑ Balsam of Peru, goldenseal, and/or tea tree oil can be applied topically to fight the infection. Goldenseal can also be taken internally to bolster the immune system.

Caution: Do not take goldenseal internally on a daily basis for more than one week at a time, as it may disturb normal intestinal flora. Do not use it during pregnancy, and use it with caution if you are allergic to ragweed.

❑ Comfrey and/or calendula salve helps to soothe itching and irritation.

RECOMMENDATIONS

❑ Diet alone cannot cure scabies. To get rid of the mites, apply permethrin cream (Elemite) or 25-percent benzyl benzoate topically to the entire body from the neck down, as directed on the label or prescribed by your physician.

❑ Thoroughly wash all bed linens used by infected individuals in hot water. A product called Rid spray, which also contains permethrin, may be recommended for treating infested clothes and bedding.

❑ Practice scrupulous personal hygiene. Avoid contact with infested persons or their clothing.

❑ To promote healing, eat plenty of foods high in zinc, such as soybeans, sunflower seeds, wheat bran, whole-grain products, yeast, and blackstrap molasses.

❑ Do not drink soft drinks or alcoholic beverages. Consume no sugar, chocolate, or junk foods.

❑ Avoid fried foods and all animal products. Use cold-pressed vegetable oils only.

CONSIDERATIONS

❑ A topical scabicide called lindane (gamma benzene hexachloride, found in Kwell) was once considered a standard treatment for scabies. In recent years, however, it has largely been replaced by permethrin, which is believed to be safer and cause fewer side effects.

❑ Scabicides are not recommended for children under the age of six or for pregnant women. In such cases, a milder sulfur solution is usually recommended.

❑ It may take one to two weeks for the itching to subside, even after treatment. An antihistamine or a cortisone cream may be recommended to provide relief. Calendula salve, cool compresses, and cool oatmeal baths are natural alternatives to those medications.

❑ Crowded, unsanitary, or institutional living conditions are conducive to the spread of scabies.

Schizophrenia

Many health care professionals divide mental illness into two basic categories: mood disorders and schizophrenic disorders. Mood disorders are generally episodic in nature, and people who suffer from them usually seem to return to normal between episodes. This is not true for most people with schizophrenia.

The characteristic symptoms of schizophrenia are disordered thinking and perception, emotional changes such as tension and/or depression, behavioral disturbances ranging from catatonia to violent outbursts, delusions, and loss of contact with reality. A person with schizophrenia often seems to withdraw into his or her own world. Hallucinations are not uncommon.

The mildest form of schizophrenic disorder is schizotypal personality disorder; the most severe is chronic deteriorating schizophrenia. While the onset of the disorder is often related to a stressful life event, the underlying cause or causes of schizophrenia are not known. There are many theories, however. Some researchers believe that schizophrenia is hereditary, and there is evidence that some cases of schizophrenia are the result of an inherited defect in body chemistry in which brain chemicals called neurotransmitters function abnormally. Others theorize that schizophrenia results from external factors, such as complications during birth, head injury, a reaction to a virus, or environmental poisons that reach and damage the brain. There is a high incidence of childhood head injuries and birth complications among people with schizophrenia. A wide range of drugs also can cause schizophrenic-type symptoms.

Yet another theory focuses on nutritional factors. There is some indication that schizophrenia may be associated with high copper levels in body tissues. When copper levels are too high, the levels of vitamin C and zinc in the body drop. This has led scientists to believe that a zinc deficiency may be at the root of the problem. Some research has linked prenatal zinc deficiency to the development of schizophrenia later in life, and the presence of high copper levels in people with schizophrenia would seem to support this theory. Zinc is an important factor in determining birth weight. A zinc deficiency also may result in damage to the pineal area of the brain, which normally contains high levels of zinc, which in turn may make an individual vulnerable to schizophrenia or other psychoses. Evidence indicates that male babies are particularly susceptible to gestational zinc deficiencies. Other clues come from the seasonality of the disorder. The incidence of schizophrenic episodes tends to peak in cold-weather months, when zinc intake tends to be lower.

Magnesium deficiency may also be a factor. Some research has shown that magnesium levels in the blood of people with active schizophrenia are lower than normal, and that the levels are higher in persons whose schizophrenia is in remission. It has been hypothesized that a type of vicious cycle may be at work here; the high level of stress experienced by those with severe psychiatric disorders may lead to magnesium deficiency, which in turn would exacerbate symptoms such as anxiety, fear, hallucinations, weakness, and physical complaints.

NUTRIENTS

SUPPLEMENT	SUGGESTED DOSAGE	COMMENTS
Essential		
Flaxseed oil	As directed on label.	To supply essential fatty acids, needed for proper brain and nerve function.
Folic acid	2,000 mcg daily.	Deficiency has been found in approximately 25 percent of those hospitalized for psychiatric disorders.
Gamma-aminobutyric acid (GABA)	As directed on label, on an empty stomach. Take with water or juice. Do not take with milk. Take with 50 mg vitamin B_6 and 100 mg vitamin C for better absorption.	Essential for brain metabolism. Aids in proper brain function. *See* AMINO ACIDS in Part One.
Garlic (Kyolic)	As directed on label.	Enhances brain function.
Ginkgo biloba		*See under* Herbs, on next page.
L-Asparagine	As directed on label.	Balances brain function.
L-Glutamic acid	As directed on label.	Helps to correct personality disorders.
L-Glutathione	As directed on label.	Deficiency can result in mental disorders.
L-Methionine	As directed on label.	Helps to counteract histamine, which is found in high levels in people with schizophrenia.
Pycnogenol or grape seed extract	As directed on label. As directed on label.	Antioxidants useful for dementia and other syndromes of the brain.
Zinc plus manganese	Up to 80 mg daily. Do not exceed 100 mg daily. Take separately from calcium.	Balances copper, often found in high concentrations in people with this disorder. Enhances action of B vitamins necessary for brain function.
Very Important		
Free-form amino acid complex	As directed on label. Take on an empty stomach.	Needed for normal brain function. Use a formula containing all the essential amino acids.
Vitamin B_3 (niacin) or niacinamide	100 mg 3 times daily. Do not exceed this amount. 1,000 mg daily.	Deficiency has been linked to schizophrenia. Injections (under a doctor's supervision) are best. *Caution:* Do not take niacin if you have a liver disorder, gout, or high blood pressure.
Raw liver extract injections plus vitamin B complex injections plus extra vitamin B_6 (pyridoxine) and vitamin B_{12}	1 cc 3 times weekly for 3 weeks, then twice weekly for 3 months. Then reduce to 1 cc once weekly. 1 cc 3 times weekly for 3 weeks, then twice weekly for 3 months. Then reduce to 1 cc once weekly. ½ cc 3 times weekly for 3 weeks, then twice weekly for 3 months. Then reduce to ½ cc once weekly. 1 cc 3 times weekly or as prescribed by physician.	To supply B vitamins and other valuable nutrients. B vitamin deficiencies are related to brain malfunction. Many people with mental disorders have found this program helpful. All injectables can be combined in a single syringe.
or vitamin B complex plus extra Vitamin B_6 (pyridoxine)	100 mg 3 times daily. 100 mg twice daily.	If injections are not available, use a sublingual form. Required by the nervous system; necessary for normal brain function.
Vitamin E emulsion or capsules	800 IU daily. Start with 200 IU daily and slowly increase to 1,000 IU daily.	An antioxidant that improves brain circulation. Emulsion form is recommended for easier assimilation and greater safety at high doses.
Important		
Coenzyme Q_{10}	100–200 mg daily.	Improves cerebral circulation.
Dimethylglycine (DMG) (Aangamik DMG from FoodScience Labs)	As directed on label.	Enhances cerebral oxygen utilization.
Essential fatty acids (primrose oil)	As directed on label 3 times daily.	Helps cerebral circulation.
Lecithin granules or capsules	1 tbsp 3 times daily, before meals. 1,200 mg 3 times daily, before meals.	Improves brain function. Contains choline and inositol. Works well with vitamin E.
L-Glutamine	1,000–4,000 mg daily, on an empty stomach. Take with water or juice. Do not take with milk. Take with 50 mg vitamin B_6 and 100 mg vitamin C for better absorption.	Needed for normal brain function. *See* AMINO ACIDS in Part One.
Vitamin C	5,000–10,000 mg daily.	Improves brain function and enhances the immune system.
Helpful		
Kelp	1,000–1,500 mg daily.	Contains balanced essential minerals.
Lithium	As prescribed by physician.	A trace mineral that helps to stabilize the mental state. Available by prescription only.
Multivitamin and mineral complex	As directed on label.	All nutrients are needed for normal brain function.
Raw thyroid glandular	As directed on label.	Reduced thyroid function results in poor cerebral function. *See* HYPOTHYROIDISM in Part Two and GLANDULAR THERAPY in Part Three.

HERBS

❑ Ginkgo biloba improves brain function and cerebral circulation, and enhances memory.

RECOMMENDATIONS

❑ Eat a high-fiber diet including plenty of fresh raw vegetables and quality protein, and try eating more frequent small meals rather than three larger ones each day. This helps to keep blood sugar levels stable, which in turn has a stabilizing influence on mood and behavior. *See* HYPOGLYCEMIA in Part Two for additional suggestions.

❑ Include the following in your diet: breast of chicken or turkey, brewer's yeast, halibut, peas, sunflower seeds, and tuna. Also eat foods rich in niacin, such as broccoli, carrots, corn, eggs, fish, potatoes, tomatoes, and whole wheat.

❑ Do not consume caffeine. It promotes the release of unwanted norepinephrine, a stimulating neurotransmitter.

❑ Avoid alcohol. Alcohol consumption depletes the body of zinc. Many psychological disorders are known to be adversely affected by zinc deficiencies.

❑ Keep environmental pressures under control. Overstimulation from strong emotions or an excessive workload can exacerbate symptoms. Also avoid understimulation.

CONSIDERATIONS

❑ A study reported in the August 29, 1992, issue of the British medical journal *The Lancet* linked city-dwelling, winter birth, and prenatal exposure to influenza to schizophrenic disorders. In addition, these factors appear to compound one another; city-born people with schizophrenia are much more likely to have been born in winter than their non-city-born counterparts.

❑ Sometimes extremely high doses of certain vitamins are needed to keep the mind functioning well.

❑ Hair analysis reveals mineral imbalances that may contribute to mental difficulties. *See* HAIR ANALYSIS in Part Three.

❑ Some experts believe that many suicides among the young may be related to undiagnosed schizophrenia.

❑ Psychiatrists found a link between schizophrenia and pellagra (vitamin B$_3$ [niacin] deficiency). (*See* PELLAGRA in Part Two.) Taking several grams of niacinamide daily (under a doctor's supervision) has been tried with good results.

❑ Undiagnosed celiac disease, caused by an intolerance to gluten, can cause symptoms similar to those of schizophrenia. Gluten intolerance can also cause severe depression. (*See* CELIAC DISEASE in Part Two.)

❑ Drug therapy is usually the medical treatment of choice for schizophrenia. However, there is no single medication that is effective in all cases. It may be necessary to try several different drugs in order to find the one that works best to keep symptoms under control. The drug lithium (Eskalith and others) is often used to treat schizophrenia, and some people who have used it have experienced improvement. If drugs are not effective by themselves, electroconvulsive therapy (ECT) may be recommended as an adjunct treatment because it accelerates the response to medication.

❑ Some cases of schizophrenia have been linked to food allergies. Many people find their symptoms improve after they fast. (*See* ALLERGIES in Part Two and FASTING in Part Three.)

Sciatica

See BACKACHE. *See also under* PREGNANCY-RELATED PROBLEMS.

Scotoma

See under EYE PROBLEMS.

Seasonal Affective Disorder (SAD)

See under DEPRESSION.

Sebaceous Cyst

Sebaceous cysts are skin growths that contain a mixture of sebum (oil) and skin proteins. They generally appear as small, slowly growing swellings on the face, scalp, or back. A whitehead is actually a tiny sebaceous cyst.

These nodules feel firm but movable, and rarely hurt unless they become infected. If infection sets in, there may be redness and swelling, and the area may become sensitive to the touch. Sebaceous cysts are benign, but they can become a site of chronic, usually bacterial, infection. With chronic infection, an abscess may form.

NUTRIENTS

SUPPLEMENT	SUGGESTED DOSAGE	COMMENTS
Very Important		
Primrose oil	1,000 mg 3 times daily.	A good healer for most skin disorders.
Vitamin B complex plus extra	As directed on label.	Anti-stress and anti-aging vitamins. Needed for healthy
vitamin B$_{12}$	100 mg 3 times daily.	skin.

467

Vitamin A	25,000 IU daily for 3 months, then reduce to 15,000 IU daily. If you are pregnant, do not exceed 10,000 IU daily.	Necessary for healing and construction of new skin tissue.
plus natural beta-carotene	As directed on label.	Used by the body to make vitamin A as needed.
Important		
Garlic (Kyolic)	2 capsules 3 times daily, with meals.	Has anti-infective properties.
Kelp	1,000–1,500 mg daily.	Supplies balanced minerals needed for good skin tone.
Zinc	50 mg daily. Do not exceed a total of 100 mg daily from all supplements.	For tissue repair. Enhances immune response. Use zinc gluconate lozenges or OptiZinc for best absorption.
Helpful		
Aloe vera		See under Herbs, below.
Superoxide dismutase (SOD)	As directed on label.	A free radical destroyer.

HERBS

❑ Aloe vera is soothing and healing. Apply pure aloe vera gel to the affected area as directed on the product label.

❑ Burdock root and red clover are powerful blood cleansers.

❑ Milk thistle aids the liver in cleansing the blood.

❑ Goldenseal extract or tea tree oil can be applied topically to fight infection.

RECOMMENDATIONS

❑ Avoid fats, especially saturated fats, and all fried foods. Also avoid alcohol, dairy products, caffeine, cheese, chocolate, cocoa, dairy products, eggs, fat, fish, meat, salt, and sugar.

❑ Follow a fasting program. See FASTING in Part Three.

❑ If the growth becomes large or infected, see your health care provider about removing it. This is usually a simple in-office procedure performed under a local anesthetic.

❑ If an antibiotic is prescribed for a severe and/or extensive infection, be sure to take an acidophilus supplement to replace necessary "friendly" bacteria.

CONSIDERATIONS

❑ See also OILY SKIN in Part Two.

Seborrhea

Seborrhea, or seborrheic dermatitis, is characterized by scaly patches of skin that result from a disorder of the sebaceous (oil-secreting) glands. Seborrhea most often oc-

curs on the scalp, face, and chest, but can appear on other parts of the body as well. It may or may not be itchy.

Seborrheic skin may be yellowish and/or greasy or dry and flaky. The scaly bumps may coalesce to form large plaques or patches. Seborrheic dermatitis can occur at any age, but is most common in infancy ("cradle cap") and middle age. The exact cause is not known, but it may be linked to nutritional deficiencies (especially a lack of biotin and vitamin A) or the effects of a yeast organism, *Pityrosporum ovale*, which normally lives in the hair follicles. Heredity and climate probably also play a role. Adult seborrheic dermatitis, which usually affects the scalp and face, is often associated with stress and anxiety. Other factors associated with an increased chance of developing seborrhea include infrequent shampooing, oily skin, obesity, Parkinson's disease, AIDS, and other skin disorders, such as acne, rosacea, and psoriasis.

Unless otherwise specified, the dosages recommended here are for adults. For a child between the ages of twelve and seventeen, reduce the dose to three-quarters the recommended amount. For a child between six and twelve, use one-half the recommended dose, and for a child under the age of six, use one-quarter the recommended amount.

NUTRIENTS

SUPPLEMENT	SUGGESTED DOSAGE	COMMENTS
Essential		
Essential fatty acids (primrose oil and Ultimate Oil from Nature's Secret are good sources)	As directed on label.	Important for many skin disorders; contains needed linoleic acid.
Tea tree oil		See under Herbs, below.
Vitamin B complex plus extra vitamin B_6 (pyridoxine)	As directed on label. 50 mg 3 times daily.	The B vitamins, especially vitamin B_6, are needed for protein metabolism, which is essential for healing and repair. Use a super-high-potency formula. A sublingual form is recommended for best absorption. Consider injections (under a doctor's supervision).
and biotin	50 mg 3 times daily.	Deficiency has been linked to seborrhea.
Zinc	50 mg daily. Do not exceed a total of 100 mg daily from all supplements.	Important for healing. Enhances immunity. Use zinc gluconate lozenges or OptiZinc for best absorption.
Important		
Concentrace from Trace Minerals Research	As directed on label.	Contains essential trace minerals to nourish the skin.
Herpanacine from Diamond-Herpanacine Associates	As directed on label.	Amino acids, vitamins, and herbs that promote skin health and remove toxins.
Pycnogenol or grape seed extract	As directed on label. As directed on label.	Powerful antioxidants that strengthen the skin to resist disease.

Vitamin A and vitamin E	Up to 50,000 IU daily. If you are pregnant, do not exceed 10,000 IU daily. 400–800 IU daily.	Deficiency may cause or contribute to seborrhea. Speeds healing. Increases oxygen intake.
or AE Mulsion Forte from American Biologics	As directed on label.	Supplies vitamins A and E in emulsion form for easier assimilation and greater safety at higher doses.
Helpful		
Acidophilus	As directed on label. Take on an empty stomach.	To replenish "friendly" bacteria. Especially important if antibiotics are prescribed.
Coenzyme Q$_{10}$	60 mg daily.	An important free radical scavenger that supplies oxygen to the cells.
Dimethylglycine (DMG) (Aangamik DMG from FoodScience Labs)	As directed on label.	Increases oxygenation of tissues.
Free-form amino acid complex	As directed on label.	For healing and repair of tissues.
Kelp	1,000–1,500 mg daily.	Contains balanced minerals. A good source of iodine.
Lecithin granules or capsules	1 tbsp 3 times daily, with meals. 1,200 mg 3 times daily, with meals.	For cellular protection.
Multivitamin and mineral complex	As directed on label.	All nutrients are necessary in balance.

HERBS

❑ Dandelion, goldenseal, and red clover, taken internally, are good for most skin disorders.

Caution: Do not take goldenseal internally on a daily basis for more than one week at a time, do not use it during pregnancy, and use it with caution if you are allergic to ragweed.

❑ Tea tree oil is a natural antiseptic and antifungal that can be applied directly to the affected area. If it is too strong, it can be diluted with an equal amount of jojoba oil (available in health food stores) or distilled water.

RECOMMENDATIONS

❑ Eat a diet composed of 50 to 75 percent raw foods and soured products such as low-fat yogurt.

❑ Avoid chocolate, dairy products, flour, fried foods, seafood, nuts, and anything containing sugar.

❑ Do not eat any foods containing raw eggs. Egg whites contain high levels of avidin, a protein that binds biotin and prevents it from being absorbed. Biotin is needed for healthy hair and skin. Eating uncooked eggs also poses a risk of *Salmonella* poisoning (*see* FOOD POISONING in Part Two).

❑ If antibiotics are prescribed, take extra B-complex vitamins and an acidophilus supplement to replace the "friendly" bacteria destroyed by the antibiotics.

❑ Try changing your hair products. Choose products without chemicals. Sometimes this helps.

❑ To minimize the frequency and severity of flare-ups, dry your skin thoroughly after bathing, and wear loose-fitting clothing made of natural fibers that "breathe."

❑ Avoid using over-the-counter ointments to treat seborrhea. This can cause an overload on the skin.

❑ Do not pick at or squeeze the affected skin.

❑ Avoid using irritating soaps, but make sure you keep the affected areas clean. Avoid greasy ointments and creams. Keep your hair clean and make sure you use a non-oily shampoo.

❑ If dietary changes and nutritional supplementation do not produce an improvement, seek the advice of a qualified health care professional.

❑ Follow a fasting program once a month. *See* FASTING in Part Three.

CONSIDERATIONS

❑ Dermatologists usually prescribe cleansing lotions containing a drying agent with sulfur and resorcinol and/or Diprosone cream from Schering.

❑ Cradle cap has been associated with food allergies. For infants, controlling food allergies plus giving supplemental biotin (if there is a deficiency) is most effective. For a child over six months old, adding liquid vitamin B complex to juice is a good way to administer the needed biotin.

❑ An absence of intestinal flora may be responsible for biotin deficiency in infants. Studies have shown that treating both the nursing mother and her infant with biotin can be successful in resolving cradle cap. For adults, treatment with biotin alone does not appear to be effective, but supplementation with biotin combined with the whole vitamin B complex and essential fatty acids produces improvement in many cases.

❑ Consumption of raw egg whites has produced seborrheic dermatitis in an experiment in rats.

❑ Some findings suggest that many skin disorders, including eczema and psoriasis, may be related to gluten allergy. A gluten-free diet may be helpful. *See* CELIAC DISEASE in Part Two for dietary suggestions.

❑ Taking supplemental vitamin B complex has been shown to be the most effective treatment in many cases.

❑ *See also* DANDRUFF and DERMATITIS in Part Two.

Seizure

See under EPILEPSY.

Senility (Senile Dementia)

Senility was once considered an inevitable consequence of aging. However, we now know that it is a physically based disease, and in fact it is not very common. It is a condition in which brain function, or certain aspects of brain function, decline to the point that mental disability results. Forgetfulness, fearfulness, depression, agitation, difficulty absorbing new information, and loss of normal emotional responses are typical. The disorder usually gets progressively worse. Complications that may occur include injuries (primarily due to falls), inadequate nutrition, constipation, and a variety of infections.

Dementia can be caused by several diseases affecting brain function. It can also result from nutritional deficiency, especially if chronic, or long-term alcohol or drug use.

Many people diagnosed as senile actually suffer from *pseudodementia*—symptoms that mimic dementia but that are actually caused by depression, deafness, brain tumors, thyroid problems, liver or kidney problems, the use of certain drugs, or other disorders. A thorough medical and psychological examination by a qualified professional, preferably a specialist in the field, is necessary for an accurate diagnosis.

Dementia is considered incurable. However, the proper diet and nutritional supplements can help. The following supplements are helpful for improving brain function. When choosing supplements, avoid heavily coated or sustained release products. These are difficult to break down. Instead, choose liquids, powders, or sublingual forms.

NUTRIENTS

SUPPLEMENT	SUGGESTED DOSAGE	COMMENTS
Essential		
Dimethylglycine (DMG) (Aangamik DMG from FoodScience Labs)	As directed on label.	Helps to maintain mental acuity and enhances immune function.
Essential fatty acids (flaxseed oil and primrose oil are good sources)	As directed on label.	Promotes brain and nerve function as well as a healthy immune system.
Free-form amino acid complex	As directed on label.	To supply protein, needed for normal brain function. Protein deficiency is common among elderly people.
Gamma-aminobutyric acid (GABA)	As directed on label, on an empty stomach. Take with water or juice. Do not take with milk. Take with 50 mg vitamin B$_6$ and 100 mg vitamin C for better absorption.	Essential for brain function and metabolism. Has a calming effect. *See* AMINO ACIDS in Part One.
Garlic (Kyolic)	As directed on label.	Enhances brain function; helps to reduce stress and anxiety.
Ginkgo biloba		*See under* Herbs, below.
L-Asparagine	As directed on label, on an empty stomach.	To maintain balance in the brain and central nervous system.
L-Phenylalanine	As directed on label, on an empty stomach.	Promotes alertness, aids memory, and helps overcome depression. *Caution:* Do not take this supplement if you are taking an MAO inhibitor drug, or if you suffer from panic attacks, diabetes, high blood pressure, or PKU.
L-Tyrosine	As directed on label, on an empty stomach.	Promotes brain function and helps fight depression. *Caution:* Do not take tyrosine if you are taking an MAO inhibitor drug, commonly prescribed for depression.
Melatonin	2–3 mg daily, taken 2 hours or less before bedtime.	Aids sleep, helps maintain equilibrium, and strengthens the immune system.
Vitamin B complex injections	1 cc once weekly or as prescribed by physician.	All B vitamins are necessary for brain and nerve health. Elderly people often have deficiencies because the ability to absorb the B vitamins declines with age. Injections (under a doctor's supervision) are best.
plus extra vitamin B$_6$ (pyridoxine)	½ cc once weekly or as prescribed by physician.	Vital for mental health and for maintaining proper electrolyte balance in the body.
plus liver extract	1 cc once weekly or as prescribed by physician.	A good source of B vitamins and other valuable nutrients.
or vitamin B complex	100 mg 3 times daily.	If injections are not available, use a sublingual form.
plus extra vitamin B$_6$ (pyridoxine)	50 mg daily.	
and vitamin B$_{12}$	2,000 mcg daily.	Needed to prevent anemia. Also prevents nerve damage and may assist memory and learning. Use a lozenge or sublingual form.
Very Important		
Choline	500 mg twice daily.	Important in brain function. Improves memory and mental capacity.
Vitamin B$_3$ (niacin)	100 mg daily. Do not exceed this amount. Take with 100 mg niacinamide to reduce flushing.	Improves cerebral circulation and lowers cholesterol levels. *Caution:* Do not take niacin if you have a liver disorder, gout, or high blood pressure.
Vitamin C	3,000–10,000 mg daily.	Reduces blood clotting tendency, improving cerebral circulation.
Vitamin E	Start with 200 IU daily and increase slowly to 600–1,000 IU daily.	Improves cerebral circulation and boosts immunity, which declines with age.
Important		
GH3 from Gero Vita	As directed on label.	Helps to promote brain function. Consider injections (under a doctor's supervision). *Caution:* Do not use GH3 if you are allergic to sulfites.
Helpful		
Multivitamin complex	As directed on label.	For necessary vitamins. Use a high-potency formula.

Coenzyme Q10	100–200 mg daily.	Free radical scavenger and immunostimulant. Increases cellular oxygen levels.
L-Glutamine	As directed on label, on an empty stomach. Take with water or juice. Do not take with milk. Take with 50 mg vitamin B6 and 100 mg vitamin C for better absorption.	Needed for normal brain function. See AMINO ACIDS in Part One.
Lecithin granules or capsules	1 tbsp 3 times daily, before meals. 1,200 mg 3 times daily, before meals.	For brain cell protection and function.
Zinc	50–80 mg daily. Do not exceed a total of 100 mg daily from all supplements.	Aids in heavy metal detoxification and enhancing immunity. Use zinc gluconate lozenges or OptiZinc for best absorption.

HERBS

❑ Anise and blue cohosh appear to sharpen brain power.

❑ Ginkgo biloba improves cerebral circulation, enhances brain function and memory, and destroys free radicals to protect brain cells. Three times a day, place ½ dropperful of alcohol-free liquid extract under your tongue and hold it there for a few minutes before swallowing. Or take 400 milligrams in capsule form three times daily.

RECOMMENDATIONS

❑ Eat a diet consisting of 50 to 75 percent raw foods, along with seeds, whole-grain cereals and breads, raw nuts, and low-fat yogurt and soured products. Eat Swiss cheese, brown rice, and plenty of fiber daily.

❑ Drink plenty of liquids, even if you are not thirsty—as we grow older, our "thirst system" does not work as well.

❑ Move the bowels daily. Oat bran, rice bran, and a high-fiber diet are important. Aerobic Bulk Cleanse (ABC) from Aerobic Life Industries, a colon cleanser, is very helpful. Enemas may be needed. See ENEMAS in Part Three.

❑ Keep active. Exercising, walking, engaging in mental activity, and doing things you enjoy, like pursuing a hobby, are important. Seek out companionship and new experiences. Some people withdraw and keep to themselves as they get older because it seems easier and/or safer, but this can lead to loneliness and depression. If getting out and about is a problem, consider investing in and learning to use a computer. There are a number of on-line services geared to seniors that can serve as a source of companionship as well as information.

❑ Protect against head injury by wearing your seat belt and by wearing protective headgear when participating in activities such as bicycle riding.

❑ Have a complete physical examination to rule out the possibility of underlying illness as a cause of symptoms.

CONSIDERATIONS

❑ Results of a study in which nearly 500 eighty-five-year-olds were screened for dementia suggested that preventable vascular problems may be responsible for as many as 50 percent of the problems with dementia. It thus seems logical that many cases of dementia may be prevented by "stroke reduction" measures—not smoking, controlling high blood pressure, pursuing chelation therapy to remove toxic metals from the body, adhering to a proper diet, and taking appropriate nutritional supplements.

❑ Studies done at the Welsh National School of Medicine and Surrey University in England found that nutritional deficiencies—specifically deficiencies of vitamin B1 (thiamine), vitamin B2 (riboflavin), vitamin B6 (pyrodixine), folic acid, vitamin C, and vitamin D—may contribute to senile dementia.

❑ Persons with atherosclerosis and high blood pressure have a higher risk of developing senility. (See ARTERIOSCLE-ROSIS/ATHEROSCLEROSIS and HIGH BLOOD PRESSURE in Part Two.)

❑ Food allergies can cause mental as well as physical symptoms. (See ALLERGIES in Part Two.)

❑ Toxic metals in the body can produce symptoms similar to those of senility. A hair analysis can reveal whether the body is incurring damage due to the presence of toxic levels of metals like aluminum and lead. (See HAIR ANALYSIS in Part Three.)

❑ See also ALUMINUM TOXICITY; ALZHEIMER'S DISEASE; and PARKINSON'S DISEASE, all in Part Two.

Sexually Transmitted Disease (STD)

There are numerous diseases that are passed on either exclusively or primarily through intimate sexual contact. These include acquired immune deficiency syndrome (AIDS), chancroid, chlamydia, gonorrhea, lymphogranuloma venereum (LGV), granuloma inguinale, genital herpes, syphilis, and trichomoniasis. Genital candidiasis also can be transmitted through sexual contact. This section deals primarily with two of the more common of these disorders, gonorrhea and syphilis.

Gonorrhea is caused by a microorganism called *Neisseria gonorrhoeae*, commonly referred to as gonococci. In women, gonorrhea often causes no symptoms. When it does, they include frequent and painful urination, vaginal discharge, abnormal menstrual bleeding, acute inflammation in the pelvic area, and rectal itching. Men with gonorrhea usually do experience symptoms, including a yellow discharge of pus and mucus from the penis and slow, difficult, and painful urination. Symptoms usually appear between two and fourteen days after sexual contact in men and between seven to twenty-one days after sexual contact in women.

Early Symptoms of Sexually Transmitted Diseases

It is important to detect sexually transmitted diseases in their early stages so that prompt treatment can begin and, in the case of some diseases, irreparable damage to the body can be prevented. Use the table below to familiarize yourself with the beginning stages of various STDs.

Disease	First Symptoms
AIDS (Acquired Immune Deficiency Syndrome)	Headache, night sweats, unexplained weight loss, fatigue, swollen lymph glands, persistent fever, oral thrush (a heavy, whitish coating on the tongue and the insides of the mouth), recurrent vaginal yeast infections, persistent diarrhea, lung infections.
Candidiasis	Itching in the genital area, pain when urinating, a thick odorless vaginal discharge.
Chlamydia	For women: a white vaginal discharge that resembles cottage cheese, a burning sensation when urinating, itching, painful intercourse. For men: a clear, watery urethral discharge. Often, however, there are no symptoms at all.
Genital herpes	Itching, burning in the genital area, discomfort while urinating, a watery vaginal or urethral discharge, weeping, fluid-filled eruptions in the vagina or on the penis.
Genital warts	Soft, cauliflower-like growths appearing either singly or in clusters in and around the vagina, anus, penis, groin, and/or scrotal area.
Gonorrhea	For women: frequent and painful urination, a cloudy vaginal discharge, vaginal itching, inflammation of the pelvic area, rectal discharge, abnormal uterine bleeding. For men: a yellowish, pus-filled urethral discharge. Often, however, there are no symptoms, especially in women.
Pelvic Inflammatory Disease (PID)	A pus-filled vaginal discharge with fever and lower abdominal pain.
Syphilis	A sore on the genitalia, rash, patches of flaking tissue, fever, sore throat, sores in the mouth or anus.
Trichomoniasis	For women: vaginal itching and pain, with a foamy, greenish or yellow foul-smelling discharge. For men: a clear urethral discharge.

If not treated, the infection can travel through the bloodstream and go into the bones, joints, tendons, and other tissues, causing a systemic illness with mild fever, achiness, inflamed joints, and, occasionally, skin lesions. At this stage, the organism is difficult to detect, and the condition is often misdiagnosed as simple arthritis. In men, complications of gonorrhea can include sterility and urethral stricture.

Syphilis is caused by a type of bacteria called *Treponema pallidum.* This disease is occasionally contracted through close physical contact such as kissing, as well as through sexual intercourse. If not treated, this illness progresses, usually over the course of many years, through three basic stages. In the first stage, a chancre—a red, painless ulcer— appears at the spot where the bacteria entered the body. In the second stage, a rash and patches of flaking tissue appear in the mouth or genital area. There may be systemic symptoms, usually mild, as well—headache, nausea, and general discomfort. If the disease progresses to its third stage (which is rare in the United States), brain damage, hearing loss, heart disease, and/or blindness can occur.

NUTRIENTS

SUPPLEMENT	SUGGESTED DOSAGE	COMMENTS
Very Important		
Acidophilus	As directed on label 3 times daily, on an empty stomach.	To restore "friendly" bacteria. Important when taking antibiotics, which are usually prescribed for STDs.
Garlic (Kyolic)	2 capsules 3 times daily.	A natural antibiotic and immune system stimulant.

Free-form amino acid complex	As directed on label.	Needed for tissue repair. Use free-form amino acids for quicker absorption and assimilation.
Vitamin C	750–2,500 mg 4 times daily.	Boosts immune function and is an antiviral agent.
Zinc	100 mg daily. Do not exceed this amount.	Important for the health of the reproductive organs. Promotes wound healing and boosts immune function to fight a broad range of microbes. Use zinc gluconate lozenges or OptiZinc for best absorption.
Important		
Colloidal silver	Use sublingually or topically as directed on label.	An antiseptic that rapidly reduces inflammation and promotes healing of lesions.
Kelp	1,000–1,500 mg daily.	Supplies balanced vitamins and minerals.
Vitamin B complex	50 mg 3 times daily.	Necessary in all cellular enzyme system functions.
Helpful		
Coenzyme Q$_{10}$	30–60 mg daily.	A powerful free radical scavenger.
Multivitamin and mineral complex	As directed on label.	All nutrients are necessary in balance. Use a high-potency formula.
Raw glandular complex plus	As directed on label.	Promotes immune function.
raw thymus glandular	As directed on label.	
Vitamin K or alfalfa	100 mcg daily.	Antibiotics destroy the intestinal bacteria that produce vitamin K, which is necessary for blood clotting. See under Herbs, below.

HERBS

❑ Alfalfa is a good source of vitamin K, which is needed for blood clotting and healing, and is depleted by antibiotics.

❑ Echinacea, goldenseal, pau d'arco, and suma may alleviate symptoms. Alternate among two or more of these herbs. Consume three cups of herbal tea daily or take herbs in capsule or extract form as directed on the product label.

Caution: Do not take goldenseal internally on a daily basis for more than one week at a time, do not use it during pregnancy, and use it with caution if you are allergic to ragweed.

❑ Hops helps to relieve pain and stress.

RECOMMENDATIONS

❑ Use a latex (not sheepskin) condom for any sexual activity until the infection has cleared completely. These diseases are highly contagious. Be aware, however, that even the use of a condom does not guarantee protection against STDs. Abstinence is the only way to avoid any chance of transmitting the infection.

❑ If you are taking penicillin or another antibiotic for a sexually transmitted disease, be sure to add some form of acidophilus to your diet to replace lost "friendly" bacteria.

CONSIDERATIONS

❑ Antibiotics are the usual treatment for both syphilis and gonorrhea. It is important to take any prescribed antibiotic for the full course, even if symptoms abate. Do not stop taking the medication early.

❑ A strain of gonococci that are resistant to both penicillin and tetracycline has spread rapidly since it was first identified in 1985. This strain is, however, curable with other antibiotics.

❑ Many health care providers consider cervical dysplasia (a precancerous condition of the cervix characterized by the formation of abnormal tissue in the cervix) to be a sexually transmitted disease. They believe that it is caused by papillomaviruses, the same viruses that cause venereal warts.

❑ Many STDs that were in decline are becoming more common. Many experts link this rise to the AIDS epidemic; AIDS increases susceptibility to disease of every kind.

❑ *See also* AIDS; CANDIDIASIS; CHLAMYDIA; HERPESVIRUS INFECTION; WARTS; and/or YEAST INFECTION, all in Part Two.

Shingles (Herpes Zoster)

Shingles is a disease caused by the varicella-zoster virus, the same virus that causes chickenpox. It affects the nerve endings in the skin. The skin of the abdomen under the ribs, leading toward the navel, is most commonly affected, but shingles can appear anywhere on the body.

Most adults have already contracted chickenpox. This common childhood disease causes a fever and a rash that itches maddeningly, but rarely does any permanent damage. However, once the varicella-zoster virus enters the body and has caused chickenpox, it doesn't go away. It may lie dormant in the spinal cord and nerve ganglia for years until activated, usually by a weakening (temporary or permanent) of the immune system. Then the varicella-zoster infection spreads to their very ends of the nerves, causing them to send impulses to the brain that are interpreted as severe pain, itching, or burning, and rendering the overlying skin much more sensitive than usual.

An attack of shingles is often preceded by three or four days of chills, fever, and achiness. There may also be pain in the affected area. Then crops of tiny blisters appear. The affected area becomes excruciatingly painful and sensitive to the touch. Other symptoms can include numbness, depression, tingling, shooting pains, fever, and headache. This phase of shingles lasts seven to fourteen days. The blisters eventually form crusty scabs and drop off.

The chance of an attack of shingles can be increased by many factors, including stress, cancer, the use of anticancer drugs, and immune system deficiency. However, serious illness is not required to activate the virus. Any type of physical or emotional stress can make one susceptible. Often, something as innocuous as a minor injury or a mild cold can lead to an attack in an otherwise healthy person. In most cases, it is never determined just what the trigger is.

Shingles strikes some 850,000 Americans each year. It can appear at any age, but is most common in people over the age of fifty, when immune function naturally begins to decline as a result of aging. Most cases of shingles run their course within a few weeks. More severe cases may last longer and require aggressive treatment. In some cases, the pain continues for months, even years, after the blisters have disappeared. This syndrome, called postherpetic neuralgia, is more likely to occur in older people. If shingles develop near the eyes, the cornea may be affected and blindness may result. About 20 percent of persons who get shingles go on to suffer a recurrence of the disease.

For people with immune deficiencies, shingles and its aftermath can be devastating. The disease is capable of affecting the internal organs, attacking even the lungs and kidneys. Disseminated shingles can cause permanent injury—including blindness, deafness, or paralysis, depending upon the area of the body that is served by the infected nerves—if it goes unchecked. Death can occur as the result of a secondary bacterial infection or viral pneumonia brought on by shingles.

NUTRIENTS

SUPPLEMENT	SUGGESTED DOSAGE	COMMENTS
Essential		
L-Lysine	500 mg twice daily, on an empty stomach. Take with water or juice. Do not take with milk. Take with 50 mg vitamin B$_6$ and 100 mg vitamin C for better absorption.	Important for healing and for fighting the virus that causes shingles. *See* AMINO ACIDS in Part One. *Caution:* Do not take this supplement for longer than 6 months at a time.
Vitamin C with bioflavonoids	2,000 mg 4 times daily.	Aids in fighting the virus and boosting the immune system.
Very Important		
Cayenne (capsicum)		*See under* Herbs, below.
Vitamin B complex	100 mg 3 times daily.	Needed for nerve health and to counteract deficiencies. Injections (under a doctor's supervision) may be necessary.
plus extra vitamin B$_{12}$	1,000 mcg twice daily.	Use a lozenge or sublingual form.
Zinc	80 mg daily for 1 week, then reduce to 50 mg daily. Do not exceed a total of 100 mg daily from all supplements.	Enhances immunity and protects against infection. Use zinc chelate lozenges for faster absorption.

Important		
Calcium plus magnesium	1,500 mg daily. 750 mg daily.	For nerve function and healing, and to combat stress. Use chelate forms.
Garlic (Kyolic)	2 capsules 3 times daily, with meals.	Excellent for building the immune system.
Vitamin A emulsion or capsules	50,000 IU daily for 2 weeks, then reduce to 25,000 IU daily. If you are pregnant, do not exceed 10,000 IU daily. 10,000 IU daily.	Boosts the immune system and protects against infection. Emulsion form is recommended for easier assimilation and greater safety at higher doses.
plus natural carotenoid complex (Betatene)	As directed on label.	To protect immune function and enhance healing.
Vitamin D	1,000 IU twice daily for 1 week, then reduce to 400 IU daily.	Aids in tissue healing and is needed for calcium absorption.
Vitamin E	400–800 IU daily. Can also open a capsule and apply the oil directly to the affected areas of skin.	Helps prevent formation of scar tissue.
Helpful		
Coenzyme Q$_{10}$	60 mg daily.	A free radical scavenger that boosts immune function.
Essential fatty acids (flaxseed oil and primrose oil are good sources)	As directed on label.	Promotes healing of skin and nerve tissue.
Grape seed extract	As directed on label.	A powerful antioxidant that protects skin cells and decreases the number of outbreaks of blisters.
Infla-Zyme Forte from American Biologics	4 tablets 3 times daily, with meals.	Has antioxidant properties and aids in proper breakdown of proteins, fats, and carbohydrates.
Maitake or shiitake or reishi	As directed on label. As directed on label. As directed on label.	Has immune-boosting and antiviral properties.
Multivitamin and mineral complex	As directed on label.	All nutrients are necessary in balance.
Wobenzym N from Marlyn Nutraceuticals	3–6 tablets 2–3 times daily, between meals.	Destroys free radicals and aids in proper breakdown and absorption of foods. Also good for inflammation.

HERBS

❑ Alfalfa, chamomile, and dandelion promote healing by helping to restore the body's normal acid/alkaline balance. Dandelion also helps to detoxify and support the liver.

Caution: Do not use chamomile on an ongoing basis, and avoid it completely if you are allergic to ragweed.

❑ Astragalus root and echinacea boost immune function.
Caution: Do not use astragalus in the presence of a fever.

❑ Cayenne (capsicum) contains a substance called capsaicin, which relieves pain and aids in healing. It also acts as a detoxifier. Cayenne is available in tablet and capsule form. Capsaicin is also the active ingredient in Zostrix, a topical cream, which is helpful for postherpetic neuralgia. Capsaicin should not be applied topically until the lesions caused by shingles have completely healed, however, or extreme burning pain can result.

❑ Goldenseal has powerful antibiotic properties and reduces infection.

Caution: Do not take this herb internally on a daily basis for more than one week at a time, do not use it during pregnancy, and use it with caution if you are allergic to ragweed.

❑ A combination of oat straw, St. Johnswort, and skullcap helps to reduce stress and itching. Mix equal amounts of oat straw, St. Johnswort, and skullcap tinctures together, and take 1 teaspoon of this mixture four times daily.

❑ Milk thistle protects the liver and promotes healthy liver function.

❑ Rose hips are high in vitamin C and are good for preventing infections on the skin.

❑ Valerian root calms the nervous system. Taken at bedtime, it acts as a sleep aid.

RECOMMENDATIONS

❑ Include in the diet brewer's yeast, brown rice, garlic, raw fruits and vegetables, and whole grains.

❑ Go on a cleansing fast. *See* FASTING in Part Three.

❑ Use bee pollen or propolis, chlorophyll, and/or kelp to fight the virus and promote healing.

Caution: Bee pollen may cause an allergic reaction in some individuals. Start with a small amount, and discontinue use if a rash, wheezing, discomfort, or other symptoms occur.

❑ Keep stress to a minimum. Stress reduces the immune system's effectiveness in fighting off infection. Studies have found that people with shingles report having recently been through stressful periods more often than other people.

❑ Avoid drafts. Allow the affected area to be exposed to sunlight for fifteen minutes each day. Wash the blisters gently when bathing, and otherwise avoid touching or scratching them.

❑ Avoid taking medications that contain acetaminophen (Tylenol, Datril, and others), as they may prolong the illness.

❑ See an ophthalmologist if the shingles appear on the forehead, near the eyes, or on the tip of the nose. Untreated ophthalmic herpes zoster can lead to vision loss.

❑ Try using essential oils. Bergamot oil, calophyllum oil (related to St. Johnswort), eucalyptus oil, geranium oil, goldenseal oil, and lemon oil can be used singly or in combination. These highly concentrated plant essences have strong antiviral properties. The best way to use them is to add a few drops of essential oil to a tablespoon of a carrier oil such as almond, peanut, or olive oil, and apply the mixture directly to the lesions at the first sign of an outbreak. In most

instances, the lesions dry up and disappear completely within three to five days after this treatment. This treatment can also be used for herpes simplex.

CONSIDERATIONS

❑ There is no known cure for shingles. Treatment focuses on shortening the acute phase of pain and rash, minimizing pain and discomfort, and attempting to prevent or minimize possible complications. Physicians often prescribe an antiviral medication called acyclovir (Zovirax), which is also used for herpes. Acyclovir often helps minimize pain as well as prevent some complications, particularly for people with compromised immune systems. If acyclovir treatment is not begun within the first few days of the onset of shingles, however, it is not usually effective. This can be a problem because early diagnosis is often difficult. Acyclovir is also relatively expensive. Pain medication, possibly a narcotic, may be necessary to ease the discomfort.

❑ Capsaicin has been attracting attention for its ability to relieve pain in persons suffering from postherpetic neuralgia. Capsaicin is not a product of chemical engineering, but a component found in plants of the same family as red peppers. Researchers in Toronto found that 56 percent of people with postherpetic neuralgia who were treated with capsaicin cream (Zostrix) for four weeks experienced significant relief of pain, and that 78 percent had at least some improvement in pain. Clinical studies suggest that capsaicin directly reduces the amount of substance P, a neurotransmitter responsible for the transmission of pain impulses. If there is a deficiency of substance P, the nerves are unable to transmit sensations of pain. Capsaicin is easy to administer—it is simply applied topically to the affected area three or four times a day. In addition, capsaicin does not interact with any other drugs or medications, which makes it an especially attractive option for elderly people, who are often taking one or more drugs on a regular basis. Capsaicin cream is sold over the counter in most drug stores and health food stores. It should not be applied until the blisters caused by shingles have healed completely, however, or extreme burning pain may result.

❑ People with compromised immune systems may be given serum or other biological products obtained from the pooled blood of people who have recently recovered from shingles to assist their own immune systems in resisting the virus. However, in this age of AIDS, such treatment has become riskier and more expensive due to screening procedures to assure safety. Physicians are now more likely to administer huge doses of antiviral drugs to try to destroy or cripple the virus.

❑ Orthomolecular physicians often administer injections of vitamin B_{12} combined with adenosine monophosphate (AMP) for shingles. This treatment, together with applications of zinc oxide and plain yogurt along the path of the affected nerve two to three times daily, can bring relief.

☐ Dimethylsulfoxide (DMSO) has been used with success to relieve the pain of shingles and promote healing of the lesions.

☐ While shingles itself is not contagious, a person with shingles may infect previously uninfected persons, particularly children, with chickenpox.

☐ If conservative measures are not effective, an antidepressant such as amitriptyline (Elavil, Endep) may be prescribed. These drugs not only ease the emotional impact of unrelenting pain, but they seem to alleviate the pain itself. They appear to do this by causing an increase in the production of endorphins, the body's own natural painkillers.

☐ Experiments are being conducted in which live chickenpox vaccine is given intravenously in an attempt to prevent shingles. Since you cannot develop shingles if you never contract chickenpox, researchers theorize that a vaccine that prevents chickenpox would therefore also prevent shingles. Detractors argue that while this approach may produce immunity in those who have never had chickenpox, the virus in the vaccine may also take refuge in the central nervous system and cause shingles years or decades later.

☐ One of the biggest obstacles to researchers in learning more about the varicella-zoster virus is the fact that there are no animals in which it can be studied; chickenpox and shingles occur only in humans, and the virus grows poorly in laboratory cultures. Nonetheless, research continues into the biology of varicella-zoster, with the hope of developing a better understanding of how the immune system controls it and perhaps finding ways to ease the suffering caused by shingles and postherpetic neuralgia.

☐ *See also* PAIN CONTROL in Part Three.

Sinusitis

Sinusitis is an inflammation of the nasal sinuses. These are four sets of open spaces within the bones of the skull that are part of the "plumbing" system of the head. There are sinuses above the eyes (frontal sinuses); to either side of the nose, inside the cheekbones (maxillary sinuses); behind the bridge of the nose (sphenoid sinuses); and in the upper nose (ethmoid sinuses). Most cases of sinusitis affect the frontal and/or maxillary sinuses, but any or all of the sinuses may be involved, and each individual tends to have problems with a particular set of sinuses. If the sinuses are too small or poorly positioned to handle the volume of mucus produced, they can become clogged. Pressure in the sinuses increases, causing pain. Sinuses that are clogged for a long time seem to invite infection.

Sinusitis can be either acute or chronic. Acute sinusitis is frequently caused by bacterial or viral infections of the nose, throat, and upper respiratory tract, such as the common cold. More than 50 percent of all cases of sinusitis are caused by

bacteria. Chronic sinusitis problems may be caused by small growths in the nose, injury of the nasal bones, smoking, and exposure to irritant fumes and smells. Allergic sinusitis may be caused by hay fever or food allergies, especially allergies to milk and dairy products. People with compromised immune systems are susceptible to fungal sinusitis, a potentially dangerous condition that requires aggressive treatment.

Symptoms of sinusitis include fever (usually low-grade, but higher in some cases), cough, headache, earache, toothache, facial pain, cranial pressure, difficulty breathing through the nose, loss of the sense of smell, and tenderness over the forehead and cheekbones. If tapping the forehead just over the eyes, the cheekbones, or the area around the bridge of the nose causes pain, the sinuses may be infected. Sometimes sinusitis produces facial swelling followed by a stuffy nose and thick discharge of mucus. The symptoms suffered by those with sinusitis can have other unpleasant effects. Postnasal drip can cause a sore throat, nausea, and bad breath; difficulty breathing can cause snoring and loss of sleep.

NUTRIENTS

SUPPLEMENT	SUGGESTED DOSAGE	COMMENTS
Very Important		
Acidophilus	As directed on label.	Replaces good bacteria in the colon. Important if antibiotics are prescribed. Use a nondairy formula.
Quercetin plus	As directed on label.	Protects against allergens and increases immunity.
bromelain or	As directed on label.	Enhances the effectiveness of quercetin.
AntiAllergy formula from Freeda Vitamins	As directed on label.	Contains quercetin, calcium pantothenate, and calcium ascorbate to provide nutritional support and reduce allergic response.
Bee pollen	Start with ½ tsp daily and increase slowly to 1 tbsp daily, taken in juice.	Increases immunity and speeds healing. *Caution:* Bee pollen may cause an allergic reaction in some individuals. Discontinue use if at any time a rash, wheezing, discomfort, or other symptom occurs.
Fenu-Thyme from Nature's Way or		*See under* Herbs, below.
PSI from Terra Maxa or		*See under* Herbs, below.
Sinus Check from Enzymatic Therapy	2 capsules 4 times daily.	A natural decongestant to help clear blocked nasal passages due to colds and sinusitis.
Flaxseed oil	As directed on label.	Reduces pain and inflammation. Enhances all body functions.
Raw thymus glandular	500 mg twice daily.	Protects immune function and health of the mucous membrane cells.

Multivitamin and mineral complex	As directed on label.	To improve overall health and assure proper nutrition.
Vitamin A	10,000 IU daily.	Enhances the immune system; protects against colds, flu, and other infections. Helps maintain the health of the mucous membranes.
plus natural beta-carotene or	15,000 IU daily.	Precursor of vitamin A.
carotenoid complex (Betatene)	As directed on label.	
Vitamin B complex	75–100 mg 3 times daily, with meals.	Helps to maintain healthy nerves and reduce stress. A sublingual form is best.
plus extra pantothenic acid (vitamin B$_5$) and	100 mg 3 times daily, with meals.	Aids in the formation of antibodies.
vitamin B$_6$ (pyridoxine)	50 mg 3 times daily, with meals.	Aids immune system function.
Vitamin C with bioflavonoids	3,000–10,000 mg daily, In divided doses.	Boosts immune function and aids in preventing infection and decreasing mucus.
Vitamin E	400–1,000 IU daily.	Improves circulation and speeds healing.
Helpful		
Coenzyme Q$_{10}$	60 mg daily.	Valuable immune system stimulant. Increases cellular oxygenation.
Dimethylsulfoxide (DMSO)	As directed on label.	Relieves pain and strengthens the immune system. Use only DMSO from a health food store.
Garlic (Kyolic)	2 capsules 3 times daily.	An immune system stimulant that helps to keep infection in check.
Proteolytic enzymes	As directed on label. Take with meals and between meals.	Destroys free radicals. Also aids in digestion of foods.
Pycnogenol or grape seed extract	As directed on label. As directed on label.	Powerful antioxidants. Reduce inflammation and the frequency of colds and flu. Neutralize allergic reactions.
Sea mussel	As directed on label.	Provides needed amino acids and aids in the functioning of the mucous membranes. Reduces inflammation.
Zinc lozenges (Ultimate Zinc-C Lozenges from Now Foods)	1 15-mg lozenge every 2–4 waking hours for 1 week. Do not exceed this amount.	Antiviral agent and immunity booster.

HERBS

❑ Anise, fenugreek, marshmallow, and red clover help to loosen phlegm and clear congestion.

❑ Bitter orange oil can be used to swab nasal passages for local relief.

❑ Cat's Claw Defense Complex from Source Naturals contains a combination of herbs designed to strengthen the body and help the body deal with outside elements.
Caution: Do not use cat's claw during pregnancy.

❑ ClearLungs from Natural Alternatives contains Chi-

nese herbal ingredients to restore free breathing, ease mucus accumulation, and enhance tissue repair.

❑ Echinacea boosts the immune system and fights viral infection.

❑ Ephedra (ma huang) helps to relieve congestion.
Caution: Do not use this herb if you suffer from anxiety, glaucoma, heart disease, high blood pressure, or insomnia, or if you are taking a monoamine oxidase (MAO) inhibitor drug for depression.

❑ Fenu-Thyme from Nature's Way Products relieves nasal and sinus congestion. Take 2 capsules three times daily. PSI from Terra Maxa is also good.

❑ Ginger root can be crushed and applied as a poultice to the forehead and nose to stimulate circulation and drainage.

❑ Goldenseal is effective in combating sinusitis. Its benefits can be enhanced by combining it with 250 to 500 milligrams of bromelain, an enzyme present in fresh pineapple. Goldenseal can be taken as a tea, or the tea can be used as an intranasal douche. Or put a dropperful of alcohol-free goldenseal extract in your mouth, swish it around for a few minutes, then swallow. Do this three times daily.
Caution: Do not take goldenseal internally on a daily basis for more than one week at a time, do not use it during pregnancy, and use it with caution if you are allergic to ragweed.

❑ Horehound helps to relieve symptoms.

❑ Mullein reduces inflammation and soothes irritation.

❑ Rose hips are a good source of vitamin C.

RECOMMENDATIONS

❑ Eat a diet consisting of 75 percent raw foods.

❑ Drink plenty of distilled water and fresh vegetable and fruit juices. Also consume plenty of hot liquids such as soups and herbal teas. These help the mucus to flow, relieving congestion and sinus pressure. Adding cayenne pepper and raw onion may bring even faster relief.

❑ Eliminate sugar from your diet. Reduce your salt intake.

❑ Do not eat dairy foods, except for low-fat soured products like yogurt and cottage cheese. Dairy products increase mucus formation.

❑ Go on a cleansing fast. *See* FASTING in Part Three.

❑ Mix a solution of 1 cup warm water, ½ teaspoon of sea salt, and a pinch of bicarbonate of soda. Use a squeeze spray bottle (available over the counter in drugstores) or an eyedropper to instil the solution in the nostrils, one side at a time. Repeat this procedure three or four times a day as necessary for relief from stuffiness.

❑ Try using a menthol or eucalyptus pack applied over the sinuses to relieve pain and swelling. Stop if the packs cause irritation.

❑ Use a vaporizer to ease breathing and clear secretions.

❑ Use steam inhalations to promote drainage and ease pressure. Boil a pot of water and add a few drops of eucalyptus oil or rosemary oil. Remove the pot from the heat and lean your face over it at a distance of about 6 inches to inhale the steam. (Be careful not to get so close that irritation or scalding results.) Place a towel over your head to capture the steam and breathe in deeply. Do this several times daily for five to ten minutes at a time. Or simply take a hot shower to help relieve the pain and pressure of sinusitis.

❑ Use warm compresses or ice packs to help relieve pain (experiment to see which works best for you).

❑ If you are taking antibiotics for a sinus infection, be sure to add an acidophilus supplement to your program. Do not take the acidophilus and the antibiotic at the same time.

❑ If you use decongestants, use them only as directed and for the prescribed amount of time. If possible, avoid using nose drops and sprays. These can become addictive and interfere with normal sinus function. In addition, drops and sprays, as well as inhalers, can shrink blood vessels in the nose, eventually causing the vessels to weaken. Moreover, withdrawal from decongestants can cause a rebound effect, in which the swelling becomes worse after use is discontinued than it was to begin with. They can also cause dangerous elevations in blood pressure. Do not use these medications if you have high blood pressure or heart problems.

❑ If sinusitis causes your eyes to become swollen, red, or itchy, or to begin tearing, try a product called OcuDyne. Made by Nutricology, this is a complex containing vitamins, minerals, antioxidants, key amino acids, active bioflavonoids, and the herbs bilberry and ginkgo biloba to protect the eyes and boost immune function.

❑ Do not use force when blowing your nose, as this forces mucus back into the sinus cavities. Instead, draw secretions to the back of the throat by sniffing, then expel them.

❑ Do not smoke, and avoid secondhand smoke. If you live in a smoggy area, consider getting an air purifier or moving to a less polluted area. The Living Air XL-15 from Alpine Industries is an air purification unit for home use. Air Supply from Wein Products is a personal air purifier. Worn around the neck, it sets up a defensive shield against microorganisms and microparticles in the air wherever you go.

❑ If you notice swelling around the eyes, consult your physician. This is a serious sign.

❑ Have regular dental examinations. Infections in the mouth can easily spread to the sinuses.

CONSIDERATIONS

❑ If nasal secretions turn clear after a week, you probably do not have an infection; if the mucus is greenish or yellowish, you probably do. If secretions are clear and you have no other symptoms of a cold, you probably have allergies.

❑ Antibiotics may be necessary to clear a bacterial infection. Always take antibiotics for the full course prescribed, even if symptoms seem to improve earlier. Stopping prematurely can lead to antibiotic-resistant bacteria and a worse infection.

❑ Sometimes physicians prescribe antibiotics even if they cannot confirm a bacterial infection. The reasoning for this is that it is very difficult to ascertain whether bacteria are causing the sinusitis, and that it may be worth it to prevent a bacterial infection from appearing later. As with any medication, it is important to know the benefits, risks, and costs of using and of not using an antibiotic.

❑ If sinus trouble is chronic and severe, and medication fails to relieve it, surgery may be needed to drain the sinuses, not only to relieve discomfort but to guard against serious consequences.

❑ Endoscopic surgery, a fairly new treatment for chronic, severe sinusitis, clears nasal passages without external incisions or scars. The procedure can be performed using local anesthesia and results in minimal pain and swelling.

❑ While they are uncommon, polyps and benign cysts that retain mucus can develop in the sinuses, especially in the large maxillary or frontal sinuses. Intrusive or malignant growths require surgical removal.

❑ Anyone suffering from unremitting sinusitis should consult a health care provider to rule out an underlying immune dysfunction. In a University of Miami study, 50 percent of chronic sinusitis patients were found to be suffering from immunological disorders.

Skin Cancer

There are several different types of skin cancer. The two most common are *basal cell carcinoma* and *squamous cell carcinoma*. Both are highly curable if treated early. The third major type of skin cancer is *malignant melanoma*, which is a more serious disease.

Basal cell carcinoma is the most common of the three major types of skin cancer. It usually occurs after the age of forty and is more prevalent in blond, fair-skinned men. Unlike many other malignant growths, it does not spread until it has been present for a long period of time. The cell damage results in an ulcerlike growth that spreads slowly as it destroys tissue. A large pearly-looking lump, most often on the face by the nose or ears, is usually the first sign. About six weeks after it appears, the lump becomes ulcerated, with a raw, moist center and a hard border that may bleed. Scabs continually form over the ulcer and then come off, but the ulcer never really heals. Sometimes basal cell carcinomas show up on the back or chest as flat sores that grow slowly.

In squamous cell carcinoma, the underlying skin cells are damaged and this leads to the development of a tumor or lump under the skin, most often on the ears, hands, face, or lower lip. The lump may resemble a wart or a small ulcerated spot that never heals. This type of skin cancer occurs most frequently in fair-skinned men over sixty years old. The risk is higher for those who have had long-term outdoor employment and for those who reside in sunny climates. Squamous cell carcinoma tends to be less invasive if it occurs on sun-damaged skin than if it occurs on skin not normally exposed to the sun, unless the lesions are found on the ears and lower lip.

Malignant melanoma is rarer than either squamous cell or basal cell carcinoma, but is much more serious. With this type of skin cancer, a tumor arises from the pigment-producing cells of the deeper layers of the skin. It is estimated that as many as half of all cases of melanoma originate in moles. People in some families seem to have a genetically based higher risk of developing melanoma. They often have odd moles, called *dysplastic nevi*, that are irregular in shape and color and can be as large as half an inch in diameter. Dysplastic nevi may be precursors to skin cancer.

If not treated at an early stage, melanoma can be life threatening, spreading through the bloodstream and lymphatic vessels to the internal organs. However, if the disease is treated early, the chances of recovery are quite good.

There are four types of melanoma, each with slightly different characteristics:

• *Superficial spreading melanoma* (SMM) is the most common type. It occurs primarily in Caucasians and more often in women than in men. An SSM lesion typically begins as a flat mole, most often on the lower legs or upper back, that develops a raised, irregular surface. As it grows, its borders usually become asymmetrical and notched.

• *Acral lentiginous melanoma* is most common among people of African and Asian descent. The lesions have flat dark-brown areas with bumpy portions that are brown-black or blue-black in color. They are most likely to appear on the palms of the hands, the soles of the feet, the nailbeds of fingers and toes, and the mucous membranes.

• *Lentigo maligna melanoma* is more common in women than in men. The lesions usually occur on the face, neck, ears, or other areas that have been heavily sun-exposed for a long period of time. This type of melanoma rarely occurs before the age of fifty, and it is usually preceded by a precancerous stage called *lentigo maligna* that appears years in advance of the melanoma.

• *Nodular melanoma* is a type of disease that attacks the underlying tissue without first spreading across the surface of the skin. It is more common in men than in women. The lesions may resemble blood blisters, and they may range in coloration from pearly white to blue-black. Nodular melanoma tends to metastasize (spread to other sites in the body) sooner than the other types of melanoma.

Overexposure to the sun's ultraviolet (UV) rays is the major factor in basal cell carcinoma, squamous cell carcinoma, and melanoma. These rays disrupt the genetic ma-

terial in the skin cells, causing tissue damage. They also harm the skin's normal repair mechanism. Normally, after UV exposure, this mechanism causes damaged cells to immediately cease reproducing, die, and be sloughed off to be replaced by new, healthy skin cells—this is why skin peels after a sunburn. If this repair system is impaired, damaged cells may continue to reproduce, and the skin becomes increasingly vulnerable to injury from subsequent exposure to UV rays. Sun exposure is not only the major cause of wrinkles; it is responsible for 90 percent of most forms of skin cancer. People who have had severe or blistering sunburns, especially in childhood, are twice as likely to develop the disease later in life. People with blond or red hair, blue or green eyes, and fair skin, who sunburn or freckle easily, are at the greatest risk for skin cancer, because they have less protective pigment in their skin.

In addition to the three major types of skin cancer, there are a number of other, less common types of cancer that affect the skin. *Mycosis fungoides* is technically a type of lymphoma (lymphatic cancer), but its main effects are on the skin. Initially, it appears as an itchy rash that may last for several years. Over time, the lesions spread, become firmer, and ulcerate. Eventually, if untreated, the disease may spread to the lymph nodes and other internal organs. Mycosis fungoides is a rare, slow-growing cancer that can be difficult to diagnose, especially early in the disease. A skin biopsy should make correct diagnosis possible.

A type of skin cancer that has become increasingly common in recent years is *Kaposi's sarcoma*. This type of cancer causes raised lesions that may be pink, red, brown, or purplish in color. They may appear anywhere on the body, but the most common sites are the legs, toes, upper torso, and mucous membranes. Kaposi's sarcoma was once a rare, very slowly progressing disease seen primarily in older men of Mediterranean descent. Since the AIDS epidemic began, however, it is no longer uncommon and is primarily associated with a poorly functioning immune system. People with AIDS tend to get a more aggressive variety of this cancer that eventually affects the lymph nodes and other internal organs.

An estimated 600,000 Americans develop some type of skin cancer each year, and over 10,000 die from the disease. In recent years, the incidence has been rising steadily, and the average age of people with skin cancer has been getting lower. Women under forty are developing the disease twice as fast as men in the same age group. Fortunately, skin cancer is quite curable when treated early. More than 90 percent of all cases of skin cancer are completely cured.

NUTRIENTS

SUPPLEMENT	SUGGESTED DOSAGE	COMMENTS
Essential		
Dimethylglycine (DMG) (Aangamik DMG from FoodScience Labs)	As directed on label.	Improves cellular oxygenation.

Coenzyme Q10	100 mg daily.	Improves cellular oxygenation.
Essential fatty acids (primrose oil)	As directed on label 3 times daily, before meals.	For cellular protection.
Garlic (Kyolic)	2 capsules 3 times daily.	Enhances immune function.
Proteolytic enzymes or Wobenzym N from Marlyn Nutraceuticals	As directed on label. Take with meals. 3–6 tablets 2–3 times daily, between meals.	Powerful free radical scavengers that also reduce inflammation and aid in proper break-down and absorption of nutrients from foods.
Selenium	200 mcg daily.	Powerful free radical scavenger. Protects against UV damage.
Superoxide dismutase (SOD)	As directed on label.	Destroys free radicals. Consider injections (under a doctor's supervision).
Vitamin A	50,000–100,000 IU daily for 10 days or for as long as you are on the program. If you are pregnant, do not exceed 10,000 IU daily.	Powerful antioxidants that destroy free radicals. Use emulsion form for easier assimilation and greater safety at high doses.
plus natural beta-carotene or carotenoid complex (Betatene)	15,000 IU daily. As directed on label.	Precursor of vitamin A.
Vitamin B complex and/or brewer's yeast	100 mg daily. 2 20-grain tablets 3 times daily.	Necessary for normal cell division and function. A good source of B vitamins.
Vitamin C with bioflavonoids	5,000–20,000 mg daily, in divided doses. See ASCORBIC ACID FLUSH in Part Three.	Powerful anti-cancer agent. Boosts immunity.
Vitamin E	Up to 1,000 IU daily.	Promotes healing and tissue repair. Use emulsion form for easier assimilation and greater safety in higher doses.

Important

Maitake or reishi or shiitake	4,000–8,000 mg daily. As directed on label. As directed on label.	These mushrooms contain substances that inhibit the growth and spread of cancerous tumors and also boost immune response.
Phytocharged nutritional supplements from Schiff	As directed on label.	Dietary supplements that protect against damage from sunlight and promote health.
Pycnogenol or grape seed extract	As directed on label. As directed on label.	Antioxidants that protect against UV-induced oxidative changes in skin.
Shark cartilage (BeneFin)	1 gm per 2 lbs of body weight daily, divided into 3 doses. If you cannot tolerate taking it orally, it can be administered rectally in a retention enema.	Has been shown to inhibit and even reverse the growth of some types of tumors. Also stimulates the immune system.
Zinc	As directed on label.	Important in activity of enzymes; cell division, growth, and repair; and proper immune function. Use zinc gluconate lozenges or zinc methionate (OptiZinc) for best absorption.

Helpful

Acidophilus	As directed on label. Take on an empty stomach.	Has an antibacterial effect on the body. Use a nondairy formula.
Aerobic 07 from Aerobic Life Industries or Dioxychlor from American Biologics	As directed on label. As directed on label.	Antimicrobial agents.
Concentrace from Trace Minerals Research	As directed on label.	To nourish skin and hair.
Dimethylsulfoxide (DMSO)	Apply topically as directed on label.	Promotes healing. Use only DMSO from a health food store.
Herpanacine from Diamond-Herpanacine Associates	As directed on label.	Contains antioxidants, amino acids, and herbs that promote skin health.
Kelp	1,000–1,500 mg daily.	For mineral balance. Use kelp in tablet form and/or eat sea vegetables.
L-Cysteine and L-methionine	As directed on label, on an empty stomach. Take with water or juice. Do not take with milk. Take with 50 mg vitamin B6 and 100 mg vitamin C for better absorption.	To detoxify harmful substances. See AMINO ACIDS in Part One.
Multienzyme complex	As directed on label. Take with meals.	To aid digestion.
Multivitamin and mineral complex	As directed on label, with meals.	All nutrients are necessary in balance. Do not use a sustained-release formula.
N-A-G from Source Naturals	As directed on label.	Supplies glucosamine, which helps in the formation of mucous membrane and connective tissues.
Para-aminobenzoic acid (PABA)	25 mg daily.	Helps to protect against skin cancer.
Raw glandular complex plus raw thymus glandular	As directed on label. As directed on label.	Stimulates glandular function, especially the thymus, an important component of the immune system.
Taurine	As directed on label.	Functions as foundation for tissue and organ repair.
Tea tree	See under Herbs, below.	
Vitamin B3 (niacin) plus choline and folic acid	100 mg daily. Do not exceed this amount. 500–1,000 mg daily. 400 mcg daily.	B vitamins that improve circulation, build red blood cells, and aid liver function. Caution: Do not take niacin if you have a liver disorder, gout, or high blood pressure.
Vitamin B12 injections or vitamin B12	As prescribed by physician. 1,000 mcg 3 times daily.	To prevent anemia. Injections (under a doctor's supervision) are best. If injections are not available, use a lozenge or sublingual form.

HERBS

❑ Alfalfa, burdock, dandelion root, horsetail, Irish moss, marshmallow root, oat straw, rose hips, and yellow dock are all beneficial for tissue repair. Rose hips are also a good source of vitamin C.

❑ Astragalus generates anticancer cells in the body and boosts the immune system.

❑ Bilberry, cayenne (capsicum), ginger, goldenseal, nettle, sarsaparilla, and turmeric stimulate the liver and help to stabilize blood composition, and may retard the proliferation of cancer cells.

❑ The seeds and peel of the Chinese cucumber inhibit cancer cells.

❑ Skin cancers may respond to treatment with poultices combining comfrey, pau d'arco, ragwort, and wood sage. See USING A POULTICE in Part Three.

❑ Essiac tea, a combination herbal remedy, has been used with good results in cancer treatment.

❑ Ginkgo biloba, pau d'arco, and curcumin (a naturally occurring pigment isolated from turmeric) are powerful antioxidants with immune-enhancing capabilities.

❑ Studies have shown that green tea has anticancer properties. Drink 4 cups daily.

❑ Tea tree oil cream, applied topically, is a natural antiseptic and antifungal that enhances healing.

RECOMMENDATIONS

❑ Eat a diet that is low in fat and high in antioxidants, such as beta-carotene-rich carrots, sweet potatoes, squash, and spinach; cruciferous vegetables such as broccoli, Brussels sprouts, cabbage, kale, and turnips; and citrus fruits.

❑ Be aware of the warning signs of skin cancer:

• An open sore that bleeds, crusts over, and does not heal properly.

• A reddish, irritated spot, usually on the chest, shoulder, arm, or leg. It may itch or hurt, or cause no discomfort.

• A smooth growth with an elevated border and an indented center. As it becomes bigger, tiny blood vessels develop on the surface.

• A shiny scarlike area that is white, yellow, or waxy, with a shiny, taut appearance.

• An enlarging, irregular, "angry-looking" lesion on the face, lips, or ears.

❑ Stay away from tanning salons. Their equipment is sometimes said to be safer than the sun because tanning beds emit ultraviolet-A (UVA) rays, the so-called cool rays, rather than the ultraviolet-B (UVB) rays, which are most often implicated in sunburn. It has been established, however, that UVA rays can cause skin cancer as well as UVB rays can. Do not be misled by claims to the contrary.

❑ Beware of new moles that appear after age forty, as well as any mole that appears unusual; is irregularly shaped or changes in size or color; is pearly white, translucent, black, or multicolored; has a ridge around the edge; spreads, bleeds, or itches; or is constantly irritated by clothing. Check for discharge from moles. Have any suspicious mole evaluated by a professional.

❑ See your health care provider if you find a growth that fits any of these descriptions. Early detection is the key to successful treatment of skin cancer.

❑ Include in the diet plenty of foods that are high in vitamin E. A diet rich in vitamin E may protect your skin against damage from UV rays. Good food sources of vitamin E include asparagus, green leafy vegetables, raw nuts, wheat germ, and organic, cold-pressed vegetable oils.

❑ To protect against skin cancer, take protective measures while in the sun. The sun's ultraviolet rays are strongest between 10:00 a.m. and 2:00 p.m. Stay out of the sun as much as possible between these hours. When spending time outdoors, wear light-colored clothing made of tightly woven material, plus a hat and sunglasses that block ultraviolet rays. Always use sunscreen. Choose a product with a sun protection factor (SPF) of 15 or higher and that specifies broad-spectrum protection. Wear sunscreen on cloudy days; nearly 85 percent of the sun's UV rays penetrate through clouds. Apply sunscreen to all exposed skin, and reapply it every three or four hours while you are outside. Be sure to protect your lips with a lip balm that has an SPF of 15, too.

❑ If you have a family history of melanoma, avoid the sun as much as possible and use a sun block every day. Keep a close watch on any moles or other skin lesions, and have them checked regularly by a physician.

❑ Avoid exposure to halogen lighting at close range. Halogen lights also emit UV radiation. The National Foundation for Cancer Research advises maintaining a distance of at least 20 inches from a 20-watt halogen bulb and 3 to 6 feet from 35- to 50-watt bulbs.

CONSIDERATIONS

❑ Skin cancer often originates in moles, but moles are not necessarily a cancer risk. They are extremely common (most people have them) and the overwhelming majority of them do not become cancerous.

❑ Medical treatment for skin cancer most often involves surgery. Excisional biopsy (removal of the growth for analysis) cures skin cancer in its early stages in about 95 percent of cases. More radical surgery may be necessary if excision is delayed, and if the growth is large, a skin graft may be necessary. Other treatments sometimes used for skin cancer include:

• Cryosurgery, a method that uses liquid nitrogen to freeze and kill the diseased tissue, which later flakes away. This type of treatment is used frequently for people with bleeding disorders and for those who cannot tolerate anesthesia.

• *Electrosurgery*, in which the cancer is scooped out with a curette (a circular blade) and an electric current burns a border around the site to kill remaining cancer cells.

• *Laser surgery*, in which a laser is used to cut away the damaged tissue and seal off surrounding blood vessels as it goes.

• *Moh's technique*, in which a surgeon shaves off cancerous tissue one thin layer at a time until healthy tissue is reached. Each layer is then examined under a microscope so that the doctor can be assured he or she has gotten all the cancer while taking a minimum of healthy skin. This surgery is most effective for recurrent cancers and for cases in which the tumor is large or the extent of the cancer is unknown.

• *Radiation therapy*, which involves training an x-ray or an electron beam on the diseased area to kill cancerous tissue. This alternative is good for cases in which surgery poses particular risks.

❑ With early detection and treatment, most people recover from skin cancer, but regular checkups are advised for at least the next five years.

❑ The Skin Cancer Foundation recommends full-body self-examination every three months. To do this, you need a full-length mirror, a hand-held mirror, and ample lighting. Look for any changes in the moles or marks on your body, using the following A-B-C-D checklist:

• **A**ssymetry. Both sides of the mole should be shaped similarly.

• **B**order. The edges of moles should be smooth, not blurred or ragged.

• **C**olor. Tan, brown, and dark brown are normal. Red, white, blue, and black are not.

• **D**iameter. Any mole that is larger than ¼ inch in diameter, or whose diameter seems to be increasing, is suspicious.

In addition to keeping track of moles, look carefully for other unusual spots or growths. Any irregularities you find should be evaluated by a dermatologist.

❑ Dry red, scaly spots on the face, neck, or the backs of the hands may be actinic, or solar, keratoses. These are lesions that result from years of overexposure to the sun, and they are considered to be precancerous. Later, these spots may become hard to the touch and grayish or brown in color. There is a prescription medication, masoprocol (Actinex), that can halt these growths without irritating the surrounding skin.

❑ The average person incurs between 50 and 80 percent of all sun exposure prior to the age of eighteen. Thus, even though skin cancer is rare in children, the childhood years have a major influence on a person's tendency to develop skin cancer later in life. An infant under the age of six months should never be exposed to direct sunlight or have sunscreen applied to his or her skin. Infants should always be dressed in protective clothing when they are outside. Sunscreen can be used on a baby over six months old (choose a PABA-free

formula, preferably one meant for young children), but sun exposure should still be limited, and the child should still be dressed in protective clothing. For toddlers and young children, limit time in the sun and apply sunscreen regularly whenever they are outdoors. Older children should be taught the importance of applying sunscreen regularly—an important lifelong habit.

❑ Certain medications may make the skin more susceptible to sun damage. These include antibiotics, antidepressants, diuretics, antihistamines, sedatives, estrogen, and acne medications such as retinoic acid. Ask your health care provider or pharmacist if any medication that you take might have such an effect.

❑ A study reported in the *Journal of the American Academy of Dermatology* found that well-educated white-collar men have the highest risk of developing melanoma. Researchers surmise that a pattern of many months of little sun exposure (a result of working indoors) with occasional overexposure and sunburn (such as that acquired at sunny resort vacations) may be responsible.

❑ The prescription medication tretinoin (Retin-A) may be able to reverse precancerous sun damage in skin. Skin care products containing alpha-hydroxy acids, which are available over the counter, may have a similar effect, although they are less potent.

❑ The U.S. Food and Drug Administration has approved for marketing as a sun protectant a line of clothing produced by Sun Precautions, Inc., of Seattle. The clothing, which carries an SPF rating of 30, is sold under the brand name Solumbra.

❑ A June 1988 article in the *British Journal of Surgery* suggested that essential fatty acids, found in such sources as primrose oil and fish oil, may be beneficial for the prevention and treatment of malignant melanoma.

❑ Preliminary research into the potential of beta-carotene, folic acid, retinoic acid, vitamin C, vitamin E, and minerals as inhibitors of skin cancer is encouraging.

❑ Garlic may be effective in fighting basal cell carcinoma by boosting the body's immune response.

❑ Skin cancer rates are still rising, despite steady sunscreen sales. One reason may be that people think that they are adequately protected and stay in the sun too long. Another is that all sunscreens protect against UVB rays, but only some protect against UVA rays. UVB rays are the "burning" rays, so a sunscreen that protects only against UVB takes away an important warning sign. Consequently, people may be overexposing themselves to UVA rays, which do not cause sunburn but have been linked to skin cancer.

❑ A worldwide rise in the incidence of skin cancer has been linked to the destruction of the earth's ozone layer. The ozone layer acts as a protective atmospheric sunscreen. As it becomes thinner and holes develop in it, more of the sun's harmful rays reach the earth.

☐ To increase awareness of the damaging potential of UV radiation, the U.S. Environmental Protection Agency and the National Weather Service have developed the following UV index and exposure guidelines for use in weather reports to help individuals evaluate the level of danger from sun exposure on any given day:

UV Index Number	Danger Level
0–2	minimal
3–4	low
5–6	moderate
7–8	high
9–10+	very high

☐ More information about skin cancer is available from the American Cancer Society at 800–227–2345 and the National Cancer Institute at 800–422–6237.

Skin Problems

See ACNE; AGE SPOTS; ATHLETE'S FOOT; BEDSORES; BOIL; BRUISING; BURNS; CANKER SORES; COLD SORES (FEVER BLISTERS); CORNS AND CALLUSES; DANDRUFF; DERMATITIS; DRY SKIN; FUNGAL INFECTION; HIVES; INSECT BITE; INTERTRIGO; LEG ULCERS; OILY SKIN; PSORIASIS; ROSACEA; SCABIES; SEBACEOUS CYST; SEBORRHEA; SKIN CANCER; SKIN RASH; SUNBURN; VITILIGO; WARTS; WRINKLING, OF SKIN. *See also under* PREGNANCY-RELATED PROBLEMS.

Skin Rash

The skin is the body's largest organ. It consists of three layers—the epidermis (outer layer), the dermis (middle layer), and the subcutaneous layer (inner layer). The skin acts as a shield between the body and the millions of foreign substances that exist in our environment. It also functions as a means of excreting toxins and other substances from the body, as the kidneys and bowels do. As a result, the skin is subject to the development of various bumps and blisters, as well as to changes in color, cracking, dryness, flaking, itching, redness, roughness, scaling, thickening, and a host of other problems.

There are many reasons for skin reactions. Some of the most common include allergies to molds, foods, chemicals, cosmetics, and other substances; insect bites; reactions to plants such as poison ivy; diaper rash; reactions to the sun and wind; reactions to drugs or alcohol; reactions to detergents; reactions to alcohol; and friction, either from two parts of the body rubbing against each other or from contact with an external agent, such as an ill-fitting shoe.

HERBS

☐ A poultice made with chaparral, dandelion, and yellow dock root benefits many types of skin rashes. *See* USING A POULTICE in Part Three.

☐ Calendula, chamomile, elder flower, and tea tree oil can be used externally as a soothing wash on rashes.

RECOMMENDATIONS

☐ For quick relief of itching and inflammation, soak a clean cloth in cool water (or, for even greater soothing effect, in comfrey tea that has cooled), wring it out, and apply it to the affected area for ten minutes. Repeat this procedure as often as necessary for relief.

☐ *See* Common Types of Rashes on page 484 to help you identify possible causes of a rash, and refer to the appropriate sections in Part Two for advice on treatment.

CONSIDERATIONS

☐ Skin rashes in children are often caused by food allergies, especially to chocolate, dairy products, eggs, peanuts, milk, wheat, fish, chicken, pork, or beef. Some experts estimate that allergies to eggs, peanuts, and milk account for as many as 75 percent of all skin rashes in children.

☐ Many doctors recommend hydrocortisone cream for minor irritations, poison ivy, itchy insect bites, and diaper rash.

☐ Allergy testing is advised, particularly for persistent rashes. (*See* ALLERGIES in Part Two.)

☐ *See also* ACNE; ALLERGIES; ATHLETE'S FOOT; CANDIDIASIS; CHEMICAL ALLERGIES; CHICKENPOX; DERMATITIS; ENVIRONMENTAL TOXICITY; FUNGAL INFECTION; GANGRENE; HERPESVIRUS INFECTION; HIVES; INSECT BITE; LUPUS; LYME DISEASE; MEASLES; MONONUCLEOSIS; PELLAGRA; POISON IVY/POISON OAK; PSORIASIS; RHEUMATIC FEVER; RINGWORM; ROSACEA; SCABIES; SEBORRHEA; SHINGLES; VITILIGO; and/or WARTS, all in Part Two.

Sleep Problems

See FATIGUE; INSOMNIA; NARCOLEPSY.

Smoking Dependency

Tobacco has been used as a mood-altering substance for centuries. It has been ingested by various means, including chewing, sniffing, and smoking. Today it is most commonly consumed by smoking cigarettes.

Tobacco smoke contains thousands of chemical constituents. The one believed to be responsible for many (if not most) of smoking's effects, as well as its extraordinary

Common Types of Rashes

The best way to approach treatment for a rash is to eliminate the underlying cause. Following are descriptions of some of the conditions most often responsible for skin rashes. This list is not exhaustive, and it is not meant as a substitute for diagnosis by a qualified health care practitioner. Any rash that persists for longer than one week, that seems to be getting worse, or that is accompanied by other symptoms, such as fever, should be evaluated by a professional.

Cause of Rash	Characteristic Features
Athlete's foot	Inflammation, scaling, cracking, and blisters on the feet, especially between the toes. Burning and/or itching may be severe.
Chickenpox	Crops of small round blisterlike pimples that crust over as they heal. Usually appears first on the torso, following a day or so of fever and headache, and then spreads to the face and extremities. Extremely itchy. Most common in children.
Dermatitis (eczema)	Patches of scaling, flaking, and thickening skin that may appear anywhere on the body. Skin color in the affected area may change. Itching is common. One type of dermatitis causes round lesions on the limbs.
Food or drug allergy	A flat pink or red rash, with possible swelling and/or itching.
Fungal infection (candida)	Moist, possibly itchy, red patches that may appear anywhere on the body, but are most common in areas where skin surfaces rub together. In babies, an inflamed, shiny diaper rash.
Herpesvirus infection	Painful fluid-filled blisters that erupt periodically around the mouth and/or genitals.
Hives	A rash that usually appears suddenly and can take the form of patches of tiny, goosebump-like spots or red, itchy welts that cover significant areas of the body—or anything in between.
Intertrigo	Sore, red, chronically damp areas, most often in the groin or underarms, the inner thighs, and under the breasts.
Lyme disease	A red, circular lesion that gradually expands as the center appears to clear up. This may be followed by a rash composed of small raised bumps on the torso. The rash may or may not be accompanied by flulike symptoms of fever, chills, and nausea.
Measles	A raised red rash that usually begins on the forehead and ears and spreads to the rest of the body. The rash usually follows several days of viral symptoms including fever, cough, sneezing, runny nose, and possibly conjunctivitis. There may be tiny red spots with white centers in the mouth as well.
Mononucleosis	A bumpy red rash accompanied by headache, achiness, low-grade fever, sore throat, and persistent fatigue.
Pellagra	An itchy, inflammatory rash, usually on the hands, face, and/or neck. Reddening of the skin is followed by the eruption of blisters, some of them large, and by crusting, peeling, and scaling. The rash may be accompanied by an inflamed and sore red tongue, diarrhea, weakness, and loss of appetite.
Poison ivy/poison oak	A red, intensely itchy rash with swelling and oozing blisters. If scratched, the rash can spread.
Psoriasis	Silvery, scaly patches that may appear anywhere on the body, but are most common on the scalp, ears, arms, legs, knees, elbows, and back. The rash follows a pattern of periodic flare-ups followed by healing. It may or may not be itchy.
Ringworm	Small, itchy round red spots that grow to be approximately ¼ inch in diameter, with scaly, slightly raised borders. They tend to clear in the center as they expand.
Rosacea	Reddening, small bumps, and pimples, usually affecting the nose and the center of the face. It resembles acne, but is chronic and is more common in middle-aged and older individuals.
Scabies	A persistent itchy rash with small red lumps that may become dry and scaly. Fine, wavy dark lines may emanate from some lumps. Most often occurs between the fingers, on the wrists and/or forearms, and on the breasts and/or genitals.
Seborrhea	Greasy yellowish, flaky patches of skin that form scales and crusts. It can appear anywhere on the body, but most often affects the scalp, face, and/or chest. It may or may not be itchy.
Shingles	Crops of tiny blisters that are extremely painful and sensitive to the touch and that eventually crust, scab, and are shed. Most common on the abdomen below the ribs, but it can occur anywhere on the body. May be preceded and/or accompanied by flulike symptoms of chills, fever, and achiness.

addictiveness, is nicotine. Nicotine acts as a stimulant on the central nervous system; when nicotine is ingested, adrenaline production increases, raising the blood pressure and heart rate. Nicotine also affects the overall metabolic rate, the regulation of body temperature, the degree of tension in the muscles, and the levels of certain hormones. These and other metabolic changes create a pleasurable sensation in the user that often—and paradoxically—is experienced as a feeling of relaxation.

This pleasurable sensation is one of the factors that makes tobacco so addictive. Another is the fact that tolerance to the effects of nicotine develops quite rapidly. That is, the dose needed to achieve the desired effect begins to rise almost immediately, encouraging you to increase the amount you smoke—which in turn increases the likelihood of addiction. Once you become addicted, your body depends on the presence of nicotine. If you then refrain from smoking, withdrawal symptoms occur. These include irritability, frustration, anger, anxiety, difficulty concentrating, restlessness, increased appetite, headache, stomach cramps, a slowed heart rate, a rise in blood pressure, and, most of all, an intense craving for nicotine.

Once the smoking habit has been acquired, it is difficult to break. Some authorities have stated that addiction to tobacco may be harder to overcome than addiction to heroin or cocaine. This is because smoking creates both physical *and* psychological dependency. It may be easier to overcome the physical addiction than the psychological dependency. Acute physical withdrawal, while unpleasant, lasts for a limited period of time, usually no more than several weeks. Long-term cravings are more likely a matter of psychological dependence, and require an ongoing effort to master. By the time an individual has become addicted to nicotine, the act of smoking itself has become a source of pleasure, and it may be so intertwined in your mind with other activities—having your morning coffee, reading the newspaper, working, socializing, whatever—that you find yourself unable to imagine engaging in these activities without a cigarette in hand. In addition, smoking provides a convenient excuse for taking a momentary break, especially during times of stress, and may help to smooth over awkward moments. Many smokers also are afraid of what might happen if they stopped; they fear withdrawal symptoms, weight gain, or a decreased ability to concentrate. All of these factors combine to make quitting difficult.

Even though it can be difficult to stop smoking, many people do it every day. There is certainly no shortage of reasons to quit. Cigarettes are a factor in approximately 17 percent of all deaths in the United States annually—that's 350,000 to 400,000 people a year. This is more than the number of deaths from alcohol, illegal drugs, traffic accidents, suicide, and homicide combined. Tobacco smoking causes an estimated one third of all cancer deaths, one fourth of fatal heart attacks, and 85 percent of deaths from chronic obstructive pulmonary disease. It accounts for at least 85 percent of lung cancer cases. Many other health problems have been linked to smoking as well, including angina, arteriosclerosis, cataracts, chronic bronchitis, colorectal cancer, diarrhea, emphysema, heartburn, high blood pressure, impotence, peptic ulcers, respiratory ailments, urinary incontinence, circulatory ailments, and cancers of the mouth and throat, especially among cigarette smokers who also consume alcohol and/or use mouthwash containing alcohol. Smoking increases the risk of catching colds and lengthens recovery time. Tobacco smoke paralyzes the cilia (hairlike protrusions lining the nose and throat), reducing their capacity to clear the passages by moving mucus—and the cold viruses trapped within it—to the outside.

Nicotine has long been known to be a deadly toxin. A single pinhead-sized drop of liquid nicotine, introduced directly into the bloodstream, would be fatal. At the doses normally ingested by smokers, nicotine makes the heart pump faster and work harder, increasing the likelihood of heart disease. It also constricts the peripheral blood vessels, contributing to circulatory disorders such as Raynaud's phenomenon and hardening of the arteries. And nicotine is not the only ingredient in cigarettes that poses a danger to health. In all, over 4,000 chemical substances have been identified as constituents of cigarette smoke, and at least 43 of these substances are known to cause cancer in humans. Cigarette smoke contains carbon monoxide, benzene, cyanide, ammonia, nitrosamines, vinyl chloride, radioactive particles, and other known irritants and carcinogens. Carbon monoxide binds to hemoglobin, interfering with the transport of oxygen throughout the body. Carbon monoxide also promotes the development of cholesterol deposits on artery walls. These two factors increase the risk of heart attack and stroke. Hydrogen cyanide causes bronchitis by inflaming the lining of the bronchi. Over the long term, smoking dramatically reduces flow of blood to the brain. Men who have smoked for years are more likely to have abnormally low penile blood pressure, which contributes to impotence. This is probably because smoking damages the blood vessels, including the tiny blood vessels that supply the penis. It also contributes to sterility; the sperm of men who smoke have less ability than that of nonsmokers to penetrate, and thus to fertilize, an egg.

Women cigarette smokers tend to experience menopause earlier, face a greater risk of osteoporosis after menopause, and have a much higher risk of developing cervical or uterine cancer. They also appear less fertile and have more difficulties during pregnancy. Smokers tend to have more miscarriages, stillbirths, and premature deliveries. Their babies often are smaller and have more health problems than babies of nonsmokers. Infants whose mothers smoke both during pregnancy and after childbirth appear to be three times as likely to die of sudden infant death syndrome (SIDS) as infants of nonsmokers.

Children whose fathers smoke also face an increase in health problems. Children of male smokers have been shown to be at a higher than normal risk of developing brain cancer and leukemia.

Smoking has a detrimental effect on nutrition. Smokers break down vitamin C about twice as fast as nonsmokers. This can deprive the body of adequate amounts of one of the most powerful and versatile antioxidants at our disposal. Other antioxidant vitamins are depleted as well. Cigarette smoke contains high concentrations of nitrogen dioxide ozone, a compound that oxidizes the antioxidant vitamins and is also known to do damage to DNA. The accelerated antioxidant usage, in combination with the DNA damage, speeds the aging process.

Finally, smoking is increasingly a social problem. More and more nonsmokers are becoming concerned about the effects of "secondhand" smoke on their own health, and justifiably so. There is a growing body of evidence that secondhand smoke may be even more dangerous than the smoke the smoker breathes. Smoking is now prohibited in many workplaces and public buildings.

The dangers of smoking are well known today, yet people continue to smoke. Why? Some people started smoking before the hazards were widely known; others start in adolescence, when people generally feel invulnerable and are more likely to engage in risk-taking behavior—especially if it seems "adult," helps them fit in with a particular social group, and/or provokes their parents. However, surveys consistently show that no matter when or why they started, most current smokers do not smoke because they want to (well over 50 percent say they wish they had never started), but because they are addicted.

The good news is that this addiction can be overcome, and that health benefits begin almost immediately. In just twenty-four hours after your last cigarette, your blood pressure and pulse rate should return to normal, as should the levels of oxygen and carbon monoxide in your blood. Within a week, your risk of heart attack begins to decrease, your senses of smell and taste improve, and breathing becomes easier.

The nutrients and dietary suggestions below are recommended to correct probable smoking-related deficiencies and damage while you work to kick the habit. They are recommended also if you cannot avoid being a passive smoker.

NUTRIENTS

SUPPLEMENT	SUGGESTED DOSAGE	COMMENTS
Essential		
Coenzyme Q10	200 mg twice daily.	Aids oxygen flow to the brain; protects heart tissue. Also acts as an antioxidant to protect cells and the lungs.
Oxy-5000 Forte from American Biologics	2 tablets 3 times daily.	A powerful antioxidant. Destroys free radicals produced in the smoke.
Vitamin C	5,000–20,000 mg daily. *See* ASCORBIC ACID FLUSH in Part Three.	Important antioxidant that protects against cell damage. Smoking drastically depletes the body of vitamin C.
Vitamin B complex	100 mg daily.	Necessary in cellular enzyme systems often damaged in smokers. Use sublingual form.
plus extra vitamin B12	1,000 mcg twice daily.	Increases energy; needed for liver function. Use a lozenge or sublingual form.
and folic acid	400 mcg daily.	Needed for the formation of red blood cells; important for healthy cell division and replication.
Vitamin E	Start with 200 IU daily and increase by 200 IU each month, up to 800 IU daily.	One of the most important antioxidants, needed to protect cells and organs from damage by the smoke.
Very Important		
Vitamin A	25,000 IU daily. If you are pregnant, do not exceed 10,000 IU daily.	Antioxidants that aid in the healing of mucous membranes.
and natural beta-carotene	15,000 IU daily.	Important for lung protection.
or carotenoid complex (Betatene)	As directed on label.	
Zinc	50–80 mg daily. Do not exceed a total of 100 mg daily from all supplements.	Important in immune function. Use zinc gluconate lozenges or OptiZinc for best absorption.
Helpful		
Body Language Super Antioxidant from Oxyfresh	As directed on label.	Contains antioxidant vitamins and herbs to protect against free radical damage.
Cell Guard from Biotec Foods	As directed on label.	Provides high levels of antioxidant enzymes for cellular health.
Dimethylglycine (DMG) (Aangamik DMG from FoodScience Labs)	As directed on label.	Detoxifies the body and helps the body maintain high energy levels.
Pycnogenol or	As directed on label.	Powerful antioxidants and free radical scavengers.
grape seed extract	As directed on label.	
Herpanacine from Diamond-Herpanacine Associates	As directed on label.	Detoxifies the body, balances the nervous system, and boosts immunity.
L-cysteine and L-methionine and L-cysteine plus	As directed on label, on empty stomach. Take with water or juice. Do not take with milk. Take with 50 mg vitamin B6 and 100 mg vitamin C for better absorption.	Potent detoxifiers that protect the lungs, liver, brain, and tissues from cigarette smoke.
glutathione	As directed on label.	Protects the liver.
Maitake	1,000–4,000 mg daily.	Inhibits carcinogenesis and protects against metastasis through the lungs.
Multivitamin and mineral complex with	As directed on label.	Necessary for immune function.
selenium	200 mcg daily.	Helps to prevent cell damage.
Raw thymus glandular	As directed on label.	A glandular that improves immune function.

HERBS

☐ Cayenne (capsicum) desensitizes respiratory tract cells to irritants from cigarette smoke.

❑ Catnip, hops, lobelia, skullcap, and/or valerian root can be used to help reduce the nervousness and anxiety that may accompany nicotine withdrawal.

Caution: Do not take lobelia internally on an ongoing basis.

❑ Dandelion root and milk thistle protect the liver against harmful toxins from cigarette smoke.

❑ Ginger causes perspiration, which helps the body to shed some of the poisons ingested through smoking. It also soothes stomach irritation occasionally experienced with the use of cayenne or lobelia.

❑ Slippery elm relieves lung congestion and coughs.

RECOMMENDATIONS

❑ Consume more asparagus, broccoli, Brussels sprouts, cabbage, cauliflower, spinach, sweet potatoes, and turnips. Eat plenty of grains, nuts, seeds, and unpolished brown rice. Millet cereal is a good source of protein. Eat wheat, oat, and bran. Also consume yellow and deep-orange vegetables such as carrots, pumpkin, squash, and yams. Apples, berries, Brazil nuts, cantaloupe, cherries, grapes, legumes (including chickpeas, lentils, and red beans), and plums are also helpful.

❑ Eat onions and garlic, or take garlic in supplement form.

❑ Drink fresh carrot juice daily as a preventive measure against lung cancer. Also drink fresh beet juice (made from both the roots and the greens) and asparagus juice. All dark-colored juices are good, as are black currants. Also beneficial is apple juice, if it is fresh. Drink fruit juices in the morning and vegetable juices in the afternoon.

❑ Cook all sprouts slightly except for alfalfa sprouts, which should be eaten raw.

❑ *Do not* consume junk foods, processed refined foods, saturated fats, salt, sugar, or white flour. Instead of salt, use a kelp or potassium substitute. If you must, use a *small* amount of blackstrap molasses or pure maple syrup as a natural sweetener in place of sugar. Use whole wheat or rye instead of white flour. Eliminate alcohol, coffee, and all teas except for herbal teas.

❑ Do not eat any animal protein except for broiled fish (up to three servings per week). *Never* eat luncheon meat, hot dogs, or smoked or cured meats. Limit your consumption of dairy products to a little low-fat yogurt, kefir, or raw cheese on an occasional basis.

❑ Do not eat any peanuts. Limit, but do not eliminate altogether, your intake of soybean products; they contain enzyme inhibitors.

❑ Keep in mind that the acute craving for a cigarette usually lasts only three to five minutes. Focusing on this fact may make it easier to wait it out. Also remember that it gets easier and easier as time goes by. When cravings strike, try taking a walk, doing some sit-ups, or engaging in any activity that can momentarily take your mind off cigarettes.

❑ To accelerate toxin elimination, *see* FASTING in Part Three, and follow the program. Take coffee enemas daily. Use cleansing enemas with lemon and water or garlic and water two or three times weekly.

❑ Drink spring or steam-distilled water only.

❑ As much as possible, avoid stress.

❑ If you take any medications, consult with your physician about the possible need for an adjustment in dosage after you quit smoking. Tobacco alters the absorption and utilization of many medications, including insulin, asthma drugs, and certain antidepressants, blood pressure medications, and painkillers.

CONSIDERATIONS

❑ The difficulty of quitting appears to be related less to how many packs a day you smoke than to how early in life you started smoking.

❑ Many people have been successful in the quest to stop smoking by going on a fast using only live juices and quality steam-distilled water. A live juice fast can quickly remove nicotine and other damaging chemicals from the body. Adhering to a five-day live juice fast can have amazing effects.

❑ There are several natural products on the market that may help you deal with withdrawal symptoms, such as Smoking Withdrawal from Natra-Bio Homeopathic.

❑ A lack of beta-carotene and the B-complex vitamins has been linked to lung and throat cancer.

❑ A study cosponsored by the British and Norwegian governments found that DNA taken from the lungs of female smokers showed significantly more damage than that taken from men. DNA damage is a marker of increased cancer risk.

❑ Smoking a pack of cigarettes a day or more triples the risk of needing surgery for a herniated disk, but quitting smoking reduces that risk, according to researchers at the Medical College of Wisconsin.

❑ According to a study reported in the *Archives of Internal Medicine,* smoking increases the risk of developing leukemia by 30 percent.

❑ A diagnostic procedure called a sputum cytology test can sometimes detect the presence of cancer before there are symptoms and before other tests show the disease. In this test, sputum coughed up from the lungs and the bronchial tubes is examined for signs of tumor cells.

❑ There are many different strategies for overcoming smoking dependency. The secret to success may be finding the approach that is right for you. *No If's, And's or Butts, The Smoker's Guide to Quitting,* by Harlan M. Krumholz and Robert H. Phillips (Avery Publishing Group, 1993), is a comprehensive and detailed guide to the many and varied strategies that have helped people to break the smoking habit. There are also a number of organizations that can provide valuable information and programs to help you quit smoking. Two of the most highly recommended are:

American Cancer Society
1599 Clifton Road
Atlanta, GA 30329
800–ACS–2345 or 404–320–3333

American Lung Association
1740 Broadway
New York, NY 10019
800–LUNG–USA or 212–315–8700

Snakebite

There are about two dozen species of poisonous snakes in the United States. The toxicity of snake venom varies from species to species. A person who has been bitten by a poisonous snake may exhibit mild to severe symptoms, which can include swelling or discoloration of the skin in the area of the bite, a racing pulse, weakness, shortness of breath, nausea, and vomiting. In extreme cases, pain and swelling can be severe, the pupils may dilate, and shock and convulsion may occur. The person may twitch and his or her speech may become slurred. In the most severe cases, paralysis, unconsciousness, and death can result.

It is worth emphasizing that the majority of snakes are *not* poisonous. Nevertheless, anyone who has been bitten by a snake should be seen by a professional immediately, because the severity of initial symptoms does not always reflect the seriousness of the bite. After appropriate medical care has been administered, taking the nutrients and following the suggestions outlined here should help alleviate pain and hasten healing.

NUTRIENTS

SUPPLEMENT	SUGGESTED DOSAGE	COMMENTS
Helpful		
A.M./P.M. Ultimate Cleanse from Nature's Secret	As directed on label.	A 2-part body cleansing program that detoxifies the organs, blood, and the channels of elimination.
Calcium and magnesium	500 mg every 4–6 hours until pain begins to ease. 1,000 mg with the first 500 mg of calcium.	To relieve pain. Acts as a sedative. Use calcium gluconate form. Works with calcium.
L-Serine	As directed on label, on an empty stomach. Take with water or juice. Do not take with milk. Take with 50 mg vitamin B$_6$ and 100 mg vitamin C for better absorption.	Helps maintain a healthy immune system and aids in the production of antibodies.
Multivitamin and mineral complex	As directed on label.	All nutrients work together to promote health.
Pantothenic acid (vitamin B$_5$)	500 mg every 4 hours for 2 days.	The anti-stress vitamin.
Vitamin C with bioflavonoids	2,000 mg every hour for 5–6 hours, up to a total of 15,000 mg.	A powerful detoxifier. Relieves pain and discomfort and fights infection.
Vitamin A	10,000 IU daily.	Enhances immunity and promotes tissue healing.
Vitamin E	600 IU daily.	Promotes healing and reduces blood pressure.
Zinc	30 mg daily.	Boosts immune function. Use zinc gluconate lozenges or OptiZinc for best absorption.

HERBS

❑ Black cohosh syrup helps to relieve pain. Take ½ to 1 tablespoon of the syrup three times daily.

❑ Poultices of comfrey, slippery elm, or white oak bark leaves and bark can be used. *See* USING A POULTICE in Part Three. Comfrey salve, plantain poultice, or plantain salve can also be used.

❑ Echinacea, taken in tea and/or capsule form, boosts the immune system.

❑ Yellow dock can be used to alleviate symptoms. Drink a cup of yellow dock tea or take 2 capsules of yellow dock every hour until the symptoms are gone.

RECOMMENDATIONS

❑ Seek medical help immediately. Until you can get professional help, remain as still as possible, preferably with the injured area just below heart level. Keep warm. Remove any constricting items such as rings and watches in case significant swelling occurs.

❑ If medical help is not available, apply a constricting band two to four inches above the bite. Keep calm and immobilize the affected area, keeping it below heart level if possible. If rapid swelling or severe pain develops, an incision can be made directly below the fang marks and suction performed. The cut should be made along the long axis of the limb with a sharp, sterilized blade. Cut just through the skin (about an eighth of an inch deep), making an incision about one-half-inch long, and then apply suction for at least thirty minutes with a suction cup, snakebite kit, or with the mouth (spit out the blood).

Caution: This procedure should be performed *only* in an extreme situation, and only if you have had some training in how to do it. Otherwise, it can cause more problems than it solves. *Never* make cuts on the head, neck, or trunk.

❑ To reduce the possibility of snakebite, always remain on paths and hiking trails when in wooded areas. Wear leather boots if walking in tall grass. Be alert. If you see a snake, do not approach it. Stay at least six feet away.

❑ Do not apply cold therapy, such as an ice pack. This can cause tissue damage.

CONSIDERATIONS

❑ A poisonous snakebite is a medical emergency. Treatment is a complex process that may include the administration of antivenin plus fluid and electrolyte replacement, the administration of oxygen, and other supportive measures.

❑ If you spend much time outdoors, a snakebite kit is a good investment. Sawyer Products of Safety Harbor, Florida, makes a kit called The Extractor that is available in many outdoor supply and camping equipment stores.

❑ Snakebite is more likely to be life-threatening for children and for elderly people.

❑ In a life-threatening situation, massive doses of vitamin C may save the victim's life. (*See* ASCORBIC ACID FLUSH in Part Three.)

❑ Most cases of snakebite occur between sunrise and sunset. Snakes are cold-blooded and are more likely to be out then, basking in the warmth of the day.

Sore Throat

Most sore throats are caused by viral infections such as the common cold. Bacterial infection, especially *Streptococcus* infection, can also be responsible. In addition, a sore throat can be caused by anything that irritates the sensitive mucous membranes at the back of the throat and mouth. Some irritants include dust, smoke, fumes, extremely hot foods or drinks, tooth or gum infections, and abrasions. Chronic coughing and excessive loud talking also irritate the throat.

An acute sore throat usually runs its course within a few days to a few weeks. Sore throats are seldom serious, but quite often are the first symptom of another disorder. Sore throats can signal a cold, flu, mononucleosis, Epstein-Barr virus, herpes simplex, as well as many childhood illnesses such as measles and chickenpox. More rarely, a sore throat may indicate chronic fatigue syndrome, diphtheria, epiglottitis, gingivitis, laryngeal cancer, or an abscess around the tonsils.

NUTRIENTS

SUPPLEMENT	SUGGESTED DOSAGE	COMMENTS
Helpful		
Acidophilus	As directed on label. Take on an empty stomach.	To replenish "friendly" bacteria. Especially important if antibiotics are prescribed.
Bee propolis	As directed on label.	Protects mucous membranes of the mouth and throat.
Garlic (Kyolic) or	2 capsules 3 times daily, with meals.	For improved immune function.
Kyo-Green from Wakunaga	As directed on label.	Contains live enzymes, amino acids, vitamins, minerals, and chlorophyll for healing.
Multivitamin and mineral complex	As directed on label.	To maintain a balance of all necessary nutrients.
Zinc lozenges (Ultimate Zinc-C Lozenges from Now Foods)	As directed on label.	For pain relief, healing, and improved immune function.
Maitake or	As directed on label.	To boost immunity and fight viral infection.
shiitake or	As directed on label.	
reishi	As directed on label.	
Natural carotenoid complex (Betatene)	As directed on label.	Provides important antioxidant protection. Enhances immunity.
Vitamin A emulsion or capsules	100,000 IU daily for 1 week, then 50,000 IU daily for 1 week, then reduce to 25,000 IU daily. If you are pregnant, do not exceed 10,000 IU daily. 50,000 IU daily, for 1 week; then 25,000 IU daily for 1 week; then reduce to 10,000 IU daily. If you are pregnant, do not exceed 10,000 IU daily.	Aids healing and potentiates immune function. Emulsion form is recommended for easier assimilation and greater safety at high doses.
Vitamin C	5,000–20,000 mg daily, in divided doses. *See* ASCORBIC ACID FLUSH in Part Three.	Has antiviral properties.
Vitamin E	600 IU daily.	Promotes healing and tissue repair.

HERBS

❑ Catnip tea enemas help to reduce fever. *See* ENEMAS in Part Three.

❑ Echinacea and goldenseal fight bacterial and viral infection.

Caution: Do not take goldenseal internally on a daily basis for more than one week at a time, do not use it during pregnancy, and use it with caution if you are allergic to ragweed.

❑ Fenugreek used as a gargle can relieve a sore throat and reduce the pain of swollen glands. Add 20 drops of extract to 1 cup water and gargle with the mixture three times daily.

❑ Lungwort soothes throat irritation. Slippery elm is very soothing for a scratchy sore throat and for mouth irritation. Licorice soothes a sore, hoarse throat.

Caution: Do not use licorice on a daily basis for more than seven days in a row. Avoid if you have high blood pressure.

❑ Marshmallow root tea soothes a scratchy, itchy throat. Raspberry leaf tea is good for easing the pain of a sore throat as well as fever blisters.

❑ Hot mullein poultices are soothing to sore throats. *See* USING A POULTICE in Part Three.

RECOMMENDATIONS

❑ If your physician prescribes antibiotics for a bacterial throat infection, eat yogurt and take an acidophilus supplement to replace the "friendly" bacteria. Do not take the acidophilus at the same time as the antibiotic, however.

❑ Liquid vitamin C, made by dissolving vitamin C powder in water or juice, is good to sip. Allow it to drip down the throat slowly.

❑ Gargle alternately with chlorophyll liquid and sea salt (½ teaspoon in a glass of warm water) every few hours.

❑ Drink plenty of liquids. Fresh juices are best.

❑ Use a mixture of raw honey and lemon juice to coat and soothe the throat.

❑ See FASTING in Part Three, and follow the program.

❑ If you smoke, stop. Smoking is a major cause of sore throats. See SMOKING DEPENDENCY in Part Two.

CONSIDERATIONS

❑ A constant tickle or chronic irritating cough can be an indication of food allergies.

❑ If sore throat recurs or lasts for longer than two weeks, you may have an underlying illness such as mononucleosis.

❑ Many sore throats and infections are contracted from bacteria on toothbrushes. Toothbrushes should be replaced once monthly and after any type of infectious illness. Between uses, store your toothbrush in hydrogen peroxide or grapefruit seed extract to kill germs (if you use hydrogen peroxide, rinse the toothbrush well before brushing).

❑ See also COMMON COLD; MONONUCLEOSIS; SINUSITIS; and TONSILLITIS, all in Part Two.

Spider Bite

The bites of spiders can be poisonous and painful. However, most spiders are not big enough to cause serious harm. A spider bite may produce numbness, redness, and swelling in the affected area, as well as generalized itching, muscular cramping, sweating, headache, dizziness, nausea, vomiting, and weakness. The bite of a black widow spider can cause severe abdominal pain that is sometimes mistaken for appendicitis.

If you suspect you have been bitten by a poisonous spider, seek medical help immediately. After appropriate medical care has been administered, taking the following nutrients should help alleviate pain and hasten healing.

NUTRIENTS

SUPPLEMENT	SUGGESTED DOSAGE	COMMENTS
Helpful		
A.M./P.M. Ultimate Cleanse from Nature's Secret	As directed on label.	Stimulates and detoxifies the organs, blood, and channels of elimination.
Colloidal silver	Apply topically as directed on label.	An antiseptic that reduces inflammation and promotes healing of skin sores.
Calcium	As directed on label.	Helps relieve pain. Use calcium gluconate form.
Dimethylglycine (DMG) Aangamik DMG from FoodScience Labs)	As directed on label.	Enhances immunity and detoxifies the body.
Flaxseed oil	As directed on label.	Reduces pain and inflammation and aids recovery.
Herpanacine from Diamond-Herpanacine Associates	As directed on label.	Promotes good skin health and detoxifies the body.
Multivitamin and mineral complex	As directed on label.	To maintain a balance of all essential nutrients.
Pycnogenol or grape seed extract	As directed on label. As directed on label.	Protect the skin, reduce inflammation, and enhance immunity.
Vitamin A plus natural carotenoid complex (Betatene)	10,000 IU daily. As directed on label.	Enhances immunity and protects the body from bacteria. Powerful antioxidants that boost the immune system.
Vitamin B complex plus extra pantothenic acid (vitamin B5)	As directed on label. 500 mg daily.	Maintains healthy nerves and skin. A sublingual form is recommended. Has anti-allergenic and anti-stress properties.
Vitamin C	1,000 mg every hour until pain and swelling subside.	Aids in detoxifying the venom and eliminating it from the body. Very important in crisis allergy situations.
Vitamin E oil	Apply topically 3–4 times daily.	Aids healing and relieves discomfort. Purchase in oil form or cut open a capsule to release the oil.
Zinc	60–90 mg daily. Do not exceed a total of 100 mg daily from all supplements.	Boosts immune response. Also acts as a natural insect repellent. Use zinc gluconate lozenges or OptiZinc for best absorption.

HERBS

❑ A tincture made from calendula buds and alcohol should be on hand for stings and other "surface" injuries. A poultice made from the fresh flower heads is also good. See USING A POULTICE in Part Three.

❑ Any of the following poultices may be beneficial:

• A combination of dandelion and yellow dock relieves itchy skin.

• Fenugreek and flaxseed mixed with slippery elm bark is useful for treating inflammation.

• Goldenseal is good for inflammations of all kinds.

• A mixture of lobelia and crushed charcoal tablets is beneficial for insect bites and most wounds.

❑ A cream containing 5 percent tea tree oil helps to heal insect bites, sunburn, cuts, rashes, and other skin irritations.

❑ Echinacea, taken in tea or capsule form, boosts the immune system.

❑ Ginkgo biloba helps to relieve muscle pains.

❑ Yellow dock purifies the blood and is beneficial for many problems affecting the skin. Drink as much yellow dock tea as you can, or take 2 capsules of yellow dock every hour until symptoms are relieved.

RECOMMENDATIONS

❑ If you suspect you have been bitten by a poisonous spider, seek professional help immediately. In the meantime, try to remain calm. If there is swelling or pain, apply a constricting band two to four inches *above* the bite. Immobilize the affected area, keeping it below heart level if possible. Lie down and keep warm. Pack ice around the wound to relieve pain and slow down the spread of the poison.

❑ If medical help is not available, try to rid the body of as much poison as possible by encouraging bleeding. This can be done by suction. *See* SNAKEBITE in Part Two.

❑ Use essential oils of basil, cinnamon, lemon, lavender, sage, savory, or thyme for their antitoxic and antivenomous properties. Apply a drop of essential oil on the sting.

CONSIDERATIONS

❑ In life-threatening cases of spider bite, injections of vitamin C and pantothenic acid (vitamin B_5), administered by a medical professional, may be invaluable.

❑ Two types of spider—the black widow and the brown recluse—are more poisonous than most and can cause a serious reaction. The bite of the black widow spider can cause spastic contractions and localized tissue death. This spider has a black body with a red hourglass shape on the main body segment. The venom of the brown recluse spider usually creates a blister encircled by red and white rings. This "bull's-eye" appearance is used to distinguish it from other spider bites.

❑ Bites from scorpions, especially those found in the southwest U.S., require emergency medical care. Scorpions can be identified by their elongated bodies and curled tails.

❑ Rattlesnake and black widow venom are similar in many respects. Treatment for a black widow bite is therefore similar to that for snakebite.

❑ *See also* BEE STING; INSECT ALLERGY; and/or SNAKEBITE in Part Two.

Sprains, Strains, and Other Injuries of the Muscles and Joints

If a muscle is stressed beyond its capability, it becomes strained. Putting undue weight on the muscles and using the muscles for prolonged periods without rest can create muscle strain. A strained muscle may go into spasms or knot up instead of relaxing normally. Localized pain (during movement), swelling, and loss of mobility occur.

If one of the ligaments, the tissues that connect bones to muscles, is wrenched or stretched excessively, the ligament may tear, causing a sprain. There is likely to be a brief sharp pain followed by rapid swelling. Soft tissue surrounding the joint may be sore and bruised. Sprains can result from unexpected movement or twisting of the affected area, or from a hard fall. The joints most often sprained are the ankle, back, fingers, knee, and wrist.

These types of injuries are common in athletes. In most cases, they heal on their own. The following supplement program can help these injuries heal.

NUTRIENTS

SUPPLEMENT	SUGGESTED DOSAGE	COMMENTS
Very Important		
Infla-Zyme Forte from American Biologics	As directed on label. Take between meals.	To destroy free radicals released during injury.
or		
Wobenzym N from Marlyn Nutraceuticals	As directed on label. Take between meals.	
Helpful		
Calcium	1,500–2,000 mg daily.	Needed for repair of connective tissue. Use *both* calcium chelate and calcium gluconate forms to assure assimilation. Very important for the skeletal system.
and		
magnesium	750–1,000 mg daily.	
Desiccated liver	As directed on label.	Aids in building healthy blood cells.
Dimethylglycine (DMG) (Aangamik DMG from FoodScience Labs)	As directed on label.	Increases tissue oxygenation.
Essential fatty acids (flaxseed oil and Ultimate Oil from Nature's Secret are good sources)	As directed on label.	Promotes cellular and cardiovascular health; improves stamina and speeds recovery.
Free-form amino acid complex	As directed on label, on an empty stomach.	To help repair and strengthen connective tissue, reduce body fat, and help increase energy.
Ginkgo biloba		*See under* Herbs, below.
Grape seed extract	As directed on label.	A powerful anti-inflammatory.
L-Leucine plus L-isoleucine and L-valine	As directed on label, on an empty stomach. Take with water or juice. Do not take with milk. Take with 50 mg vitamin B_6 and 100 mg vitamin C for better absorption.	Branched-chain amino acids that promote the healing of bones, skin, and muscle tissue. *See* AMINO ACIDS in Part One.
Neonatal Multi-Gland from Biotics Research	As directed on label.	To stimulate healing of connective tissue.
or		
B Cell Formula from Ecological Formulas	As directed on label.	

Multivitamin and mineral complex	As directed on label.	To promote good health, nutritional balance, and tissue repair.
Potassium	99 mg daily.	Vital for tissue repair.
Silica	500 mg daily.	Supplies silicon, needed for connective tissue repair and calcium absorption.
Vitamin A plus	10,000 IU daily.	Enhances immunity and aids in protein utilization.
natural carotenoid complex (Betatene)	As directed on label.	Powerful antioxidants that boost the immune system.
Vitamin B complex	100 mg daily.	All the B vitamins are important during stressful situations. Use a high-potency formula.
plus extra pantothenic acid (vitamin B5)	500 mg daily.	The most important anti-stress vitamin.
Vitamin C	5,000–20,000 mg daily, in divided doses. See ASCORBIC ACID FLUSH in Part Three.	An antioxidant required for tissue growth and repair. Calcium ascorbate is the best form to use for these injuries.
Vitamin E	400–1,000 IU daily.	A free radical scavenger.
Zinc	50 mg daily. Do not exceed a total of 100 mg daily from all supplements.	Important in tissue repair. Use zinc gluconate lozenges or OptiZinc for best absorption.

HERBS

☐ Fenugreek and flaxseed powder can be combined with slippery elm bark to make a poultice for swelling. *See* USING A POULTICE in Part Three.

☐ Poultices made from goldenseal are good for reducing inflammation.

☐ Mustard poultices are good for swelling and can relax tense muscles.

☐ Once you begin alternating cold and hot treatments (*see under* Recommendations, below), combine turmeric and a little hot water to make a paste. Apply this mixture to the injured area with a gauze dressing. This treatment helps to reduce swelling. It is also good for bruising.

RECOMMENDATIONS

☐ After the initial cold therapy, alternate between hot and cold treatments every twenty minutes to help relieve pain. *Do not* use heat immediately following an injury.

☐ Consume plenty of juices made from fresh raw vegetables, including beets, garlic, and radishes. Raw vegetables are high in valuable vitamins and enzymes.

Sports and Nutrition

Glucose is the body's main fuel. It is stored in the muscles and the liver in the form of glycogen, a related compound that is readily converted into glucose as needed. The amount of glycogen available to the muscles is a key factor in how much activity you can perform without becoming tired—in other words, in physical strength and fitness. A high-intensity workout is possible only as long as glycogen is available in sufficient quantities.

The main source of energy in the diet is carbohydrates, because these compounds are quickly converted into glucose. A diet high in complex carbohydrates is thus the most beneficial for building the glycogen stores necessary for vigorous activity. This is why many athletes engage in a practice known as "carbohydrate loading" in the day or days before competition.

The second source of energy used to power the muscles is body fat. After about twenty minutes of exercise, the body begins to release stored fatty acids and use them as a source of fuel. It is primarily body fat, not dietary fat, that is used for this purpose.

Although fats can supply energy for muscular activity, a high-fat diet is not recommended. Both fats and carbohydrates, if consumed in excess, are converted into body fat, but dietary fat can be converted to body fat more easily than carbohydrates can. Moreover, the link between fat consumption and cardiovascular disease is well known,

and while regular exercise decreases the likelihood of heart disease, it does not make you immune to it.

Proteins are needed to build muscle and for tissue repair, but they are not an important source of cellular energy. Only if there are insufficient amounts of carbohydrates and fats available will the body use protein for energy. If this happens, losses of lean tissue and muscle occur. In addition, if the body is forced to break down protein for energy, this can result in the buildup of toxic levels of ammonia, a byproduct of protein metabolism. The need for protein does *not* increase with exercise; while you burn more carbohydrates and fats exercising than you do sitting at a desk, you do not normally burn more protein. Also, excessive protein intake increases elimination of urine by the body. This may cause dehydration and hinder performance and endurance. You may faint if you become dehydrated. Because excess protein is not stored, it puts a strain on the liver and kidneys. The consumption of too much protein can damage the kidneys and interfere with calcium metabolism.

The following supplements and guidelines outlined here are designed to enhance athletic performance and promote good health in anyone involved in physical conditioning. Most of the supplements listed can be found both individually and in combination products. Always read product labels carefully to ensure that you do not exceed the recommended amounts.

NUTRIENTS

SUPPLEMENT	SUGGESTED DOSAGE	COMMENTS
Essential		
Dimethylglycine (DMG) (Aangamik DMG from FoodScience Labs)	As directed on label.	Use before and during workouts to increase oxygen supply to the cells.
Gamma-amino-butyric acid (GABA)	As directed on label, on an empty stomach. Take with water or juice. Do not take with milk. Take with 50 mg each of vitamins B$_6$ and C for better absorption.	A potentiator of growth hormone; also produces an analgesic effect. See AMINO ACIDS in Part One.
L-Glutamine	As directed on label, on an empty stomach.	Promotes building of lean tissue and prevents wasting of muscle mass. See AMINO ACIDS in Part One.
L-Leucine plus L-isoleucine and L-valine	As directed on label, on an empty stomach. As directed on label, on an empty stomach. As directed on label, on an empty stomach.	Branched-chain amino acids that protect muscles and act as fuel (see AMINO ACIDS in Part One). Often found together in a single supplement.
L-Proline	As directed on label, on an empty stomach.	Required for the formation and maintenance of muscle and connective tissue.
Multivitamin and mineral complex or Wellness Formula from Source Naturals	As directed on label. As directed on label.	To ensure optimum health and supply all needed nutrients.
Important		
Body Language Super Antioxidant from Oxyfresh	As directed on label.	To protect the body from free radical damage.
Calcium and magnesium	1,000 mg daily. 500 mg daily.	For healthy heart and bones. Clears lactic acid from body. Use calcium lactate form. For proper muscle tone. Use magnesium oxide form.
Chromium picolinate	200 mcg daily.	Stabilizes blood sugar and increases energy levels.
Coenzyme Q$_{10}$	60–100 mg daily.	Increases tissue oxygenation.
Infla-Zyme Forte from American Biologics	As directed on label.	Beneficial for muscle aches, pain, swelling, and overexertion.
Potassium	99 mg daily.	Needed to replace potassium lost through sweat during exercise.
Vitamin C with bioflavonoids and rutin	3,000 mg daily.	Increases energy. Powerful antioxidants crucial for tissue repair.
Vitamin E plus selenium	400–1,000 IU daily. Do not exceed 600 IU daily if you are also taking octocasonal. 200 mcg daily.	Supplies oxygen to the cells and increases energy levels. Works synergistically with vitamin E.

Helpful		
Bee pollen	1,000 mg daily.	Increases energy and endurance. Caution: Bee pollen may cause an allergic reaction in some individuals. Discontinue use if a rash, wheezing, discomfort, or other symptom occurs.
Boron	3 mg daily. Do not exceed this amount.	Needed for proper calcium uptake.
Creatine	As directed on label.	A safe way to extend "work time" of muscles, thereby adding muscle mass.
Desiccated liver	As directed on label.	Increases energy. Use liver from organically raised beef.
Garlic (Kyolic)	2 capsules 3 times daily.	For energy and detoxification.
Glucose polymers	As directed on label.	Complex carbohydrate formulation to increase energy.
Inosine	As directed on label.	Promotes the manufacture of ATP, the prime source of energy at the cellular level.
Iron or Floradix Iron + Herbs from Salus Haus	As directed by physician. Take with 100 mg vitamin C for better absorption. As directed on label.	For hemoglobin production. Caution: Do not take iron unless anemia is diagnosed. A natural, nontoxic source of iron, which is vital for endurance. Deficiency is common among athletes.
Kelp	150 mg daily.	High in iodine.
L-Arginine and L-ornithine plus L-lysine	250 mg each daily, on an empty stomach. Take with water or juice. Do not take with milk. Take with 50 mg vitamin B$_6$ and 100 mg vitamin C for better absorption. 250 mg daily, on an empty stomach.	Use these amino acids in place of steroids; they stimulate the release of growth hormone, which helps to burn fat and build muscle tissue. See AMINO ACIDS in Part One. To maintain proper amino acid balance.
Multienzyme complex with amylase and betaine hydrochloride (HCl) and lipase and papain and trypsin	As directed on label 3 times daily, with meals.	For complete digestion and absorption of nutrients.
Muscle Octane from Anabol Naturals or Whey to Go from Solgar	As directed on label. As directed on label.	A blend of amino acids and vitamins to protect the muscles and provide fuel. A blend of whey protein and free-form amino acids to enhance muscle maintenance and metabolism.

L-Carnitine	500 mg daily.	Carries fat to the muscles for energy.
Manganese	10 mg daily. Take separately from calcium.	Helps the body incorporate calcium into the skeletal structure.
Octacosanol	1,000 mg daily.	Improves endurance by increasing oxygen utilization during exercise.
Omega-3 essential fatty acids	As directed on label.	Lowers cholesterol and triglyceride levels.
RNA complex	As directed on label.	For tissue and organ repair.
Silica	25–100 mg daily.	Needed for normal growth and bone repair.
Vanadyl sulfate	As directed on label.	Regulates the actions of insulin and carbohydrate metabolism.
Vitamin A plus	10,000 mg daily.	To destroy free radicals formed during exercise.
natural beta-carotene or	15,000 mg daily.	
carotenoid complex (Betatene)	As directed on label.	
Vitamin B complex plus extra	50 mg 3 times daily, with meals.	Increases energy and helps relieve stress during exercise.
vitamin B_3 (niacin)	100 mg daily. Do not exceed this amount.	Increases supply of oxygen to muscle tissue. *Caution:* Do not take niacin if you have a liver disorder, gout, or high blood pressure.
and pantothenic acid (vitamin B_5) and	100 mg daily.	Reduces stress on the body.
vitamin B_6 (pyridoxine) and	50 mg 3 times daily.	Increases metabolism of fat and carbohydrates in the muscles.
vitamin B_{12} and	1,000–2,000 mcg daily.	Increases energy. Use a lozenge or sublingual form.
folic acid	800 mcg daily.	
Vitamin D	1,000 IU daily.	Important in calcium metabolism.
Zinc	50 mg daily. Do not exceed a total of 100 mg daily from all supplements.	For stress and tissue repair and to replace zinc lost during exercise. Deficiency leads to fatigue, decreased alertness, and may result in injury. Use zinc gluconate form.

HERBS

❑ Dong quai, ephedra, ginseng, gotu kola, pau d'arco, and suma are energy boosters. They can be taken in tea or in pill form. Ginseng also aids in physical conditioning.

Caution: Do not use ephedra if you suffer from anxiety, glaucoma, heart disease, high blood pressure, or insomnia, or if you are taking a monoamine oxidase (MAO) inhibitor drug for depression. Do not use ginseng if you have high blood pressure.

❑ Fenugreek tea helps to regulate insulin production and blood sugar levels.

❑ Horsetail aids in physical conditioning.

❑ St. Johnswort can be used topically to relieve muscle spasms and joint pain.

❑ Sarsaparilla and saw palmetto are herbs that can be used to help boost testosterone levels naturally.

❑ White willow is a natural analgesic that can be used to relieve aches and pains from overexertion.

RECOMMENDATIONS

❑ Creatine and chromium picolinate supplements can be taken to help boost muscle mass and aid in fat metabolism.

❑ Consume solid foods no later than four hours before competition or vigorous exercise.

❑ Drink fluids before, during, and after exercising, regardless of whether or not you feel thirsty. This helps to prevent dehydration and muscle cramping. You lose moisture when you inhale and exhale vigorously during exercise, even in the winter. In fact, you can lose 25 percent more fluids in the winter due to the cold. A half-and-half combination of unsweetened juice and water is beneficial.

❑ Limit roughage consumption before exercising. It requires energy to digest, and will make you feel full and sluggish.

❑ Avoid the following foods before a workout: bananas, celery, grapes, peaches, and shrimp. Some people have experienced severe reactions to these foods after exercising.

❑ After a workout, allow your body temperature to cool to normal before taking a shower. Providing for a cool-down period can prevent abnormal muscle contractures and cramping, and even heart attack.

❑ Always stretch and warm up your muscles before exercising to avoid injury. Before the muscles have been worked, they are at a temperature of approximately 98°F and are stiff. After a five-minute warm-up, their temperature rises several degrees and they loosen up.

❑ If you are over thirty-five, have any kind of chronic health problem or doubts about your fitness, or have been sedentary for some time, consult your physician before embarking on an exercise program.

❑ If you have a heart problem, do not lift weights. When you lift, you stop breathing for a moment and the muscles in the chest and abdomen tighten, exerting undue pressure on the lungs and heart. Circulation to the brain and heart also decreases.

❑ Do not use steroids in an attempt to boost athletic performance. In men, the long-term use of these drugs can lead to osteoporosis, shrinkage of the testicles, cancer, sterility, and breast enlargement; in women, they can result in shrinkage of the breasts, excess facial and body hair, breast cancer, and deepening of the voice. Anabolic steroids may also cause heart attacks. Use sarsaparilla and saw palmetto instead (*see under* Herbs, above).

❑ If you have glaucoma, a heart disorder, a hernia, circulatory disease, or spinal instability, or if you take anticoagulants or aspirin on a regular basis, do not use gravity boots and a back swing.

CONSIDERATIONS

❑ Dimethylsulfoxide (DMSO), a byproduct of wood processing, is a liquid that can be applied topically to relieve pain, reduce swelling, and promote healing of injuries.

Note: Only DMSO from a health food store should be used. Commercial-grade DMSO such as that found in hardware stores is not suitable for healing purposes. The use of DMSO may result in a garlicky body odor. This is temporary and is not a cause for concern.

❑ If you have food allergies, exercise may increase the absorption of the allergenic food by the body, resulting in a more severe reaction to it.

❑ Fasting can improve your overall health by giving your body a chance to repair and cleanse itself. Regular training while fasting stimulates anabolic pathways and protein synthesis in muscle cells, and prevents loss of lean body mass. *See* FASTING in Part Three.

❑ Apply cold packs to the injured area immediately, especially if a sprain may be involved. Cold helps to reduce swelling and inflammation. If possible, elevate the injured area. Apply cold for ten minutes and remove it for ten minutes. Repeat this cycle for at least sixty to ninety minutes following the injury. Thereafter, apply cold intermittently for another twenty-four to thirty-six hours, keeping the injury elevated as much as possible.

❑ If there is significant swelling, call your physician right away or go to a hospital emergency room to have the injury evaluated. Especially with injuries to the wrists and ankles, it is wise to have x-rays taken to make sure no bones have been broken.

❑ To provide support, use an elastic bandage to wrap the sprained part for two to four weeks following the injury. Make sure that the bandage allows adequate circulation. Refrain from using or putting weight on the injured area until it no longer causes pain to do so and the swelling has gone down.

❑ Soaking the affected area in warm or hot water may help relieve prolonged pain; however, do not do so until the swelling subsides, at least two days after the injury.

❑ To prevent sprains and strains, do stretching exercises both before and after exercise and other physical activity.

CONSIDERATIONS

❑ Aromatherapy can be helpful. Cold compresses made with essential oils of camphor, chamomile, eucalyptus, lavender, and/or rosemary are good. Add 10 drops or so of essential oil to 1 quart of cool water and use the mixture to make the compresses.

❑ Clay poultices can be used to treat sprains and fractures. (*See* USING A POULTICE in Part Three.)

❑ The risk of injury to the muscles and joints is higher in contact sports than in other types of activity.

❑ *See also* BRUISING and FRACTURE, both in Part Two.

❑ *See also* PAIN CONTROL in Part Three.

STD

See SEXUALLY TRANSMITTED DISEASE.

Stomach Flu

See under INFLUENZA.

Strained Muscle

See under SPRAINS, STRAINS, AND OTHER INJURIES OF THE MUSCLES AND JOINTS.

Streptococcus Infection

See under KIDNEY DISEASE; MENINGITIS; RHEUMATIC FEVER; SORE THROAT; TONSILLITIS.

Stress

The term "stress" refers to any reaction to a physical, mental, or emotional stimulus that upsets the body's natural balance. Stress is an unavoidable part of life. It can result from many things, both physical and psychological. Pressures and deadlines at work, problems with loved ones, the need to pay the bills, and getting ready for the holidays are obvious sources of stress for many people. Less obvious sources include everyday encounters with crowds, noise, traffic, pain, extremes of temperature, and even welcome events such as starting a new job or the birth or adoption of a child. Overwork, lack of sleep, physical illness, excessive alcohol consumption, and smoking are common physical factors that put stress on the body. Some people create their own stress; whether there is anything objectively wrong in their lives or not, they find things to worry about.

Some people handle stress well. Others are very negatively influenced by it. Stress can cause fatigue, chronic headaches, irritability, changes in appetite, memory loss, low self-esteem, withdrawal, tooth-grinding, cold hands, high blood pressure, shallow breathing, nervous twitches, lowered sexual drive, insomnia or other changes in sleep patterns, and/or gastrointestinal disorders. Stress creates an excellent breeding ground for illness. Researchers estimate that stress contributes to as many as 80 percent of all major illnesses, including cardiovascular disease, cancer, endocrine and metabolic disease, skin disorders, and infectious ailments of all kinds. Many psychiatrists believe that the majority of back problems—one of the most common adult ailments in the United States—are related to stress. Stress is also a common precursor of psychological difficulties such as anxiety and depression.

While stress is often viewed as a mental or psychological problem, it has very real physical effects. The body responds to stress with a series of physiological changes that include increased secretion of adrenaline, elevation of blood pressure, acceleration of the heartbeat, and greater tension in the muscles. Digestion slows or stops, fats and sugars are released from stores in the body, cholesterol levels rise, and the composition of the blood changes slightly, making it more prone to clotting. Almost all body functions and organs react to stress. The pituitary gland increases its production of adrenocorticotropic hormone (ACTH), which in turn stimulates the release of the hormones cortisone and cortisol. These have the effect of inhibiting the functioning of disease-fighting white blood cells and suppressing the immune response. This complex of physical changes is called the "fight or flight" response, and is apparently designed to prepare one to face an immediate danger. Today, most of our stresses are not the result of physical threats, but the body still responds as if they were.

The increased production of adrenal hormones is responsible for most of the symptoms associated with stress. It is also the reason that stress can lead to nutritional deficiencies. Increased adrenaline production causes the body to step up its metabolism of proteins, fats, and carbohydrates to quickly produce energy for the body to use. This response causes the body to excrete amino acids, potassium, and phosphorus; to deplete magnesium stored in muscle tissue; and to store less calcium. Further, the body does not absorb ingested nutrients well when under stress. The result is that, especially with prolonged or recurrent stress, the body becomes at once deficient in many nutrients and unable to replace them adequately. Many of the disorders that arise from stress are the result of nutritional deficiencies, especially deficiencies of the B-complex vitamins, which are very important for proper functioning of the nervous system, and of certain electrolytes,

which are depleted by the body's stress response. Stress also promotes the formation of free radicals that can become oxidized and damage body tissues, especially cell membranes.

Many people attribute their stress-related symptoms to "nerves," and in fact stress usually does affect the parts of the body that are related to the nervous system first, especially through the digestive organs. Symptoms of stress-related digestive disorders may be a flare-up of an ulcer or irritable bowel syndrome. If stress that produces such symptoms is not handled properly, then more serious illnesses may result.

Stress can be either acute or long-term. Long-term stress is particularly dangerous. A state of continual stress eventually wears out the body. Because of its effect on immune response, stress increases susceptibility to illness and slows healing.

NUTRIENTS

SUPPLEMENT	SUGGESTED DOSAGE	COMMENTS
Essential		
ACES + Zinc from Carlson Labs	2 capsules daily.	Contains beta-carotene, selenium, and vitamins C and E, which work together as antioxidants to disarm damaging free radicals caused by stress.
Gamma-aminobutyric acid (GABA) (GABA Plus from Twinlab)	750 mg twice daily. Take with 50 mg inositol and 500 mg niacinamide to enhance effectiveness.	Acts as a tranquilizer and is important for proper brain function (*see* AMINO ACIDS in Part One).
Vitamin B complex injections plus extra vitamin B$_6$ (pyridoxine) and vitamin B$_{12}$	1 cc weekly or as prescribed by physician. ½ cc weekly or as prescribed by physician. 1 cc weekly or as prescribed by physician.	All B vitamins are necessary for health and proper functioning of the nervous system. Intramuscular injections (under a doctor's supervision) give fast results.
and/or vitamin B complex	100 mg daily.	Take oral supplements either in addition to injections or alone, if injections are unavailable. Use a sublingual form.
plus extra pantothenic acid (vitamin B$_5$)	500 mg daily.	An anti-stress vitamin needed by the thymus gland.
Vitamin C with bioflavonoids	3,000–10,000 mg daily.	Essential to adrenal gland function. Stress depletes the adrenal gland hormones, the anti-stress hormones.
Very Important		
Anti-Stress Enzymes from Biotec Foods	As directed on label.	Enzymes that remove toxic wastes and restore balance and equilibrium to the system.
L-Tyrosine	500 mg twice daily, during the day and at bedtime. Take with water or juice on an empty stomach. Do not take with milk. Take with 50 mg vitamin B$_6$ and 100 mg vitamin C for better absorption.	Helps reduce stress on the body. An effective and safe sleeping aid. Also good for depression. *See* AMINO ACIDS in Part One. *Caution:* Do not take this supplement if you are taking an MAO inhibitor drug.

Calcium and magnesium	2,000 mg daily. 1,000 mg daily.	Lost when stress is present. Use calcium chelate form. Deficiency is common in highly stressed individuals, and can result in anxiety, fear, and even hallucinations.
Melatonin	Start with 1.5 mg daily, taken 2 hours or less before bedtime. If this is not effective, gradually increase the dosage until an effective level is reached (up to 5 mg daily).	A natural hormone that promotes sound sleep; helpful if stress leads to occasional sleeplessness.
Helpful		
Fiber (oat bran and psyllium husks are good sources)	As directed on label. Take separately from other supplements and medications.	For bowel cleansing and improved bowel function. Stress often causes diarrhea and/or constipation.
Free-form amino complex	As directed on label.	To supply protein, which is used rapidly by the body at stressful times. Use a formula containing both essential and nonessential amino acids.
Lecithin granules or capsules	1 tbsp 3 times daily, with meals. 2,400 mg 3 times daily, with meals.	For cellular protection and brain function.
L-Lysine	As directed on label. Take with 50 mg vitamin C and 1 15-mg zinc gluconate lozenge (Ultimate Zinc-C Lozenges from Now Foods).	For cold sores, often an early indicator of stress. Reduces stress so it is better handled. *Caution:* Do not take for longer than 6 months at a time.
Maitake	As directed on label.	An adaptogen that helps the body adapt to stress and normalizes body fuctions.
Multivitamin and mineral complex with		Especially necessary during stress.
natural beta-carotene and	25,000 IU daily.	An important antioxidant.
potassium and	99 mg daily.	To replace potassium lost due to excretion during stress.
selenium	200 mcg daily.	A potent antioxidant that decreases anxiety attacks.
Raw adrenal and raw thymus glandulars	As directed on label. As directed on label.	To stimulate the adrenal and thymus glands, important in the body's stress reaction.
Vitamin E	400–600 IU daily. Take with meals.	Needed for immune function. Acts as a powerful antioxidant.
Zinc	50 mg daily. Do not exceed a total of 100 mg daily from all supplements.	Needed for immune function and to protect the cells from free radical damage. Use zinc gluconate lozenges or OptiZinc for best absorption.

HERBS

❑ Bilberry prevents destruction, mutation, and premature death of cells throughout the body.

❑ Ginkgo biloba aids in proper brain function and good circulation.

❑ Milk thistle cleanses and protects the liver, and has antioxidant properties.

❑ Many plants produce their own antioxidants, which they use as protection against environmental stresses. Specific herbs tend to protect specific parts of the body. However, because of their strong antioxidant properties, most have important influences on other parts of the body as well. For a robust anti-stress tonic, mix ½ teaspoon of any three of the herbs listed below and steep in 2 cups of almost-boiling distilled water, or use alcohol-free extracts mixed in water.

• Catnip is an effective anti-stress herb that also causes drowsiness.

• Chamomile is a gentle relaxant. It is a good nerve tonic, soothing to the digestive tract, and a pleasant sleep aid. *Caution:* Do not use this herb on an ongoing basis and avoid it completely if you are allergic to ragweed.

• Dong quai, rehmannia, and schizandra support the kidneys, adrenal glands, and central nervous system. These organs are among the most susceptible to the effects of stress.

• Hops helps to ease nervousness, restlessness, and stress. It also decreases the desire for alcohol.

• Kava kava relaxes the mind as well as the entire body.

• Passionflower is calming, and is a potent addition to any anti-stress formula.

• Polygala root and sour jujube seed are powerful Chinese herbs known to soothe and calm the spirit.

• Skullcap is good for nervous disorders. It also relieves headaches and aids sleep.

• Valerian keeps the nervous system from being overwhelmed. It also is a powerful sleep aid when taken at bedtime, and helps to ease stress-related headaches.

RECOMMENDATIONS

❑ Eat a diet composed of 50 to 75 percent raw foods. Fresh fruits and vegetables not only supply valuable vitamins and minerals, but are rich in compounds called flavonoids, many of which scavenge and neutralize dangerous free radicals.

❑ Avoid processed foods and all foods that create stress on the system, such as artificial sweeteners, carbonated soft drinks, chocolate, eggs, fried foods, junk foods, pork, red meat, sugar, white flour products, foods containing preservatives or heavy spices, and chips and similar snack foods.

❑ Eliminate dairy products from your diet for three weeks. Then reintroduce them slowly—and watch for returning symptoms of your "nervous" condition.

❑ Limit your intake of caffeine. Caffeine contributes to nervousness and can disrupt sleep patterns.

❑ Avoid alcohol, tobacco, and mood-altering drugs. While these substances may offer temporary relief from stress, they do nothing to really address the problem and they are harmful to your health. The stress will still be there the next day.

❑ Follow a monthly fasting program. *See* FASTING in Part Three.

❑ Get regular exercise. Physical activity can clear your mind and keep stress under control. Some people like to run or walk by themselves, while others prefer team sports or group workouts. Any type of exercise will do the trick, as long as it is *regular*. Exercising once a month will not do much to relieve stress.

❑ Learn to relax. Relaxation is often difficult for people suffering from the effects of stress, but it is necessary. A technique called *progressive relaxation* can be helpful. This involves tightening and relaxing the major muscle groups one at a time, being aware of each sensation. Start at your feet and work up to your head. Tense the muscles for a count of ten, concentrating on the tension, then let the muscles go lax and breathe deeply, enjoying the sensation of release.

❑ Get sufficient sleep each night. This may be difficult, because stress can keep you up at night (unless you are one of those people who welcomes sleep as an escape), but it is very important. The less sleep you get, the more stress will affect you, the more your immune system will weaken, and the greater your chance of becoming ill will be.

❑ Try meditation. Many people find that regular meditation helps them to relax and handle stress. Meditation does not have to have spiritual or religious connotations. For example, you can meditate on a word such as "peace," "calm," "relax," or "warm." Or you may find it helpful to meditate on a pleasant person, place, or event. It is good to have a store of pleasant thoughts to draw on during stressful times. While meditation can have some short-term benefits, it is more effective when practiced on a daily basis. Try meditating twice a day for ten to twenty minutes each time.

❑ Practice deep breathing. This can be done when facing a stressful situation—at home, at work, in your car, or elsewhere. Holding your breath is also good for relieving stress. Inhale deeply with your mouth closed, hold your breath for a few seconds (do not wait until you are uncomfortable), then exhale slowly through your mouth, with your tongue placed at the top of your teeth, next to the gum line. Do this four or five times, or until the tension passes.

❑ Monitor your internal conversations. The way we talk to ourselves has a lot to do with how we feel about ourselves and our environments. Telling yourself things like "I should be able to handle this better," or "I shouldn't have let that idiot cut me off in traffic," or "I'll never get the hang of this computer" only adds to the stressfulness of situations, and does nothing to resolve them. Learn to listen for—and then make yourself stop—these futile inner conversations.

❑ Identify the sources of stress in your life. This can be an important first step in managing stress. Take a stress inventory periodically to help you understand what is causing you problems. You can use the following list of major stressors as a starting point:

- Death of a spouse or other close family member.
- Divorce.
- Death of a close friend.
- Legal separation from spouse.
- Job loss.
- Major injury.
- New marriage.
- Scheduled surgery.
- Change in family member's health.
- Serious trouble at work.
- Increased responsibility at work or at home.
- Sexual problems.
- Change of jobs.
- Child leaving home.
- Change in residence.
- Major change in diet.
- Vacation.
- Allergies.

Remember that this list is not exhaustive and that different people react to the same events differently.

❑ Take a day off—that's what weekends are for. Take a drive, listen to music, go to the beach or lake, read—whatever you find rewarding and relaxing. Try to keep your thoughts in the present during this time so that you do not think about whatever it is that is causing the stress.

❑ Pursue a hobby. Hobbies are great for relieving stress. Take the time to do what you enjoy. Don't feel guilty about spending time doing something for yourself. Your health is worth it.

❑ Avoid hassles. Identify the things that are making you feel stressed out and either eliminate them from your life or prepare yourself to cope with them. If rush-hour traffic causes you stress, see if you can change your work hours slightly to avoid it. If that isn't possible, join a carpool or listen to a book on tape or a favorite piece of music.

❑ Do not repress or deny your emotions. This only compounds stress. Admit your feelings and accept them. Keeping strong feelings bottled up only causes them to resurface later as illness. Don't be afraid to cry. Learning to cry can help you to manage stress. Crying can relieve anxiety and let loose bottled-up emotions.

❑ Work on creating a stress-free home environment. Keep the noise level down—noise contributes to stress. Turn down the radio, stereo, and television. Throw rugs and wall hangings absorb noise, and are good additions to decor. Color is another important element of your environment to consider. Certain colors are much more calming and soothing than others (*see* COLOR THERAPY in Part Three). Also, use as much natural lighting in your home as possible. Unnatural fluorescent lighting can be especially aggravating.

❑ Investigate aromatherapy. This is the art of using highly concentrated distilled plant essences, called essential oils, for healing purposes. Essential oils affect both the mind and the body by means of olfactory stimulation of the brain. Essential oils that are particularly good for relieving stress include chamomile, bergamot, sandalwood, lavender, and sweet marjoram. Add 10 to 20 drops of one or more of these oils to a warm bath and relax in the tub, or simply dab a couple of drops of oil on a tissue or handkerchief and inhale the aroma periodically during the day. *Aromatherapy for Vibrant Health and Beauty* by Roberta Wilson (Avery Publishing Group, 1995) is a practical, user-friendly guide to exploring this healing art.

❑ Try not to take life too seriously. Learn to laugh.

❑ If stress-related symptoms become chronic or recurrent, consult your doctor to rule out an underlying illness.

❑ If you feel you simply cannot handle the stresses in your life, consider seeking outside help. It may be worth it to consult a qualified counselor or other practitioner who can help you to handle your problems and learn effective stress-reduction techniques. It is often enlightening and beneficial to talk with someone who can offer an objective response, whether a trusted friend or a professional counselor.

CONSIDERATIONS

❑ A study done at the University of Washington Medical School rated stressful situations according to their negative effects on physical and mental health. Rated highest was the death of a spouse. Divorce is next, followed by such circumstances such getting married, personal illness, and so on. The study found that the more stressful situations a person is experiencing, the greater the chance of illness.

❑ Research has shown that the hormone dehydroepiandrosterone (DHEA) can help people to cope with stress. (*See* DHEA THERAPY in Part Three.)

❑ Evidence shows that stress can trigger reactions to allergens and make allergic symptoms more severe.

❑ Stress can aggravate certain skin disorders, such as psoriasis and skin cancer, by damaging immune cells in the skin. The damage is done by a chemical released when nerve cells respond to stress.

❑ Dr. Hans Selye, stress expert and author of *Stress Without Distress*, said that it is not stress that is harmful—it is *distress*. Distress occurs when unresolved emotional stress is prolonged and not dealt with in a positive way.

❑ A group of Dutch researchers studied a group of eighty people for a period of six months. They found that individuals with high levels of stress had fewer than half the antibodies in their systems that subjects under less stress did.

❑ Kombucha tea may be helpful for people under stress. It is revitalizing and detoxifying, and helps to boost the immune system. (*See* MAKING KOMBUCHA TEA in Part Three.)

❑ In a study done at the University of Pennsylvania, people who considered themselves chronic worriers found that they could reduce their anxiety levels by setting aside a specific time to worry each day. They reserved thirty minutes each day to worry and did not permit themselves to worry at other times.

❑ Heavy metal intoxication and food allergies can both cause symptoms that mimic those of stress. A hair analysis can reveal heavy metal poisoning. (*See* HAIR ANALYSIS in Part Three; *see also* ALLERGIES in Part Two.)

❑ The symptoms of hypoglycemia may mimic those of stress. (*See* HYPOGELYCEMIA in Part Two.)

❑ *See also* ANXIETY DISORDER and DEPRESSION in Part Two.

Stretch Marks

See under PREGNANCY-RELATED PROBLEMS.

Stroke

See under ARTERIOSCLEROSIS/ATHEROSCLEROSIS; CARDIOVASCULAR DISEASE.

Stye

See under EYE PROBLEMS.

Substance Abuse

See ALCOHOLISM; DRUG ADDICTION; SMOKING DEPENDENCY.

Sunburn

Sunburn is caused by excessive exposure to the sun's ultraviolet (UV) rays. The amount of exposure required to cause a burn depends on the individual, the geographical location, the time, and the atmospheric conditions.

Most sunburns are first-degree burns that cause the skin to become red, warm, and tender to the touch. Depending on the severity of the burn and the individual's skin type, the burn may subsequently "cool" into a suntan or thin layers of skin may peel off. A more serious sunburn can be a second-degree burn, causing extreme reddening, swelling, pain, and even blisters. This is a sign that the burn has gone deeper than just the surface layer of the skin and has caused damage and the release of fluids from cells in the lower layers of the skin. This results in eruptions and breaks in the skin where bacteria and other infectious organisms can enter. In the most severe cases, the burn may be accompanied by chills, fever, nausea, and/or delirium.

Fair-skinned people are more prone to sunburn than darker skinned individuals, but no matter what your skin color, you will burn if you get enough exposure. Symptoms do not necessarily appear while you are in the sun; they may begin from one hour to twenty-four hours after sun exposure, and usually reach their peak in two to three days.

Today, the effects of sun exposure are becoming an increasing concern because of the decline in the earth's ozone layer. The ozone layer screens out the most harmful ultraviolet rays, but it is becoming steadily thinner all over the world, and holes that fluctuate in size have developed in various places. This state of affairs increases the likelihood of sunburn as well as the incidence of skin cancer.

NUTRIENTS

SUPPLEMENT	SUGGESTED DOSAGE	COMMENTS
Important		
Cell Guard from Biotec Foods	As directed on label.	Provides high levels of antioxidants to protect and nourish the cells.
Coenzyme Q10	60 mg daily.	Free radical scavenger that also increases the supply of oxygen to the cells.
Colloidal silver	Apply topically as directed on label.	Antiseptic to prevent infection. Subdues inflammation and promotes healing.
Concentrace from Trace Minerals Research	As directed on label.	Nourishes the skin by providing needed trace minerals.
Dimethylglycine (DMG) (Aangamik DMG from FoodScience Labs)	As directed on label.	Increases tissue oxygenation.
Free-form amino acid complex	As directed on label.	To supply protein, needed for tissue repair.
Herpanacine from Diamond-Herpanacine Associates	As directed on label.	Promotes skin health, detoxifies the body, and enhances immunity.
L-Cysteine	500 mg daily, on an empty stomach. Take with water or juice. Do not take with milk. Take with 50 mg vitamin B6 and 1,500 mg vitamin C.	Promotes healing of burns.
Multivitamin and mineral complex	As directed on label.	All nutrients are necessary in balance.
Potassium	99 mg daily.	Potassium lost through sunburn must be replaced.
Vitamin C with bioflavonoids	10,000 mg daily and up.	Needed for tissue repair and healing. Also reduces scarring. Use calcium ascorbate form.
Vitamin A and vitamin E	100,000 IU daily for 2 weeks, then reduce to 50,000 IU daily until healed. If you are pregnant, do not exceed 10,000 IU daily. Start with 100 IU daily and increase slowly to 1,600 IU daily until healed.	To destroy free radicals released by sun exposure and aid in tissue repair and healing.
or AE Mulsion Forte from American Biologics	As directed on label.	Contains vitamins A and E in emulsion form, which enters the system more rapidly. Allows for easier assimilation and greater safety at higher doses.
plus natural carotenoid complex (Betatene)	As directed on label.	Free radical scavengers and immune enhancers.
Helpful		
All-Purpose Bactericide Spray from Aerobic Life Industries	Apply topically as directed on label.	Destroys bacteria on the skin, reducing the possibility of infection.
Aloe vera		*See under* Herbs, below.
Calcium and magnesium	2,000 mg daily. 1,000 mg daily.	Necessary for proper pH balance and potassium utilization. Also reduces stress on tissues.
Essential fatty acids (primrose oil and Ultimate Oil from Nature's Secret are good sources)	As directed on label.	Needed for tissue healing.
Silica or horsetail	As directed on label.	Supplies silicon, needed for repair of skin tissue. *See under* Herbs, below.
Vitamin B complex plus extra vitamin B6 (pyridoxine) and para-aminobenzoic acid (PABA)	100 mg daily, with meals. 50 mg 3 times daily, with meals. 25 mg daily, with meals.	Important for tissue healing, especially for serious burns. A sublingual form is best. Needed for protein metabolism. Good for protecting the skin.
Vitamin E oil or ointment	Once the burn has cooled and healing has begun, apply topically to the affected area 3–4 times daily.	Promotes healing and helps prevent scarring. Purchase in oil or ointment form, or open a capsule to release the oil.
Zinc	100 mg daily for 1 month; then reduce to 50 mg daily. Do not exceed 100 mg daily.	Boosts the immune system and aids in tissue healing. Use zinc gluconate lozenges or OptiZinc for best absorption.

HERBS

❑ Aloe vera is a remarkably effective treatment for any kind of burn. It is even used in the burn units of some hospitals. Aloe relieves discomfort, speeds healing, and also helps to moisturize the skin and relieve dryness. Gently apply a thin layer of aloe vera gel to the sunburned area. Reapply it every hour until the pain is gone. Pulp taken directly from inside the fresh plant is best. If you use a commercial aloe product, make sure to choose one that contains no mineral oil, paraffin waxes, alcohol, or coloring.

❑ Apply a salve of calendula flowers and St. Johnswort to badly burned areas. These two herbs have antiseptic properties, act as a painkiller for burns, and promote healing of skin wounds.

❑ An herbal bath can help minimize the stinging and pain of sunburn. Add 6 cups of chamomile tea or 6 drops of chamomile oil to a lukewarm tubful of water. Soak in the bath for thirty minutes or more. Lavender oil is also good and can be used in place of chamomile oil if you wish.

❑ Make a large pot of strong comfrey or gotu kola tea and let it cool. Soak sterile cotton gauze in the tea to make a compress and apply it to the affected area. Leave the compress in place for up to thirty minutes.

Note: Comfrey is recommended for external use only.

❑ Horsetail is a good source of silica, which is beneficial for tissue repair.

❑ A cream containing at least 5 percent tea tree oil helps to heal sunburn and other skin irritations.

RECOMMENDATIONS

❑ Eat high-protein foods for tissue repair, and raw fruits and vegetables to supply needed vitamins and minerals.

❑ Drink plenty of fluids; sunburn dehydrates the body.

❑ For immediate relief of sunburn pain, use cool-water compresses or cold clay poultices. *See* USING A POULTICE in Part Three. Or dissolve 1 pound of baking soda in a tubful of cool water, and soal in the bath for about thirty minutes. The herbal treatments described above are also excellent for relieving pain and stinging.

❑ Strictly avoid any further sun exposure until the burn is completely healed.

❑ When it comes to sunburn, prevention is better than cure. While most sunburns are minor burns that heal on their own, a history of sunburn is strongly linked to the development of skin cancer. Take precautions to prevent yourself from getting sunburned:

• Avoid spending time outdoors between the hours of 10:00 a.m. and 3:00 p.m.

• When you do spend time outdoors, wear a sun hat, protective clothing, and sunglasses that specify UV protection. The best type of clothing is made of light-colored, light-weight, tightly woven material.

• Always use a sunscreen with a sun protection factor (SPF) of 15 or higher. Apply the sunscreen to all exposed areas of skin. Reapply it frequently, at least every three to four hours, more often if you are swimming or perspiring.

• Add to your sunscreen the contents of 1 capsule each of vitamin A, vitamin C, vitamin E, and selenium to help prevent free radical damage to the skin. After sunning, add these antioxidants to whatever skin cream you use for added protection and to aid in preventing wrinkles.

• Don't neglect your lips. The lips also are susceptible to sunburn. Use a sun protection product designed for the lips as well as a sunscreen for your face and body. Choose a formula containing natural ingredients such as aloe vera and vitamin E. Your health food store should carry such products in handy stick form.

• Do not rely on the weather to judge how strong the sun is. Cloudy or hazy days do not afford protection against sunburn; approximately 80 percent of the sun's ultraviolet rays pass through clouds. Reflections from water, metal, sand, or snow may increase—even double—the amount of ultraviolet rays you absorb. Take the same precautions on cloudy or hazy days that you do on bright, sunny days.

• To prevent dehydration, drink plenty of water while spending time in the sun.

❑ If you desire a tan, start with only fifteen-minute periods of sun exposure, and increase your exposure slowly, adding no more than fifteen more minutes at a time. This helps to prevent burning and results in a longer-lasting tan.

❑ If you take any medications, ask your physician or pharmacist if they may increase your sensitivity to the sun.

CONSIDERATIONS

❑ Tretinoin (vitamin A acid), the active ingredient in the prescribed medication Retin-A, is sometimes prescribed to help to repair skin that has been damaged by sun exposure. However, the use of tretinoin renders the skin significantly more vulnerable to additional sun damage. If you use this medication, you should *always* use a high-SPF sun block and avoid sun exposure as much as possible. This product should not be used during pregnancy, as it may cause birth defects.

❑ For a severe burn, a physician may prescribe silver sulfadiazine (Silvadene) cream and/or antibiotics to prevent infection, debridement to remove dead tissue, and/or hydrotherapy to loosen dead skin. Depending on the location and extent of the burn, physical therapy may be prescribed to keep muscles flexible. Muscle contracture can result from overlying skin damage and contraction.

❑ Berlock dermatitis is a heightened reaction to the sun caused by oil of bergamot, a common ingredient in perfumes, pomades, and colognes.

Sweating

See under PREGNANCY-RELATED PROBLEMS.

Swimmer's Ear

See under EAR INFECTION.

Temporomandibular Joint Syndrome

See TMJ SYNDROME.

Tendinitis

See under BURSITIS.

Thrombophlebitis

Phlebitis means inflammation of a vein. This problem usually occurs in the extremities and in particular the legs. If the inflammation is associated with the formation of a thrombus (a blood clot) in the vein, the condition is called *thrombophlebitis.*

Thrombophlebitis can be either superficial or deep. It is considered superficial if it affects a subcutaneous vein, one of the veins near the skin's surface. In superficial thrombophlebitis, the affected vein can be felt (it feels harder than normal), and may be seen as a reddish line under the skin, with localized swelling, pain, and tenderness to the touch. If there is widespread vein involvement, the lymphatic vessels (thin-walled vessels carrying fluid from the tissues to the bloodstream) may become inflamed. Superficial thrombophlebitis is a relatively common disorder. A superficial clot may be brought about by trauma, infection, standing for long periods of time, lack of exercise, and intravenous drug use. Pregnancy, varicose veins, obesity, and smoking increase the risk of superficial vein thrombophlebitis. Thrombophlebitis may also be associated with environmental sensitivities or allergies. Diagnosis of the condition is usually based on physical findings and/or a medical history indicating an increased risk.

Deep thrombophlebitis (known also as deep venous thrombosis, or DVT) affects the intermuscular or intramuscular veins further below the skin's surface. DVT is a much more serious condition than superficial thrombophlebitis because the veins affected are larger and located deep within the musculature of the leg. These are the veins responsible for the transport of 90 percent of the blood that flows back to the heart from the legs. Symptoms of DVT may include pain, warmth, swelling, and/or bluish discoloration of the skin of the affected limb. These symptoms are sometimes (but not often) accompanied by fever and chills. The pain is typically felt as a deep soreness that is worse when standing or walking and that gets better with rest, especially with the leg elevated. The veins directly under the skin may become dilated and more visible.

The primary risk associated with DVT is a sharp restriction in blood flow through the veins that can result in chronic venous insufficiency, a condition characterized by swelling, increased pigmentation, dermatitis, and ulceration of the affected leg. DVT can even be life threatening if a blood clot breaks off from the venous lining and travels through the bloodstream to the heart, lung, or brain, where it may lodge in a blood vessel and cut off circulation to those vital organs. However, despite its potential seriousness, DVT can be completely without symptoms. Indeed, nearly half of all people who have it have no symptoms. In order to make a definitive diagnosis of DVT, a doctor must rule out a number of other disorders, including cellulitis and occlusive arterial disease. Diagnosis is based on the results of medical tests, including Doppler ultrasonography (ultrasound) and plethysmography, a test that can detect reduced or restricted blood flow in the affected area.

The reason or reasons for the formation of clots in the veins are often unknown. In most cases, clots are probably the result of a minor injury to the inside lining of a blood vessel. If the vessel lining receives a microscopic tear, for instance, this initiates clotting—a normal part of the body's repair processes. Platelets clump together to protect the injured area, and a series of biochemical events is initiated that results in the transformation of fibrinogen, a circulating blood protein, into strands of insoluble fibrin, which are deposited to form a net that traps blood cells, plasma, and yet more platelets. The result is a blood clot. Other possible causes of deep thrombus formation include abnormal clotting tendencies; poor circulation; certain types of cancer; and Behçet's syndrome, a condition affecting the small blood vessels that predisposes an individual to the formation of clots. Factors that increase the risk of DVT include recent childbirth, surgery, trauma, the use of birth control pills, and prolonged bed rest (some studies indicate that up to 35 percent of hospital patients develop DVT).

Anyone can get thrombophlebitis, but the disorder occurs more frequently in women than in men. The risk of developing DVT increases dramatically after the age of forty and triples with each additional twenty years.

NUTRIENTS

SUPPLEMENT	SUGGESTED DOSAGE	COMMENTS
Important		
Acetyl-L-carnitine	500 mg daily.	Protects the brain and blood vessels from fat accumulation.
Coenzyme Q10	100–200 mg daily.	Improves circulation and protects the heart.
Flaxseed oil or Ultimate Oil from Nature's Secret	2 tsp daily. As directed on label.	To supply essential fatty acids that minimize blood clot formation and keep veins and arteries soft and pliable, promoting cellular and cardiovascular health.
Garlic (Kyolic)	2 capsules 3 times daily, with meals.	Improves circulation and thins the blood.

Heart Science from Source Naturals	As directed on label.	Contains powerful antioxidants and artery lining protectors.
Magnesium plus calcium	1,000 mg daily. 1,500 mg daily.	A natural blood thinner that reduces abnormal clotting. Works with magnesium.
L-Cysteine and L-methionine	500 mg each daily, on an empty stomach. Take with water or juice, not milk. Take with 50 mg vitamin B6 and 100 mg vitamin C for better absorption.	Protects and preserves cells; prevents accumulation of fat in the blood vessels. See AMINO ACIDS in Part One.
Lecithin granules or capsules	1 tbsp 3 times daily, before meals. 1,200 mg 3 times daily, before meals.	Fat emulsifier; to increase circulation.
L-Histidine	500 mg daily.	Important blood vessel dilator.
Pycnogenol or grape seed extract	50 mg 3 times daily. As directed on label.	Antioxidants that restore flexibility to arterial walls and reduce the risk of blood vessel disease and thrombophlebitis.
Vitamin C with bioflavonoids	4,000–8,000 mg daily.	Aids circulation and reduces clotting tendencies. Bioflavonoids prevent bruising and promote healing.
Vitamin E	Start with 400 IU daily and increase slowly to 1,600 IU daily. If you have a clotting disorder or high blood pressure, start with 100 IU daily and increase slowly to 400 IU daily.	Thins the blood and reduces platelet "stickiness." Emulsion form is recommended for easier assimilation and greater safety at high doses.
Zinc	50 mg daily. Do not exceed a total of 100 mg daily from all supplements.	Aids in healing of ulcers and boosts immune function. Needed to maintain proper concentration of vitamin E in the body. Use zinc gluconate lozenges or OptiZinc for best absorption.
Helpful		
Advanced Carotenoid Complex from Solgar	As directed on label.	Contains antioxidants, immune enhancers, free radical scavengers, potential cancer fighters, and heart disease protectors.
Body Language Super Antioxidant from OxyFresh	As directed on label.	Protects the body from free radical damage, environmental stresses, and pollutants.

HERBS

❑ Alfalfa, pau d'arco, red raspberry, rosemary, and yarrow are antioxidant herbs that improve blood oxygenation.

❑ Butcher's broom improves circulation.

❑ Cayenne (capsicum) thins the blood, eases blood pressure, and improves circulation. It can also be combined with ginger, plantain, and witch hazel in a poultice and applied directly on the affected area.

❑ Hawthorn leaf or berry protects the heart.

❑ Ginger, skullcap, and valerian root dilate the blood vessels and aid circulation.

❑ Ginkgo biloba improves circulation and brain function, and is a powerful antioxidant.

❑ Leg ulcers can be treated with alcohol-free goldenseal extract. Moisten a sterile piece of gauze with a dropperful of extract and place it over the affected area.

RECOMMENDATIONS

❑ Eat plenty of fresh fruits and vegetables; raw nuts and seeds; soybean products; and whole grains.

❑ Reduce your consumption of red meat. Better yet, eliminate it from your diet.

❑ Do not consume any dairy products, fried or salty foods, or processed or partially hydrogenated vegetable oils.

❑ Get regular moderate exercise. Walking, swimming, and other exercise improves circulation and prevents sluggishness in the veins, lessening the tendency to form clots.

❑ Take alternating hot and cold sitz baths, or apply alternating hot and cold compresses using the herbs recommended above. See SITZ BATH in Part Three.

❑ Lie on a padded slant board with your feet higher than your head for fifteen minutes a day. This is particularly helpful if you stand on your feet a lot.

❑ Ask your pharmacist about special elastic support stockings (antiembolism stockings) to improve circulation.

❑ If you smoke, stop. Smoking constricts the blood vessels, resulting in poor circulation and weakened blood flow. This is especially important if you are taking birth control pills. See SMOKING DEPENDENCY in Part Two.

❑ Avoid wearing tight-fitting clothing that cuts off circulation, such as knee socks with tight bands and girdles.

❑ If you experience a swollen, painful vein that does not disappear within two weeks, talk to a health professional.

❑ If you are confined to bed, move your legs as much as possible to counteract pooling of the blood in the veins. Clean your legs daily to remove germs that can cause infection. Avoid using products that can dry your skin. Contact your health care provider if you notice any redness or swelling in the legs—these may be signs of infection.

❑ If you develop leg ulcers, keep the ulcers clean and germ-free to prevent infection. Follow your physician's recommendations concerning proper care for your ulcers, and be forewarned that leg ulcers may take three months to a year to heal. See LEG ULCERS in Part Two.

CONSIDERATIONS

❑ Superficial thrombophlebitis is usually treated by elevating the affected limb; warm moist compresses; and bed rest. A doctor may also prescribe anti-inflammatory drugs.

❑ Some studies have shown that low doses of aspirin (less than one regular tablet per day) may be as effective as stronger anticoagulants in treating DVT.

❑ DVT is a potentially serious health problem and hospi-

503

talization may be recommended. An anticoagulant such as heparin or warfarin (Coumadin) is usually given, both intravenously and orally. Surgery may be needed to tie off the affected vein to prevent the clot from traveling to the lungs, a condition known as a pulmonary embolism. Recovery time varies, depending on the severity of the disease.

❑ Behçet's syndrome is a chronic multisystem disease distinguished by thrombophlebitis, plus arthritis, iritis, uveitis, and ulceration of the mouth and genitalia. This disease is found worldwide, but is most common in young men of eastern Mediterranean and eastern Asian descent. Persons with Behçet's syndrome should avoid needle punctures, as these can induce inflammatory skin lesions.

❑ *See also* CIRCULATORY PROBLEMS and LEG ULCERS, both in Part Two.

Thrush

See under FUNGAL INFECTION.

Thyroid Problems

See HYPERTHYROIDISM; HYPOTHYROIDISM.

Tic Douloureux

See under HEADACHE.

Tinnitus

See under HEARING LOSS.

TMJ Syndrome

An estimated 10 million Americans suffer from temporomandibular joint (TMJ) syndrome, a condition in which the temporomandibular joint does not function properly. This is the joint that connects the temporal bone (the bone that forms the sides of the skull) with the mandible (the jawbone). This painful affliction produces pain in the muscles and joints of the jaw that sometimes radiates to the face, neck, and shoulder. There may also be difficulty opening the mouth all the way, and clicking, grinding, and popping

noises may occur during chewing and movement of the joint. Headaches, toothaches, dizziness, feelings of pain and pressure behind the eyes, pain and ringing in the ears, and difficulty opening and closing the jaw normally are other possible symptoms.

The jaw joint is embedded in an intricate web of nerves and muscle. The force of chewing (something we do a lot of) and of clenching or gritting the teeth creates enormous tension and pressure in that region of the face. The cartilage disk that cushions the joint may become displaced or wear out. This causes the bones of the temporomandibular joint to rub against one another, rather than gliding smoothly past each other. In some instances, a misalignment of the jaw and teeth prevents smooth operation of the joint.

The most common underlying causes of TMJ are stress and a poor bite, together with clenching and grinding of the teeth (bruxism), especially at night. TMJ can also be caused by bad posture, habits such as cradling the telephone between the shoulder and jaw, repeated or hard blows to the jaw or chin, or whiplash. Poor dental work and orthodontia may aggravate the problem, as can habits such as gum chewing, thumb-sucking, and chewing exclusively on one side of the mouth. A common contributing factor is hypoglycemia; people tend to clench and grind their teeth more when their blood sugar is low.

To diagnose TMJ, a physician may use x-rays and a technique called arthrography, in which an opaque dye is injected into the joint and then viewed with fluoroscopy.

A correct diet and the proper supplements, possibly in conjunction with other treatment, are valuable for TMJ and often solve the problem.

TMJ SELF-TEST

Place your little fingers in your ears so that hearing is obstructed. Then slowly and steadily open and close your jaw. If at any point you hear a clicking, popping, and/or grinding noise, the jaw joints may be out of alignment, and examination by a professional experienced in diagnosing and treating TMJ is advisable.

NUTRIENTS

SUPPLEMENT	SUGGESTED DOSAGE	COMMENTS
Essential		
Calcium and magnesium	2,000 mg daily. 1,500 mg daily, in divided doses, after meals and at bedtime.	For proper muscular function and calming effect. Prevents bone softening and relieves stress. Use chelate forms.
Vitamin B complex plus extra pantothenic acid (vitamin B$_5$)	100 mg 3 times daily. 100 mg twice daily.	Anti-stress vitamins. Sublingual forms are recommended for best absorption.
Helpful		
Coenzyme Q$_{10}$	60 mg daily.	Improves oxygenation of affected tissues.

L-Tyrosine	500 mg daily. Take at bedtime on an empty stomach with water or juice. Do not take with milk. Take with 50 mg vitamin B₆ and 500 mg vitamin C for better absorption.	Improves the quality of sleep and relieves anxiety and depression. *See* AMINO ACIDS in Part One. *Caution:* Do not take tyrosine if you are taking an MAO inhibitor drug.
Multivitamin and mineral complex	As directed on label.	For balanced nutrients. A hypoallergenic product is best.
Vitamin C	4,000–8,000 mg daily.	Combats stress and is necessary in adrenal gland function. Also necessary for healing and repair of connective tissue.

HERBS

❑ Blue violet, catnip, chamomile, hops, lobelia, skullcap, kava, thyme, red raspberry, passionflower, valerian root, and wild lettuce have calming and anti-stress properties.

Caution: Do not use chamomile regularly, as ragweed allergy may result. Avoid it completely if you are allergic to ragweed. Do not take lobelia internally on an ongoing basis.

❑ SP-14 Valerian Blend from Solaray Products combats stress and is also beneficial.

RECOMMENDATIONS

❑ Eat a diet including lightly steamed vegetables, fresh fruits, whole-grain products, white fish, skinless chicken and turkey, brown rice, and homemade soups and breads.

❑ Avoid high-stress foods: all forms of sugar, all white flour products, all junk foods, candy, colas, potato chips, pies, and fast foods.

❑ Do not consume any foods or beverages containing caffeine. As a stimulant, caffeine can increase tension, which often aggravates the problem. Also avoid taking over-the-counter medications containing decongestants, which can have a similar effect.

❑ Do not consume alcoholic beverages. These are a common contributing factor in bruxism (tooth-grinding), which can cause or aggravate TMJ.

❑ If you work at a desk, check your posture periodically throughout the day. Do not lean over the desk; keep your back comfortably straight, with your ears not too far in front of your shoulders. Try to keep your head aligned so that your cheekbones are over your collarbone.

❑ Sleep on your back to give your back, shoulder, and neck muscles plenty of rest. Do not sleep on your side or lie on your stomach with your head turned to the side. Avoid propping your head at a sharp angle to read or watch television in bed.

❑ Fast at least once a month to give the body and jaws a rest. *See* FASTING in Part Three.

❑ Do not chew gum. Avoid overly chewy foods such as red meat and bagels.

❑ Experiment with heat and cold therapy, and use hot or cold packs—whichever works best—for relief of pain, especially pain in the neck and shoulders.

❑ Be wary of any practitioner who rigidly adheres to one single approach in treating TMJ. A multidisciplinary team is a better choice. If possible, seek help from practitioners associated with a university dental or medical school.

CONSIDERATIONS

❑ TMJ is often treated with a special bite plate that is worn at night to prevent tooth-clenching and compression of the joint, and to correct the bite.

❑ Stress management, combined with heat and muscle relaxants, often relieves the symptoms of TMJ.

❑ Physical therapy is becoming a widely recognized, viable treatment for TMJ. This may involve jaw and tongue exercises to retrain stressed muscles and/or the use of a transcutaneous nerve stimulation (TENS) unit; ultrasound, which promotes tissue healing; and electrogalvanic stimulation, which helps relax muscles. These types of therapy should be prescribed in conjunction with an exercise and stress-reduction program.

❑ Some TMJ sufferers have been helped by biofeedback readings taken from the masseter muscle (the muscle that opens and closes the jaw). This treatment, combined with relaxation techniques such as controlled breathing, has proved effective.

❑ TMJ has become a much misdiagnosed and overtreated disorder. People with ambiguous pain in various parts of their bodies (such as menstrual cramps) have been misdiagnosed as having TMJ, for example. Some health care practitioners have voiced concern that TMJ may be providing inadequately trained or even disreputable practitioners with an opportunity to take advantage of patients. According to an article published in the February 1993 issue of the *New York State Journal of Medicine*, TMJ is an area in which "dental quackery" is quite common.

❑ Orthodontists, dentists, physical therapists, and many other "specialists" now offer treatments for TMJ. However, it is estimated that 90 percent of all cases of TMJ respond to simple, inexpensive treatments, such as those recommended in this section. It therefore makes sense to try such measures *before* investing in expensive medical or dental treatment.

❑ TMJ is not the only disorder that can cause jaw pain. Another possible cause is rheumatoid arthritis. In this disorder, the symptoms are more severe in the morning and tend to ease somewhat as the day goes on (*see* ARTHRITIS in Part Two). This is not usually the case with TMJ. A displaced disk can also cause jaw pain. Treatment for this disorder involves realigning the ligaments with a plastic splint.

❑ *See also* BRUXISM and STRESS, both in Part Two.

Tonsillitis

Tonsillitis is an inflammation of the tonsils, small organs composed of lymphatic tissue located on either side of the entrance to the throat. The inflammation is typically caused by bacteria, usually *Streptococcus*, but may also be caused by viral infection. Symptoms include sore throat, difficulty swallowing, hoarseness, coughing, and redness, pain, and swelling of the tonsils. Other possible symptoms include headache, earache, fever and chills, nausea and vomiting, nasal obstruction and discharge, and enlarged lymph nodes throughout the body.

This disorder is most common in children, but it can occur at any age. In adults, it may be a sign that the body's resistance to disease is lower than it should be. An improper diet that is high in refined carbohydrates and low in protein and other nutrients may also predispose one to developing tonsillitis. Some people have repeated bouts of tonsillitis, and it can become a chronic condition. In general, the more repeated bouts of tonsillitis a person has, the more difficult it is to cure. Each time the tonsils become inflamed, scar tissue accumulates on the tonsils.

NUTRIENTS

SUPPLEMENT	SUGGESTED DOSAGE	COMMENTS
Important		
Vitamin C	5,000–20,000 mg daily. See ASCORBIC ACID FLUSH in Part Three.	To fight infection and boost the immune response.
Zinc lozenges (Ultimate Zinc-C Lozenges from Now Foods)	1 15-mg lozenge every 2–3 waking hours for 3 days, then reduce to 1 lozenge 4 times daily until healed.	An immunostimulant that aids healing.
Helpful		
Acidophilus	As directed on label. Take on an empty stomach.	Necessary if antibiotics are prescribed.
Chlorophyll	Use as a gargle as directed on label.	Has an antibiotic effect and can heal irritations in the mouth and throat. Use a liquid form.
Cod liver oil	As directed on label.	Aids immune response and healing of tissue.
Colloidal silver	As directed on label.	Subdues inflammation and promotes healing.
Maitake or	As directed on label.	Mushrooms with immune-boosting and antiviral properties.
shiitake or	As directed on label.	
reishi	As directed on label.	
Proteolytic enzymes	As directed on label. Take between meals.	Aids in reducing inflammation.
Vitamin A	10,000 IU daily for 3 days, then reduce to 5,000 IU daily.	Needed for repair of tissue. Aids healing. Emulsion form is recommended for easier assimilation.
Vitamin B complex plus extra pantothenic acid (vitamin B$_5$)	50 mg 3 times daily, with meals. 100 mg daily.	To help maintain a healthy mouth and throat. Plays a role in the production of the formation of antibodies and aids in the utilization of other vitamins.
and vitamin B$_6$ (pyridoxine)	50 mg daily.	Helps reduce swelling.
Vitamin E	400 IU daily.	Destroys free radicals and enhances the immune system.

HERBS

❑ Catnip tea enemas are good for reducing fever. *See* ENEMAS in Part Three.

❑ Chamomile relieves fever, headaches, and pain.
Caution: Do not use this herb on an ongoing basis, as ragweed allergy may result. Avoid it completely if you are allergic to ragweed.

❑ ClearLungs from Natural Alternatives is an herbal combination that helps to strengthen the immune system, enhances tissue repair, and controls inflammation.

❑ Echinacea fights infection and boosts the immune system. Make echinacea tea and drink as much of it as you can.

❑ A hot infusion made from equal parts of dried elder flower, peppermint, and yarrow eases the pain of tonsillitis. Drink this throughout the day.

❑ Hot mullein poultices are soothing. *See* USING A POULTICE in Part Three.

❑ Pau d'arco is a natural antibiotic and potentiates immune function. It is also a powerful antioxidant.

❑ Sage tea, made with a bit of alum, can be used as a gargle. It can also be prepared with hot malt vinegar and taken orally in 2– to 3–ounce doses.
Caution: Do not use sage if you suffer from any type of seizure disorder.

❑ For sore throat, take alcohol-free extract of goldenseal or St. Johnswort. Place 6 drops or ½ dropperful of extract under your tongue and leave it there for a few minutes before swallowing. Do this four times daily for three days.
Caution: Do not take goldenseal internally on a daily basis for more than one week, do not use it while pregnant or breastfeeding, and use it with caution if you are allergic to ragweed.

❑ Thyme reduces fever, headaches, and mucus. It is good for chronic respiratory problems and sore throat.

RECOMMENDATIONS

❑ Use a warm saltwater gargle. Dissolve ½ teaspoon of salt in 1 cup of warm water and gargle with the mixture three times a day to help reduce swelling, relieve pain, and remove mucus.

❑ Do not smoke, and avoid secondhand smoke. Tobacco smoke irritates the throat.

For relief of tonsillitis pain, inhale essential oils of bergamot, lavender, tea tree, thyme, benzoin, and lemon.

❑ If you have a sore throat that does not improve within two weeks, consult your health care provider to determine what type of sore throat you have.

❑ If your physician prescribes antibiotics for bacterial tonsillitis, eat yogurt and take an acidophilus supplement to replace the "friendly" bacteria. Do not take the acidophilus at the same time as the antibiotic, however.

❑ Rest and drink plenty of fluids.

CONSIDERATIONS

❑ A cleansing juice fast for three days with vegetable broth can be helpful. (*See* FASTING in Part Three.)

❑ If an abscess develops, surgical drainage may be required.

❑ If tonsillitis becomes recurrent or chronic, tonsillectomy (removal of the tonsils) may be recommended. In the past, doctors removed tonsils on a very frequent basis. Today we know that the tonsils are important for the proper functioning of the immune system. Tonsils should not be removed unless absolutely necessary.

Tooth Decay

Tooth decay rivals the common cold as the most prevalent human disorder. It is not a natural process, as many people believe, but a bacterial disease. Bacteria in the mouth combine with mucus and food debris to create a sticky mass called plaque that sticks to the surfaces of the teeth. The bacteria in the plaque feed on ingested sugars and produce an acid that leaches calcium and phosphate from the teeth. Gradually, if the sticky deposits are not removed, the teeth erode—first the enamel (the outer layer) and then the dentin (the body of the tooth). If unchecked, decay can progress even further, into the pulp that contains the nerve in the center of the tooth, resulting in a toothache. Infection may result, leaving the tooth vulnerable to abscess.

Tooth decay depends on three factors: the presence of bacteria, the availability of sugars for the bacteria to feed on, and the vulnerability of tooth enamel. Poor nutrition and poor oral hygiene are probably the main factors behind most cavities. In particular, people who consume large quantities of refined carbohydrates—especially sticky-textured foods that cling to tooth surfaces—or who snack frequently without cleaning their teeth afterwards are much more likely to have a problem with tooth decay. There are also some people who, for reasons not yet understood, seem to have unusually acidic saliva and/or higher than normal levels of bacteria present in their mouths, and they too are more prone to cavities.

Tooth decay normally causes no symptoms until it is rather far advanced. Then the tooth may become sensitive to heat, cold, and the consumption of sugar. In later stages, a toothache may occur.

NUTRIENTS

SUPPLEMENT	SUGGESTED DOSAGE	COMMENTS
Important		
Acidophilus	As directed on label.	Important if taking antibiotics; protects "friendly" bacteria in the colon.
Calcium and	1,500 mg daily.	Necessary for strong, healthy teeth.
magnesium	750 mg daily.	Needed to balance with calcium.
L-Tyrosine	As directed on label, on an empty stomach. Take with water or juice. Do not take with milk. Take with 50 mg vitamin B_6 and 500 mg vitamin C for better absorption.	Use for relief of pain and anxiety. *See* AMINO ACIDS in Part One. *Caution:* Do not take this supplement if you are taking an MAO inhibitor drug.
VitaCarte from Phoenix Biolabs	As directed on label.	Contains bovine cartilage, which accelerates wound healing and reduces inflammation.
Vitamin A	10,000 IU daily.	Important for healing and for tooth formation.
Vitamin B complex	As directed on label.	Helps maintain healthy nerves and gums. A sublingual type is best.
Vitamin C	3,000 mg daily.	Protects against infection and inflammation. *Do not* use a chewable form, as this may erode tooth enamel.
Vitamin D	400 mg daily.	Needed for absorption of calcium and healing of gum tissue.
Vitamin E	600 IU daily.	Promotes healing.
Helpful		
Multivitamin and mineral complex	As directed on label.	All nutrients are needed in balance.
Zinc	30 mg daily. Do not exceed a total of 100 mg daily from all supplements.	Boosts immune function. Use zinc gluconate lozenges or OptiZinc for best absorption.

HERBS

❑ Calendula, chamomile, peppermint, and yarrow are natural anti-inflammatories.

❑ Clove oil is helpful for toothache pain. Apply 1 or 2 drops to the affected tooth with a cotton swab as needed. If you find the clove oil too strong, dilute it with olive oil.

❑ Alcohol-free goldenseal extract can be used as an antibacterial mouthwash. If inflammation is present, place a few drops of goldenseal extract on a piece of sterile cotton and apply it to the affected area at bedtime. Leave the cotton in place overnight. Do this for three consecutive nights to destroy bacteria and reduce inflammation.

❑ Kava kava, St. Johnswort, white willow bark, and wintergreen have analgesic properties. White willow bark is also an anti-inflammatory.

RECOMMENDATIONS

❑ Eat plenty of raw fruits and vegetables. These contain minerals that help to keep the saliva from becoming too acidic.

❑ Avoid carbonated soft drinks. These are high in phosphates, which promote the loss of calcium from the tooth enamel.

❑ Practice good oral hygiene. Brush your teeth after eating and floss between the teeth daily. This is the only way to remove cavity-causing plaque. There are also mouth rinses available to enhance the plaque-removing power of brushing and flossing.

❑ Do not use chewable vitamin C supplements, which can erode tooth enamel. Tablets or powders designed for swallowing do not pose this danger.

❑ To ease the pain of toothache or abscess until you can see your dentist, rinse the affected area with warm salt water (add ½ teaspoon of salt to 8 ounces of warm water).

CONSIDERATIONS

❑ Regularly scheduled dental checkups are recommended at least once yearly.

❑ At present, the only known way to stop tooth decay once it has started is to remove the decayed area and cover it with some type of filling. Many different materials are used to fill cavities. The most common is the "silver" amalgam filling. Amalgam formulas vary, but virtually all contain about 50 percent mercury, a toxic heavy metal. There are other filling choices, however, including gold and ceramic-based materials called composites. You may wish to discuss concerns about filling materials with your dentist before treatment.

❑ Many dentists recommend routine fluoride treatments to prevent cavities, especially for children. Fluoride is a substance derived from the element fluorine. Fluorine is a deadly chemical, but fluoride is not believed to be dangerous in small amounts. However, a government investigation of 156 cancer deaths over three years suggests that fluoride accumulates in the body and may eventually cause cancer or other illnesses. Animal and human epidemiology studies conducted on fluoride have so far not been conclusive as to whether or not fluoride is a carcinogen.

Tooth-Grinding

See BRUXISM.

Toxicity

See ALUMINUM TOXICITY; ARSENIC POISONING; CADMIUM TOXICITY; CHEMICAL POISONING; COPPER TOXICITY; ENVIRONMENTAL TOXICITY; FOOD POISONING; LEAD POISONING; MERCURY TOXICITY; NICKEL TOXICITY.

Tuberculosis

Tuberculosis (TB) is a highly contagious disease caused by the bacteria *Mycobacterium tuberculosis*. It is primarily a disease of the lungs, but it can affect any body organ, including the bones, kidneys, intestines, spleen, and liver. One of the most lethal among infectious diseases, TB is found throughout the world. Although it has a long history, modern medical knowledge of this disorder was not acquired until late in the nineteenth century. Early medical literature described it as *phthisis* or "consumption."

TB is usually spread by infected airborne droplets that are coughed up by individuals with the active disease and then inhaled by susceptible persons. Once inhaled, the bacteria normally lodge in the lungs. The body may successfully battle the infection at this point. If the immune system is not functioning optimally, however, or if another onslaught of the bacteria reaches the lungs, chances are the bacteria will multiply and proceed to liquefy and destroy lung tissue. Tuberculosis may also be contracted from contaminated food or from milk that has not been pasteurized. In such cases, the primary focus of the infection usually is in the digestive tract. This type of tuberculosis is more common in developing countries. It is very rare in the Western world.

Symptoms of TB may be slow in developing and initially resemble those of influenza—general malaise, coughing, loss of appetite, night sweats, chest pain, and low-grade fever. At first, the cough may be nonproductive, but as the disease progresses, increasing amounts of sputum are produced. As the condition worsens, fever, night sweats, chronic fatigue, weight loss, chest pain, and shortness of breath may occur, and the sputum may become bloody. In advanced cases, TB of the larynx can occur, making it impossible to speak above a whisper. Chest x-ray, sputum culture, and a tuberculin skin test may be used to diagnose the disease.

Not so long ago, the medical community expected TB to become more of a curiosity than a serious public health problem. Antibiotic regimens that could successfully combat the disease had been developed, and living standards had risen so that the poor nutrition and inadequate hygienic standards that had once helped TB to spread and flourish were no longer prevalent. Yet after decades of declining TB rates, the U.S. Centers for Disease Control and Prevention reported that between 1985 and 1991, there was an 18-percent *increase* in active TB infections in the United States. Other authorities likewise report that TB is once again on the rise. Worse, new strains of TB have been appearing that are resistant to conventional antibiotic treatment.

TB now appears to be more pernicious and virulent than ever. Several factors that have come into play have contributed to TB's comeback. First, to be successful against TB, antibiotic treatment must usually be taken every day for about one year after the initial diagnosis. The symptoms, however, improve much sooner. Researchers have documented thousands of cases in which people discontinue treatment after the symptoms are gone but before the infection itself is under control. This results in the most susceptible of the TB bacteria being killed off, while the most antibiotic-resistant bacteria remain alive—and proceed to produce new generations that resist conventional treatment. Other important factors in the resurgence of TB are the AIDS epidemic (HIV infection increases susceptibility to infectious illness of every type) and the rising numbers of people living in circumstances that are conducive to the spread of the disease, including homeless shelters and prisons. The deepening poverty and crowded living conditions in our inner cities also provide ideal conditions for TB to spread and thrive. Increased immigration to the United States from the world's poorer countries and more world travel in general may play a role as well.

Unlike many infectious illnesses, TB is a chronic disease, and it is debatable whether an absolute cure can ever be achieved. In many if not most cases, some tubercle bacilli appear to remain in the lung in a dormant state even after the disease has been treated and its progress arrested. Relapses can then occur at any time, usually in response to lowered immunity. This can result from stress, increasing age, poor nutrition, steroid therapy, infection, a chronic disease such as diabetes, or anything else that impairs the functioning of the immune system. The risk of contracting TB is highest among African-American and Hispanic men between the ages of twenty-five and forty-four; individuals who have had TB in the past; persons with multiple sex partners; recent immigrants from Mexico and from countries in Africa, South America, and Asia; drug and alcohol users; residents in institutions such as mental health facilities and nursing homes; persons who have undergone gastrectomy (surgical removal of all or part of the stomach); and individuals with weakened immune systems, especially those with HIV or AIDS.

NUTRIENTS

SUPPLEMENT	SUGGESTED DOSAGE	COMMENTS
Very Important		
Garlic (Kyolic)	2 capsules 3 times daily, with meals.	Acts as a natural antibiotic; keeps infection in check and stimulates immune function.
AE Mulsion Forte from American Biologics	As directed on label, to supply 200,000 IU vitamin A daily. If you are pregnant, do not exceed 10,000 IU daily.	To supply vitamins A and E, vital for healing of lung tissue and protection against free radicals. This emulsion form is easily assimilated and is safe at high doses.
or vitamin A plus	25,000 IU daily. If you are pregnant, do not exceed 10,000 IU daily.	
natural carotenoid complex (Betatene) plus	25,000 IU daily.	
vitamin E	400–800 IU daily.	
Coenzyme Q_{10}	75 mg daily.	Helps carry oxygen to tissues for healing.
Colloidal silver	As directed on label.	An antiseptic that subdues inflammation and heals lesions.
Free-form amino acid complex	As directed on label.	Needed for tissue repair. Free-form amino acids are rapidly absorbed and assimilated by the body.
Grape seed extract	As directed on label.	A powerful antioxidant that enhances immunity.
L-Cysteine and L-methionine	500 mg each twice daily, on an empty stomach. Take with water or juice. Do not take with milk. Take with 50 mg vitamin B_6 and 1,500 mg vitamin C for better absorption and prevention of cysteine kidney stones.	To protect the lungs and liver by detoxifying harmful toxins. See AMINO ACIDS in Part One.
Selenium	200 mcg daily.	Protects against free radicals and promotes a healthy immune system.
Vitamin B complex	100 mg 3 times daily.	Needed for production of red blood cells and antibodies. Aids in utilization of oxygen. Use a high-stress formula. Injections (under a doctor's supervision) may be necessary. If injections are not available, use a sublingual form.
plus extra pantothenic acid (vitamin B_5) and	100 mg 3 times daily.	The anti-stress vitamin.
vitamin B_6 (pyridoxine) plus	50 mg 3 times daily.	Some drugs used to fight TB can cause a deficiency of this vitamin.
brewer's yeast	1–2 tsp daily. Take in juice or water.	Reduces inflammation and boosts immunity.
Vitamin C	5,000–20,000 mg daily, in divided doses. See ASCORBIC ACID FLUSH in Part Three.	Strengthens immune response and promotes healing.
Vitamin D	Start with 1,000 IU daily and decrease slowly to 400 IU daily over the course of 1 month.	Essential for utilization of calcium and phosphorus. People with TB need sunlight daily and/or vitamin D for healing.
Vitamin E	Start with 400 IU daily and increase slowly to 1,600 IU daily over the course of 1 month.	Powerful free radical scavenger. Protects the lung tissues and provides oxygen to the cells. Emulsion form is recommended for easier assimilation and greater safety at high doses.

Important		
ACES + Zinc from Carlson Labs	As directed on label. Do not exceed 100 mg zinc daily from all sources.	A formula that fights free radicals with enzymes and antioxidants.
ClearLungs from Natural Alternatives		*See under* Herbs, below.
CTR Support from PhysioLogics	As directed on label.	To diminish damage caused by inflammation.
Essential fatty acids (Ultimate Oil from Nature's Secret is a good source)	As directed on label.	Important in formation of all cells, including lung tissue.
Glutathione	500 mg daily, on an empty stomach.	Protects the lungs and cells from oxidant damage.
Kelp	2,000–3,000 mg daily.	For a natural supply of minerals. Rich in iodine.
L-Serine	500 mg daily, on an empty stomach. Take with water or juice. Do not take with milk. Take with 50 mg vitamin B6 and 100 mg vitamin C for better absorption.	Helps the body maintain immune function. *See* AMINO ACIDS in Part One.
Multienzyme complex plus proteolytic enzymes	As directed on label. Take with meals. As directed on label. Take between meals.	Needed to keep inflammation down, to digest essential nutrients, and to improve absorption.
Multimineral complex with boron and calcium and magnesium and silica	3 mg daily. Do not exceed this amount. 1,000 mg daily. 750 mg daily. 25–100 mg daily.	All nutrients are needed for strength and healing. Take with meals. Use a high-potency formula. Do not use a sustained-release formula.
Multivitamin complex	As directed on label.	To provide a balance of needed nutrients.
Oxy-5000 Forte from American Biologics	As directed on label.	An antioxidant with superoxide dismutase (SOD).
Zinc	50–80 mg daily. Do not exceed a total of 100 mg daily from all supplements.	Promotes immune function and healing. Use zinc gluconate lozenges or OptiZinc for best absorption.

HERBS

❑ Butcher's broom, calendula, cayenne (capsicum), chamomile, peppermint, and yarrow have anti-inflammatory properties.

❑ Elecampane, ephedra, goldenseal root, horehound, licorice, lobelia, marshmallow root, mullein, myrrh gum, and thyme have decongestant and expectorant properties.

❑ A combination echinacea and pau d'arco tea is beneficial. Echinacea is a powerful antioxidant and bolsters the immune system; pau d'arco benefits the body by cleansing the blood and acting as an antibacterial agent, as well as possessing anti-tumor agents. Drink 3 cups of this tea daily. Or combine echinacea tincture with equal parts of tinctures

of elecampane and mullein, and take 1 teaspoon of this mixture three times daily.

❑ ClearLungs from Natural Alternatives is a Chinese herbal formula that relieves bronchial and lung congestion.

RECOMMENDATIONS

❑ If you suspect you may have tuberculosis, or that you may have been exposed to it, see your health care provider. Prompt, proper treatment is essential.

❑ Follow the prescribed treatment regimen exactly. If any medications cause side effects, contact your physician. *Do not* discontinue taking the medications on your own.

❑ To promote healing, eat a diet consisting of at least 50 percent raw vegetables and fruits. Eat two fertilized eggs daily. Also eat alfalfa sprouts, fish, fowl, pomegranates, raw cheeses, raw seeds and nuts, whole grains, and garlic.

❑ Drink fresh pineapple and carrot juice and a "green drink" daily. Drink fresh raw potato juice; potato juice contains compounds called protease inhibitors, which block carcinogens and prevent cell mutation. *See* JUICING in Part Three.

❑ Make purée of steamed asparagus in a blender. Refrigerate and take 4 tablespoons twice a day with meals. Asparagus stimulates immune function and is anticarcinogenic.

❑ Make kefir, buttermilk, and fresh sugar-free yogurt a part of your daily diet. Also take an acidophilus supplement for as long as you are taking antibiotics, to relieve stress on the gastrointestinal tract and enhance nutrient absorption. Do not take the acidophilus at the same time as the antibiotic.

❑ Do not smoke or consume alcohol or recreational drugs. All of these affect the ability of the immune system to fight infection. Smoking is even more dangerous than usual in the presence of a lung infection.

❑ Avoid stress. Rest, sunshine, and fresh air are most important. A dry climate is recommended.

CONSIDERATIONS

❑ People infected with TB should not use cortisone preparations. Cortisone supresses immune function and makes the infection more difficult to treat.

❑ Vaccines and drugs cannot control TB if poor lifestyle practices are followed. Cleanliness, proper nutrition, and good hygiene are vital in combating this disease.

❑ Experts estimate that up to 90 percent of the population may have encountered the tubercle bacillus sometime in their lives, but in the majority of cases, the immune system successfully fights off a full-blown infection. People who do not defeat it outright often carry the germ in a dormant state, sometimes for decades, before immunity weakens and the bacteria begin replicating and infect the host.

❑ The Air Supply personal air purifier from Wein Products is a small unit worn around the neck. It sets up an invisible pure air shield against microorganisms (such as viruses, bacteria, and mold) and microparticles (including dust, pollen, and pollutants) in the air. It also eliminates vapors, smells, and harmful volatile compounds in the air. The Living Air XL-15 unit from Alpine Industries is an ionizing unit good for purifying the air in the home or workplace.

❑ The tubercle bacillus has an incredible capacity for reproduction. A single organism is capable of producing billions of descendants within one month.

❑ The American Lung Association estimates that tuberculosis affects approximately 14 in every 100,000 persons in the United States. The World Health Organization has singled out TB as a "global health emergency."

❑ Persons who are HIV positive are likely to have tuberculosis as well at some point. A study by the Florida Department of Health and Rehabilitative Services found that 83.2 percent of the people with AIDS in Florida had had TB as well.

❑ The Bacillus Calmette-Guerin vaccine (BCG), which consists of a weakened form of tubercle bacilli, can be used for vaccination against tuberculosis. Many medical authorities believe BCG is an effective preventive measure against TB, while others have serious doubts about its safety. It is widely used in some countries, but not in the U.S.

Tumor

A tumor is a swelling or abnormal growth of tissue that has no useful function in the body. Tumors may be either benign or malignant (cancerous). Benign tumors are isolated growths that can occur anywhere in the body. They generally do not pose a threat to health, do not spread to other parts of the body, and do not grow back if they are removed. Polyps and uterine fibroids are examples of benign tumors.

Unlike benign tumors, malignant tumors are usually a serious, even life-threatening, health problem. They tend to grow uncontrollably, interfere with normal metabolic or organ functioning, and spread to other parts of the body. They are also likely to recur after surgical removal.

Environmental factors and diet seem to play an important role in the development of tumors of all types. Tumors have been known to decrease in size and even disappear in response to dietary changes and supplementation with vitamins and minerals. The suggestions here are designed to enhance immune function and suppress the growth of tumors—both benign and malignant.

NUTRIENTS

SUPPLEMENT	SUGGESTED DOSAGE	COMMENTS
Important		
Coenzyme Q10	100 mg daily.	Promotes immune function; carries oxygen to the cells.
Garlic (Kyolic)	2 capsules 3 times daily, with meals.	May help to reduce the size of tumors.
Maitake	As directed on label.	Strengthens the body and improves overall health; has immunostimulant properties that inhibit tumor growth.
and/or shiitake	As directed on label.	Has a powerful anti-tumor action; reverses T cell suppression caused by tumors.
Proteolytic enzymes or	As directed on label.	To help the immune system and aid in the breakdown of undigested foods.
Infla-Zyme Forte from American Biologics or	As directed on label.	
Wobenzym N from Marlyn Nutraceuticals	As directed on label.	
Shark cartilage (BeneFin)	1 gm per 2 lbs of body weight daily, divided into 3 doses. If you cannot tolerate taking it orally, it can be administered in a retention enema.	Has been shown to inhibit and even reverse the growth of some types of tumors. Also stimulates the immune system.
Vitamin C	3,000–10,000 mg daily, in divided doses.	Promotes immune function.
Zinc	30–80 mg daily. Do not exceed a total of 100 mg daily from all supplements.	Promotes a healthy immune system and wound healing, and helps maintain the proper concentration of vitamin E in the blood. Use zinc gluconate lozenges or OptiZinc for best absorption.
Helpful		
Kelp	1,000–1,500 mg daily.	Promotes immune function. Supplies balanced minerals.
L-Arginine	500 mg daily, on an empty stomach. Take with water or juice. Do not take with milk. Take with 50 mg vitamin B6 and 100 mg vitamin C for better absorption.	Retards tumor growth by enhancing immune function. See AMINO ACIDS in Part One.
and L-cysteine	500 mg daily, on an empty stomach. Take with 1,500 mg vitamin C to prevent cystine kidney stones.	Detoxifies harmful toxins, protects the body against radiation, and acts against carcinogens.
plus glutathione	500 mg daily, on an empty stomach.	Helps reduce side effects of chemotherapy and protect the liver.
plus taurine	500 mg daily, on an empty stomach.	Used in some clinics for treatment of breast cancer.
Lecithin granules or capsules	1 tbsp 3 times daily, with meals. 1,200 mg 3 times daily, with meals.	An important component of healthy cell membranes.
Multivitamin and mineral complex	As directed on label, with meals.	For necessary vitamins and minerals. Use a high-potency formula.
Primrose oil or flaxseed oil or salmon oil	1,000 mg 3 times daily, before meals. As directed on label. As directed on label.	To supply essential fatty acids, specifically useful for breast tumors.
Raw thymus glandular	As directed on label.	Stimulates the thymus gland, which is important for immune function. See GLANDULAR THERAPY in Part Three.

Vitamin A	25,000 IU daily. If you are pregnant, do not exceed 10,000 IU daily.	Powerful immunostimulants and antioxidants. Emulsion forms are recommended for easier assimilation and greater safety at higher doses.
plus natural carotenoid complex (Betatene) plus	25,000 IU daily.	
vitamin E	Start with 400 IU daily and increase slowly to 800 IU daily.	
or ACES + Selenium from Carlson Labs	As directed on label.	Supplies vitamin C in addition to vitamins A and E and selenium.
Vitamin B complex	As directed on label.	Vital in intracellular metabolism and normal cell multiplication. A sublingual type is best.
plus brewer's yeast	As directed on label.	A good source of B vitamins.
Vitamin B$_6$ (pyridoxine)	50 mg 3 times daily.	Required for normal cell growth and brain and nervous system function. Enhances immunity. Consider injections (under a doctor's supervision).
plus pantothenic acid (vitamin B$_5$)	100 mg daily.	An anti-stress vitamin that plays a role in hormone and antibody production, energy production, vitamin production, and in treating depression and anxiety.

HERBS

❑ Cat's claw boosts the immune system and has anti-tumor properties. Cat's Claw Defense Complex from Source Naturals is a combination of cat's claw and other herbs, plus antioxidant nutrients such as beta-carotene, N-acetylcysteine, vitamin C, and zinc.

Caution: Do not use cat's claw during pregnancy.

❑ Many people with external tumors have responded well to poultices made from comfrey, pau d'arco, ragwort, and wood sage. *See* USING A POULTICE in Part Three.

❑ For breast lumps, try using poultices made of poke root, which is effective in combating glandular swelling. *See* USING A POULTICE in Part Three.

Note: Poke root is recommended for external use only.

❑ Other beneficial herbs include barberry, dandelion, pau d'arco, and red clover. Essiac tea and Jason Winters Tea are also good. These herbs purify the blood, stimulate liver activity, act as natural antibiotics, and generally help healing.

Caution: Do not use barberry during pregnancy.

RECOMMENDATIONS

❑ Eat a diet consisting of 50 percent raw fruits and vegetables. Nuts, seeds, whole grains, and low-fat yogurt and yogurt products should be included. Do not consume animal protein, dairy products (except for yogurt), processed and packaged foods, salt, sugar, white flour, or white flour products. *See* CANCER in Part Two and follow the recommended diet.

❑ *See* FASTING in Part Three and follow the program.

CONSIDERATIONS

❑ Although benign tumors are generally limited in growth, they usually should be removed; a small percentage may later become malignant.

❑ Malignant tumors must be treated as early as possible. Depending on the site and size of the tumor, surgical removal, chemotherapy, and/or radiation therapy may be recommended. *See* CANCER in Part Two.

❑ Iron deficiency has been linked to the development of tumors. However, iron supplements should be taken only if tests show a deficiency. People with cancer should *not* take supplemental iron.

❑ Scientists of the University of California–Los Angeles School of Medicine have found that sodium linoleate, which contains linoleic acid (an essential fatty acid), has the ability to fight cancer cells in the laboratory.

❑ Studies done in Japan suggest that taking garlic supplements may help reduce the size of tumors.

❑ *See also* BREAST CANCER; CANCER; FIBROCYSTIC DISEASE OF THE BREAST; FIBROIDS; POLYPS; PROSTATE CANCER; SKIN CANCER; and/or WARTS, all in Part Two.

Ulcer

See BEDSORES; CANKER SORES; LEG ULCERS; PEPTIC ULCER. *See also under* EYE PROBLEMS.

Ulcerative Colitis

Ulcerative colitis is a chronic disorder in which the mucous membranes lining the colon become inflamed and develop ulcers, causing bloody diarrhea, pain, gas, bloating, and, at times, hard stools. The colon muscles then have to work harder to move these hardened stools through the colon. This can cause the mucous lining of the colon wall to bulge out into small pouchlike projections called diverticula. This usually occurs in the lower left section of the large intestine that is called the *sigmoid* ("S-shaped") colon, although it can occur in any part of the colon. *Enteritis* and *ileitis* are types of inflammation of the small intestine often associated with colitis.

Ulcerative colitis can range from relatively mild to severe. Common complications are diarrhea and bleeding. A rarer complication is toxic megacolon, in which the intestinal wall weakens and balloons out, threatening to rupture.

The cause or causes of most cases of colitis are unknown, but possible contributing factors include poor eating habits, stress, and food allergies. Colitis can also be caused by infectious agents such as bacteria. This type of colitis is often associated with the use of antibiotics, which alter the normal bowel flora and permit microorganisms that are normally held in check to proliferate. The symptoms can range from simple diarrhea to the more severe type of symptoms associated with ulcerative colitis.

NUTRIENTS

SUPPLEMENT	SUGGESTED DOSAGE	COMMENTS
Essential		
Proteolytic enzymes	As directed on label. Take between meals.	Vital for proper digestion of proteins and helps to control inflammation.
plus multienzyme complex with pancreatin	As directed on label. Take after meals.	Anti-inflammatory enzymes. Use a formula that is high in pancreatin and low in hydrochloric acid (HCl).
Very Important		
Acidophilus or Bio-Bifidus from American Biologics or Kyo-Dophilus from Wakunaga	As directed on label twice daily, on an empty stomach.	To normalize the intestinal bacteria. If you have a milk intolerance, use a nondairy formula.
Aerobic Bulk Cleanse (ABC) from Aerobic Life Industries or psyllium husks	1 tbsp in water or juice on an empty stomach in the morning. Drink it down quickly, before it thickens. Take separately from other supplements and medications. As directed on label.	To keep the colon walls clean of toxic wastes.
Alfalfa		*See under* Herbs, below.
Free-form amino acid complex	As directed on label twice daily, on an empty stomach.	To supply needed protein.
L-Glutamine	500 mg twice daily, on an empty stomach. Take with water or juice. Do not take with milk. Take with 50 mg vitamin B$_6$ and 100 mg vitamin C for better absorption.	A major metabolic fuel for the intestinal cells; maintains the villi, the absorption surfaces of the intestines. *See* AMINO ACIDS in Part One.
Vitamin A and vitamin E	25,000 IU daily. If you are pregnant, do not exceed 10,000 IU daily. Up to 800 IU daily.	An antioxidant that protects the mucous membranes and aids in healing. An antioxidant that promotes healing. Deficiency has been associated with bowel cancer.
Vitamin B complex	50–100 mg daily, in divided doses.	Essential for the breakdown of fats, protein, and carbohydrates and for proper digestion. Use a hypoallergenic formula.
Helpful		
Aerobic 07 from Aerobic Life Industries or	As directed on label twice daily.	Provides stabilized oxygen to the colon and destroys unwanted bacteria.
Dioxychlor from American Biologics	10–20 drops sublingually 1–2 times daily.	An important antibacterial, antifungal, and antiviral agent.
Essential fatty acids (flaxseed or primrose oil)	As directed on label.	Important in cell formation. Protects the lining of the colon.

Garlic (Kyolic)	2 capsules 3 times daily, with meals.	A natural antibiotic that has a healing effect on the colon.
Glucosamine sulfate or N-Acetylglucosamine (N-A-G from Source Naturals)	As directed on label. As directed on label.	An important component in the protective mucous secretions of the digestive tract.
Multimineral complex with calcium and chromium and magnesium and zinc	As directed on label.	Malabsorption of these essential minerals is a problem with colitis. Calcium also is needed for the prevention of cancer, which may occur due to constant irritation. Use a high-potency formula.
Raw thymus glandular	500 mg twice daily.	Important in immune function. *See* GLANDULAR THERAPY in Part Three.
VitaCarte from Phoenix BioLabs	As directed on label.	Contains pure bovine cartilage, which can be effective in improving ulcerative colitis.
Vitamin C with bioflavonoids	3,000–5,000 mg daily, in divided doses.	Needed for immune function and healing of mucous membranes. Use a buffered form.

HERBS

❑ Aerobic Bulk Cleanse (ABC) from Aerobic Life Industries contains healing herbs that cleanse the colon. Take it mixed with half fruit or vegetable juice and half aloe vera juice, before meals.

Note: Always take this product separately from other supplements and medications.

❑ Alfalfa, taken in capsule or liquid form, supplies vitamin K and chlorophyll, needed for healing. Take it as directed on the product label three times daily.

❑ Aloe vera aids in healing the colon, thereby easing pain. Drink ½ cup of aloe vera juice in the morning and again at bedtime.

❑ Chamomile, dandelion, feverfew, papaya, red clover, slippery elm, and yarrow extract or tea are beneficial for colitis, as is pau d'arco tea.

Caution: Do not use chamomile on an ongoing basis, and avoid it completely if you are allergic to ragweed. Do not use feverfew during pregnancy.

❑ Lobelia tea is good to drink. Also use it as an enema for inflammation of the colon; it gives quick relief. *See* ENEMAS in Part Three.

Caution: Do not take lobelia internally on an ongoing basis.

RECOMMENDATIONS

❑ Do not wear clothing that is tight around the waist.

❑ For acute pain, try drinking a large glass of water. This aids in flushing out particles caught in the crevices of the colon, relieving pain.

Diet for Colitis

Ulcerative colitis can be an extremely painful and even temporarily disabling condition. Diet is probably the most significant factor in achieving and maintaining remission. Shari Lieberman, nutritionist and author, recommends the following dietary guidelines for people with colitis:

• The most important thing to do is keep a daily record of what you eat and what symptoms you experience. This way you can see which foods have aggravated or improved your condition. Some people are sensitive only to certain foods, such as yeast products, wheat products, or dairy products. By checking your daily record, you can see which food or foods have caused flare-ups or made you feel better.

• Eat a low-carbohydrate, high-vegetable-protein diet. Include alfalfa or barley in the diet. Baked or broiled fish, chicken, and turkey (without the skin) are acceptable sources of protein.

• Eat lots of vegetables. If you cannot tolerate raw vegetables, steam them.

• Eat a high-fiber diet. Oat bran, brown rice, barley and other whole grains, lentils, and related products such as rice cakes are good. Be sure grains are well cooked.

• Keep fats and oils out of your diet, and stay away from high-fat milk and cheeses. Fats and oils exacerbate the diarrhea that comes with colitis.

• Include garlic in the diet for its healing and antibiotic properties.

• Eat cooked foods broiled or baked, not fried or sautéed. Avoid sauces made with butter.

• Avoid carbonated soft drinks, spicy foods, and anything containing caffeine. These substances irritate the colon. Also avoid red meat, sugar, and processed foods.

• Try soy-based cheese instead of dairy cheese; try soymilk or rice milk instead of cow's milk. If you do eat dairy foods, use nonfat types. If you have a lactose intolerance, try lactose-free milk. Many lactose-intolerant people can tolerate low-fat yogurt.

• Drink plenty of liquids—at least eight 8-ounce glasses of water daily to make up for the fluid lost with diarrhea. Carrot and cabbage juices and "green drinks" are also good. Or add chlorophyll liquid to juices.

• Do not eat fruit on an empty stomach. Eat it at the end of a meal instead. Fruit juices should be diluted with water and taken during or after meals.

❑ During a flare-up, consume only soft foods until the pain has subsided. Put oat bran or steamed vegetables through a blender. Add 1 tablespoon of oat or rice bran daily to cereals and juice to add the bulk needed for cleansing the colon. Or add 1 tablespoon of Aerobic Bulk Cleanse to juice and drink it on an empty stomach upon arising.

❑ Try eating junior baby foods for two weeks. Baby foods are easy to digest. Earth's Best baby foods are organic and are available in many health food stores and supermarkets. While on the baby food diet, take extra fiber such as glucomannan. Glucomannan should be taken one-half to one hour before meals with a large glass of liquid.

Note: Always take supplemental fiber separately from other supplements and medications.

❑ Do stretching exercises and take proteolytic enzymes to improve digestion.

❑ Use cleansing enemas made with 2 quarts of lukewarm water. This helps to rid the colon of undigested foods and relieve pain. Use wheatgrass juice as a retention enema. For severe gas and bloating, use an *L. bifidus* enema. *See* ENEMAS in Part Three.

❑ For long-term management of ulcerative colitis and to prevent flare-ups, *see* Diet for Colitis, above, and follow the suggestions there.

❑ *See* FASTING in Part Three, and follow the program once a month.

CONSIDERATIONS

❑ A food sensitivity test is advised for anyone who suffers from colitis. We have seen many people with colitis do well once they make changes in their diet and lifestyle.

❑ When magnesium is given intravenously with vitamin B6, it relaxes the muscles in the walls of the bowels and can control an attack of spastic colon.

❑ Vitamin K deficiency has been linked to gastrointestinal disorders and ulcerative colitis. Vitamin K is found in alfalfa and dark green leafy vegetables. Sulfa drugs and mineral oil deplete vitamin K.

❑ If serious complications arise and all other treatments have failed, surgery may be required.

❑ Colloidal silver is a natural broad-spectrum antiseptic that fights infection, subdues inflammation, and promotes healing. It is a clear golden liquid composed of 99.9-percent pure silver particles approximately 0.001 to 0.01 micron ($\frac{1}{1,000,000}$ to $\frac{1}{100,000}$ millimeter) in diameter suspended in pure water. Colloidal silver can be taken by mouth, administered intravenously, or applied topically.

❑ The earliest signs of ulcerative colitis sometimes mimic the symptoms of arthritis—achiness and joint pain. These symptoms may or may not be accompanied by the abdominal discomfort typical of colitis. If you start experiencing arthritis-like symptoms, it may be beneficial to change your diet and see if improvement results. *See* Diet for Colitis on page 514.

☐ Anyone who has had ulcerative colitis for at least five years—even if it is mild or inactive for a long time—should undergo regular colonoscopy, since people with this disease run a much greater risk of developing colon cancer than the general population. A colonoscopy is an examination performed with a long, flexible instrument that allows a physician to see inside the length of the colon.

☐ *See also* DIVERTICULITIS and MALABSORPTION SYNDROME in Part Two.

Underweight

Some people are thinner than average all their lives, and are perfectly healthy that way. For others, however, underweight may be associated with health problems. This is particularly true if the condition results from unintended, perhaps sudden, weight loss. Unintended weight loss can result from a malabsorption problem; intestinal parasites; certain types of cancer; a colon disorder such as Crohn's disease, ulcerative colitis, or diverticulitis; or a chronic illness such as diabetes, chronic diarrhea, or hyperthyroidism. Surgery, stress, or trauma, such as the loss of a loved one, can also contribute to sudden weight loss.

Underweight can also be caused by treatments such as cancer chemotherapy and radiation therapy, whose side effects include nausea, vomiting, and loss of appetite. An individual who is underweight but believes he or she weighs too much may be suffering from an eating disorder. People with AIDS often suffer from what is known as "wasting syndrome," in which they become more and more emaciated as the disease progresses.

Weight loss may in turn cause nutritional deficiencies that further impair health and complicate recovery. Two age groups for whom undernutrition is a special problem are the very young and the very old. Malnutrition in childhood, especially in infancy, can have permanent effects because it interferes with normal growth and development. Children also have less in the way of nutritional reserves in their bodies to draw upon if intake or absorption of nutrients is inadequate. At the other end of the life span, many elderly people find themselves less and less interested in eating as time goes by, and reduced financial resources may add to the incentive to skip meals. As a result, older people have an increased risk of becoming malnourished.

The suggestions in this section are intended for people who require nutritional rehabilitation. They may also be useful for people who have higher than normal nutritional requirements, such as people who have hepatitis or are undergoing cancer treatment, those who are recovering from burns or trauma, and women who are pregnant or nursing.

NUTRIENTS

SUPPLEMENT	SUGGESTED DOSAGE	COMMENTS
Essential		
Raw liver extract	As directed on label.	Excellent source of B vitamins and minerals. Use a liquid form for easily assimilation.
Vitamin A plus	10,000 IU daily.	Antioxidants that enhance immunity and aid in fat storage.
natural carotenoid complex (Betatene)	As directed on label.	Essential for protein utilization.
Vitamin B complex	100 mg daily, with meals.	Increases the appetite and aids in digestion of fats, carbohydrates, and protein. Use a sublingual form for best absorption. Injections (under a doctor's supervision) may be necessary.
Vitamin C	3,000 mg daily.	Helps prevent cancer, protects against infection, and enhances immunity.
Vitamin E	600 IU daily.	A powerful antioxidant that helps prevent cancer and inhibits the formation of free radicals.
Zinc	80 mg daily. Do not exceed this amount.	Improves the senses of taste and smell. Use zinc gluconate lozenges or OptiZinc for best absorption.
Important		
Essential fatty acids (Ultimate Oil from Nature's Secret is a good source)	As directed on label.	A most important element of the diet.
Free-form amino acid complex	As directed on label.	To supply needed protein in a form that is readily available and easily metabolized. Use a formula containing all the essential amino acids.
Garlic (Kyolic)	2 capsules 3 times daily, with meals.	Provides protection against free radicals. Contains many essential nutrients.
Infla-Zyme Forte from American Biologics or	4 tablets 3 times daily, with meals.	Aids in the proper breakdown of proteins, fats, and carbohydrates for better absorption of foods.
Wobenzym N from Marlyn Nutraceuticals	3–6 tablets 2–3 times daily, between meals.	Destroys free radicals and aids in proper breakdown and absorption of foods.
Quercetin	As directed on label.	Aids in preventing reactions to certain foods, pollens, and other allergens. Increases immunity.
plus bromelain	As directed on label.	Enhances effectiveness of quercetin.
Helpful		
Brewer's yeast	As directed on label.	Stimulates the appetite and supplies B vitamins.
Floradix Iron + Herbs from Salus Haus	As directed on label.	Increases appetite and helps digestion.
Multienzyme complex	As directed on label.	Aids digestion.

| Multivitamin and mineral supplement | As directed on label. | To supply a balance of all needed vitamins and minerals. Use a high-potency formula. |
| Spiru-tein from Nature's Plus | As directed on label. Take between meals. | A safe protein supplement. |

HERBS

❑ Alfalfa, blessed thistle, caraway, cayenne (capsicum), celery, dill, fennel, hyssop, and lady's mantle all work to stimulate the appetite.

❑ Fenugreek and ginseng have long been used as appetite stimulants and digestive aids, especially for elderly people.

Caution: Do not use ginseng if you have high blood pressure.

RECOMMENDATIONS

❑ If you think you may be underweight, and particularly if you are experiencing unintended weight loss, have a complete medical examination to check for an underlying physical disorder. You may have a health problem that requires treatment. Be concerned about an infant or young child who suddenly seems to stop gaining weight normally.

❑ Eat a diet consisting of at least 300 grams of complex carbohydrates, 100 grams of protein, and 2,500 to 3,000 calories a day. Include starchy vegetables, such as potatoes and beans, as well as grains, turkey, chicken, fish, eggs, avocados, olive oil, safflower oil, raw cheeses, nuts, and seeds. Eat only whole-grain breads, pasta, crackers, and hot and cold cereals. For infants, mashed bananas are good.

❑ Eat nondairy soy-based cream soups. Soymilk can be used in the same ways as cow's milk. Cream soups are usually higher in protein and calories than broth soups and should be used as tolerated.

❑ Drink herbal teas, fruit and vegetable juices, and mineral water.

❑ Eat frequent but small meals and snacks, and eat them slowly. If you are undernourished, you may lose your appetite if confronted with large amounts of food at one sitting. You can always have additional servings if you are still hungry after the first.

❑ Do not eat fried or junk foods for extra calories. Instead, eat these high-calorie snacks between meals or before bedtime: raw cheese; banana soy pudding; turkey, chicken, or tuna sandwiches with cheese; raw nuts; rice crackers with nut butter; yogurt; yogurt fruit shakes; carob soymilk; almond milk; buttermilk; custard; nuts; and avocados.

❑ Eliminate from the diet coffee, tea, and anything else (such as soft drinks) that contains caffeine.

❑ If possible, get regular moderate exercise. Walking and similar activities are good. Moderate exercise helps in the assimilation of nutrients and in increasing the appetite. Avoid strenuous exercise.

❑ Eat in relaxed surroundings. Do not try to eat when you are upset or nervous.

❑ If you smoke, stop.

❑ Investigate the possibility of food allergies. (*See* ALLERGIES in Part Two.) Avoid any foods you think you may be allergic to.

❑ If other people comment on your thinness but you feel you actually could stand to lose weight, consider professional evaluation for an eating disorder. *See* ANOREXIA NERVOSA and/or BULIMIA in Part Two.

CONSIDERATIONS

❑ Consideration of the appearance and smell of the food, as well as the eating environment, is important when trying to stimulate a poor appetite.

❑ The color red helps to stimulate taste buds. (*See* COLOR THERAPY in Part Three.)

❑ *See also* APPETITE, POOR.

Urinary Tract Infections

See CYSTITIS; KIDNEY DISEASE; VAGINITIS.

Uterine Prolapse

See PROLAPSE OF THE UTERUS.

Uveitis

See Dimness or Loss of Vision *under* EYE PROBLEMS.

Vaginitis

The symptoms of vaginitis, or inflammation of the mucous membranes lining the vagina, include a burning and/or itching sensation and abnormal vaginal discharge. Vaginitis may be caused by bacterial or fungal infection, vitamin B deficiency, intestinal worms, or irritation from excessive douching or the use of such products as deodorant sprays. Infectious vaginitis is often caused by trichomonas, gonococci, or other sexually transmitted organisms. Other factors, such as poor hygiene and tight, nonporous clothing, may contribute to the problem. Pregnancy, diabetes, and the use of antibiotics disturb the body's natural balance, creating an environment in which infectious organisms can thrive. Oral contraceptives also can produce vaginal inflammation.

Atrophic vaginitis is a condition primarily found in post-menopausal women and those whose ovaries have been surgically removed. This disorder can result in the formation of adhesions and a high susceptibility to infection. Common symptoms include itching or burning, painful intercourse, and a thin, watery discharge, occasionally tinged with blood.

NUTRIENTS

SUPPLEMENT	SUGGESTED DOSAGE	COMMENTS
Very Important		
Acidophilus	As directed on label 3 times daily, with meals.	To replenish normal "friendly" bacteria.
Biotin	300 mcg 3 times daily.	Inhibits yeast.
Essential fatty acids	As directed on label.	Aids healing.
Garlic (Kyolic)	1 capsule 3 times daily, with meals.	Has antifungal properties.
Vitamin B complex	50–100 mg 3 times daily, with meals.	Often deficient in people with vaginitis. Use a high-potency formula.
Yeast•Gard from Lake Consumer Products	As directed on label.	Excellent antifungal agent. Reduces pain.
Helpful		
Colloidal silver	As directed on label.	A broad-spectrum antibiotic that subdues inflammation and promotes healing.
Kyo-Dophilus from Wakunaga	Open up 3 capsules and dissolve in 1 qt warm water with 6 drops tea tree oil added to use as a douche.	Replenishes "friendly" bacteria.
L-Isoleucine and L-leucine and L-lysine	As directed on label, on an empty stomach. Take with water or juice. Do not take with milk. Take with 50 mg vitamin B₆ and 100 mg vitamin C for better absorption.	Good for fighting herpes and for tissue repair and healing of skin lesions. *See* AMINO ACIDS in Part One.
N-A-G from Source Naturals	As directed on label.	Amino acid compound. Forms the basis of complex molecular structures that are key parts of mucous membrane tissue.
Oxy C-2 Gel from American Biologics	As directed on label.	A useful antibacterial, antiviral, and antifungal.
Vitamin A and vitamin E	50,000 IU daily. If you are pregnant, do not exceed 10,000 IU daily. 400 IU daily.	Powerful antioxidants that aid healing.
Vitamin B complex	As directed on label.	Regulates metabolism and promotes good health.
Vitamin B₆ (pyridoxine)	50 mg 3 times daily.	Especially important if using estrogen cream for treatment of atrophic vaginitis.
Vitamin C	2,000–5,000 mg daily.	Important immune system stimulant. Necessary for tissue healing.
Vitamin D with calcium and magnesium	1,000 mg daily. 1,500 mg daily. 1,000 mg daily.	To relieve stress. Women need extra supplements of these nutrients at this time.
Zinc	30 mg daily. Do not exceed a total of 100 mg daily from all supplements.	To increase immunity and promote proper utilization of vitamin A. Also reduces severity of herpes outbreaks. Use zinc gluconate lozenges or OptiZinc for best absorption.

HERBS

❑ Douche with infusions made from antiseptic herbs such as calendula, echinacea, garlic, goldenseal, fresh plantain, St. Johnswort, or tea tree oil, along with herbs such as comfrey leaves, to soothe irritation. Echinacea and goldenseal can also be taken orally.

Note: Comfrey is recommended for external use only. Do not take goldenseal internally on a daily basis for more than one week at a time, do not use it during pregnancy, and use it with caution if you are allergic to ragweed.

❑ Calendula and vitamin A vaginal suppositories are soothing and healing to irritated tissues. Goldenseal suppositories are useful for all types of infection.

❑ Meno-Fem from Prevail Corporation is a combination of traditional herbs and nutrients designed to combat the symptoms of menopause. It is helpful for vaginitis related to hormonal imbalance.

❑ Tea tree oil is good for vaginitis. Topical tea tree oil cream is effective against fungal infection, herpes blisters, warts, and other types of infection. Tea tree oil suppositories have been used successfully for vaginal yeast infections.

RECOMMENDATIONS

❑ Eat plain yogurt that contains live yogurt cultures, or apply yogurt directly to the vagina. This can help fight infection and soothe inflammation. Also consume brown rice, millet, and acidophilus.

❑ Consume fiber daily. Oat bran is a good source.

❑ Eat a diet that is fruit-free, sugar-free, and yeast-free. Avoid aged cheeses, alcohol, chocolate, dried fruits, fermented foods, all grains containing gluten (wheat, oats, rye, and barley), ham, honey, nut butters, pickles, raw mushrooms, soy sauce, sprouts, sugar in any form, vinegar, and all yeast products. Also eliminate citrus and acidic fruits (oranges, grapefruits, lemons, tomatoes, pineapple, and limes) from your diet until the inflammation subsides. Then add them back slowly.

❑ Keep clean and dry. Wear white cotton underwear, which absorbs moisture and allows air to circulate. Avoid tight clothing and synthetic fabrics. Change into dry clothing as soon as possible after swimming. Do not spend prolonged periods of time in a wet bathing suit.

☐ To relieve itching, open a vitamin E capsule and apply the oil to the inflamed area. Or use vitamin E cream.

☐ Add 3 cups of pure apple cider vinegar to bath water to treat vaginitis. Soak in the tub for twenty minutes, allowing the water to flow into the vagina.

☐ Do not use corticosteroids or oral contraceptives until your condition improves. Oral contraceptives can upset the balance of microorganisms in the body.

☐ Do not use sweet-smelling douches. If douching provides relief, you can douche with plain warm water, water with 2 acidophilus capsules added, or plain yogurt. You can also add 1 teaspoon of fresh garlic juice.

☐ Avoid taking iron supplements until the inflammation subsides. Infectious bacteria require iron for growth. If a bacterial infection is present, the body naturally "hides" iron by storing it in the liver, spleen, and bone marrow to inhibit the growth of the bacteria.

☐ Drink steam-distilled water only.

CONSIDERATIONS

☐ Physicians often prescribe the drug ketoconazole (Nizoral) for vaginitis, with no apparent adverse side effects. Clotrimazole (Gyne-Lotrimin, Mycelex, and others), which is available without a prescription, is also used.

☐ Atrophic vaginitis is often treated with prescription estrogen ointments. The use of these products increases the body's need for vitamin B6. Vaginal absorption of synthetic estrogen may be dangerous.

☐ Natural progesterone cream applied to the vagina is beneficial for atrophic vaginitis.

☐ *See also* BLADDER INFECTION; CANDIDIASIS; KIDNEY DISEASE; and/or YEAST INFECTION, all in Part Two.

Varicose Veins

Blood pulses through the arteries, powered by the beating of the heart, to provide nutrients and oxygen to the body tissues. It returns to the heart by means of the veins. Like the arteries, the veins are tube-shaped vessels in graduated sizes, but unlike the arteries, the veins have tiny valves on their inner walls to prevent the blood from flowing backward, toward the arteries. If the valves do not work properly, circulation is impaired and blood accumulates in the veins, stretching them. The result is varicose veins—abnormally enlarged, bulging, often bluish and lumpy-looking veins. These prominent veins are often accompanied by dull, nagging aches and pains. Swelling, leg sores, itching, leg cramps, and a feeling of heaviness in the legs are characteristic of varicose veins.

Because lack of circulation contributes to the formation of varicose veins, they are more common in people who sit or stand in one position for prolonged periods of time, people who habitually sit with their legs crossed, and those who lack proper regular exercise. Excess weight, heavy lifting, and pregnancy put increased pressure on the legs, increasing the likelihood of developing varicose veins. Constipation, phlebitis, heart failure, liver disease, and abdominal tumors can also play a role in the formation of varicose veins. A deficiency of vitamin C and bioflavonoids (mainly rutin) can weaken the collagen structure in the vein walls, which can lead to varicose veins. A tendency toward varicose veins may also run in families.

Most cases of varicose veins do not pose a serious problem and can be managed with simple home measures. In some cases, however, if varicose veins are not treated properly, complications such as bleeding under the skin, deep-vein blood clots, an eczema-like condition near the affected veins, or ulcerated spots near the ankles may occur.

NUTRIENTS

SUPPLEMENT	SUGGESTED DOSAGE	COMMENTS
Very Important		
Coenzyme Q10	100 mg daily.	Improves tissue oxygenation, increases circulation, and enhances immunity.
Dimethylglycine (DMG) (Aangamik DMG from FoodScience Labs)	50 mg 3 times daily.	Improves oxygen utilization in the tissues.
Essential fatty acids (Ultimate Oil from Nature's Secret is a good source)	As directed on label.	Reduces pain and helps to keep blood vessels soft and pliable.
Glutathione	As directed on label.	Protects the heart, veins, and arteries from oxidant damage.
Pycnogenol or grape seed extract	As directed on label. As directed on label.	Stimulate blood circulation, boost immunity, neutralize free radicals, and strengthen connective tissue, including that of the cardiovascular system.
Vitamin C plus bioflavonoid complex plus extra rutin	3,000–6,000 mg daily. 100 mg daily. 50 mg 3 times daily.	Aids circulation by reducing blood clotting tendencies. To promote healing and prevent bruising. A potent noncitrus bioflavonoid that helps maintain the strength of blood vessels.
Important		
Vitamin E	Start with 400 IU daily and slowly increase to 1,000 IU daily.	Improves circulation and aids in preventing heavy feeling in the legs.
Helpful		
Aerobic Bulk Cleanse (ABC) from Aerobic Life Industries	As directed on label. Take separately from other supplements and medications.	Keeping the colon clean is important.
Brewer's yeast	As directed on label.	Contains needed protein and B vitamins.

Lecithin granules or capsules	1 tbsp 3 times daily, with meals. 1,200 mg 3 times daily, with meals.	Fat emulsifier that aids circulation.
Multivitamin and mineral complex	As directed on label.	To maintain a balance of all necessary nutrients.
Vitamin A plus natural carotenoid complex (Betatene)	10,000 IU daily. As directed on label.	To enhance immunity, protect the cells, and slow the aging process.
Vitamin B complex plus extra vitamin B$_6$ (pyridoxine) and vitamin B$_{12}$	50–100 mg 3 times daily, with meals. 50 mg daily. 300–1,000 mcg daily.	B vitamins are needed to help in digestion of foods. Sublingual forms are best for all the B vitamins.
Vitamin D plus calcium and magnesium	1,000 mg daily, at bedtime. 1,500 mg daily, at bedtime. 750 mg daily, at bedtime.	This combination helps to relieve leg cramps. Use calcium chelate form.
Zinc	80 mg daily.	Aids healing.

HERBS

❑ Butcher's broom, ginkgo biloba, gotu kola, and hawthorn berries improve circulation in the legs.

❑ Horse chestnut makes a good treatment for the discomfort of varicose veins. Mix ½ teaspoon of horse chestnut powder with 2 cups of water, and moisten a sterile cotton gauze cloth with the mixture. Rub the cloth gently over the affected area. This is soothing to inflamed veins. Witch hazel can also be used this way to reduce discomfort.

❑ Bathing your legs or other affected area in white oak bark herb tea three times a day helps to stimulate blood flow. Simmer (but do not boil) a strong tea and use the tea to make compresses. Apply the compresses to affected areas.

RECOMMENDATIONS

❑ Eat a diet that is low in fat and refined carbohydrates and includes plenty of fish and fresh fruits and vegetables.

❑ Make sure that your diet contains plenty of fiber to prevent constipation and keep the bowels clean.

❑ Avoid animal protein, processed and refined foods, sugar, ice cream, fried foods, cheeses, peanuts, junk foods, tobacco, alcohol, and salt.

❑ Maintain a healthy weight and get regular moderate exercise. Walking, swimming, and bicycling all promote good circulation. Change your daily routine to allow more time for exercise and movement for your legs.

❑ Wear loose clothing that does not restrict blood flow. It is a good idea to wear supportive elastic stockings; these help to support the varicose veins and prevent them from becoming more swollen.

❑ Avoid long periods of standing or sitting. Take rest periods several times during the day to elevate your legs above heart level. Avoid crossing your legs, doing heavy lifting, and putting any unnecessary pressure on your legs.

❑ After bathing, apply castor oil directly over the problem veins and massage the oil into your legs from the feet up.

❑ To help improve circulation and ease pain, fill a tub with cold water. Stand in the water and simulate walking.

❑ Avoid scratching the itchy skin above varicose veins. This can cause ulceration and bleeding.

CONSIDERATIONS

❑ Some physicians treat varicose veins by injecting a sodium tetradecyl sulfate (saline) solution into the affected vein and applying compression bandages for a period of time. The solution fuses the vein walls together permanently, closing the defective vein. The body compensates for lost vessels by finding an alternate route for blood flow.

❑ Spider veins are chronically dilated capillaries near the surface of the skin. They are harmless and rarely cause any problems, although distressing for cosmetic reasons.

❑ Hemorrhoids are actually varicose veins of the anus or rectum. Symptoms of hemorrhoids include rectal itching, pain, and blood in the stool. (*See* HEMORRHOIDS in Part Two.)

❑ Dimethylsulfoxide (DMSO) has been used to relieve the swelling and pain of severe varicose veins. This liquid, a byproduct of wood processing, is applied topically to the affected area as needed. Only DMSO from a health food store should be used for therapeutic purposes.

❑ The symptoms of varicose veins are similar to those of thrombophlebitis. In addition, the chances of developing varicose veins increase greatly if you suffer from thrombophlebitis. (*See* THROMBOPHLEBITIS in Part Two.)

❑ *See also* CIRCULATORY PROBLEMS in Part Two.

❑ *See also under* PREGNANCY-RELATED PROBLEMS in Part Two.

Venereal Disease

See SEXUALLY TRANSMITTED DISEASE.

Vertigo

Vertigo is a sensation of dizziness, faintness, or lightheadedness that results from an impaired sense of balance and equilibrium. The term comes from *vertere*, the Latin verb meaning "to turn," and is usually due to an inner ear problem. A person suffering from vertigo may feel that he or she is sinking or falling and/or that the room and objects in it are spinning around. In some cases, the individual may feel that he or she is spinning, too. Vertigo is sometimes accompanied by nausea and hearing loss.

Vertigo occurs when the central nervous system receives conflicting messages from the inner ear, eyes, muscles, and skin pressure receptors. This may result from a variety of causes, including brain tumors, high or low blood pressure, allergies, head injuries, inadequate or interrupted supply of oxygen to the brain, anemia, viral infection, fever, the use of certain drugs, nutritional deficiencies, neurological disease, psychological stress, changes in atmospheric pressure, blockage of the ear canal or eustachian tube, middle ear infections, or excess wax in the ear. Poor cerebral circulation also can cause dizziness and the inability to maintain balance. Poor cerebral circulation may be due to either the narrowing of the blood vessels that supply the brain (arteriosclerosis), pinched blood vesels in the neck (cervical osteoarthritis), or a disorder such as diabetes or anemia.

Because of the effects of aging on the body, older people are more prone than others to experience vertigo. The body maintains a sense of balance through a complex mechanism involving both the inner ears and visual input. Within the canals of the inner ears, there are structures called *otoliths*, which are minute calcium carbonate crystals that press upon the hairlike cells that line the inner membranes. Gravity acts on the otoliths so that they shift in response to head movements. This bends the fiber cells, which, in turn, transmit signals to the brain. The brain then uses these signals to calculate the positioning of the head. As people age, tiny bits of debris may accumulate in the inner ears and press against the hair cells, resulting in false signals being sent to the brain. This can interfere with the sense of balance and result in vertigo. In addition, with increasing age, nerve impulses require more time to travel from the eyes to the brain and spinal cord. This can cause dizziness and loss of balance upon sudden movement.

Dizziness is not synonymous with vertigo. Anyone may occasionally experience a feeling of lightheadedness, dizziness, unsteadiness, or the sensation of feeling faint. Those with low blood pressure may have this feeling upon rising quickly from a sitting or lying position. In some cases, dizziness can be a warning sign of a heart attack, stroke, concussion, or brain damage.

NUTRIENTS

SUPPLEMENT	SUGGESTED DOSAGE	COMMENTS
Very Important		
Dimethylglycine (DMG) (Aangamik DMG from FoodScience Labs)	As directed on label.	Increases oxygen supply to the brain.
Vitamin B₃ (niacin)	100 mg 3 times daily. Do not exceed this amount.	Improves cerebral circulation and lowers cholesterol. *Caution:* Do not take niacin if you have a liver disorder, gout, or high blood pressure.
Vitamin B complex plus extra vitamin B₆ (pyridoxine) and vitamin B₁₂	100 mg 3 times daily, with meals. 50 mg daily. 300–1,000 mcg daily.	B vitamins are necessary for normal brain and central nervous system function. Consider injections (under a doctor's supervision) for better absorption. If injections are not available, use sublingual forms.
Vitamin C	3,000–10,000 mg daily, in divided doses.	An antioxidant that also improves circulation.
Vitamin E	Start with 200 IU daily and increase slowly to 400–800 IU daily.	Improves circulation.
Important		
Choline and inositol and/or	As directed on label 3 times daily.	Necessary in nerve function.
lecithin	As directed on label.	Helps to prevent hardening of the arteries and improve brain function.
Coenzyme Q₁₀	100–200 mg daily.	Improves circulation to the brain.
Ginkgo biloba		*See under* Herbs, below.
Vitamin A	10,000 IU daily.	Enhances immunity and acts as an antioxidant.
Zinc	30 mg daily. Do not exceed a total of 100 mg daily from all supplements.	Promotes a healthy immune system and helps maintain vitamin E levels. Use zinc gluconate lozenges or OptiZinc for best absorption.
Helpful		
Brewer's yeast	½ tsp daily for 3 days, then increase to 1 tbsp daily.	Contains balanced B vitamins.
Calcium and magnesium	1,500 mg daily. 750 mg daily.	Important in maintaining regular nerve impulses. To help prevent dizziness.
Kelp	1,000–1,500 mg daily.	For necessary balanced minerals and vitamins.
Melatonin	1.5–5 mg daily, taken 2 hours or less before bedtime.	Helps to maintain equilibrium.
Multivitamin and mineral complex	As directed on label.	For necessary balance of vitamins and minerals.

HERBS

❑ Butcher's broom and cayenne (capsicum) help improve circulation.

❑ Dandelion tea or extract is very good for high blood pressure.

❑ Ginger relieves dizziness and nausea.

❑ Ginkgo biloba improves circulation and improves brain function by increasing the supply of oxygen to the brain. Take 120 mg of ginkgo biloba extract daily.

RECOMMENDATIONS

❑ Avoid making rapid or extreme movements and rapid changes in body position.

Limit your total sodium intake to less than 2,000 milligrams per day. Too much sodium can disrupt the workings of the inner ear.

Avoid alcohol, caffeine, nicotine, and all fried foods.

To subdue dizziness, sit in a chair with your feet flat on the floor and stare at a fixed object for a few minutes.

If you begin to experience dizziness soon after taking new medication, assume that the problem is drug related. Discuss the problem with your physician or pharmacist.

If vertigo is a recurring problem, consult your health care provider. It may be a sign of an underlying problem that requires treatment.

CONSIDERATIONS

Persons who have vertigo sometimes experience a phenomenon called nystagmus, involuntary rapid or jerky eye movements. It may occur spontaneously or as a result of changing positions.

Air contains less oxygen at altitudes high above sea level. Lower oxygen levels can cause mild, temporary dizziness or lightheadedness.

Certain activities, such as taking amusement park rides, watching action movies, sailing, or playing virtual-reality video games, may bring on vertigo or dizziness. In such cases, symptoms dimish soon after the activity ceases.

Viral Infection

See AIDS; BLADDER INFECTION; BRONCHITIS; CHICKENPOX; COLD SORES; COMMON COLD; CROUP; DIARRHEA; EAR INFECTION; FEVER; GERMAN MEASLES; HEPATITIS; HERPESVIRUS INFECTION; INFLUENZA; MEASLES; MENINGITIS; MONONUCLEOSIS; MUMPS; PANCREATITIS; PNEUMONIA; REYE'S SYNDROME; SHINGLES; SORE THROAT; TONSILLITIS; WARTS. See also under EYE PROBLEMS.

Vitiligo

Vitiligo, also called leukoderma, is a skin condition characterized by chalky white patches of skin surrounded by a dark border. The spots can be few or many; they may be tiny or cover the body. They usually appear on both sides of the body in approximately the same place, and they do not hurt or itch. These spots occur because, for some reason, the cells that normally produce the skin pigment melanin are absent. If the affected area is on the scalp, the hair that grows from it is likely to be white as well.

The underlying cause of vitiligo is not known, but it can run in families and may be related to an autoimmune prob-

lem. A thyroid gland malfunction may be involved as well. Vitiligo can also occur after physical trauma to the skin. The unpigmented spots are a concern primarily for cosmetic reasons and are highly vulnerable to sunburn.

NUTRIENTS

SUPPLEMENT	SUGGESTED DOSAGE	COMMENTS
Very Important		
Vitamin B complex	50 mg and up, 3 times daily.	Needed for proper skin tone and texture. Helps to combat stress. A sublingual form is recommended.
plus extra pantothenic acid (vitamin B5) and	300 mg daily, in divided doses.	The anti-stress vitamin. Important in skin pigmentation. Sublingual form is best.
para-aminobenzoic acid (PABA)	100 mg and up, 3 times daily.	Aids in stopping discoloration of the hair. Consider injections (under a doctor's supervision).
Important		
Essential fatty acids (primrose oil and Ultimate Oil from Nature's Secret are good sources)	As directed on label.	Stimulates hormone function and contains all the needed essential fatty acids.
Helpful		
Ageless Beauty from Biotec Foods	As directed on label.	Protects the skin from free radical damage.
Calcium and magnesium	1,000 mg daily. 500 mg daily.	Deficiency contributes to fragility of the skin. Needed to balance with calcium.
Multivitamin and mineral complex	As directed on label.	To maintain a balance of all essential nutrients.
Silica	As directed on label.	Important for developing skin's strength and elasticity; stimulates collagen formation.
Vitamin A plus natural carotenoid complex (Betatene)	10,000 IU daily. As directed on label.	To promote healing and construction of new skin tissue.
Vitamin C with bioflavonoids	3,000–5,000 mg daily, in divided doses.	Necessary for the formation of collagen, a protein that gives skin its flexibility. Also fights free radicals and strengthens the capillaries that feed the skin.
Vitamin E	Start with 400 IU daily and increase slowly to 800 IU daily.	Protects against free radicals that can damage the skin.
Zinc plus copper	50 mg daily. Do not exceed a total of 100 mg daily from all supplements. 3 mg daily.	For tissue strength and repair. Use zinc gluconate lozenges or OptiZinc for best absorption. Needed for collagen production and healthy skin. Also needed to balance with zinc.

HERBS

The use of picrorrhiza (an Indian herb used in Ayurvedic medicine) has been shown to reduce the number and size of unpigmented skin patches.

RECOMMENDATIONS

❑ Consult a nutritionally oriented physician for vitamin B complex plus PABA injections (*see under* Nutrients, above). This treatment is often effective.

❑ Always apply a sunscreen with a sun protection factor (SPF) of 15 or higher to any unpigmented areas. They have no natural protection against the sun's ultraviolet rays.

CONSIDERATIONS

❑ Vitiligo sometimes responds to the use of PABA and magnesium. Small spots of pigment appear gradually, like freckles. The spots gradually merge until normal color is restored. Some people with vitiligo have prematurely gray or white hair. A small percentage of such people treated with PABA and magnesium have experienced a return of both skin and hair to the original color.

❑ Vitiligo lesions may be de-emphasized by the use of commercial cosmetics that cover the affected area with an opaque, waterproof layer. DermaBlend is one widely available product.

❑ Creams containing fluorinated steroids may be prescribed to stimulate repigmentation of the skin.

❑ For persons with widespread vitiligo, bleaching of the unaffected skin with hydroquinone (a weak but safe depigmenting agent) may be recommended. This is done to minimize the difference in color between pigmented and depigmented areas.

❑ An article in *Let's Live* magazine reported on a new treatment in which healthy pigment cells were transplanted into the affected area. These transplants were successful in all but one case and none of the recipients rejected the transplantation of healthy pigment cells.

❑ GH3 cream from Gero Vita International has given good results for many skin problems. This face cream is for adult use only.

Warts

Warts are small growths on the skin that are caused by human papillomaviruses (HPV). There are at least sixty known types of HPV. Warts may appear singly or in clusters, and most are benign, although several types of warts have been linked to an increased likelihood of cancer. This section addresses three types of warts: common warts, plantar warts, and genital warts.

Common warts can be found anywhere on the body, but are most common on the hands, fingers, elbows, forearms, knees, face, and the skin around the nails. Most often, they often occur on skin that is continually exposed to friction, trauma, or abrasion. They can also occur on the larynx (the

voice box) and cause hoarseness. Common warts may be flat or raised, dry or moist, and have a rough and pitted surface that is either the same color as or slightly darker than the surrounding skin. They can be as small as a pinhead or as large as a small bean. Highly contagious, the virus that causes common warts is acquired through breaks in the skin. It may be contracted by going barefoot in a locker room or other public area, or by using another persons's comb or hair brush. Common warts can spread if they are picked, trimmed, bitten, or touched. Warts on the face can spread as a result of shaving. Common warts typically do not cause pain or itching.

Plantar warts occur on the soles of the feet and the undersides of the toes. They are bumpy white growths that may resemble calluses, except that they can be tender to the touch and often bleed if the surface is trimmed. They also often have an identifiable hard center. Plantar warts do not tend to spread to other parts of the body.

Genital warts are soft, moist growths found in and around the vagina, anus, penis, groin, and/or scrotum. In men, they can grow in the urethra as well. They are usually pink or red in color and resemble tiny heads of cauliflower. Genital warts most often occur in clusters, but they can appear singly as well. They are sexually transmitted and are highly contagious; because the warts do not usually appear until three months or more after an individual becomes infected with the HPV that causes them, the virus can be spread before the carrier is even aware that he or she has it. Two of the strains of HPV that cause genital warts have been associated with cancer of the cervix; five strains of HPV are seen in nearly all surface cancers of the cervix, vagina, vulva, anus, penis, and perianal area. An infant can contract warts by being exposed to genital warts during the birth process.

NUTRIENTS

SUPPLEMENT	SUGGESTED DOSAGE	COMMENTS
Very Important		
Vitamin B complex	50 mg 3 times daily.	Important in normal cell multiplication.
Vitamin C	4,000–10,000 mg daily.	Has powerful antiviral capacity.
Important		
L-Cysteine	500 mg twice daily, on an empty stomach. Take with water or juice. Do not take with milk. Take with 50 mg vitamin B$_6$ and 100 mg vitamin C for better absorption.	Supplies sulfur, needed for prevention and treatment of warts. *See* AMINO ACIDS in Part One.
Vitamin A	100,000 IU daily for 1 month, then 50,000 IU daily for 1 month, then reduce to 25,000 IU daily for 1 month or until warts disappear. If you are pregnant, do not exceed 10,000 IU daily.	Needed for normalizing skin and epithelial membranes. Use emulsion form for easier assimilation and greater safety at higher doses.

Vitamin E	400–800 IU daily. Can be applied topically; cut open capsule to release oil. Apply to warts daily.	Improves circulation and promotes tissue repair and healing.
Zinc	50–80 mg daily. Do not exceed a total of 100 mg daily from all supplements.	Increases immunity against viruses. Use zinc gluconate lozenges or OptiZinc for best absorption.
Helpful		
Multivitamin and mineral complex	As directed on label.	Needed for normal cell division.
Shiitake or reishi	As directed on label. As directed on label.	Has antiviral properties.

HERBS

❑ Aloe vera gel; myrrh; oils of clove, tea tree, or wintergreen; and tinctures of black walnut, chickweed, goldenseal, and pau d'arco have all been used externally to treat warts. Place a small dab of one on the wart two or three times daily until the wart is gone. If irritation occurs, dilute the oil or extract with distilled water or cold-pressed vegetable oil.

RECOMMENDATIONS

❑ To remove common warts, try one or more of the following remedies:

• Crush a garlic clove and apply the garlic directly on the wart. Cover it with a bandage and leave it in place for twenty-four hours. Blisters should then form and the wart should fall off in about a week.

• Apply a paste made from castor oil and baking soda to the wart. Put the mixture on each night and cover it with a bandage. This may remove the wart in three to six weeks.

❑ Increase the amount of sulfur-containing amino acids in your diet by eating more asparagus, citrus fruits, eggs, garlic, and onions. Desiccated liver tablets are also good.

❑ If you suspect you may have genital warts, see your health care provider promptly. This is especially important for women, because genital warts have been linked to cervical cancer. An immediate Pap test is advised.

❑ Keep genital warts dry. After bathing, use a hair dryer on a low setting to dry the area. Do not rub or irritate it. Wear only cotton underwear. Do not have sexual intercourse until the warts are completely healed.

❑ Do not cut or burn a wart off yourself. These are procedures that must be done by a qualified health care provider.

CONSIDERATIONS

❑ Plantar warts may not require treatment. However, if a wart is painful and interferes with walking, treatment is warranted. Several treatment sessions may be necessary to eliminate them, but doctors can usually eradicate even the most stubborn plantar warts.

❑ Adequate daily vitamin C intake is most important in maintaining effective immunity against the viruses that cause warts.

❑ People who take medications to suppress the immune system, such as those who have received organ transplants or who have certain autoimmune disorders, are more prone to develop warts.

❑ Most common warts disappear within a year or two, even without treatment. Unless a common wart becomes bothersome, there is no need to do anything about it.

❑ Commonly used medical treatments for common and plantar warts include fulguration (using electric current to destroy wart tissue); freezing with liquid nitrogen; and topical applications of various types of acid. Some physicians have achieved good results using the drug bleomycin (Blenoxane) to treat warts. It is injected or applied locally.

❑ Common warts can be treated with a mild acid solution such as salicylic acid. It is thought that the acid weakens the walls of the wart enough to allow some of the virus to enter the bloodstream, causing the production of antibodies that eventually attack and destroy the warts. Removal does not allow the body to build up immunity to the virus.

❑ There are a variety of treatments for genital warts, but none is a perfect cure and all have side effects. Treatment falls into three categories: prescription topical preparations that destroy wart tissue; surgical methods to remove wart tissue; and biological approaches that target the virus.

❑ Laser treatment is proving more effective in treating genital warts than chemicals or conventional surgery. Lasers remove them completely (other treatments only reduce size). Treatment is performed on an outpatient basis, and usually prevents recurrences and transmission during sex.

❑ A study on the injection of interferon alfa directly into genital warts found this treatment to be successful approximately 36 percent of the time. Interferon alfa is a powerful antiviral substance. However, using this treatment for large numbers of warts may be too uncomfortable and expensive.

❑ Women who have been diagnosed with genital warts should have a vaginal and uterine Pap smear every six months, as these warts are associated with an increased risk of cervical cancer.

Weakened Immune System

Modern conventional medicine battles disease directly by means of drugs, surgery, radiation, and other therapies, but true health can be attained only by maintaining a healthy, properly functioning immune system. It is the immune system that fights off disease-causing microorganisms and that engineers the healing process. The immune system is the key to fighting every kind of insult to the body, from that little shaving nick to the myriad of viruses that seem to abound these days. Even the aging process may be more closely related to the functioning of the immune system than to the passage of time.

Weakening of the immune system results in increased susceptibility to virtually every type of illness. Some common signs of impaired immune function include fatigue, listlessness, repeated infections, inflammation, allergic reactions, slow wound healing, chronic diarrhea, and infections that represent an overgrowth of some normally present organism, such as oral thrush, systemic candidiasis, or vaginal yeast infections. It is estimated that healthy adults in our society have an average of two colds a year. Persons who have significantly more colds and infectious illnesses than that are likely to have some problem with immune function. By understanding some of the basic elements of the immune system and how they work, plus the overall role the immune system plays in your health, you can take responsibility for your own health.

In its simplest terms, the task of the immune system is to identify those things that are "self" (that naturally belong in the body) and those that are "nonself" (foreign or otherwise harmful material), and then to neutralize or destroy that which is nonself. The immune system is unlike other bodily systems in that it is not a group of physical structures but a system of complex interactions involving many different organs, structures, and substances, among them white blood cells, bone marrow, the lymphatic vessels and organs, specialized cells found in various body tissues, and specialized substances, called serum factors, that are present in the blood. Ideally, all of these components work together to protect the body against infection and disease.

The human immune system is functional at birth, but it does not yet function well. In large part this is because immunity is something that develops as the system matures and the body learns to defend itself against different foreign invaders, termed antigens. The immune system has the ability to learn to identify, and then to remember, specific antigens that have been encountered. It does this through two basic means, known as *cell-mediated immunity* and *humoral immunity*.

In cell-mediated immunity, white blood cells called T lymphocytes identify and then destroy cancerous cells, viruses, and microorganisms like bacteria and fungi. The T lymphocytes, or T cells, mature in the thymus gland (hence the "T" designation). This is where they learn to recognize what is "self," and therefore should be tolerated, and what is "nonself," and therefore should be destroyed. The thymus, a small gland located behind the top of the breastbone, is a major gland of the immune system. In the thymus, each T cell is programmed to identify one particular type of invading enemy. Not all prospective T cells make a successful passage through the thymus. Those whose programming is imperfect (for instance, those that mistakenly identify "self" as "nonself") are eliminated. The ones that do make it are released into the bloodstream to search out and destroy antigens that correspond to their programming. They attack the antigens in part through the secretion of proteins called cytokines. Interferon is one of the better known types of cytokines.

Humoral immunity involves the production of antibodies. These are not cells, but special proteins whose chemical structures are formed to match the surfaces of specific antigens. When they encounter their specific antigens, antibodies either damage the invasive cells or alert the white blood cells to attack. The antibodies are produced by another group of white blood cells, the B lymphocytes, which are manufactured by and mature in the bone marrow. When a B lymphocyte is presented with a particular antigen, it engineers an antibody to match it and stores a blueprint of the invader so that it can initiate the production of antibodies in case of a subsequent exposure, even if a long period of time elapses in between. For this system to work, each B cell must come into existence prepared to produce an almost infinite variety of different antibodies, so that it can match whatever antigen it is presented with. This is made possible by a mechanism known as "jumping genes." Inside the B cells, the genes that determine the chemical structure of the protein to be produced can be shuffled around and linked up in an astronomical number of different combinations. As a result, any B cell is capable of producing an antibody molecule to match virtually any foreign invader. It is the phenomenon of humoral immunity that makes immunization possible.

Because of their crucial role in all aspects of immunity, both cell-mediated and humoral, white blood cells are considered the body's first line of defense. White blood cells are larger than red blood cells. In addition, they can move independently in the bloodstream and are able to pass through the cell walls. This enables them to travel quickly to the site of an injury or infection. There are different categories of white blood cells, each of which performs a specific function. These include:

- *Granulocytes.* There are three types of granulocytes:
  1. *Neutrophils,* the most abundant type of white blood cell, whose function is to ingest and destroy microorganisms such as bacteria.
  2. *Eosinophils,* which ingest and destroy antigen-antibody combinations (formed when antibodies intercept antigens) and also moderate hypersensitive (allergic) reactions by secreting an enzyme that breaks down histamine. High levels of eosinophils in the blood are often present in individuals with allergic disorders, presumably because the body is attempting to tame the allergic reaction.
  3. *Basophils,* which secrete compounds such as heparin or histamine in response to contact with antigens.
- *Lymphocytes.* The lymphocytes are responsible for the development of specific immunities. Three important types of lymphocytes are T cells, B cells and NK cells:

1. *T cells* undergo maturation in the thymus gland and play a major role in cell-mediated immunity.

2. *B cells* mature in the bone marrow and are responsible for the production of antibodies.

3. *NK (natural killer) cells* destroy body cells that have become infected or become cancerous.

• *Monocytes.* The largest cells in the blood, monocytes act as the "garbage collectors" of the body. They engulf and digest foreign particles as well as damaged or aging cells, including tumor cells. After spending about twenty-four hours circulating in the bloodstream, most monocytes enter the tissues and perform similar functions there. At this point, they are known as macrophages.

Another important component of immunity is the lymphatic system. This is a system of organs (including the spleen, the thymus, the tonsils, and the lymph nodes) and fluid, called lymph, that circulates through the lymphatic vessels in the body and also bathes the body's cells. The lymphatic system provides a kind of continuous cleansing that operates at the cellular level. It is through the lymphatic system that fluid from the spaces between cells is drained, taking with it waste products, toxins, and other debris from the tissues. The lymph flows through the lymph nodes, where the macrophages filter out the undesirables, and from it there returns to the venous circulation.

Marvelous as it is, the immune system can work as it should only if it is cared for properly. This means getting all the right nutrients and providing the right environment, plus avoiding those things that tend to depress immunity. Many elements of the environment we live in today compromise our immune systems' defensive abilities. The chemicals in the household cleaners we use; the overuse of antibiotics and other drugs; the antibiotics, pesticides, and myriad additives present in the foods we eat; and exposure to environmental pollutants all place a strain on the immune system. Another factor that adversely affects the immune system is stress. Stress results in a sequence of biochemical events that ultimately suppresses the normal activity of white blood cells and places undue demands on the endocrine system, as well as depleting the body of needed nutrients. The result is impaired healing ability and lowered defense against infection.

Proper immune function is an intricate balancing act. While inadequate immunity predisposes one to infectious illness of every type, it is also possible to become ill as a result of an immune response that is too strong or directed at an inappropriate target. Many different disorders, including allergies, lupus, pernicious anemia, rheumatic heart disease, rheumatoid arthritis, and, possibly, diabetes, have been linked to inappropriate immune system activity. Consequently, they are known as autoimmune, or "self-attacking-self," disorders.

While much is known about the functioning of the immune system, much more remains to be learned; only in the past ten to fifteen years have many facets of it begun to be studied and understood by physicians and researchers. The field of immunology (the study of the immune system) is one of the fastest growing fields in medicine today.

The program of supplements outlined here is designed to strengthen the immune system, whether it is damaged as a result of disease, stress, inadequate nutrition, poor living habits, chemotherapy, or a combination of one or more of these factors.

NUTRIENTS

SUPPLEMENT	SUGGESTED DOSAGE	COMMENTS
Acetyl-L-carnitine	As directed on label.	An energy carrier, metabolic facilitator, and cell membrane protectant. Protects the heart.
Acidophilus	As directed on label. Take on an empty stomach.	Restores important bacteria to the intestinal tract.
Aerobic 07 from Aerobic Life Industries or	9 drops twice daily, taken in water.	For tissue oxygenation. Kills harmful bacteria and viruses.
Dioxychlor from American Biologics	As directed on label.	
Béres Drops Plus from BDP America	As directed on label.	Contains minerals and trace elements that boost and nourish the immune system.
Body Language Super Antioxidant from Oxyfresh	As directed on label.	To protect the body from free radical damage, environmental stresses, and pollutants.
Bovine colostrum	As directed on label.	Contains immunoglobulins and antibody-stimulating factors. Enhances immunity.
Coenzyme Q10	100 mg daily.	Supports the immune system. An oxygen enhancer to protect the cells and heart function.
Essential fatty acids (Ultimate Oil from Nature's Secret is a good source)	As directed on label.	A most important element in the diet. Necessary for a healthy immune system.
Free-form amino acid complex	As directed on label, on an empty stomach.	Protein that is broken down into a form the body can use. Use a formula containing all the essential amino acids.
Garlic (Kyolic)	2 capsules 3 times daily.	Stimulates the immune system.
Glutathione	As directed on label.	Inhibits the formation of free radicals; aids in red blood cell integrity; protects immune cells.
Kelp	2,000–3,000 mg daily.	Supplies a balance of minerals needed for immune system integrity.
Kyo-Green from Wakunaga	As directed on label.	Supplies nutrients and chlorophyll needed for tissue repair, and cleanses the blood. Important in immune response.
L-Arginine and L-ornithine	As directed on label, on an empty stomach. Take with water or juice. Do not take with milk. Take with 50 mg vitamin B6 and 100 mg vitamin C for better absorption.	To enhance the immune system and retard the growth of tumors and cancer. Necessary for the immune system. *See* AMINO ACIDS in Part One.

L-Cysteine and L-methionine plus L-lysine	500 mg each twice daily, on an empty stomach.	To destroy free radicals and viruses and protect the glands, especially the liver. *See* AMINO ACIDS in Part One.
Lecithin granules or capsules	1 tbsp 3 times daily, with meals. 1,200 mg 3 times daily, with meals.	Aids in cellular protection.
Maitake or shiitake or reishi	As directed on label. As directed on label. As directed on label.	Mushrooms that build immunity and fight viral infections and cancer.
Manganese	2 mg daily.	Necessary for proper immune function. Works with the B vitamins to provide a general feeling of well-being.
Proteolytic enzymes or Infla-Zyme Forte from American Biologics or Wobenzym N from Marlyn Nutraceuticals	As directed on label. 4 tablets 3 times daily, with meals. 3–6 tablets 2–3 times daily, between meals.	To aid in proper breakdown of proteins, fats, and carbohydrates for better absorption of nutrients. Destroys free radicals and aids in proper breakdown and absorption of foods.
Pycnogenol and/or grape seed extract	As directed on label 3 times daily, with meals. As directed on label.	A unique bioflavonoid that is a potent antioxidant and immune enhancer. One of the most potent antioxidants; protects the cells.
Quercetin plus bromelain	As directed on label. As directed on label.	Helps to prevent reactions to certain foods, pollens, and other allergens. Increases immunity. Enhances effectiveness of quercetin.
Raw thymus glandular plus multiglandular complex with raw spleen glandular	As directed on label. As directed on label. As directed on label.	To enhance T cell production. Glandulars from lamb source are best.
Selenium	200 mcg daily.	Important free radical destroyer.
Squalene (shark liver oil)	As directed on label.	Aids in rebuilding and functioning of cells; has anticancer properties.
Superoxide dismutase (SOD) plus dimethylglycine (DMG) (Aangamik DMG from FoodScience Labs)	As directed on label. As directed on label.	To improve oxygenation of tissues.
Taurine Plus from American Biologics	As directed on label.	An antioxidant and immune regulator necessary for white blood cell activation and neurological function.
Vitamin A plus natural carotenoid complex (Betatene)	10,000 IU daily. As directed on label.	Needed for proper immune function. Powerful antioxidants, free radical scavengers, and immune enhancers. May protect against cancer and heart disease.

Vitamin B complex plus extra vitamin B6 (pyridoxine) and vitamin B12 plus raw liver extract	100 mg 3 times daily, with meals. 50 mg 3 times daily. 1,000–2,000 mcg daily. As directed on label.	Anti-stress vitamins, especially important for normal brain function. Consider injections (under a doctor's supervision). If injections are not available, use a sublingual form. Vitamins B6 and B12 potentiate amino acids and are necessary for best absorption of amino acids and for proper functioning of enzymes in the body. A good source of B vitamins and iron. Consider injections (under a doctor's supervision).
Vitamin C with bioflavonoids	5,000–20,000 mg daily, in divided doses. *See* ASCORBIC ACID FLUSH in Part Three.	An important antioxidant that decreases susceptibility to infection.
Vitamin E	400 IU daily.	An antioxidant that is an integral part of the body's defense system. Use emulsion form for easier assimilation.
Multivitamin and mineral complex	As directed on label.	All vitamins and minerals are necessary in balance. Use a high-potency formula.
Zinc plus copper	50–80 mg daily. Do not exceed this amount. 3 mg daily.	Very important for the immune system. Use zinc chelate form. Needed to balance with zinc.

HERBS

❑ Astragalus boosts the immune system and generates anticancer cells in the body. It is also a powerful antioxidant and protects the liver from toxins.

Caution: Do not take this herb in the presence of a fever.

❑ Bayberry, fenugreek, hawthorn, horehound, licorice root, and red clover all enhance the immune response.

Caution: If overused, licorice can elevate blood pressure. Do not use this herb on a daily basis for more than seven days in a row. Avoid if you have high blood pressure.

❑ Black radish, dandelion, and milk thistle help to cleanse the liver and the bloodstream. The liver is *the* organ of detoxification and must function optimally.

❑ Boxthorn seed, ginseng, suma, and wisteria contain germanium, a trace element that aids immune function and has anticancer properties.

Caution: Do not use ginseng if you have high blood pressure.

❑ Echinacea boosts the immune system and enhances lymphatic function.

❑ Ginkgo biloba is good for the brain cells, aids circulation, and is a powerful antioxidant.

❑ Goldenseal strengthens the immune system, cleanses the body, and has antibacterial properties.

Caution: Do not take goldenseal internally on a daily basis for more than one week at a time, do not use it during pregnancy, and use it with caution if you are allergic to ragweed.

❑ St. Johnswort is a natural blood purifier and fights viruses such as HIV and Epstein-Barr virus.

❑ Ligustrum (known in Chinese herbology as *nu zhen zi*) increases bone marrow production of lymphocytes as well as their maturation into T cells. It is beneficial for thymus and spleen health and inhibits tumor growth.

❑ Picrorrhiza, an Indian herb used in Ayurvedic medicine, is a powerful immunostimulant that boosts all aspects of immune function.

RECOMMENDATIONS

❑ Take an inventory of the factors that may be compromising your immune system and take steps to correct them. Two of the most common immune suppressors include stress and an incorrect diet, especially a diet high in fat and refined processed foods.

❑ Supply your immune system with adequate amounts of nutrients that promote proper immune function. Some of the most valuable include:

• Vitamin A is the anti-infection vitamin. If used properly and in moderate doses, vitamin A is rarely toxic and is very important in the body's defense system.

• Vitamin C may be the single most important vitamin for the immune system. It is essential for the formation of adrenal hormones and the production of lymphocytes. It also has a direct effect on bacteria and viruses. Vitamin C should be taken with bioflavonoids, natural plant substances that enhance absorption and reinforce the action of this vitamin.

• Vitamin E interacts with vitamins A and C and the mineral selenium, acting as a primary antioxidant and scavenger of toxic free radicals. Vitamin E activity is an integral part of the body's defense system.

• Zinc boosts the immune response and promotes the healing of wounds when used in appropriate doses (100 milligrams or less daily). It also helps to protect the liver. Doses over 100 milligrams per day may actually depress immune function, however.

❑ Begin a diet of fresh fruits and vegetables (preferably raw) plus nuts, seeds, grains, and other foods that are high in fiber.

❑ Include in the diet chlorella, garlic, and pearl barley. These foods contain germanium, a trace element beneficial for the immune system. Also add kelp to the diet, in the form of giant red kelp or brown kelp. Kelp contains iodine, calcium, iron, carotene, protein, riboflavin, and vitamin C, which are necessary for the immune system's functional integrity.

❑ Consume "green drinks" daily.

❑ Avoid animal products, processed foods, sugar, and soda.

❑ Follow a fasting program once a month to rid your body of toxins that can weaken the immune system. *See* FASTING in Part Three.

❑ Use spirulina, especially while fasting. Spirulina is a naturally digestible food that aids in protecting the immune system. It supplies many nutrients needed for cleansing and healing.

❑ Be sure to get sufficient sleep. As much as possible, avoid stress.

❑ Get regular moderate exercise (but don't overdo it). Exercise reduces stress and elevates mood, which has a positive effect on immune response. In addition, T lymphocyte production is stimulated by exercise.

❑ Avoid overeating.

❑ Do not smoke or consume beverages containing alcohol or caffeine.

❑ Do not take any drugs except for those prescribed by your physician.

CONSIDERATIONS

❑ Marijuana use weakens the immune system. Delta-9 tetrahydrocannabinol (THC), the most active compound in marijuana, alters the normal immune response, making the white blood cells 35 to 40 percent less effective than normal.

❑ Mercury amalgam dental fillings have been linked to a weakened immune system. Toxic metals suppress the immune system. A hair analysis can be used to check for heavy metal intoxication. (*See* MERCURY TOXICITY in Part Two and HAIR ANALYSIS in Part Three.)

❑ A person's mental state can suppress his or her immune system. A positive frame of mind is important in building up the immune system. (*See* ANXIETY DISORDER; DEPRESSION; and/or STRESS in Part Two.)

❑ An underactive thyroid results in immune deficiency. (*See* HYPOTHYROIDISM in Part Two.)

❑ Food allergies and adverse food reactions can place stress on the immune system. (*See* ALLERGIES in Part Two.)

❑ Research has shown that dehydroepiandrosterone (DHEA), a hormone, may enhance the functioning of the immune system. (*See* DHEA THERAPY in Part Three.)

❑ Human growth hormone (HGH) is another naturally occurring hormone that strengthens the immune system. Treatment with HGH requires the supervision of a physician. (*See* GROWTH HORMONE THERAPY in Part Three.)

❑ *See also* AIDS in Part Two.

Weight Problems

See ANOREXIA NERVOSA; APPETITE, POOR; BULIMIA; OBESITY; UNDERWEIGHT.

Wilson's Disease

Wilson's disease is a rare inherited disorder that affects approximately 1 in 30,000 persons worldwide. In persons with Wilson's disease, the body is unable to metabolize the trace element copper as it should, with the result that excess copper accumulates in the brain, kidneys, liver, and the corneas of the eyes. This causes organ damage and other complications, including neurological problems and psychotic behavior. Untreated, Wilson's disease leads to brain damage, cirrhosis of the liver, hepatitis, and, ultimately, death. Fortunately, early detection and treatment of the disease can minimize the symptoms and complications and possibly even prevent them altogether.

Symptoms of Wilson's disease may include bloody vomit; difficulty speaking, swallowing, and/or walking; drooling; an enlarged spleen; jaundice; loss of appetite; loss of coordination; progressive fatigue and/or weakness; progressive intellectual impairment; psychological deterioration manifested as personality changes and/or bizarre behavior; rigidity, spasms, or tremors of the muscles; swelling and/or fluid accumulation in the abdomen; and unexplained weight loss. Sometimes the first sign is the development of a pigmented ring, known as a Kayser-Fleischer ring, at the outer margin of the cornea, which may be detected during a routine eye examination. In the advanced stages of the disease, symptoms due to chronic active hepatitis or cirrhosis may appear, menstrual cycles may cease, and an individual may experience chest pains, heart palpitations, lightheadedness, pallor, and shortness of breath as a result of exertion.

Although persons with Wilson's disease are born with the disorder, symptoms are rarely seen before the age of six and most often do not appear until adolescence or even later. However, to prevent complications, treatment is required whether symptoms have appeared or not. Diagnosis is usually based on a study of individual and family medical history plus blood tests to determine levels of ceruloplasmin (a copper-carrying protein in the blood) and to check for anemia, plus a urine test to reveal elevated levels of copper in the urine. A liver biopsy to evaluate the amount of copper in liver tissue may be done to confirm the diagnosis.

NUTRIENTS

SUPPLEMENT	SUGGESTED DOSAGE	COMMENTS
Very Important		
Vitamin C	As directed on label.	Protects against inflammation, anemia, and hepatitis, and reduces copper levels in the body. Use an esterified form.
Iron	As directed by physician. Take with 100 mg vitamin C for better absorption.	To correct and protect against anemia. *Caution:* Do not take iron unless anemia is diagnosed.
Multivitamin and mineral complex with	As directed on label.	A balance of all nutrients is essential for healing.
potassium and	99 mg daily.	Necessary for proper muscle contraction.
selenium	200 mcg daily.	Needed for proper adrenal gland function.
Vitamin A plus	10,000 IU daily.	Powerful antioxidants that also enhance immunity.
beta-carotene	15,000 IU daily.	
Vitamin B complex plus extra	75 mg 3 times daily,	Protects the liver and is needed for proper brain function.
vitamin B6 (pyridoxine)	50 mg daily.	Helps to prevent damage to the nervous system and guard against anemia. Also combats fluid retention.
Vitamin E	600 IU daily. Take separately from iron.	Promotes normal healing and prevents cell damage.
Zinc	75 mg daily. Do not exceed this amount.	Decreases copper levels and enhances immunity. Zinc balances copper in the body.
Important		
Acetyl-L-Carnitine	As directed on label.	Protects liver and heart function.
Advanced Carotenoid Complex from Solgar	As directed on label.	Contains powerful free radical scavengers and immune enhancers.
Calcium and	1,500–2,000 mg daily.	Minerals that work together to prevent muscle spasms.
magnesium	750–1,000 mg daily.	
Coenzyme Q10	As directed on label.	A powerful antioxidant that also increases circulation and energy.
Flaxseed oil	As directed on label.	To supply essential fatty acids, which are vital for brain and nerve function and enhance immunity.
Free-form amino acid complex	As directed on label, on an empty stomach.	Necessary for protein synthesis. Use a formula containing all the essential amino acids.
Gamma-aminobutyric acid (GABA)	As directed on label, on an empty stomach.	Essential for proper brain function. Also has a tranquilizing effect. *See* AMINO ACIDS in Part One.
L-Arginine and L-ornithine	As directed on label, on an empty stomach. Take at bedtime with water or juice. Do not take with milk. Take with 50 mg vitamin B6 and 100 mg vitamin C for better absorption.	To aid in liver and kidney detoxification. *See* AMINO ACIDS in Part One.
plus L-cysteine	As directed on label, on an empty stomach.	Reduces the body's absorption of copper.
Milk thistle		*See under* Herbs, below.
Pycnogenol and/or grape seed extract	As directed on label.	Powerful antioxidants that lessen mental deterioration.

HERBS

☐ Burdock, dandelion, milk thistle, and suma cleanse and support the liver and help to fight fatigue.

❑ Alfalfa, ginkgo biloba, gotu kola, kava, lobelia, parsley, oat straw, periwinkle, and skullcap are good for overall good health and the functioning of the brain and nervous system.

Caution: Do not take lobelia internally on an ongoing basis.

❑ Astragalus, echinacea, and pau d'arco are helpful for fatigue.

Caution: Do not use astragalus in the presence of a fever.

❑ Black radish and red clover strengthen the liver.

❑ Cat's claw is an anti-inflammatory, antioxidant, immune system enhancer, and internal cleanser. Cat's Claw Defense Complex from Source Naturals is a good source of this herb and also contains other beneficial ingredients.

Caution: Do not use cat's claw during pregnancy.

❑ Cayenne (capsicum) eases blood pressure, fights fatigue, and helps support the nervous system.

❑ Goldenseal is helpful if symptoms include difficulty swallowing, and it can ease fatigue as well. Licorice is also beneficial for swallowing difficulties, as is gargling with thyme tea.

Caution: Do not take goldenseal internally on a daily basis for more than one week at a time, do not use it during pregnancy, and use it with caution if you are allergic to ragweed. Do not use licorice on a daily basis for more than seven days in a row, and avoid if you have high blood pressure.

❑ St. Johnswort is beneficial for the nervous system and also helps to overcome fatigue and difficulty swallowing.

❑ Siberian ginseng is a tonic herb that helps reduce fatigue and supports brain and nervous system function.

Caution: Do not use this herb if you have hypoglycemia, high blood pressure, or a heart disorder.

❑ Valerian root is calming, and is good for the brain and nervous system. It can also be beneficial for swallowing difficulties.

RECOMMENDATIONS

❑ Increase your consumption of onions and garlic. These foods contain sulfur, which helps to rid the body of copper.

❑ Eat fresh (not canned) pineapple frequently. It contains bromelain, an enzyme that helps to keep down swelling and inflammation.

❑ Have the copper level of your drinking water tested. Look in the yellow pages of your local telephone directory or consult your state's environmental agency for laboratories that can do this type of testing. If your tap water contains more than 1 part per million of copper, drink quality bottled water instead (steam-distilled is best) or check the pipes in your home; if you can determine that all or most of the copper in your water is coming from the pipes, it may be worthwhile to replace them with copper-free ones.

❑ If you take a multivitamin and/or mineral supplement, be sure to choose a formula that does *not* contain copper.

❑ Eliminate from the diet foods high in copper. These include broccoli, chocolate, enriched cereals, molasses, mushrooms, nuts, organ meats, and shellfish, as well as avocados, beans and other legumes, egg yolks, oats, raisins, soybeans, and whole grains.

❑ Do not use copper cooking vessels or other utensils.

CONSIDERATIONS

❑ Wilson's disease can be neither prevented nor cured. With appropriate management, however, the prognosis is excellent.

❑ Anyone with a family history of Wilson's disease should undergo diagnostic testing—the sooner the better, and whether or not symptoms are present—so that treatment, if necessary, may begin as soon as possible.

❑ Treatment of Wilson's disease is a lifelong proposition. Most often, it involves taking penicillamine (Cuprimine, Depen), a drug that removes copper from the body by increasing its excretion in the urine. Possible side effects of this drug include deficiencies of vitamin B_6 (pyridoxine) and iron. A person with a sensitivity to penicillamine may be given a steroid such as prednisone (Deltasone and others) in addition, or the drug trientine (Syprine) may be prescribed instead. This medication also chelates copper so that it can be eliminated from the body.

❑ Some doctors prescribe high doses of zinc in place of, or in conjunction with, conventional drugs to keep copper levels under control. Zinc naturally balances with copper in the body.

❑ Regardless of the treatment regimen, regular checkups are required to monitor possible side effects from medication and to check the level of copper in the urine.

❑ Elevated copper levels in the body result in the depletion of vitamin C and zinc. Persons with Wilson's disease therefore always require a higher that normal intake of these nutrients.

❑ Wilson's disease is not the only cause of elevated levels of copper in the body. Toxic levels of copper can also accumulate in the body as a result of excessive exposure to the metal. If a person with elevated copper levels has normal liver function and no corneal abnormalities, it is likely that the toxicity is due to something other than Wilson's disease. In addition, copper toxicity as a result of excessive copper ingestion can be demonstrated by hair analysis, whereas persons with Wilson's disease do not exhibit elevated levels of copper in the hair.

❑ *See also* COPPER TOXICITY in Part Two.

Wilson's Syndrome

See under HYPOTHYROIDISM.

Worms

Worms are parasites that live in the gastrointestinal tract. The most common types of worms are roundworms (including hookworms, pinworms, and threadworms) and tapeworms. Roundworms are contagious intestinal parasites that are shaped like earthworms but smaller in size. They can easily be seen with the naked eye. Pinworms are white, threadlike worms about a third of an inch long. Tapeworms vary in length from an inch up to thirty feet and can survive for up to twenty-five years in the body. In the United States, pinworm infestation in young children is by far the most prevalent parasitic worm problem.

Depending on the type of worm involved and the severity of the infestation, the individual may experience abdominal pain, loss of appetite and weight, diarrhea, anemia, colon disorders, and/or rectal itching. The latter is especially likely to happen at night, when the worms tend to migrate outside of the anus in the warmth of the bed. Worm larvae may or may not be noticeable in the stool. In some cases, there may be no perceptible symptoms at all.

Worm infestation results in poor absorption of essential nutrients, and in some cases loss of blood, from the gastrointestinal tract. It can therefore lead to such deficiency-related disorders as anemia and growth problems. Malabsorption resulting from parasitic infection makes one susceptible to many diseases because it results in diminished immune function.

Worms can be contracted through a variety of mechanisms, including improper disposal of human or animal waste, walking barefoot on contaminated soil, and ingestion of eggs or larvae from uncooked or partially cooked meat. In some cases, eggs may become airborne and be inhaled.

Parasites are more common than most people suppose, and they can be behind many ills, including colon disorders. They are more common in children than in adults. They are also common in people with AIDS, chronic fatigue syndrome, candidiasis, and many other disorders. Unfortunately, physicians often do not check for worm infestation.

NUTRIENTS

SUPPLEMENT	SUGGESTED DOSAGE	COMMENTS
Important		
Acidophilus	As directed on label.	Restores normal intestinal flora.
Essential fatty acids (Ultimate Oil from Nature's Secret is a good source)	As directed on label.	Helps to protect the gastrointestinal tract.
Garlic (Kyolic)	2 capsules 3 times daily, with meals. A fresh clove of garlic can also be put in the shoes to be absorbed through the skin.	Has antiparasitic properties.
Black walnut		*See under* Herbs, below.
Multivitamin and mineral complex	As directed on label.	To promote overall health and proper nutrition. All nutrients are needed by persons with these disorders.
Pumpkin		*See under* Herbs, below.
Vitamin B complex plus extra vitamin B$_{12}$	50 mg 3 times daily, with meals. 1,000–2,000 mcg twice daily.	To prevent anemia associated with parasitic infestation. Use sublingual forms to assure absorption.
Vitamin C	3,000 mg daily.	Protects against infection and enhances immune function.
Zinc	50 mg daily. Do not exceed a total of 100 mg daily from all supplements	Promotes a healthy immune system and proper wound healing.

HERBS

❑ Aloe vera juice, taken twice daily as directed on the product label, has an alkalinizing and anti-inflammatory effect.

❑ Black walnut extract destroys many types of worms. Take black walnut extract on an empty stomach three times per day.

❑ Butternut bark, fennel seed, flaxseed, licorice root, and senna leaf are good for bowel and colon cleansing.

Caution: If overused, licorice can elevate blood pressure. Do not use this herb on a daily basis for more than seven days in a row. Avoid if you have high blood pressure.

❑ Calendula ointment or witch hazel can be used to help relieve anal itching and irritation.

❑ Cascara sagrada, ficus, gentian root, mugwort, rhubarb root, slippery elm, thyme, and wormwood are effective against many types of worms.

Caution: Do not use wormwood during pregnancy. It is not recommended for long-term use. It can be habit-forming.

❑ Cayenne (capsicum), garlic, and turmeric help to strengthen the immune system.

❑ Grapefruit seed extract is very effective for destroying parasites. It can be taken internally and is also good for washing vegetables before eating (mix 10 drops of extract in 2 quarts of water) to remove any bacteria or parasites.

❑ Pinkroot works well against roundworms.

❑ Pumpkin extract contains zinc and aids in expelling worms.

RECOMMENDATIONS

❑ Eat a high-fiber diet consisting primarily of raw vegetables and whole grains.

❑ Eat pumpkin seeds, sesame seeds, and figs (or fig juice) on an empty stomach three times per day. This can be combined with the black walnut extract mentioned under Herbs, above.

530

❑ Drink only filtered or bottled steam-distilled water.

❑ Monitor your intake and output of fluids, and replace fluids as needed.

❑ Eliminate *all* sugar, refined carbohydrates, fruits (except figs and pineapples), and pork and pork products from the diet until the worms have been completely eradicated. Worms thrive on sugar.

❑ For tapeworms, fast for three days on raw pineapple. *See* FASTING in Part Three. The bromelain in pineapple destroys tapeworms.

❑ For pinworms, eat bitter melon, a cucumber-shaped vegetable found in Asian markets. This is effective against pinworms and is a good immune system strengthener. Eat one or two melons a day for seven to ten days. Do this again after two months to ensure that the infestation has not returned.

❑ *Never* eat meat, fish, or poultry that is not fully cooked or that has been left out at room temperature for too long (*see* FOOD POISONING in Part Two).

❑ Maintain meticulous personal hygiene. Avoid scratching the anal area, and wash your hands frequently, scrubbing well under the fingernails. If children are affected, teach them proper hygiene as well.

❑ Wash underwear, bed linens, and towels after each use in very hot water with chlorine bleach added, if possible. Change linens and towels daily.

❑ For a severe infestation, use high colonics (also known as colonic irrigation). This procedure is usually performed in a professional office. If this treatment is not available, follow the procedure for colon cleansing described in this book. *See* COLON CLEANSING and ENEMAS, both in Part Three. A product called 10-Day Colon Cleanse from Aerobic Life Industries is also recommended.

CONSIDERATIONS

❑ Worm infestations can be persistent and stubborn. It may be necessary to treat all members of the household to finally eradicate the parasites. All family members should be examined for possible infection. In addition, it is a good idea to compile a list of people who have been in close contact with the affected individual and advise them to seek the evaluation and advice of a health care provider.

❑ Doctors treat most types of worms with prescription medications such as mebendazole (Vermox) or thiabendazole (Mintezol), or with pyrantel pamoate (Antiminth), which is available over the counter. Creams or ointments may be prescribed to relieve anal itching and irritation.

❑ Some sushi has been found to be contaminated with a wormlike parasite called anisakis, which can cause illness similar to Crohn's disease if ingested. This parasite is a tightly coiled, clear worm, about one-half to three-quarters inch in length. It commonly embeds itself in herring and other fish. Fortunately, an experienced sushi chef can spot this parasite easily, so its presence in sushi is relatively rare.

❑ The risk of parasitic infection is increased by travel to places with inadequate public sanitation, personal hygiene levels, and/or food handling practices.

❑ Because of the generalized nutritional deficiency associated with this disorder, good nutrition is vital. Foods high in protein and iron are particularly important.

Wrinkling of Skin

Wrinkles form when the skin loses its elasticity. As long as the skin is supple, any creasing of the skin disappears as soon as you stop making the expression that caused it. But skin that has lost its suppleness retains the lines formed by smiling or frowning, for instance, even after you have assumed a more neutral expression. Over time, these lines deepen into wrinkles.

Some amount of wrinkling is a result of aging and is probably inevitable; no matter what you do, you will develop some lines if you simply live long enough. The first signs of wrinkles usually appear in the delicate tissue around the eyes—smile lines or "crow's feet." The cheeks and lips show damage next. As we age, our skin becomes both thinner and dryer, both of which contribute to the formation of wrinkles. But other factors help to determine both the rate and the extent of wrinkling, including diet and nutrition, muscle tone, habitual facial expressions, stress, proper skin care (or lack thereof), exposure to environmental pollutants, and lifestyle habits such as smoking. Heredity probably also plays a role.

The most important factor of all is sun exposure, which not only dries out the skin but also leads to the generation of free radicals that can damage skin cells. The sun is your skin's worst enemy. It is estimated that 90 percent of what we think of as signs of age are actually signs of overexposure. Furthermore, overexposure does not necessarily mean sunbathing or sunburn; approximately 70 percent of sun damage is incurred during such everyday activities as driving and walking to and from your car. The ultraviolet-A (UVA) rays that do this damage are present all day long and in all seasons. Worse, the effects of the sun are cumulative, although they may not be obvious for many years.

NUTRIENTS

SUPPLEMENT	SUGGESTED DOSAGE	COMMENTS
Very Important		
Primrose oil or black currant seed oil	1,000 mg 3 times daily. As directed on label.	Good healers for dermatitis, acne, and most other skin disorders. These oils contain linoleic acid, which is needed by the skin.

Vitamin A	25,000 IU daily for 3 months, then reduce to 15,000 IU daily. If you are pregnant, do not exceed 10,000 IU daily.	Necessary for healing and construction of new skin tissue.
plus natural carotenoid complex (Betatene)	As directed on label.	Antioxidants and vitamin A precursors.
Vitamin B complex plus extra vitamin B$_{12}$	As directed on label. 300–1,000 mcg daily.	Anti-stress and anti-aging vitamins. Sublingual forms are best.

Important		
Kelp	1,000–1,500 mg daily.	Supplies balanced minerals needed for good skin tone.
Selenium	200 mcg daily.	An antioxidant that works synergistically with vitamin E.
Silica	As directed on label.	Important for skin strength and elasticity. Stimulates collagen formation.
Vitamin C with bioflavonoids	3,000–5,000 mg daily, in divided doses.	Necessary for the formation of collagen, a protein that gives the skin its flexibility. Also fights free radicals and strengthens the capillaries that feed the skin.
Vitamin E	Start with 400 IU daily and increase slowly to 800 IU daily.	Protects against free radicals that can damage the skin and contribute to aging.
Zinc plus copper	50 mg daily. Do not exceed a total of 100 mg daily from all supplements. 3 mg daily.	For tissue strength and repair. Use zinc gluconate lozenges or OptiZinc for best absorption. Needed for collagen production and healthy skin. Also needed to balance with zinc.

Helpful		
Ageless Beauty from Biotec Foods	As directed on label.	Protects the skin from free radical damage.
Aloe vera		See under Herbs, below.
Calcium and magnesium	1,500 mg daily. 750 mg daily.	Deficiency contributes to fragility of the skin. Needed to balance with calcium.
Collagen cream	Apply topically as directed on label.	Good for very dry skin. A nourishing cream.
Elastin cream	Apply topically as directed on label.	Helps smooth existing wrinkles. Prevents formation of new ones.
Flaxseed oil capsules or liquid or Ultimate Oil from Nature's Secret	1,000 mg daily. 1 tsp daily. As directed on label.	To supply needed essential fatty acids.
GH3 cream from Gero Vita	Apply topically as directed on label.	Excellent for the prevention of wrinkles. Also good for any discoloration of the skin.
Glucosamine sulfate or N-Acetylglucosamine (N-A-G from Source Naturals)	As directed on label. As directed on label.	Important for the formation of healthy skin and connective tissue.
Herpanacine from Diamond-Herpanacine Associates	As directed on label.	Contains antioxidants, amino acids, and herbs that promote skin health.
Pycnogenol	As directed on label.	A free radical scavenger that also strengthens collagen.

Superoxide dismutase (SOD)	As directed on label.	A free radical destroyer. Also good for brown age spots.
Tretinoin (Retin-A)	As prescribed by physician.	Removes fine lines and smooths out wrinkles; also excellent for age spots, precancerous lesions, and sun-damaged skin. Available by prescription only. Takes around 6 months to show results.
Vitamin D	400 IU daily.	Deficiency can contribute to aging of the skin.

HERBS

☐ Alfalfa, burdock root, chamomile, horsetail, oat straw, and thyme are all good for general nourishment of the hair, skin, and nails.

☐ Aloe vera has soothing, healing, and moisturizing properties. Apply pure aloe vera gel to dry skin as directed on the product label.

☐ Other herbs that are beneficial for skin tone include borage seed, flaxseed, ginger root, lemongrass, parsley, and pumpkin seed.

RECOMMENDATIONS

☐ Eat a well-balanced diet that includes many and varied fruits and vegetables, preferably raw, to provide your skin with the nutrients it needs. Also eat whole grains, seeds, nuts, and legumes.

☐ Drink at least 2 quarts of water every day, even if you do not feel thirsty. This helps to keep the skin hydrated and to flush away toxins, discouraging the formation of wrinkles.

☐ Obtain fatty acids from cold-pressed vegetable oils. Avoid saturated and animal fats.

☐ Do not smoke, and avoid alcohol and caffeine. All of these substances dry out the skin, making it more vulnerable to wrinkling. In addition, the smoking habit means pursing one's lips hundreds of times each day. The creases that form when you inhale from a cigarette often develop into wrinkles at a comparatively early age.

☐ No matter what your age or skin type, protect yourself from the sun. Always apply a sunscreen with a sun protection factor (SPF) of at least 15 to all exposed areas of skin, especially your face, regardless of the season or the weather. Sun exposure is the single greatest source of skin damage.

☐ Get regular exercise. Like other organs of the body, skin gets its nourishment from the bloodstream. Exercise increases the circulation of blood to the skin.

☐ Exercise your face. Sit in a chair and extend your jaw in an exaggerated chewing motion. Stretch the muscles under your chin and the front of your neck. Lying on a slant board for fifteen minutes a day is also good.

☐ Avoid alcohol-based toning products. Use witch hazel or an herbal/floral water instead.

❑ Pay attention to your facial expressions. If you find yourself squinting, raising your eyebrows, or making some other potentially wrinkle-inducing expression over and over again, you can make a conscious effort to stop.

❑ Practice good skin care and keep your skin well lubricated, especially if it is dry. *See* DRY SKIN in Part Two.

❑ Avoid using harsh soaps or solid cleansing creams such as cold cream on your face. Use natural oils such as avocado oil instead to remove dirt and old makeup. Apply it gently to your face and rinse it off with warm water. E•Gem Skin Care Soap from Carlson Laboratories is also good. Use a facial sponge or loofah several times a week to remove dead, dry skin cells and stimulate circulation.

❑ After cleansing your skin, apply a moisturizing lotion, preferably while the skin is still damp. Vitamin A Moisturizing Gel from Derma-E Products is a good nongreasy moisturizer that is quickly absorbed and diminishes the appearance of fine lines. It is available in health food stores.

❑ Open a capsule of ACES + Zinc from Carlson Labs and add the contents to your moisturizing cream before applying. This will help protect the skin from free radical damage. Do the same with your sunscreen.

❑ Do not apply heavy oils around the eye area before going to bed. This may cause eyes to be puffy in the morning.

❑ Limit your use of cosmetics, and choose the ones you do use carefully. Do not share your cosmetics, and replace them every three months.

CONSIDERATIONS

❑ Selecting good skin care products can be confusing. We recommend that you seek out products containing natural ingredients, and avoid those that contain petrolatum, mineral oil, or any hydrogenated oils. Some good ingredients to look for in skin care products include the following:

• *Allantoin,* a soothing agent derived from comfrey.

• *Alpha-hydroxy acids,* natural fruit acids that encourage the shedding of dead surface skin cells and the formation of fresh, new skin cells.

• *Aloe vera,* which is rich in nutrients and softens the skin.

• *Arnica,* an herb with astringent and skin-soothing properties.

• *Burdock,* an herb that helps the body eliminate poisons from the skin.

• *Calendula,* an herb that promotes skin cell formation and stimulates tissue growth, and also soothes and softens sensitive skin.

• *Chamomile,* an anti-inflammatory, antibacterial herb that is good for sensitive skin.

• *Collagen,* a protein found in healthy young skin tissue.

• *Comfrey,* an herb that aids healing and soothes chapped, irritated, or blemished skin.

• *Cucumber,* which contains amino and organic acids that cool and refresh the skin and tighten the pores.

• *Essential fatty acids* (including linoleic, linolenic, and arachadonic acids), which smooth rough skin, protect against moisture loss, and prevent invasion by free radicals.

• *Ginkgo biloba,* an antioxidant that helps skin stay younger looking.

• *Glycerine,* a soap byproduct that attracts and holds moisture in the skin.

• *Ivy,* an herb that stimulates circulation and aids other ingredients in penetrating the skin.

• *Liposomes,* microscopic bubbles that deliver active ingredients deep into the skin.

• *Panthenol (provitamin B5),* a nutrient that builds moisture and soothes irritation.

• *Retinoic acid,* a form of vitamin A that smooths skin, promotes cell renewal, and improves circulation to the skin.

• *Sage,* an herb with astringent properties that can help relieve dry, itchy skin.

• *Witch hazel,* a natural astringent that tones the skin.

• *Yarrow,* an astringent herb that acts as an anti-inflammatory and tightens and firms saggy skin.

❑ There are many excellent home facial treatments that can help with specific skin problems. Some of the best include:

• *To add color to sallow skin,* mash ½ cup or so of strawberries in a blender and apply them to your face. Leave them on for ten minutes, then rinse with tepid water.

• *To alleviate puffiness in the eye area,* place cool cucumber slices over your eyes for ten minutes or more, as needed.

• *To cleanse the pores,* rub mashed tomato over your face.

• *To help protect your skin from free radical damage,* add a few drops of green tea extract to your lotions, astringents, and other beauty products.

• *To moisturize your skin,* mash together grapes (a natural source of collagen and alpha-hydroxy acids) with enough honey to make a paste, and apply the mixture to your face as a mask. Leave it in place for twenty to thirty minutes while you relax, then rinse it off.

• *To remove dead surface skin cells and improve skin texture,* gently rub a small handful dry short-grain rice against your face for a few minutes. This technique has been used by Japanese women for centuries.

• *To soften and nourish the skin,* mash half of an avocado and apply it to your face. Leave it on until it dries, then rinse off with warm water. Avocado contains essential fatty acids and other nutrients that help prevent premature wrinkling.

• *To tighten and refine pores,* whip up the white of an egg with a pinch of alum and apply it to your face as a mask. After fifteen to twenty minutes, rinse it off with lukewarm water.

Xerophthalmia

See under EYE PROBLEMS.

Yeast Infection (Yeast Vaginitis)

When a fungus such as *Candida albicans* overgrows and infects the vagina, the result is a type of vaginitis commonly called a yeast infection. Because candida is part of the body's normal flora, almost every woman has a yeast infection at some time in her life. The most common yeast infection symptoms include local irritation, a large amount of white, cheesy discharge, and intense itching and burning. The skin around the vagina may be sore and appear red.

Yeast infections are common during pregnancy, when the acidity and sugar content of vaginal secretions are altered. Oral contraceptives, which have a similar effect on the body, also can lead to the development of yeast infections. Intrauterine devices (IUDs) can create a more favorable environment for fungal growth by decreasing normal vaginal secretions. Because fungi such as *C. albicans* thrive in the presence of sugar, women with diabetes are more susceptible to yeast infections. The use of antibiotics often leads to yeast infections because antibiotics not only kill infectious bacteria, but also destroy the "good" bacteria in the body that normally keep the growth of organisms such as candida in check. Yeast infections can also be sexually transmitted. This may be why some women suffer from chronic and/or recurrent yeast infections. Some women are especially vulnerable to yeast infections following their menstrual periods, due to changes in the vaginal environment from menstrual flow and cyclical hormonal changes. Other factors that can contribute to vaginal yeast infections include allergies, nutritional deficiencies, improper hygiene, and the consumption of refined carbohydrates.

NUTRIENTS

SUPPLEMENT	SUGGESTED DOSAGE	COMMENTS
Essential		
Biotin	300 mcg 3 times daily.	Inhibits yeast.
Bovine colostrum	As directed on label.	Boosts immunity and normalizes intestinal flora.
Essential fatty acids (Ultimate Oil from Nature's Secret is a good source)	As directed on label.	Enhances immunity, speeds recovery, and reduces pain.
Garlic (Kyolic)	2 capsules 3 times daily, with meals.	Fights the infecting organism.
Vitamin C	2,000–5,000 mg daily.	Improves immunity.

Yeast•Gard from Lake Consumer Products	As directed on label.	Destroys yeast and soothes irritated tissue.
Very Important		
Multivitamin and mineral complex	As directed on label.	To maintain a balance of all necessary nutrients in the body.
Vitamin A plus natural carotenoid complex (Betatene) plus vitamin E or	50,000 IU daily. If you are pregnant, do not exceed 10,000 IU daily. As directed on label. 400 IU daily.	Powerful free radical scavengers that aid vaginal healing.
AE Mulsion Forte from American Biologics	As directed on label.	Supplies vitamins A and E in emulsion form for easier assimilation.
Zinc	30 mg daily. Do not exceed a total of 100 mg daily from all supplements.	Enhances immunity and promotes healing. Use zinc gluconate lozenges or OptiZinc for best absorption.
Helpful		
Acidophilus	As directed on label. Take on an empty stomach.	Restores normal vaginal bacterial balance. Use a nondairy formula if you are allergic to milk.
Dioxychlor from American Biologics	5 drops in water twice daily.	Helps to prevent yeast infections. Use this product if the infections are recurrent.
Free-form amino acid complex	As directed on label.	Needed for repair of tissue. Use a formula containing all the essential amino acids.
Vitamin B complex plus extra vitamin B6 (pyridoxine)	100 mg daily. 50 mg 3 times daily.	Yeast infection can lead to vitamin B deficiency. Use a yeast-free formula. A sublingual form is best. Aids in antibody production and promotes immune function.
Vitamin D plus calcium and magnesium	400 IU daily. 1,500 mg daily. 750 mg daily.	Women need extra amounts of these nutrients when the body is fighting infection.

HERBS

❑ Aloe vera is helpful for infections and is known for its healing effects. Aloe vera gel can be applied topically to relieve itching. Aloe vera juice can be taken internally or used as a douche.

❑ Barberry has remarkable infection-fighting properties.

❑ Calendula, goldenseal, marshmallow root, usnea, and yarrow can all be used in douche form to fight a yeast infection. Make a strong tea using one or more of these herbs and douche with it twice daily for one week.

❑ Tea tree oil is effective against fungal infections and herpes, and has a healing effect. It is especially beneficial when used as a douche. Tea tree oil suppositories, used with alternating hot and cold sitz baths, are also effective. *See* SITZ BATH in Part Three.

❑ Chamomile destroys fungi.

❑ Cinnamon and dandelion inhibit the growth of the fungus *Candida albicans.*

Caution: Do not use cinnamon in large quantities during pregnancy.

❑ Echinacea has antifungal properties and enhances the functioning of the immune system. It can be taken internally or used as a douche.

❑ Pau d'arco contains a natural antibacterial agent and has a healing effect. It can be taken in capsule form or made into a tea and used as a douche.

RECOMMENDATIONS

❑ Include low-fat yogurt and soured products such as kefir and buttermilk in your diet. Yogurt and soured products contain microorganisms called *lactobacilli,* which are normally present in the bowel and vagina, and which actually destroy the fungus. To be effective, yogurt must contain active live cultures. Homemade yogurt is best. Yogurt makers are relatively inexpensive and are easy to use.

❑ Do not eat sugar, fruit, refined carbohydrates, or sweets of any kind until the infection has healed. Fungus multiplies in a sugary environment. Also avoid alcohol, aged cheeses, fermented foods, mushrooms, and yeast and yeast products.

❑ Avoid all dairy products except for low-fat yogurt and other soured products.

❑ Maintain the health of your immune system. Get proper rest, eat a healthy diet, and get regular moderate exercise. Avoid stress and antibiotics.

❑ Try douching with 2 capsules of garlic or with fresh garlic juice in a quart of warm water. Alternate this treatment with acidophilus douches. Open 2 acidophilus capsules and add them either to 1 quart of warm water or to plain yogurt. The garlic fights infection, while the acidophilus helps to restore normal flora and acid balance.

❑ Try using garlic suppositories. Peel a clove of garlic and wrap it in a piece of sterile gauze. Lubricate the suppository with pure organic vegetable oil and insert it in the vagina, making sure to leave a "tail" of gauze protruding externally. Maintain this treatment for three days, changing suppositories every twelve hours.

❑ Keep the vaginal area clean and dry. After bathing, hold a blow dryer (set on cool) 6 to 8 inches from the vaginal area until thoroughly dried. Wear loose-fitting cotton clothing and white cotton underwear to allow for free circulation of air.

❑ To replace "friendly" bacteria and reestablish normal intestinal flora, use a *L. bifidus* retention enema. *See* ENEMAS in Part Three.

❑ Launder clothing in unscented detergent, and avoid fabric softeners. Cotton underwear can be microwaved to destroy yeast. Wet the garment, wring it out well, and microwave it on high for 30 seconds.

❑ Avoid contact with any potentially irritating chemicals. This means avoiding colored and/or scented toilet paper, perfumes, deodorants, dyed underwear, "feminine hygiene sprays," and commercial sexual lubricants.

CONSIDERATIONS

❑ Many health care providers recommend clotrimazole (Gyne-Lotrimin, Mycelex, and others) or miconazole (Monistat and others) for yeast infections. Long available only by prescription, these medications are now available over the counter in drugstores as vaginal suppositories and creams. Like any topical medication, these can cause irritation and/or allergic reactions in susceptible individuals.

❑ Some physicians prescribe a more powerful antifungal, ketoconazole (Nizoral), particularly for stubborn infections. This drug is taken orally. Oral ketoconazole has been associated with some cases of liver toxicity, and its use must be carefully monitored by a physician.

❑ A newer treatment for yeast infections is terconazole (Terazol), which is specific for candida infection. It appears to be highly effective and cause few side effects.

❑ Routine douching is not necessary for personal hygiene. Douching is best reserved for therapeutic purposes, as excessive douching may actually help promote infection. If you do use douches from time to time, it is better to use a solution of 2 tablespoons of apple cider vinegar in a quart of water rather than commercial preparations.

❑ A study done at Cornell University showed that boric acid powder capsules were effective 98 percent of the time against yeast infections.

Note: Boric acid capsules should *not* be confused with boric acid crystals.

❑ Women who have chronic and/or unusually persistent vaginal candidiasis should be checked for diabetes and for immune system dysfunction, such as that caused by cancer or HIV infection.

❑ *See also* CANDIDIASIS; FUNGAL INFECTION; and VAGINITIS, all in Part Two.

PART THREE

REMEDIES AND THERAPIES

INTRODUCTION

In Part Two, various treatment programs were recommended for each of the health problems discussed. Part Three explains how to implement these remedies and therapies. It describes when each treatment can be beneficial, and, when appropriate, offers instructions for effective use. You can choose from among the more traditional remedies, such as juicing, fasting, and poultices, or from more conventional treatments, such as hyperbaric oxygen therapy. These remedies can be used in conjunction with a healthy diet and supplementation program. After learning about the available treatments, you will be able to choose the options that are most suitable for you.

Acupressure

See under PAIN CONTROL.

Acupuncture

See under PAIN CONTROL.

Ascorbic Acid Flush

Because vitamin C (ascorbic acid) promotes the healing of wounds and protects the body from bacterial infection, allergens, and other pollutants, it is often beneficial to flush the body with ascorbic acid. This therapy can help treat chemical allergies and chemical poisoning, arsenic and radiation poisoning, influenza, and sprains, and it can help prevent other illnesses, including cancer and AIDS.

PROCEDURE FOR ADULTS

Place 1,000 milligrams of ascorbic acid in a cup of water or juice. To make this drink, use ascorbic acid in the form of either esterified vitamin C, such as Ester-C, or a buffered product, such as calcium ascorbate. Take every half hour, keeping track of how much has been taken, until diarrhea results. Count the number of teaspoons needed to produce diarrhea. Subtract 1 from this amount, and take the resulting ascorbic acid drink every four hours for one to two days. During therapy, make sure the stool retains a tapioca-like consistency. If it again becomes watery, decrease dosage as necessary. Repeat therapy once a month.

PROCEDURE FOR INFANTS AND CHILDREN

Place 250 milligrams of ascorbic acid in a cup of water or juice, using an esterified vitamin C product, such as Ester-C, or a buffered product, such as calcium ascorbate. Give to the child every hour until a stool of tapioca-like consistency is produced. If the child or infant does not produce this stool within 24 hours, increase dose to 500 milligrams every hour, and keep the child on this schedule for one or two days. *Do not exceed 500 milligrams per hour.* Children should be given treatment only under medical supervision.

NUTRIENTS

SUPPLEMENT	SUGGESTED DOSAGE	COMMENTS
Very Important		
Multivitamin and mineral complex	As directed on label.	To replace any lost vitamins and minerals during therapy.

Biofeedback

See under PAIN CONTROL.

Blood Purification

Blood is composed of four components: plasma, the watery, colorless liquid in which the other components float; red blood cells; white blood cells; and platelets. Through these components, the blood performs several life-sustaining functions. The red blood cells transport oxygen to the cells. The platelets are needed for the blood-clotting process. The white blood cells destroy bacteria and other disease-producing organisms. In addition, blood transports nutrients to the cells and carries away wastes; transports hormones from the endocrine glands to other parts of the body; helps regulate the amounts of acids, bases, salts, and water in the cells; and helps regulate body temperature. If any of these functions is impaired, the consequences can have a direct bearing on your health.

There are several ways in which the functions carried out by the blood may be hampered. First, hundreds of chemicals—ranging from gases such as carbon monoxide to toxic metals such as lead to natural substances such as fat—can find their way into the blood and impair its function. These foreign substances enter the body through the air we breathe, the water we drink, the food we eat, and the surfaces with which we come in contact through our skin. Because these substances act on the blood in different ways, the adverse effects they produce may vary widely.

Second, the performance of the blood may be hampered by a lack of specific nutrients. A classic example is an iron deficiency that results in anemia. However, there are many nutrients that the blood requires on a daily basis if it is to perform normally.

Finally, genetics can play a role in creating blood disorders. Sickle cell anemia and hemophilia are two common examples of such disorders.

Blood purification techniques can act in two ways. Some help draw foreign substances out of the body, while others provide important nutrients to help restore the blood's normal structure and maximize its performance.

PROCEDURE

Blood purification is achieved through the use of a special fast. Once you have decided to follow a blood purification program, it is vital to choose an appropriate time for the fast. Consider that fasting requires the conservation of energy. Therefore, avoid fasting on a week when, for instance, you are moving your office or participating in a sports event. Also keep in mind that the cold-weather months are not an ideal time for a fast, as some of the heat you need to withstand the cold is created during the digestive process. Most important is the need to be mentally prepared. If you are "psyched up" for the fast, it is the right time to fast.

Once you have chosen the time for the fast and have prepared yourself mentally, you can begin to prepare yourself physically. For one week prior to the fast, follow a raw vegetable diet, including lots of "green drinks." Chlorophyll, obtained from tablets or fresh juice, "pre-cleanses" the body, making the fast less of a shock to your system.

While on the fast, consume only steam-distilled water; juices; and dandelion, milk thistle, licorice root, yellow dock root, burdock root, or red clover tea or extract. Drink at least 8 to 10 cups of distilled water daily to aid in cleansing and to help carry toxins out of the body. The best juices for blood purification are lemon juice, beet juice, carrot juice, and the juices of all leafy greens. Leafy green juices are particularly important because they supply chlorophyll, an essential part of any blood purification therapy. Chlorophyll not only cleanses the blood of impurities, but also builds up the blood with important nutrients, promotes regularity, and inhibits cellular damage from radiation. This makes chlorophyll helpful in the treatment of many disorders. Wheatgrass, barley, and alfalfa juices are all rich in chlorophyll.

Stay on the fast for three days, or as directed by your health-care provider. Once you have completed the fast, avoid white flour and all sugars—substances that are highly refined and hard to digest. The stress placed on your body by such foods can "undo" all of the good accomplished by the fast. Ideally, these foods should be avoided all of the time. At the very least, eliminate them—as well as heated fats and oils—for at least one month after your fast.

NUTRIENTS

SUPPLEMENT	SUGGESTED DOSAGE	COMMENTS
Very Important		
Chlorophyll tablets or	As directed on label.	Cleanses and refurbishes red blood cells. Aids immune system function.
liquid	As directed on label. Take with juice.	
Important		
Cell Guard from Biotec Foods	As directed on label.	A good antioxidant formula.
Helpful		
A.M./P.M. Ultimate Cleanse from Nature's Secret	As directed on label.	A 2-part system that helps stimulate and detoxify the organs, blood, and channels of elimination.
Kyo-Green from Wakunaga	As directed on label.	Good for the liver and the colon. Contains wheatgrass and barley grass.

HERBS

❑ Echinacea cleanses the lymph glands.

❑ Barberry, black radish, eyebright, lobelia, milk thistle, Oregon grape, pau d'arco, wild yam, and yellow dock cleanse and detoxify the liver and the endocrine system. You can use these herbs independently or in any combination.

Caution: Do not take lobelia internally on an ongoing basis. Do not use Oregon grape during pregnancy.

❑ Borage seed, chamomile, dandelion, ginkgo biloba, and sarsaparilla help to restore the acid/alkaline balance to the bloodstream. Ginkgo biloba is also a powerful antioxidant.

Caution: Do not use chamomile on an ongoing basis, as ragweed allergy may result. Avoid it completely if you are allergic to ragweed.

❑ Burdock, dandelion, hawthorn, licorice, pau d'arco, red clover, rhubarb, sage, shiitake mushroom, and Siberian and other ginsengs detoxify and cleanse the blood. These herbs can be used independently or in any combination.

Caution: Do not use licorice on a daily basis for more than seven days in a row, and avoid it completely if you have high blood pressure. Do not use sage if you have any kind of seizure disorder. Do not use Siberian ginseng if you have hypoglycemia or a heart disorder. Do not use any type of ginseng if you have high blood pressure.

❑ Goldenseal cleanses the mucous membranes.

Caution: Do not take this herb internally on a daily basis for more than one week at a time, as it may disturb normal intestinal flora. Do not use it during pregnancy, and use it with caution if you are allergic to ragweed.

Considerations

❑ *See also* FASTING in Part Three.

Chelation Therapy

Chelation (pronounced *key-LAY-shun*) therapy is a safe, nonsurgical treatment used to rid the body of excess toxins, particularly metals. Chelating agents used in this therapy are available in over-the-counter formulas that can be taken orally at home, and in intravenous solutions that must be administered under the supervision of a physician. These chelators draw out toxic metals and other harmful substances that impair body function, and help the body eliminate these toxins via the kidneys. Oral chelating agents can often prevent problems from occurring by restoring circulation to the body's tissues. If serious health problems already exist, intravenous therapy is usually necessary.

Chelation therapy is used to treat a variety of health problems. First, chelating agents are used to bind with heavy toxic metals such as cadmium, lead, and mercury—substances that enter our body through food, water, and other means—and excrete these metals from the body. As certain minerals accumulate in the body, they interact with other minerals, promoting the actions of some and inhibiting the actions of others. Lead, for instance, has been shown to inhibit the actions of calcium, iron, and potassium, all of which are important nutrients. When chelating agents are used to eliminate toxic metals such as lead from the body, essential nutrients are better able to do their job.

Chelation therapy is also used in the treatment of atherosclerosis and other circulatory disorders, as well as in the treatment of gangrene, which often is the result of poor circulation. In atherosclerosis, deposits of cholesterol, fats, and other substances collect on the walls of large and medium-sized arteries in the form of hard plaque. It has been found that calcium acts as the "glue" that holds the atherosclerotic plaque together. Chelating agents bind with this calcium and carry it out of the body, breaking up the plaque deposits, unclogging the arteries, and permitting more normal blood flow.

ORAL CHELATION THERAPY

Oral chelating agents offer a safe, convenient alternative for persons who are at risk for circulatory problems or problems caused by toxic metal accumulation. Among the many disorders that may be helped by chelation therapy are multiple sclerosis, Parkinson's disease, Alzheimer's disease, and arthritis. Despite reservations voiced by many in the medical establishment, many severely disabled, high-risk individuals have reported dramatic improvement in arterial circulation after chelation treatment.

Procedure

The following chelating agents can be used to prevent many degenerative illnesses, and can often alleviate the symptoms of existing conditions. These agents can be purchased in the combinations shown below in health food stores and drugstores. Follow package directions regarding dosage.

- Alfalfa, fiber, rutin, and selenium.
- Calcium and magnesium chelate with potassium.
- Chromium, garlic, pectin, and potassium.
- Coenzyme Q10.
- Copper chelate, iron, sea kelp, and zinc chelate.

In addition, the following supplements can act as oral chelating agents to rid the body of excess minerals.

NUTRIENTS

SUPPLEMENT	SUGGESTED DOSAGE	COMMENTS
Aangamik DMG from FoodScience Labs	200 mg daily.	Increases available oxygen and prevents cellular and tissue oxidation.
Alfalfa liquid or tablets	Double the amount directed on the label.	Detoxifies the liver and and alkalizes the body. Chelates toxic substances from the body.
Apple pectin and rutin	As directed on label. As directed on label.	To bind with unwanted toxic metals and remove them from body through the intestinal tract.

Calcium plus magnesium	1,500 mg daily. 700–1,000 mg daily.	Replaces calcium lost by using chelating substances. Use calcium citrate form. Displaces calcium within the cells of the artery walls.
Coenzyme Q10	60–90 mg daily.	Improves circulation, lowers blood pressure, and acts as a chelating agent.
Garlic (Kyolic)	2 capsules twice daily, with meals.	A good chelating agent and detoxifier.
L-Cysteine and L-methionine	500 mg each twice daily, on an empty stomach. Take with water or juice. Do not take with milk. Take with 50 mg vitamin B6 and 100 mg vitamin C for better absorption.	Two of the most important natural dietary chelators.
L-Lysine plus glutathione	500 mg each daily.	Aids in detoxifying harmful toxins and metals. Powerful free radical scavengers and antioxidants that remove unwanted substances from the body. Caution: Do not take lysine longer than 6 months at a time.
Selenium	200 mcg daily.	A powerful free radical scavenger.
Vitamin A plus natural beta-carotene or carotenoid complex	25,000 IU daily. If you are pregnant, do not exceed 10,000 IU daily. 25,000 IU daily. As directed on label.	To aid in excreting toxic substances. Use emulsion forms for easier assimilation.
Vitamin B complex plus extra vitamin B3 (niacin) and pantothenic acid (vitamin B5) and vitamin B12	100 mg 3 times daily. 50 mg 3 times daily. 50 mg 3 times daily. 200 mcg 3 times daily.	B vitamins aid in protecting the body from harmful substances and are needed for all cellular functions. Caution: Do not take niacin if you have a liver disorder, gout, or high blood pressure.
Vitamin C with bioflavonoids	5,000–15,000 mg daily, in divided doses.	Powerful chelating agents and immunostimulants.
Vitamin E	Start with 600 IU daily and increase slowly to 1,000 IU daily.	Removes toxic substances and destroys free radicals. Emulsion form is recommended for easier assimilation and greater safety at higher doses.

Recommendations

❑ Follow a diet designed to treat heart disease and/or high cholesterol. Avoid fried foods; dairy products; mayonnaise, oils, and other fats; red meat; processed and fast foods; salt; and gravies. Drink only steam-distilled water. Eat as many fiber-rich foods as possible. Oats, brown rice, and wheat bran are all good sources of fiber. See CARDIOVASCULAR DISEASE and HIGH CHOLESTEROL in Part Two for more information.

❑ Add a high-protein drink to your diet, or take the essential amino acids in supplement form. A deficiency of any one essential amino acid will reduce the effectiveness of all the others.

❑ Increase your intake of manganese by eating Brazil nuts, pecans, barley, buckwheat, whole wheat, and dried split peas. Manganese is an important chelating agent when consumed in manganese-rich foods. It is a major factor in blocking calcium from entering the cells of the arterial lining.

❑ Incorporate onions into your daily meals. Onions produce a natural chelating effect in the body, and tend to decrease the "clotting power" of blood.

❑ When using chelation therapy, make sure to replace any essential minerals that might be displaced by chelating agents. Alfalfa, iron, kelp, and zinc supplements are recommended. Use a natural source of iron, such as blackstrap molasses or Floradix Iron + Herbs from Salus Haus.

❑ If taking zinc supplements, eat sulfur-rich foods, like garlic, onions, and legumes. Zinc inhibits the action of sulfur.

INTRAVENOUS CHELATION THERAPY

Intravenous chelation therapy is often used to remove calcified, hardened plaque from the arterial walls, improving circulation. When used under the care of a physician, this procedure can be a safe alternative to vascular surgery. This therapy is also used to remove heavy metals, such as lead, from the body. Most serious illnesses require repeated injections of the agents.

The most common chelating agent now used in intravenous therapy is ethylenediaminetetraacetic acid (EDTA). A strong substance, EDTA attracts lead, strontium, and many other metals, as well as calcium. Although there is controversy surrounding the use of this agent, it has not been found to be toxic when used correctly.

Prior to beginning a course of EDTA chelation therapy, you must undergo a thorough physical examination. This includes a series of laboratory tests, including evaluations of cholesterol, blood, kidney function, liver function, glucose, and electrolytes. In addition, an electrocardiogram and chest x-ray are routinely performed. Other studies often assess vitamin B_{12} and mineral status. Typically, kidney function studies are repeated several times during the course of chelation therapy. Blood studies may have to be repeated, too, depending on the initial laboratory results.

The course of chelation therapy varies from person to person, but a typical course includes two treatments per week, each of three hours' duration. In addition to EDTA, physicians frequently administer supplements—including vitamin C, magnesium, and trace minerals—with the intravenous infusion, depending on the individual's particular illness and the results of the laboratory studies.

Recommendations

❑ While undergoing EDTA chelation therapy, be sure to take supplemental vitamins and minerals, particularly zinc, chromium, and the B-complex vitamins. This is important, as chelation agents are known to bind with and remove certain vitamins and minerals from the body. During therapy, take these supplements as directed in NUTRITION, DIET, AND WELLNESS in Part One.

Considerations

❑ When supervised by a qualified physician, EDTA intravenous chelation therapy is safe and causes few side effects.

❑ A 1989 study, published in the *Journal of Advancement in Medicine,* used EDTA to treat 3,000 people with coronary artery disease and other vascular problems. Nearly 90 percent experienced significant improvement.

❑ Hair analysis is an excellent means of determining the concentration of minerals in the body. (*See* HAIR ANALYSIS in Part Three.)

❑ There are over 150 doctors in the United States who are certified by the American Board of Chelation Therapy as approved chelation therapists. For information on the approved physicians in your area, you can contact one of the following groups:

The American College of Advancement
  in Medicine (ACAM)
P.O. Box 3427
Laguna Hills, CA 92654
800–532–3688 or 714–583–7666

Perlmutter Health Center
800 Goodlette Road, Suite 270
Naples, FL 33940
941–649–7400

Chiropractic

See under PAIN CONTROL.

Colon Cleansing

Retained debris in the colon leads to the absorption of toxins, resulting in systemic intoxication (poisoning). Symptoms of this condition can include mental confusion, depression, irritability, fatigue, gastrointestinal irregularities, and even allergic reactions such as hives, sneezing, and coughing. Many nutritionists and researchers believe that this toxicity can eventually lead to more serious disorders. Colon cleansing can rid the colon of debris, and help prevent and treat a variety of health problems.

PROCEDURE

The best means of removing toxins and wastes from the body is a fast. This should be the first step in any colon cleansing program. (*See* FASTING in Part Three.) In addition to following a fast, use a wheatgrass, fresh lemon juice, garlic, or coffee enema. (*See* ENEMAS in Part Three.) If bowel problems or related symptoms are chronic, repeat this program once monthly.

The following supplements aid in cleansing the colon.

NUTRIENTS

SUPPLEMENT	SUGGESTED DOSAGE	COMMENTS
Very Important		
Fiber (ground flaxseeds, oat bran, and psyllium seed husks are good sources)	1 capsule or 1 teaspoon 4 times daily. Take separately from other supplements and medications.	Essential for a clean colon. Not habit forming.
Important		
Acidophilus or Kyo-Dophilus from Wakunaga	As directed on label. Take on an empty stomach. As directed on label. Take on an empty stomach.	Restores the normal "friendly" bacteria in the colon. If you are allergic to dairy products, use a nondairy formula.
Aloe vera juice	½ cup 3 times daily.	Heals colon inflammation. Use a pure form.
Bio-Bifidus from American Biologics	As directed on label. For fast results, also use as an enema (do this only once).	Replaces the bowel flora.
Helpful		
A.M./P.M. Ultimate Cleanse from Nature's Secret	As directed on label.	An excellent detoxification program.
Apple pectin	As directed on label.	Source of quality fiber. Helps to detoxify heavy metals.
Kyo-Green from Wakunaga or ProGreens from Nutricology or wheatgrass juice or capsules	As directed on label. As directed on label. As directed on label. As directed on label.	To assist in keeping the colon clear of toxic debris and aid in healing of an inflamed colon.
Sonne's #7 from Sonne Organic Foods	As directed on label.	An intestinal cleanser. Contains liquid bentonite, which absorbs and eliminates toxins.
Vitamin C	6,000–20,000 mg daily, in divided doses. *See* ASCORBIC ACID FLUSH in Part Three.	Protects the body from pollutants. Use a buffered or esterified form.

HERBS

❑ Aloe vera, calendula, and peppermint help to restore the acid/alkaline balance of the colon and promote healing.

❑ Burdock, echinacea, horsetail, and licorice have detoxifying properties. Licorice also supports the organs.
Caution: If overused, licorice can elevate blood pressure. Do not use this herb on a daily basis for more than seven days in a row. Avoid it completely if you have high blood pressure.

❑ Barberry, butternut bark, cascara sagrada, flaxseed, red raspberry, rhubarb, and senna can be used to flush the colon and release waste.
Caution: Do not use barberry during pregnancy.

❑ Boneset, elecampane, fenugreek, lobelia, and yarrow loosen and flush mucus from the intestines.
Caution: Do not use lobelia on an ongoing basis.

❑ Fennel restores the acid/alkaline balance of the colon, promotes healing, flushes the colon, and releases waste.

❑ Garlic eliminates parasites.

❑ Marshmallow restores the acid/alkaline balance of the colon, promotes healing, and loosens and flushes mucus from the intestines.

❑ Pau d'arco restores the acid/alkaline balance of the colon, promotes healing, and has detoxifying properties.

❑ Slippery elm soothes inflammation and cleanses excess waste from the colon. For quick relief, use slippery elm tea as an enema.

RECOMMENDATIONS

❑ Eat only raw foods for two weeks, and then maintain a diet of 50 percent raw foods, including plenty of sprouts and raw vegetables.

❑ Drink at least eight 8-ounce glasses of water each day, even if you are not thirsty. Insufficient liquid intake promotes hard stools, which can stay in the colon for weeks or even months, causing symptoms such as headache, fatigue, and depression, and resulting in a toxic bloodstream.

❑ Avoid saturated fats, sugar, and highly processed foods. Avoid oils and fried foods until the colon returns to normal and the stools are normal. Use olive oil, canola oil, or essential fatty acids sparingly during this cleansing period. Dairy products should be avoided because they create excess mucus in the colon. This diet helps to maintain a clean colon.

❑ If you have a blood sugar problem, avoid sweet fruits.

❑ Upon arising and at bedtime, drink the juice of a fresh lemon squeezed into a cup of warm water to cleanse the bloodstream and detoxify and neutralize the system.

❑ Each morning, take a brisk walk and drink fresh carrot and apple juice, "green drinks," or fresh pineapple and papaya juice.

❑ Make a colon-cleansing drink by mixing 1 tablespoon of bentonite with 1 teaspoon of psyllium seed, ½ cup of apple juice, ½ cup of aloe vera juice, and ½ cup of steam-distilled water. Take this mixture once daily until the colon is clean and not foul smelling.

❑ Use a fiber supplement such as psyllium seed on a daily basis. Mix the supplement with water or juice, and drink it immediately, as the mixture thickens quickly. Avoid fiber supplements in capsule and pill form.

Color Therapy (Chromotherapy)

The effects of color on our moods, health, and way of thinking have been studied by scientists for years. Even an individual's preference for one color over another may be related to the way that color makes the individual feel.

Color can be described as light—visible radiant energy—of certain wavelengths. Photoreceptors in the retina, called cones, translate this energy into colors. The retina contains three kinds of cones: one for blue, one for green, and one for red. We perceive other colors by combining these colors.

According to Dr. Alexander Schauss, director of the American Institute for Biosocial Research in Tacoma, Washington, when the energy of color enters our bodies, it stimulates the pituitary and pineal glands. This in turn affects the production of certain hormones, which in turn affect a variety of physiological processes. This explains why color has been found to have such a direct influence on our thoughts, moods, and behavior—an influence that many experts believe is distinctly separate from psychological and cultural factors. Remarkably, color seems to have an effect even on blind people, who are thought to sense color as a result of energy vibrations created within the body.

Clearly, the colors you choose for your clothes and for your home, office, car, and other surroundings can have a profound effect on you. Colors have been known to ease stress, to fill you with energy, and even to alleviate pain and other physical problems. This idea, it should be noted, is far from new. In fact, the "color your world" concept is part of the ancient Chinese design technique *Feng Shui.*

When selecting a color to effect a change in mood or to relieve discomfort, it is vital to choose the color suited to your particular objective. For instance, blue has a relaxing, calming effect. Blue lowers the blood pressure, the heart rate, and respiration. In one study, children prone to aggressive behavior became calmer when placed in a blue classroom. Blue has also been found to make people in hot and humid environments feel cooler. To help relieve the pain of ulcers, back problems, rheumatism, and inflammatory disorders, surround yourself with blue, and focus your mind on the body part you want to heal while looking at the color. One good place to do this is in the countryside, where the blue of the sky and the water can impart a feeling of calming "oneness" with the universe.

As another of nature's most abundant colors, green, like blue, has a soothing and relaxing effect on the body as well as the mind. People who are depressed or anxious can benefit from green surroundings. Green also helps nervous disorders, exhaustion, heart problems, and cancer. When you are ill, try sitting on a hillside or by a green pasture, and focus on the body part you want to heal. Green may also be a good environmental color for the dieter.

Like blue and green, violet creates a peaceful environment. Violet also suppresses the appetite, and is good for scalp and kidney problems and for migraine headaches.

The color red stimulates, excites, and warms the body. Red increases the heart rate, brain wave activity, and respiration. The color of passion and energy, red is also good for impotence and frigidity, as well as for anemia, bladder infections, and skin problems. Those who have poor coordination should avoid wearing the color red. In addition, people suffering from hypertension (high blood pressure) should avoid rooms with a red decor, as this can cause their blood pressure to rise. Conversely, red has a good effect on those with hypotension (low blood pressure).

Pink has a soothing effect on the body, relaxing the muscles. Because it has been found to have a tranquilizing effect on aggressive and violent people, pink is often used in prisons, hospitals, and juvenile and drug centers. Those suffering from anxiety or withdrawal symptoms can benefit from pink surroundings. Pink is also a good color for the bedroom, where it can help evoke feelings of romance.

Orange is the color of choice for stimulating the appetite and reducing fatigue. Use this color—in orange place mats and tablecloths, for instance—to encourage a finicky eater, or to pique the appetite of a person who is ill. This color should be avoided by those who are trying to lose weight. If you are feeling tired or run down, try wearing an orange garment to lift your energy level. General weakness, allergies, and constipation may also improve.

Yellow is the most memorable of all the colors. Whenever you want to remember something, jot it down on yellow paper. This color also raises the blood pressure and increases the pulse rate, but to a lesser degree than red does. As the color of sunshine, yellow has an energizing effect; it can help relieve depression. A chromotherapist may use the color to treat muscle cramps, hypoglycemia, overactive thyroid, and gallstones.

Black is a "power" color. Try wearing black clothes for a feeling of strength and self-confidence. Black also suppresses the appetite. If you want to lose weight, cover your dining table with a black tablecloth.

DHEA Therapy

The most abundant hormone found in the bloodstream, dehydroepiandrosterone (DHEA) is produced by the adrenal glands, which sit atop the kidneys. Much like human growth hormone (HGH) and melatonin—two other hormones now known to have anti-aging properties—DHEA is produced abundantly during youth, with production peaking around age twenty-five. After this, though, production wanes. By the age of eighty, people are thought to have only 10 to 20 percent of the DHEA they had at twenty.

Research has shown that DHEA has many functions in

the body pertaining to health and longevity. Among other things, it helps to generate the sex hormones estrogen and testosterone; increases the percentage of muscle mass; decreases the percentage of body fat; and stimulates bone deposition, thereby helping to prevent osteoporosis. As the production of DHEA declines with age, the structures and systems of the body appear to decline with it. This leaves the body vulnerable to various cancers, including cancer of the breast, prostate, and bladder, as well as to atherosclerosis, high blood pressure, Parkinson's disease, diabetes, nerve degeneration, and other age-related conditions.

Research suggests that DHEA replacement therapy can have a number of highly beneficial effects. In a 1986 study based on twelve years of research involving 242 middle-aged and elderly men, small doses of DHEA appeared to be linked with a 48-percent reduction in death from heart disease, and a 36-percent reduction in death from other causes. In a twenty-eight-day study, DHEA therapy enabled men to lose 31 percent of mean body fat without changing body weight. DHEA is thought to have caused this loss of fat by blocking an enzyme that is known to produce fat tissue and promote cancer cell growth. In another study, middle-aged and elderly men taking DHEA for one year experienced a markedly greater sense of well-being, including a better ability to cope with stress, increased mobility, decreased pain, and higher quality sleep. Research also indicates that DHEA supplements can help prevent cancer, arterial disease, multiple sclerosis, and Alzheimer's disease; treat lupus and osteoporosis; enhance the activity of the immune system; and improve memory. Laboratory studies in animals have indicated that DHEA can increase life span by as much as 50 percent.

DHEA comes both in nonprescription-strength pills and capsules, and in higher-dosage prescription-strength pills and capsules. Most of the DHEA that you can buy is made in laboratories from substances extracted from wild yams, the most common substance being *diosgenin*. Also available are extracts of the wild yams that have *not* been processed into DHEA, but which the body may convert into DHEA.

DHEA therapy should be undertaken with caution. Some physicians believe that high doses of DHEA suppress the body's natural ability to synthesize the hormone. Animal studies have indicated that high doses can also lead to liver damage. For this reason, while undergoing DHEA replacement therapy, it is important to take supplements of the antioxidants vitamin C, vitamin E, and selenium to prevent oxidative damage to the liver.

Enemas

Over time, toxic wastes can accumulate in the colon and liver, and then circulate throughout the body via the bloodstream. A clean and healthy colon and liver, then, are essential for the health of all the organs and tissues of the body.

There are two types of enemas—the retention enema and the cleansing enema. The primary action of the retention enema, which is held in the body for about fifteen minutes, is to help rid the liver of impurities. The cleansing enema, which is retained for only a few minutes, is used to flush out the colon.

When using any enema, keep in mind that they should never be used if there is rectal bleeding. In such a case, contact a physician immediately.

If you experience tension or spasms in the bowel while using an enema, try using warmer water—99°F is a good temperature—to help relax the bowel. If the bowel is weak or flaccid, try using colder water—75°F to 80°F—to help strengthen it.

After using any enema, be sure to wash and sterilize the tip of the enema bag.

THE COFFEE RETENTION ENEMA

When used as a retention enema—an enema that is held in the body for a specified period of time—coffee does not go through the digestive system, and does not affect the body as a coffee beverage does. Instead, the coffee solution stimulates both the liver and the gallbladder to release toxins, which are then flushed from the body.

A coffee retention enema is quite helpful during a serious illness, after hospitalization, and after exposure to toxic chemicals. This enema can also be used during fasts to relieve the headaches sometimes caused by a fast-induced release of toxins.

Procedure

To make the coffee enema solution, place 2 quarts of steam-distilled water in a pan, and add 6 heaping tablespoons of ground coffee (do not use instant or decaffeinated). Boil the mixture for fifteen minutes, cool to a comfortable temperature, and strain. Use only 1 pint of the strained coffee at a time, and refrigerate the remainder in a closed jar.

Place 1 pint of the enema solution in an enema bag. Do not use petroleum jelly to lubricate the tip of the enema bag. Instead, use vitamin E oil (buy it in oil form or pierce the end of a vitamin E capsule and squeeze the liquid onto the tip). The liquid will both ease insertion and have a healing effect on the anus and the lining of the colon, if these areas are inflamed. Aloe vera may also be used for this purpose.

The best position to assume when receiving the enema is "head down and rear up." After the liquid has been inserted, roll onto your right side and hold the solution in your body for fifteen minutes before allowing the fluid to be expelled. Do not roll from side to side.

Do not be concerned if the liquid is not expelled after fifteen minutes. Simply stand up and move around as usual until you feel the urge to expel the liquid.

Recommendations

☐ To maximize the benefits of this or any other retention enema, use a cleansing enema first.

☐ Do not abuse coffee enemas by using them too often. Use them only once daily while following a program for a specific disorder, unless you are being treated for cancer. People with cancer may need up to three enemas a day. You may also use coffee enemas occasionally as needed.

☐ Remember that excessive use of coffee enemas over six months or more may deplete the body's stores of iron, as well as other minerals and vitamins, causing anemia. Do not use coffee enemas for longer than four to six weeks at a time. If you develop anemia during treatment—or whenever you use this enema daily for a long period of time—be sure to take desiccated liver tablets as directed on the label.

☐ If you have cancer, AIDS, or another serious illness, or if you have a malabsorption problem, add 1 cc of B-complex vitamins or 2 cc of injectable liver extract, plus a dropperful of liquid kelp or sea water concentrate (found in health food stores), to the enema solution. If you are unable to locate injectable forms of these supplements, open 2 capsules of a B-complex supplement and add the contents to the enema solution, making sure it dissolves before use. Used daily, these supplements replace any lost B vitamins, help rebuild the liver, and provide an extra boost of energy.

☐ To kill unwanted bacteria in the colon—or for any type of colon disorder, including diarrhea and constipation—add 5 drops of either Aerobic 07 from Aerobic Life Industries or Dioxychlor from American Biologics to the enema solution.

THE *L. BIFIDUS* RETENTION ENEMA

This retention enema, which should be used only three to six times a year, is helpful in cases of candidiasis and other yeast infections, and in cases of severe gas and bloating. When gas is the problem, the *L. bifidus* enema may provide relief within minutes. This remedy may also be beneficial when high colonics have been used or when antibiotics have been taken over long periods of time—practices that can kill the body's "friendly" bacteria. The *L. bifidus* enema replaces this flora, helping the body fight yeast infections and improving digestion. In fact, this enema can be useful during any severe illness.

Procedure

To make the *L. bifidus* enema solution, place 6 ounces of Digesta-Lac from Natren (found in health food stores) in 1 quart of lukewarm steam-distilled water. (Be sure to avoid using very cold or very warm water.) Kyo-Dophilus from Wakunaga may also be used (empty the contents of 6 to 8 capsules into the water), although the Digesta-Lac works best. Mix until formula is dissolved. Use only 1 pint of the solution at a time, and refrigerate the remainder in a jar.

For best results, use a plain water enema before using the *L. bifidus* enema, as this makes it easier to retain the *L. bifidus* solution for the necessary period of time. After expelling the plain water enema, place 1 pint of the *L. bifidus* solution in an enema bag. Do not use petroleum jelly to lubricate the tip of the enema bag. Instead, use vitamin E oil (buy it in oil form or pierce the end of a vitamin E capsule and squeeze the liquid onto the tip). The liquid will both ease insertion and have a healing effect on the anus and the lining of the colon, if these areas are inflamed. Aloe vera may also be used for this purpose.

The best position to assume when receiving the enema is "head down and rear up." After the liquid has been inserted, roll onto your right side and hold the solution in your body for fifteen minutes before allowing the fluid to be expelled. Do not roll from side to side.

Do not be concerned if the liquid is not expelled after fifteen minutes. Simply stand up and move around as usual until you feel the urge to expel the liquid.

THE LEMON JUICE CLEANSING ENEMA

The lemon juice enema is an excellent means of cleansing the colon of fecal matter and other impurities and of detoxifying the system. This enema also balances the pH of the colon, and is useful whenever cleansing of the colon is desired, as well as for colon disorders, such as constipation.

Procedure

To make the solution for the lemon enema, add the juice of 3 lemons to 2 quarts of lukewarm steam-distilled water. (Be sure to avoid using either very cold or very warm water.) If desired, add 2 droppersful of liquid kelp to boost the mineral content of the solution.

Place all of the solution in an enema bag. Do not use petroleum jelly to lubricate the tip of the enema bag. Instead, use vitamin E oil (buy it in oil form or pierce the end of a vitamin E capsule and squeeze the liquid onto the tip). The liquid will both ease insertion and have a healing effect on the anus and the lining of the colon, if these areas are inflamed. Aloe vera may also be used for this purpose.

The best position to assume when receiving the enema is "head down and rear up." After the liquid has been inserted, roll onto your back, and finally roll over and lie on your left side. As you are doing this, massage your colon to help loosen any fecal matter. Start on your right side and gradually move your fingers up toward the bottom of your rib cage, then across your abdomen and down the left side.

Note that 2 quarts is a lot of liquid. If you experience any pain during insertion, stop the flow of the enema bag and, remaining in the same position, take deep breaths until the pain subsides. Then resume the enema flow. If you expel the liquid before all of it has been inserted, simply begin the process over again. If pain persists, discontinue the enema procedure.

Hold the solution in your body for three or four minutes before allowing it to be expelled. After two or three such sessions, you will find it easier to insert and hold the liquid.

Recommendations

❑ If you have trouble with constipation, use the lemon juice enema once a week, and the coffee retention enema once a week. The bowels will shortly move on their own, the colon will be clean, and the stool will not be foul-smelling.

❑ If you suffer from colitis, use the lemon juice enema once a week. Any time pain from colitis is experienced, this enema will quickly relieve the discomfort.

❑ If allergic to lemons, prepare the enema solution with 1 to 2 ounces of wheatgrass or garlic juice in place of the lemon juice, or fill the enema bag with plain steam-distilled water.

THE CATNIP TEA ENEMA

Catnip tea enemas are a good way to bring a high fever down quickly and keep it down. These also relieve constipation and congestion, which keep fever up. When body temperature goes above 102°F (103°F in children over two), take a cleansing catnip tea enema. Repeat the procedure every four to six hours, and continue taking the enemas twice daily as long as fever persists. Catnip tea enemas should *not* be used by children under two years of age.

Procedure

To make the solution for the catnip tea enema, place about 8 tablespoons of fresh or dried catnip leaves in a glass or enameled pot. (If you are using bagged catnip tea, use the amount recommended on the package to make 1 quart of tea.) In a separate pot, bring 1 quart of steam-distilled water to a boil. Remove the water from the heat and pour it over the herbs. Cover the pot and let the tea steep for five to ten minutes. Then strain out the catnip and allow the tea to cool to a comfortable, slightly warm temperature.

Place all of the solution in an enema bag. Do not use petroleum jelly to lubricate the tip of the enema bag. Instead, use vitamin E oil (buy it in oil form or pierce the end of a vitamin E capsule and squeeze the liquid onto the tip). The liquid will both ease insertion and have a healing effect on the anus and the lining of the colon, if these areas are inflamed. Aloe vera may also be used for this purpose.

The best position to assume when receiving the enema is "head down and rear up." If you experience any pain during insertion, stop the flow of the enema bag and, remaining in the same position, take deep breaths until the pain subsides. Then resume the enema flow. If you expel the liquid before all of it has been inserted, simply begin the process over again. If pain persists, discontinue the enema procedure.

After the liquid has been inserted, roll onto your back, and finally roll over and lie on your left side. As you are doing this, massage your colon to help loosen any fecal matter. Start on your right side and gradually move your fingers up toward the bottom of your rib cage, then across your abdomen and down the left side. Hold the solution in your body for three or four minutes before expelling it.

Exercise

The closest thing to a "magic bullet" for maintaining youth and optimal health is a well-balanced combination of exercise and proper nutrition. The entire body benefits from this formula, both physically and psychologically.

Regular exercise improves digestion and elimination, increases endurance and energy levels, promotes lean body mass while burning fat, and lowers overall blood cholesterol while increasing the proportion of "good" cholesterol (HDL) to "bad" cholesterol (LDL). (*See* Understanding Cholesterol on page 326.) Exercise also reduces stress and anxiety, which are contributing factors to many illnesses and conditions. In addition to the physical benefits, studies have shown that regular exercise elevates mood, increases feelings of well-being, and reduces anxiety and depression.

The power of exercise in maintaining health was underscored by the continuing Aerobics Center Longitudinal Study, which was designed to examine the effects of different fitness levels. According to its 1996 report, published in the *Journal of the American Medical Association*, low fitness may pose as great a risk to health as smoking, and a greater risk than high cholesterol, high blood pressure, or obesity. It was reported that smokers who are moderately physically fit, but have high blood pressure and high cholesterol, live longer than nonsmokers who are healthy but sedentary. Moderate fitness, it was stated, can be achieved in ten weeks through many different forms of exercise, including daily sessions of walking, bicycling, or even gardening.

Exercise includes a variety of movements and different activities. *Recreational exercise* is meant for enjoyment and relaxation, while *therapeutic exercise* is intended to alleviate or prevent a particular problem. Sometimes an exercise can be both recreational and therapeutic. Take swimming, for example. With careful attention to arm and shoulder movements, swimming can meet both the recreational and therapeutic needs of someone who has arthritis of the shoulder.

There are a number of exercise types, each of which has a specific purpose:

• *Aerobic or endurance exercise* improves the body's capacity to use fuel and oxygen. Swimming, bicycle riding, jogging, and power walking are examples of this type of exercise. The body's cardiovascular system benefits through increased blood supply to the muscles and enhanced oxygen delivery throughout the body. Just twenty minutes a day of sustained aerobic activity can lower blood pressure and strengthen heart function.

• *Range-of-motion exercise* helps maintain a joint's complete movement by putting a body part through its maximum available range of motion. Extending and moving one's arms in wide circular motions is an example of this. Some degree of flexibility is required to perform range-of-motion exercises, so stretching is recommended beforehand.

• *Strengthening exercise* helps a muscle's ability to contract and do work. Doing sit-ups, for example, is a way of strengthening abdominal muscles.

One exercise rarely achieves two goals. For instance, a strengthening exercise will not significantly affect endurance, and range-of-motion exercises will not necessarily improve strength. A total exercise program must consider the individual's goals and include activities designed to achieve those goals.

Exercise should not be looked at as a chore. Try to select activities that you enjoy and look forward to doing. Whatever you choose, start out slowly, listen to your body, and gradually increase the intensity and duration of your workout.

A word of caution: If you are over thirty-five and/or have been sedentary for some time, consult with your health care provider before beginning any new exercise program.

Fasting

Over time, toxins build up in the body as the result of the pollutants in the air we breathe, the chemicals in the food and water we consume, and other means. Periodically, the body seeks to rid itself of these toxins, and releases them from the tissues. The toxins then enter the bloodstream, causing the body to experience a "low" or "down" cycle. During such a cycle, you may suffer from headaches, diarrhea, or depression. Fasting is an effective and safe method of helping the body detoxify itself and move through this low cycle with greater speed and fewer symptoms. In fact, fasting is recommended for any illness, as it gives the body the rest it needs to recover. Acute illnesses, colon disorders, allergies, and respiratory diseases are most responsive to fasting, while chronic degenerative diseases are the least responsive. By relieving the body of the work of digesting foods, fasting permits the system to rid itself of toxins while facilitating healing.

But fasting is helpful not just in times of poor health or during the body's low cycles. By fasting regularly, you give all of your organs a rest, and thus help reverse the aging process and live a longer and healthier life. During a fast:

• The natural process of toxin excretion continues, while the influx of new toxins is reduced. This results in a reduction of total body toxicity.

• The energy usually used for digestion is redirected to immune function, cell growth, and eliminatory processes.

• The immune system's workload is greatly reduced, and the digestive tract is spared any inflammation due to allergic reactions to food.

• Due to a lowering of serum fats that thins the blood, tissue oxygenation is increased and white blood cells are moved more efficiently.

• Fat-stored chemicals, such as pesticides and drugs, are released.

• Physical awareness and sensitivity to diet and surroundings are increased.

Due to these effects of fasting, a fast can help you heal with greater speed; cleanse your liver, kidneys, and colon; purify your blood; help you lose excess weight and water; flush out toxins; clear the eyes and tongue; and cleanse the breath. It is recommended that you fast at least three days a month, and follow a ten-day fast at least twice a year.

Depending on the length of the fast, it accomplishes different things. A three-day fast helps the body rid itself of toxins and cleanses the blood. A five-day fast begins the process of healing and rebuilding the immune system. A ten-day fast can take care of many problems before they arise and help to fight off illness, including the degenerative diseases that have become so common in our chemically polluted environment.

Certain precautions should be taken during fasts. First, *do not* fast on water alone. An all-water fast releases toxins too quickly, causing headaches and worse. Instead, follow the live-juice diet detailed below, as this both removes toxins and promotes healing by supplying the body with vitamins, minerals, and enzymes. Such a fast is also more likely to lead to a continued healthy diet once the fast is over, as it will accustom you to the taste of raw vegetables and the vitality that this diet promotes. Second, whenever you fast for more than three days, do so only under the supervision of a qualified health-care professional. If you have diabetes, hypoglycemia, or another chronic health problem, even short fasts should be supervised by a doctor. Pregnant and lactating women should *never* fast.

A final word of advice: It took years to wear your body down, and it will take time to build it back up to its peak condition. But believe that it can be done. Then, whenever you start to feel unwell, fast and feel better!

PROCEDURE

To prepare for the fast, eat only raw vegetables and fruits for two days. This will make the fast less of a shock to the system.

While on the fast, consume at least eight 8-ounce glasses of steam-distilled water a day, plus pure juices and up to 2 cups of herbal tea a day. Dilute all juices with the water, adding about 1 part water to 3 parts juice. Do not drink orange or tomato juice, and avoid all juices made with sweeteners or other additives.

The best juice to use during your fast is fresh lemon juice.

Add the juice of one lemon to a cup of warm water. Fresh apple, beet, cabbage, carrot, celery, and grape juices are also good, as are "green drinks," which are made from green leafy vegetables. These green drinks are excellent detoxifiers. Raw cabbage juice is particularly good for ulcers, cancer, and all colon problems. Just be sure to drink the cabbage juice as soon as it is prepared. As this juice sits, it loses its vitamin content.

Follow the juice-water-and-tea fast with a two-day diet of raw fruits and vegetables. The desired effects of the fast can be ruined by eating cooked foods immediately afterward. Because both the size of the stomach and the amount of secreted digestive juices may decrease during fasting, the first meals after a fast should be frequent and small.

HERBS

❑ Herbal teas may be consumed throughout the fast, once or twice per day. Try the following teas:

• Use alfalfa, burdock, chamomile, dandelion, milk thistle, red clover, and rose hips tea to rejuvenate the liver and cleanse the bloodstream.

Caution: Do not use chamomile on an ongoing basis, as ragweed allergy may result. Avoid it completely if you are allergic to ragweed.

• Drink 2 parts pau d'arco and echinacea tea mixed with 1 part unsweetened cranberry juice. Used four times a day, this will rebuild the immune system, aid in bladder function, and rid the colon of unwanted bacteria.

• Use peppermint tea for its calming and strengthening effect on the nerves, and for indigestion, nausea, and flatulence.

• Use slippery elm tea for inflammation of the colon. This tea also is beneficial when used as an enema solution.

❑ Take 2 capsules of garlic twice a day. If you prefer a liquid supplement, add the garlic oil to a cup of water. Garlic supplements may be taken on a daily basis before, during, and after a fast to promote overall health, aid in the healing process, and rid the colon of many types of parasites.

RECOMMENDATIONS

❑ If you must have something to eat during the fast, eat a piece of watermelon. Always eat watermelon by itself, with no additional foods. You can also try applesauce—fresh, not canned—made in a blender or food processor. Leave the skin on the apples, and do not cook them.

❑ Take a fiber supplement on a daily basis before and after your fast, but not during the fast. To promote cleansing of the colon before and after your fast, be sure to make extra fiber a part of your daily diet. Bran, especially oat bran, is an excellent source of fiber. Try to avoid supplements containing wheat bran, as they may be irritating to the colon wall. Another good fiber source is Aerobic Bulk Cleanse (ABC) from Aerobic Life Industries. To use this colon cleanser, mix it with half George's Aloe Vera Juice from

Warren Laboratories, and half natural cranberry juice. This mixture adds fiber and has a healing and cleansing effect also. Psyllium seed husks and ground flaxseed are other good-quality fiber products. Be certain to accompany any fiber capsule with a large glass of water, because the capsules expand and soak up a good deal of water.

❑ Do not chew gum while on the fast. The digestive process starts when chewing prompts the body to secrete enzymes into the gastrointestinal tract. If there is no food in the stomach for the enzymes to digest, trouble occurs.

❑ If desired, take spirulina during the fast. Spirulina is high in protein and contains a wide range of vitamins and minerals, plus chlorophyll for cleansing. If you are using tablets, take 5 tablets three times daily. If you are using powder, take 1 teaspoon three times daily, mixing the powder with a cup of juice.

❑ If you have hypoglycemia, never fast without also using a protein supplement. Spirulina, described above, is a good choice. Make sure the spirulina is of good quality, has been laboratory tested, and has been cleaned before processing. Kyo-Green from Wakunaga is also valuable. Before starting any fast, consult a qualified health care professional.

❑ If you are over sixty-five, or if you need daily supplements for another reason, continue taking your vitamin and mineral supplements during the fast. Older people need certain vitamins and minerals daily. When you are drinking juices, reduce the dosage of supplements that you take.

❑ If desired, before, during, and after your fast, use Kyo-Green from Wakunaga of America and ProGreens from Nutricology. These products contain all the nutrients needed to aid in the healing process. If used during the fast, these products should replace a cup of "green drink."

❑ During a fast, as toxins are released from your body, you may experience fatigue; body odor; dry, scaly skin; skin eruptions; headaches; dizziness; irritability; anxiety; confusion; nausea; coughing; diarrhea; dark urine; dark, foul-smelling stools; body aches; insomnia; sinus and bronchial mucus discharge; and/or visual or hearing problems. These symptoms are not serious, and will quickly pass. To alleviate any of these symptoms, use a daily lemon juice enema to cleanse the colon, and a daily coffee enema to rid the liver of impurities. *See* ENEMAS in Part Three.

❑ During your fast, be sure to get adequate rest. If necessary, try napping during the day to recharge your batteries.

❑ If desired, before, during, and after your fast, use Desert Delight from Aerobic Life Industries. This product, which contains cranapple, papaya, and aloe vera juice, helps keep the colon clean, and also supports kidney and bladder function, aids digestion, and has a healing effect on ulcers. If used during the fast, substitute this product for a cup of juice.

❑ To make an excellent juice for healing many illnesses, juice together 3 carrots, 3 kale leaves, 2 stalks celery, 2 beets, 1 turnip, ¼ pound spinach, ½ head of cabbage, ¼ bunch of parsley, ¼ of an onion, and ½ clove of garlic. If you don't have a juicer, place the vegetables in a pure vegetable broth and gently boil them, adding no seasonings. A cup of this juice may be substituted for any other juice while fasting. Save the vegetables from the broth to eat after your fast. Remember that no solid food is allowed during the fast.

❑ During a fast, as toxins are released from your body, you will probably experience a coated tongue and an unpleasant taste in your mouth. To relieve this problem, try rinsing your mouth with fresh lemon juice.

❑ If desired, before, during, and after your fast, use Daily Detox Tea from Houston International to help the bloodstream and organs eliminate toxins. If used during the fast, this product should replace a cup of herbal tea.

❑ If you are a denture wearer, keep your dentures in your mouth throughout the fast to prevent shrinkage of the gums.

❑ While fasting, continue your normal daily routine, including moderate exercise. Avoid any strenuous exercise.

❑ Be aware that when you fast during a low phase, you help your body experience the "up" phase of the cycle—a period during which you feel great. This occurs because the body has been cleansed of impurities. However, when you start to pollute your body again, the toxins once again begin to build up, and, in time, you will again have a low phase. When this occurs, the fast should be repeated.

❑ Before, during, and after your fast, use dry-brush massages to help rid the skin of toxins and dead cells. Perform the massage with a *natural* bristle brush that has a long handle, so that you can reach your back. Always brush toward the heart—from wrist to elbow, elbow to shoulder, ankles to knees, knees to hips, and so on. This massage will flake away large amounts of dead skin, freeing the pores of impediments, and, in turn, helping the skin to excrete poisons. It will also greatly improve circulation. *Do not* use this technique on areas of the body affected by acne, eczema, or psoriasis. Also avoid brushing areas that are broken or recently scarred, or that have protruding varicose veins.

Glandular Therapy

The glandular system is both complex and important. Virtually all body functions—from digestion to reproduction to growth—depend on a healthy glandular system.

To a large degree, the health of the glands, like the health of any organs of the body, can be greatly improved by adequate vitamin and mineral supplementation. Glandular therapy, the use of concentrated forms of various raw animal glands, can also improve the health of specific glands.

Turn-of-the-century endocrinologists hypothesized that

Maintaining a Healthy Glandular System

A gland is an organ that manufactures and releases fluids and other substances into the body for the body's use. The function of these fluids is so wide-ranging that virtually all body processes depend on a healthy glandular system. An imbalance or malfunction of any one glandular substance or gland can create tremendous problems throughout the body.

Glands fall into two categories: the exocrine glands and the endocrine glands. The exocrine glands, each of which secretes a specialized substance, open onto a surface of an organ or other structure through a duct. Examples of such glands are the salivary glands of the mouth, and the sweat and oil glands of the skin. Other exocrine glands can be found in the kidneys, the mammary glands, and the digestive tract. These glands perform a variety of functions. The salivary glands, for instance, secrete saliva, which aids in the digestion of food, while the sweat glands help rid the body of waste products.

Unlike the exocrine glands, the endocrine glands are ductless, and thus secrete the substances they produce—specifically, hormones—directly into the bloodstream. Examples of these glands include the adrenal glands, found atop the kidneys; the gonads, found in the reproductive organs; the pancreas, found behind the stomach; the pituitary gland, found at the base of the brain; the thyroid and parathyroid glands, found in the neck; and the thymus gland, found below the thyroid. The pineal gland,

which is attached to the brain, is also thought to be an endocrine gland.

By secreting hormones—chemicals that start or control the activity of an organ or group of cells—the endocrine glands help regulate practically all body functions. For instance, the pancreas secretes insulin, an important regulator of sugar metabolism. The female gonads, called the ovaries, produce hormones like estrogen, which aids the development of secondary sex characteristics, prepares the walls of the uterus to receive a fertilized egg, and performs many other important functions. The thymus secretes thymosin, a hormone that is critical to proper immune system function. The pituitary gland, which is often called the "master gland," regulates the functions of the other glands, and also produces a hormone that stimulates body growth. It should be noted that the pituitary gland, like many of the other endocrine glands, produces more than one hormone. Similarly, some hormones, such as estrogen, are secreted by more than one gland.

Like all organs, the glands need nutritional support, especially when stress depletes the body's stores of nutrients. Glandulars—concentrated forms of various animal glands—are one means of improving the health of the glands. In addition, nutritional supplements can help maintain the health of these glands, and thereby ensure proper functioning of the glandular system.

NUTRIENTS

SUPPLEMENT	SUGGESTED DOSAGE	COMMENTS
Very Important		
Kelp	Up to 200 mg daily.	Rich in minerals and the element iodine, which are necessary for thyroid function.
L-Arginine	500 mg daily.	Increases the size and activity of the thymus gland.
L-Glycine	500 mg daily.	Essential for the health of the thymus gland, spleen, and bone marrow.
L-Tyrosine	500 mg daily.	Important to the health and function of the adrenal, thyroid, and pituitary glands.
Manganese	As directed on label. Take separately from calcium.	Crucial to the production of thyroxine, the hormone that regulates the metabolic process. This nutrient is stored and used by the liver, kidneys, pancreas, lungs, prostate gland, and brain.
Vitamin A plus natural beta-carotene and other carotenoids	As directed on label. As directed on label.	Nutrients that nourish the thymus gland and increase antibody production. All organs with duct systems require these nutrients.
Vitamin B complex plus extra vitamin B₂ (riboflavin) and pantothenic acid (vitamin B₅)	100 mg twice daily. 50 mg 3 times daily. 50 mg 3 times daily.	B vitamins work best when all are taken together. Especially important if you are under stress. Vital to the health of the entire glandular system, especially the adrenal glands. *The* anti-stress vitamin.
Vitamin C	1,500 mg daily.	Important for adrenal function, and should be taken when using L-cysteine to prevent formation of cystine kidney stones.
Zinc	50 mg daily. Do not exceed 100 mg daily from all supplements.	Needed by the immune system, and for thymus and pancreas health. Especially important for the sex glands (gonads).
Important		
Lecithin granules or capsules	1 tsp 3 times daily, before meals. 1,200 3 times daily, before meals.	All cells and organs have lecithin surrounding them for protection. Also helps cleanse the liver.
Raw thymus glandular plus multiglandular complex	As directed on label. As directed on label.	To stimulate immune function and aid glandular function. A sublingual form is best.
Helpful		
Selenium	As directed on label.	Nourishes the liver and pancreas.
Essential fatty acids (flaxseed oil, primrose oil, and salmon oil are good sources)	As directed on label.	Needed to nourish the glands.
L-Cysteine and L-methionine plus glutathione	500 mg each daily, on an empty stomach. Take with water or juice. Do not take with milk. Take with 50 mg vitamin B₆ and 100 mg vitamin C for better absorption.	Aid in detoxifying glands of harmful pollutants. Also necessary for insulin production, and act as powerful antioxidants.
Silica or horsetail or oat straw	500 mg twice daily.	To supply silicon, a trace mineral that aids in healing the glands and tissues. *See under* Herbs, below. *See under* Herbs, below.
Superoxide dismutase (SOD) or Cell Guard from Biotec Foods	As directed on label, on an empty stomach. Take with a large glass of water. As directed on label.	A potent detoxifier that also transports oxygen for healing in the glandular system. An antioxidant complex that contains SOD.
Vitamin E	400–800 IU daily.	Rids the body of toxic substances when combined with vitamin C and selenium.

HERBS

❑ Black cohosh, black radish extract, goldenseal, licorice, lobelia, mullein, and red clover, taken in tea form, help strengthen and rebuild the liver, and restore glandular balance.

Caution: Do not take goldenseal internally on a daily basis for more than one week at a time, do not use it during pregnancy, and use it with caution if you are allergic to ragweed. Do not use licorice on a daily basis for more than seven days in a row, and avoid it completely if you have high blood pressure. Do not take lobelia on an ongoing basis, and do not take it in capsule form.

❑ Burdock helps rid the body of toxins.

❑ Cedar stimulates pancreatic function.

❑ Celery seed and hydrangea are diuretics that can be used to stimulate the kidneys.

❑ Chicory, milk thistle, and stillingia root stimulate and cleanse the liver.

❑ Dandelion stimulates and cleanses the liver. It also stimulates bile production, thereby benefiting the spleen and improving the health of the pancreas.

❑ Echinacea cleanses and strengthens the kidneys, liver, pancreas, and spleen.

❑ Horsetail and oat straw are good sources of silicon, which aids in healing, and are also high in calcium. They can be taken in tea or capsule form.

❑ Parsley is a diuretic that stimulates kidney function. It also helps strengthen and rebuild the liver, and maintain glandular balance.

❑ Safflower flowers encourage the pancreas to manufacture insulin.

❑ Uva ursi is a diuretic that stimulates kidney function. It also has a germicidal effect, and thereby destroys any bacteria that may be present. It is a tonic for a weakened liver, kidneys, and other glands.

❑ Gentian contains elements that are known to normalize the functions of the thyroid gland.

RECOMMENDATIONS

❑ *See* BLOOD PURIFICATION in Part Three and follow the instructions.

❑ Use alfalfa, beet, black radish, and dandelion juice for cleansing the liver, which is the largest gland in the body. *See* JUICING in Part Three.

❑ Use olive oil and lemon juice (3 tablespoons of olive oil mixed with the juice of a fresh lemon), plus plenty of pure apple juice, to stimulate the gallbladder and help excrete bile and even small gallstones. *See* GALLBLADDER DISORDERS in Part Two.

❑ *See* FASTING in Part Three and follow the program once monthly to allow glands time to heal and rest.

❑ *See* HYPOTHYROIDISM in Part Two and follow the temperature self-test to determine how well your thyroid gland is functioning.

CONSIDERATIONS

❑ When toxic substances circulate through the bloodstream due to poor eating habits, the use of drugs, or other factors, the presence of these substances is reflected in the lymphatic system. The lymph glands act as a filter, removing poisons from the body.

❑ *See also* GLANDULAR THERAPY in Part Three.

---

glandulars worked by providing nutrients the body lacked. Once supplied with the missing nutrients, the malfunctioning organ was able to repair itself and function properly.

In the 1930s, Dr. Royal Lee, a pioneering biochemical researcher, began his own work with glandulars, and developed a different explanation for the substances' effectiveness—an explanation that has been supported by more recent research. Dr. Lee hypothesized that the organs were malfunctioning not because of missing nutrients, but because the body was attacking its own organs. This attack—which may be compared to the immune system's attack of a transplanted organ, although it is milder in nature—impairs organ function, causing chronic health problems. Glandulars, said Lee, neutralize such attacks, allowing the organs to heal themselves.

Some of the most important glandulars are the following:

- Raw adrenal gland.
- Raw brain.
- Raw heart.
- Raw kidney.
- Raw liver.
- Raw lung.
- Raw mammary gland.
- Raw ovary.
- Raw pancreas.
- Raw pituitary gland.
- Raw spleen.
- Raw thymus.
- Raw thyroid gland.

Care should be taken in the purchase of glandulars. Many glandular products are byproducts of the meat-processing industry, and are taken from adult animals that show the effects of aging and exposure to toxins. This impairs the quality of the glandular. For best results, make sure that the glandulars you buy come from young, organically raised free-range animals that have not received hormones.

Growth Hormone Therapy

Human growth hormone (HGH) is secreted by the pituitary gland in the brain. Like all hormones, HGH works to regulate the activities of vital organs, and thus helps maintain health throughout the body. HGH was originally called a growth hormone because it is produced in greatest amounts during adolescence, when growth is most rapid. HGH does indeed help control growth. Because of the link between this hormone and the growth process, HGH therapy was first used to treat children who were failing to grow normally because of a deficiency of this hormone. Without HGH therapy, these children would have become dwarfs; with it, their growth was normal.

However, it has been found that HGH regulates more than just growth. Tissue repair, healing, cell replacement, organ health, bone strength, brain function, enzyme production, and the health of nails, hair, and skin all require adequate amounts of HGH. In addition, this hormone strengthens the immune system and helps the body resist oxidative damage.

Unfortunately, after adolescence, levels of HGH begin to decline at a rate of about 14 percent per decade. As production of the hormone decreases, so does the function of all vital organs. Because of this correlation between declining HGH production and aging, another application of HGH therapy has developed: the use of the hormone to reverse or retard age-related symptoms of physical and mental decline, and to treat some non-age-related disorders as well. It is this newer use of HGH therapy that we are concerned with in this discussion.

According to reports in scientific literature, benefits from HGH replacement therapy include a reversal of declining pulmonary function, decreased body fat, increased capacity to exercise, increased bone mass in people with osteoporosis, and the improvement or reversal of many other age-related symptoms and disorders. HGH has also been shown to strengthen the immune system and to improve the quality of life for people with AIDS by treating "wasting syndrome"—severe weight and muscle loss. People receiving HGH have reported a general enhancement of health and well-being, including a more positive outlook.

Although HGH injections may be self-administered, therapy must be prescribed and supervised by a physician. This is particularly important in light of the fact that as the therapy promotes tissue repair and other processes, the need for many nutrients increases. Therefore, treatment should include the supplementation of various vitamins, minerals, and, in some cases, other hormones.

As long as the dosage remains low—4 to 8 international units of the hormone per week—HGH therapy appears to be free of significant side effects. Those side effects that do occur usually pass as the body adjusts to the therapy.

RECOMMENDATIONS

❑ Avoid the consumption of excessively sweet foods, as it results in a blood sugar level that is counterproductive to the release and utilization of HGH. High-sugar foods should especially be avoided before going to bed, as the primary supply of HGH is released during sleep.

❑ Avoid eating immediately before exercising. Although vigorous exercise usually stimulates the production of HGH, blood sugar levels must be stable during exercise for HGH release to take place.

❑ To stimulate the body's production of HGH, take the amino acid arginine, which has been shown to encourage HGH manufacture. This amino acid is best taken in supplement form (500 milligrams daily), as foods that are high in arginine also contain amino acids that inhibit its ability to reach the pituitary gland, the site of HGH release.

CONSIDERATIONS

❑ The use of some brands of HGH has resulted in the production of antibodies to growth hormone.

❑ For information about other anti-aging hormones, *see* Melatonin under NATURAL FOOD SUPPLEMENTS in Part One, and DHEA THERAPY in Part Three.

Guided Imagery

See under PAIN CONTROL.

Hair Analysis

Hair analysis offers an accurate assessment of the concentration of minerals in the body—those that are toxic in any amount, those that are essential, and those that are needed in small amounts, but toxic in larger amounts. By allowing early detection of toxic substances such as mercury, lead, cadmium, and aluminum, hair analysis makes it possible to identify and treat toxicity before overt symptoms appear; and by showing levels of minerals such as calcium, it makes it possible to identify and treat a range of nutritional deficiencies well before health problems become serious.

Before the technique of hair analysis was developed, medical practitioners who were interested in the concentration of trace elements in the body had to rely on urine and serum sampling. Unfortunately, these tests have been shown to be inaccurate. They simply do not reflect the concentration of minerals in the cells and organs, but instead show the level of *circulating* minerals. The correlation between mineral concentrations in the internal organs of the body and concentrations in hair has been found to be much more reliable. In fact, hair analysis has been found to be such an accurate measure of substance exposure that it is often used to detect drug use.

Hair analysis begins with the removal of a small amount of hair, usually from the nape of the neck. Because harsh chemical treatment of the hair through coloring, bleaching, and permanent-waving can result in inaccuracies, a pubic hair specimen may be used instead. The hair sample is chemically washed and stripped of all substances found on it. A specific amount (by weight) of the resulting sample is then dissolved in a known volume of acid. Finally, using a method of chemical analysis called atomic absorption photospectrometry, each mineral is isolated and measured on a parts-per-million (ppm) basis.

Hair analysis also provides a relatively permanent record of mineral concentrations, which can be analyzed by computer to determine the correlation between various elements in the hair. Treatment of any identified problems, using chelation therapy and/or other programs, can then be designed and implemented before the condition becomes irreversible. (*See* CHELATION THERAPY in Part Three.) Later, follow-up hair analyses can be compared with the initial results to learn the effectiveness of the treatment.

The table on page 554 lists the minerals that can be measured through hair analysis. Next to each element is its symbol. In addition, the table shows the way in which each mineral interacts with other elements. In the case of lead, for instance, note that the presence of lead does not promote the action of any other mineral (second column). On the other hand, lead does inhibit the action of calcium, iron, and potassium (third column)—all important nutrients. Finally, the action of lead itself is inhibited by the presence of selenium and zinc (fourth column).

Your health care professional should be able to help you obtain an analysis of your hair. Do be sure that the laboratory you are dealing with is a reputable one. Questions you might ask about the lab include: Does the laboratory conform to the standards set by the American Society of Elemental Testing Laboratories, or the Hair Analysis Standardization Board? How long has this laboratory been in business? How old is the equipment being used? How experienced is the staff?

INTERACTION OF MINERALS

Mineral Name	Elements Promoted by Mineral	Elements Inhibited by Mineral	Inhibitors of the Mineral
Aluminum (Al)	P	F	
Arsenic (As)	Co, I	Se	
Beryllium (Be)		Mg	
Cadmium (Cd)		Cu	Zn
Calcium (Ca)	Fe, Mg, P	Cu, F, Li, Mn, Zn	Cr, Pb, S
Chlorine (Cl)*			
Chromium (Cr)		Ca	
Cobalt (Co)	As, F	Fe, I	
Copper (Cu)	Fe, Mo, Zn	P	Ag, Ca, Cd, Mn, S
Fluorine (F)		Mg	Al, Ca
Iodine (I)	As, Co, G		
Iron (Fe)	Ca, Cu, K, Mn, P		Co, Mg, Pb, Zn
Lead (Pb)		Ca, Fe, K	Se, Zn
Lithium (Li)		Na	Ca
Magnesium (Mg)	Ca, K, P	Fe	Mn
Manganese (Mn)	Cu, Fe, K, P	Mg	Ca
Mercury (Hg)*			
Molybdenum (Mo)	Cu, S	P	N
Nickel (Ni)*			
Nitrogen (N)		Mo	
Phosphorus (P)	Al, Be, Ca, Fe, Mg, Mn, Zn	Na	Cu, Mo
Potassium (K)	Fe, Mg, Mn, Na		Pb
Selenium (Se)		Cd, Pb	As, S
Silver (Ag)		Cu	
Sodium (Na)	K		Li, P
Sulfur (S)	Mo	Ca, Cu, Se	Zn
Zinc (Zn)	Cu, P	Cd, Fe, Pb, S	Ca

*Mineral interactions have not been documented.

Heat and Cold Therapy

See under PAIN CONTROL.

Hydrotherapy

Hydrotherapy—the therapeutic use of water, steam, and ice—has been used for centuries to effectively treat injuries and a wide range of illnesses. Treatment techniques include baths (full body and specific body parts), compresses, showers, sitz baths, steam baths, and whirlpools. Hospitals, clinics, and spas worldwide use forms of hydrotherapy as safe and effective methods for treating such conditions as AIDS, back pain, bronchitis and other respiratory problems, cancer, hypertension, muscle pain and inflammation, and rheumatoid arthritis. Hydrotherapy is also useful in treating the discomfort caused by spinal trauma.

There are three categories of external hydrotherapy: hot water, cold water, and alternating hot and cold water. *Hot water* stimulates the immune system and increases circulation, helping to relieve the body of toxins. By soothing nerves, hot water calms and relaxes the body. *Cold water,* which constricts blood vessels, is effective in reducing inflammation. Cold-water treatments are also used to reduce fever. *Alternating hot- and cold-water* treatments have been found to alleviate upper respiratory congestion and stimulate organ function through improved circulation.

Many hydrotherapy techniques for a range of conditions can be effectively performed at home. For instance, muscular pain and swelling caused by a sprain or strain respond favorably to an immediate application of cold. An ice pack, applied continually (up to twenty minutes on, followed by twenty minutes off) during the initial twenty-four hours following a trauma, can reduce swelling and provide relief.

Sitz baths, in which the pelvis is immersed in water, increase blood flow in the pelvic region and help to relieve problems in that area. Hot-water sitz baths are commonly used for the treatment of inflamed hemorrhoids, painful ovaries and testicles, muscular disorders, prostate disorders, and uterine cramps. Cold-water sitz baths are used to treat constipation, impotence, inflammation, sore muscles, and vaginal discharge. Alternating hot- and cold-water sitz baths are helpful in relieving abdominal disorders, blood poisoning, congestion, foot infection, headaches, muscle disorders, neuralgia, and swollen ankles. (*See* SITZ BATH in Part Three.)

Other effective hydrotherapy methods include simple, soothing baths and showers, body wraps, foot and hand baths, steam inhalation, and hot and/or cold compresses.

Although many hydrotherapy methods can be performed at home, certain treatments such as hyperthermia, neutral baths, and whirlpool baths, are available only in clinics or hospitals. These treatments must be performed under the careful supervision of a licensed therapist or other health care provider:

• *Hyperthermia.* Fever stimulates the body's immune system to produce the antibodies necessary for fighting certain illnesses. Hyperthermia is a hot-immersion bath used to induce fever in those who cannot achieve one naturally. This hydrotherapy method has been used effectively in the treatment of AIDS, cancer, and upper respiratory infections.

• *Neutral bath.* This therapy, in which the body is submerged to the neck in warm water (92°F to 98°F), helps to soothe the body. Neutral baths are effective in calming nervousness and emotional upsets, reducing joint swelling, and helping the body rid itself of toxins.

• *Whirlpool bath.* Used effectively in treating muscle and joint injuries, whirlpool baths are also used to soothe burns and to stimulate circulation in those with paralysis.

If you are interested in locating a hydrotherapy facility in your area, check with your local hospital. You can also look in the yellow pages of your local telephone directory under "Health Resorts" or "Physical Therapists."

A word of caution: If you have any health-related problems or conditions, be sure to consult with your health care provider before beginning *any* hydrotherapy treatment. All of the treatments presented in this section are recommended for those who are in generally good health.

Hypnotherapy

See under PAIN CONTROL.

Hyperbaric Oxygen Therapy

All human tissues and organs need oxygen in order to function. Hyperbaric oxygen therapy (HBOT) is the administration of oxygen at high atmospheric pressure. This saturates the body with oxygen, increasing the total available amount. HBOT is useful in the treatment of a variety of conditions that are associated with an insufficient amount of oxygen in part or all of the body.

HBOT is administered by placing the individual being treated in a special chamber that delivers pure oxygen at three times the normal atmospheric pressure. In most cases, the entire chamber is pressurized for treatment, and then depressurized before the person is removed. In some cases, oxygen is delivered by mask, making pressurization and depressurization unnecessary.

In the United States, HBOT is most commonly used in cases of trauma, including burns, wounds, injuries from motor vehicle accidents, carbon monoxide poisoning, acute cyanide poisoning, smoke inhalation, and the death of tissues from radiation therapy. HBOT is also used to treat skin grafts that are failing to take, gangrene, decompression sickness, and certain cases of blood loss and anemia. When used after surgery, HBOT has been shown to greatly im-

prove early healing in a majority of cases. It has also been used to bring near-drowning victims out of comas, and it has proved to be a valuable adjunctive treatment for people who have opportunistic infections resulting from immunosuppression, as occurs in people with HIV and AIDS.

In other countries, HBOT has been widely used to treat people who have had strokes and those afflicted with alcoholism, drug addiction, arterial and vascular disorders, and multiple sclerosis. While the therapy has occasionally been used to treat such problems in the U.S., at this time, many of these applications are still controversial among American practitioners. Nevertheless, HBOT is now being used by both conventional and alternative physicians, and continues to gain acceptance for new applications.

Although HBOT is strictly controlled for safety, it may not be appropriate for all individuals. People with a history of emphysema, middle ear infection, or spontaneous pneumothorax (accumulation of air in the chest cavity) may encounter problems with this therapy.

Juicing

Fruits and vegetables are excellent sources of a wide range of vitamins, minerals, and other nutrients, including phytochemicals—compounds that have been shown to combat cancer. Since more of the healthful substances found in fruits and vegetables are being discovered all the time, no supplement pill can contain all of these compounds. Also, because each plant appears to produce particular phytochemicals that work against cancer in particular ways, it is suggested that a rich assortment of fruits and vegetables be included in the diet. It is also recommended that you consume two glasses of live juices a day for health maintenance. Four glasses a day is recommended if you want to speed healing and recovery from illness.

Juicing is an excellent means of adding fruits and vegetables to your diet. Since juice contains the whole fruit or vegetable—except for the fiber, which is the indigestible part of the plant—it contains virtually all of the plants' health-promoting components. Because fresh juices are made from *raw* fruits and vegetables, all of the components remain intact. Vitamin C and other water-soluble vitamins can be damaged by overprocessing or overcooking. Enzymes, which are proteins needed for digestion and other important functions, can also be damaged by cooking. Fresh juice, however, provides all of the plants' healthful ingredients in a form that is easy to digest and absorb. In fact, it has been estimated that fruit and vegetable juices can be assimilated in twenty to thirty minutes.

Ideally, the juices recommended in this book should be made fresh in your kitchen and consumed immediately. Many commercial juices are heat-treated to lengthen shelf life. As just discussed, this process can destroy important

Preparing Produce for Juicing

Juicing is an easy way to make delicious drinks that can boost your health and help you treat a number of disorders. By following these guidelines, you will ensure that your juices are as pure, nutrient-rich, and appetizing as possible:

• Whenever possible, buy and use organically grown produce—produce that is grown without the use of pesticides and other harmful chemicals. This prevents chemical residues from ending up in your juice.

• If you are unable to obtain organically grown fruits and vegetables, peel or thoroughly wash the produce, using a vegetable brush to remove chemical residues and waxes. Most health food stores carry vegetable washes that will help remove any residues.

• When purchasing potatoes for juicing, avoid those with a green tint, and be sure to remove any sprouts or eyes. The chemical solanine, which gives the potato its green cast, can cause diarrhea, vomiting, and abdominal pain.

• When using organically grown produce, feel free to leave the skin on in most cases. Do remove the skin, though,

before juicing apricots, grapefruits, kiwis, oranges, papayas, peaches, and pineapples. The skins of oranges and grapefruits are quite bitter, and also contain a toxic substance that should not be consumed in large amounts. Because kiwis and papayas are tropical fruits, their skins are likely to contain residues of the harmful sprays often used in foreign countries, where some chemicals outlawed in the United States may still be legal. The skins of pineapples are too thick to be processed by most juicers.

• When juicing fruits, leave in small seeds, except when using apples. Apple seeds actually contain cyanide, a toxic substance. Because of their size and hardness, all pits *must* be removed.

• Juice most produce with stems and leaves intact. However, remove carrot and rhubarb greens, as they contain toxic substances.

• When using soft fruits that contain very little water—avocados, bananas, and papayas, for instance—purée the fruits in a blender rather than using a juicer. Then stir the purée into other juices.

---

nutrients. In addition, preservatives may have been added. Even pure, freshly made juices can lose some of their nutrients by being allowed to sit for long periods of time. By buying the best produce available, properly preparing it for juicing, and processing it in your own juicer, you will produce the most healthful, nutrient-rich drinks possible.

The individual entries in Parts Two and Three recommend the use of specific juices for the treatment of specific disorders. It is helpful, though, to be familiar with the three categories into which juices generally fall: green juices, vegetable juices, and fruit juices.

GREEN JUICES OR "GREEN DRINKS"

Green juices cleanse the body of pollutants and have a rejuvenating effect. Made from a variety of green vegetables, green juices are rich in chlorophyll, which helps to purify the blood, build red blood cells, detoxify and heal the body, and provide the body with fast energy.

Green juices can be made with alfalfa sprouts, cabbage, kale, dandelion greens, spinach, and other green vegetables, including wheatgrass. Wheatgrass juice is particularly important in any cancer treatment, especially when radiation therapy is involved.

To sweeten and dilute your green juices, try adding fresh carrot and apple juice. (No other fruit juices should be added.) Steam-distilled water is another good addition.

Although green juices have great health benefits, they should be consumed in moderation. Try drinking about 8 to 10 ounces a day. The following is an excellent "green drink":

Ageless Cocktail

4–5 carrots
3 sprigs fresh parsley
1 large handful spinach
1 large handful kale
1 beet, including tops
1 clove garlic, peeled

1. Thoroughly wash all vegetables, peeling the carrots and beet if they were not grown organically. Cut the vegetables into pieces small enough to fit into the juicer.

2. Process the vegetables in the juicer, and drink immediately.

VEGETABLE JUICES

Fresh vegetable juices are restorers and builders. They boost the immune system, remove acid wastes, and balance the metabolism. They also aid in the control of obesity by removing excess body fat.

Among the most healthful and delicious of the vegetable juices are beet, cabbage, carrot, celery, cucumber, kale, parsley, turnip, spinach, watercress, and wheatgrass juice. Carrot juice is probably the most popular of the juices, and is packed with beta-carotene, the vitamin A precursor that helps fight cancer. Because carrots are the sweetest of the vegetables, their juice is not just delicious on its own, but is great for mixing with other vegetables to increase their appeal. On the other hand, strong-flavored vegetables—broccoli, celery, onions, parsley, rutabaga, and turnips, for instance—should be used in small amounts only.

Garlic is a great addition to vegetable drinks. Before juicing, drop the garlic into vinegar for 1 minute to destroy any bacteria and mold on its surface. To avoid irritating the lining of the intestinal tract, use only 1 fresh garlic clove in 2 glasses of juice.

For the greatest health benefits, use many different vegetables when making your juices. That way, you will provide your body with a variety of important nutrients. The recipes that follow are just two of the many healthful vegetable juice drinks that you might want to try.

Potassium/Raw Potato Juice

1 pound potatoes
1 carrot or 1 stalk celery (optional)
6–8 ounces steam-distilled water

1. Scrub the potatoes well, and cut out any eyes.

2. Cut each potato in half. Cut the peel from the potato, making sure to keep about ½ inch of potato on the peel. Set aside the potato center for another use.

3. Cut the potato skins into small enough pieces to fit into the juicer. If desired, wash the carrot or celery, peeling the carrot if it was not grown organically. Cut into pieces.

4. Process the vegetables in the juicer. Add the water, and drink immediately. Do not allow to stand.

Cabbage Juice for Ulcers

¼–½ head cabbage
1 apple or 2 carrots
¼ cup steam-distilled water

1. Thoroughly wash the vegetables and fruit, peeling the apple or carrots if they were not grown organically. Cut the produce into small enough pieces to fit into the juicer.

2. Process the vegetables and fruit in the juicer. Add the water, and drink immediately. Do not allow to stand.

FRUIT JUICES

Fruit juices help cleanse the body and nourish it with important nutrients, including cancer-fighting antioxidants.

Although any fruit can be juiced, certain juices are particularly healthful and delicious. One favorite cleansing juice is watermelon. To make this refreshing drink, place a whole piece of watermelon—with the rind intact—in the juicer. Other delicious juices can be made with apples, apricots, bananas, berries, citrus fruits, kiwi, melons, pears—with just about any fruit that you want to use.

You can enjoy fruit juices at any time of the day. About 10 to 12 ounces per day is recommended. The following is just one of the delicious fruit juice drinks you can make at home.

Kiwi Deluxe

1 firm kiwi, peeled
1 small bunch red grapes
1 green apple

1. Wash all of the fruit thoroughly, peeling the apple if it was not grown organically. Cut the fruit into small enough pieces to fit into the juicer.

2. Process the fruit in the juicer. Pour over ice, and drink.

Making Kombucha Tea

Kombucha tea is made from the kombucha tea "mushroom," a large, flat, pancake-shaped fungus-like growth. Technically, the kombucha is *not* a mushroom, nor is it purely a fungus. Rather, it is part lichen, part bacterium xylinum, and part natural yeast culture. When placed in a mixture of ordinary sugar and tea for seven to ten days, the kombucha produces both a winey-tasting health-restoring tea and a new "baby" kombucha.

The history of kombucha tea can be traced back 2,000 years to China, Russia, Japan, and Korea. Over time, it has been been used as a curative in many regions, primarily in Manchuria and Russia. Russian scientists studied the fungus during the 1950s, 1960s, and 1970s. According to the Moscow Central Bacteriological Institute, kombucha tea, when properly made, contains a number of substances important for good health, including gluconic acid, which impedes the progression of viral infections and can dissolve gallstones; hyaluronic acid, a component of connective tissue; chondroitin sulfate, a component of cartilage; and mucoitin-sulfuric acid, a component of the stomach lining and the vitreous humor of the eye. The beverage also contains vitamins B_1 (thiamine), B_2 (riboflavin), B_3 (niacin), B_6 (pyridoxine), and B_{12}; folic acid; lactic acid; dextrogyral; and usnic acid, a substance with strong antibacterial and antiviral effects.

According to researchers and to anecdotal evidence, kombucha tea is a potent immune system booster, and can be an important part of treatment for acne, aging skin, AIDS, arteriosclerosis (hardening of the arteries), arthritis, asthma, bronchitis, cancer, candidiasis, chronic fatigue, constipation, diabetes, diarrhea and other digestive disorders, hair loss, hemorrhoids, high cholesterol, hypoglycemia, incontinence in both men and women, kidney and gallstone disorders, menopausal problems, multiple sclerosis, premenstrual syndrome, prostate problems, psoriasis, and weight problems. It is also said to greatly increase energy, and to promote a general feeling of well-being.

Many people prepare kombucha tea at home, as the tea-making process is both easy and inexpensive. However, kombucha tea beverages are available commercially in health food stores, and are just as effective and nutritious as homemade brews. The one drawback to the commercial products is that some have a sour taste due to the longer fermentation process. The longer process does not, however, affect the product's potency. Also available are extracts and tinctures made from the pressed fungus. These products are handy when traveling, and are particularly effective for motion sickness.

There is some debate regarding the best time to consume kombucha tea. Most proponents of the tea feel that it should be poured off after four to six days, and then allowed to sit in a container for another three days before being consumed. Russian researchers have concluded that the antibiotic activity is at its highest level on the seventh and eighth days. Be aware that if left to brew too long—for over a month—the tea will turn to vinegar. While you would not want to drink this vinegar as a beverage, you can use it just as you would use any other vinegar.

PROCEDURE

The preparation of kombucha tea is a simple process that requires only a small amount of equipment and ingredients. Before following this procedure, be sure to remove your rings, as metal should never touch the "mushroom." To prevent contamination, make sure that your utensils and work area are scrupulously clean. Also keep in mind that ingredient substitutions should *never* be made. For instance, a reduction of the amount of sugar or the substitution of brown sugar for white could adversely affect the health of the fungus. White sugar is essential to its survival.

Keep in mind that tobacco smoke can kill your kombucha. If you must smoke, do so outside. Better yet, quit.

After using one kombucha "mushroom" for some time, environmental stresses may affect the organism, causing the tea to taste flat. When this happens, use green tea, rather than black, to make the growing medium, and use the tea from a "livelier" fungus until the old one is restored.

To make the tea, you will need:

3 quarts distilled water
1 cup refined white sugar
4 tea bags (green or black tea only)
4 ounces newly harvested kombucha tea or 4 ounces apple cider vinegar
1 large kombucha "mushroom"
6-quart glass or enamel pot
4-quart glass bowl
1 square of cheesecloth
6-inch rubber band
Wooden or plastic spoon

1. Place the water in the glass or enamel pot over high heat. (Do not use an aluminum pot.) Add the sugar, and boil for 5 minutes.

2. Remove the pot from the heat. Add the tea bags to the pot, and steep for 10 minutes. Wash your hands, and remove and discard the tea bags.

3. Pour the tea into the glass bowl (do not use crystal, metal, ceramic, or plastic), and allow it to reach room temperature. Add the harvested Kobucha tea or vinegar.

4. Place the mushroom smooth side up in the "growing" tea. Cover the bowl with the cheesecloth, and secure the cloth with the rubber band.

5. Place the bowl in a dark, quiet, ventilated place with a temperature between 70°F and 90°F. (A shelf in the kitchen is an ideal place.) Allow the bowl to remain there for 7 to 10 days. Do not refrigerate.

6. After 7 to 10 days, remove the "mushrooms" with a wooden or plastic spoon. Note that a "baby" kombucha is now growing on top of the original kombucha. Separate the baby from the mother by gently pulling them apart with clean hands.

7. Using the cloth as a strainer, pour the new tea from the bowl into a glass bottle, leaving some space at the top of the bottle. (Do not store the tea in plastic, as chemicals can leach out of the container into the tea.) Store in the refrigerator, and drink 4 ounces 3 times a day, before or after meals. (Do not drink more than the recommended amount.) Use the 2 "mushrooms" and part of the newly harvested tea to make more tea.

If you are unable to obtain a kombucha tea "mushroom" from a friend, you can get a mushroom and growing kit from Laurel Farms of Studio City, California. Prepared kombucha tea beverages, capsules, and extracts can be obtained from Pronatura, Inc., located in Niles, Illinois. (*See* MANUFACTURER AND DISTRIBUTOR INFORMATION in the Appendix.)

Light Therapy

The body's circadian rhythm—its inner clock—is regulated by the pineal gland. Affected by the absence or presence of light, the pineal gland is responsible for controlling such bodily functions as hormone production, body temperature, and the timing of sleep. Disturbances in the circadian rhythm can lead to depression as well as insomnia and other sleep disorders. The use of natural sunlight and various forms of light therapy has been effective in reestablishing the body's natural rhythm.

Natural sunlight contains the full-wavelength spectrum needed for maintaining health. It triggers the impulses that regulate most bodily functions. Artificial lighting—incandescent and fluorescent—lacks the complete balanced spectrum found in sunlight. Without certain wavelengths, the body cannot absorb some nutrients. Inadequate exposure to proper light can contribute to or worsen such illnesses and conditions as fatigue, depression, stroke, hair loss, suppressed immune function, cancer, hyperactivity, osteoporosis, and Alzheimer's disease.

A variety of light therapies has been used effectively in the treatment of a number of disorders. Some of the most common therapies are:

• *Bright Light Therapy*. This therapy involves the use of bright white light that ranges in intensity from 2,000 to 5,000 lux. (A lux is equal to the light of one candle: the average indoor light ranges from 50 to 500 lux.) Bright light therapy has proven helpful in treating cases of bulimia, sleep phase syndrome (a condition in which the person cannot fall asleep until the middle of the night), and irregular menstrual cycles.

• *Cold Laser Therapy*. Utilizing a low-intensity beam of laser light that stimulates the natural healing process at a cellular level, cold laser therapy has proven effective in the treatment of pain, trauma, and orthopedic myofascial syndrome. It has also been used in dentistry, dermatology, and neurology.

• *Full-Spectrum Light Therapy*. Exposure to natural sunlight and other forms of full-spectrum light is effective in relieving a number of disorders, including depression, hyperactivity, hypertension, insomnia, migraines, and premenstrual syndrome. Sunlight has long been used to treat babies with jaundice. Full-spectrum light, as well as bright white light, is effective in the treatment of seasonal affective disorder (SAD). Common symptoms of SAD, which is also called the "winter blues," are depression, fatigue, overeating, and lowered libido.

• *Photodynamic Light Therapy*. This therapy involves injecting light-absorbing dye into specific types of malignant tumors, then exposing the tumors to certain light. The dye absorbs the light, causing a chemical reaction that, in turn, kills the cancer cells.

• *Syntonic Optometry*. In this treatment, colored light is applied directly into the eyes to intensify the control centers of the brain that regulate various body functions. Syntonic optometry has been useful in treating pain, inflammation, headaches, and traumatic brain injuries.

• *Ultraviolet Light Therapy*. Ultraviolet light therapies are used to treat illnesses such as asthma and cancer, as well as conditions like high cholesterol and premenstrual syndrome. The sun's UVA rays, which have longer wavelengths than UVB and UVC rays, are considered the least harmful. There are a variety of ultraviolet light therapies. *UVA-1 therapy* isolates a portion of the UVA wavelength. It is used in the treatment of systemic lupus erythematosus. *Hemoirradiation therapy* involves removing an amount of blood (up to a pint) from the body, irradiating it with ultraviolet light, then reinjecting it. This therapy has been used successfully in treating asthma, blood poisoning, cancer, infections, rheumatoid arthritis, and symptoms stemming from AIDS. Patients with vitiligo and psoriasis can benefit from the treatment of *PUVA light therapy* (psoralen UV-A). First, patients are injected with psoralen, a light-sensitive drug; then they are exposed to UV light.

Further information on light therapies is available from the Environmental Health & Light Research Institute, 16057 Tampa Palms Boulevard, Suite 227, Tampa, FL 33647; telephone 800–544–4878.

Massage

See under PAIN CONTROL.

Meditation

See under PAIN CONTROL.

Music and Sound Therapy

Music therapy is the controlled use of music in the treatment of physical, mental, or emotional disorders. A variety of problems—including depression, high blood pressure, asthma, migraines, ulcers, and a range of physical disabilities—are currently treated with music. In general, the nature of the problem dictates the precise form of the therapy. For some problems, specific musical pieces are played for the person being treated. In other instances, individuals actively participate in rhythm bands, group singing, individual or group music lessons, or music-accompanied physical activities.

Music has been shown to have various therapeutic capabilities. When played for individuals or groups with mental or emotional problems or with stress-related ailments, music can reduce anxiety and lessen irritability. In work with blind people, music has facilitated the development of better auditory perception. As a part of physical therapy, music has been used to stimulate or regulate movement. Also as a means of physical therapy, the playing of instruments has been employed both for its psychological benefits, such as greater self-confidence, and for its physical benefits, such as the strengthening of weak mouth and lip muscles.

Music is not the only type of sound that has been found to have therapeutic value. For many years, environmental sounds—the sound of a running stream, a waterfall, or bird songs, for instance—have been used by therapists and psychologists as a means of treatment. These sounds, it appears, can do much to relieve stress and lift depression.

Anyone can take advantage of the ability of music and other sounds to induce relaxation, with or without professional guidance. Soft music and soothing sounds, used alone or with relaxation techniques, can effectively alleviate stress, relax muscles, and evoke a positive mood. Researchers suggest that these sounds promote the production of endorphins, the body's own painkillers, and can thereby also help in the control of pain. In some cases, of course—when music is to be applied to physical therapy, for instance—an experienced practitioner should be consulted.

Pain Control

Pain is a message sent by the body to the brain, signaling that disease, injury, or strenuous activity has caused trouble in some area. Without pain, you would remain unaware of many problems—from torn ligaments to appendicitis—until the disorders became serious. At low levels, pain can motivate you to rest the injured area so that tissues can be repaired and additional damage can be prevented. When severe, pain can motivate you to seek treatment as well.

Not all pain, though, appears to serve a useful function. While *acute pain*, the pain described above, can alert us to a problem that needs immediate attention, in some cases pain lasts long after an injured area has healed. In other instances, pain may be caused by recurring backache, migraines and other headaches, arthritis, and other disorders. Referred to as *chronic pain*—which may be defined as pain that occurs, continually or intermittently, for more than six months—this pain may signal an ongoing problem that cannot be eliminated through treatment. In such a case, pain management often becomes the treatment goal.

For some people, pain is cyclical—pain produces anxiety and this anxiety intensifies the pain. Fear and anticipation of the physical problem can also heighten the pain, leading to feelings of depression and helplessness. When experiencing such pain, it is natural to limit one's activities. This can lead to a "chronic pain cycle," which can adversely affect one's confidence and self-esteem.

Being aware of the chronic pain cycle as well as understanding its psychological effects can help you avoid being drawn into it:

1. The cycle generally begins with prolonged periods of rest and inactivity, causing a loss in physical strength, endurance, and flexibility. As a result, you may begin to lose confidence in your ability to do things, causing a lowering of personal goals.

2. Inability to perform usual activities at home or work is likely to promote feelings of frustration, and you may begin perceiving yourself as unproductive. This sense of lowered self-esteem may further lead to depression.

3. During times when the pain subsides or is more tolerable than usual, you may overexert yourself in an effort to prove to yourself and others that you can still do the things you did before the chronic pain began.

4. As a result of the overexertion, the pain often returns and may be more severe than before. You may find yourself unable to finish tasks or accomplish goals. Discouraged and in pain, you begin limiting your activities, and the cycle begins again.

One way to keep from getting caught up in the chronic pain cycle is through pain management. Often, the reduction of physical pain can prevent the cycle from starting.

There are a variety of treatments that can help alleviate pain. Some do so on a purely physical level, perhaps by interrupting the pain process or desensitizing nerve endings. Others approach pain control on a psychological level, by affecting the mind's perception of the pain. In the treatment of pain, however, there often is no clear-cut separation of the physical and the psychological. Just as a physical reduction of pain may decrease anxiety and improve outlook, so can the mind be used to relax muscles and effect other physical changes that then reduce symptoms.

The following sections are meant to introduce you to some of the many pain-control techniques now available. Depending on the cause of your pain, the level of your pain, and your own treatment preferences, you may want to try one or more of these techniques. While some of these approaches, like the use of hot and cold packs, can easily be used on your own; other techniques, like biofeedback, require at least initial training by a qualified practitioner; and some, like chiropractic, must be performed by a professional. When possible, get referrals from your health care provider or from friends. If a reputable pain clinic is available to you, this can be a wonderful resource—one that offers a range of practitioners experienced in using a variety of pain-control techniques. Make sure that the professional you consult has successfully treated a condition such as yours. Try to obtain the names of others who have used this practitioner and speak to them about their therapies.

ACUPUNCTURE

This ancient Chinese practice is based on the belief that health is determined by *chi*, the vital life energy that flows through every living thing. This energy is thought to move through the body along pathways called meridians, each of which is linked to a specific organ. If the flow of energy is balanced, the individual enjoys good health. If something interrupts this flow, however, various problems, including pain, can result. Acupuncture is used to restore proper energy flow, and, as a result, good health.

In acupuncture treatment, the acupuncturist inserts thin needles at specific points in the body. Although slight discomfort may occasionally be felt upon insertion of the needle, the treatment is virtually painless. The needles may be left in place for anywhere from a few minutes to half an hour. To support the acupuncture therapy, the practitioner may recommend taking herbs in the form of teas and capsules, and may also suggest specific lifestyle changes and exercises. Relief may be experienced after only one treatment, or after a series of treatments.

Although used for a variety of health problems, including addictions and mental disorders, in the United States, acupuncture is perhaps most commonly used to relieve pain, including backache and migraine headaches. Studies have indicated that acupuncture may stimulate the production of endorphins, the body's own painkillers. Completely safe, acupuncture has no known side effects.

For more information on acupuncture and a list of practitioners in your area, you can contact the following organizations:

American Association of Oriental Medicine
433 Front Street
Catasauqua, PA 18032
610–433–2448

Sitike Counseling Center
1211 Old Mission Road
San Francisco, CA 94080
415–589–9305

ACUPRESSURE

Based on the same beliefs that are the foundation of acupuncture (see the above discussion), acupressure—also known as "contact healing"—is actually the older of the two methods. Acupressure and the healing art of shiatsu (a massage technique) are commonly referred to as "acupuncture without needles." Like acupuncture, acupressure seeks to restore health by restoring the normal flow of *chi*, the life energy that flows through the body along pathways called meridians. While acupuncture uses the insertion of needles to promote energy flow, acupressure uses finger and hand pressure. During pressure stimulation, neurotransmitters, which help to inhibit the reception and transmission of pain, are released.

Acupressure is a safe, simple, and inexpensive treatment. Although it may be performed by a skilled practitioner, because of the treatment's noninvasive nature, acupressure may also be performed by the individual for the immediate relief of pain. In fact, a number of self-acupressure techniques, including Acu-Yoga, *Do-In*, and *Tui Na*, can help you control pain through finger pressure, massage, body positioning, and a variety of other means.

More information on acupressure is available from the Acupressure Institute, 1533 Shattuck Avenue, Berkeley, CA 94709; telephone 510–845–1059.

BIOFEEDBACK

Biofeedback combines a variety of relaxation methods such as guided imagery and meditation with the use of instruments that monitor the individual's responses. Over time, this teaches you to consciously regulate a number of your own *autonomic functions*—heart rate, blood pressure, and other processes previously believed to be involuntary. By consciously regulating these functions, you can control a number of problems, including pain.

During a biofeedback session, electrodes connected to a monitoring unit are taped or otherwise painlessly attached to the skin. The machine may measure any one of a number of things, including skin temperature, pulse, blood pressure, muscle tension, and brain wave activity. As you use various techniques, such as relaxation, to create the desired response—lower blood pressure, for instance—the machine, through sound or images, provides moment-by-moment feedback on your progress. Eventually, with the practitioner's help, you should become able to effect the desired response without the use of the machine.

Although biofeedback has been successfully used to help control a wide range of health problems, it is perhaps best known for its use in the treatment of headaches. In a large number of cases, biofeedback has been successfully used to avert the onset of migraines. It has also been used to treat injuries, as well as to relieve the pain of TMJ syndrome.

It should be noted that biofeedback only measures stress; it does not cure it. Sessions should be conducted in conjunction with other therapies under the watchful eye of a qualified health care practitioner.

If you are considering biofeedback training, you can contact the following organizations for a list of certified practitioners in your area:

Association for Applied Psychophysiology
  and Biofeedback
10200 West 44th Avenue, Suite 304
Wheat Ridge, CO 80033
303–422–8436

Center for Applied Psychophysiology
Menninger Clinic
P.O. Box 829
Topeka, KS 66601–08829
913–273–7500

CHIROPRACTIC

Chiropractic is a form of treatment that seeks to eliminate pain—and, in some cases, other problems—through the manipulation of the spinal column. Chiropractors believe that if the spinal vertebrae are properly aligned, impulses from the brain are able to travel freely along the spinal cord to the various organs, maintaining healthy function throughout the body. If a misalignment of the spine occurs, however, the normal flow of impulses is disrupted, resulting in pain as well as other physical disorders. Chiropractors seek to return the spine's alignment to its normal, healthy state. This permits the nervous system to regain normal function, allowing the body to heal itself and eliminate the pain.

After the chiropractor locates any spinal misalignments, chiropractic adjustment is used to reestablish normal function. This adjustment may involve touch; active motion, in which the patient bends and stretches in specific ways; and passive movement, in which the doctor assists the patient's movements. A hand-held rubber-tipped instrument may be used to gently manipulate the vertebrae. Some chiropractors support adjustment therapy with applications of heat and cold, electrical stimulation, nutrition, and other natural therapies. Chiropractic does not use drugs or surgery.

The U.S. Department of Health and Human Services lists spinal manipulation as a "proven treatment" for low back pain. Chiropractic therapy is also used to treat arthritis, bursitis, and a variety of other disorders, including many nonpainful ailments.

GUIDED IMAGERY

Much research has indicated that bodily functions previously thought to be totally beyond conscious control can be modified using psychological techniques. Guided imagery, a technique that has grown in popularity in the last several years, uses this mind-body connection to help people cope with a variety of disorders, including pain.

Researchers have established a link between negative emotions and lowered immune function. Conversely, they have found a connection between positive emotions and a healthy immune response. Guided imagery—the mind thinking in pictures—is an effective tool for eliminating negative thoughts and replacing them with positive ones.

Through guided imagery, the mind conjures up mental pictures or scenes in order to better direct the body's energy. You can, for instance, close your eyes and visualize the pain as a sharp knife in the affected body area. Then you can imagine that the knife is being withdrawn, and that a cooling, soothing cream is being applied to the area. Through imagery, people with cancer commonly visualize the cancer cells in their bodies as weak and their white "fighter" cells as strong and destructive. In other instances, people have found that, rather than visualizing the pain, focusing on a pleasant scene, such as a beautiful day at the beach, promotes relaxation and substantially controls pain.

Used successfully in the treatment of rheumatoid arthritis, cancer, and other illnesses, guided imagery has also been shown to reduce stress, slow the heart rate, and stimulate the immune system. Taught properly, guided imagery can be an effective form of self-care; however, it is not meant to replace your doctor or prescribed medication. Rather, it can be used to enhance your prescribed course of treatment.

More information on this mind-body healing technique is available from The Academy of Guided Imagery, P.O. Box 2070, Mill Valley, CA 94942; telephone 800–726–2070.

HEAT AND COLD THERAPY

Hot and cold packs are simple-to-use pain-control tools that have been widely employed for many years. When applied singly or in combination, these techniques often provide relief not only from the pain itself, but, in some cases, from any accompanying swelling.

Heat

Pain from backaches, arthritis, and similar disorders often responds well to heat therapy. By increasing the temperature in selected areas of the body, this treatment enhances blood circulation and helps muscles to relax, reducing stiffness and increasing mobility.

Heat can be applied to the affected area through a number of means, including hot water bottles and electric heating pads. Often, moist heat works better than dry heat. Some electric heating pads are capable of producing moist heat, as are some gel packs. Hot showers and wet towels are other means of concentrating moist heat on a painful area. Poultices can also be effective and, for certain disorders, sitz baths are helpful. (*See* USING A POULTICE and SITZ BATH in Part Three.)

Use all forms of heat therapy with caution. Monitor the intensity of the heat and the duration and frequency of the treatment. Do not allow yourself to fall asleep while using an electric heating pad. Regardless of the heat source, a good rule of thumb is twenty minutes on, and twenty minutes off. After removing the heat, firmly rub or massage the affected area. This will both dissipate the heat and help relieve tension. Do not massage the area if it is inflamed or has just sustained a serious injury. And never massage the area if you have phlebitis or other vascular problems.

Counterirritants

A variety of over-the-counter topical products, such as capsaicin cream, Ben-Gay, and Icy Hot, can be used in lieu of a heat pack to treat localized pain. As counterirritants, these products stimulate blood flow to the affected area, acting much like heat. While such products may be relatively convenient and easy to use, they should be used with discretion. Do not apply anything but ordinary clothing to an area that has been treated with a counterirritant. Heating pads placed over treated areas can increase the medication's rate of absorption into the skin, thus causing serious damage.

Cold

Because of its ability to prevent swelling, cold packs are often the treatment of choice directly following a strain, sprain, or other injury. In such cases, cold packs alone should be used during the first twenty-four to thirty-six hours. Cold packs can also help relieve certain types of chronic pain.

Ice packs are probably the most common means of applying cold. These packs can simply be applied to the painful area, or they can be rubbed on the area using a circular motion for five to seven minutes. Lower back pain seems to be particularly responsive to ice rubs. Cold gel packs, which are kept in the freezer between uses, are also effective, and, because of their pliable consistency, are often more comfortable than ice packs.

Like heat therapy, cold therapy should be used with caution. Wrap ice packs and gel packs in a towel before applying them to the affected area. Then apply the packs for no more than twenty minutes at a time.

Heat and Cold

In some cases, alternating hot and cold treatments work best. For a painful and stiff neck, for instance, try using a warm shower to relieve tension. After the shower, use a five- to seven-minute ice massage to reduce swelling and further relieve pain.

Experimentation is the best way to discover whether heat, cold, or alternating heat and cold best relieves your discomfort. If several applications of one type of treatment—say, heat—do not provide any relief, try the opposite treatment. If your pain persists, and especially if you are not sure of its cause, consult your health care provider.

HERBS

Many herbs have been used for centuries for their pain-relieving properties. Some of the best include:

• Angelica, black haw, cramp bark, kava kava, rosemary, and valerian root are good for pain related to cramps and muscle spasms.

• A tea made of blue violet, catnip, chamomile, gotu kola, licorice, rosemary, white willow, or wood betony is effective in relieving tension and nerve pain. DLPA complex by Nature's Plus, containing white willow bark plus DL-phenylalanine and bromelain, is a good natural pain reliever.

Caution: Do not use chamomile on an ongoing basis, and avoid it completely if you are allergic to ragweed. Do not use licorice on a daily basis for more than seven days in a row, and avoid it completely if you have high blood pressure. Do not take a product containing phenylalanine if you are pregnant or nursing a baby; if you take an MAO inhibitor drug; or if you suffer from panic attacks, diabetes, or phenylketonuria (PKU). If you have high blood pressure, start with the lowest dosage and monitor your blood pressure before increasing the dose.

• Capsaicin, an ingredient in cayenne (capsicum), can provide pain relief when regularly applied to the affected area. Now available in Zostrix, an over-the-counter topical cream, capsaicin is thought to relieve pain by limiting the production of a neural pain transmitter called substance P. Although the application of capsaicin may cause a burning sensation at first, repeated use keeps nerves from replenishing their supply of substance P, so that pain is not transmitted to the brain. In studies, capsaicin has been used to control the pain of postherpetic neuralgia, diabetic neuropathy, rheumatoid arthritis, osteoarthritis, and cluster headaches. Cayenne may also help to alleviate pain if taken orally.

• Hops, kava kava, passion flower, valerian root, wild lettuce, and wood betony have muscle-relaxing properties, and may help to relieve lower back pain.

• Essential oils of jasmine, juniper, lavender, peppermint, rose, rosemary, and thyme have been effective in the treatment of a variety of types of pain.

• Migraine Pain Reliever from Natural Care is an herbal blend that has been effective in relieving migraines.

• Fresh papaya juice and/or fresh pineapple is highly recommended for the treatment of inflammation, heartburn, ulcers, back pain, and digestive disorders.

• Saffron has been found to be effective in treating abdominal pain after childbirth.

HYPNOTHERAPY

Like meditation and visualization, hypnotherapy is a method by which a qualified physician or therapist can induce a positive mental state in an individual. The therapist attempts to quiet the person's conscious mind to make the unconscious mind more accessible. Hypnosis is designed to generate a state of deep relaxation in which there is a heightened receptivity to suggestion through the calm repetition of words and statements. Once an individual is in this state, the practitioner provides simple verbal suggestions that help the mind block the awareness of pain and replace it with a more positive feeling, such as a feeling of warmth. If the pain is the result of an earlier injury, the practitioner may also help the individual more clearly remember the incident—a practice that often helps alleviate anxiety and thus reduce pain.

Hypnotherapy enhances positive imagery, helps to reduce anxiety, and induces a deep level of relaxation. During a hypnotic state, the mind is highly focused and fully aware of the situation, enabling the person to concentrate without being distracted. During hypnosis, breathing and pulse rate slow down and blood pressure may drop.

No one can be forced into hypnosis. You must be a willing participant in the process. Good rapport between therapist and client is important.

Hypnosis has been used successfully to control back pain, joint pain, burn pain, and the pain of migraines and other headaches. This technique can be a valuable self-help tool, as you can learn to hypnotize yourself whenever you need it. However, self-hypnosis must first be learned from a licensed psychologist, a certified hypnotherapist, or another professional with experience in hypnotherapy.

MASSAGE

Massage, which falls under the category of bodywork, involves the manipulation of muscles and other soft tissues. It is beneficial in treating a wide range of conditions, including muscle spasms and pain, soreness from injury, and headaches. Massage works to relieve pain in a number of ways: by promoting muscle relaxation; by increasing lymphatic circulation, and thereby reducing inflammation; by breaking up scar tissue and adhesions; by promoting blood flow through the muscles; and by promoting drainage of the sinus fluids.

Massage is not advisable for everyone. Those with a history of phlebitis, high blood pressure, or any other vascular disorder should not receive any type of deep muscle massage performed with strong pressure. Always check with a physician before receiving deep muscle massage. Massage should not be performed on inflamed areas or on individuals with malignant or infectious conditions.

A variety of massage therapies are currently in use. Each is based on a different theory and utilizes specific techniques. The following bodywork systems represent some of those most widely used:

• *Deep Tissue Massage.* Used to release chronic muscular tension, deep tissue massage is applied with greater pressure and on deeper muscles than classic Swedish massage. It generally focuses on a specific problem area.

• *Esalen Massage.* This massage technique attempts to bring about a sense of well-being through deep and beneficial states of consciousness. Esalen massage focuses on the mind and body as a whole. It is a hypnotic method that uses slow, rhythmic movements to bring about a general state of relaxation.

• *The Feldenkrais Method.* The idea of "self-image" is central to the theory and technique of this method. Through exercise and "touch," the therapist helps eliminate negative muscle patterns and the feelings and thoughts associated with them. This method uses two approaches: *Awareness through Movement* and *Functional Integration.* Awareness through Movement employs a group approach in which the participants are guided through a slow, gentle sequence designed to replace old movement patterns with new ones. Functional Integration is an individualized approach that uses hands-on touch and movement. The Feldenkrais Method differs from most other types of massage in that there is no attempt to alter the body's structure. Rather, it is through touch that the practitioner attempts to communicate a sense of improved self-image and movement.

• *Neuromuscular Massage.* This form of deep tissue massage concentrates on a specific muscle. Through the use of concentrated finger pressure, sensitive "trigger points" are released and blood flow is increased.

• *Rolfing or Structural Integration.* This method is based on the belief that function is improved when body parts are properly aligned. Through manipulation of connective tissue linking muscles to bones, the therapist attempts to restore fuller movement, resulting in a more balanced body.

• *Shiatsu.* Literally meaning "finger pressure" in Japanese, this Oriental massage technique focuses on acupressure points to restore and maintain health. Through firm, rhythmic pressures applied to specific points for three to ten seconds each, the Shiatsu therapist attempts to unblock the energy that flows through the acupuncture meridians.

• *Sports Massage.* A combination of kneading, passive stretching, and range of deep-tissue motions, sports massage is designed to ease muscle strain and promote flexibility. It is most effective when applied before or after exercising.

• *Swedish Massage.* This technique, developed by Peter Hendricks Ling in the early 1800s, uses kneading, stroking, tapping, and shaking to induce the body to relax. Swedish massage can also relieve soreness and swelling, as well as promote rehabilitation after an injury.

So numerous are your massage choices that before making a decision, you might wish to visit your local library. There, resources will familiarize you with what is available, and help you either learn techniques of self-massage, or choose the type of massage therapist who can best provide the help you need.

For further information about massage therapy, you can contact the following organizations:

The American Massage Therapy Association
820 Davis Street, Suite 100
Evanston, IL 60201
312–761–2682

Esalen Institute
Big Sur, CA 93920
408–667–3000

Feldenkrais Guild
P.O. Box 489
Albany Trail, OR 97321
503–926–0981

International Rolf Institute
P.O. Box 1868
Boulder, CO 80306
303u449–5903

MEDICATION

Several over-the-counter medications are available to help you control your pain. Two of the simplest nonnarcotic pain relievers are acetylsalicylic acid (aspirin) and acetaminophen (found in Tylenol, Datril, and many other products). Both of these medications can help relieve mild to moderate pain. Aspirin can also reduce swelling and inflammation. If you take aspirin for pain relief, you should also take supplements of vitamin C, as this nutrient has been shown to make the effects of the analgesic last longer.

Nonsteroidal anti-inflammatory drugs, another type of nonnarcotic analgesic, may also be helpful in the relief of aches and pains. These products include ibuprofen (Advil, Nuprin, and others), ketoprofen (Orudis), and naproxen sodium (Aleve).

Although over-the-counter analgesics are generally regarded as safe, discretion should be exercised in their use. If you take acetaminophen, be sure to avoid the consumption of alcohol, as this can both decrease the effectiveness of the drug and cause damage to the liver. If you take aspirin, be aware that it may affect the stomach. More important, you should *never* give aspirin to a child, especially a child with a cold or flulike symptoms. Regardless of the pain reliever being used, you should never take more than the dosage directed on the label without first consulting your health care provider. Virtually any medication can cause problems when used inappropriately.

MEDITATION

Meditation, which has been practiced for thousands of years, is an effective means of treating stress and managing pain. Broadly defined, meditation is an activity that calms the mind and keeps it focused on the present. In the meditative state, the mind is not cluttered with thoughts or memories of the past, nor is it concerned with future events.

There are hundreds of meditation techniques, most of which fall into one of two categories: *concentrative* and *mindfulness*. During concentrative meditation, attention is focused on a single sound, an object, or one's breath, to bring about a calm, tranquil mind. One simple, common technique involves sitting or lying comfortably in a quiet environment, closing your eyes, and focusing attention on your breath as you inhale through your nose for a count of three, then exhale through your mouth for a count of five. This focus on your breathing rhythm — slow, deep, regular breaths—allows your mind to become tranquil and aware.

During mindfulness meditation, the mind becomes aware of but does not react to the wide variety of sensations, feelings, and images tied in with a current activity. By sitting quietly and allowing the images of your surroundings to pass through your mind without reacting to or becoming involved with them, you can attain a calm state of mind.

Much research has been done on transcendental meditation (TM). TM brings about a state of deep relaxation in which the body is totally at rest, but the mind is highly alert. Studies show that meditation, especially TM, is effective in controlling anxiety, enhancing the immune system, and reducing conditions such as high blood pressure. Meditation has also been used successfully to treat chronic pain and to control substance abuse.

Meditation is an effective self-care technique that can be a useful part of your health care program. However, it is not an alternative to recommended medical treatment.

RELAXATION TECHNIQUES

Once pain occurs—whether from injury or another source—your psychological reaction to it can have a profound effect on the duration and intensity of the pain. In some people, pain is cyclical; pain produces anxiety and tension, and tension intensifies pain. In the case of disorders such as migraines, tension can be a significant cause of the initial pain. By releasing tension, relaxation techniques can greatly reduce certain types of pain and actually prevent some pain from occurring.

A variety of relaxation techniques are available, including biofeedback, deep breathing, guided imagery, meditation, progressive relaxation, and yoga. These techniques facilitate deep relaxation and reduce stress. The advantage of relaxation therapy is that you can easily master these methods, either on your own or with the help of a professional, and then use them whenever they are needed.

TENS UNIT THERAPY

Transcutaneous electric nerve stimulation (TENS) units can be helpful in dealing with localized pain, and are widely used both in doctors' offices and physiotherapy clinics. TENS therapy can also be performed at home.

With this technique, electrodes are placed on the skin and joined to the TENS unit with wires. Electric signals are then sent to the nerve endings, blocking pain signals before they reach the brain. It is believed that these signals may also stimulate the production of endorphins, the body's natural painkillers. TENS therapy is not considered painful, although some people report feelings of mild discomfort.

Pain relief from TENS therapy can be long- or short-term in nature. Because the treatments are safe and have no known side effects, they can be repeated as necessary.

Using a Poultice

A poultice is made of a soft, moist substance that is mixed to the consistency of a paste, and then spread on or between layers of cloth. The cloth is then placed on a body surface. Poultices act by increasing blood flow, relaxing tense muscles, soothing inflamed tissues, or drawing toxins from an infected area. Thus, they can be used to relieve the pain and inflammation associated with abscesses; boils; bruises; carbuncles; fibrocystic disease; fractures; enlarged glands in the neck, breast, or prostate; leg ulcers; sprains; sunburn; tumors; and ulcerated eyelids. They are also used to break up congestion, draw out pus, and remove embedded particles from the skin.

PROCEDURE

An herbal poultice may be made with dried or fresh herbs. The two types of poultices are prepared in slightly different ways. (For information on choosing the best herbal poultice for your condition, as well as cautions regarding the use of specific herbs, *see* Types of Poultices in this section.)

Preparing a Dried Herb Poultice

If you are using dried herbs, use a mortar and pestle to grind the herbs to a powder. Place the herbs in a bowl, and add enough warm water to make a thick paste that can be easily applied. Make a quantity sufficient to cover the affected area. The ratio of ground herbs to water will vary according to the herb being used. Add the water in small increments, just until the mixture is thick but not stiff.

Arrange a clean piece of gauze, muslin, linen, or white cotton sheeting on a clean, flat surface. The material should be large enough to cover the affected area completely. Spread the herbal paste over the cloth. Cleanse the affected area with hydrogen peroxide, and place the poultice over the area. Wrap a towel or plastic wrap around the poultice to prevent the soiling of clothes or sheets. Use a pin or other fastener to secure the poultice in place.

Preparing a Fresh Herb Poultice

If using fresh herbs for your poultice, place 2 ounces of the whole herb—about ½ cup—and 1 cup of water in a small saucepan. Simmer for 2 minutes. Do not drain.

Arrange a clean piece of gauze, muslin, linen, or white cotton sheeting on a clean, flat surface. The material should be large enough to cover the affected area completely. Pour the herbal solution over the cloth. Cleanse the affected body part with hydrogen peroxide, and place the poultice over the area. Wrap a towel or plastic wrap around the poultice to prevent the soiling of clothes or sheets. Use a pin or other fastener to secure the poultice in place.

Treatment Duration

Herbal poultices should be kept in place for one to twenty-four hours, as needed. During this period, you may experience a throbbing pain as the poultice draws out infection and neutralizes toxins. When the pain subsides, you will know that the poultice has accomplished its task and should be removed. Apply fresh poultices as needed until the desired level of healing has been reached. Wash the skin thoroughly after each poultice is removed.

TYPES OF POULTICES

By making your poultice with the appropriate herbs or other substances, you will help ensure that the treatment is effective. Herbs commonly used in poultices are listed below, along with the conditions for which they are appropriate. Note that when the mixture used to make the poultice contains an irritant, such as mustard, it should not come into direct contact with the skin, but should be placed between pieces of cloth.

• Chaparral, dandelion, and yellow dock can be used to treat skin disorders such as acne, eczema, itchy or dry skin, psoriasis, and rashes. You can use one herb, or combine two or three. The greatest benefit will be obtained from using all three. Use chaparral only if you grow it yourself or purchase it from a reputable organic grower.

• Elderberry can relieve pain associated with hemorrhoids.

• Fenugreek, flaxseed, and slippery elm can be combined to treat inflammation. Slippery elm can also be used alone for the inflamed gangrenous sores often associated with diabetes, and for leg ulcers. The use of a slippery elm poultice upon the appearance of sores and ulcers can help prevent gangrene. Slippery elm can also be combined with lobelia to treat abscesses, blood poisoning, and rheumatism.

• Goldenseal is good for inflammations of all kinds.

• Lobelia and charcoal (available in health food stores) can be combined and used to treat insect bites, bee stings, and almost all wounds. Lobelia can be combined with slippery elm to treat abscesses, blood poisoning, and rheumatism.

• Mullein is used for inflamed hemorrhoids, lung disorders, mumps, tonsillitis, and sore throat. To make the poultice, mix 4 parts mullein with 1 part hot vinegar and 1 part water.

• Mustard is beneficial for inflammation, lung congestion, and swelling, and can help relax tense muscles. Because mustard is an irritant, place the mixture between two pieces of cloth, rather than placing it in direct contact with the skin.

• Onion is good for ear infections, and for boils and sores that have difficulty healing. To make this poultice, place finely chopped onion between two pieces of cloth, rather than placing it in direct contact with the skin.

• Pau d'arco, ragwort, and wood sage can be combined and used to treat tumors and external cancers.

• Poke root is good for an inflamed or sore breast.

• Sage, like poke root, can help relieve breast inflammation and soreness.

Sitz Bath

As a form of hydrotherapy—the use of hot and cold water, steam, and ice to restore and maintain health—the sitz bath increases blood flow to the pelvic and abdominal areas, and thus can help reduce inflammation and otherwise alleviate a variety of problems. Sitz baths can use hot or cold water only, or can alternate heat and cold. Hot sitz baths are particularly helpful for such disorders as hemorrhoids, muscular disorders, painful ovaries and testicles, prostate problems, and uterine cramps. Cold sitz baths are helpful in the treatment of constipation, impotence, inflammation, muscle disorders, and vaginal discharge. Alternating hot and cold sitz baths can help relieve abdominal disorders, blood poisoning, congestion, foot infection, headaches, muscle disorders, neuralgia, and swollen ankles.

PROCEDURE

To prepare a sitz bath, fill a tub or basin so that the water covers the hips and reaches the middle of the abdomen. If possible, place the water in a basin that will allow you to immerse just the pelvic and abdominal regions. In this case, you can fill another basin with water that is a few degrees warmer, and immerse your feet in it while sitting in the sitz bath. If no suitable basins are available, place the sitz bath water in a bathtub. You may wish to cover your body with a sheet or blanket to increase your comfort.

As discussed above, the temperature of the water should vary according to the type of illness you are treating. When using a hot sitz bath, the bathtub or basin should be filled with water of about 110°F. (Make sure that the temperature of the water does not exceed 120°F.) You might want to make the water 90°F to 100°F at the beginning of the bath, and then gradually increase the temperature to 110°F. As already mentioned, your feet can be immersed in slightly hotter water. You might wish also to apply a cold compress to your forehead, as the compress will make it easier for you to withstand the heat of the bath. (Make sure that the sitz bath, foot bath, and cold compress are all prepared ahead of time.)

Stay in the bath for twenty to forty minutes. After the moist heat of the bath has soothed the area being treated, you can further stimulate the body by taking a quick cold shower or simply splashing your body with cool water. Then towel yourself dry.

When using a cold sitz bath, fill the bathtub or basin with ice water. Stay in the cold bath for thirty to sixty seconds only. By no means should you stay in the water for more than sixty seconds, as this added time will provide no additional benefits, and may even be harmful. Then towel yourself dry.

When using alternating hot and cold baths, fill one basin with water of about 110°F, and a second basin with ice water. Immerse yourself first in the hot sitz bath, and remain there for three to four minutes. Then move to the cold sitz bath, and remain there for thirty to sixty seconds. Repeat this two to four times, and towel yourself dry.

A word of caution: If you have any health related problems or conditions, be sure to consult with your health care provider before using any type of sitz bath.

Steam Inhalation

Steam inhalation therapy is helpful for relieving the congestion of bronchitis, the common cold, and a variety of other respiratory and sinus conditions. Steam inhalation opens up congested sinuses and lung passages, allowing you to discharge mucus, breathe more easily, and heal faster. To make the steam, you may use water only, or you may add dried or fresh herbs or herbal oils to enhance the effects of the treatment.

PROCEDURE

To provide the steam for the inhalation treatment, you may place the hot water in either a sink or a pot. In most cases, you can choose whichever method you find most convenient and comfortable. But if you are using fresh or dried herbs, you should use a glass or enameled pot, rather than the sink, to hold the water.

Using a Sink

If using your bathroom sink to hold the water, fill the sink with very hot water. If desired, add 2 to 5 drops of herbal oil. Keep the water hot and steaming during the treatment by allowing a small, continuous trickle of hot water to flow into the basin. (The overflow outlet of your sink should prevent the water from spilling over.) As the water becomes diluted, add a few more drops of the herbal oil as needed.

Hold your head over the sink, and breathe in the steam. Usually, five to ten minutes of steam should be sufficient to clear your congestion. In some cases, you may choose to extend the session. Keep your face far enough from the water so that the steam does not irritate or burn your skin. This is particularly important when a child is being treated, as a child's skin is more sensitive to heat.

Using a Pot

If you choose to use a pot to hold the water, and you are using fresh or dried herbs, be sure to select glass or enameled cookware only. This is important, as a metal pot can cause herbs to lose some of their medicinal properties. If you are using water only, any type of pot is appropriate.

Fill a wide pot with water, and bring it to a boil. Then remove the pot from the heat source, and place it on a heatproof pad or cutting board at a convenient height for the inhalation treatment.

Once the water stops bubbling, if desired, add fresh or dried herbs or several drops of essential oil to the water. Allow the water to cool slightly. Then hold your head over the pot, and breathe in the steam. Capture the steam by draping a towel over your head and the pot, creating a "tent." Usually, five to ten minutes of steam should be sufficient to clear your congestion. In some cases, you may choose to extend the session. Keep your face far enough from the water so that the steam does not irritate or burn your skin. This is particularly important when a child is being treated, as a child's skin is more sensitive to heat.

Whichever method you use, after each steam inhalation treatment, take several deep, full breaths to clear lung congestion. Repeat the therapy as needed.

HERBS

❑ Coltsfoot, comfrey, elecampane, ephedra, eucalyptus, fennel, fenugreek, horseradish, licorice, lobelia, lungwort, mullein, pleurisy root, thyme, vervain, and yerba santa are expectorants that facilitate the excretion of mucus from the throat, lungs, and sinuses. These herbs may be used singly, in combination with one another, or in combination with the demulcent herbs listed below.

❑ Burdock, chickweed, coltsfoot, Irish moss, lungwort, marshmallow, mullein, peach bark, and slippery elm are demulcents—substances that soften and relieve irritation of the mucous membranes. These herbs may be used singly, in combination with one another, or in combination with the expectorant herbs listed above.

Preparing for and Recovering From Surgery

Although few people enjoy the prospect of surgery, sometimes surgery is the best available means of improving the quality of life or extending life. After you have been informed of all your options and have decided that surgery is the only viable alternative, use the nutritional guidelines provided in the table below to prepare for the surgery. (For more information on making the decision to have surgery, see the inset on that subject in this section.) By taking these nutrients both before and after surgery, you will support the healing process and lessen postsurgical discomfort and pain. Make sure that your diet is well balanced and healthy. Remember that your general health *after* surgery partly depends on your general health *before* surgery.

NUTRIENTS

SUPPLEMENT	SUGGESTED DOSAGE	COMMENTS
Acidophilus	As directed on label 3 times daily.	To stabilize the intestinal bacterial flora if antibiotics are used. Use a high-potency powdered form.
Coenzyme Q$_{10}$	60 mg daily.	A free radical destroyer that improves tissue oxygenation.
Essential fatty acids (salmon oil and Ultimate Oil from Nature's Secret are good sources)	As directed on label.	Important for proper cell growth and healing of all tissues.
Free-form amino acid complex	As directed on label.	Aids in collagen synthesis and wound healing. Is a readily available form of protein, easily absorbed by the body.
Garlic (Kyolic)	2 capsules 3 times daily.	A natural antibiotic that enhances immune function.
L-Cystine	500 mg twice daily.	Speeds healing of wounds.
L-Glutamine	500 mg 3 times daily and at bedtime.	Speeds healing of wounds.
L-Lysine	500 mg daily.	Speeds healing of wounds and aids collagen formation. *Caution:* Do not take lysine for longer than 6 months at a time.
Multivitamin complex with vitamin A and natural beta-carotene	As directed on label.	Provides necessary vitamins and minerals. Vitamin A is needed for protein utilization in tissue repair, and is a free radical scavenger.
Vitamin K	As directed on label.	This important vitamin is needed for blood clotting.
Vitamin C	6,000–10,000 mg daily, in divided doses.	Aids in tissue repair and healing of wounds. Vital in immune function. Use a buffered form.
Vitamin E	Beginning the day after surgery, take 600 IU daily. Do *not* take any vitamin E during the 2 weeks before surgery, as it thins the blood.	Improves circulation and repairs tissues.
Vitamin E oil	After the stitches are removed and healing has begun, apply topically to the area of the incision 3 times daily.	Promotes healing and reduces scar formation. Purchase in oil form or cut open a capsule to release the oil.
Zinc plus	50 mg daily.	Important for tissue repair. Look for a supplement that contains all of these nutrients.
calcium and	1,500 mg daily.	
magnesium and	As directed on label.	
silica and	As directed on label.	
vitamin D	400 IU daily.	

HERBS

❑ Herbal teas are highly recommended before and after surgery. Try the following teas:

• Echinacea enhances immune system function.

• Goldenseal is a natural antibiotic and helps to prevent infection.

Caution: Do not take this herb internally on a daily basis for more than one week at a time, as it may disturb normal intestinal flora. Do not use it during pregnancy, and use it with caution if you are allergic to ragweed.

• Milk thistle protects the liver from the toxic buildup of drugs and chemicals resulting from surgical procedures.

• Pau d'arco is a natural antibacterial herb. It enhances healing, cleanses the blood, and aids in the prevention of candidiasis.

• Rose hips are a good source of vitamin C and enhance healing.

RECOMMENDATIONS

❑ Consult with your physician about minimally invasive surgery, also called laparoscopic, "keyhole," and "band-aid" surgery. This type of procedure—involving one or more small incisions rather than a large one—does less damage to the skin, muscles, and nerves than does conventional "open" surgery. It also involves a shorter hospital stay and less recovery time. Be aware that such procedures can be used for certain surgeries only.

❑ If you are overweight and have sufficient time to diet before surgery, try to gradually lose the extra weight. Studies show that excess weight can increase both the difficulty of performing surgery and the length of the recovery time. It has also been linked to an increased likelihood of postoperative infection.

Making the Decision to Have Surgery

In the United States, millions of operations are performed annually. Many of these may be unnecessary. Before choosing surgery, explore all other means of treating the problem. Make sure that any surgical recommendation is given by a board-certified surgeon; you want to feel confident that the surgeon is qualified to perform the type of surgery you need. Get a second opinion, and possibly even a third one. You will be better able to decide on the best form of treatment if you are well informed. Don't be afraid to ask your doctor questions.

Your physician should address the following concerns:

• How will the surgery improve your quality of life and/or your chances for survival?

• Are there other forms of treatment that might be used instead of surgery?

• What are the risks of the surgery?

• What percentage of the operations performed of this type are successful?

• What physical changes will result from this operation, and what improvements can you expect?

• How long is the recovery period?

• What is the cost of the operation?

It is also wise to consult with your health insurance provider regarding coverage for the procedure.

❑ If you smoke, stop. Smoking delays healing and interferes with the actions of certain drugs.

❑ Make sure your doctor and those who will care for you are aware of any allergies you have to drugs, chemicals, or foods.

❑ Ask your surgeon if there is anything that you can do to prepare for the surgery. In addition to the surgeon's recommendations, avoid taking vitamin E supplements, aspirin, and all compounds containing aspirin for two weeks prior to surgery. These substances thin the blood.

❑ Make sure your doctor and those who will care for you are aware of any supplements and medications—including natural medicines—you take regularly.

❑ Because blood transfusions are sometimes required during surgery, speak to your doctor about the possibility of storing your own blood for use during the operation. By using your own blood, you will avoid the risk of contracting hepatitis or the AIDS virus. Remember that even disease-free blood can cause reactions such as rashes if not perfectly matched. Your doctor will tell you if you need to take iron supplements a week before the first blood collection. Arrange the appointments so that the last time you give blood is at least four days before the surgery. (Whole blood can be stored for thirty-five days.)

❑ Many operations require that the patient be shaved. If this is necessary, tell the surgeon that you prefer to be shaved the day of surgery. Studies show that the infection rate is lower for patients who are shaved the day of surgery when compared with those who are shaved the night before.

❑ Add fiber to your diet. It ensures better intestinal tract function.

❑ Check with your surgeon before using any treatments at home prior to surgery. If the surgeon concurs, take two cleansing enemas using the juice of a fresh lemon before entering the hospital. It is important to have a clean colon prior to surgery. Taking a half glass of George's Aloe Vera Juice (from Warren Laboratories) in the morning and before bedtime will help to keep your colon clean. Take a bottle of this remedy with you to the hospital. It tastes like spring water and needs no refrigeration.

❑ Many hospitals employ massage with therapeutic essential oils to promote relaxation and relieve the inevitable stress of the presurgical period. If your hospital does not practice this therapy, make arrangements for a qualified massage therapist who is knowledgeable about aromatherapy to give you a massage prior to surgery.

❑ Keep a positive attitude about your surgery, and look forward to getting out of bed and back to normal as soon as possible. The sooner you get out of bed, the better your chances of avoiding postoperative infection.

❑ After surgery, don't overwork your body by eating highly processed foods. Try to consume at least 8 cups of liquids each day, including distilled water, herbal teas, juices, and protein drinks. The appetite is often poor after surgery, and large meals can be overwhelming. Try eating five to seven small, light, nutritious meals a day.

❑ After surgery, exercise caution when engaging in strenuous activity such as lifting. Most doctors advise patients to avoid lifting anything in excess of 10 pounds for two weeks after surgery. Ask your doctor when you can begin light exercise, which has been shown to aid circulation and speed physical recovery. Also ask if there are any specific exercises that can aid your recovery.

CONSIDERATIONS

❑ After major surgery, people generally experience a rapid breakdown of skeletal muscle, which increases any feelings of weakness. In studies in which the amino acid glutamine was added to postsurgical intravenous solutions, muscle breakdown rates were greatly diminished.

❑ Nicholas Cavarocchi, M.D., of Temple University recommends that patients be given 2,000 international units of vitamin E twelve hours prior to heart surgery. This amount of vitamin E lowers free radical levels in the blood. This is recommended only under a physician's supervision.

❑ Some foods interfere with the actions of certain medications. Milk, dairy products, and iron supplements may interfere with some forms of antibiotics. Acidic fruits, such as oranges, pineapples, and grapefruits, can inhibit the action of penicillin and aspirin. *See* Substances That Rob the Body of Nutrients on page 240 for a list of the nutrients that are lost with the use of different drugs.

❑ Postsurgical depression is not uncommon. A healthy dietary program can help fight depression.

❑ Remember: It takes the body a few weeks to recover from the trauma of surgery. During this period, hormonal imbalances are corrected and the rate of metabolism is adjusted. Most incisions close within two days and heal within a week to the point that the skin will hold together under normal stress and body movement. However, you should obtain your doctor's approval before engaging in any exercise, or lifting anything over 10 pounds in weight.

Therapeutic Liquids

The benefits of vegetables and grains are discussed throughout this book. This section offers two recipes that provide these benefits in broths that have healing properties.

The first of the broths derives its healthful properties—including its high potassium content—from potatoes and other vegetables. When purchasing potatoes, choose ones that do not have a green tint. The chemical solanine, which gives the potato its green cast, can interfere with nerve impulses and cause diarrhea, vomiting, and abdominal pain. Use Potato Peeling Broth as a nutritious drink when fasting. This broth is also good for heart disorders.

The second broth—Barley Water—has healing and for-

tifying properties, and is useful during convalescence from many different illnesses. You can also add powdered slippery elm to the water to make a drink that is not only nourishing, but also soothing to the throat and digestive tract.

Many other therapeutic liquids can also be made from vegetables and grains, as well as from fruits. To learn about nutritious juices, *see* JUICING in Part Three.

Potato Peeling Broth

3 potatoes
1 carrot, sliced
1 celery stalk, sliced
2 quarts steam-distilled water
1 onion, sliced and/or 3 cloves garlic, peeled

1. Scrub the potatoes well, and cut out any eyes.
2. Cut the potatoes in half. Cut the peel from the potatoes, making sure to keep about ½ inch of potato with the peel. Set aside the potato centers for another use.
3. Place the potato peelings, carrot, and celery in a large pot. Cover with the water. Add the onion and/or garlic to taste, and boil for about 30 minutes.
4. Cool the broth. Strain out and discard the vegetables, and serve the broth as desired.

Barley Water

1 cup barley
3 quarts steam-distilled water

1. Place the barley and the water in a large pot, and boil for about 3 hours.
2. Cool the broth. Strain out and discard the barley, and serve the broth as desired.

TENS Unit Therapy

See under PAIN CONTROL.

APPENDIX

Glossary

absorption. Nutritionally, the process by which nutrients are absorbed through the intestinal tract into the bloodstream to be used by the body. If nutrients are not properly absorbed, nutritional deficiencies can result.

acetic acid. A weak inorganic acid that is the active ingredient in vinegar; a 4- to 5-percent solution of acetic acid in water makes vinegar.

acid. Any of a class of compounds that share certain basic chemical characteristics. Acids have low pH, are usually sour to the taste, and, in their pure form, are often corrosive. They can be either organic or inorganic compounds. Acids found in plant tissues (especially fruits) tend to prevent the secretion of fluids and shrink tissues.

acute illness. An illness that comes on quickly and may cause relatively severe symptoms, but is of limited duration.

adaptogen. A term for a substance, usually an herb, that produces suitable adjustments in the body. Adaptogens tend to normalize body functions, and when the job is completed, they are eliminated or incorporated into the body without side effects. Some beneficial adaptogens include garlic, ginseng, echinacea, ginkgo, goldenseal, and pau d'arco.

adrenal gland. One of a pair of glands situated atop the kidneys. The adrenal glands are the source of the stress hormones epinephrine (adrenaline) and cortisol, among others.

AIDS. Acquired immune deficiency syndrome.

allergen. A substance that provokes an allergic response.

allergy. An inappropriate response by the immune system to a normally harmless substance. Allergies can affect any of the body's tissues. Hay fever is a common type of allergy.

amino acid. Any of twenty-two nitrogen-containing organic acids from which proteins are made.

anabolic compound. A substance that allows the conversion of simple nutritive material into complex materials that are part of living tissue during the constructive phase of metabolism.

analgesic. Tending to relieve pain, or a substance that relieves pain.

anemia. A deficiency in the blood's ability to carry oxygen to the body tissues.

anesthetic. Causing loss of sensation, or a substance that causes the loss of sensation, especially the ability to feel pain.

angina. Angina pectoris. A syndrome of chest pain with sensations of suffocation, typically brought on by exertion and relieved by rest.

antacid. A substance that neutralizes acid in the stomach, esophagus, or the first part of the duodenum.

antibiotic. Tending to destroy or inhibit the growth of microorganisms, especially bacteria and/or fungi; or a substance that has this property.

antibody. A protein molecule made by the immune system that is designed to intercept and neutralize a specific invading organism or other foreign substance.

antigen. A substance that can elicit the formation of an antibody when introduced into the body.

antihistamine. A substance that interferes with the action of histamines by binding to histamine receptors in various body tissues (*see* histamine).

antioxidant. A substance that blocks or inhibits destructive oxidation reactions. Examples include vitamins C and E, the minerals selenium and germanium, the enzymes catalase and superoxide dismutase (SOD), coenzyme Q_{10}, and some amino acids.

arrhythmia. *See* cardiac arrhythmia.

arteriosclerosis. A circulatory disorder characterized by a thickening and stiffening of the walls of large and medium-sized arteries, which impedes circulation.

artery. A blood vessel through which blood is pumped from the heart to all the organs, glands, and other tissues of the body.

ascorbate. A mineral salt of vitamin C. Taken as nutritional supplements, ascorbates are less acidic (and therefore less irritating) than pure ascorbic acid, and also provide for better absorption of both the vitamin C and the mineral.

ascorbic acid. The organic acid more commonly known as vitamin C.

atherosclerosis. The most common type of arteriosclerosis, caused by the accumulation of fatty deposits in the inner linings of the arteries.

autoimmune disorder. Any condition in which the immune system reacts inappropriately to the body's own tissues and attacks them, causing damage and/or interfering with normal functioning. Examples include Bright's disease, diabetes, multiple sclerosis, rheumatoid arthritis, and systemic lupus erythematosus.

autologous transfusion. A transfusion of one's own blood that has been collected and kept for later use.

bacteria. Single-celled microorganisms. Some bacteria can cause disease; other ("friendly") bacteria are normally present in the body and perform such useful functions as aiding digestion and protecting the body from harmful invading organisms.

benign. Literally, "harmless." Used to refer to cells, especially cells growing in inappropriate locations, that are not malignant (cancerous).

beta-carotene. A substance the body uses to make vitamin A.

bile. A bitter, yellowish substance that is released by the liver into the intestines for the digestion of fats.

biofeedback. A technique for helping an individual to become conscious of usually unconscious body processes, such as heartbeat or body temperature, so that he or she can gain some measure of control over them, and thereby learn to manage the effects of various disorders, including acute back pain, migraines, and Raynaud's disease.

bioflavonoid. Any of a group of biologically active flavonoids. They are essential for the stability and absorption of vitamin C. Although they are not technically vitamins, they are sometimes referred to as vitamin P.

biopsy. Excision of tissue from a living being for diagnosis.

blood count. A basic diagnostic test in which a sample of blood is examined and the number of red blood cells, white blood cells, and platelets determined; or the results of such a test.

blood-brain barrier. A mechanism involving the capillaries and certain other cells of the brain that keeps many substances, especially water-based substances, from passing out of the blood vessels to be absorbed by the brain tissue.

bronchi. The two main branches of the trachea (windpipe) that lead to the lungs.

capillaries. Tiny blood vessels (their walls are about one cell thick) that allow the exchange of nutrients and wastes between the bloodstream and the body's cells.

carbohydrate. Any one of many organic substances, almost all of them of plant origin, that are composed of carbon, hydrogen, and oxygen, and serve as the major source of energy in the diet.

carcinogen. An agent that is capable of inducing cancerous changes in cells and/or tissues.

cardiac. Pertaining to the heart.

cardiac arrhythmia. An abnormal heart rate or rhythm.

carotene. A yellow to orange pigment that is converted into vitamin A in the body. There are several different forms, including alpha-, beta-, and gamma-carotene.

CAT scan. Computerized axial tomography scan. A computerized x-ray scanning procedure used to create a three-dimensional picture of the body, or part of the body, for the purpose of detecting abnormalities.

cauterization. A technique used to stop bleeding that involves applying electrical current, a laser beam, or a chemical such as silver nitrate directly to a broken blood vessel.

cell. A very small but complex organic unit consisting of a nucleus, cytoplasm, and a cell membrane. All living tissues are composed of cells.

cellulose. An indigestible carbohydrate found in the outer layers of fruits and vegetables.

cerebral. Pertaining to the brain.

chelation. A chemical process by which a larger molecule or group of molecules surround or enclose a mineral atom.

chelation therapy. The introduction of certain substances into the body so that they will chelate, and then remove, foreign substances such as lead, cadmium, arsenic, and other heavy metals. Chelation therapy can also be used to reduce or remove calcium-based plaque from the linings of the blood vessels, easing the flow of blood to vital organs and tissues.

chemotherapy. Treatment of disease by the use of chemicals (such as drugs), especially the use of chemical treatments to combat cancer.

chiropractic. A system of healing based on the belief that many disorders result from misalignments (called subluxations) of the spinal vertebrae and other joints. Chiropractors primarily treat illness by using physical manipulation techniques to bring the body into proper alignment and thus restore normal health and functioning.

chlorophyll. The pigment responsible for the green color of plant tissues. It can be taken in supplement form as a source of magnesium and trace elements.

cholesterol. A crystalline substance that is soluble in fats and that is produced by all vertebrates. It is a necessary constituent of cell membranes, and facilitates the transport and absorption of fatty acids. Excess cholesterol, however, is a potential threat to health.

chronic illness. A disorder that persists or recurs over an extended period, often for life. Chronic illnesses can be as relatively benign as hay fever or as serious as multiple sclerosis.

citric acid. An organic acid found in citrus fruits. Often used to lower the pH of cosmetic products, to bring them closer to the natural pH of the skin.

clotting factor. One of several substances, especially vitamin K, that are present in the bloodstream and are important in the process of blood clotting.

cobalt 60. A radioactive form of the element cobalt that is widely used in radiation therapy.

co-carcinogen. An agent that acts with another to cause cancer.

coenzyme. A molecule that works with an enzyme to enable the enzyme to perform its function in the body. Coenzymes are necessary in the utilization of vitamins and minerals.

cold-pressed. A term used to describe food oils that are extracted without the use of heat in order to preserve nutrients and flavor.

colic. Sharp abdominal pains that result from spasm or obstruction of certain organs or structures, especially the intestines, uterus, or bile ducts.

colonoscope. An instrument for examining the colon.

complete protein. A source of dietary protein that contains a full complement of the eight essential amino acids.

complex carbohydrate. A type of carbohydrate that, owing to its chemical structure, releases its sugar into the body relatively slowly and also provides fiber. The carbohydrates in starches and fiber are complex carbohydtates. Also called *polysaccharides.*

complication. A secondary infection, reaction, or other negative event that makes recovery from illness more difficult and/or longer.

congenital. Present from birth, but not necessarily inherited.

contraceptive. Tending to prevent conception, or a device, substance, or method used to prevent pregnancy.

contusion. A bruise; an injury in which the skin is not broken.

convulsion. A seizure characterized by intense, uncontrollable contraction of the voluntary muscles that results from abnormal cerebral stimulation.

coryza. The nasal symptoms of the common cold.

cruciferous. Literally, "cross-shaped." A term used to refer to a group of vegetables—including broccoli, Brussels sprouts, cabbage, cauliflower, turnips, and rutabagas—that have characteristic cross-shaped blossoms and that contain substances that may help to prevent colon cancer.

cystoscope. Instrument used to examine the urinary bladder.

dementia. A permanent acquired impairment of intellectual function that results in a marked decline in memory, language ability, personality, visuospatial skills, and/or cognition (orientation, perception, reasoning, abstract thinking, and calculation). Dementia can be either static or permanent, and can result from many different causes.

demulcent. Soothing, especially to mucous membranes.

dermis. The layer of skin that lies underneath the epidermis. Blood and lymphatic vessels and the glands that secrete perspiration and sebum are all found in the dermis.

detoxification. The process of reducing the buildup of various poisonous substances in the body.

disorientation. The loss of a normal relationship to one's surroundings; the inability to comprehend time, people, and place.

diuretic. Tending to increase urine flow, or a substance that promotes the excretion of fluids.

DNA. Deoxyribonucleic acid. Substance in the cell nucleus that genetically contains the cell's genetic blueprint and determines the type of life form into which a cell will develop.

echocardiogram. A diagnostic test that uses ultrasound to detect structural and functional abnormalities of the heart.

edema. Retention of fluid in the tissues that results in swelling.

EDTA. Ethylenediaminetetraacetic acid. An organic molecule used in chelation therapy.

EEG. Electroencephalogram. A test used to measure brain wave activity.

EKC (or ECG). Electrocardiogram. A test that monitors heart function by tracing the conduction of electrical impulses associated with heart activity.

electrolyte. Soluble salts dissolved in the body's fluids. Electrolytes are the form in which most minerals circulate in the body. They are so named because they are capable of conducting electrical impulses.

ELISA. Enzyme-linked immunoadsorbent assay. A test that determines the presence of a particular protein, such as an antibody, by detecting the presence of an enzyme that is linked to that protein.

embolus. A loose particle of tissue, a bloot clot, or a tiny air bubble that travels through the bloodstream and, if it lodges in a narrowed portion of a blood vessel, can block blood flow.

emulsion. A combination of two liquids that do not mix with each other, such as oil and water; one substance is broken into tiny droplets and is suspended within the other. Emulsification is the first step in the digestion of fats.

endemic. Native to or prevalent in a particular geographic region. Often used to describe diseases.

endocrine system. The system of glands that secrete hormones into the bloodstream. Endocrine glands include the pituitary, thyroid, thymus, and adrenal glands, as well as the pancreas, ovaries, and testes.

endorphin. One of a number of natural hormonelike substances found primarily in the brain. One function of endorphins is to suppress the sensation of pain, which they do by binding to opiate receptors in the brain.

endoscope. Instrument for examining the interior of a hollow organ.

enteric. Pertaining to the small intestines.

enzyme. One of many specific protein catalysts that initiate or speed chemical reactions in the body without being consumed.

epidemic. An extensive outbreak of a disease, or a disease occurring with an unusually high incidence at certain times and places.

epidermis. The outer layer of the skin.

Epstein-Barr virus (EBV). A virus that causes infectious mononucleosis and that may cause other health problems as well, especially in people with compromised immune systems.

erythema. Reddening, especially of the skin.

essential. A term for nutrients needed for building and repair that cannot be manufactured by the body, and that therefore must be supplied in the diet. At present, there are some forty-two known essential nutrients.

excision. Surgical cutting away and/or removal of tissue.

fat-soluble. Capable of dissolving in the same organic solvents as fats and oils.

fatty acid. Any one of many organic acids from which fats and oils are made.

FBS. Fasting blood sugar. The level of glucose present in a blood sample drawn at least eight hours after the last meal.

fiber. The indigestible portion of plant matter. Fiber is an important component of a healthy diet because it is capable of binding to toxins and escorting them out of the body.

flatulence. Excessive amounts of gas in the stomach or other parts of the digestive tract.

flavonoid. Any of a large group of crystalline compounds found in plants.

free radical. An atom or group of atoms that is highly chemically reactive because it has at least one unpaired electron. Because they join so readily with other compounds, free radicals can attack cells and can cause a lot of damage in the body. Free radicals form in heated fats and oils, and as a result of exposure to atmospheric radiation and environmental pollutants, among other things.

free radical scavenger. A substance that removes or destroys free radicals.

fungus. One of a class of organisms that includes yeasts, mold, and mushrooms. A number of fungal species, such as *Candida albicans*, are capable of causing severe disease in immunocompromised hosts.

gastritis. Inflammation of the stomach lining.

gastroenteritis. Inflammation of the mucous lining of the stomach and the intestines.

gastrointestinal. Pertaining to the stomach, small and large intestines, colon, rectum, liver, pancreas, and gallbladder.

genetic. Inherited.

gingivitis. Inflammation of the gums surrounding the teeth.

gland. An organ or tissue that secretes a substance(s) for use elsewhere in the body rather than for its own functioning.

globulin. A type of protein found in the blood. Certain globulins contain disease-fighting antibodies.

glucose. A simple sugar that is the principal source of energy for the body's cells.

gluten. A protein found in many grains, including wheat, rye, barley, and oats.

glycogen. A polysaccharide (complex carbohydrate) that is the main form in which glucose is stored in the body, primarily in the liver and muscles. It is converted back into glucose as needed to supply energy.

hair analysis. A method of determining the levels of minerals, including both toxic metals and essential minerals, in the body by measuring the concentrations of those minerals in the hair. Unlike mineral levels in the blood, those in the hair reflect the person's status over several preceding months.

heavy metal. A metallic element whose specific gravity (a measurement of mass as compared with the mass of water or hydrogen) is greater than 5.0. Some heavy metals, such as arsenic, cadmium, lead, and mercury, are extremely toxic.

hematocrit. The percentage of blood (by volume) that is composed of red blood cells.

hematoma. A bulge or swelling that is filled with blood. Hematomas are usually the result of a blunt injury or other trauma that causes a blood vessel under the skin to break.

hemicellulose. An indigestible carbohydrate resembling cellulose, found in plant cell walls, that absorbs water.

hemoglobin. The iron-containing red pigment in the blood that is responsible for the transport of oxygen.

hemorrhage. Profuse or abnormal bleeding.

hepatic. Pertaining to the liver.

hepatitis. A general term for inflammation of the liver. It can result from infection or exposure to toxins.

herbal therapy. The use of herbal combinations for healing or cleansing purposes. Herbs can be used in tablet, capsule, tincture, or extract form, as well as in baths and poultices.

hernia. A condition in which part of an internal organ protrudes, inappropriately, through an opening in the tissues that are supposed to contain it.

histamine. A chemical released by the immune system that acts on various body tissues. It has the effect of constricting the smooth bronchial tube muscles, dilating small blood vessels, allowing fluid to leak from various tissues, and increasing the secretion of stomach acid.

HIV. Human immunodeficiency virus. The virus that causes AIDS.

Hodgkin's disease. A type of lymphoma (cancer of the lymphatic system).

homeopathy. A medical system based on the belief that "like cures like"—that is, that illness can be cured by taking a *minute* dose of a substance that, if taken by a healthy person, would produce symptoms like those being treated. Homeopathy employs a variety of plant, animal, and mineral substances in very small doses to stimulate the body's natural healing powers and to bring the body back into balance.

hormone. One of numerous essential substances produced by the endocrine glands that regulate many bodily functions.

host. An organism in or on which another organism lives and from which the invading organism obtains nourishment.

hyaluronic acid. An organic acid known as the most effective natural skin moisturizer. It is present in human skin, and is able to hold 500 times its own weight in water.

hydrochloric acid. A strong, corrosive inorganic acid that is produced in the stomach to aid in digestion.

hydrogenation. A chemical process used to turn liquid oils into more solid form by bombarding the oil molecules with hydrogen atoms. Hydrogenation destroys the nutritional value of the oil and also results in the formation of potentially cis- and trans-fatty acids, strangely altered fatty acid molecules that do not occur in nature.

hypercalcemia. The presence of abnormally high amounts of calcium in the blood.

hypertension. High blood pressure. Generally, hypertension is defined as a regular resting pressure over 140/90.

hypoallergenic. Having a low capacity for inducing hypersensitive (allergic) reactions.

hypocalcemia. The presence of abnormally low amounts of calcium in the blood.

hypotension. Low blood pressure.

hypothalamus. A portion of the brain that regulates many aspects of metabolism, including body temperature and the hunger response.

idiopathic. Term describing a disease of unknown cause.

immune globulin. A protein that functions as an antibody in the body's immune response. Immune globulins are manufactured by certain white blood cells and found in body fluids and on mucous membranes.

immune system. A complex system that depends on the interaction of many different organs, cells, and proteins. Its chief function is to identify and eliminate foreign substances such as harmful bacteria that have invaded the body. The liver, spleen, thymus, bone marrow, and lymphatic system all play vital roles in the proper functioning of the immune system.

immunity. The condition of being able to resist and overcome disease or infection.

immunodeficiency. A defect in the functioning of the immune system. It can be inherited or acquired, reversible or permanent. Immunodeficiency renders the body more susceptible to illness of every type, especially infectious illnesses.

immunology. The branch of medical science that deals with the functioning of the immune system.

immunotherapy. Treatment of disease by using techniques to stimulate or strengthen the immune system.

incubation period. The period of time between exposure to an infectious disease and the appearance of symptoms, during which the infection is developing.

infection. Invasion of body tissues by disease-causing organisms such as viruses, protozoa, fungi, or bacteria.

infestation. An invasion of the body by parasites such as insects, worms, or protozoa.

inflammation. A reaction to illness or injury characterized by swelling, warmth, and redness.

inguinal. Pertaining to the groin.

insomnia. The inability to sleep.

insulin. A hormone produced by the pancreas that regulates the metabolism of glucose (sugar) in the body.

interaction. A phenomenon that occurs when two or more substances affect one another's activity or combine to create a different effect than any of them would have on its own. Any substance introduced into the body can potentially interact with another substance or substances already present. Drugs, foods, herbs, minerals, and vitamins can all interact with one another.

interferon. A protein produced by the cells in response to viral infection that prevents viral reproduction and is capable of protecting uninfected cells from viral infection. There are different types of interferon, designated alpha, beta, and gamma.

intestinal flora. The "friendly" bacteria present in the intestines that are essential for the digestion and metabolism of certain nutrients.

intolerance. Nutritionally, the inability to digest a particular food, usually due to a lack or deficiency of certain enzymes.

intravenous (IV) infusion. The use of a needle inserted in a vein to assist in fluid replacement or the giving of medication.

ischemia. The condition of being starved for blood. Ischemia affecting the heart or brain can cause a heart attack or stroke.

IU. International unit. A measure of potency based on an accepted international standard. Dosages of vitamin A and E supplements, among others, are usually measured in international units. Because this is a measurement of potency, not weight or volume, the number of milligrams in an international unit varies, depending on the substance being measured.

lactase. An enzyme that converts lactose into glucose and galactose. It is necessary for the digestion of milk and milk products.

lactic acid. An acid that results from anaerobic glucose metabolism. It is present in certain foods, including certain fruits and sour milk (when milk becomes sour, this means that some of the lactose, or milk sugar, it contained has been converted into lactic acid). Lactic acid is also produced in the muscles during anaerobic exercise. It is the buildup of lactic acid that causes muscle fatigue during strenuous activity. Synthetic lactic acid is used in food products as a flavoring and preservative.

lactobacilli. Any of a number of species of bacteria that are capable of transforming lactose (milk sugar) into lactic acid through fermentation. Lactobacilli are naturally present in the colon, and are sometimes referred to as "friendly" bacteria because they aid in digestion and fight certain disease-causing microorganisms. The two species of lactobacilli most commonly available in supplement form are *L. acidophilus* and *L. bifidus*.

laser. Light amplification by stimulated emission of radiation. An instrument that focuses highly amplified light waves. Lasers are used in surgical procedures, especially eye surgery.

lecithin. A mixture of phospholipids that is composed of fatty acids, glycerol, phosphorus, and choline or inositol. All living cell membranes are largely composed of lecithin.

leukemia. Cancer of the blood-producing tissues, especially the bone marrow and lymph nodes, resulting in an over-abundance of white blood cells. It can be either acute (most common in children) or chronic (most common in adults). It is similar in certain respects to Hodgkin's disease.

limbic system. A group of deep brain structures that, among other things, transmit the perception of pain to the brain and generate an emotional reaction to it.

lipid. Substances found in nature that are soluble in the same organic solvents as fats and oils are. Important nutritional lipids include choline, gamma-linolenic acid, inositol, lecithin, and linoleic acid.

lipoprotein. A type of protein molecule that incorporates a lipid. Lipoproteins act as agents of lipid transport in the lymph and blood.

lipotropic. Any of a number of substances that help to prevent the accumulation of abnormal or excessive amounts of fat in the liver, control blood sugar levels, and enhance fat and carbohydrate metabolism. Commonly used lipotropics include choline, inositol, and methionine.

lymph. A clear fluid derived from blood plasma that circulates throughout the body, is collected from the tissues, and flows through the lymphatic vessels, eventually returning to the blood circulation. Its function is to nourish tissue cells and return waste matter to the bloodstream.

lymph nodes. Organs located in the lymphatic vessels that act as filters, trapping and removing foreign material. They also form lymphocytes, immune cells that develop the capacity to seek out and destroy specific foreign agents.

lymphadenopathy. Enlargement of a lymph node or nodes as a result of the presence of a foreign substance or disease. This condition is often referred to as "swollen glands."

lymphocyte. A type of white blood cell found in lymph, blood, and other specialized tissues, such as the bone marrow and tonsils. There are several different categories of lymphocytes, designated B-lymphocytes, T-lymphocytes, and null (or non-B, non-T) lymphocytes. These cells are crucial components of the immune system. B-lymphocytes are primarily responsible for antibody production, whereas the T-lymphocytes are involved in the direct attack against invading organisms. It is the T-helper cell, a subtype of T-lymphocyte, that is the primary cell infected and destroyed by human immunodeficiency virus (HIV), the virus that causes AIDS.

lymphokine. Any of a group of substances produced by the cells of the immune system when exposed to antigens. They are not antibodies, but rather perform such functions as stimulating the production of additional lymphocytes and activating other immune cells.

lymphoma. Cancer of the lymphatic tissues.

macrobiotics. A dietary approach adapted from Far Eastern philosophy whose basic principle consists of balancing the yin and yang energies of foods. Yin foods, such as water, are expansive; yang foods, such as salt or meat, are contractile. For the most part, the macrobiotic diet consists of whole grain cereals, millet, rice, soups, and vegetables, with beans and supplementary foods depending on the individual and the condition. Different conditions are considered either yin or yang, so the macrobiotic program must be adapted to each individual.

malabsorption. Nutritionally, a defect in the absorption of nutrients from the intestinal tract into the bloodstream.

malignant. Literally, "evil." Used to refer to cells or groups of cells that are cancerous and likely to spread.

mammography. An x-ray examination of the breast.

melanoma. A malignant tumor originating from pigment cells in the deep layers of the skin.

menopause. The cessation of menstruation, caused by a sharp decrease in the production of the sex hormones estrogen and progesterone. Menopause usually occurs after the age of forty-five or following the removal of the female reproductive organs.

metabolism. The physical and chemical processes necessary to sustain life, including the production of cellular energy, the synthesis of important biological substances, and degradation of various compounds.

metabolite. A substance produced as a result of a metabolic process.

microgram. A measurement of weight equivalent to $\frac{1}{1,000}$ of a milligram.

milligram. A measurement of weight equivalent to $\frac{1}{1,000}$ of a gram (a gram is equal to approximately $\frac{1}{28}$ of an ounce).

mineral. An inorganic substance required by the body in small quantities.

MRI. Magnetic resonance imaging. A technique used in diagnosis that combines the use of radio waves and a strong magnetic field to produce detailed images of the internal structures of the body.

mucous membranes. Membranes that line the cavities and canals of the body that communicate with the air. Examples include the membranes lining the inside of the mouth, nose, anus, and vagina.

naturopathy. A form of health care that uses diet, herbs, and other natural methods and substances to cure illness. The goal is to produce a healthy body state without the use of drugs by stimulating innate defenses.

neuropathy. A complex of symptoms caused by abnormalities in motor or sensory nerves. Symptoms may include tingling or numbness, especially in the hands or feet, followed by gradual, progressive muscular weakness.

neurotransmitter. A chemical that transmits nerve impulses from one nerve cell to another. Major neurotransmitters include acetylcholine, dopamine, gamma-aminobutyric acid, norepinephrine, and serotonin.

nucleic acid. Any of a class of chemical compounds found in all viruses and plant and animal cells. Ribonucleic acid (RNA) and deoxyribonucleic acid (DNA), which contain the genetic instructions for every living cell, are two principal types.

nutraceutical. A food- or nutrient-based product or supplement designed and/or used for a specific clinical and/or therapeutic purpose.

nutrient. A substance that is needed by the body to maintain life and health.

occult blood test. A test that detects the presence of blood in bodily excretions such as stool, sputum, or urine. It is most often used in screening for cancer.

oncologist. A cancer specialist.

oncology. The medical specialty dealing with cancer.

organic. A term used to describe foods that are grown without the use of synthetic chemicals, such as pesticides, herbicides, and hormones.

osteopathy. A system of medicine based on the belief that the body is a vital mechanical organism whose structural and functional integrity are coordinated and interdependent, and that disturbances in the musculoskeletal system can therefore cause disorders elsewhere in the body. Because of this philosophy, although osteopaths can prescribe drugs and perform surgery, they are more likely to recommend physical therapy or musculoskeletal manipulation as the treatment of first choice.

osteoporosis. A disorder in which minerals leach out of the bones, rendering them progressively more porous and fragile.

oxidation. A chemical reaction in which oxygen reacts with another substance, resulting in a chemical transformation. Many oxidation reactions result in some type of deterioration or spoilage.

Pap test. Microscopic examination of cells collected from the vagina and cervix to test for signs of cancer.

parasite. An organism that lives on or in another organism and obtains nourishment from it.

pH. Potential of hydrogen. A scale used to measure the relative acidity or alkalinity of substances. The scale runs from 0 to 14. A pH of 7 is considered neutral; numbers below 7 denote increasing acidity and numbers above 7 denote increasing alkalinity.

pharyngitis. Sore throat.

phenylketonuria (PKU). An inherited disorder caused by a lack of an enzyme necessary to convert the amino acid phenylalanine into another amino acid, tyrosine, so that excesses can be eliminated from the body. A buildup of excess phenylalanine in the blood can lead to neurological disturbances and mental retardation.

phytochemical. Any one of many substances present in fruits and vegetables that have various health-promoting properties. Some phytochemicals appear to protect against certain types of cancer.

pituitary. A gland located at the base of the brain that secretes a number of different hormones. Pituitary hormones regulate growth and metabolism by coordinating the actions of other endocrine glands.

placebo. A pharmacologically inactive substance, primarily used in experiments to provide a basis for comparison with pharmacologically active substances.

plaque. An unwanted deposit of a certain substance on tissues, often with the potential to cause some type of health problem. The buildup of plaque in the arteries is a leading cause of cardiovascular disease; plaque deposits on the teeth can lead to gum disease; Alzheimer's disease is associated with the accumulation of characteristic plaques in brain tissue.

precancerous lesion. Abnormal tissue that is not malignant, but that may be in the process of becoming so.

prognosis. A forecast as to the likely course and/or outcome of a disorder or condition.

prostaglandin. Any of a number of hormonelike chemicals that are made in the body from essential fatty acids and that have important effects on target organs. They influence the secretion of hormones and enzymes, and are important in regulating the inflammatory response, blood pressure, and blood clotting time.

protein. Any of many complex nitrogen-based organic compounds made up of different combinations of amino acids. Proteins are basic elements of all animal and vegetable tissues. Biological substances such as hormones and enzymes also are composed of protein. The body makes the specific proteins it needs for growth, repair, and other functions from amino acids that are either extracted from dietary protein or manufactured from other amino acids.

proteolytic enzymes. Enzymes that break down dietary proteins, yet do not attack the proteins that make up the normal cells of the body. Proteolytic enzymes may have value in fighting cancer and other diseases. Cancer cells have a type of protein coating; theoretically, if this coating is destroyed by proteolytic enzymes, the white blood cells would be able to attack the cancer cells and destroy them.

pruritus. Itching.

pulmonary. Pertaining to the lungs.

purulent. Containing or causing the production of pus.

radiation. Energy that is emitted or transmitted in the form of waves. The term is often used to refer to radioactivity; however, radioactivity is a specific type of radiation that comes from the decay of unstable atoms.

radiation therapy. A type of treatment, most often used for cancer, that involves the use of ionizing radiation, including Roentgen rays, radium, or other radioactive substances to destroy specific areas of tissue. Also called *radiotherapy*.

RAST. Radioallergosorbent test. A blood test that measures levels of specific antibodies produced by the body's immune system, used to test for allergic reactions.

RDA. Recommended daily allowance. The amount of a vitamin or other nutrient that should be consumed daily in order to prevent nutritional deficiency. RDAs are determined by the U.S. Food and Drug Administration.

red blood cell. A blood cell that contains the red pigment hemoglobin and transports oxygen and carbon dioxide in the bloodstream.

remission. Lessening or reversal of the signs and symptoms of disease. This term is used particularly of serious and/or chronic illnesses such as cancer and multiple sclerosis.

renal. Pertaining to the kidneys.

retinoic acid. Vitamin A acid. A form of retinoic acid is the active ingredient in the medication Retin-A.

retrovirus. A type of virus that has RNA as its core nucleic acid and contains an enzyme called *reverse transcriptase* that permits the virus to copy its RNA into the DNA of infected cells, in effect taking over the cells' genetic machinery. Human immunodeficiency virus (HIV), the virus that causes AIDS, is a retrovirus. Retroviruses are also known to cause certain types of cancer in animals, and are suspected of causing forms of leukemia and lymphoma in humans.

RNA. Ribonucleic acid. A complex protein found in plant and animal cells. RNA carries coded genetic information from DNA, in the cell nucleus, to protein-producing cell structures called ribosomes, where these instructions are translated into the form of protein molecules—the basic component of all living tissue.

saturated fat. A fat that is solid at room temperature. Most saturated fats are of animal origin, although a few, such as coconut oil and palm oil, come from plants.

saturation. With regard to fats, the term "saturation" refers to the chemical structure of the fatty acid molecules, specifically the number of hydrogen atoms present. Fat molecules that cannot incorporate any additional hydrogen atoms are said to be *saturated*; those that could incorporate one additional hydrogen atom are referred to as *monounsaturated*; and those that could incorporate two or more additional hydrogen atoms are referred to as *polyunsaturated*.

scratch test. A procedure in which a small amount of a suspected allergen is applied to a lightly scratched area of skin to test for an allergic reaction.

sebum. The oily secretion produced by glands in the skin.

secondary infection. An infection that develops after and is made possible by the presence or effect of a previous infection, inflammation, or other condition, but that is not necessarily directly caused by it.

seizure. A sudden, brief episode characterized by changes in consciousness, perception, muscular motion, and/or behavior. A convulsion is a type of seizure.

serotonin. A neurotransmitter found principally in the brain that is considered essential for relaxation, sleep, and concentration.

serum. The fluid portion of the blood.

simple carbohydrate. A type of carbohydrate that, owing to its chemical structure, is rapidly digested and absorbed into the bloodstream. Glucose, lactose, and fructose are examples of simple carbohydrates.

sorbic acid. An organic acid used as a food preservative.

steroid. One of a group of fat-soluble organic compounds with a characteristic chemical composition. A number of different hormones, drugs, and other substances—including cholesterol—are classified as steroids.

stroke. An attack in which the brain is suddenly deprived of oxygen as a result of interrupted blood flow. If it continues for more than a few minutes, brain damage and even death may result.

sublingual. Literally, "under the tongue." Sublingual medications and supplements often look like tablets or liquids meant for swallowing, but they are designed to be held in the mouth while the active ingredient is absorbed into the bloodstream through the mucous membranes.

symptom. An alteration in normal feeling or functioning experienced as a result of a bodily disorder.

syncope. Temporary loss of consciousness; fainting.

syndrome. A group of signs and symptoms that together are known or presumed to characterize a disorder.

synergy. An interaction between two or more substances in which their action is greater when they are together than the sum of their individual actions would be.

systemic. Pertaining to the entire body.

T cell. A type of lymphocyte that is a crucial part of the immune system.

teratogen. An agent that causes malformation of a developing embryo or fetus.

therapy, alternative. The treatment of disease by means other than conventional medical, pharmacological, and surgical techniques.

thrombus. An obstruction in a blood vessel.

thrush. A fungal infection caused by *Candida albicans* that is characterized by small whitish spots on the tongue and the insides of the cheeks. It occurs most often in infants and in persons with compromised immune systems.

topical. Pertaining to the surface of the body.

toxicity. The quality of being poisonous. Toxicity reactions in the body impair bodily functions and/or damage cells.

toxin. A poison that impairs the health and functioning of the body.

trace element. A mineral required by the body in extremely small quantities.

tremor. Involuntary trembling.

triglyceride. A compound consisting of three fatty acids plus glycerol. Triglycerides are the form in which fat is stored in the body, and are the primary type of lipid in the diet.

tumor. An abnormal mass of tissue that serves no function. Tumors are usually categorized as either benign or malignant (cancerous).

type A personality. A personality that tends to be impatient and aggressive. Persons with type A personalities tend to have stronger stress reactions, and may be more susceptible to cardiovascular disease.

type B personality. A personality that tends to be relaxed and patient, and less reactive to stress. Those with type B personalities may be less prone to develop stress-related illnesses such as high blood pressure and heart disease.

ultrasound. Ultra-high-frequency sound waves. Ultrasound technology is used in a number of different medical diagnostic and treatment tools.

unsaturated fat. Any of a number of dietary fats that are liquid at room temperature. Unsaturated fats come from vegetable sources and are good sources of essential fatty acids. Examples include flaxseed oil, sunflower oil, safflower oil, and primrose oil.

urticaria. Hives.

vaccine. A preparation administered to achieve immunity against a specific agent by inducing the body to make antibodies to that agent. A vaccine may be a suspension of living or dead microorganisms, or a solution of an allergen or viral or bacterial antigens.

vascular. Pertaining to the circulatory system.

vein. One of the blood vessels that returns the blood from the body tissues to the heart.

venom. A poisonous substance produced by an animal, such as certain snakes and insects.

virus. Any of a vast group of minute, often disease-causing, structures composed of a protein coat and a core of DNA and/or RNA. Because they are incapable of reproducing on their own (they must reproduce inside the cells of an infected host), viruses are not technically considered living organisms. Unlike bacteria, viruses are not affected by antibiotics.

visualization. A technique that involves consciously using the mind to influence the health and functioning of the body. Also called creative visualization.

vital signs. Basic indicators of an individual's health status, including pulse, breathing, blood pressure, and body temperature.

vitamin. One of approximately fifteen organic substances that are essential in small quantities for life and health. Most vitamins cannot be manufactured by the body, and so need to be supplied in the diet.

water-soluble. Capable of dissolving in water.

white blood cell. A blood cell that functions in fighting infection and in wound repair.

withdrawal. The process of adjustment that occurs when the use of a habit-forming substance to which the body has become accustomed is discontinued.

yeast. A type of single-celled fungus. Certain types of yeast can cause infection, most commonly in the mouth, vagina, or gastrointestinal tract. Common yeast infections include vaginitis and thrush.

Manufacturer and Distributor Information

Below are the manufacturers and distributors of some of the brand-name products mentioned in this book, plus their addresses and phone numbers. This information is provided to enable you to contact these companies to order or to obtain further information about their products. None of the manufacturers or distributors mentioned has had any connection with the production of this book. Rather, we list these companies because we believe their products to be effective and of high quality. Be aware that addresses and telephone numbers are subject to change.

Abkit Inc.
207 East 94th Street, 2nd Floor
New York, NY 10128
800–226–6227 212–860–8358
CamoCare Facial Therapy; Natureworks Marigold Ointment.

Aerobic Life Industries
3045 South 46th Street
Phoenix, AZ 85040
800–798–0707 602–968–0707
Aerobic 07; Aerobic Bulk Cleanse (ABC); All-Purpose Bactericide Spray; Burn Gel; China Gold; Desert Delight; 45 Day Cleanse for Colon, Blood and Lymph; Homozon; 10-Day Colon Cleanse.

AIM International
3904 East Flamingo Avenue
Nampa, ID 83687
800–456–2462
Barleygreen.

AkPharma, Inc.
P.O. Box 111
Pleasantville, NJ 08232
800–732–6441 609–645–5100
Beano.

Alacer Corporation
14 Morgan
Irvine, CA 92718–2003
800–854–0249 714–751–9660
E•mergen•C.

Aller//Guard Corporation
40 Cindy Lane
Ocean, NJ 07712–7248
X-MITE powder.

Allergy Research Group
400 Preda Street
San Leandro, CA 94577
800–545–9960
Chronoset.

Alpine Air of America
220 Reservoir
Needham Heights, MA 02194
800–628–2209
Living Air XL-15.

American Biologics
1180 Walnut Avenue
Chula Vista, CA 91911
800–227–4473 619–429–8200
AE Mulsion Forte; Bio-Bifidus; Bio Rizin; Dioxychlor; GE-132; Infla-Zyme Forte; Oxy-5000 Forte; Oxy C-2 Gel; Panoderm I; Selenium Forte; Taurine Plus.

Anabol Naturals
1550 Mansfield Street
Santa Cruz, CA 95062
800–426–2265 408–479–1403
Muscle Octane.

Anurex Labs
P.O. Box 414760
Miami, FL 33141
305–757–7733
Cryotherapy device for hemorrhoids.

Apollo Light Systems, Inc.
369 South Mountainway Drive
Orem, UT 84058
800–545–9667 801–226–2370
Brite Lite III.

Bayer Corporation
P.O. Box 3100
Elkhart, IN 46515
800–248–2637
Glucometer Elite; Glucometer Encore.

BDP America, Inc.
4045 Sheridan Avenue, Suite 363
Miami Beach, FL 33140
800–294–8787 305–673–3164
Béres Drops Plus.

Bio Nutritional
41 Bergen Line Avenue
Westwood, NJ 07675
201–666–2300
Eugalan Forte.

Bioforce of America, Ltd.
122 Smith Road
Kinderhook, NY 12106
800–645–9135 518–758–6060
Bio-Strath; Echinaforce Extract.

Biotec Food Corp
4614 Kilquea Avenue, Suite 553
Honolulu, HI 96826
800–788–1084
Ageless Beauty; Anti-Stress Enzymes; Cell Guard.

Biotics Research
8122 East Fulton
Ada, MI 49301
800–437–1298 616–676–3380
Bio-Cardiozyme Forte; Cytozyme-F; Cytozyme-M; Intenzyme Forte; Neonatal Multi-Gland; Osteo-B-plus.

Boiron
6 Campus Boulevard, Building A
Newtown Square, PA 19073
800–BLU–TUBE 610–325–7464
Homeopathic remedies.

CamoCare
See Abkit Inc.

Carlson Laboratories, Inc.
15 College Drive
Arlington Heights, IL 60004
800–323–4141 708–255–1600
ACES + Zinc; Amino-LIV; E•Gem Skin Care Soap; Key-E suppositories.

CC Pollen Company
3627 East Indian School Road, Suite 209
Phoenix, AZ 85018
800–875–0096 602–957–0096
Aller Bee-Gone.

Clean Water Revival Inc.
85 Hazel Street
Glen Cove, NY 11542
800–444–3563 516–674–2441
Ceramic water filtration systems.

Country Life
101 Corporate Drive
Hauppauge, NY 11788
516–231–1031
Nutritional supplements.

Derma-E Products Inc.
9400 Lurline Avenue, #C-1
Chatsworth, CA 91311
818–718–1420 800–521–3342
*Vitamin A Moisturizing Gel; Wrinkle
Treatment Oil.*

Diamond-Herpanacine Associates
P.O. Box 544
Ambler, PA 19002
215–542–2981
Herpanacine; Healthy Horizons.

Eclectic Institute
14385 SE Lusted Road
Sandy, Oregon 97055
800–332–HERB
*Organic herbs, herbal extracts, nutritional
supplements.*

**Ecological Formulas/Cardiovascular
Research**
1061 Shary Circle
Concord, CA 94518
800–888–4585 510–827–2636
*B Cell Formula; Buffered Vitamin C Powder;
Caprystatin; Essential Fatty Acid Complex;
Free-Form Amino Acid Crystals; Orithrush;
Quercitin-C; Tri-Salts.*

En Garde Health Products
7702 Balboa Boulevard, Building #10
Van Nuys, CA 91406
818–901–8505
DynamO2.

Enzymatic Therapy
825 Challenger Drive
Green Bay, WI 54311
800–783–2286 414–469–1313
*Derma-Klear; Grape Seed (PCO) Phytosome;
Kidney-Liver Complex #406; Liquid Liver
Extract #521; Lung Complex #407; Sinu
Check; ThymuPlex #398; Vira-Plex #135.*

E'Ola Products
3879 South River Road
St. George, UT 84790
800–748–6020 801–634–9444
Smart Longevity.

Esteem Products
12826 SE 40th Lane, Suite 200
Bellevue, WA 98006
800–255–7631 206–562–1281
Diet Esteem Plus.

Ethical Nutrients
971 Calle Negocio
San Clemente, CA 92673
800–668–8743 800–621–6070
Bone Builder; Bone Builder With Boron.

Flora
P.O. Box 950
Lynden, WA 98264
800–446–2110
Herbal extracts.

FoodScience Laboratories
20 New England Drive
Essex Junction, VT 05453
800–874–9444 802–878–5508
*Aangamik DMG; Energy Now; Glucosamine
Plus.*

Forest Pharmaceuticals, Inc.
2510 Metro Boulevard
St. Louis, MO 63043
314–569–3610
Armour Thyroid Tablets.

Freeda Vitamins and Pharmacy
36 East 41st Street
New York, NY 10017
800–777–3737 212–685–4980
AntiAllergy; FemCal; Ferrous fumarate.

Futurebiotics
145 Rice Field Lane
Hauppauge, NY 11788
800–367–5433
*Colloidal mineral supplements; Fiber Plus
Cholestatin; Megavital Forte.*

Gaia Herbs, Inc.
12 Lancaster County Road
Harvard, MA 01451
800–831–7780 508–772–5400
Saw Palmetto Supreme.

Gero Vita International
520 Washington Street, #391
Marina Del Ray, CA 90292
800–825–8482
GH3; Prostata.

Green Foods Corporation
318 North Graves Avenue
Oxnard, CA 93030
805–983–7470
Green Magma.

Health from the Sun
P.O. Box 840
Sunapee, NH 03782
800–447–2229
Sanhelio's Circu Caps.

Heart Foods Company
2235 East 38th Street
Minneapolis, MN 55407
612–724–5266
Herbal supplements; cayenne products.

Henkel Corporation
5325 South Ninth Avenue
LaGrange, IL 60525
708–579–6150
Betatene.

Holistic Health Services
513 North F Street
Livingston, MT 59047
406–222–1261
Nutritional holistic products.

Houston International, LLC
1719 West University, Suite 187
Tempe, AZ 85281
800–255–2690 602–437–0127
Daily Detox Tea.

Hybrivet Systems
P.O. Box 1210
Framingham, MA 01701
800–262–LEAD 508–651–7881
LeadCheck Aqua; LeadCheck Swabs.

Hyland's / P&S Laboratories
Div. of Standard Homeopathic Company
210 West 131 Street
Los Angeles, CA 90061
800–624–9659 213–321–4284
Poison Ivy/Oak Tablets.

**International Reforestation Suppliers
(Terra Tech)**
2100 West Broadway
Eugene, OR 97402
800–321–1037 541–345–0597
Lil Sucker.

Jarrow Formulas Inc.
1824 South Robertson Boulevard
Los Angeles, CA 90035
800–726–0886 310–204–6936
Colostrum Specific.

Johnson & Johnson
1001 US Highway 202
Raritan, NJ 08869–0610
800–421–6736
Advanced Care Cholesterol Kit.

Juice Plus
KELCO
931 Goodstein Drive
Casper, WY 82601
800-455-1740
Nutritional supplements/antioxidants.

KAL Nutrition Supplements
c/o Nutraceutical Corporation
1104 Country Hills Drive, Suite 300
Ogden, UT 84403
800–669–8877
Bone Defense; Virility Two.

LactAid, Inc.
7050 Camp Hill Road
Fort Washington, PA 19034–2299
800–LACTAID
LactAid.

Lake Consumer Products
625 Forest Edge Drive
Vernon Hills, IL 60061
800–635–3696
Yeast•Gard.

Lane Labs-USA, Inc.
172 Broadway
Woodcliff Lake, NJ 07675
800–526–3001 201–391–8600
BeneFin Shark Cartilage.

Laurel Farms
P.O. Box 2896
Sarasota, FL 34230
941–351–2233
Kombucha "mushrooms" and growing kits.

Lifestar International, Inc.
301 Vermont Street
San Francisco, CA 94103
800–858–7477
Salute Santé Grapeseed Oil.

Marlyn Nutraceuticals
14851 North Scottsdale Road
Scottsdale, AZ 85254
800–462–7596
Wobenzym N.

MegaFood
P.O. Box 325
Derry, NH 03038
800–258–5014
Nutritional supplements.

Metagenics
800–692–9400.
Ultra Clear Sustain. Products available through health care professionals only.

Miller Pharmacal Group, Inc.
350 Randy Road, #2
Carol Stream, IL 60188
800–323–2935 708–871–9557
Proteolytic enzymes.

Montana Naturals International, Inc.
19994 Highway 93
Arlee, MT 59821
800–872–7218 406–726–3214
Royal jelly.

National Enzyme Company
P.O. Box 128
Forsyth, MO 65653–0128
800–825–8545 417–546–4796
Plant-derived digestive enzyme products.

Natra-Bio Homeopathic
P.O. Box 1596
Ferndale, WA 98248
800–232–4005 206–384–5656
Homeopathic remedies.

Natren
3105 Willow Lake
Westlake Village, CA 91361
800–992–3323
Bifido Factor; Digesta-Lac; Gy-na-tren; Lifestart; Megadophilus; Trenev Trio.

Natrol, Inc.
20731 Marilla Street
Chatsworth, CA 91311
800–326–1570 818–701–9966
Ester C Plus Bioflavonoids.

Nature's Answer
75 Commerce Drive
Hauppauge, NY 11788
800–645–5720 516–231–5522
Slumber.

Nature's Herbs (A Twinlab Company)
600 East Quality Drive
American Fork, UT 84003
800–437–2257 801–763–0700
Bronc-Ease.

Nature's Plus
548 Broadhollow Road
Melville, NY 11747
800–645–9500 800–525–0200 516–293–0030
Bromelain; Fuel for Thought; Candida Forte; Detoxygen; Liv-R-Actin; Ocu-Care; Spiru-tein; Ultra Hair; Ultra Nails.

Nature's Products
2525 Davie Road
Davie, FL 33317
800–752–7873 305–474–9049
EPA Pure/300; EPA Pure/1200.

Nature's Secret
5485 Conestoga Court
Boulder, CO 80301
800–525–9696 303–546–6306
A.M./P.M. Ultimate Cleanse; Ultimate Fiber; Ultimate Oil.

Nature's Way Products
10 Mountain Springs Parkway
Springville, UT 84663
800–962–8873 801–489–1500
Fenu-Thyme; KB Formula; Nutralax 2; Primadophilus; Silent Night.

Natureworks
See Abkit Inc.

New Chapter, Inc.
Brattleboro, VT 05301
800–543–7279 802–257–0018
Mainstream; Neo-Flora; Tum-Ease.

Now Foods
550 Mitchell Road
Glendale Heights, IL 60139
800–999–8069 708–545–9098
Joint Support; Ultimate Zinc-C Lozenges.

Nutramax Laboratories, Inc.
5024 Campbell Boulevard
Baltimore, MD 21236
800–925–5187 410–931–4000
Cosamin.

NutriCology Inc.
400 Preda Street
San Leandro, CA 94577
800–545–9960 510–639–4572
ProGreens.

Nutrition 21
1010 Turquoise Street, Suite 335
San Diego, CA 92109
619–488–1021
Mineral supplements.

Omega-Life, Inc.
15355 Woodbridge Road
Brookfield, WI 53005
800–328–3529 414–786–2070
Fortified Flax.

Omega Nutrition
1924 Franklin Street
Vancouver, BC Z5L IR2
Canada
800–661–3529
Organic oil products.

Optimal Nutrients
1163 Chess Drive, Suite F
Foster City, CA 94404
800–966–8874
Coenzyme Q10.

Oxyfresh USA, Inc.
P.O. Box 3723
Spokane, WA 99220
800–999–9551 509–924–4999
Body Language Essential Green Foods; Body Language Super Antioxidant.

Para Laboratories/Queen Helene
100 Rose Avenue
Hempstead, NY 11550
800–645–3752 516–538–4600
Batherapy; Footherapy.

Parametric Associates, Inc.
10934 Lin-Valle Drive
St. Louis, MO 63123
800–747–1601 314–892–0988
Brain Alert; Calcium-Collagen Complex; Cardio-Power; Cold & Sinus; Digest-All; D-Yeast; Fat Metabolizer; Fatigue Free; Female Harmony; G.O.U.T.; Male Formula; Mobility; Multiple "Plus"; Nutra-Mune; Para-Cleans; Pure & Regular; Stress Free; Super Antioxidant; and Sweet Dreams.

Pep Products, Inc.
3130 North Commerce Court
P.O. Box 8002
Castle Rock, CO 80104
800–833–8737 303–688–6633
PEP Formula.

Pharmaceutical Purveyors of Oklahoma
1725 North Portland
Oklahoma City, OK 73107
800–234–1091 405–943–1091
Perfect B.

PhysioLogics
6565 Odell Place
Boulder, CO 80301
800–765–6775
Coloklysis-7; CTR Support. Products available through health care professionals only.

PhytoPharmica
825 Challenger Drive
Green Bay, WI 54311
800–553–2370
Glucosamine Sulfate; Glucosamine Sulfate Complex.

Planetary Formulas
23 Janis Way
Scotts Valley, CA 95066
408–438–1700
Triphala.

Prevail Corporation
2204-8 NW Birdsdale
Gresham, OR 97030
800–248–0885
Acid-Ease; Meno-Fem; Osteo Formula; Sinease.

Primary Source
1150 Post Road
Fairfield, CT 06430
800–667–1538
OPC-85.

Probiologic Inc.
8707 148th Avenue NE
Redmond, WA 98052
800–678–8218 206–881–8218
Capricin.

Progressive Research Labs, Inc.
9396 Richmond, Suite 514
Houston, TX 77063
800–877–0966
Diabetic Nutrition Rx.

Prolongevity
P.O. Box 229120
Hollywood, FL 33022–9120
800–841–5433 954–766–8433
Cognitex.

Pronatura, Inc.
6211-A West Howard Street
Niles, IL 60714
800–555–7580
Kombucha tea, capsules, and extract.

Pure-Gar, Inc.
P.O. Box 98813
Tacoma, WA 98498
800–537–7695 206–582–6421
Nutritional supplements.

RidgeCrest Herbals, Inc.
1151 South Redwood Road, Suite 106
Salt Lake City, UT 84104
800–242–4649 801–978–9633
ClearLungs.

Salus Haus
158 Business Center Drive
Corona, CA 91720
800–446–2110
Floradix Iron and Iron + Herb Formulas.

Schiff Products
1960 South 4250 West
Salt Lake City, UT 84104
Phytocharged nutritional supplements.

Solaray Products
1104 Country Hill Drive, Suite 412
Ogden, UT 84403
800–669–8877 801–626–4900
SP-6 Cornsilk Blend; SP-8 Hawthorn Motherwort Blend; SP-14 Valerian Blend.

Solgar Vitamin Company, Inc.
500 Willow Tree Road
Leonia, NJ 07605
201–944–2311
BeneFin Shark Cartilage; Earthsource Greens & More; MaxEPA.

Sonne Organic Foods
P.O. Box 2160
Cottonwood, CA 96022
916–347–5868
Sonne's #7.

Source Naturals
P.O. Box 2118
Santa Cruz, CA 95063
800–777–5677 408–438–6851
Activated Quercetin; Calcium Night; Coenzymate B Complex; GlucosaMend; Heart Science; N-A-G; Proangenol 100; Proanthodyn; Urban Air Defense; Vital Eyes.

Spectrum Naturals
133A Copeland
Petaluma, CA 94952
707–778–8900
Flaxseed oil.

Sun Precautions
2815 Wetmore Avenue
Everett, WA 98201
800–882–7860
Solumbra clothing.

The SunBox Company
19217 Orbit Drive
Gaithersburg, MD 20879
800–548–3968 301–869–5980
Dawn Simulator.

Synergy Plus/International Vitamins
500 Halls Mill Road
Freehold, NJ 07728–8811
800–666–8482 908–308–9793
Bone Support; Capralin.

Terra Maxa, Inc.
3301 West Central Avenue
Toledo, OH 43606
800–783–7817 419–385–3001
PSI.

Thompson Nutritional Products
851 Broken Sound Parkway, NW
Boca Raton, FL 33487
800–421–1192
Life Guard.

Threshold Enterprises
23 Janis Way
Scotts Valley, CA 95066
800–777–5677
Vitamin and mineral supplements.

Thursday Plantation
P.O. Box 5613
Montecito, CA 93150
800–848–8966 805–963–2297
Tea tree oil.

Tom's of Maine
P.O. Box 710
Kennebunk, ME 04043
207–985–2944
Tom's of Maine Natural Toothpaste and other natural body care products.

Trace Minerals Research
1990 West 3300 South
Ogden, UT 84401
800–624–7145 801–731–6051
Concentrace; Arth-X.

Tri-Sun International
2230 Cape Cod Way
Santa Ana, CA 92703
800–387–4786
Jason Winters Tea.

Twinlab
2120 Smithtown Avenue
Ronkonkoma, NY 11779
800–645–5626 516–467–3140
GABA Plus; OcuGuard.

UniTea Herbs
P.O. Box 8005, #318
Boulder, CO 80306–8005
303–443–1248
SensualiTea.

Urohealth Corporation
3050 Redhill Avenue
Costa Mesa, CA 92626
800–328–1103
Snap Gauge.

Wakunaga of America Company, Ltd.
23501 Madero
Mission Viejo, CA 92691–2764
800–421–2998 714–855–2776
Be Sure; Ginkgo Biloba Plus; Kyo-Dophilus; Kyo-Green; Kyolic Garlic.

Warren Laboratories, Inc.
12603 Executive Drive, Suite 806
Stafford, TX 77477
800–232–2563 713–240–2563
George's Aloe Vera Juice.

Wein Products Inc.
Air Supply.
Distributed by:
Breath Free Products
1750 Ocean Boulevard.
Suite 305
Long Beach, CA 90802
888–434–8313

Health and Medical Organizations

The following is a list of organizations that can provide assistance for specific disorders and situations. The services offered by these organizations vary. Some provide information only; others offer various types of referrals, support groups, and even access to medical or social services. In most cases, the organizations' areas of interest are obvious from their names. Where this is not the case, a brief description of the organization's focus is offered. Be aware that addresses and telephone numbers are subject to change.

AIDS Action Committee
131 Clarendon Street
Boston, MA 02116
617–437–6200

Alcoholics Anonymous
475 Riverside Drive, 11th Floor
New York, NY 10115
212–870–3400

Alexander Graham Bell Association for the Deaf
3417 Volta Place NW
Washington, DC 20007–2778
202–337–5220

Alzheimer's Association
919 North Michigan Avenue, Suite 1000
Chicago, IL 60611
800–272–3900
312–335–8700

American Academy of Allergy and Immunology
611 Wells Street
Milwaukee, WI 53202
800–822–ASMA

American Academy of Child and Adolescent Psychology
3615 Wisconsin Avenue NW
Washington, DC 20016
202–966–7300

American Academy of Dermatology
930 North Meacham Road
P.O. Box 4014
Schaumburg, IL 60168
708–330–0230

American Anorexia/Bulimia Association (AABA)
293 Central Park West, Suite 1R
New York, NY 10024
212–501–8351

American Apitherapy Society
P.O. Box 54
Hartland Four Corners, VT 05049
802–436–2708

American Association of Sex Educators, Counselors, and Therapists
435 North Michigan Avenue, Suite 1717
Chicago, IL 60611
312–644–0828

American Association on Mental Retardation (AAMR)
444 North Capitol Street NW, Suite 846
Washington, DC 20001–1512
800–424–3688 202–387–1968

American Board of Chelation Therapy
1407–B North Wells
Chicago, IL 60601
800–356–2228 312–787–2228

American Brain Tumor Research Assn.
2720 River Road, Suite 146
Des Plains, IL 60018
708–827–9910

American Cancer Society
1599 Clifton Road
Atlanta, GA 30329
800–ACS–2345

American Celiac Society
58 Musano Court
West Orange, NJ 07052
201–325–8837

American College of Advancement in Medicine (ACAM)
P.O. Box 3427
Laguna Hills, CA 92654
800–532–3688 714–583–7666
Provides a list of chelation therapists.

American Council for Headache Education (ACHE)
875 Kings Highway, Suite 200
Woodbury, NJ 08096
800–255–ACHE

American Council of the Blind
1155 15th Street NW, Suite 720
Washington DC 20005
800–424–8666 202–467–5081 (Monday to
Friday, 3:00 to 5:30 p.m. Eastern time)

American Dental Association
211 East Chicago Avenue
Chicago, IL 60611
312–440–2500

American Diabetes Association
1660 Duke Street
Alexandria, VA 22314
800–232–3472 703–549–1500

Alliance of Genetic Support Groups
35 Wisconsin Circle, Suite 440
Chevy Chase, MD 20815
800–336–4363 301–652–5553

American Fertility Society
1209 Montgomery Highway
Birmingham, AL 35216
205–978–5000

American Foundation for AIDS Research (AMFAR)
733 Third Avenue, 12th Floor
New York, NY 10017
212–682–7440

American Foundation for the Blind
11 Penn Plaza
New York, NY 10001
800–232–5463

American Genetic Association
P.O. Box 39
Buckeystown, MD 21717
301–695–9292

American Heart Association
7272 Greenville Avenue
Dallas, TX 75231
214–373–6300

American Industrial Hygiene Association
475 Wolf Ledges Parkway
Akron, OH 44311
216–762–7294

American Kidney Fund (AKF)
6110 Executive Boulevard, Suite 1010
Rockville, MD 20852
800–638–8299 301–881–3052

American Liver Foundation
1425 Pompton Avenue
Cedar Grove, NJ 07009
800–223–0179 291–256–2550

American Lung Association
1740 Broadway
New York, NY 10019
800–LUNG–USA

American Medical Association (AMA)
515 North State Street
Chicago, IL 60610
312–464–5000

American Mental Health Foundation
1049 Fifth Avenue
New York, NY 10028
212–737–9027

American Pain Society
5700 Old Orchard Road
Skokie, IL 60077
708–966–5595

American Parkinson Association
1250 Hylan Boulevard
Staten Island, NY 10305
800–223–2732

American Sleep Disorders
1610 14th Street, Suite 300
Rochester, MN 55901
507–287–6006

American Society of Cataract and Refractive Surgery
3702 Pender Drive, Suite 250
Fairfax, VA 22030
703–591–2220

American Speech-Language-Hearing Assn.
10801 Rockville Pike
Rockville, MD 20852
800–638–TALK 301–897–5700

American Tinnitus Association
P.O. Box 5
Portland, OR 97207
503–248–9985

Amyotrophic Lateral Sclerosis (ALS) Society
21021 Ventura Boulevard, Suite 321
Woodland Hills, CA 91364
800–782–4747 818–340–7500

Anorexia Nervosa and Associated Disorders
P.O. Box 7
Highland Park, IL 60035
847–831–3438

Anorexia Nervosa and Related Eating Disorders (ANRED)
P.O. Box 5102
Eugene, OR 97405
503–344–1144

Anxiety Disorders Association of America
6000 Executive Boulevard, Suite 513
Rockville, MD 20852
301–231–9350

Arthritis Foundation
1314 Spring Street NW
Atlanta, GA 30309
800–283–7800

Asbestos Victims of America
P.O. Box 559
Capitola, CA 95010
408–476–3646

Association for the Education and Rehabilitation of the Blind and Visually Impaired
206 North Washington Street, Suite 320
Alexandria, VA 22314
703–548–1884

Asthma and Allergy Foundation of America
1717 Massachusetts Avenue NW, Suite 305
Washington, DC 20036
800–7–ASTHMA 202–466–7643 (Monday to Friday, 9:00 a.m. to 5:00 p.m. Eastern time)

Attention Deficit Disorder Association
P.O. Box 972
Mentor, OH 44061
800–487–2282

Autism Society of America
7910 Woodmont Avenue, Suite 650
Bethesda, MD 20814
301–657–0881

Brain Injury Association
1776 Massachusetts Avenue NW, Suite 100
Washington, DC 20036
800–444–6443
202–296–6443

Brain Research Foundation
208 South LaSalle Street, Suite 1426
Chicago, IL 60604
312–782–4311

Cancer Information Service
National Cancer Institute
Building 31, Room 10A24
9000 Rockville Pike
Bethesda, MD 20892
800–4–CANCER

Cancer Treatment Centers of America
Midwestern Regional Medical Center
2501 Emmaus Avenue
Zion, IL 60099
800–FOR–HELP 708–872–4561
Offers information on alternatives for the diagnosis and effective treatment of cancer.

Celiac Disease Foundation
13251 Ventura Boulevard, Suite 3
Studio City, CA 91604–1838
818–990–2354

Center for the Treatment of Eating Disorders
c/o Harding Hospital
445 East Granville Road
Worthington, OH 43085
614–846–2833

Centers for Disease Control and Prevention (CDC)
1600 Clifton Road NE
Atlanta, GA 30333
404–332–4555

CHILDHELP USA
6463 Independence Avenue
Woodland Hills, CA 91367
800–422–4453
Provides help for abused children.

Children of Aging Parents (CAPS)
1609 Woodburne Road, Suite 302A
Levittown, PA 19081
215–945–6900

Children with Attention-Deficit Disorders
499 Northwest 70th Avenue, Suite 101
Plantation, FL 33317
305–587–3700

Choice in Dying
200 Varick Street, 10th floor
New York, NY 10014–4810
212–366–5540

Chronic Fatigue and Immune Dysfunction Syndrome (CFIDS) Foundation
P.O. Box 220398
Charlotte, NC 28222–0398
800–442–3437

Crohn's and Colitis Foundation of America
386 Park Avenue South, 17th floor
New York, NY 10016–8804
800–343–3637 212–685–3440

Cystic Fibrosis Foundation (CFF)
6931 Arlington Road, Suite 2000
Bethesda, MD 20814
800–344–4823 301–951–4422

Do It Now Foundation
P.O. Box 27568
Tempe, AZ 85285–7568
602–491–0393
Publishes substance abuse and behavioral health information.

Dogs for the Deaf
10175 Wheeler Road
Central Point, OR 97502
503–826–9220

Endometriosis Association
8585 North 76th Place
Milwaukee, WI 53223
800–992–ENDO (United States)
800–426–2END (Canada)

The Epilepsy Foundation of America
4351 Garden City Drive
Landover, MD 20785–2267
800–213–5821 301–577–0100

Feingold Association of the United States
P.O. Box 6550
Alexandria, VA 22306
703–768–3287
Provides information on the effects of food and food additives on health, behavior, and learning.

Fertility Research Foundation
1430 Second Avenue, Suite 103
New York, NY 10021
212–744–5500

Food Allergy Network
4744 Holly Avenue
Fairfax, VA 22030–5647
703–691–3179

Foundation for Glaucoma Research
490 Post Street, Suite 830
San Franciso, CA 94102
415–986–3162

Gay Men's Health Crisis (GMHC)
129 West 20th Street
New York, NY 10011–3629
212–807–6655 TTY 212–645–7470
*Provides information and services relating
to HIV and AIDS.*

Guiding Eyes for the Blind
611 Granite Springs Road
Yorktown Heights, NY 10598
800–942–0149 914–245–4024

Help for Incontinent People
P.O. Box 544
Union, SC 29379
803–579–7900

Herpes Resource Center
P.O. Box 13827
Research Triangle Park, NC 27709
919–361–8488

**Human Growth Disorder
Foundation**
7777 Leesberg Pike
Falls Church, VA 22043
800–451–6434 703–883–1773

Immune Deficiency Foundation
P.O. Box 586
Colombia, MD 21045
410–461–3127

Impotence Foundation
P.O. Box 60260
Santa Barbara, CA 93160
800–221–5517

**Institute for the Psychology
of Air Travel**
25 Huntington Avenue, Suite 300
Boston, MA 02116
617–437–1811

**Institute for the Study of Anorexia
and Bulimia**
1 West 91st Street
New York, NY 10024
212–595–3449

**International Association
for Medical Assistance to Travelers**
736 Center Street
Lewiston, NY 20402
716–754–4883

International Diabetes Center
3800 Park Nicollet Boulevard
Minneapolis, MN 55416
612–927–3393

International Tremor Foundation
360 West Superior
Chicago, IL 60610
312–733–1893

Interstitial Cystitis Association
P.O. Box 1553
Madison Square Station
New York, NY 10159
212–674–1454

Juvenile Diabetes Foundation
120 Wall Street, 19th Floor
New York, NY 10005
800–533–2873 212–785–9500

Learning Disabilities of America (LDA)
4156 Library Road
Pittsburgh, PA 15234
412–341–1515

Leukemia Society of America
733 Third Avenue
New York, NY 10017
212–573–8484

The Living Bank
P.O. Box 6725
Houston, TX 77265
800–528–2971 713–961–9431
*Provides information and maintains registry of
donated organs, tissues, bones, and bodies for
transplants or research.*

Lung Line Information Service
National Jewish Hospital
1400 Jackson Street
Denver, CO 80226
800–222–5864 303–355–5864

Lupus Foundation of America
4 Research Place, Suite 180
Rockville, MD 20850–3226
800–558–0121 301–670–9292

Lyme Borreliosis Foundation
P.O. Box 462
Tolland, CT 06084
203–525–2000

March of Dimes National Foundation
1275 Mamaroneck Avenue
White Plains, NY 10605
914–428–7100

Medic Alert Foundation
2323 Colorado Avenue
Turlock, CA 95381–1009
800–432–5378 800–344–3226 209–668–3333
*Maintains files on individuals who wear a
medical bracelet to provide information in case
of an emergency.*

Mothers Against Drunk Driving (MADD)
511 John Carpenter Freeway, Suite 700
Irving, TX 75062–8187
800–438–MADD

Multiple Sclerosos Foundation
6350 North Andrews Avenue
Fort Lauderdale, FL 33309
800–441–7055

Muscular Dystrophy Association
3561 East Sunrise Drive
Tucson, AZ 85718
800–572–1717

Myasthenia Gravis Foundation
222 South Riverside Plaza
Suite 1540
Chicago, Il 60606
800–541–5454

Narcolepsy Institute
Montefiore Medical Center
111 East 210th Street
Bronx, NY 10467
718–920–6799

National Aging Information Center
500 E Street SW, Suite 910
Washington, DC 20024–2710
202–554–9800

National Alopecia Areata Foundation
714 C Street, Suite 216
San Rafael, CA 94901
415–456–4644

**National Association for the
Visually Handicapped**
3201 Balboa Street
San Francisco, CA 94121
415–221–3201

National Association of the Deaf
814 Thayer Avenue
Silver Spring, MD 20910
301–587–1788

**National Association of People With
AIDS (NAPWA)**
1413 K Street NW, Suite 700
Washington, DC 20005
202–898–0414

National Asthma Center Lung Line
1400 Jackson Street
Denver, CO 80206
800–222–LUNG

National Burn Victim Foundation
32–34 Scotland Road
Orange, NJ 07050
201–676–7700

**National Chronic Pain Outreach
Association**
7979 Old Georgetown Road, Suite 100
Bethesda, MD 20814
301–652–4948

**National Clearinghouse for Alcohol
and Drug Information**
11426–28 Rockville Pike, Suite 200
Rockville, MD 20847–2345
800–729–6686 301–443–6500

National Council on Aging
409 Third Street SW, 2nd Floor
Washington, DC 20024
202–479–1200

National Council on Alcoholism
12 West 21st Street
New York, NY 10010
800–622–2255

National Diabetes Information Clearinghouse (NDIC)
1 Information Way
Bethesda, MD 20892–3560
301–654–3327

National Digestive Diseases Information Clearinghouse
2 Information Way
Bethesda, MD 20892–3570
301–654–3810

National Down Syndrome Congress
1605 Chantilly Drive, Suite 250
Atlanta, GA 30324
800–232–NDSC

National Down Syndrome Society (NDSS)
666 Broadway
New York, NY 10012
800–221–4602 212–460–9330

National Eating Disorders Organization
6655 South Yale
Tulsa, OK 74136
918–481–4044

National Eye Institute (NEI)
National Institutes of Health
Building 31, Room 6A32
31 Center Drive, MSC 2510
Bethesda, MD 20892–2510
301–496–5248

National Foundation for Depressive Illness
P.O. Box 2257
New York, NY 10116
800–248–4344

National Headache Foundation
5252 North Western Avenue
Chicago, IL 60625
800–843–2256

National Health Information Center
P.O. Box 1133
Washington, DC 20013–1133
800–336–4797
301–565–4167

National Heart, Lung, and Blood Institute
Information Center
P.O. Box 30105
Bethesda, MD 20824–0105
301–251–1222

National Hemophilia Foundation (NHF)
110 Greene Street, Suite 303
New York, NY 10012
212–219–8180

National Hospice Organization
1901 North Moore Street, Suite 901
Arlington, VA 22209
703–243–5900

National Institute of Allergies and Infectious Diseases
National Institutes of Health
Building 31, Room 7A50
9000 Rockville Pike
Bethesda, MD 20892
301–496–5717

National Institute of Diabetes and Digestive and Kidney Diseases (NIDDK)
National Institutes of Health
Building 31, Room 9A04
31 Center Drive MSC 2560
Bethesda, MD 20892–2560
301–496–3583

National Institute of Mental Health (NIMH)
5600 Fishers Lane
Rockville, MD 20857
800–64–PANIC 301–443–4513

National Institute on Aging
Alzheimer Education Referral Center
P.O. Box 8250
Silver Spring, MD 20907–8250
800–438–4380

National Institute on Alcohol Abuse and Alcoholism
6000 Executive Boulevard, Suite 409
Rockville, MD 20892–7003
301–443–3860

National Institute on Drug Abuse
5600 Fishers Lane
Rockville, MD 20857
301–443–6245

National Kidney Foundation
30 East 33rd Street, Suite 1100
New York, NY 10016
800–622–9010

National Library Service for the Blind and Physically Handicapped
Library of Congress
1291 Taylor Street NW
Washington, DC 20542
202–707–5100

National Mental Health Association
1021 Prince Street
Alexandria, VA 22314
800–969–6642

National Multiple Sclerosis Society
733 Third Avenue
New York, NY 10017
800–344–4867 212–986–3240

National Neurofibromatosis Foundation
95 Pine Street, 16th Floor
New York, NY 10005
800–323–7938 212–344–6633

National Organization for Rare Diseases
100 Route 37
P.O. Box 8923
New Fairfield, CT 06812–8923
800–999–NORD

National Organization for Seasonal Affective Disorder
P.O. Box 40133
Washington, DC 20016

National Osteoporosis Foundation
2100 M Street NW, Suite 602
Washington, DC 20037
800–223–9994

National Parkinson's Foundation (NPF)
1501 NW 9th Avenue
Miami, FL 33136
800–327–4545 305–547–6666

National Pediculosis Association
P.O. Box 149
Newton, MA 02161
617–449–NITS

National Pesticide Telecommunications Network (NPTN)
Agricultural Chemistry Extension
333 Weiniger
Corvallis, OR 97331–6502
800–858–7378
Provides information on health hazards of and safety precautions against pesticides.

National Psoriasis Foundation
6600 SW 92nd Avenue, Suite 300
Portland, OR 97223
800–723–9166 503–244–7404

National Reye's Syndrome Foundation
426 North Lewis
P.O. Box 829
Bryan, OH 43506
800–233–7393

National Rosacea Society
220 South Cook Street, Suite 201
Barrington, IL 60010
708–382–8971

National Safety Council
444 North Michigan Avenue
Chicago, IL 60611
312–527–4800

National Sjögren's Syndrome Association
P.O. Box 42207
Phoenix, AZ 85080-2207
800–395–NSSA

National Society to Prevent Blindness
500 East Remington Road
Schaumburg, IL 60173
708–843–2020

National Stroke Association
8480 East Orchard Road, Suite 1000
Englewood, CO 80111–5105
800–STROKES

Nursing Home Information Service Center
National Council of Senior Citizens
1331 F Street, Suite 500
Washington, DC 20004–1171
202–347–8800

Obsessive-Compulsive Anonymous
P.O. Box 215
New Hyde Park, NY 10041
516–741–4901

Parkinson Support Group of America
11376 Cherry Hill Road, Suite 204
Beltsville, MD 20705
301–937–1545

Parkinson's Education Program
3900 Birch Street, Suite 105
Newport Beach, CA 92660
800–344–7872

Planned Parenthood Federation of America
810 Seventh Avenue
New York, NY 10019
212–541–7800

PMS Access
P.O. Box 9362
Madison, WI 53715
800–222–4767 608–833–4767

Premenstrual Syndrome Action
P.O. Box 16292
Irvine, CA 92713
714–854–4407

Project Inform
1965 Market Street, Suite 220
San Francisco, CA 94103
800–822–7422
Provides information to help educate people with HIV and their health care providers about treatment.

Recovery of Male Potency
27177 Lahser, Suite 101
Southfield, MI 48034
810–357–1314

Retinitis Pigmentosa Foundation
11350 McCormick Road
Executive Plaza One, Suite 800
Hunt Valley, MD 21031–1014
800–683–5555

Scleroderma Federation
P.O. Box 910
Lynnfield, MA 01940
508–535–6600

Scoliosis Association
P.O. Box 811705
Boca Raton, FL 33481–1705
800–800–0669

Self-Help for Hard of Hearing People
7910 Woodmont Avenue, Suite 1200
Bethesda, MD 20814
301–657–2248

SIDS Resource Center
8201 Greensboro Drive, Suite 600
McLean, VA 22102
703–821–8955, extension 249

Simon Foundation
P.O. Box 815
Wilmette, IL 60091
800–622–9010
Provides information on dealing with incontinence.

Sjögren's Syndrome Foundation
333 North Broadway, Suite 2000
Jericho, NY 11753
516–933–6365

Skin Cancer Foundation
245 Fifth Avenue, Suite 2402
New York, NY 10016
212–725–5176

The Speech Foundation of America
P.O. Box 11749
Memphis, TN 38111
901–452–0995

Spina Bifida Association of America (SBAA)
4590 MacArthur Boulevard NW, Suite 250
Washington, DC 20007 4226
800–621–3141 202–944–3285

The Stroke Foundation, Inc.
898 Park Avenue
New York, NY 10021
212–734–3461

Sudden Infant Death Syndrome Alliance
53 West Jackson, Suite 1601
Chicago, IL 60604
800–432–7437

Support Source
P.O. Box 245
Swarthmore, PA 19081
610–544–3605
Provides information on care for elderly persons.

Thyroid Foundation of America
Ruth Sleeper Hall - RSL 350
40 Parkman Street
Boston, MA 12114–2698
800–832–8321

United Cerebral Palsy Association
1660 L Street NW, Suite 700
Washington, DC 20036
800–872–5827

United Ostomy Association
36 Executive Park, Suite 120
Irvine, CA 92714
800–826–0826 714–660–8624

United Parkinson Foundation
800 North Washington Road
Chicago, IL 60607
312–733–1893

Water Quality Association
4151 Naperville Road
Lisle, IL 60532
708–505–0160
Provides information on types of water and methods of water treatment.

Wilson's Syndrome Foundation
P.O. Box 539
Summerfield, FL 34492
800–621–7006

Y-ME National Breast Cancer Organization
212 West Van Buren Street
Chicago, IL 60607
800–221–2141

Health and Medical Hot Lines

The hot lines listed below provide information, help, and support for people with various illnesses and for those in emergency situations. All calls are confidential.

AIDS Hot Line
English: 800–342–AIDS (all times)
Spanish: 800–344–7432 (8:00 a.m.–2:00 p.m. Eastern time)
TTY: 800–243–7889 (Monday–Friday, 10:00 a.m.–10:00 p.m. Eastern time)
Offers information and educational services on HIV- and AIDS-related topics. Also provides medical and support-group referrals. Sponsored by the Centers for Disease Control and Prevention.

Alcohol and Drug Helpline
800–252–6465

American Anorexia/Bulimia Association
212–501–8351
Provides information on eating disorders, as well as referrals and outreach programs for those affected by such disorders.

American Kidney Fund
800–638–8299 301–881–3052
Assists kidney patients unable to pay for treatment.

Cancer Information Service
800–4–CANCER
Provides information on cancer treatment and prevention. Sponsored by the National Cancer Institute.

Cancer Treatment Centers of America
800–FOR–HELP 708–872–4561
Offers information on alternatives for the diagnosis and effective treatment of cancer.

Center for Nutrition and Dietetics Consumer Hot Line
800–366–1655

Child Abuse Hot Line
800–422–4453
Provides twenty-four-hour service that offers counseling facilities and provides reporting agencies for victims of child abuse.

Cocaine Hot Line
800–COCAINE
Provides referrals to hospitals, counseling centers, and doctors specializing in cocaine treatment.

Dial a Hearing Test
800–222–EARS
800–345–EARS (Pennsylvania)

Hearing Aid Helpline
800–521–5247

Impotence Foundation
800–221–5517
Offers information on impotence and other male and female dysfunctions. Also provides professional advice and referrals.

The Living Bank
800–528–2971 713–961–9431
Provides information and maintains registry of donated organs, tissues, bones, and bodies for transplants or research.

Lung Line Information Service
800–222–5864 303–355–5864
Provides information on respiratory diseases and immune disorders. Specialists available to answer specific questions.

Meat and Poultry Hotline
800–535–4555
Provides information to help consumers prevent food-borne illness through proper food handling.

Medic Alert Foundation
800–432–5378 800–344–3226 209–668–3333
Maintains files on individuals who wear a medical bracelet to provide information in case of an emergency.

Medicare Hot Line
800–638–6833
Provides up-to-date information on medicare-related topics.

National Institute on Drug Abuse
301–443–6245
Provides referrals for drug-abuse prevention programs.

Pesticide Telecommunications Network
800–858–7378
Provides information on health hazards of and safety precautions against pesticides.

Poison Control Center
See listing of local emergency numbers on page 432.

Project Inform
800–822–7422
415–558–9051 (San Francisco area)
Offers a national HIV-treatment hotline to update people on the latest treatment news—and to debunk the latest in treatment hype.

Prostate Information Hot Line
800–543–9632

Runaway Hot Line
800–231–6946
Accepts calls from runaways. Offers free bus ride home, forwards messages to home, and provides referrals for medical aid and shelter.

Sexually Transmitted Diseases Hot Line
800–227–8922

Suggested Reading

The following list of books is provided for those who wish to explore a particular topic further. The books mentioned here are good sources of further information.

Airola, Paavo. *Cancer Causes, Prevention, and Treatment: The Total Approach.* Phoenix, AZ: Health Plus Publishers, 1972.

Airola, Paavo. *How to Get Well.* Phoenix, AZ: Health Plus Publishers, 1974.

Airola, Paavo. *How to Keep Slim, Healthy, and Young With Juice Fasting.* Phoenix, AZ: Health Plus Publishers, 1971.

Airola, Paavo. *Hypoglycemia: A Better Approach.* Phoenix, AZ: Health Plus Pub., 1977.

Aladjem, Henrietta. *Understanding Lupus.* New York: Scribner, 1986.

Antol, Marie Nadine. *Healing Teas.* Garden City Park, NY: Avery Publishing Group, 1996.

Appleton, Nancy. *Lick the Sugar Habit.* Garden City Park, NY: Avery Publishing Group, 1996.

Astor, Stephen. *Hidden Food Allergies.* Garden City Park, NY: Avery Publishing Group, 1989.

Atkins, Robert C. *Dr. Atkins' Nutritional Breakthrough.* New York: W Morrow & Co., 1981.

Balch, James F., and Phyllis A. Balch. *Prescription for Dietary Wellness.* Greenfield, IN: P.A.B. Books, Inc., 1995.

Barnes, Broda O., and Lawrence Galton. *Hypothyroidism: The Unsuspected Illness.* New York: Cromwell, 1976.

Becker, Robert O., and Gary Selden. *Body Electric: Electromagnetism and the Foundation of Life.* New York: William Morrow & Co., 1987.

Bland, Jeffrey. *Medical Applications of Clinical Nutrition.* New Canaan, CT: Keats Pub., 1983.

Bland, Jeffrey. *Your Health Under Seige: Using Nutrition to Fight Back.* Greene, 1982.

Blauer, Stephen. *The Juicing Book.* Garden City Park, NY: Avery Publishing Group, 1989.

Bliznakov, Emile, and Gerry Hunt. *The Miracle Nutrient: Coenzyme Q10.* New York: Bantam Books, 1987.

Brighthope, Ian. *The AIDS Fighters.* New Canaan, CT: Keats Publishing, 1988.

Brinkley, Ginny, Linda Goldberg, and Janice Kukar. *Your Child's First Journey.* Garden City Park, NY: Avery Publishing Group, 1989.

Buist, Robert. *Food Chemical Sensitivity.* Garden City Park, NY: Avery Publishing Group, 1988.

Cabot, Sandra. *Smart Medicine for Menopause.* Garden City Park, NY: Avery Publishing Group, 1995.

Check, William A., and Ann G. Fettner. *The Truth About AIDS: Evolution of an Epidemic.* New York: Holt, Rinehart & Winston, 1985.

Clare, Sally, and David Clare. *Creative Vegetarian Cookery.* Dorset, England: Prism Press, 1988.

Crook, William G. *The Yeast Connection*, rev. ed. New York: Vintage Books, 1986.

Davidson, Paul. *Are You Sure It's Arthritis?* New York: Macmillan Publishing Co., 1985.

Davis, Adelle. *Let's Eat Right to Keep Fit.* New York: Harcourt Brace Jovanovich, Inc., 1970.

de Haas, Cherie. *Natural Skin Care.* Garden City Park, NY: Avery Publishing Group, 1989.

Donsbach, Kurt W. *Dr. Donsbach's Guide to Good Health.* Long Shadow Books, 1985.

Editors of *East West Journal. Shopper's Guide to Natural Foods.* Garden City Park, NY: Avery Publishing Group, 1988.

Edwards, Linda. *Baking for Health.* Garden City Park, NY: Avery Publishing Group, 1988.

Erasmus, Udo. *Fats and Oils.* Vancouver: Alive Press, 1987.

Evans, Gary. *Chromium Picolinate: Everything You Need to Know.* Garden City Park, NY: Avery Publishing Group, 1996.

Evans, Richard A. *Making the Right Choice: Treatment Options in Cancer Surgery.* Garden City Park, NY: Avery Publishing Group, 1995.

Feingold, Ben F. *Why Your Child Is Hyperactive.* New York: Random House, 1985.

Feingold, Helene, and Ben Feingold. *The Feingold Cookbook for Hyperactive Children and Others With Problems Associated With Food Additives and Salicylates.* New York: Random House, 1979.

Fink, John. *Third Opinion: An International Directory to Alternative Therapy Centers for the Treatment and Prevention of Cancer.* Garden City Park, NY: Avery Publishing Group, 1997.

Fujita, Takuo. *Calcium and Your Health.* Tokyo: Japan Publications, 1987.

Fulder, Stephen. *The Ginger Book.* Garden City Park, NY: Avery Publishing Group, 1996.

Fulder, Stephen. *The Ginseng Book.* Garden City Park, NY: Avery Publishing Group, 1996.

Germann, Donald R. *The Anti-Cancer Diet.* New York: Wyden Books, 1977.

Gittleman, Ann Louise. *Guess What Came to Dinner: Parasites and Your Health.* Garden City Park, NY: Avery Publishing Group, 1993.

Gregory, Scott J., and Bianca Leonardo. *They Conquered AIDS!* True Life Publications, 1989.

Griffith, H. Winter. *Complete Guide to Symptoms, Illness and Surgery for People Over 50.* Los Angeles: The Body Press, 1992.

Heidenry, Carolyn. *Making the Transition to a Macrobiotic Diet.* Garden City Park, NY: Avery Publishing Group, 1988.

Heinerman, John. *Aloe Vera, Jojoba & Yucca.* New Canaan, CT: Keats, 1982.

Howard, Mary Ann. *Blueprint for Health.* Grand Rapids, MI: Zondervan Publishing House, 1985.

Howell, Edward. *Enzyme Nutrition.* Garden City Park, NY: Avery Publishing Group, 1987.

Huggins, Hal A. *It's All in Your Head.* Garden City Park, NY: Avery Publishing Group, 1993.

Jacobson, Michael. *Safe Food: Eating Wisely in a Risky World.* Washington, DC: Living Planet Press, 1991.

Krumholz, Harlan M., and Robert H. Phillips. *No If's, And's or Butts, The Smoker's Guide to Quitting.* Garden City Park, NY: Avery Publishing Group, 1993.

Kushi, Aveline, and Wendy Esko. *The Macrobiotic Cancer Prevention Cookbook.* Garden City Park, NY: Avery Publishing Group, 1987.

Kushi, Michio, with Edward Esko. *The Macrobiotic Approach to Cancer.* Garden City Park, NY: Avery Publishing Group, 1991.

Kushi, Michio. *The Macrobiotic Way.* Garden City Park, NY: Avery Publishing Group, 1993.

Lance, James W. *Migraine and Other Headaches.* New York: Scribner, 1986.

Lane, I. William, and Linda Comac. *Sharks Don't Get Cancer: How Shark Cartilage Could Save Your Life.* Garden City Park, NY: Avery Publishing Group, 1992.

Lane, I. William, and Linda Comac. *Sharks Still Don't Get Cancer.* Garden City Park, NY: Avery Publishing Group, 1996.

Lerman, Andrea. *The Macrobiotic Community Cookbook.* Garden City Park, NY: Avery Publishing Group, 1989.

Levenstein, Mary Kerney. *Everyday Cancer Risks and How to Avoid Them.* Garden City Park, NY: Avery Publishing Group, 1992.

Levitt, Paul, and Elissa Guralnick. *The Cancer Reference Book.* New York: Paddington Press, 1979.

Livingston-Wheeler, Virginia, and Edmond G. Addleo. *The Conquest of Cancer: Vaccines and Diet.* New York: Franklin Watts, 1984.

Messina, Mark, and Virginia Messina, with Ken Setchell. *The Simple Soybean and Your Health.* Garden City Park, NY: Avery Publishing Group, 1994.

Mindell, Earl. *Unsafe at Any Meal.* New York, NY: Warner Books, 1986.

Moss, Ralph. *Cancer Therapy: The Independent Consumer's Guide to Non-Toxic Treatment & Prevention.* Equinox Press, 1995.

Olkin, Sylvia Klein. *Positive Pregnancy Fitness.* Garden City Park, NY: Avery Publishing Group, 1987.

Ott, John N. *Light, Radiation, and You: How to Stay Healthy.* Old Greenwich, CT: Devin-Adair Publishers, 1982.

Passwater, Richard A. *Supernutrition.* New York: Dial Press, 1985.

Passwater, Richard A., and Elmer Cranton. *Trace Elements, Hair Analysis and Nutrition.* New Canaan, CT: Keats Publishing, 1983.

Pauling, Linus. *Vitamin C and the Common Cold.* San Francisco: W.H. Freeman & Co., 1970.

Pearsall, Paul. *Superimmunity: Master Your Emotions and Improve Your Health.* New York: McGraw-Hill, 1987.

Pfeiffer, Carl. *Nutrition and Mental Illness: An Orthomolecular Approach to Balancing Body Chemistry.* Rochester, VT: Inner Traditions, 1988.

Pfeiffer, Carl. *Zinc and Other Micro-Nutrients.* New Canaan, CT: Keats, 1978.

Phillips, Robert H. *Coping With Osteoarthritis.* Garden City Park, NY: Avery Publishing Group, 1989.

Phillips, Robert H. *Coping With Prostate Cancer.* Garden City Park, NY: Avery Publishing Group, 1994.

Podell, Ronald M. *Contagious Emotions: Staying Well When Your Loved One Is Depressed.* New York: Pocket Books, 1993.

Randolph, Theron G. *Human Ecology and Susceptibility to the Chemical Environment.* Springfield, IL: Charles C. Thomas, 1981.

Rapp, Doris J. *Allergies and the Hyperactive Child.* New York: Sovereign Books, 1979.

Sahelian, Ray. *DHEA: A Practical Guide.* Garden City Park, NY: Avery Publishing Group, 1996.

Selye, Hans. *Stress Without Distress.* Philadelphia: J.B. Lippincott Co., 1974.

Shelton, Herbert M. *Fasting Can Save Your Life,* rev. ed. Natural Hygeine, 1981.

Shute, Wilfrid. *Dr. Wilfrid E. Shute's Complete Updated Vitamin E Book.* New Canaan, CT: Keats Publishing, 1975.

Smith, Lendon. *Feed Your Kids Right: Dr. Smith's Program for Your Child's Total Health.* New York: McGraw-Hill, 1979.

Steinman, David, and Samuel S. Epstein. *The Safe Shoppers Bible.* New York: Macmillan, 1995.

Teitelbaum, Jacob. *From Fatigued to Fantastic.* Garden City Park, NY: Avery Publishing Group, 1996.

Treben, Maria. *Health from God's Garden: Herbal Remedies for Glowing Health and Glorious Well-Being.* Rochester, VT: Thorsons Publishers, 1987.

Wade, Carlson. *Carlson Wade's Amino Acids Book.* New Canaan, CT: Keats Publishing, 1985.

Walker, Morton. *The Chelation Way.* Garden City Park, NY: Avery Publishing Group, 1990.

Walters, Richard. *Options: The Alternative Cancer Therapy Book.* Garden City Park, NY: Avery Publishing Group, 1993.

Warren, Tom. *Beating Alzheimer's.* Garden City Park, NY: Avery Publishing Group, 1991.

Weber, Marcea. *Macrobiotics and Beyond.* Garden City Park, NY: Avery Publishing Group, 1989.

Weber, Marcea. *Whole Meals.* Dorset, England: Prism Press, 1983.

Weiner, Michael A. *Maximum Immunity.* Boston: Houghton Mifflin Co., 1986.

Wigmore, Ann. *Be Your Own Doctor: A Positive Guide to Natural Living,* rev. ed. Garden City Park, NY: Avery Publishing Group, 1983.

Wigmore, Ann. *Recipes for Longer Life.* Garden City Park, NY: Avery Publishing Group, 1982.

Wigmore, Ann. *The Wheatgrass Book.* Garden City Park, NY: Avery Publishing Group, 1985.

Wigmore, Ann. *Why Suffer?* rev. ed. Garden City Park, NY: Avery Publishing Group, 1984.

Williams, Roger J., and Dwight K. Kalita. *A Physician's Handbook on Orthomolecular Medicine.* New Canaan, CT: Keats Publishing, 1979.

Williams, Xandria. *What's in My Food?* Dorset, England: Prism Press, 1988.

Wilson, Roberta. *Aromatherapy for Vibrant Health and Beauty.* Garden City Park, NY: Avery Publishing Group, 1995.

Wlodyga, Ronald R. *Health Secrets From the Bible.* Triumph Publishers, 1979.

Woessner, Candace, Judith Lauwers, and Barbara Bernard. *Breastfeeding Today.* Garden City Park, NY: Avery Publishing Group, 1988.

Zand, Janet, Rachel Walton, and Bob Rountree. *Smart Medicine for a Healthier Child.* Garden City Park, NY: Avery Publishing Group, 1994.

Ziff, Sam. *Silver Dental Fillings: The Toxic Timebomb.* Santa Fe, NM: Aurora Press, 1984.

About the Authors

Phyllis Balch is a certified nutritional consultant who received her certification from the American Association of Nutritional Consultants in 1980. For over two decades, Phyllis has sought the answers to how the body maintains health and which alternative methods work best for natural healing. Her interest in natural foods led to the establishment of *Good Things Naturally*, a health foods store.

During her many years of counseling Dr. Balch's patients on nutrition, Phyllis has emphasized the importance of each individual's responsibility for maintaining his or her own health. This belief is the underlying basis of her writings, which include various newspaper columns, magazine articles, and the books *Prescription for Nutritional Healing* and *Prescription for Dietary Wellness*.

Phyllis Balch continues to study nutritionally based therapies, procedures, and treatments both here and abroad. A highly sought-after lecturer, she appears on television and radio talk shows throughout the United States and Canada.

Dr. James Balch is a graduate of Indiana University's School of Medicine. He completed his surgical residency at Indiana University Medical Center, specializing in urology. Following a two-year tour of duty in the United States Navy, Dr. Balch established a private practice as a urologist. He is presently a member of the American Medical Association, is board certified in the American Board of Urology, and is a fellow in the American College of Surgeons. Dr. Balch received a masters degree in theology from Martin University in Indianapolis in August 1996.

During the past seventeen years, Dr. Balch has helped patients to assume a portion of responsibility for their own well-being. This philosophy is reflected in his newspaper column and his radio broadcast. Through the years, Dr. Balch has appeared on numerous television and radio shows throughout North America.